Global HIV/AIDS Medicine

This book is dedicated to the visionary leaders of the Academic Alliance for AIDS Care in Africa, a model for care-based professional training and research as an indispensable means of ending the AIDS pandemic.

Global HIV/AIDS Medicine

Edited by

Paul A. Volberding, MD
Marvin Sleisenger Professor of Medicine and Vice
Chair Department of Medicine
University of California San Francisco
Chief, Medical Service
San Francisco Veterans Affairs Medical Center
San Francisco, CA, USA

Merle A. Sande, MD
Professor of Medicine, Universixty of Washington
School of Medicine
President, Academic Alliance for AIDS Care and
Prevention in Africa
USA

Warner C. Greene, MD, PhD
Director, Gladstone Institute of Virology and Immunology
Nick and Sue Hellman Endowed Professor of
Translational Biology
Professor of Medicine, Microbiology and Immunology
University of California San Francisco
San Francisco, CA, USA

Joep M. A. Lange, MD, PhD
Center for Poverty-Related
Communicable Diseases
International AIDS Therapy Evaluation Center
University of Amsterdam
Amsterdam, The Netherlands

Associate Editor

Joel E. Gallant, MD, MPH
Professor of Medicine and Epidemiology
Johns Hopkins University School of Medicine
Baltimore, MD, USA

Assistant Editor

Carrie Clark Walsh, ELS
Principal Editor
University of California San Francisco
San Francisco CA, USA

SAUNDERS

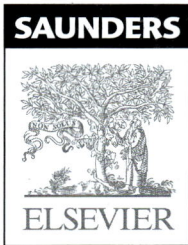

ELSEVIER

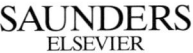

SAUNDERS
ELSEVIER

An imprint of Elsevier Inc
© 2008, Elsevier Inc. All rights reserved.

Chapter 69 © Tony Barnett.
The material in Chapter 63 is in the public domain and may be used and reprinted without special permission; citation of the source, however, is appreciated.

First published 2008

ISBN *978-1-4160-2882-6*

British Library Cataloguing in Publication Data
A catalogue record for this book is available from the British Library

Library of Congress Cataloging in Publication Data
A catalog record for this book is available from the Library of Congress

Notice

Medical knowledge is constantly changing. Standard safety precautions must be followed, but as new research and clinical experience broaden our knowledge, changes in treatment and drug therapy may become necessary or appropriate. Readers are advised to check the most current product information provided by the manufacturer of each drug to be administered to verify the recommended dose, the method and duration of administration, and contraindications. It is the responsibility of the practitioner, relying on experience and knowledge of the patient, to determine dosages and the best treatment for each individual patient. Neither the Publisher nor the author assume any liability for any injury and/or damage to persons or property arising from this publication.

The Publisher

Printed in China

Working together to grow libraries in developing countries

www.elsevier.com | www.bookaid.org | www.sabre.org

ELSEVIER | BOOK AID International | Sabre Foundation

Last digit is the print number: 9 8 7 6 5 4 3 2 1
Commissioning Editor: Karen Bowler
Development Editor: Marsha Bell
Project Manager: Cheryl Brant
Design Manager: Stewart Larking
Illustration Manager: Bruce Hogarth
Illustrator: Richard Prime
Marketing Manager(s) (UK/USA): Clara Toombs/Paul Leese

The Editors acknowledge the generous and unrestricted gift from Pfizer Global Health.

Contents

Preface xi

List of Contributors xiii

SECTION ONE **Epidemiology and Biology of HIV Infection**

CHAPTER 1 The Global Epidemiology of HIV/AIDS.. 1
Kevin M. DeCock

CHAPTER 2 The Origins and Diversification of HIV 13
Michael Worobey

CHAPTER 3 Molecular Biology of HIV: Implications for New Therapies............... 23
Warner C. Greene
B. Matija Peterlin

CHAPTER 4 The Immune Response to HIV 39
Clive M. Gray
Bruce Walker

CHAPTER 5 Viral and Host Determinants of HIV-1 Disease Progression 51
Hanneke Schuitemaker
Angélique B. van't Wout

CHAPTER 6 Acute HIV Infection 63
Anthony D. Kelleher
David A. Cooper

CHAPTER 7 Biology of HIV-1 Transmission.. 75
Julie Overbaugh

CHAPTER 8 The Design of a Global AIDS Vaccine 81
John R. Mascola
Richard A. Koup

SECTION TWO **Prevention, Diagnosis, and Treatment of HIV Infection**

CHAPTER 9 HIV Prevention.. 91
Helene D. Gayle

CHAPTER 10 Laboratory Testing for HIV Infection...101
James C. Shepherd
Oliver Laeyendecker
Thomas C. Quinn

CHAPTER 11 Testing and Counseling 111
Rhoda Wanyenze
Primo Madra
Allan Ronald

CHAPTER 12 New HIV Drug Development 123
Ferdinand W. N. M. Wit
Joep M. A. Lange
Paul A. Volberding

CHAPTER 13 Overview of Antiretroviral Therapy...135
Paul A. Volberding

CHAPTER 14 Development and Transmission of HIV Drug Resistance 149
Mark A. Wainberg
Marco Petrella

CHAPTER 15 Clinical Implications of HIV Fitness and Virulence 161
Jason D. Barbour
Steven G. Deeks

CHAPTER 16 Pharmacology of Antiretroviral Drugs 171
Concepta Merry
Charles W. Flexner

CHAPTER 17 Complications Resulting from Antiretroviral Therapy for HIV
Infection 181
David Nolan
Simon Mallal
Peter Reiss

CHAPTER 18 HIV Immune Reconstitution Inflammatory Syndrome......................193
Paul R. Bohjanen
David R. Boulware

CHAPTER 19 Adherence to HIV Antiretroviral Therapy in Resource-limited
Settings...207
Jayne Byakika-Tusiime
Catherine Orrell
David Bangsberg

SECTION THREE **Diseases Associated with HIV Infection**

CHAPTER 20 Oral Complications of HIV Infection...215
John S. Greenspan
Deborah Greenspan

CHAPTER 21 Ocular Manifestations 227
James P. Dunn

CHAPTER 22 Global HIV and Dermatology 237
Toby Maurer

CHAPTER 23 Gastrointestinal Disorders in HIV..251
Michael H. Serlin
Douglas Dieterich

CHAPTER 24 Primary Neurological Manifestation of HIV/AIDS 261
David B. Clifford
Mesfin Teshome Mitike

CHAPTER 25 Psychiatric Barriers and the International AIDS Epidemic 271
Alex Thompson
Jessica L. Long
Andrew Angelino
Glenn Treisman

CHAPTER 26 Cardiovascular Complications of HIV Infection 279
James H. Stein

CHAPTER 27 Endocrine Complications of HIV Infection 287
Melissa E. Weinberg
Joan C. Lo
Carl Grunfeld
Morris Schambelan

CHAPTER 28 Renal Complications of HIV Infection 299
Jula K. Inrig
Lynda A. Szczech
Trevor E. Gerntholtz
Paul E. Klotman

CHAPTER 29 *Pneumocystis* Pneumonia.. 309
J. Lucian Davis
Laurence Huang

CHAPTER 30 Other HIV-related Pneumonias.. 323
John G. Bartlett

CHAPTER 31 HIV-associated Tuberculosis 333
Edward C. Jones-López
David J. Cennimo
Jerrold J. Ellner

CHAPTER 32 Disseminated *Mycobacterium avium* Complex and other
Atypical Mycobacterial Infections.. 355
Mark A. Jacobson

CHAPTER 33 *Candida* in HIV Infection... 365
Emma Devitt
William G. Powderly

CHAPTER 34 Cryptococcosis and Other Fungal Infections (Histoplasmosis
and Coccidioidomycosis) in HIV-infected patients 375
Kathleen R. Page
Richard Chaisson
Merle A. Sande

CHAPTER 35 Infection due to *Penicillium marneffei* 393
Khuanchai Supparatpinyo
Thira Sirisanthana

CHAPTER 36 AIDS-associated Toxoplasmosis 399
Carlos S. Subauste
Jose G. Montoya
Jack S. Remington

CHAPTER 37 Hepatitis Virus Infections 415
Marion Peters
Oren K. Fix

CHAPTER 38 *Bartonella* Infections in HIV-infected Individuals.............................. 425
Jane E. Koehler

CHAPTER 39 Management of Herpesvirus Infections (Cytomegalovirus,
Herpes Simplex Virus, and Varicella-Zoster Virus) 437
W. Lawrence Drew
Kim S. Erlich

CHAPTER 40 HIV-associated Neoplasia 463
Lawrence D. Kaplan

SECTION FOUR **Prevention and Management in Resource-rich Settings**

CHAPTER 41 Managing HIV Infection in Children and Adolescents.......................475
Andrew T. Pavia

CHAPTER 42 Special Issues Regarding Women with HIV Infection 487
Meg D. Newman

CHAPTER 43 Prevention of Mother-to-Child Transmission of HIV-1 497
Lynne M. Mofenson

CHAPTER 44 HIV Disease Among Substance Users: Treatment Issues 513
R. Douglas Bruce
Frederick L. Altice
Gerald Friedland

CHAPTER 45 Models of Care: HIV Care in the Urban USA 527
Richard D. Moore
Jeanne C. Keruly

CHAPTER 46 Antiretroviral Therapy of Drug-resistant HIV 537
Marianne Harris
P. Richard Harrigan
Julio S. G. Montaner

CHAPTER 47 Complementary and Alternative Medicine 547
Jason Tokumoto
Donald I. Abrams

CHAPTER 48 The HIV-infected International Traveler 555
Malcolm John

SECTION FIVE **Prevention and Management in Resource-poor Settings**

CHAPTER 49 HIV Transmission and its Prevention in Africa 565
Catherine Hankins
Steffanie Strathdee
Salim Abdool Karim

CHAPTER 50 HIV Transmission and its Prevention in Asia 577
Stephen Kerr
Kiat Ruxrungtham

CHAPTER 51 HIV Transmission and its Prevention in Eastern Europe 587
Kasia Malinowska-Sempruch

CHAPTER 52 Vaginal Microbicides Against HIV 595
Zeda F. Rosenberg
Mark Mitchnick
Paul Coplan

CHAPTER 53 Implications and Management of Malnutrition 603
Heather Southwell

CHAPTER 54 Antiretroviral Therapy in Resource-poor Settings: Challenges,
Research Priorities, Opportunities 615
Joep M. A. Lange
Elly Katabira
Papa Salif Sow

CHAPTER 55 Antiretroviral Treatment and Follow-up of HIV-infected Children
in Resource-limited Settings 621
Sibyl Geelen
Philippa Musoke

CHAPTER 56 Epidemiology, Natural History and Treatment of HIV-2
Infections 637
Maarten F. Schim van der Loeff

CHAPTER 57 Affordable CD4 T-cell Enumeration and HIV/AIDS Viral Load
Monitoring in Resource-poor Settings 649
Tobias F. Rinke de Wit

CHAPTER 58 Essential Medicines for HIV/AIDS 661
Hans V. Hogerzeil

CHAPTER 59 Pharmacoeconomics of HIV/AIDS Treatment 667
Máirín Ryan

CHAPTER 60 Logistics and Models of Implementing HAART in
Resource-constrained Settings... 677
Ernest Darkoh-Ampem

CHAPTER 61 Universal Access to Antiretroviral Therapy: The Brazilian
Experience 695
Mauro Schechter
Marie Charles

CHAPTER 62 Surveillance of Antiretroviral Drug Resistance in
Resource-poor Settings 703
Inge Derdelinckx
Charles Boucher

CHAPTER 63 Post-exposure Prevention... 711
Adelisa L. Panlilio
Denise M. Cardo

CHAPTER 64 Selected NGOs Active in HIV and Web Links 725
Sahai Burrowes
Laurence Peiperl

CHAPTER 65 Etiology and Management of Diarrhea in HIV-infected
Patients and Impact on Antiretroviral Therapy........................ 737
Oluma Y. Bushen
Richard L. Guerrant

CHAPTER 66 Malaria and HIV Infection 747
Feiko O. ter Kuile
James A. G. Whitworth

CHAPTER 67 The Role of Unsterile Injections in the HIV Pandemic..................... 755
Ernest Drucker
Cristian Apetrei
Robert Heimer
Preston Marx

SECTION SIX **Economic and Social Consequences of the HIV Epidemic**

CHAPTER 68 The Economic Impact of HIV/AIDS in Developing Countries:
Systematic Under-estimation 769
Jean-Paul Moatti
Bruno Ventelou

CHAPTER 69 The Long Wave of HIV/AIDS: A Special Case of Pathogen–
Host–Environment Interactions 779
Tony Barnett

CHAPTER 70 The Growing Problem of AIDS Orphans... 787
Theo Sowa

CHAPTER 71 International Funding Mechanisms for AIDS Care and
Prevention 793
Mabel van Oranje

Index 801

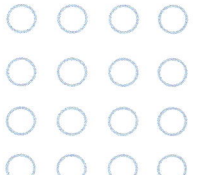

The first edition of this book's predecessor, *The Medical Management of AIDS*, appeared in 1988, at a time when care for even the most economically privileged sought to ameliorate but not reverse what was then an invariably fatal disease. The epidemic in less advantaged areas such as Africa was barely mentioned, and antiretroviral therapy, primarily zidovudine monotherapy, had only modest benefit.

The next six editions of *The Medical Management of AIDS* saw great changes. By 1999, when the sixth edition appeared, multi-drug antiretroviral regimens had begun to reverse AIDS mortality trends in the US and other resource-rich countries, and had been shown to dramatically decrease transmission from infected women to their infants. The incidence of formerly common opportunistic infections and malignancies had decreased, and HIV infection was increasingly seen as a chronic, albeit still serious, disease. Still, in 1999, almost no one dared hope that similar benefits could be achieved in Africa, Asia, or other resource-constrained regions.

Much has changed by this edition's publication in 2007. Antiretroviral regimens have become more convenient, less toxic, and, in resource-limited settings, often much less expensive. Generic and off-patent production along with pharmaceutical subsidies and governmental distribution are allowing millions of patients access to potent treatment. Although huge challenges remain, hope is now possible for those areas most in need in confronting the scourge of HIV along with tuberculosis, malaria, and the crushing poverty and gender inequalities that serve as the stage on which the epidemic often unfolds.

The editors of the prior volume hope that this book's re-birth as *Global HIV/AIDS Medicine* addresses both the hope of newer treatment and the challenges that remain to be addressed for this hope to be realized globally. Additional editors have brought new expertise to the book's leadership, and many new authors and topics make this the first textbook aimed at a comprehensive approach to the management of what is truly a global problem. The editors hope that this effort can play a valuable role in extending the incredible advances of HIV/AIDS therapy to the many millions still in desperate need.

Paul A. Volberding, Merle A. Sande
Warner C. Greene, Joep M. A. Lange, Joel E. Gallant

Donald I. Abrams MD
Director of Clinical Programs
Osher Center for Integrative
Medicine
Professor of Clinical Medicine
University of California San
Francisco
San Francisco, CA
USA

Frederick L. Altice MD
Associate Professor of Medicine
Yale University AIDS Program
Yale University
New Haven, CT
USA

Andrew Angelino MD
Assistant Professor
Department of Psychiatry and
Behavioural Sciences
The Johns Hopkins University
School of Medicine,
Baltimore, MD
USA

Cristian Apetrei MD, PhD
Associate Professor
Department of Microbiology
Tulane National Primate
Research Center
Covington, LA
USA

David Bangsberg MD, MPH
Associate Professor of Medicine
Department of Medicine
University of California San
Francisco
San Francisco, CA
USA

Jason D. Barbour PhD, MHS
Assistant Professor of Medicine
Positive Health Program
San Francisco General Hospital
University of California San
Francisco
San Francisco, CA
USA

**Tony Barnett BA (Hons), MA
(Econ), PhD**
ESRC Professorial Research
Fellow
LSE Health
London School of Economics
London
UK

John G. Bartlett MD
Professor of Medicine
Division of Infectious Diseases
The John Hopkins University
School of Medicine
Baltimore, MD
USA

Paul R. Bohjanen MD, PhD
Associate Professor of
Microbiology and Medicine
Department of Microbiology
University of Minnesota
Minneapolis, MN
USA

Charles Boucher MD, PhD
Department of Virology
Eijkman-Winkler Institute
University Medical Center
Utrecht
Utrecht , The Netherlands

**David R. Boulware MD, MPH,
DTMH**
Assistant Professor of Medicine
Department of Medicine
Division of Infectious Diseases
and International Medicine
University of Minnesota
Minneapolis, MN
USA

R. Douglas Bruce MD, MA
Clinical Instructor of Medicine
Yale University AIDS Program
Yale School of Medicine
New Haven, CT
USA

Sahai Burrowes MALD
International Projects Manager
Center for HIV Information
University of California San
Francisco
San Francisco, CA
USA

Oluma Y. Bushen MD
Associate Director
Tulane University Technical
Assistance Program
Addis Ababa
Ethiopia

**Jayne Byakika-Tusiime
BPharm, MSc**
PhD Candidate and
Epidemiologist
University of California Berkeley
Berkeley, CA
USA

Denise M. Cardo MD
Director
Division of Healthcare Quality
Promotion
Centers for Disease Control and
Prevention
Atlanta, GA
USA

David J. Cennimo MD
Chief Medical Resident
Department of Medicine
New Jersey Medical School
Newark, NJ
USA

Richard E. Chaisson MD
Professor of Medicine,
Epidemiology and International
Health
Johns Hopkins University
Baltimore, MD
USA

Marie Charles MD, MIA
Chair & CEO, International
Center for Equal Healthcare
Access
Henry Crown Fellow
The Aspen Institute
Adjunct Professor, Columbia
University, School of
International and Public Affairs
New York, NY
USA

David B. Clifford MD
Melba and Forest Seay Professor
of Clinical Neuropharmacology
Department of Neurology
Washington University School of
Medicine
St Louis, MO
USA

David A. Cooper MD, DSc
Professor of Medicine
National Centre in HIV
Epidemiology and Clinical
Research
University of New South Wales
Darlinghurst, NSW
Australia

Paul Coplan MSc, DSc, MBA
Senior Director, Risk
Management
Global Safety Surveillance,
Epidemiology and Labeling
Wyeth Pharmaceuticals
Worldwide
Collegeville, PA
USA

**Ernest Darkoh-Ampem MD,
MPH, MBA**
Chairman and Founding Partner
BroadReach Healthcare
Washington, DC
USA

J. Lucian Davis MD
Clinical Instructor
Division of Pulmonary and
Critical Care Medicine and HIV/
AIDS Division
San Francisco General Hospital
University of California San
Francisco
San Francisco, CA
USA

**Kevin M. DeCock MD, FRCP,
DTM&H**
Director, HIV/AIDS Program
World Health Organization
Geneva
Switzerland

Steven G. Deeks MD
Associate Professor of Medicine
Positive Health Program
San Francisco General Hospital
University of California San
Francisco
San Francisco, CA
USA

Inge Derdelinckx MD, PhD
Associate Professor
Department of Virology
Eijkman Winkler Institute
University Medical Center
Utrecht
The Netherlands

Emma Devitt MB BCh
Special Lecturer in Medicine
Medical Professorial Unit
University College Dublin/Mater
Hospital
Dublin
Ireland

Douglas Dieterich MD
Professor of Medicine
Department of Medicine
Mount Sinai School of Medicine
New York, NY
USA

W. Lawrence Drew MD, PhD
Director, Clinical Virology
Laboratory
Professor, Laboratory Medicine
and Medicine
Medical Center at Mount Zion
University of California San
Francisco
San Francisco, CA
USA

Ernest Drucker PhD
Professor of Epidemiology and
Social Medicine
Montefiore Medical Center
Albert Einstein College of
Medicine
New York, NY
USA

James P. Dunn MD
Associate Professor of
Ophthalmology
The Wilmer Eye Institute
John Hopkins School of Medicine
Baltimore, MD
USA

Jerrold J. Ellner MD
Professor and Chair
Department of Medicine
New Jersey Medical School
Newark, NJ
USA

Kim S. Erlich MD
Assistant Clinical Professor of
Medicine
University of California San
Francisco
San Francisco, CA
USA

Oren K. Fix MD, MSc
Assistant Professor of Medicine
Division of Gastroenterology
University of Washington
Medical School
Seattle, WA
USA

Charles W. Flexner MD
Professor of Medicine,
Pharmacology and Molecular
Sciences, and International
Health
Division of Clinical
Pharmacology
Johns Hopkins University
Baltimore, MD
USA

Gerald Friedland MD
Professor of Medicine and
Epidemiology and Public Health
Director, AIDS Program
Yale New Haven Hospital
Yale School of Medicine
New Haven, CT
USA

Helene D. Gayle MD, MPH
President and Chief Executive
Officer
CARE USA
Atlanta, GA
USA

Sibyl Geelen MD, PhD
Senior Consultant
Pediatric Infectious Disease
Specialist
Center for Poverty-related
Communicable Diseases-
PharmAccess Foundation
Amsterdam
Department of Pediatric
Infectious Diseases
University Medical Center
Utrecht
The Netherlands

Trevor E. Gerntholtz MD
Dumisani Mzamane African
Institute of Kidney Disease
Chris Hani Baragwanath
Hospital
Soweto
South Africa

Clive M. Gray MSc, PhD
Chief Specialist Scientist
Head of HIV Immunology
HIV Immunology AIDS Research
Unit
National Institute for
Communicable Diseases
Johannesburg
South Africa

Warner C. Greene MD, PhD
Director, Gladstone Institute of
Virology and Immunology
Nick and Sue Hellman Endowed
Professor of Translational Biology
Professor of Medicine,
Microbiology and Immunology
University of California San
Francisco
San Francisco, CA
USA

Deborah Greenspan BDS, DSc, FDSRCS
Leland and Gladys Barber
Distinguished Professor and
Interim Chair
Department of Orofacial Sciences
School of Dentistry
University of California San
Francisco
San Francisco, CA
USA

John S. Greenspan BSc, BDS, PhD, FRC Path, ScD(hc), FDSRCS (Eng)
Professor and Dean for Research
School of Dentistry
Director
AIDS Research Institute
School of Medicine
University of California San
Francisco
San Francisco, CA
USA

Carl Grunfeld MD, PhD
Professor of Medicine
Metabolism and Endocrine
Sections
University of California San
Francisco
San Francisco, CA
USA

Richard L. Guerrant MD
Thomas H. Hunter Professor of
International Medicine
Division of Infectious Diseases
and International Health
Director, Center for Global
Health,
University of Virginia
Charlottesville, VA
USA

Catherine Hankins MD, MSc, FRCP(C)
Chief Scientific Adviser and
Associate Director
Policy, Evidence and Partnerships
UNAIDS
Geneva
Switzerland

P. Richard Harrigan PhD
Director
Research Labs
British Columbia Centre for
Excellence in
HIV/AIDS
Vancouver, BC
Canada

Marianne Harris MD
Clinical Research Advisor
AIDS Research Programme
St Paul's Hospital
Vancouver, BC
Canada

Robert Heimer PhD
Professor of Epidemiology and
Public Health
Department of Epidemiology and
Public Health
Yale University School of
Medicine
New Haven, CT
USA

Hans V. Hogerzeil MD, PhD, DSc, FRCP(Edin)
Director
Medicines Policy and Standards
World Health Organization
Geneva
Switzerland

Laurence Huang MD
Associate Professor of Medicine
Chief, AIDS Chest Clinic
HIV/AIDS Division and Division
of Pulmonary and Critical Care
Medicine
Department of Medicine
San Francisco General Hospital
University of California San
Francisco
San Francisco, CA
USA

Jula K. Inrig MD
Instructor in Medicine
Division of Nephrology
Department of Medicine
Duke University Medical Center
Durham, NC
USA

Mark A. Jacobson MD
Professor of Medicine in
Residence
Positive Health Program
University of California San
Francisco
San Francisco, CA
USA

Malcolm John MD, MPH
Assistant Clinical Professor
Director, 360: The Positive Care
Center at USCF
Division of Infectious Diseases-
Department of Medicine
University of California San
Francisco
San Francisco, CA
USA

Edward C. Jones-López MD, MS
Assistant Professor of Medicine
Division of Infectious Diseases
and Center for Emerging
Pathogens
New Jersey Medical School
Newark, NJ
USA

Lawrence D. Kaplan MD
Professor of Medicine
University of California San
Francisco
San Francisco, CA
USA

Elly Katabira MD
Deputy Dean for Research
Faculty of Medicine
Makerere University Medical
School
Kampala
Uganda

Salim Abdool Karim MBChB, PhD
Director
Centre for the AIDS Programme
of Research
South Africa
Professor in Clinical
Epidemiology
Columbia University
Adjunct Professor in Medicine
Cornell University
New York, NY
USA

Anthony D. Kelleher PhD, MB BS, MD
Associate Professor of Medicine
National Centre in HIV
Epidemiology and
Clinical Research
University of New South Wales
Darlinghurst, NSW
Australia

Stephen J. Kerr BPharm, MIPH, PhD
Biostatistician
HIV Netherlands Australia
Thailand Resarch collaboration
(HIV-NAT)
Bangkok
Thailand
Senior Lecturer
National Centre in HIV
Epidemiology and Clinical
Research
University of New South Wales
Sydney
Australia

Jeanne C. Keruly MS, CRNP
Assistant Professor of Medicine
Department of Medicine
Johns Hopkins University School
of Medicine
Baltimore, MD
USA

Paul E. Klotman MD
Professor and Chair
Division of Nephrology
Mount Sinai School of Medicine
New York, NY
USA

Jane E. Koehler MA, MD
Professor of Medicine
Division of Infectious Diseases
University of California San
Francisco
San Francisco, CA
USA

Richard A. Koup MD
Chief, Immunology Laboratory
Vaccine Research Center
National Institute of Allergy and
Infectious Diseases
Bethesda, MD
USA

Oliver Laeyendecker MS, MBA
Research Assistant
Division of Infectious Diseases
Department of Medicine
Johns Hopkins School of
Medicine
Baltimore, MD
USA

Joep M. A. Lange MD, PhD
Center for Poverty-Related
Communicable Diseases
International AIDS Therapy
Evaluation Center
University of Amsterdam
Amsterdam, The Netherlands

Joan C. Lo MD
Assistant Professor of Medicine
Division of Endocrinology
San Francisco General Hospital
University of California San
Francisco
San Francisco, CA
USA

Jessica L. Long MD
Johns Hopkins School of
Medicine, MS IV
JH Bloomberg School of Public
Health, MPH Candidate
Baltimore, MD
USA

Primo Madra MD, PhD
National Program Officer
UNFPA – Uganda Country Office
Kampala
Uganda

**Kasia Malinowska-Sempruch
MSW**
Program Director
International Harm Reduction
Development Program (IHRD)
Open Society Institute
New York, NY
USA

**Simon Mallal MB BS, FRACP,
FRCPA**
Professor of Clinical Immunology
and Infectious Diseases
Centre for Clinical Immunology
and Biomedical Statistics
Royal Perth Hospital
Perth, WA
Australia

Preston Marx PhD
Chair, Division of Microbiology
and Professor of Tropical
Medicine
Tulane National Primate
Research Center
Covington, LA
USA

John R. Mascola MD
Deputy Director
Vaccine Research Center
National Institute of Allergy and
Infectious Diseases
Bethesda, MD
USA

Toby Maurer MD
Associate Professor
Department of Dermatology
University of California San
Francisco
San Francisco, CA
USA

**Concepta Merry MB, PhD, MSc,
MRCPI**
Clinical Researcher
University of Makerere
Kampala
Uganda

Mark Mitchnick MD
Chief Scientific Consultant
International Partnership for
Microbicides
East Hampton, NY
USA

Mesfin Teshome Mitike MD
Assistant Professor
Department of Internal Medicine
Faculty of Medicine
Addis Ababa University
Addis Ababa
Ethiopia

Jean-Paul Moatti PhD
Professor of Health Economics
University of Mediterranean &
INSERM
Marseilles
France

Lynne M. Mofenson MD
Chief, Pediatric, Adolescent and
Maternal AIDS Branch
National Institute of Child Health
and Human Development
Rockville, MD
USA

Julio S. G. Montaner MD
Professor of Medicine & Chair of
AIDS Research
University of British Columbia
AIDS Research Program
St Paul's Hospital
Vancouver, BC
Canada

Jose G. Montoya MD
Associate Professor of Medicine,
Division of Infectious Diseases
and Geographical Medicine
Stanford University School of
Medicine
Stanford, CA
USA

Richard D. Moore MD
Professor of Medicine
Department of Medicine
John Hopkins University School
of Medicine
Baltimore, MD
USA

Philippa Musoke MB, ChB
Consultant Paediatrician
Paediatrics Department
Mulago Hospital
Kampala
Uganda

Meg D. Newman MD
Associate Professor of Clinical
Medicine
Positive Health Program at San
Francisco General Hospital
University of California San
Francisco
San Francisco, CA
USA

David Nolan MB BS, FRACP
Centre for Clinical Immunology
and Biomedical Statistics
Royal Perth Hospital and
Murdoch University
Perth, WA
Australia

Catherine Orrell MBChB, MMed
Clinical Trials Manager
Infectious Diseases Unit
UCT Lung Institute
University of Cape Town
Cape Town
South Africa

Julie Overbaugh PhD
Member, Division of Human
Biology
Fred Hutchinson Cancer
Research Center
Seattle, WA
USA

Kathleen R. Page MD
Instructor of Medicine
Division of Infectious Diseases
Johns Hopkins University School
of Medicine
Baltimore, MD
USA

Adelisa L. Panlilio MD, MPH
Medical Epidemiologist
Department of Healthcare
Quality Promotion
Centers for Disease Control and
Prevention
Atlanta, GA
USA

Andrew T. Pavia MD
Professor of Pediatrics and
Medicine
Chief, Division of Pediatric
Infectious Diseases
University of Utah Health
Sciences Center
Salt Lake City, UT
USA

Laurence Peiperl MD
Associate Professor of Clinical
Medicine
University of California San
Francisco
San Francisco, CA
USA

B. Matija Peterlin MD
Professor of Medicine,
Microbiology and Immunology
Rosalind Russell Medical
Research Center
University of California San
Francisco
San Francisco, CA
USA

Marion Peters MD
Chief of Hepatology Research
Professor of Medicine
Division of Gastroenterology
University of California San
Francisco
San Francisco, CA
USA

Marco Petrella
Neurochem Inc.
Québec
Canada

William G. Powderly MD, FRCPI
Professor of Medicine
Head, School of Medicine
University College Dublin School
of Medicine
Dublin
Ireland

Thomas C. Quinn MD, MSc
Director
Johns Hopkins Center for Global
Health
Professor of Medicine,
International Health,
Epidemiology, and Molecular
Microbiology and Immunology
Johns Hopkins Medical
Institutions
Associate Director for
International Research
Division of Intramural Research
National Institute of Allergy and
Infectious Diseases
National Institutes of Health
Bethesda, MD
USA

Peter Reiss MD, PhD
Professor of Medicine
Department of Infectious
Diseases, Tropical Medicine and
AIDS
Academic Medical Center
Amsterdam
The Netherlands

Jack S. Remington MD
Professor Emeritus
Department of Medicine
Division of Infectious Diseases
and Geographic Medicine
Stanford University School of
Medicine
Marcus A. Krupp Research Chair
and Chairman
Department of Immunology and
Infectious Diseases Research
Institute
Palo Alto Medical Foundation
Palo Alto, CA
USA

Tobias F. Rinke de Wit PhD
Professor of Sustainable
Diagnostics
PharmAccess Foundation
Center for Poverty-related
Communicable Diseases
Academic Medical Center –
University of Amsterdam
Amsterdam
The Netherlands

Allan Ronald OC, FRSC, MD, FRCPC, MACP
Distinguished Professor Emeritus
Department of Internal Medicine
University of Manitoba
Winnipeg, MB
Canada

Zeda F. Rosenberg ScD
Chief Executive Officer
International Partnership for
Microbicides
Silver Spring, MD
USA

Kiat Ruxrungtham MD, MSc
Professor of Medicine
Department of Medicine
Chulalongkorn University
Bangkok
Thailand

Máirín Ryan BSc(Pharm), Dip Clin Pharm, Dip Health Econ, PhD
Lecturer in Pharmacoeconomics
National Centre for
Pharmacoenconomics
Trinity College
Dublin
Ireland

Merle A. Sande MD
Professor of Medicine, University
of Washington School of
Medicine
President, Academic Alliance for
AIDS Care and Prevention in
Africa
USA

Morris Schambelan MD
Professor of Medicine
Associate Chair for Clinical and
Translational Research
University of California San
Francisco
San Francisco, CA
USA

Mauro Schechter MD, PhD
Professor of Infectious Diseases
University Federal do Rio de
Janeiro
Rio de Janeiro
Brazil

Maarten F. Schim van der Loeff MD, MSc, PhD
Senior Epidemiologist
Center for Poverty-related
Communicable Diseases
Academic Medical Center –
University of Amsterdam
Amsterdam
The Netherlands

Hanneke Schuitemaker PhD
Professor in Virology, Viro-
pathogenesis of AIDS
Department of Clinical Viro-
Immunology
University of Amsterdam
Amsterdam
The Netherlands

Michael H. Serlin MD
Interim Chair of the Special
Services/HIV Department
Attending, Department of
Medicine
Division of Infectious Diseases
North General Hospital
Instructor, Department of
Medicine
Mount Sinai School of Medicine
New York, NY
USA

James C. Shepherd MD, PhD
Adjunct Assistant Professor
Division of Infectious Diseases
Johns Hopkins School of
Medicine
Baltimore, MD
USA

Thira Sirisanthana MD
Department of Medicine
Chiang Mai University Hospital
Chiang Mai
Thailand

Heather Southwell MS, RD
Research Dietitian
San Francisco VA Medical Center
San Francisco, CA
USA

Papa Salif Sow MD
Professor of Infectious Diseases
Dakar University Teaching
Hospital
Dakar
Senegal

Theo Sowa
Social Development Specialist
London
UK

James H. Stein MD
Associate Professor of Medicine
Cardiovascular Medicine
Division
University of Wisconsin School of
Medicine and Public Health
Madison, WI
USA

Steffanie Strathdee PhD
Professor and Harold Simon
Chair
Division of International Health
and Cross Cultural Medicine
University of California School of
Medicine
Adjunct Professor
John Hopkins Bloomberg School
of Public Health
USA

Carlos S. Subauste MD
Associate Professor
Departments of Ophthalmology
and Medicine
Case Western Reserve University
School of Medicine
Cleveland, OH
USA

Khuanchai Supparatpinyo MD
Associate Professor
Department of Medicine
Faculty of Medicine,
Chiang Mai University Hospital
Chiang Mai
Thailand

Lynda A. Szczech MD, MSCE
Assistant Professor
Division of Nephrology
Department of Medicine,
Duke University Medical Center
Durham, NC
USA

Feiko O. ter Kuile MD, PhD
Senior Clinical Lecturer
Tropical Child Health
Liverpool School of Tropical
Medicine
Liverpool
UK

Alex Thompson MD, MBA
Acting Instructor and Senior
Research Fellow
Department of Psychiatry and
Behavioral Sciences
Johns Hopkins University School
of Medicine
Baltimore, MD
USA

Jason Tokumoto MD
Assistant Clinical Professor of
Medicine
National HIV/AIDS Clinicians'
Consultation Center
San Francisco General Hospital
University of California San
Francisco
San Francisco, CA
USA

Glenn Treisman MD, PhD
Associate Professor
Department of Psychiatry and
Behavioral Sciences
Johns Hopkins University School
of Medicine
Baltimore, MD
USA

Mabel van Oranje MSc
International Advocacy Director
Open Society Institute
London
UK

Angélique B. van't Wout PhD
Senior Investigator
Department of Clinical Viro-
Immunology
Sanquin Research
Amsterdam
The Netherlands

Bruno Ventelou PhD
Senior Researcher
Centre for National Scientific
Research
University of Mediterranean &
INSERM
Marseilles
France

Paul A. Volberding MD
Marvin Sleisenger Professor of
Medicine and Vice Chair
Department of Medicine
University of California San
Francisco, Chief, Medical Service
San Francisco Veterans Affairs
Medical Center,
San Francisco, CA
USA

Mark A. Wainberg PhD
Professor of Medicine and
Microbiology
Director McGill University AIDS
Centre
Montreal, QC
Canada

Bruce Walker MD
Professor of Medicine
Harvard Medical School
Director
Harvard Center for AIDS
Research
Boston, MA
USA

Rhoda Wanyenze MBChB, MPH
Program Manager
Mulago-Mbarara Teaching
Hospitals' Joint AIDS Program
Makerere University Faculty of
Medicine
Kampala
Uganda

Melissa E. Weinberg, MD
Fellow in Endocrinology
University of California San
Francisco
San Francisco, CA
USA

**James A. G. Whitworth MD,
FRCP, FFPH, DTM&H**
Head of International Activities
Wellcome Trust
London
UK

**Ferdinand W. N. M. Wit MD,
PhD**
Director, Science and Medical
Affairs
International Antiviral Therapy
Evaluation Center (IATEC)
Amsterdam
The Netherlands

Michael Worobey PhD
Assistant Professor
Ecology and Evolutionary
Biology
University of Arizona
Tucson, AZ
USA

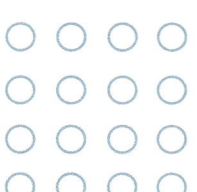

CHAPTER 1

The Global Epidemiology of HIV/AIDS

Kevin M. DeCock

Introduction

Of all problems in global health, few have had as devastating an impact in recent times as HIV/AIDS, and few are as unequally distributed across the world's population. Two different types of human immunodeficiency virus (HIV), HIV-1 and HIV-2, affect humans. Considerable evidence exists favoring the hypothesis that HIV-1 in humans arose from cross-species transmission of an agent in chimpanzees, and HIV-2 from cross-species transmission from sooty mangabees.[1-3]

Three groups of HIV-1 have been recognized: groups M, N, and O. The great majority of the world's infections are with HIV-1 group M viruses, of which some 10 different subtypes ('clades') exist. Subtype B predominates in the USA and the Americas, Europe, and Australia. Subtype C has spread rapidly throughout much of southern Africa and parts of India.[4] In some parts of the world, such as West Africa, recombinant viruses are especially prevalent, e.g. AG. In general, when people speak of 'HIV,' it is assumed they are referring to HIV-1. Groups O and N viruses are essentially restricted to Central Africa.

HIV-2 is less transmissible than HIV-1, possibly because viral load is lower throughout much of its natural history.[5] HIV-2 is largely restricted to West Africa, but has been recognized in individual cases across all continents. It has been seen more frequently in countries with sizeable West African immigrant populations such as France, as well as in Portugal and former Portuguese colonies.[6]

There is little evidence to suggest that different subtypes of HIV-1 have different transmissibility or natural history.[7] Subtypes are of interest because of insights their different distribution can give about epidemic spread; because of the theoretical but uncertain possibility that eventual HIV vaccines may have unequal protective efficacy for different clades; and because performance of diagnostics may not be equal for all subtypes. Figure 1.1 shows the relative importance of different HIV-1 subtypes in different parts of the world.

Transmission of HIV[8]

Transmission of HIV may occur from person to person through heterosexual and male-to-male sexual intercourse; through exposure to contaminated blood (blood transfusion, sharing of contaminated injection equipment for intravenous drug use, needlesticks from infected sources, etc.); and from mother-to-child, including through breast-feeding.[8]

Whatever the route of transmission, the quantity of virus in the exposure affects the probability of transmission. Thus, persons with advanced HIV disease and those recently infected, both of whom have high viral loads, may be especially prone to transmit infection. Blood transfusion is a highly efficient means of transmission because of the high viral burden in an infected unit. Additional factors may influence the likelihood of transmission such as the presence of other sexually transmitted infections, but especially ulcerative conditions, increasing viral load in genital fluids and thus transmissibility. Although the risk of infection following a contaminated needlestick injury is low (estimated

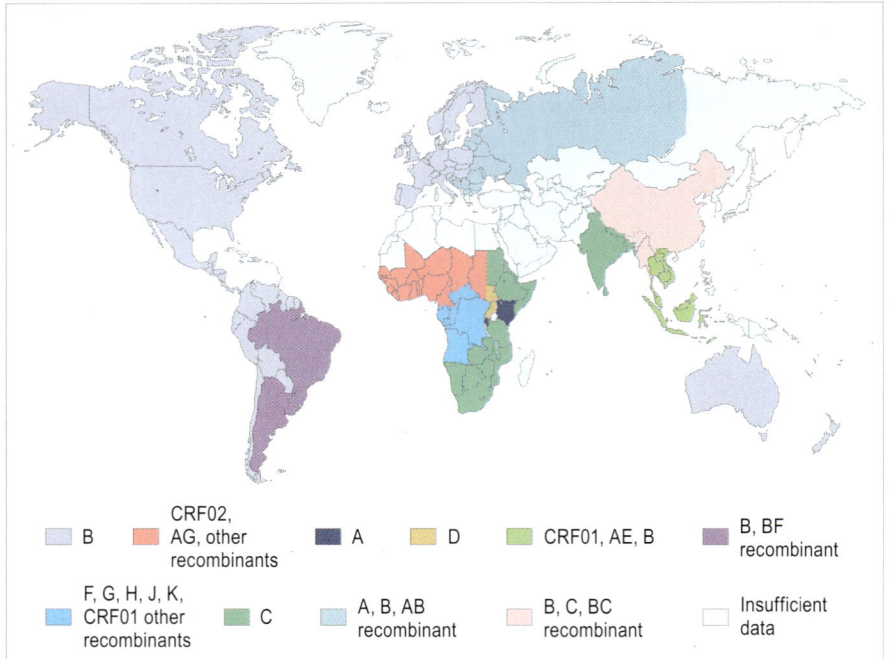

Figure 1.1 Global distribution of HIV-1 subtypes and recombinants. (First published in the IAVI report. Data source: Francine McCutcheon, Henry M. Jackson.)

at 0.003), this is increased in cases of deep injection, if the needle was used for venous or arterial puncture, if blood contamination of the needle was evident, and if the source patient had end-stage disease. Concerning mother-to-child transmission, viral load is the principal risk factor for determining the likelihood of transmission. For breast-feeding women, exclusive breast-feeding may be associated with lower risk of transmission than mixed-feeding. Duration of breast-feeding also affects the risk of transmission, although most infections occur early on.

The Global Burden of HIV/AIDS

The cumulative total of HIV infections and deaths since the beginning of the pandemic exceeds 60 million and 25 million, respectively.[9] At end-2005, the Joint United Nations Programme on HIV/AIDS (UNAIDS) and the World Health Organization (WHO) estimated that there were some 40.3 million adults living with HIV (Fig. 1.2), with some 4.9 million new HIV infections and 3.1 million AIDS deaths occurring in that calendar year.

How the Burden of HIV/AIDS is Measured[10]

Figure 1.3 illustrates the cycle of HIV disease, with the rate of water flowing through the open faucet representing the incidence of HIV infections (the number of new infections per unit population per unit time); the level of water in the first receptacle the prevalence of HIV infection (the proportion of people infected with HIV); the outflow of water from the first receptacle the incidence of AIDS; the level in the second receptacle the prevalence of AIDS; and the final outflow rate the mortality from AIDS (deaths per unit population per unit time). Each of these important parameters can be measured directly in one way or another.

Historically, public health surveillance in industrialized countries focused on monitoring the incidence of AIDS, which was made a reportable disease after it was first recognized. In the USA, major revisions of the original case definition were undertaken in 1985, 1987 and 1993.[11] Once a test for HIV became available, the reporting of persons diagnosed with HIV was possible but was slow to be adopted. HIV case-reporting became more urgent after the intro-

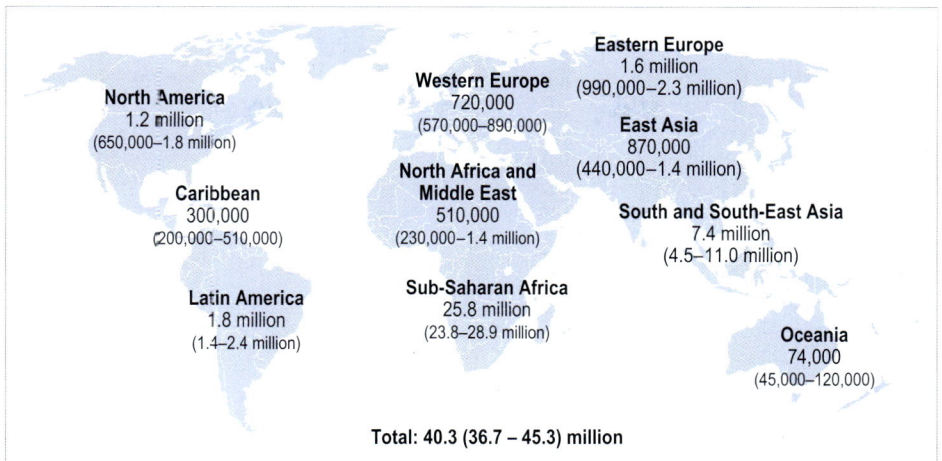

Figure 1.2 Global burden of HIV/AIDS, end-2005. (Reproduced with kind permission from UNAIDS.[9])

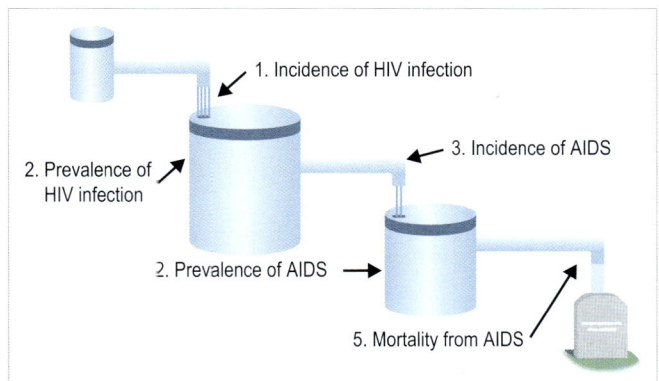

Figure 1.3 The cycle of HIV disease.

duction of highly active antiretroviral therapy since disease progression was no longer predictable and AIDS case reports became less representative of transmission trends. HIV prevalence was monitored through surveys in groups at risk, such as men who have sex with men (MSM) attending sexually transmitted infections (STI) clinics, injecting drug users at drug treatment clinics, and others. AIDS mortality in industrialized countries is monitored through the reliable vital registration and death certification systems that exist in such countries.

HIV incidence was previously estimated through back-calculation in which modeling is used to apply the known natural history of HIV infection to observed AIDS surveillance data, reconstructing the HIV incidence trends that would have been necessary to produce observed disease patterns.[12] The advent of highly active antiretroviral therapy (HAART), which delays progression of HIV infec-

tion to AIDS, has rendered this technique no longer possible. Other ways of measuring HIV incidence include direct measurement in cohorts or persons testing repeatedly in facilities such as drug treatment or STI clinics, or through use of newly developed serologic testing approaches that allow recognition of recently acquired HIV infections.[13] Concern has arisen that the latter approaches may be overestimating incidence in some settings.

In developing countries, a clinical case definition for AIDS was introduced to allow surveillance that did not require sophisticated laboratory support (Boxes 1.1, 1.2), but limited sensitivity of the definition and under-reporting have limited the effectiveness of AIDS surveillance in resource-poor settings.[14] Excellent data have been obtained by extensive use of unlinked anonymous testing among sentinel groups such as pregnant women attending antenatal clinics, in which left over blood collected for other

3

Box 1.1[14]

Expanded WHO case definition for AIDS surveillance

For the purposes of AIDS surveillance an adult or adolescent (>12 years of age) is considered to have AIDS if a test for HIV antibody gives a positive result, and one or more of the following conditions are present:

- 10% body weight loss or cachexia, with diarrhea or fever, or both, intermittent or constant, for at least 1 month, not known to be due to a condition unrelated to HIV infection
- Cryptococcal meningitis
- Pulmonary or extrapulmonary tuberculosis
- Kaposi's sarcoma
- Neurological impairment that is sufficient to prevent independent daily activities not known to be due to a condition unrelated to HIV infection (for example, trauma or cerebrovascular accident)
- Candidiasis of the oesophagus (which may be presumptive diagnosis based on the presence of oral candidiasis accompanied by dysphagia)
- Clinically diagnosed life-threatening or recurrent episodes of pneumonia, with or without etiologic confirmation
- Invasive cervical cancer.

Box 1.2

WHO case definition for AIDS surveillance

For the purpose of AIDS surveillance, an adult or adolescent (>12 year of age) is considered to have AIDS if at least two of the following major signs are present in combination with at least one of the minor signs listed below, and if these signs are not known to be due to a condition unrelated to HIV infection.
 Major signs:

- Weight loss ≥10% of body weight
- Chronic diarrhea for more than 1 month
- Prolonged fever for more than 1 month (intermittent or constant)

 Minor signs:

- Persistent cough for more than 1 month[a]
- Generalized pruritic dermatitis
- History of herpes zoster
- Oropharyngeal candidiasis
- Chronic progressive or disseminated herpes simplex infection
- Generalized lymphadenopathy.

The presence of either generalized Kaposi's sarcoma or cryptococcal meningitis is sufficient for the diagnosis of AIDS for surveillance purposes.

[a]For patients with tuberculosis, persistent cough for more than 1 month should not be considered as a minor sign.

purposes such as syphilis testing has personal identifiers removed before being tested for HIV infection.[10,15] This has allowed consistent data to be collected across different countries with monitoring of trends by age. Several countries in Africa have undertaken population-based HIV prevalence studies, sometimes in the context of regular demographic and health surveys, and these have tended to show lower prevalence than among pregnant women.[15,16] Data from antenatal serosurveillance have been adjusted to account for urban-rural differences (urban prevalence tends to be higher than rural) and male-female differences (women in Africa tend to have higher prevalence than men) so as to generate estimates of HIV prevalence in the general population.

The weakness of vital registration systems in developing countries has limited the use of AIDS mortality. Some autopsy and mortuary-based studies have given insight into proportional rates of AIDS mortality, occasionally allowing extrapolation to minimum AIDS-specific mortality rates.[17] In general, international estimates of AIDS incidence and mortality have been made though modeling from HIV prevalence data, an activity conducted through the

Joint United Nations Programme on HIV/AIDS (UNAIDS) and the World Health Organization.[9]

HIV/AIDS in the Americas

United States[18]

The USA, the country where in 1981, cases of AIDS were first recognized, has the most severe HIV/AIDS epidemic in the industrialized world. Although AIDS incidence trends have become less representative of trends in HIV transmission since the use of HAART became widespread in 1996, AIDS incidence remains a powerful indicator of the burden of disease (Fig. 1.4). Through 2004, a cumulative total of 918 286 cases of AIDS was reported, and in 2004 alone, there were 44 615 reported cases of AIDS in adults and adolescents, 73% in males and 27% in females, for a population-based rate of 15 per 100 000. The number of reported cases in children in 2004 was 122.

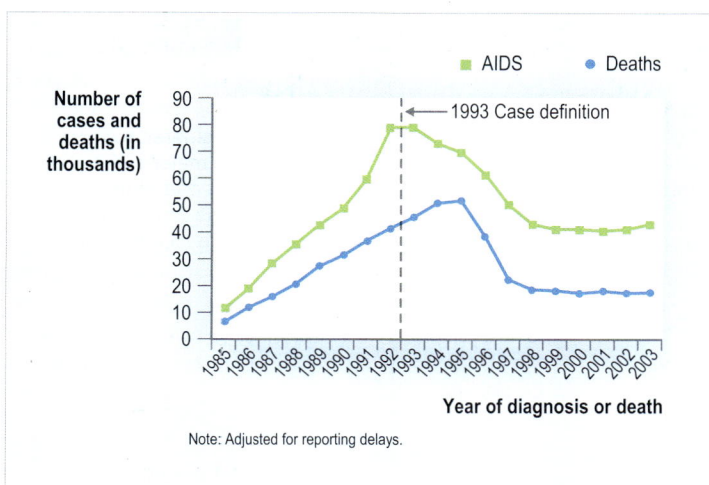

AIDS ■   Deaths ●

1993 Case definition

Number of cases and deaths (in thousands)

Year of diagnosis or death

Note: Adjusted for reporting delays.

Figure 1.4 Estimated number of AIDS cases and deaths among adults and adolescents with AIDS – USA, 1985–2003.

There is now increased emphasis on the reporting of HIV infections, but such reports cannot indicate alone whether acquisition of infection was recent or remote in time. Reported HIV infections are influenced by HIV transmission trends as well as testing uptake, and AIDS trends now reflect testing uptake and access and response to treatment.

The total estimated number of people living with HIV infection in the USA at the end of 2003 was estimated to be between 1 039 000 and 1 185 000. It is estimated that every year, approximately 40 000 new HIV infections occur; a number that has been stable since the early 1990s. A total of 35 states or territories, representing approximately 61% of the US epidemic, have integrated HIV and AIDS reporting systems since at least 2000, whereas AIDS data are available from all states and territories. New reports of HIV/AIDS from these 35 areas declined slightly between 2001 and 2004, whereas the prevalence of HIV/AIDS increased.

Table 1.1 compares descriptive features of persons reported with HIV stratified by AIDS status (with and without AIDS), those without AIDS being more indicative of recently acquired infection (and/or greater uptake of HIV testing). Persons reported with AIDS tended to be older, and were more often male injecting drug users, male heterosexuals, and black or Hispanic than persons reported with HIV alone. Among persons with HIV alone, a greater proportion was contributed by young persons and female heterosexuals compared with persons diagnosed with AIDS. As illustrated by the greater proportion of persons with HIV alone whose transmission category was male-to-male sex, it is not possible to

Table 1.1 Proportional distribution of characteristics of persons reported with HIV infection, with and without AIDS, USA – 2003 (35 areas)[9]

	Without AIDS (%)	With AIDS (%)
Age (years)		
<13	0.7	0.3
13–24	15.3	5.7
>24	84.0	94.0
Sex		
Male	69.9	74.8
Female	30.1	25.2
Race/ethnicity		
Black	50.4	51.2
White	29.6	28.6
Hispanic	18.5	18.8
Asian	1.0	0.9
Native American	0.5	0.4
Transmission category		
Men		
Male-male sex	64.6	57.2
IDU	13.8	17.5
Both	5.1	5.1
Heterosexual	16.0	19.1
Other	0.5	0.9
Women		
Heterosexual	78.0	75.2
IDU	20.4	22.2
Other	1.6	2.6

be certain whether these proportional differences reflect trends in HIV transmission or uptake of HIV testing, or both. They can suggest, however, which groups are benefiting least from early diagnosis and treatment, and where HIV transmission may be most intense.

Figure 1.5 illustrates the distribution of HIV/AIDS cases by sex and transmission category, and Figure 1.6 trends in the numbers of affected persons by race/ethnicity. Figure 1.7 illustrates progress towards the elimination of pediatric HIV disease as a result of programs to prevent the transmission of HIV from mother-to-child. These trends in the USA, with disproportionate impact among minority populations, increasing heterosexual transmission, continued, intense transmission among MSM, stable or declining transmission through injection drug use, and greatly reduced transmission to infants, are broadly representative of the recent history of HIV/AIDS in the rest of the industrialized world.

The Rest of the Americas[9]

The Caribbean is the most heavily affected region of the world after sub-Saharan Africa, with approximately 300 000 people living with HIV at the end of 2005. Haiti is the single most affected country, but HIV prevalence has exceeded 2% in several other countries, including the Bahamas, Belize, Guyana, and Trinidad and Tobago. Transmission is predominantly heterosexual. Injecting drug use is relatively more important in Puerto Rico and Bermuda than in other parts of the region.

Latin America has approximately 1.8 million persons living with HIV; Brazil accounting for at

least one-third of cases. Epidemiology in Latin America is diverse, with all routes of transmission, and especially male-to-male sex, being represented, but to differing extents in different countries. Guatemala and Honduras have epidemics in which national adult HIV prevalence exceeds 1%. Brazil's epidemic has increasingly affected heterosexual populations, women, the poor, and people of color. Brazil is best known as the single developing country that from early on guaranteed free treatment to persons living with HIV/AIDS, with consequent effects of reduced mortality. Argentina has suffered a well publicized outbreak of hospital-based multidrug resistant tuberculosis involving HIV-infected persons.

HIV/AIDS in Europe[19–21]

A total of 52 countries in the WHO European Region report on HIV and AIDS to the European Centre for the Epidemiological Monitoring of AIDS in Paris. Data are presented by the Centre within three geographic areas, the West, the Centre, and the East, though sub-totals are also available for the 25 countries making up the European Union. As in the USA, emphasis on HIV reporting has increased since 1996 when antiretroviral therapy began to make AIDS case reports less reflective of underlying HIV trends. Even within the three geographic areas, surveillance practices by country vary widely and data are not always comparable. HIV reports must be interpreted with caution because changes in reporting practices, testing behaviors, and underlying incidence trends cannot be differentiated. In 2004, a total of 71 755

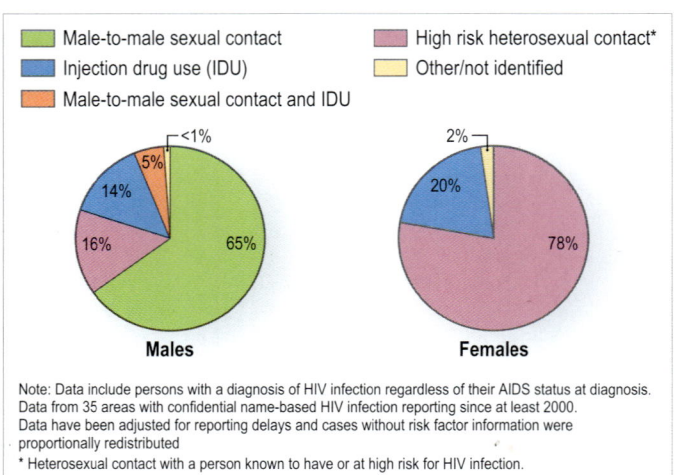

Figure 1.5 Proportion of HIV/AIDS cases among adults and adolescents by sex and transmission category – USA, 2004 (35 areas).

Legend:
- Male-to-male sexual contact
- Injection drug use (IDU)
- Male-to-male sexual contact and IDU
- High risk heterosexual contact*
- Other/not identified

Males: <1%, 5%, 14%, 16%, 65%

Females: 2%, 20%, 78%

Note: Data include persons with a diagnosis of HIV infection regardless of their AIDS status at diagnosis. Data from 35 areas with confidential name-based HIV infection reporting since at least 2000. Data have been adjusted for reporting delays and cases without risk factor information were proportionally redistributed
* Heterosexual contact with a person known to have or at high risk for HIV infection.

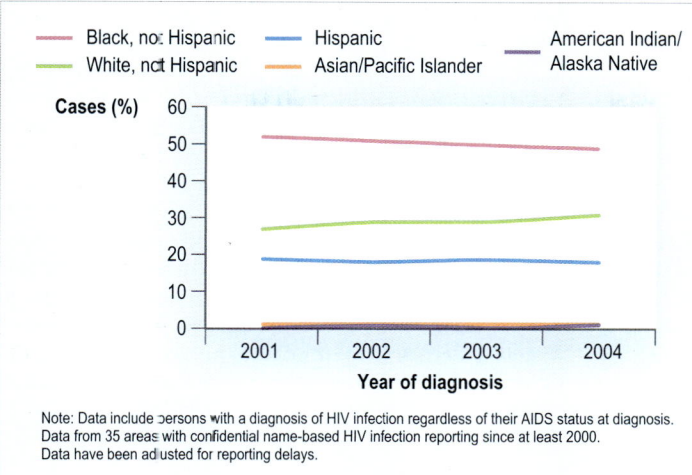

Figure 1.6 Proportion of HIV/AIDS cases among adults and adolescents by race/ethnicity – USA, 2001–2004 (35 areas).

Note: Data include persons with a diagnosis of HIV infection regardless of their AIDS status at diagnosis. Data from 35 areas with confidential name-based HIV infection reporting since at least 2000. Data have been adjusted for reporting delays.

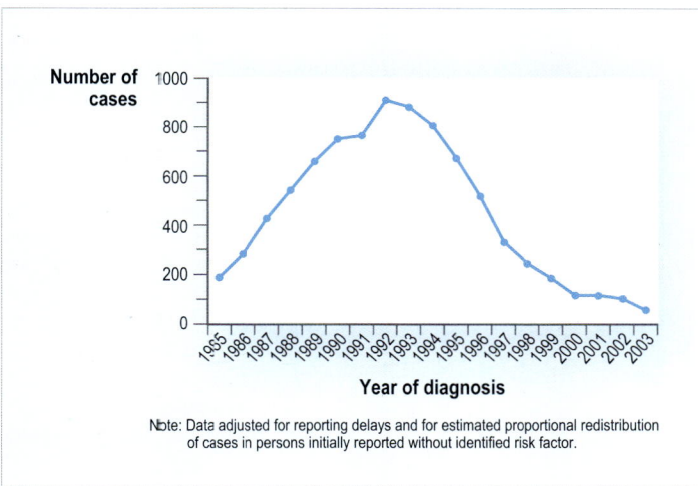

Figure 1.7 Estimated number of perinatally acquired AIDS cases by year of diagnosis – USA, 1985–2003.

Note: Data adjusted for reporting delays and for estimated proportional redistribution of cases in persons initially reported without identified risk factor.

HIV infections were reported, 70% from the East, 28% from the West, and 2% from the Centre.

West

The number of reported cases of HIV has increased substantially in recent years, especially because of increased reports from the UK. A total of 20 229 newly diagnosed HIV infections were reported in 2004. Recent epidemiologic trends have included increased numbers of cases resulting from heterosexual contact, reversal of previous declines in reports among MSM, and a decline in numbers of reports among injection drug users. Heterosexual

contact accounted for 56% of reports, but this proportion is heavily influenced by the frequency of African immigrants in this category.

Portugal, which has suffered a severe epidemic among injecting drug users, has the highest HIV reporting rate (281 per million), with Luxembourg, Switzerland, and the UK reporting rates above 100 per million. Data from some of the more heavily affected countries, however, such as France, Spain, and Italy, were incomplete. Data for this part of the world have been profoundly impacted by migration patterns; over one-quarter of new HIV diagnoses and almost half of heterosexual cases of HIV infection are Africans. A particularly sharp increase in the number of HIV reports has occurred in recent years in the UK, reflecting on-going transmission among MSM as well as increased diagnoses among African immigrants.

In 2004, 7199 AIDS cases were reported, with the highest incidence (80 per million) in Portugal. The dominant exposure category was heterosexual contact, accounting for 47% of cases, compared with 28% for injecting drug use and 23% male-to-male sex. The most frequent indicator diseases were tuberculosis and *Pneumocystis carinii* pneumonia, each reported in almost one-quarter of adult cases. Some 2252 AIDS deaths were reported in 2004, less than the number of new reports of HIV infections or AIDS, indicating that the prevalence of persons living with HIV/AIDS continues to increase.

Centre

The countries of the central European region have a low prevalence of HIV, and only 1597 new HIV diagnoses were reported in 2004. In order of importance, reported exposure categories were heterosexual contact (50% of cases), injecting drug use (22% of cases), and homosexual or bisexual contact (21% of cases). Poland and Romania were the countries with the greatest number of reported cases, accounting for half of the cases in the Centre, but their population-based rates were still lower than in any country in the western region.

AIDS incidence is also low, with 599 cases diagnosed in the region in 2004. Romania has the highest AIDS incidence, reflecting heterosexual HIV transmission as well as the legacy of extensive nosocomial transmission of HIV to infants and children in the late 1980s and early 1990s. The principal AIDS indicator disease is tuberculosis.

East

HIV infections increased steeply in the East during the late 1990s and early 2000s, peaking in 2001 when more than 100 000 HIV newly diagnosed infections were reported, and declining since 2002. A total of 49 929 new diagnoses were reported in 2004, 40% of them in females, and 60% in persons under 30 years of age. Injecting drug use accounted for 65% of infections and heterosexual contact for 34% of cases. The highest rate of reported infection is in Estonia (568 per million), and three countries, Estonia, the Russian Federation, and Ukraine account for 90% of all cases in the East. As a result of increasing heterosexual transmission, an increasing number of infections are being reported in infants and children in this region.

The inevitable epidemic of AIDS is now following the recent HIV epidemic, and in 2004, the East's AIDS incidence rate exceeded that of the West for the first time. A total of 3057 AIDS cases were reported in 2004, although data, including from the Russian Federation, are incomplete. The majority of AIDS cases were in males (72%) and injection drug users (77%). As elsewhere, AIDS cases reflect earlier rather than current HIV transmission patterns. Tuberculosis was the commonest AIDS indicator disease, accounting for over half of cases. AIDS deaths are increasing with the emergence of AIDS itself.

HIV/AIDS in Asia[9,22]

Approximately 8.3 million persons in Asia were estimated to be infected with HIV by the end of 2005, almost one-quarter of them women. Some countries such as Thailand were affected early on and their experience attracted great international attention. HIV is now emerging as a problem in yet others, including in Indonesia and parts of China. Finally, in a number of Asian countries, such as Pakistan and Bangladesh, HIV remains rare. Because Asia's population is so large, even low rates of infection can account for large numbers of infected persons. This applies especially to India and China, whose combined populations approach 2.5 billion people, four times the population of sub-Saharan Africa. The extent to which HIV/AIDS spreads in these two countries will profoundly influence the long-term history of the pandemic.

HIV infection in Asia has been driven by commercial sex and injecting drug use. Thailand's experience exemplifies how commercial sex led to an epidemic of HIV infection, with men acquiring HIV from female commercial sex workers and then transmitting the infection to their regular partners. Thailand also clearly illustrated the effectiveness of prevention, by requiring and vigorously implementing '100% condom use' in the context of commercial sex transactions. HIV infection rates in sentinel groups of men such as military recruits fell, as they did among pregnant women, and today Thailand's estimated adult HIV prevalence is well under 2%. A comparable experience occurred in Cambodia, where prevention interventions have resulted in a reduction in the use of commercial sex, increased condom use, and reduced incidence of other sexually transmitted infections.

Much less success has been achieved with curbing the transmission of HIV through injecting drug use, which can lead to very high levels of prevalence in a very short time. In many Asian cities, the prevalence of HIV infection in injecting drug users exceeds 50%. Although the sexual and injecting drug user-associated epidemics were introduced separately into Thailand and involved different subtypes of HIV-1, there is increasing overlap between these phenomena since many drug users sell sex to meet their living and drug-using requirements. In addition, many drug injectors, the majority of whom are male, have stable sexual partners. These high risk behaviors, commercial sex and injecting drug use, provide the opportunity for HIV to seep into general, low risk populations.

A neglected phenomenon increasing HIV risk is that of male-to-male sex in Asia.[23] While some male-to-male sex occurs in the context of commercial sex, some of it by injecting drug users, an epidemic of HIV infection in indigenous Thai MSM has been described, with a reported prevalence in such men of 17%. This was the first clear description of such an epidemic outside of the industrialized world that was not associated with contact with foreigners or tourists.

HIV infection is well established throughout China, concentrated among commercial sex workers and injecting drug users. The estimated number of infected persons in China is close to one million. A highly publicized outbreak contributing to this number occurred among rural commercial blood donors (i.e. persons who sold their blood) who became infected through exposure to contaminated blood collecting equipment.

India has a larger and more diverse epidemic, with over 5 million estimated infections, more than any country in the world other than South Africa. Injecting drug users and their partners are most affected in northern states, with antenatal prevalence approaching 5% in some cities. Elsewhere, commercial sex has been the major factor behind HIV spread. As elsewhere, some male-to-male sex occurs but its contribution to the overall epidemic is likely to be low.

HIV/AIDS in Africa[9]

While home to only just over 10% of the world's population, sub-Saharan Africa accounts for almost two-thirds of the world's HIV infections. In 2005, it was estimated that some 25.8 million Africans were living with HIV, 3.2 million became infected, and 2.4 million HIV-infected persons died. Sub-Saharan Africa accounts for over three-quarters of the world's HIV-infected women, and over 80% of the world's HIV-infected children and AIDS orphans. Although HIV infection rates tend to be higher in urban than rural areas, the virus has essentially penetrated all over the continent.

HIV transmission in Africa is predominantly heterosexual in nature, explaining the large numbers of women as well as men infected, and the consequent epidemic of HIV/AIDS in children. The very highest rates of infection, in excess of 80%, have been found in commercial sex workers in different parts of the continent. Unsafe blood transfusion has been estimated to cause up to 10% of HIV infections in Africa, a problem which is eminently addressable through technological intervention. Despite controversy around the importance of contaminated injection equipment as a means of transmission of HIV, consensus is that needles play little role in epidemic spread.[24] Male-to-male sex does occur in Africa, although it is generally a taboo; although inadequately studied, it is not considered epidemiologically important. Injecting drug use is increasing in some countries, such as in Kenya, but remains rarer than in other regions of the world.

HIV/AIDS by Region

Marked regional variations occur, with southern Africa most heavily affected (Fig. 1.8). Antenatal HIV prevalence in this region has risen dramatically since the early 1990s to levels few thought possible. Botswana, Lesotho, Swaziland, and Namibia have all reported HIV prevalence levels in pregnant women exceeding 30%. Since national estimates of prevalence are derived from multiple surveillance sites, this means that in some settings prevalence even exceeds 50%. South Africa has the highest number of people in the world living with HIV, over 5 million. Overall HIV prevalence in pregnant women in 2004 was 29.5%. There is no evidence yet of a decline in infection rates in the most heavily affected countries of the southern African region; very recently, slight declines have been reported from Zimbabwe.

East Africa was affected earlier than southern Africa and several countries, most strikingly Uganda but also Kenya and some others, have shown a decline in their rates of HIV infection. The national rate of infection in Kenya is estimated to be about 7% and most countries in this region have prevalence rates below 15%. The precipitous decline in HIV

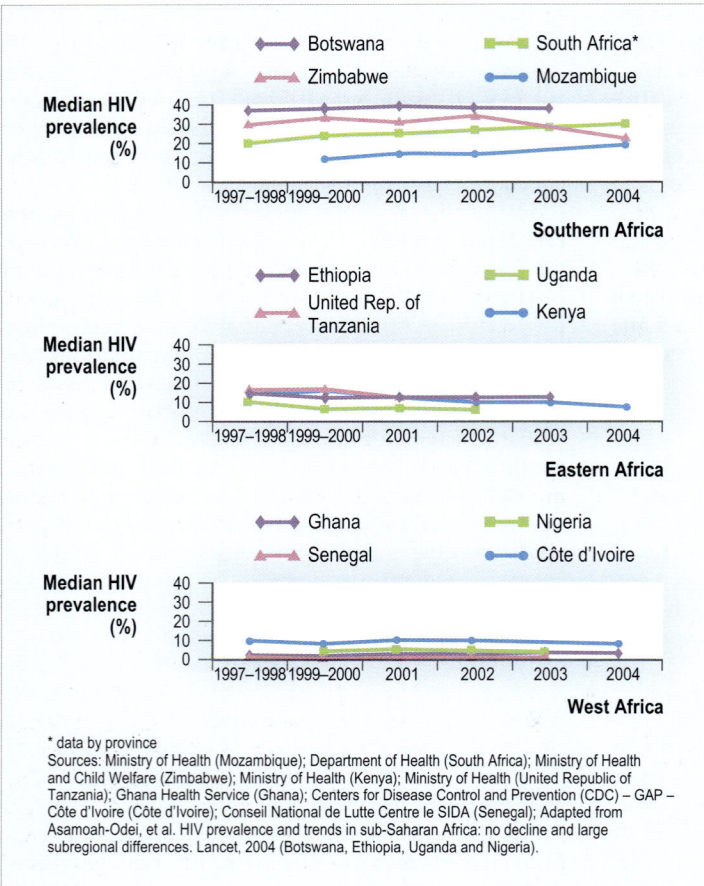

Figure 1.8 Trends in HIV prevalence in pregnant women in sub-Saharan Africa. (Reproduced with kind permission from UNAIDS.[9])

* data by province
Sources: Ministry of Health (Mozambique); Department of Health (South Africa); Ministry of Health and Child Welfare (Zimbabwe); Ministry of Health (Kenya); Ministry of Health (United Republic of Tanzania); Ghana Health Service (Ghana); Centers for Disease Control and Prevention (CDC) – GAP – Côte d'Ivoire (Côte d'Ivoire); Conseil National de Lutte Centre le SIDA (Senegal); Adapted from Asamoah-Odei, et al. HIV prevalence and trends in sub-Saharan Africa: no decline and large subregional differences. Lancet, 2004 (Botswana, Ethiopia, Uganda and Nigeria).

infection rates in Uganda since the mid-1990s have aroused much speculation as to their cause. An important feature, true also in Kenya, is that at some point deaths began to exceed new infections. More accurate surveillance practices and laboratory work may have contributed to lowering estimates, as well as behavior change. The Ugandan experience has been widely interpreted as demonstrating the efficacy of the ABC strategy (Abstinence; Be faithful; Condoms for those who cannot abstain or be faithful to one partner) although many factors were likely involved, including high mortality.

The prevalence of HIV infection in Central and West Africa is generally lower than in East and southern Africa, though some countries (Cameroon, Central African Republic, Cote d'Ivoire) stand out as exceptions. The Democratic Republic of Congo is interesting because despite the longstanding presence of HIV there, infection having been shown as far back as 1959, prevalence has remained stable

at a relatively low rate. The higher rate in Cote d'Ivoire, around 10% in pregnant women, is likely related to its importance as a regional hub for trade and employment. Spread has increased in Nigeria, Africa's most populous country, which is accounting for an increasing proportion of African infections.

Impact of the Epidemic in Africa[25]

The direct effect of the epidemic, especially in countries with the highest rates of infection, is to cause huge increases in mortality, with consequent reduction in life expectancy due to increased adult as well as child mortality. Directly measured life expectancy in a rural part of western Kenya where the adult prevalence of HIV infection is approximately 20–25% is now 38 years, and a number of southern African countries report national life expectancies below 40 years, representing the loss of two or more decades of life. The demographic structure of the population changes under such conditions, with increased deaths in young children and young adults, the groups most affected by HIV. Further consequences are the epidemic of orphans, expected to approach 20 million by 2010, significant socioeconomic losses and increases in family poverty, and negative impact on food production and food security. A medical consequence is a serious secondary epidemic of tuberculosis whose incidence has increased several times in many African countries over the past decade. In some southern African countries, tuberculosis incidence is more than 100 times that in the USA.

Epidemiologic Heterogeneity[25,26]

HIV/AIDS in Women and Children

One of the striking features of high prevalence countries is the high ratio of infections in women compared with men, especially among youth. Overall, the female:male infection ratio in Africa is about 1.3, although in the 15–24 year age groups three to six times as many women as men are infected. In Kenya, the overall ratio is a surprising 1.9.[16] The reasons are biological, male-to-female transmission probably being more efficient than female-to-male, as well as social.

The epidemic in children is eroding gains in life expectancy that were won over several decades through investment in maternal and child health. Since approximately 35–45% of children born to breast-feeding, HIV-infected women, acquire the infection, prevalence rates in children are lower than in adults, including hospitalized patients. Approximately 35% and 52%, respectively, of HIV-infected children in Africa die by the ages of 1 or 2 years.[27]

Reasons for Heterogeneity[25,26]

Why HIV/AIDS is so severe in Africa compared with elsewhere, and why such marked regional variations occur are incompletely understood. Like other infectious diseases, HIV/AIDS epidemiology reflects the interaction between the viral agent, the human host, and the environment. Mathematically, epidemic spread is determined by the basic reproductive rate, the number of secondary infections generated from one primary case, which depends on the rate of partner change, transmissibility, and the duration of infectiousness.

A well known study[26] aimed at elucidating differences between high and low prevalence settings in Africa concluded that biological rather than behavioral factors were predominant determinants of epidemic severity, particularly rates of genital herpes and male circumcision. Genital herpes has been consistently found to approximately double the risk of acquiring HIV, and male circumcision to halve the risk in men.[28,29] For a sexually transmitted infection like HIV, behavior must be important but in high prevalence settings any sexual contact with a person of unknown serostatus is potentially dangerous. Sexual networks and whether sexual relationships across a society are predominantly consecutive or concurrent are important but poorly studied issues. While biological reasons exist to explain the lesser spread of HIV-2 than HIV-1,[5] there is no good epidemiologic evidence supporting the concept that particular subtypes of HIV-1 determine HIV/AIDS epidemiology.[7]

The Status of the Global Response[30]

The first international response to the pandemic occurred in 1986, when the WHO established its Special (later the Global) Programme on AIDS. The Joint United Nations Programme on HIV/AIDS (UNAIDS) was set up in 1995 to coordinate international efforts, bringing together different agencies of the United Nations. Substantially increased funding has been made available in the last few years, under different initiatives including the US President's Emergency Plan for AIDS Relief (PEPFAR), the World Bank's Multi-Country AIDS Programme (MAP), the Global Fund to Fight AIDS, Tuberculosis, and Malaria, and WHO's Three by Five initiative. The WHO initiative and PEPFAR have a strong focus on the provision of treatment to HIV-infected persons in developing countries.

Global efforts to combat the pandemic have substantially increased in the past few years, and the dichotomy of treatment in the industrialized world but not in the more heavily affected South is finally being addressed. There is a danger that the welcome efforts to expand treatment may neglect prevention efforts, and that treatment availability may increase risk behavior. Africa will remain the global epicenter for HIV/AIDS for the foreseeable future, but epidemic expansion in Eastern Europe and Asia, especially in India and China, may profoundly affect future epidemiology. The long-term future of the pandemic is uncertain and at this time, infection and death for many more tens of millions of people seems inevitable.[31]

References

1. Hahn BH, Shaw GM, DeCock KM, et al. AIDS as a zoonosis: scientific and public health implications. Science 2000; 287:607–614.

2. Sharp PM, Shaw GM, Hahn BH. Simian immunodeficiency virus infection of chimpanzees. J Virol 2005; 79:3891–3902.

3. Lemey P, Pybus OG, Wang B, et al. Tracing the origin and history of the HIV-2 epidemic. PNAS 2003; 100:6588–6592.

4. Osmanov S, Pattou C, Walker N, et al. WHO Network for HIV isolation and characterization. Estimated global distribution and regional spread of HIV-1 genetic subtypes in the year 2000. J Acquir Immune Defic Syndr 2002; 29:184–190.

5. DeCock KM, Adjorlolo G, Ekpini E, et al. Epidemiology and transmission of HIV-2. Why there is no HIV-2 pandemic. JAMA 1993; 270:2083–2086.

6. Van der Loef S, Aaby P. Towards a better understanding of the epidemiology of HIV-2. AIDS 1999; 13:S69–S84.

7. Hu DJ, Buve A, Baggs, et al. What role does HIV-1 subtype play in transmission and pathogenesis? An epidemiological perspective. AIDS 1999; 13:873–881.

8. Ambroziak J, Levy JA. Epidemiology, natural history, and pathogenesis of HIV infection. In: Holmes KK, Sparling PF, Mardh P-A, et al., eds. Sexually transmitted diseases. 3rd edn. New York: McGraw-Hill; 1999:251–258.

9. UNAIDS. AIDS epidemic update: December 2005. Geneva: UNAIDS/WHO; 2005.

10. Diaz T, DeCock KM, Brown T, et al. New strategies for HIV surveillance in resource-constrained settings: An overview. AIDS 2005; 19:S1–S8.

11. Fleming PL, Ward JW, Janssen RS, et al. Guidelines for human immunodeficiency virus case surveillance, including monitoring for human immunodeficiency virus infection and acquired immunodeficiency syndrome. MMWR 1999; 48:1–27.

12. Rosenberg PS, Biggar RJ. Trends in HIV incidence among young adults in the United States. JAMA 1998; 279:1894–1899.

13. Janssen RS, Satten GA, Stramer SL, et al. New testing strategy to detect early HIV-1 infection for use in incidence estimates and for clinical and prevention purposes. JAMA 1998; 280:42–48.

14. World Health Organization. WHO case definitions for AIDS surveillance in adults and adolescents. Wkly Epidemiol Rec (WHO) 1994; 69:273–280.

15. Boerma JT, Ghys PD, Walker N. Estimates of HIV-1 prevalence from national population-based surveys as a new gold standard. Lancet 2003; 362:1929–1931.

16. Central Bureau of Statistics (CBS) [Kenya], Ministry of Health (MOH) [Kenya], and ORC Macro. Kenya Demographic and Health Survey 2003. Calverton: CBS, MOH, and ORC Macro; 2004.

17. DeCock KM, Barrere B, Diaby L, et al. AIDS: the leading cause of adult death in the West African city of Abidjan, Cote d'Ivoire. Science 1990; 249:793–796.

18. Centers for Disease Control and Prevention. HIV/AIDS surveillance report, 2004. Vol. 16. Atlanta: US Department of Health and Human Services, Centers for Disease Control and Prevention; 2005.

19. EuroHIV. HIV/AIDS Surveillance in Europe. End-year report 2004. Saint Maurice: Institut de veille sanitaire; 2004: No. 71.

20. Hamers FF, Downs AM. HIV in central and eastern Europe. Lancet 2003; 361:1035–1044.

21. Hamers FF, Downs AM. The changing face of the HIV epidemic in western Europe: what are the implications for public health policies? Lancet 2004; 364:83–94.

22. Ruxrungtham K, Brown T, Phanuphak P. HIV/AIDS in Asia. Lancet 2004; 364:69–82.

23. Griensven F van, Thanprasertsuk S, Jommaroeng R, et al. Evidence of a previously undocumented epidemic of HIV infection among men who have sex with men in Bangkok, Thailand. AIDS 2005; 19:521–526.

24. Schmid G, Buvé A, Mugyenyi P, et al. Eliminating unsafe injections is important, but will have little impact on HIV transmission in sub-Saharan Africa. Lancet 2004; 363:482–488.

25. Buvé A, Bishikwabo-Nsarhaza K, Mutangadura G. The spread and effect of HIV-1 infection in sub-Saharan Africa. Lancet 2002; 359:2011–2017.

26. Carael M, Holmes K, eds. The multicentre study of factors determining the different prevalences of HIV in sub-Saharan Africa. AIDS 2001; 15:Suppl 4.

27. Newell ML, Coovadia H, Cortina-Borja M, et al. Mortality of infected and uninfected infants born to HIV-infected mothers in Africa: a pooled analysis. Lancet 2004; 364:1236–1243.

28. Wald A, Link K. Risk of human immunodeficiency virus infection in herpes simplex virus type-2 seropositive persons: a meta-analysis. J Infect Dis 2002; 185:45–52.

29. Weiss H, Quigley MA, Hayes R. Male circumcision and risk of HIV infection in sub-Saharan Africa: a systematic review and meta-analysis. AIDS 2000; 14:2361–2370.

30. Behrman G. The invisible people. New York: Free Press; 2004.

31. AIDS in Africa. Three scenarios to 2025. Geneva: UNAIDS; 2005.

CHAPTER 2

The Origins and Diversification of HIV

Michael Worobey

Introduction

Human immunodeficiency virus (HIV) is not one but several, related viruses that have crossed into the human population on multiple occasions from non-human primate reservoir species in Africa. Only one such lineage, the 'main' group of HIV type 1 (HIV-1 group M), has reached pandemic proportions; it accounts for more than 99% of the more than 40 million HIV infections and has a global distribution. The other HIVs, though relatively minor, hold important clues about the nature of the origins and diversification of this important group. This chapter will begin with a broad scope, surveying the primate lentivirus radiation and placing the various HIV groups within it. It will then focus specifically on the genesis of HIV-1 group M, summarizing when, where, and how this most important HIV variant originated, diversified, and spread around the world. An important goal of this chapter will be to bring into sharp relief the biological meaning and medical relevance of the various levels of HIV genetic diversity commonly recognized ('types,' 'groups,' 'subtypes,' and so on). Understanding what such classifications do and do not represent, is critical to any rational approach to exploiting knowledge about viral evolution in order to combat HIV/AIDS.

The Deep Roots of HIV

Phylogenetic trees, reconstructed using the remarkably rich historical information stamped onto the genomes of these viruses, have emerged as the pre-eminent tools for reconstructing the history of HIV and simian immunodeficiency virus (SIV). The genealogical patterns that emerge from phylogenies provide not only an invaluable historical record, but also a window through which we can glimpse the medically relevant evolutionary and epidemiological processes that generated the patterns. Gene trees also offer a framework for systematizing the extensive genetic diversity of HIV and related viruses into a coherent classification scheme. With any organism's classification, however, there is a danger of becoming fixated on *pattern* rather than *process*, and HIV is no exception. Some of the potential pitfalls of doing so are discussed below.

AIDS was first recognized in the USA in the early 1980s,[1] and the discovery of HIV followed soon after.[2] It is now clear, however, that HIV emerged decades earlier, from naturally infected primates on another continent.[3] Figure 2.1 illustrates the relationships between the different variants of HIV (red branches) and related viruses that have been discovered in a large number of African monkeys and apes. To date, at least 36 species of non-human primates have shown evidence of infection by SIV,[4] every one of which is restricted in range to sub-Saharan Africa. Since the primate lentiviruses form a single, distinct clade on the mammalian lentivirus phylogeny, and given that no primates outside of Africa appear to be infected, SIV evidently had its origin in an African monkey at some point sufficiently deep in time to account for its spread throughout most of the continent, and into most of the (catarrhine) primate species there.

The precise nature of the timescale is still open to question. Remarkably, there is as yet no definitive

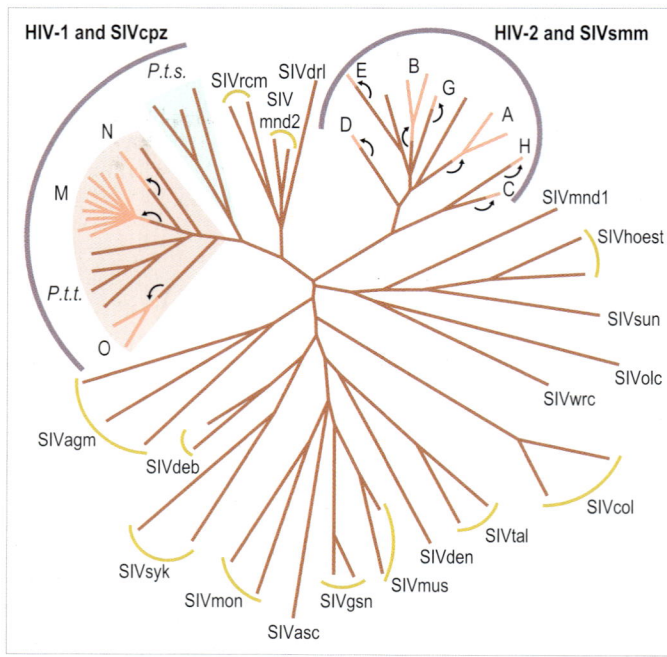

Figure 2.1 Maximum likelihood phylogenetic tree of SIV and HIV partial *pol* gene sequences. The sequence alignment was downloaded from the Los Alamos National Laboratories HIV database (www.hiv.lanl.gov) and reconstructed under the HKY85 model of nucleotide substitution with gamma distributed among-site rate heterogeneity. The scale bar represents 5% genetic distance. SIVcpz strains recovered from *Pan troglodytes troglodytes* (*P.t.t.*) are shaded in pink, while those from *P. t. schweinfurthii* (*P.t.s.*) are shaded in green. A small arrow leading to a lighter pink branch indicates inferred cross-species transmission leading to an HIV group. The abbreviations and species names are as follows: SIVsmm, sooty mangabey; SIVmnd1 and SIVmnd2, mandrill; SIVlhoest, L'Hoest's monkey; SIVsun, sun-tailed monkey; SIVolc, olive colobus; SIVwrc, western red colobus; SIVtal, talapoin; SIVden, Dent's mona; SIVmus, mustached guenon; SIVgsn, greater spot-nosed monkey; SIVasc, red-tailed monkey; SIVmon, mona monkey; SIVsyk, Sykes's monkey; SIVdeb, De Brazza's monkey; SIVagm, African green monkey (this includes SIVgri, grivet; SIVtan, tantalus monkey; SIVver, vervet monkey); SIVcpz, common chimpanzee; SIVrcm, red-capped mangabey; SIVdrl, drill.

evidence that would narrow the possible range even within three orders of magnitude. Comparisons of primate and virus phylogenies have led to suggestions that some SIVs have co-diverged with their hosts, as the animals split into new species from their common ancestors. This would place a time scale measured in the millions of years to get back to the most recent common ancestor (MRCA) of the SIVs. (To visualize this, picture the evolutionary tree depicted in Figure 2.1 as a snapshot of an exploding firework, with the ancestral virus at its center and the contemporary sequences at the tips of the branches emanating from it; the center is the point in evolutionary time we are trying to date.) On the other hand, detailed studies of SIV evolutionary rates make it hard to conceive of dates older than a few thousand years for the SIV MRCA.[5] Extrapolations from the rapid short-term evolutionary rates observed in lentiviruses[6] suggest that, for SIV lineages that diverged more than even a few thousand years ago, the molecular evidence of shared ancestry ought to have become overwritten by a succession of nucleotide substitutions.

There are a couple of possible ways this conundrum could be sorted out. Either long-term rates of SIV are slower than our best current nucleotide substitution models allow, or the viruses did not actually co-speciate with their hosts after all. If the latter turns out to be the case, the pattern of closely-related hosts having closely-related viruses might be explained not by co-divergence but, instead, by cross-species transmission events occurring preferentially between closely-related hosts.[7] Recent studies of genes involved in innate immunity, such as APOBEC3G,[8] suggest the sort of mechanism that could have generated such a pattern of correspondence.

HIV/SIV Nomenclature

Of the dozens of species with naturally occurring SIV, only two, the common chimpanzee (*Pan troglodytes*) and the sooty mangabey (*Cercocebus atys*), are known to have acted as reservoirs of HIV. HIV type 1 (HIV-1) is the designation given to forms of the human virus linked to the SIV from *P. troglodytes* (SIVcpz), while HIV type 2 (HIV-2) denotes human viruses related to the sooty mangabey virus (SIVsmm). Inspection of the SIV/HIV phylogenetic tree shows that, within both SIVcpz and SIVsmm, more than one cross-species transmission event has occurred. The key observation here is that HIV lineages intermingle on the tree with SIV lineages. HIV-1 groups N and M are both more closely related to some of the SIVcpz viruses on the tree than they are to HIV-1 group O, whose lineage branched off the main trunk at an earlier point. In other words, HIV-1 group M shared a most recent common ancestor with a chimpanzee virus, not with HIV-1 group O. Likewise, HIV-2 group E is the 'sister' group to one SIVsmm strain, and HIV-2 group A is the sister group of another. If there had been only a single transmission from each reservoir species to humans, we would expect the human viruses to fall into single clusters (or monophyletic clades, in the jargon of phylogenetics) – one for HIV-1 and one for HIV-2. This is not the case.

Recombination, whereby genes from separate strains are combined into a new, chimeric viral genome within a dually infected host, complicates these phylogenetic inferences somewhat. For example, HIV-1 group N,[9] though closely related to HIV-1 group M in the *pol* region (Fig. 2.1), apparently arose from a recombination event: some of its genome is much more distantly related to group M.[10] Such complications aside, each lineage depicted in bold in Figure 2.1 is thought to have arisen from an independent cross-species transmission, and hence each of these groups is thought to be more closely related to either an SIVcpz or an SIVsmm than to the other groups in its type.

So, while the two different *types* of HIV denote the two different primate reservoirs that have served as sources of human infection, the various *groups* within each type represent independent introductions from primate to human. Within HIV-1, three such events are inferred, giving rise to HIV-1 groups M, O ('outlier'),[11] and N ('new').[9] Within HIV-2, eight independent transmissions are indicated, corresponding to HIV-2 groups A through H.[3,12] Earlier studies of HIV-2 used the term *subtype* for these lineages, but this usage has given way to the use of the term *group* in order to bring HIV-2 nomenclature in line with the more widely cited (if slightly less logical) HIV-1 conventions.[12] The goal of the change was to emphasize the biological parallel between the different lineages of HIV-1 and HIV-2 that arose via unique zoonotic origins. In this sense, HIV nomenclature reflects the evolutionary processes driving observed patterns of genetic diversity rather well.

The term *subtype*, in turn, is used within HIV-1 group M. Each of the nine branches in the M group in Figure 2.1 represents one of the recognized subtypes (A to D, F to H, J, K). Different subtypes dominate in different regions. For example, subtype B accounts for most infections in Europe and the Americas, subtype C predominates in southern African countries like South Africa, as well as in India, and subtype D is common in east Africa. The unfortunate fact that *subtypes* are nested within *groups*, rather than *types*, in this naming scheme, owes to the fact that the use of the term predates the discovery of HIV-1 group O, at which point the new designation of *group* had to be wedged between *type* and *subtype*. The system of naming HIVs and SIVs has thus evolved over time as the full diversity of natural SIV infections in African primates was revealed, and as new, distinct lineages of HIV have been discovered.

As hinted above, recombination plays a large role in the evolution of both SIV and HIV.[13] The existence of clear recombinants, with genomes that are mosaics of distinct lineages, has led to the introduction of a formal system for recognizing them.[14] These *circulating recombinant forms* (CRFs) represent virus populations that have diversified from a single, ancestral strain generated by recombination between two or more of the recognized M group subtypes.[14] The 'missing' subtypes, E and I, have been re-classified as CRFs after detailed analysis of their genomes revealed that they had recombinant origins.[14] Some CRFs are the dominant HIV-1 group M strain in some locales (e.g. CRF01 in Thailand, CRF02 in Nigeria).

There is also abundant evidence of recombination among the SIVs of different primate species, and even between HIV-1 groups M and O.[15] Most notably, the progenitor of HIV-1, SIVcpz, turns out to be a recombinant between the SIVs of red-capped mangabeys and greater spot-nosed monkeys, two prey species of the chimpanzee.[16] All strains of HIV-1 are thus ultimately recombinant in origin, their genomes a mosaic of two monkey viruses, trafficked through an ape intermediary.

In summary, the primate lentivirus phylogenetic tree and the system of HIV nomenclature reflect some key evolutionary insights. First, SIVs are naturally found in a variety of sub-Saharan African primates and this region is hence the cradle of HIV. Second, despite the many primates infected, and frequent opportunities for human exposure, as far as is known SIV has only crossed successfully into humans from chimpanzees and sooty mangabeys, but has crossed multiple times from each, a curious pattern for which no definitive explanation has been proposed. Finally, the virus that first appeared on the medical world's radar in high risk populations in the USA made an extraordinary journey there: from African monkeys, then to the apes that preyed upon them, then onto human beings in central Africa and beyond.

Where did HIV Enter the Human Population?

Using the geographic distributions of the primate species that have spawned HIV variants it has been possible to infer, with remarkable precision, the specific areas in Africa where the various HIV-1 and HIV-2 groups originated. HIV-2 was the first to give up its secrets, and by the early 1990s it was clear that different groups of HIV-2 were independently derived from SIVsmm, the SIV variant endemic in the sooty mangabey monkeys of West Africa.[17] HIV-2 is endemic to the same region, and is only rarely detected elsewhere. Although HIV-2 accounts for relatively few infections compared with HIV-1, many more cross-species transmissions involving this virus have been detected, with eight groups (A–H) currently recognized. Only two of these, groups A and B, appear to have established themselves as endemic human infections. In all the other cases, the 'group' is in fact comprised of a single patient infected with an HIV-2 variant that is sufficiently genetically divergent from the others that it was likely acquired independently. Some or all of these may represent evolutionary 'dead ends.'[18] In some cases, the human virus bears a surprisingly close resemblance to SIVsmm infecting free-living or pet sooty mangabeys from the same local area,[18,19] strong evidence of repeated independent cross-species transmission.

The geographical origins of HIV-1 have taken longer to piece together, but it now seems clear that all three HIV-1 groups can be traced to a single subspecies of chimpanzee, *P. troglodytes troglodytes*, the 'central' chimpanzee, whose range encompasses southern Cameroon, Central African Republic, Equatorial Guinea, Gabon, and the Republic of Congo (Congo-Brazzaville).[3,10,20,21] Although both the central chimpanzee and the 'eastern' subspecies, *P. t. schweinfurthii*, are naturally infected with SIVcpz, the viruses recovered from the two chimpanzee lineages form distinct clades on the SIV phylogenetic tree (Fig. 2.1), indicating that they have been evolving in isolation for a considerable time.

Crucially, each of the three instances of cross-species transmission from chimpanzees to humans (HIV-1 groups M, N, and O), is phylogenetically linked to the SIVcpz of the *P. t. troglodytes* chimpanzee (the blue shaded clade in Fig. 2.1). No known variant of HIV-1 has emerged from the eastern chimpanzee (green shaded clade in Fig. 2.1). HIV-1 groups N and O are both endemic to Cameroon, within the

range of *P. t. troglodytes,* and neither has spread substantially beyond this presumptive region of origin. Group O exhibits about 0.4% prevalence in Cameroon,[22] while group N is exceedingly rare, with less than 10 positive individuals identified to date.[23] Despite the relative rarity of these groups, their pathogenic profile appears indistinguishable from group M's,[22] an indication that *pathogenic* potential and *epidemic* behavior of AIDS viruses are not necessarily coupled.[12] Given the very different properties of the three groups of HIV-1 in terms of rate of spread through human host populations, it is tempting to speculate that their pathogenic properties may owe more to their common genetic heritage, as close relatives descended from SIVcpz, than to convergent evolutionary trajectories once they entered humans. The recent discovery of the first rare variant of HIV-2 known to cause immunosuppression lends support to this notion,[12] but future studies will be required to further clarify the ground rules of the evolution of HIV pathogenicity.

The geographical source of the main group of HIV-1 has been somewhat obscured by its global spread, but the available evidence links it to the same region. First of all, it falls soundly within the same clade as groups O and N, among the diverse viruses of the *P. t. troglodytes* chimpanzees – powerful evidence that it emerged from within their range.[10] Furthermore, since group O is actually *basal* to the M/N part of the phylogenetic tree (i.e. its SIVcpz precursor branched off prior to the point at which the M and N precursors diverged from their common ancestor; Fig. 2.1), the most parsimonious solution to the puzzle is that the M group crossed into the human population in the same area. That group N is a recombinant virus, part of whose genome derives from an M-like 'parental' strain of SIVcpz,[10] is further, subtle yet damning evidence placing the M-group ancestor at the same scene.

Much more direct evidence linking HIV-1 group M to Cameroon is now available, however. By screening non-invasively-collected fecal samples from the region, Beatrice Hahn and colleagues have identified several closely related SIVcpz strains from wild-living Cameroonian chimpanzees, viruses that are remarkably similar to group M, and which form a well-supported cluster with it on phylogenetic trees (B. Hahn, personal communication). These *P. t. troglodytes* SIVs bear the genetic fingerprint of being descendents of a close relative of the very SIVcpz strain that crossed into humans and went on to become the pandemic AIDS virus.

When did HIV Enter the Human Population?

It has been said that RNA viruses represent a 'moving target,' and the point is well taken. HIV has been measured directly and found to have an error rate as high as 10^{-4} mutations per site and two to three recombination events per genome per replication cycle. The high error rate of its reverse transcriptase, plus its high replication rate, mean that mutations rapidly arise and accumulate, making HIV one of the fastest evolving organisms in nature.

Generally, the longer the time span since two HIV sequences diverged from a common ancestor, the greater the number of nucleotide differences we expect when we compare their homologous gene sequences. Although different regions of the genome evolve at different rates,[24] and a strict 'molecular clock' is often rejected with HIV molecular data sets,[6] this observation means that illuminating inferences about the timing of HIV evolution can often be culled from alignments of gene sequences.

Estimates of the time to the most recent common ancestor of each of the four most prevalent HIV groups have been inferred using phylogenetic trees and maximum likelihood and/or Bayesian statistical methods.[6,24,25] Behind the sophisticated mathematical models used for such inferences lies a simple concept: if viral nucleotide sequences diverge from each other by, say, 1% per year after they split from a common ancestor, then a pair of sequences that differ by, say, 30% must have diverged about 30 years ago. The tricks with HIV are (1) to correct for multiple changes at the same site – a particular concern with fast-evolving organisms, (2) to calibrate the 'molecular clock,' and (3) to account adequately for the inherent 'sloppiness' of the clock and any potential methodological biases. Fortunately, we can calibrate the clock simply by watching HIV evolve in real time: samples collected over a span of several years will reveal the rate at which substitutions accrue, with early-sampled sequences tending to have short branches (less change) and late-sampled sequences tending to have longer branch lengths (more change). As for dealing with the noisy phylogenetic signal, it is important to consider appropriate confidence intervals around estimated divergence dates. A recent study of HIV-1 group O, for example, estimated that its most recent common ancestor existed in 1920, but with a wide confidence interval (1890–1940).[24] The best estimate for group M is 1931 (1915–1941),[6] while those for HIV-2 groups A and B are 1940 (1924–1956) and 1945 (1931–1959), respectively.[25] And although the specter of unaccounted-for recombination biasing such estimates looms over such analyses,[26] there is surprisingly little indication that it systematically affects divergence date inferences in one direction or the other.[24]

Inferences from more or less contemporary sequences, though, are not the only source of information about historical landmarks in HIV evolution. Arguably the most important HIV-1 sequence published to date is that of ZR59, recovered from an archival blood sample taken from an adult male in 1959 in what is now the Democratic Republic of the Congo.[27] The few hundred nucleotides sequenced from this strain showed not only that the main group of HIV-1 was already circulating in the human population at this early date, but also, more importantly, that this group of viruses must have been circulating for some considerable time *before* this point: the strain falls far enough away from the putative ancestral virus that the most recent common ancestor of the M group must have existed many years prior to 1959. This provides crucial, independent evidence that the ancestor of group M existed long before 1959.

HIV/AIDS: Collateral Damage from Unsafe Medical Practices?

The phylogenetic position of the 1959 sequence is, on its own, enough to argue convincingly against the controversial theory that HIV-1 group M had its origins in experimental polio vaccines allegedly prepared using SIV-contaminated chimpanzee tissue, then administered across central Africa in the late 1950s.[28] Perhaps more than any other modern human disease, AIDS has inspired impassioned debate about the circumstances surrounding its origins and spread, and the 'Oral Polio Vaccine/AIDS' (OPV/AIDS) hypothesis has been one of the most controversial explanations. While the idea was worthy of careful consideration since – at least in later incarnations – it correctly implicated chimpanzees as the source if HIV-1 group M, several lines of evidence have argued strongly against it. First there is the 'disconnect' between the inferred M group divergence date (around 1930) and the earliest use of the experimental vaccines (1957), a discrepancy in timing that, as explained in the next section, cannot be resolved by invoking a separate introduction for each subtype.[29] There is also the geographical evidence discussed above: all forms of HIV-1, including the M group, evidently evolved from a *P. t. troglodytes*

SIVcpz ancestor. The chimpanzees implicated in the OPV/AIDS theory were collected from the Democratic Republic of the Congo. Such *P. t. schweinfurthii* chimpanzees, including ones collected near Kisangani (the strain marked with an asterisk in Fig. 2.1), where the polio vaccine work was centered, are infected by a distant cousin of HIV-1 group M,[21,30] one that is not a plausible M group precursor.

The fact that SIVcpz is a recombinant of two monkey SIVs is also very telling since it puts the lie to the woolly notion that non-natural circumstances such as mass vaccinations are somehow required for the successful transmission of SIV from one species to the next.[28] In fact, the non-human primate SIVs tell a very different story, one where transmission between species is a common, perhaps even dominant, evolutionary process. Recombination events imply a history of cross-species transfers among not only chimpanzees, red-capped mangabeys, and greater spot-nosed monkeys,[16] but also others, including green monkeys (*C. sabeus*). Cross-species transmission must also have introduced at least one of the two distinct mandrill SIVs (Fig. 2.1).[31] Moreover, several species, including patas monkeys, yellow baboons, and chacma baboons, have acquired SIV from local African green monkeys with which they interact.[32] In spite of claims to the contrary,[28,33] the phylogenetics of SIV and HIV indicate that primate lentiviruses have the capacity to cross species boundaries and establish new epidemics naturally.

It follows from this observation, and from the pre-1950 divergence dates for all the epidemic forms of HIV, that the rapid growth of unsterile injections in Africa beginning in the 1950s was not the key to the establishment of HIV, as has been proposed.[33] When considering the emergence of HIV, it is helpful to decompose the process into factors promoting the establishment of HIV as a human-to-human infection, and those favoring the subsequent spread of a virus that has become established. A plethora of 'dirty needles' may have helped *spread* groups A, B, M, and O in Africa in the 1950s and later, but the *establishment* of each – the transmission of the ancestral SIV into the first human host, and the initial human-to-human transmission of each nascent HIV – appears to have occurred earlier. Iatrogenic infection is not currently the dominant mode of HIV transmission in sub-Saharan Africa,[34,35] and may never have been, but this is not to say that it is not a serious concern. Even if it accounts for only 5% of HIV incidence there, then there are presumably more medically infected HIV-positive Africans than there are HIV-positive Americans in the entire US

epidemic. Such is the magnitude of the HIV/AIDS epidemic in the hardest hit region.

The Meaning of Genetic Diversity within HIV-1 Group M

Given the attention paid to them, it is of clear medical importance to understand the nature of the HIV-1 group M subtypes. Recognizing certain lineages as 'subtypes' has certainly aided the tracking of epidemiologically important lineages across the globe.[14] But parsing the huge amount of genetic diversity within the main group of HIV-1 into subtypes has also imbued them with an undeserved status. Are they well-defined biological entities with intrinsic, medically meaningful properties? Is it a sound idea, for example, to pursue *subtype*-specific vaccines against different portions of global HIV-1 M variation (as opposed to broader or narrower phylogenetic criteria)? Answering such fundamental questions requires careful differentiation between pattern and process.

Figure 2.2 shows a phylogenetic tree encompassing the global diversity of group M strains. Below the tree are two schematic phylogenies showing the phylogenetic pattern observed when only sequences from outside of the group M epicenter are analyzed (left), versus the pattern obtained when sequences from the putative source population are added (right). The labels indicate recognized subtype/CRF designations. The crucial point here is that the subtypes within group M are artifacts of 'founder' effects and biased sampling.[29,36] The 'subtypiness' of group M, with distinct clades separated by long internal branches reflective of independent evolutionary history, only arises on phylogenies reconstructed with sequences sampled *outside* of the central African source of the pandemic. When samples from the source population are included, the gaps between the subtypes fill in and largely disappear (lower right schematic). So do the subtypes.[29]

The 'source' population is represented in Figure 2.2 by HIV sequences sampled in the Democratic Republic of the Congo (DRC), the country with the most extensive M-group genetic diversity described to date[37] and the longest evidence of the presence of the virus.[27] It is the best-sampled central African country,[37] but whether or not its M group diversity is uniquely rich remains to be seen. M- group genetic diversity on the other side of the Congo River, in Brazzaville (Republic of Congo), is also extensive.[38]

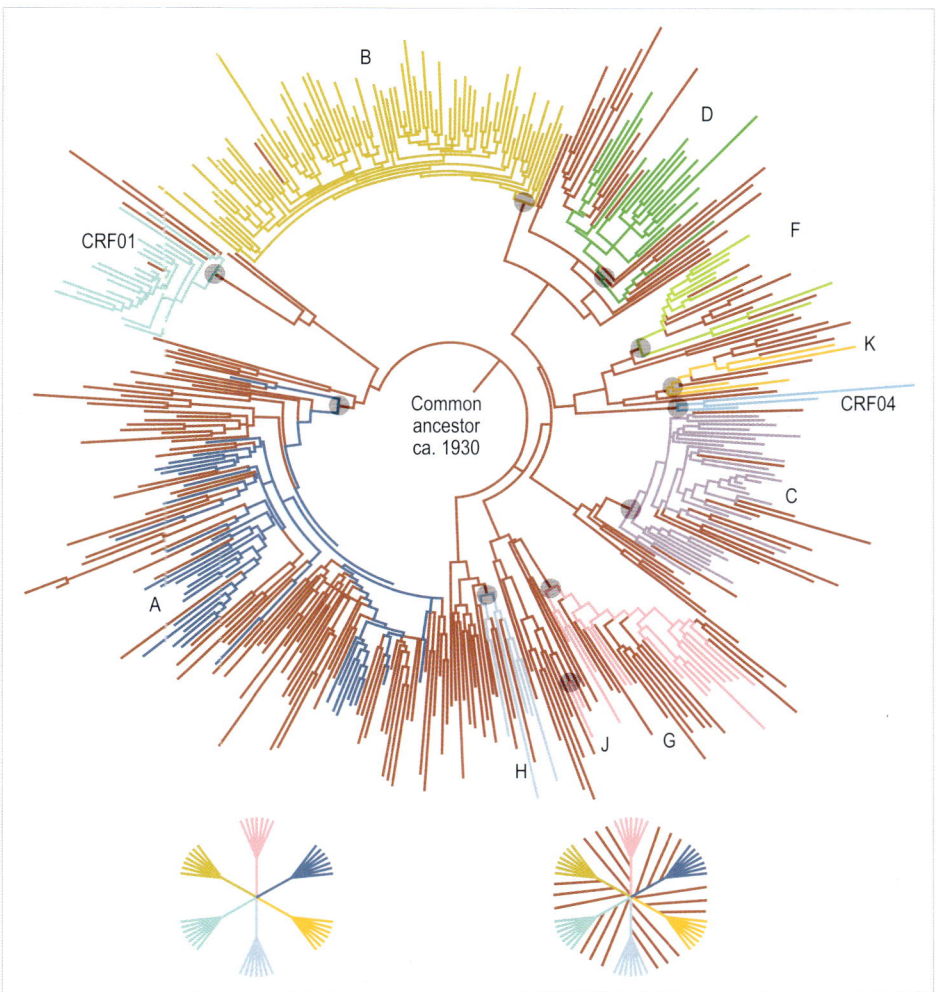

Figure 2.2 A maximum likelihood phylogenetic tree of HIV-1 group M (top) plus schematic representations of the M group subtypes (below) The phylogeny is courtesy of Andrew Rambaut and is based on partial *env* gene (V2–V5) sequences collected both within the Democratic Republic of the Congo (red branches)[29,37] and outside the DRC (other branches) (www.hiv.lanl.gov . The branches radiating from the center are drawn to scale. The ancestor of each subtype/CRF is marked with a circle. Several DRC strains fall basal to these points, and the much more extensive diversity of group M lineages encountered in the DRC indicates that this region has experienced a long, continuous epidemic.

Although the sampling in the Congo-Brazzaville study was far less intensive, the same pattern emerges from the phylogenies: there is a preponderance of unclassifiable strains and strains that fell *basal* to the subtypes as defined by global diversity. Describing such basal lineages as *members* of these subtypes misses the point. The subtypes only have meaning outside of this epicenter region, and these basal lineages already existed before the 'birth' of the subtype (i.e before some strain was exported out of the source region and began a chain of infections

elsewhere, in relative isolation). The lack of a clear distinction between strains in this part of the group M phylogeny underscores the lack of intrinsic biological properties uniting members of a subtype (Fig. 2.3).

Conclusion

Although it is clear that it would be naïve to treat subtypes as 'immunotypes,' rational vaccine design

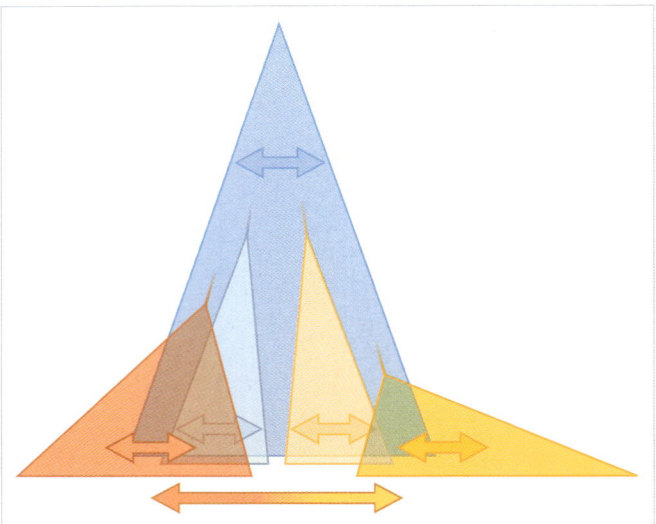

Figure 2.3 A schematic diagram of the processes underlying the phylogenetic patterns observed in HIV-1 group M. Time/divergence increases down the vertical axis; number of infected hosts is represented on the horizontal axis; arrows depict recombination. Several successful lineages (smaller triangles) trace their ancestry back to the source population (large triangle). This source population derives from a single infected host (apex), and has been evolving as a continuous epidemic, hence the lack of clear subtypes.[29] In addition to nucleotide substitution, recombination occurs regularly within all the populations (arrows)[26] but will be most conspicuous within the source with its full range of diversity, and between contemporary, divergent strains (bottom arrow). Early, complex recombinants reflect the special legacy of recombination in the ancestral zone where the most divergent strains have always co-circulated and recombined. Small triangles correspond both to subtypes and circulating recombinants forms (e.g. CRF02 in Nigeria). In each instance, a founder effect has occurred such that one strain has been exported outside the geographical range of the source population and has initiated an epidemic elsewhere. (Adapted from Worobey M. The occurrence and impact of viral recombination. D.Phil thesis, 2001: University of Oxford, UK.)

(to highlight one important medical example) demands much more detailed information about the precise relationship between HIV genetic diversity and human biology. How many future HIV vaccines will be required to protect people in an HIV-diverse country like the DRC? One? Ten? Or is the notion of an effective, protective vaccine perhaps doomed to failure? We simply cannot say at the moment. In light of the fact that wild-type HIV-infected individuals are eventually unable to protect against even the most *local* level of phylogenetic diversity – the swarm of strains that replicate within their own bodies – we cannot currently rule out this sobering possibility. Without such fundamental knowledge about the consequences of HIV genetic variation, it is difficult to make informed decisions about how best to allocate research dollars among the different methods of control.

The rapid evolution of HIV has left behind a record of the virus's past, and reconstructing the circumstances of its origins and emergence has been a major triumph, one that has yielded key insights into the public health risks posed by SIV and HIV. A more difficult challenge still confronts us: fully discerning the medically relevant aspects of past, current, and future HIV genetic diversity and then translating such knowledge into successful therapeutic and preventative control measures. With virtually every existing and potential medical approach, there is an urgent need to come to grips not only with the remarkable diversity of currently circulating strains of HIV, but also with the relentless onslaught of new genetic variation that will be generated by these viruses in future months, years and decades.

References

1. Gottlieb MS, Schanker HM, Fan PT, et al. Pneumocystis pneumonia – Los Angeles. MMWR 1981; 30:250–252.
2. Barre-Sinoussi F, Chermann JC, Rey F, et al. Isolation of a T-lymphotrophic retrovirus from a patient at risk for acquired immune-deficiency syndrome (AIDS). Science 1983; 220:868–871.

3. Hahn BH, Shaw GM, DeCock KM, et al. AIDS – AIDS as a zoonosis: Scientific and public health implications. Science 2000; 287:607–614.

4. Bibollet-Ruche F, Bailes E, Gao F, et al. New simian immunodeficiency virus infecting De Brazza's monkeys (Cercopithecus neglectus): Evidence for a Cercopithecus monkey virus clade. J Virol 2004; 78:7748–7762.

5. Sharp PM, Bailes E, Gao F, et al. Origins and evolution of AIDS viruses: estimating the time-scale. Biochem Soc Trans 2000; 28:275–282.

6. Korber B, Muldoon M, Theiler J, et al. Timing the ancestor of the HIV-1 pandemic strains. Science 2000; 288:1789–1796.

7. Charleston MA, Robertson DL. Preferential host switching by primate lentiviruses can account for phylogenetic similarity with the primate phylogeny. Syst Biol 2002; 51:528–535.

8. Turelli P, Trono D. Editing at the crossroad of innate and adaptive immunity. Science 2005; 307:1061–1065.

9. Simon F, Mauclere P, Roques P, et al. Identification of a new human immunodeficiency virus type 1 distinct from group M and group O. Nat Med 1998; 4:1032–1037.

10. Gao F, Bailes E, Robertson DL, et al. Origin of HIV-1 in the chimpanzee *Pan troglodytes troglodytes*. Nature 1999; 397:436–441.

11. Gurtler LG, Hauser PH, Eberle J, et al. A new subtype of human immunodeficiency virus type 1 (MVP-5180) from Cameroon. J Virol 1994; 68:1581–1585.

12. Damond F, Worobey M, Campa P, et al. Identification of a highly divergent HIV type 2 and proposal for a change in HIV type 2 classification. AIDS Res Hum Retroviruses 2004; 20:666–672.

13. Peeters M. Recombinant HIV sequences: Their role in the global epidemic. In: Theoretical Biology and Biophysics Group, eds. HIV sequence compendium. Los Alamos: Los Alamos National Laboratory; 2000:39–54.

14. Robertson DL, Anderson JP, Bradac JA, et al. HIV-1 nomenclature proposal. Science 2000; 288:55–57.

15. Takehisa J, Zekeng L, Ido E, et al. Human immunodeficiency virus type 1 intergroup (M/O) recombination in Cameroon. J Virol 1999; 73:6810–6820.

16. Bailes E, Gao F, Bibollet-Ruche F, et al. Hybrid origin of SIV in chimpanzees. Science 2003; 300:1713–1713.

17. Gao F, Yue L, White AT, et al. Human infection by genetically diverse SIVsm-related HIV-2 in West Africa. Nature 1992; 358:495–499.

18. Chen ZW, Telfer P, Gettie A, et al. Genetic characterization of new west African simian immunodeficiency virus SIVsm: Geographic clustering of household-derived SIV strains with human immunodeficiency virus type 2 subtypes and genetically diverse viruses from a single feral sooty mangabey troop. J Virol 1996; 70:3617–3627.

19. Chen ZW, Luckay A, Sodora DL, et al. Human immunodeficiency virus type 2 (HIV-2) seroprevalence and characterization of a distinct HIV-2 genetic subtype from the natural range of simian immunodeficiency virus-infected sooty mangabeys. J Virol 1997; 71:3953–3960.

20. Santiago ML, Roderburg CM, Kamenya S, et al. SIVcpz in wild chimpanzees. Science 2002; 295:465–465.

21. Worobey M, Santiago ML, Keele BF, et al. Origin of AIDS – Contaminated polio vaccine theory refuted. Nature 2004; 428:820–820.

22. Ayouba A, Mauclere P, Martin PMV, et al. HIV-1 group O infection in Cameroon, 1986–1998. Emerging Infect Dis 2001; 7:466–467.

23. Roques P, Robertson DL, Souquiere S, et al. Phylogenetic characteristics of three new HIV-1 N strains and implications for the origin of group N. AIDS 2004; 18:1371–1381.

24. Lemey P, Pybus OG, Rambaut A, et al. The molecular population genetics of HIV-1 group O. Genetics 2004; 167:1059–1068.

25. Lemey P, Pybus OG, Wang B, et al. Tracing the origin and history of the HIV-2 epidemic. Proc Natl Acad Sci USA 2003; 100:6588–6592.

26. Worobey M. A novel approach to detecting and measuring recombination: New insights into evolution in viruses, bacteria, and mitochondria. Mol Biol Evol 2001; 18:1425–1434.

27. Zhu TF, Korber BT, Nahmias AJ, et al. An African HIV-1 sequence from 1959 and implications for the origin of the epidemic. Nature 1998; 391:594–597.

28. Hooper E. The river: a journey back to the source of HIV and AIDS. London: Penguin; 1999.

29. Rambaut A, Robertson DL, Pybus OG, et al. Human immunodeficiency virus – Phylogeny and the origin of HIV-1. Nature 2001; 410:1047–1048.

30. Santiago ML, Lukasik M, Kamenya S, et al. Foci of endemic simian immunodeficiency virus infection in wild-living eastern chimpanzees (*Pan troglodytes schweinfurthii*). J Virol 2003; 77:7545–7562.

31. Souquiere S, Bibollet-Ruche F, Robertson DL, et al. Wild Mandrillus sphinx are carriers of two types of lentivirus. J Virol 2001; 75:7086–7096.

32. Bibollet-Ruche F, GalatLuong A, Cuny G, et al. Simian immunodeficiency virus infection in a patas monkey (*Erythrocebus patas*): Evidence for cross-species transmission from African green monkeys (*Cercopithecus aethiops sabaeus*) in the wild. J Gen Virol 1996; 77:773–781.

33. Marx PA, Alcabes PG, Drucker E. Serial human passage of simian immunodeficiency virus by unsterile injections and the emergence of epidemic human immunodeficiency virus in Africa. Philos Trans R Soc Lond Ser 2001; 356:911–920.

34. Schmid GP, Buve A, Mugyenyi P, et al. Transmission of HIV-1 infection in sub-Saharan Africa and effect of elimination of unsafe injections. Lancet 2004; 363:482–488.

35. Walker PR, Worobey M, Rambaut A, et al. Sexual transmission of HIV in Africa. Other routes of infection are not the dominant contributor to the African epidemic. Nature 2003; 422:679–679.

36. Rambaut A, Posada D, Crandall KA, et al. The causes and consequences of HIV evolution. Nat Rev Genet 2004; 5:52–61.

37. Vidal N, Peeters M, Mulanga-Kabeya C, et al. Unprecedented degree of human immunodeficiency virus type 1 (HIV-1) group M genetic diversity in the Democratic Republic of Congo suggests that the HIV-1 pandemic originated in Central Africa. J Virol 2000; 74:10498–10507.

38. Taniguchi Y, Takehisa J, Bikandou B, et al. Genetic subtypes of HIV type 1 based on the vpu/env sequences in the Republic of Congo. AIDS Res Hum Retroviruses 2002; 18:79–83.

CHAPTER 3

Molecular Biology of HIV: Implications for New Therapies

Warner C. Greene

B. Matija Peterlin

Introduction

Sharply curbing the expanding global HIV epidemic requires more effective approaches to decrease the horizontal and vertical spread of this pathogenic retrovirus coupled with the broader use of existing and likely new antiretroviral therapies. These interventions must be deployable in the developing world, where HIV is hitting the hardest. Understanding the dynamic interplay of HIV with its cellular host cell forms the foundation for success in this endeavor. In the following sections, we review our current understanding of the HIV life cycle highlighting promising future points of attack.

HIV Entry

The 9 kilobase HIV RNA encodes nine genes yielding 15 distinct proteins. Compared with other retroviruses, HIV is genetically complex. Investigations over the past several years yielded informative insights into the function of each of HIV's individual gene products, many of which could form potential targets for new therapies (Fig. 3.1). To productively infect a cell, HIV must introduce its genetic material into the cytoplasm. HIV entry requires the initial binding or attachment of the HIV envelope protein to CD4 receptors on the surface of target cells. The rational development of inhibitors of HIV attachment has been propelled by structural studies unraveling the 'lock and key' assembly of trimeric gp120

Env spikes present on virions with CD4 receptors residing on the surface of the target cells.[1] The insertion of a key phenylalanine residue in the outer portion of the CD4 protein into a recessed pocket in gp120 produces a very high-affinity interaction of these two proteins.

BMS 488043 is a promising second-generation attachment inhibitor that blocks the insertion of this CD4 residue into this pocket of gp120. Protein-based approaches to interrupting the gp120-CD4 interaction are also being developed. For example, PRO 542, a tetravalent fusion protein containing the D1 and D2 domains of human CD4 and the heavy – and light – chain constant regions of human IgG2, has shown promise as an attachment inhibitor in phase I and phase II testing.[2,3]

In addition, TNX-355 corresponds to a humanized anti-CD4 IgG4 monoclonal antibody that specifically reacts with a conformational epitope in the D2 domain of CD4 that is induced by gp120 binding. This antibody blocks subsequent Env engagement of the HIV chemokine co-receptors.[4] However, both of these protein-based attachment inhibitors require parenteral administration.

The second phase of HIV entry involves the engagement of the HIV co-receptors. The initial binding of trimeric gp120 to CD4 induces a conformational change in the envelope that promotes binding of the virion to a specific subset of chemokine co-receptors. These receptors contain seven membrane-spanning domains and normally help hematopoietic cells to migrate down specific chemokine gradients to sites of inflammation. Although

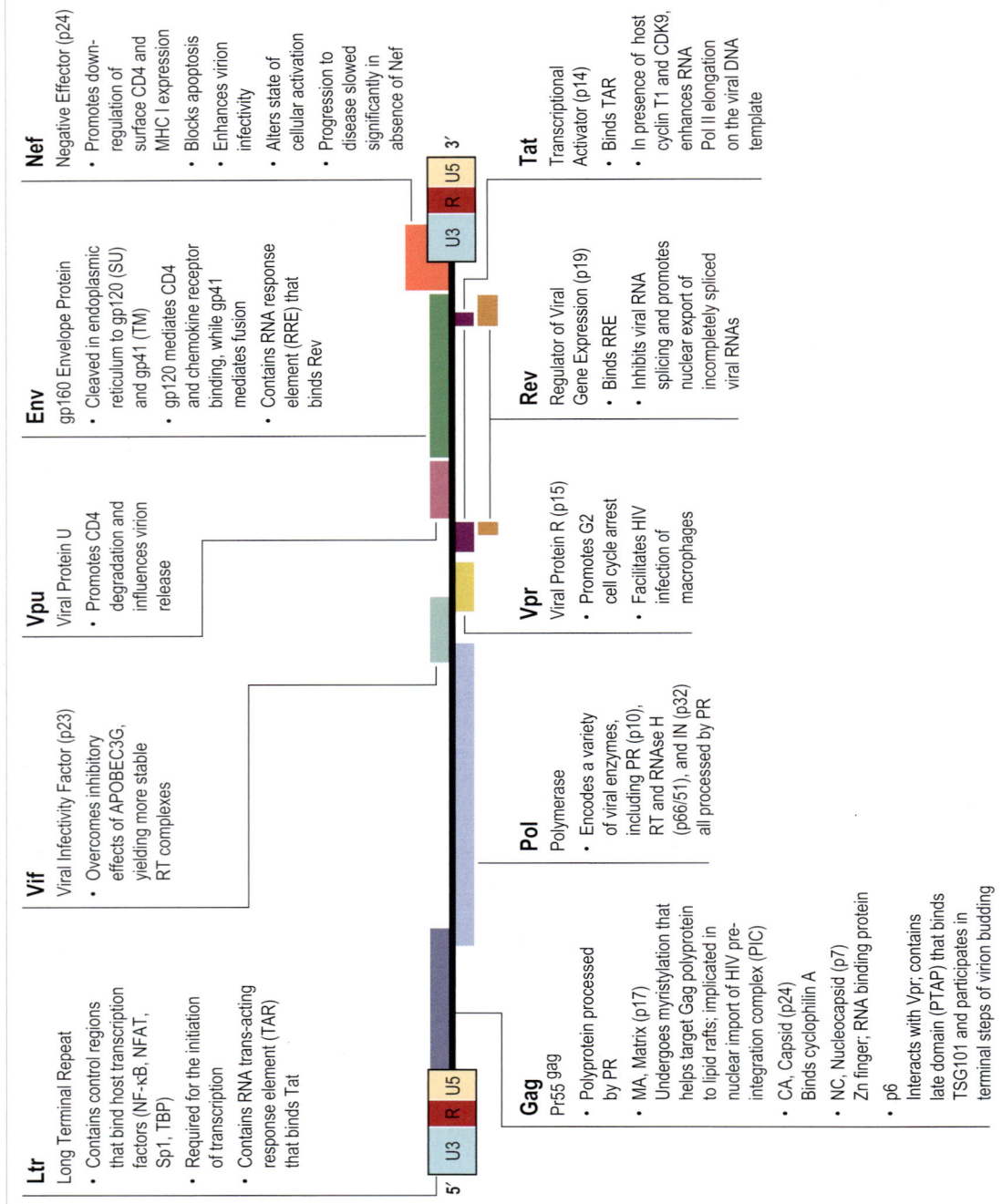

Figure 3.1 An overview of the organization of the ~9-kilobase genome of the HIV provirus and a summary of the functions of its nine genes encoding 15 different proteins.

Ltr
Long Terminal Repeat
• Contains control regions that bind host transcription factors (NF-κB, NFAT, Sp1, TBP)
• Required for the initiation of transcription
• Contains RNA trans-acting response element (TAR) that binds Tat

Gag
Pr55 gag
• Polyprotein processed by PR
• MA, Matrix (p17) Undergoes myristylation that helps target Gag polyprotein to lipid rafts; implicated in nuclear import of HIV pre-integration complex (PIC)
• CA, Capsid (p24) Binds cyclophilin A
• NC, Nucleocapsid (p7) Zn finger; RNA binding protein
• p6 Interacts with Vpr; contains late domain (PTAP) that binds TSG101 and participates in terminal steps of virion budding

Vif
Viral Infectivity Factor (p23)
• Overcomes inhibitory effects of APOBEC3G, yielding more stable RT complexes

Pol
Polymerase
• Encodes a variety of viral enzymes, including PR (p10), RT and RNAse H (p66/51), and IN (p32) all processed by PR

Vpu
Viral Protein U
• Promotes CD4 degradation and influences virion release

Vpr
Viral Protein R (p15)
• Promotes G2 cell cycle arrest
• Facilitates HIV infection of macrophages

Env
gp160 Envelope Protein
• Cleaved in endoplasmic reticulum to gp120 (SU) and gp41 (TM)
• gp120 mediates CD4 and chemokine receptor binding, while gp41 mediates fusion
• Contains RNA response element (RRE) that binds Rev

Rev
Regulator of Viral Gene Expression (p19)
• Binds RRE
• Inhibits viral RNA splicing and promotes nuclear export of incompletely spliced viral RNAs

Nef
Negative Effector (p24)
• Promotes down-regulation of surface CD4 and MHC I expression
• Blocks apoptosis
• Enhances virion infectivity
• Alters state of cellular activation
• Progression to disease slowed significantly in absence of Nef

Tat
Transcriptional Activator (p14)
• Binds TAR
• In presence of host cyclin T1 and CDK9, enhances RNA Pol II elongation on the viral DNA template

these receptors signal through G proteins,[5] such signaling is not required for HIV infection. A total of 12 different chemokine receptors have been shown to function as HIV co-receptors in cultured cells, but only two, CCR5 and CXCR4, are normally used *in vivo*.[5] CCR5 binds macrophage-tropic, non-syncytium-inducing (R5-tropic) viruses, which are associated with mucosal and intravenous transmission of HIV infection. CXCR4 binds T-cell-tropic, syncytium-inducing (X4) viruses, which generally emerge only during the later stages of disease.[6] Utilization of CXCR4 is associated with accelerated disease progression but only occurs in about half of patients infected with HIV.

A naturally occurring deletion of 32 base pairs in the CCR5 gene[7,8] is present in approximately 13% of individuals of northern European descent. This mutation gives rise to a truncated form of the CCR5 receptor that never reaches the cell surface. Emphasizing the key role of CCR5 in horizontal transmission, individuals homozygous for this CCR5 Δ32mutation (~2% of the Caucasian population) are almost completely resistant to HIV infection.[7,8] This 'experiment of nature' propelled pharmaceutical development of small molecules that prevent HIV interaction with CCR5. Within only 7 years after the discovery of HIV co-receptors, several small-molecule antagonists of CCR5, including Schering D, UK 427–857, GW873140, and TAK 220, have entered advanced clinical testing in humans. Protein-based CCR5 inhibitors are also being explored. For example, PRO 140 is a humanized IgG4 monoclonal antibody that binds to CCR5 and blocks HIV infectivity. Interest has also focused on using modified versions of the chemokine RANTES, a natural ligand for CCR5, to block HIV infection. A key unanswered concern is whether blockade of CCR5 will promote an earlier switch to CXCR4 co-receptor utilization by HIV. As noted, such a switch could lead to more rapid clinical deterioration since many more CD4 T cells express CXCR4 than CCR5.

Both CD4 and chemokine co-receptors for HIV are found disproportionately within lipid signaling rafts located within the cell membrane.[9] These cholesterol- and sphingolipid-enriched microdomains likely provide a better environment for membrane fusion possibly because HIV virions bud from such lipid rafts and acquire similar lipids.[10] Removing cholesterol from virions, producer cells, or target cells greatly decreases the infectivity of HIV.[11] Studies currently are underway exploring whether cholesterol-depleting compounds might be efficacious as topically applied microbicides to inhibit HIV transmission at mucosal surfaces. The

development of effective microbicides would be an exceptionally valuable approach in efforts to prevent HIV transmission. CCR5 inhibitors could also formulate for topical administration as microbicides.

The third phase of HIV entry is virion fusion. The binding of surface gp120, CD4, and the chemokine co-receptors generates a sharp conformational change in gp41, the second HIV envelope protein.[12] Assembled as a trimer on the virion membrane, this coiled-coil protein springs open, projecting three peptide fusion domains that 'harpoon' the lipid bilayer of the target cell. The gp41 trimers then fold back on themselves, forming a hairpin structure. The recently approved T20 fusion inhibitor acts by preventing the formation of this hairpin structure that is essential for successful fusion. The fusion reaction leads to intracytoplasmic insertion of the HIV viral core.[12]

HIV virions also enter cells by endocytosis. However, this form of entry does not lead to productive viral infection likely because the internalized virions are inactivated within acidified endosomes. However, a special form of endocytosis associated with facilitated infection of CD4 T cells has been described in dendritic cells. These cells normally process and present antigens to immune cells, and many dendritic cells express a specialized attachment receptor termed DC-SIGN[13] or closely related C-type lectin receptors. DC-SIGN binds HIV gp120 with high affinity but does not trigger the conformational changes in Env required for fusion. Rather, virions bound to DC-SIGN may be internalized into a vesicular compartment that does not lead to viral inactivation. Rather, these vesicles containing viable HIV virions are transported back to the cell surface after the dendritic cell has matured and migrated to regional lymph nodes, where it engages T cells.[14] Indeed, these virus-laden vesicles may selectively accumulate at the immunological synapse formed between dendritic cells and CD4 T cells. Thus, these dendritic cells expressing DC-SIGN or related C-type lectin receptors may act as 'Trojan horses' that facilitate the spread of HIV from mucosal surfaces to lymphatic organs in the absence of productive infection of the dendritic cell itself. However, more recent studies suggest that immature dendritic cells present at mucosal surfaces are particularly susceptible to fusion and productive infection by R5-tropic but not X4-tropic viruses. It is possible that local production of new R5-tropic virions could play a key role in the preferential horizontal transmission of this type of HIV. Further, the degree to which surface-bound versus internalized virions in dendritic cells is responsible for virion transfer to CD4 T cells remains to be defined.

Early Cytoplasmic Events

Once inside the cell, the virion undergoes 'uncoating', probably while still associated with the plasma membrane (Fig. 3.2). This process is poorly understood but appears to involve phosphorylation of the matrix protein by a mitogen-activated protein (MAP) kinase[15] and additional actions of cyclophilin A[16] and the viral proteins Nef[17] and Vif.[18] Nef can bind to a universal proton pump, V-ATPase,[19] which could facilitate uncoating by inducing local changes in pH in a manner similar to that of the M2 protein of influenza.[20] Nef may also help the viral cores penetrate the formidably dense cortical actin network that exists beneath the plasma membrane of cells.[21] After the viral core is uncoated, the viral reverse transcription complex is liberated and begins the conversion of viral RNA into double stranded DNA.[22] This complex includes the diploid viral RNA genome, tRNA(Lys) primer, reverse transcriptase, integrase, matrix, nucleocapsid, viral protein R (Vpr), and various host proteins. It docks with actin microfilaments.[23] This interaction, mediated by the phosphorylated matrix, is required for the commencement of efficient reverse transcription. A variety of nucleoside (AZT, ddI, ddC, and 3TC), nucleotide (tenofovir), and non-nucleoside (nevirapine) inhibitors of the HIV reverse transcriptase are widely used in the clinic. Indeed, targeting of the viral reverse transcriptase represents one of the most successful strategies for impairing HIV growth.

Effective reverse transcription yields the HIV preintegration complex (PIC), composed of double-stranded viral cDNA, integrase, matrix, Vpr, reverse transcriptase, and the high mobility group DNA-binding protein HMGI(Y).[24] The PIC may move toward the nucleus by sliding down microtubules.[25] Adenovirus and herpes simplex virus 1 similarly dock to microtubules and use dynein, the microtubule-associated molecular motor, for cytoplasmic transport. This finding suggests that many viruses utilize these cytoskeletal structures for directional movement. How the switch from actin microfilaments to microtubules is orchestrated remains unknown.

Recent studies have revealed a mechanism by which the target cell defends itself against the HIV intruder.[26,27] Within 30 min of infection, select host proteins including the integrase interactor 1 (also known as INI-1, SNF5, or BAF47), a component of the SWI/SNF complex, and PML, a protein present in promyelocytic oncogenic domains, translocate from the nucleus into the cytoplasm[27] (Fig. 3.2). Addition of arsenic trioxide sharply blocks PML movement and enhances the susceptibility of cells to HIV infection, raising the possibility that the normal function of PML is to oppose HIV infection.[27] The binding of integrase to integrase interactor 1 may be a viral adaptation that recruits additional components of the chromatin remodeling machinery. Whether these complexes alter the site of viral integration or improve subsequent proviral gene expression is not known.

Crossing the Nuclear Pore

Unlike most animal retroviruses, HIV can infect non-dividing cells, such as terminally differentiated macrophages.[28] This requires an ability of the viral PIC to cross intact nuclear membranes. With a Stokes radius of approximately ~28 nm resembling the size of a ribosome,[29] the PIC is about twice as large as the maximal diameter of the central aqueous channel of the nuclear pore. It seems likely that the 3 μm contour length of viral DNA must undergo significant compaction, and the import process must involve considerable molecular gymnastics.

One of the more controversial areas of HIV research involves the identification of key viral proteins that mediate the nuclear import of the PIC. Integrase,[30] matrix,[31] and Vpr[32] have each been implicated (Fig. 3.2). Because plus-strand synthesis is discontinuous in reverse transcription, a triple helical DNA domain or 'DNA flap' is produced[33] that may bind a host protein containing a nuclear targeting signal. Matrix encodes a canonical nuclear localization signal that is recognized by importin-α and -β, which are key components in the classical nuclear import pathway. However, recent studies have questioned the contributions of the nuclear import signal in integrase as well as the DNA flap to the nuclear uptake of the PIC.[34] The HIV Vpr gene product[35] contains at least three non-canonical nuclear targeting signals. Vpr may bypass the importin system altogether, perhaps mediating the direct docking of the PIC with one or more components of the nuclear pore complex. The multiple nuclear targeting signals within the PIC, which could involve unidentified cellular factors, may also function in a cooperative manner or play larger roles individually in different target cells. For example, while Vpr is not needed for HIV infection of non-dividing, resting T cells,[36] it markedly enhances viral infection occurring in non-

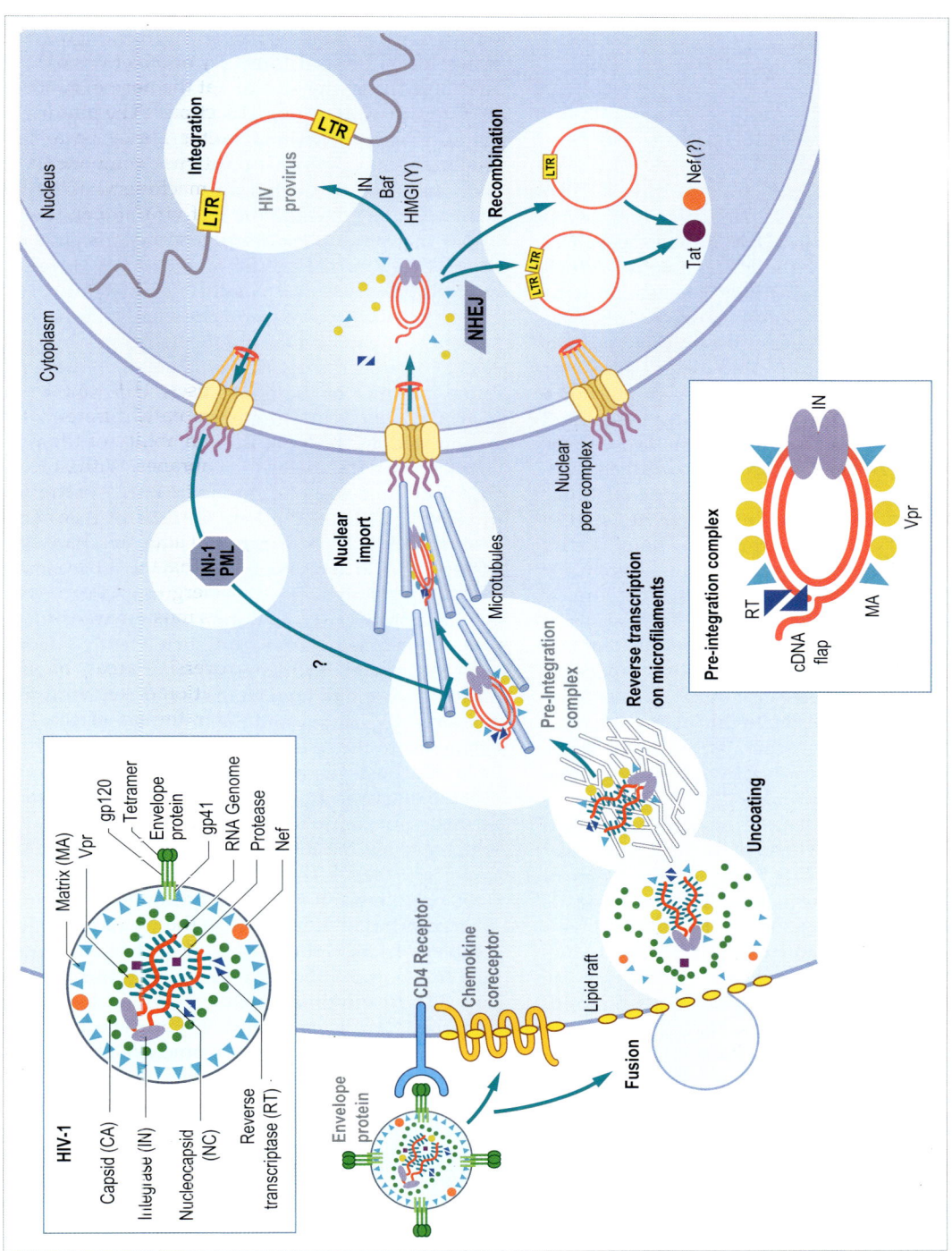

Figure 3.2 Schematic description of early events occurring after HIV infection of a susceptible target cell. Interactions between gp120, CD4, and chemokine receptors (CCR5 or CXCR4) lead to gp41-mediated fusion, which is followed by virion uncoating, reverse transcription of the RNA genome, nuclear import of the viral pre-integration complex, and integration of the double-stranded viral cDNA into the host chromosome, thus establishing the HIV provirus.

dividing macrophages.[37] The finding that both matrix[38] and Vpr[35] shuttle between the nucleus and cytoplasm likely ensures their availability for incorporation into new virions.

Integration

Once inside the nucleus, the viral PIC can establish a functional provirus (Fig. 3.2). Effective integration of the double-stranded viral DNA into the host chromosome is mediated by the HIV integrase, which binds the ends of the viral DNA.[24] The host proteins HMGI(Y) and barrier to autointegration (BAF) are required for efficient integration, although their precise functions remain unknown.[39] Integrase removes nucleotides from viral ends, producing a two-base recess and thereby correcting the ragged ends generated by the terminal transferase activity of reverse transcriptase.[24] It also catalyzes the subsequent joining reaction that establishes the HIV provirus within the chromosome. Recent studies indicate that HIV integration preferentially occurs in actively transcribed genes.[40] The search for effective integrase inhibitors has been frustratingly slow. However, promising advances have occurred recently. Merck and Shinogi identified naphthyridine (L-870,81) and diketoacid (S-1360) compounds, respectively, that interfere with integrase-mediated strand transfer, the final step in the integration reaction.[41] Both have advanced into early clinical trials. Hopefully, effective integrase inhibitors will soon join the HIV therapeutic ranks.

Not all PICs that enter the nucleus result in a functional provirus. The ends of the viral DNA may be joined to form a 2-LTR (long terminal repeat) circle or the viral genome may undergo homologous recombination yielding a single LTR circle. Finally, the viral DNA may autointegrate into itself, producing a rearranged circular structure. Although some circular forms may direct the synthesis of the transcriptional transactivator Tat and Nef, none produces infectious virus.[42] The non-homologous end joining system may form 2-LTR circles to protect the cell.[43] This system is responsible for rapid repair of double-strand breaks, which minimizes the number of free DNA ends within the cell, thereby preventing an apoptotic response. A single double-strand break detected within a cell is sufficient to induce G1 cell-cycle arrest. The ability of the free ends of the viral DNA to mimic such double-strand chromosomal breaks may contribute to the direct cytopathic effects observed with HIV.

Transcriptional Events

Integration can lead to latent or transcriptionally active forms of viral infection.[44] The chromosomal environment at the site of viral integration likely helps shape transcriptional activity of the provirus.[45] For example, proviral integration into repressed heterochromatin might favor the generation of latent proviruses (Fig. 3.3). Other causes of post-integration latency for HIV include the relative absence of activators that bind to the transcriptional enhancer in the HIV LTR or the failure of Tat to act. However, multiple proviruses are usually integrated into a cell, and one is likely to be transcriptionally active. This fact may explain why the number of latently infected cells[46,47] in infected patients is so small. However, it is the presence of these latently infected cells that has undermined early attempts to eradicate the virus in infected individuals despite administration of effective antiviral therapy for several years. Memory CD4 T cells correspond to one latently infected set of cells. Because of the long half-life of these cells (>44 months), it is estimated that antiretroviral therapy would have to be administered for more than 60 years to achieve depletion of virus in this cellular pool. Clearly, new approaches to the difficult task of purging the virus from such latently infected cells are needed. Such approaches critically depend on improving our understanding of the molecular basis for HIV latency and the full range of cells harboring latent proviruses.

In the host genome, the 5′ LTR functions like other eukaryotic transcriptional units. It contains downstream and upstream promoter elements, which include the initiator (Inr), TATA-box (T), and three Sp1 sites.[48] These regions help position the RNA polymerase II (RNAPII) at the site of initiation of transcription and assemble the pre-initiation complex. Transcription begins but the polymerase fails to elongate efficiently along the viral genome (Fig. 3.3). In the process, short non-polyadenylated transcripts are synthesized, which are stable and persist in cells due to the formation of an RNA stem loop called the transactivation response (TAR) element.[49] Slightly upstream of the promoter is the transcriptional enhancer, which in HIV-1 binds nuclear factor κB (NF-κB), nuclear factor of activated T cells (NFAT), and Ets family members.[50] NF-κB and NFAT re-localize to the nucleus after cellular activation. NF-κB is liberated from its cytoplasmic inhibitor, IκB, by stimulus-coupled phosphorylation, polyubiquitylation, and proteasomal degradation of the inhibitor.[51] NFAT is dephosphorylated by calci-

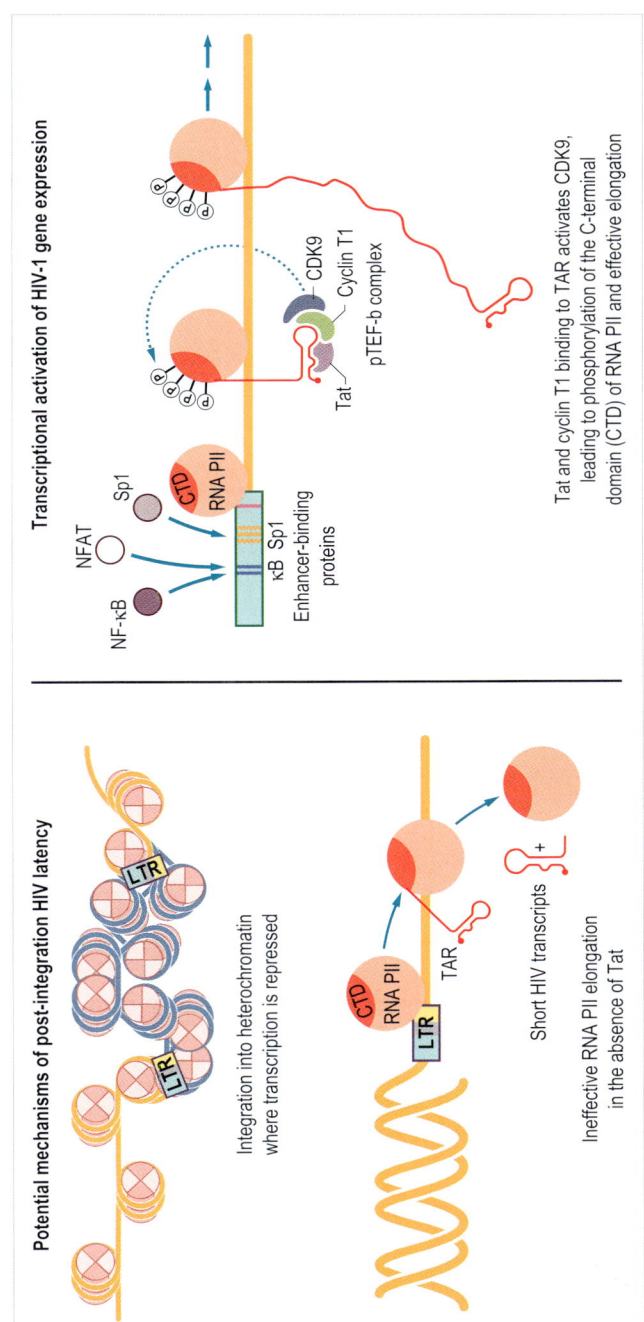

Figure 3.3 A summary of two different mechanisms potentially underlying post-integration HIV latency contrasted with the central role of Tat in promoting productive infection of target cells.

neurin (a reaction inhibited by cyclosporin A) and, after its nuclear import, assembles with AP1 to form the fully active transcriptional complex.[52] NF-κB, which is composed of p50 and p65 (RelA) subunits, increases the rates of both initiation and elongation of viral transcription.[53] Since NF-κB is activated after several antigen-specific and cytokine-mediated events, it may play a key role in rousing transcriptionally silent proviruses.

Tat is responsible for markedly increasing the rate of viral gene expression. With cyclin T1 (CycT1), it binds TAR and recruits the cellular cyclin-dependent kinase 9 (Cdk9) to the HIV LTR[54] (Fig. 3.3). In the positive transcription elongation factor b (P-TEFb) complex, Cdk9 phosphorylates the C-terminal domain of RNAPII, which marks the transition from initiation to elongation of eukaryotic transcription.[55] Other targets of P-TEFb include negative transcription elongation factors (N-TEF), such as the DRB-sensitivity inducing (DSIF) and negative elongation (NELF) factors.[55] In the absence of Tat, the HIV LTR functions as a very poor promoter because it so effectively binds these negative transcription factors *in vivo*. An arginine-rich motif (ARM) within Tat binds to the 5' bulge region in TAR. A shorter ARM in cyclin T1, which is also called the Tat-TAR recognition motif (TRM), engages the central loop of TAR.[54] These regions form a high-affinity RNA-binding unit that is required for Tat transactivation. In the presence of the complex between Tat and P-TEFb, the RNAPII becomes a highly efficient elongating complex. Because murine CycT1 contains a cysteine at position 261, the complex between Tat and murine P-TEFb binds TAR weakly.[56] Thus, Tat transactivation is severely compromised in murine cells. Cdk9 also must be autophosphorylated on several serines and threonines near its C-terminus for productive interactions between Tat, P-TEFb, and TAR.[57] Additionally, basal levels of P-TEFb may be low in resting cells or only weakly active due to the interaction between P-TEFb and 7SK RNA.[58] All of these events could contribute to post-integration latency.

Expression of Viral Genes

Transcription of the viral genome results in more than a dozen different HIV-specific transcripts.[59] Some are processed co-transcriptionally and, in the absence of inhibitory RNA sequences (IRS), transported rapidly into the cytoplasm.[60] These multiply spliced transcripts encode Nef, Tat, and Rev, the 'early' expressed genes of HIV. Other singly spliced or unspliced viral transcripts remain in the nucleus and are relatively stable. These viral transcripts encode the structural, enzymatic, and accessory proteins and represent genomic RNAs that are needed for the assembly of fully infectious virions.

Incomplete splicing likely results from suboptimal splice donor and acceptor sites in viral transcripts. In addition, the regulator of virion gene expression, Rev, may inhibit splicing by its interaction with alternate splicing factor/splicing factor 2 (ASF/SF2)[61] and its associated p32 protein.[62]

Transport of the incompletely spliced viral transcripts to the cytoplasm depends on an adequate supply of Rev.[60] Rev is a small shuttling protein that binds a complex RNA stem loop termed the Rev response element (RRE), which is located in the Env gene. Rev binds first with high affinity to a small region of the RRE termed the stem loop IIB[63] (Fig. 3.4). This binding leads to the multimerization of Rev on the remainder of the RRE. In addition to a nuclear localization signal, Rev contains a leucine-rich nuclear export sequence (NES).[60] Of note, the study of Rev was the catalyst for the identification of such NES's in many cellular proteins and of the complex formed between CRM1/exportin-1 and this sequence.[60]

This Rev-CRM1/exportin assembly critically depends on yet another host factor, RanGTP. Ran is a small guanine nucleotide-binding protein that switches between GTP- and GDP-bound states. RanGDP is found predominantly in the cytoplasm because it is expressed in this cellular compartment. Conversely, the Ran nucleotide exchange factor, RCC1, which charges Ran with GTP, is expressed predominantly in the nucleus. The inverse nucleocytoplasmic gradients of RanGTP and RanGDP produced by the subcellular localization of these enzymes likely plays a major role in determining the directional transport of proteins into and out of the nucleus. Outbound cargo is only effectively loaded onto the CRM1/exportin-1 in the presence of RanGTP. However, when the complex reaches the cytoplasm, GTP is hydrolyzed to GDP, upon which the bound cargo is released. The opposite relationship regulates the nuclear import by importins-α and -β, where nuclear RanGTP stimulates cargo release.[60]

For HIV infection to spread, a balance between splicing and transport of incompletely spliced viral mRNA species must be achieved. If splicing is too efficient, then only the multiply spliced transcripts appear in the cytoplasm. Although required, these regulatory proteins are insufficient to support full viral replication. However, if splicing is markedly impaired, adequate synthesis of Tat, Rev, and Nef will not occur. In many non-primate cells, HIV transcripts may be overly spliced, thus producing a block to viral replication in these hosts.[64]

Replicating New Viruses

In contrast to Tat and Rev, which act directly on viral RNA structures, Nef reshapes the environment of the infected cell to optimize viral replication[5] (Fig. 3.4). The absence of Nef in infected monkeys and humans is associated with much slower clinical progression to AIDS.[65,66] This increase in virulence caused by Nef appears to be associated with its ability to affect signaling cascades, including the activation of T-cell antigen receptor,[67] and to decrease the expression of CD4 on the cell surface.[68,69] Nef also promotes the production and release of more infectious virions.[70,71] Effects of Nef on the PI3-K signaling cascade – which involve the guanine nucleotide exchange factor Vav, the small GTPases Cdc42 and Rac1, and p21-activated kinase PAK – cause profound cytoskeletal rearrangements and alter downstream effector functions.[72] Indeed, Nef and viral structural proteins colocalize in lipid rafts.[71,73] Two other HIV proteins assist Nef in downregulating expression of CD4.[74] gp120 binds CD4 in the endoplasmic reticulum, slowing its export to the plasma membrane,[75] and Vpu binds the cytoplasmic tail of CD4, promoting recruitment of TrCP and Skp1p (Fig. 3.5). These events target CD4 for ubiquitylation and proteasomal degradation before it reaches the cell surface.[76]

Nef reduces the immunological response to HIV infections directly and indirectly. In T cells, Nef activates the expression of FasL, which induces apoptosis in bystander cells that express Fas,[77] thereby killing cytotoxic T cells that could eliminate HIV-1 infected cells. It reduces the expression of MHC I determinants on the cell surface[78] (Fig. 3.4) and so decreases the immunological visibility of infected cells to CD8 cytotoxic T cells. However, Nef does not decrease the expression of HLA-C[79] so that the infected cells are not recognized and killed by natural killer cells.

Nef also inhibits apoptosis. It binds to and inhibits the intermediate apoptosis signal regulating kinase-1 (ASK-1)[80] that functions in the Fas and TNFR death signaling pathways and stimulates the phosphorylation of Bad, leading to its sequestration by 14-3-3 proteins[81] (Fig. 3.4). Nef also binds and inhibits p53.[82] Via these different mechanisms, Nef prolongs the life of the infected cell, thereby optimizing viral replication.

Other viral proteins also participate in the modification of the environment in infected cells. Rev-dependent expression of Vpr induces the arrest of proliferating infected cells at the G2/M phase of the cell cycle.[83] Since the viral LTR is more active during G2, this arrest likely enhances viral gene expression.[84] These cell-cycle arresting properties involve localized defects in the structure of the nuclear lamina that lead to dynamic, DNA-filled herniations that project from the nuclear envelope into the cytoplasm[85] (Fig. 3.4). Intermittently, these herniations rupture, causing the mixing of soluble nuclear and cytoplasmic proteins.

Assembly and Budding of HIV Virions

New virions are assembled at the plasma membrane (Fig. 3.5). Each virion consists of roughly 1500 Gag and 100 Gag-Pol polyproteins,[86] two copies of the viral RNA genome, and Vpr.[87] Several proteins participate in the assembly process, including Gag-Pol, and Gag polyproteins as well as Nef and Env. A human ATP-binding protein, HP68 (previously identified as an RNase L inhibitor), likely acts as a molecular chaperone, facilitating conformational changes in Gag needed for the assembly of these capsids.[88] The Gag polyproteins are subject to myristylation,[89] and thus preferentially associate with cholesterol- and glycolipid-enriched membrane microdomains.[90] Virion budding occurs through these specialized regions in the lipid bilayer, yielding virions with cholesterol-rich membranes. This lipid composition likely favors release, stability, and fusion of virions with the subsequent target cell.[10]

The budding reaction involves the action of several proteins, including the 'late domain'[91] sequence (PTAP) present in the p6 portion of Gag (Fig. 3.5).[92] The p6 protein also appears to be modified by ubiquitylation. The product of the tumor-suppressor gene 101 (TSG101) binds the PTAP motif of p6 Gag and also recognizes ubiquitin through its ubiquitin enzyme 2 (UEV) domain.[93,94] The TSG101 protein normally associates with other cellular proteins in the vacuolar protein-sorting pathway to form the ESCRT-1 complex that selects cargo for incorporation into the multivesicular body (MVB).[95] The MVB is produced when surface patches on late endosomes bud away from the cytoplasm and fuse with lysosomes, releasing their contents for degradation within this organelle. In the case of HIV, TSG101 appears to be 'hijacked' for the budding of virions into the extracellular space away from the cytoplasm.

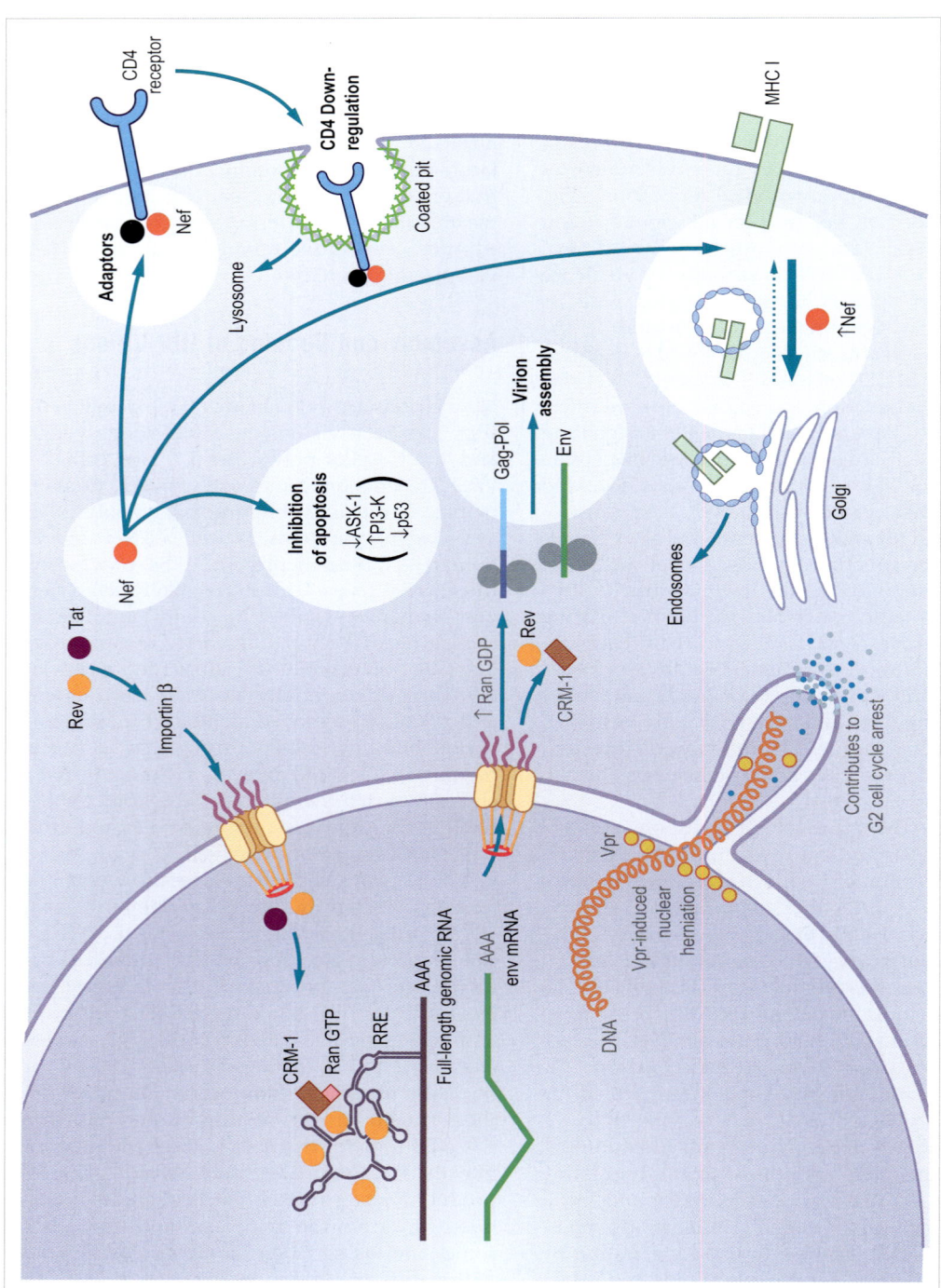

Figure 3.4 A summary of late events in the HIV-infected cell that culminates in the assembly of new infectious virions. Highlighted are the roles of various viral proteins in optimizing the intracellular environment for viral replication, including downregulation of CD4 and MHC I and inhibition of apoptosis by Nef, and the induction of G2 cell cycle arrest by Vpr. A key action of the HIV Rev protein in promoting nuclear export of incompletely spliced viral transcripts that encode the structural and enzymatic proteins as well as the viral genome of new virions is also illustrated.

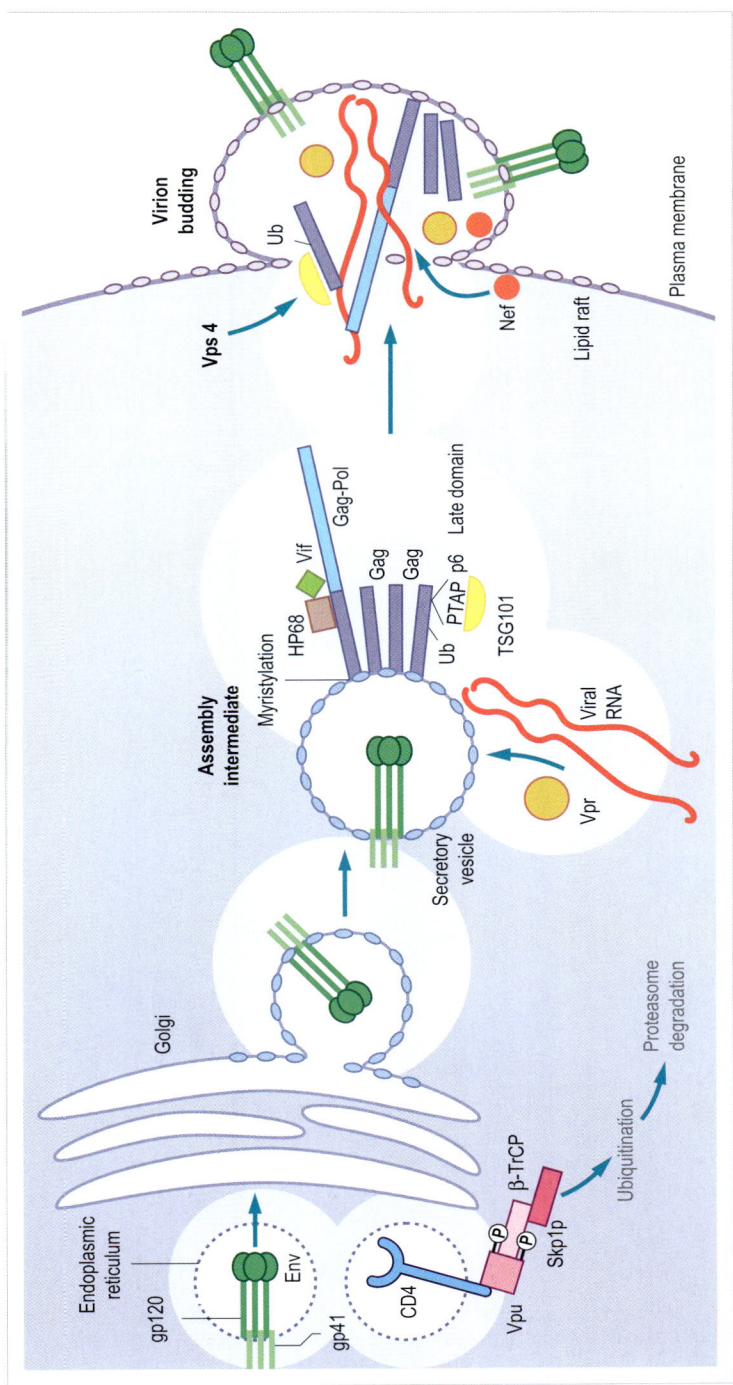

Figure 3.5 Late steps in the assembly of new virions. Components of vesicular protein sorting machinery, TSG101 and Vps4, have critical roles in the terminal phases of virion budding. Although virion assembly occurs principally at the plasma membrane, the involvement of these vesicular sorting proteins raises the possibility that virion assembly may be initiated on secretory vesicles that are destined for the plasma membrane. The final phase of virion release likely involves viral 'hijacking' and retargeting the process of budding away from the cytoplasm that normally occurs in the multivesicular body.

Antiviral Host Factors

APOBEC3G

In primary CD4 T lymphocytes, Vif plays a key but poorly understood role in the assembly of infectious virions. In the absence of Vif, normal levels of virus are produced, but these virions are noninfectious, displaying an arrest at the level of reverse transcription in the subsequent target cell. Heterokaryon analyses involving the fusion of non-permissive cells (require Vif for viral growth) and permissive cells (support the growth of Vif-deficient viruses) have revealed that Vif overcomes the effects of a natural inhibitor of HIV replication.[96,97] Recently this factor, initially termed CEM15/APOBEC3G, was identified[98] and shown to share homology a family of RNA editing/DNA mutator enzymes with cytidine deam-

inase activity. More recent studies have shown that APOBEC3G is incorporated into budding HIV virions in the absence of Vif.[99,100] When these virions infect the next target cells, APOBEC3G deaminates dC in the single-stranded minus strand viral DNA producing dU at these sites.[101] These viral DNAs are either degraded by the combined action uracil N-glycosylase and apurinic-apyrimidinic endonuclease or plus strand DNA is synthesized, producing dG→dA hypermutations and possibly introducing of multiple stop codons in normally open reading frames. Vif circumvents these antiviral activities of APOBEC3G by targeting the antiviral enzyme for both accelerated degradation in proteasomes and decreased synthesis[99,102,103] (Fig. 3.6). In terms of the accelerated degradation, Vif both binds to APO-BEC3G and a specific E3 ligase complex that mediates polyubiquitylation of APOBEC3G, marking it for proteasomal degradation.[104] These combined

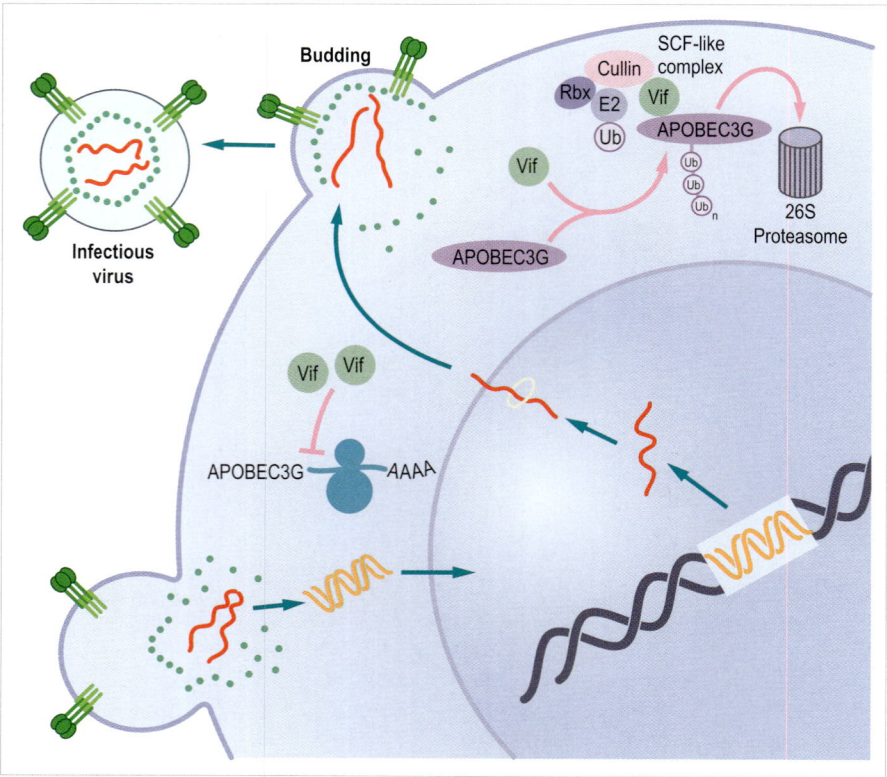

Figure 3.6 Mechanism by which HIV Vif circumvents the antiviral action of APOBEC3G. Vif depletes intracellular APOBEC3G both by promoting polyubiquitylation and proteasome mediated degradation of this enzyme and by partially blocking APOBEC3G mRNA translation. These combined effects lead to essentially complete depletion of APOBEC3G in the virus producing cells thus making APOBEC3G unavailable for virion incorporation. Vif-induced degradation of APOBEC3G involves recruitment of a specific E3 ligase complex that targets APOBEC3G for polyubiquitylation. Small molecules interfering with the binding of Vif to APOBEC3G or Vif binding to the E3 ligase represent promising new targets for future drug discovery.

effects lead to the depletion of intracellular APOBEC3G in the virus-producing cell thus the enzyme is not available for virion incorporation. The assembly of Vif with APOBEC3G and Vif-induced degradation of the antiretroviral enzyme forms an intriguing new target for antiviral drug development. The goal is to identify small molecules that would interfere with APOBEC3G degradation thereby preserving the intracellular levels of the enzyme and making it available for incorporation into the virion. APOBEC3G is then capable of unleashing its potent DNA-mutating effects during the next round of reverse transcription.

More recent studies have revealed that another intriguing antiviral function of APOBEC3G. Resting CD4 T cells express an enzymatically active low molecular weight form of APOBEC3G. This cellular form of the enzyme functions as a potent post-entry restriction factor for HIV infection of these cells. When resting CD4 T cells are activated, the antiviral function of APOBEC3G is lost due to its recruitment into an inactive high molecular weight RNA-protein complex, making these cells highly permissive for productive viral infection.[105]

TRIM5α

HIV fails to replicate in most nonhuman primate cells (chimpanzee and gibbon ape cells are notable exceptions). HIV entry occurs normally in these 'non-permissive' primate cells, but a block prior to reverse transcription occurs. This block stems from an inhibitory action of the Lv-1 gene (lentivirus susceptibility) product that somehow targets the HIV capsid protein, perhaps by blocking effective uncoating of the virus. In an exciting recent study, the Lv-1 gene product was identified as the tripartite motif 5α protein, or TRIM5α.[106] TRIM5α contains four interesting protein domains: a zinc-binding ring finger, a B box that also binds zinc, a coiled-coil region (SPRY domain) that mediates protein aggregation in the cytoplasm, and a B30.2 (SPRY) domain that is involved in protein-protein interactions. When levels of rhesus TRIM5α are decreased by RNA interference, HIV replication in these cells is greatly increased. In contrast to the inhibitory effects of rhesus TRIM5α, human TRIM5α does not impair HIV replication.

With a greater understanding of how rhesus TRIM5α acts, it may be possible to develop small molecules that transform the highly related human TRIM5α into an effective inhibitor of HIV replication. The success of this approach will critically depend on deciphering precisely how rhesus TRIM5α achieves its inhibitory effects. Leading possibilities include the potential action of rhesus TRIM5α as an ubiquitin ligase or as an inhibitor of sumoylation. Alternatively, rhesus TRIM5α may help stabilize the viral core by interacting with human cyclophilin A bound to the HIV capsid protein. This promises to be a fertile area for future research that hopefully will be translatable into new HIV therapies.

Conclusion and Perspective

The global AIDS pandemic continues to expand. Advances in antiretroviral therapies have slowed its advance in the industrialized world, but due to lack of wide availability, have had less impact in the developing world. Because of its high rate of mutation, HIV is able to refine and optimize its interactions with various host proteins and pathways, thereby promoting its growth and spread. The virus ensures that the host cell survives until the viral replicative cycle is completed. Possibly even more damaging, HIV establishes stable latent forms that support the chronic nature of infection. Eradication of the virus appears unlikely until effective methods are developed to purge these latent viral reservoirs.

Basic science will clearly play a leading role in future attempts to solve the mysteries of viral latency and replication. A small-animal model that recapitulates the pathogenic mechanisms of HIV is sorely needed to study the mechanisms underlying viral cytopathicity. Such cell death is not only limited to infected targets but also involves uninfected bystander cells.[46] Murine cells do not support efficient assembly or release of Gag.[47] Currently, this defect represents a major impediment to the successful development of a rodent model of AIDS.

Proposed mechanisms for HIV killing of T cells include the formation of giant cell syncytia through the interactions of gp120 with CD4 and chemokine receptors,[107] the accumulation of unintegrated linear forms of viral DNA, the proapoptotic effects of the Tat,[108] Nef,[109] and Vpr[110] proteins, and the adverse effects conferred by the metabolic burden that HIV replication[111] places on the infected cell. Of note, expression of Nef alone as a transgene in mice recapitulates many of the clinical features of AIDS, including immunodeficiency and loss of CD4-positive cells.[112] Finally, future therapies will likely target viral proteins other than its enzymes, namely reverse transcriptase, protease, and integrase. Clinical trials are already under way with small molecules or small peptides that block the binding of HIV to surface chemokine receptors and a peptide that interrupts the machinery of fusion is already in clinical use. Although only under preclinical evaluation, small chemicals capable of interfering with Tat transactivation[113] and Rev-dependent nuclear export of viral transcripts are under study.[114] As a proof of principle, dominant-negative mutants of Tat, Rev, and Gag proteins have been shown to block viral replication. By increasing the number of antiviral compounds available that target different steps in the viral replicative cycle and by ensuring that these drugs can be deployed in developing countries, we should be positioned better to extend survival, to improve the quality of life for infected individuals and to inhibit the spread of AIDS.

Acknowledgements

We thank Gary Howard and Stephen Ordway for editorial support, John Carroll for graphics preparation, Robin Givens for administrative support, and the National Institutes of Health (R01 AI45234, R01 CA86814, P01 HD40543), the UCSF California AIDS Research Center (CC02-SF-002), and the J. David Gladstone Institutes for funding support. (This chapter was adapted and updated from a prior review published in *Nature Medicine* 2002; 8:673–680.)

References

1. Kwong PD, Wyatt R, Robinson J, et al. Structure of an HIV gp120 envelope glycoprotein in complex with the CD4 receptor and a neutralizing human antibody. Nature 1998; 393:648–659.
2. Jacobson JM, Israel RJ, Lowy I, et al. Treatment of advanced human immunodeficiency virus type 1 disease with the viral entry inhibitor PRO 542. Antimicrob Agents Chemother 2004; 48:423–429.
3. Jacobson JM, Lowy I, Fletcher CV, et al. Single-dose safety, pharmacology, and antiviral activity of the human immunodeficiency virus (HIV) type 1 entry inhibitor PRO 542 in HIV-infected adults. J Infect Dis 2000; 182:326–329.
4. Kuritzkes DR, Jacobson J, Powderly WG, et al. Antiretroviral activity of the anti-CD4 monoclonal antibody TNX-355 in patients infected with HIV type 1. J Infect Dis 2004; 189:286–291.
5. Doms RW, Trono D. The plasma membrane as a combat zone in the HIV battlefield. Genes Dev 2000; 14:2677–2688.
6. Scarlatti G, Tresoldi E, Bjorndal A, et al. In vivo evolution of HIV-1 co-receptor usage and sensitivity to chemokine-mediated suppression. Nat Med 1997; 3:1259–1265.
7. Liu R, Paxton WA, Choe S, et al. Homozygous defect in HIV-1 coreceptor accounts for resistance of some multiply-exposed individuals to HIV-1 infection. Cell 1996; 86:367–377.
8. Martinson JJ, Chapman NH, Rees DC, et al. Global distribution of the CCR5 gene 32-basepair deletion. Nat Genet 1997; 16:100–103.
9. Kozak SL, Heard JM, Kabat D. Segregation of CD4 and CXCR4 into distinct lipid microdomains in T lymphocytes suggests a mechanism for membrane destabilization by human immunodeficiency virus. J Virol 2002; 76:1802–1815.
10. Campbell SM, Crowe SM, Mak J. Lipid rafts and HIV-1: from viral entry to assembly of progeny virions. J Clin Virol 2001; 22:217–227.
11. Liao Z, Cimakasky LM, Hampton R, et al. Lipid rafts and HIV pathogenesis: host membrane cholesterol is required for infection by HIV type 1. AIDS Res Hum Retroviruses 2001; 17:1009–1019.
12. Chan DC, Kim PS. HIV entry and its inhibition. Cell 1998; 93:681–684.
13. Geijtenbeek TB, Kwon DS, Torensma R, et al. DC-SIGN, a dendritic cell-specific HIV-1-binding protein that enhances trans-infection of T cells. Cell 2000; 100:587–597.
14. Kwon DS, Gregorio G, Bitton N, et al. DC-SIGN-mediated internalization of HIV is required for trans- enhancement of T cell infection. Immunity 2002; 16:135–144.
15. Cartier C, Sivard P, Tranchat C, et al. Identification of three major phosphorylation sites within HIV-1 capsid. Role of phosphorylation during the early steps of infection. J Biol Chem 1999; 274:19434–40.
16. Franke EK, Yuan HE, Luban J. Specific incorporation of cyclophilin A into HIV-1 virions. Nature 1994; 372:359–362.
17. Schaeffer E, Geleziunas R, Greene WC. Human immunodeficiency virus type 1 Nef functions at the level of virus entry by enhancing cytoplasmic delivery of virions. J Virol 2001; 75:2993–3000.
18. Ohagen A, Gabuzda D. Role of Vif in stability of the human immunodeficiency virus type 1 core. J Virol 2000; 74:11055–11066.
19. Lu X, Yu H, Liu SH, et al. Interactions between HIV1 Nef and vacuolar ATPase facilitate the internalization of CD4. Immunity 1998; 8:647–656.
20. Takeda M, Pekosz A, Shuck K, et al. Influenza a virus M2 ion channel activity is essential for efficient replication in tissue culture. J Virol 2002; 76:1391–1399.
21. Campbell EM, Nunez R, Hope TJ. Disruption of the actin cytoskeleton can complement the ability of Nef to enhance human immunodeficiency virus type 1 infectivity. J Virol 2004; 78:5745–5755.
22. Karageorgos L, Li P, Burrell C. Characterization of HIV replication complexes early after cell-to-cell infection. AIDS Res Hum Retroviruses 1993; 9:817–823.
23. Bukrinskaya A, Brichacek B, Mann A, et al. Establishment of a functional human immunodeficiency virus type 1 (HIV-1) reverse transcription complex involves the cytoskeleton. J Exp Med 1998; 188:2113–2125.
24. Miller MD, Farnet CM, Bushman FD. Human immunodeficiency virus type 1 preintegration complexes: studies of organization and composition. J Virol 1997; 71:5382–5390.
25. McDonald D, Vodicka MA, Lucero G, et al. Visualization of the intracellular behavior of HIV in living cells. J Cell Biol 2002; 159:441–452.
26. Bell P, Montaner LJ, Maul GG. Accumulation and intranuclear distribution of unintegrated human immunodeficiency virus type 1 DNA. J Virol 2001; 75:7683–7691.
27. Turelli P, Doucas V, Craig E, et al. Cytoplasmic recruitment of INI1 and PML on incoming HIV preintegration complexes: interference with early steps of viral replication. Mol Cell 2001; 7:1245–1254.
28. Weinberg JB, Matthews TJ, Cullen BR, et al. Productive human immunodeficiency virus type 1 (HIV-1) infection of nonproliferating human monocytes. J Exp Med 1991; 174:1477–1482.
29. Pemberton LF, Blobel G, Rosenblum JS. Transport routes through the nuclear pore complex. Curr Opin Cell Biol 1998; 10:392–399.
30. Gallay P, Hope T, Chin D, et al. HIV-1 infection of nondividing cells through the recognition of integrase by the importin/karyopherin pathway. Proc Natl Acad Sci USA 1997; 94:9825–9830.
31. Bukrinsky MI, Haggerty S, Dempsey MP, et al. A nuclear localization signal within HIV-1 matrix protein that governs infection of non-dividing cells. Nature 1993; 365:666–669.

32. Heinzinger NK, Bukinsky MI, Haggerty SA, et al. The Vpr protein of human immunodeficiency virus type 1 influences nuclear localization of viral nucleic acids in nondividing host cells. Proc Natl Acad Sci USA 1994; 91:7311–7315.

33. Zennou V, Petit C, Guetard D, et al. HIV-1 genome nuclear import is mediated by a central DNA flap. Cell 2000; 101:173–185.

34. Dvorin JD, Bell P, Maul GG, et al. Reassessment of the roles of integrase and the central DNA flap in human immunodeficiency virus type 1 nuclear import. J Virol 2002; 76:12087–12096.

35. Sherman MP, Noronha CM de, Heusch MI, et al. Nucleocytoplasmic shuttling by human immunodeficiency virus type 1 Vpr. J Virol 2001; 75:1522–1532.

36. Eckstein DA, Sherman MP, Penn ML, et al. HIV-1 Vpr enhances viral burden by facilitating infection of tissue macrophages but not nondividing CD4+ T cells. J Exp Med 2001; 194:1407–1419.

37. Vodicka MA, Koepp DM, Silver PA, et al. HIV-1 Vpr interacts with the nuclear transport pathway to promote macrophage infection. Genes Dev 1998; 12:175–185.

38. Dupont S, Sharova N, DeHoratius C, et al. A novel nuclear export activity in HIV-1 matrix protein required for viral replication. Nature 1999; 402:681–685.

39. Chen H, Engelman A. The barrier-to-autointegration protein is a host factor for HIV type 1 integration. Proc Natl Acad Sci USA 1998; 95:15270–15274.

40. Schroder AR, Shinn P, Chen H, et al. HIV-1 integration in the human genome favors active genes and local hotspots. Cell 2002; 110:521–529.

41. Billich A. S-1360 Shionogi-GlaxoSmithKline. Curr Opin Investig Drugs 2003; 4:206–209.

42. Wu Y, Marsh JW. Selective transcription and modulation of resting T cell activity by preintegrated HIV DNA. Science 2001; 293:1503–1506.

43. Li L, Olvera JM, Yoder KE, et al. Role of the non-homologous DNA end joining pathway in the early steps of retroviral infection. Embo J 2001; 20:3272–3281.

44. Adams M, Sharmeen L, Kimpton J, et al. Cellular latency in human immunodeficiency virus-infected individuals with high CD4 levels can be detected by the presence of promoter-proximal transcripts. Proc Natl Acad Sci USA 1994; 91:3862–3866.

45. Jordan A, Defechereux P, Verdin E. The site of HIV-1 integration in the human genome determines basal transcriptional activity and response to Tat transactivation. Embo J 2001; 20:1726–1738.

46. Finkel TH, Tudor-Williams G, Banda NK, et al. Apoptosis occurs predominantly in bystander cells and not in productively infected cells of HIV- and SIV-infected lymph nodes. Nat Med 1995; 1:129–134.

47. Bieniasz PD, Cullen BR. Multiple blocks to human immunodeficiency virus type 1 replication in rodent cells. J Virol 2000; 74:9868–9877.

48. Taube R, Fujinaga K, Wimmer J, et al. Tat transactivation: a model for the regulation of eukaryotic transcriptional elongation. Virology 1999; 264:245–253.

49. Kao SY, Calman AF, Luciw PA, et al. Anti-termination of transcription within the long terminal repeat of HIV-1 by tat gene product. Nature 1987; 330:489–493.

50. Jones KA, Peterlin BM. Control of RNA initiation and elongation at the HIV-1 promoter. Annu Rev Biochem 1994; 63:717–743.

51. Karin M, Ben-Neriah Y. Phosphorylation meets ubiquitination: the control of NF-[kappa]B activity. Annu Rev Immunol 2000; 18:621–663.

52. Crabtree GR. Generic signals and specific outcomes: signaling through Ca2+, calcineurin, and NF-AT. Cell 1999; 96:611–614.

53. Barboric M, Nissen RM, Kanazawa S, et al. NF-kappaB binds P-TEFb to stimulate transcriptional elongation by RNA polymerase II. Mol Cell 2001; 8:327–337.

54. Wei P, Garber ME, Fang SM, et al. A novel CDK9-associated C-type cyclin interacts directly with HIV-1 Tat and mediates its high-affinity, loop-specific binding to TAR RNA. Cell 1998; 92:451–462.

55. Price DH. P-TEFb, a cyclin-dependent kinase controlling elongation by RNA polymerase II. Mol Cell Biol 2000; 20:2629–2634.

56. Garber ME, Wei P, KewalRamani VN, et al. The interaction between HIV-1 Tat and human cyclin T1 requires zinc and a critical cysteine residue that is not conserved in the murine CycT1 protein. Genes Dev 1998; 12:3512–3527.

57. Garber ME, Mayall TP, Suess EM, et al. CDK9 autophosphorylation regulates high-affinity binding of the human immunodeficiency virus type 1 tat-P-TEFb complex to TAR RNA. Mol Cell Biol 2000; 20:6958–6969.

58. Yang Z, Zhu Q, Luo K, et al. The 7SK small nuclear RNA inhibits the CDK9/cyclin T1 kinase to control transcription. Nature 2001; 414:317–322.

59. Saltarelli MJ, Hadziyannis E, Hart CE, et al. Analysis of human immunodeficiency virus type 1 mRNA splicing patterns during disease progression in peripheral blood mononuclear cells from infected individuals. AIDS Res Hum Retroviruses 1996; 12:1443–1456.

60. Cullen BR. Retroviruses as model systems for the study of nuclear RNA export pathways. Virology 1998; 249:203–210.

61. Powell DM, Amaral MC, Wu JY, et al. HIV Rev-dependent binding of SF2/ASF to the Rev response element: possible role in Rev-mediated inhibition of HIV RNA splicing. Proc Natl Acad Sci USA 1997; 94:973–978.

62. Luo Y, Yu H, Peterlin BM. Cellular protein modulates effects of human immunodeficiency virus type 1 Rev. J Virol 1994; 68:3850–3856.

63. Malim MH, Tiley LS, McCarn DF, et al. HIV-1 structural gene expression requires binding of the Rev trans-activator to its RNA target sequence. Cell 1990; 60:675–683.

64. Malim MH, Cullen BR. Rev and the fate of pre-mRNA in the nucleus: implications for the regulation of RNA processing in eukaryotes. Mol Cell Biol 1993; 13:6180–6189.

65. Kestler HW 3rd, Ringler DJ, Mori K, et al. Importance of the nef gene for maintenance of high virus loads and for development of AIDS. Cell 1991; 65:651–662.

66. Deacon NJ, Tsykin A, Solomon A, et al. Genomic structure of an attenuated quasi species of HIV-1 from a blood transfusion donor and recipients. Science 1995; 270:988–991.

67. Simmons A, Aluvihare V, McMichael A. Nef triggers a transcriptional program in T cells imitating single-signal T cell activation and inducing HIV virulence mediators. Immunity 2001; 14:763–777.

68. Khan IH, Sawai ET, Antonio E, et al. Role of the SH3-ligand domain of simian immunodeficiency virus Nef in interaction with Nef-associated kinase and simian AIDS in rhesus macaques. J Virol 1998; 72:5820–5830.

69. Glushakova S, Munch J, Carl S, et al. CD4 down-modulation by human immunodeficiency virus type 1 Nef correlates with the efficiency of viral replication and with CD4 (+) T-cell depletion in human lymphoid tissue ex vivo. J Virol 2001; 75:10113–10117.

70. Lama J, Mangasarian A, Trono D. Cell-surface expression of CD4 reduces HIV-1 infectivity by blocking Env incorporation in a Nef- and Vpu-inhibitable manner. Curr Biol 1999; 9:622–631.

71. Zheng YH, Plemenitas A, Linnemann T, et al. Nef increases infectivity of HIV via lipid rafts. Curr Biol 2001; 11:875–879.

72. Geyer M, Fackler OT, Peterlin BM. Structure–function relationships in HIV-1 Nef. EMBO Rep 2001; 2:580–585.

73. Wang JK, Kiyokawa E, Verdin E, et al. The Nef protein of HIV-1 associates with rafts and primes T cells for activation. Proc Natl Acad Sci USA 2000; 97:394–399.

74. Chen BK, Gandhi RT, Baltimore D. CD4 down-modulation during infection of human T cells with human immunodeficiency virus type 1 involves independent activities of vpu, env, and nef. J Virol 1996; 70:6044–6053.

75. Crise B, Buonocore L, Rose JK. CD4 is retained in the endoplasmic reticulum by the human immunodeficiency virus type 1 glycoprotein precursor. J Virol 1990; 64:5585–5593.

76. Margottin F, Bour SP, Durand H, et al. A novel human WD protein, h-beta TrCp, that interacts with HIV-1 Vpu connects CD4 to the ER degradation pathway through an F-box motif. Mol Cell 1998; 1:565–574.

77. Xu XN, Laffert B, Screaton GR, et al. Induction of Fas ligand expression by HIV involves the interaction of Nef with the T cell receptor zeta chain. J Exp Med 1999; 189:1489–1496.

78. Collins KL, Chen BK, Kalams SA, et al. HIV-1 Nef protein protects infected primary cells against killing by cytotoxic T lymphocytes. Nature 1998; 391:397–401.

79. Le Gall S, Erdtmann L, Benichou S, et al. Nef interacts with the mu subunit of clathrin adaptor complexes and reveals a cryptic sorting signal in MHC I molecules. Immunity 1998; 8:483–495.

80. Geleziunas R, Xu W, Takeda K, Ichijo H, et al. HIV-1 Nef inhibits ASK1-dependent death signalling providing a potential mechanism for protecting the infected host cell. Nature 2001; 410:834–838.

81. Wolf D, Witte V, Laffert B, et al. HIV-1 Nef associated PAK and PI3-kinases stimulate Akt-independent Bad-phosphorylation to induce anti-apoptotic signals. Nat Med 2001; 7:1217–1224.

82. Greenway AL, McPhee DA, Allen K, et al. Human immunodeficiency virus type 1 Nef binds to tumor suppressor p53 and protects cells against p53-mediated apoptosis. J Virol 2002; 76:2692–2702.

83. Jowett JB, Planelles V, Poon B, et al. The human immunodeficiency virus type 1 vpr gene arrests infected T cells in the G2 + M phase of the cell cycle. J Virol 1995; 69:6304–6313.

84. Goh WC, Rogel ME, Kinsey CM, et al. HIV-1 Vpr increases viral expression by manipulation of the cell cycle: a mechanism for selection of Vpr in vivo. Nat Med 1998; 4:65–71.

85. Noronha CM de, Sherman MP, Lin HW, et al. Dynamic disruptions in nuclear envelope architecture and integrity induced by HIV-1 Vpr. Science 2001; 294:1105–1108.

86. Wilk T, Gross I, Gowen BE, et al. Organization of immature human immunodeficiency virus type 1. J Virol 2001; 75:759–771.

87. Freed EO. HIV-1 gag proteins: diverse functions in the virus life cycle. Virology 1998; 251:1–15.

88. Zimmerman C, Klein KC, Kiser PK, et al. Identification of a host protein essential for assembly of immature HIV-1 capsids. Nature 2002; 415:88–92.

89. Gottlinger HG, Sodroski JG, Haseltine WA. Role of capsid precursor processing and myristoylation in morphogenesis and infectivity of human immunodeficiency virus type 1. Proc Natl Acad Sci USA 1989; 86:5781–5785.

90. Ono A, Freed EO. Plasma membrane rafts play a critical role in HIV-1 assembly and release. Proc Natl Acad Sci USA 2001; 98:13925–13930.

91. Garnier L, Parent LJ, Rovinski B, et al. Identification of retroviral late domains as determinants of particle size. J Virol 1999; 73:2309–2320.

92. Strack B, Calistri A, Accola MA, et al. A role for ubiquitin ligase recruitment in retrovirus release. Proc Natl Acad Sci USA 2000; 97:13063–13068.

93. Garrus JE, Schwedler UK von, Pornillos OW, et al. Tsg101 and the vacuolar protein sorting pathway are essential for HIV-1 budding. Cell 2001; 107:55–65.

94. VerPlank L, Bouamr F, LaGrassa TJ, et al. Tsg101, a homologue of ubiquitin-conjugating (E2) enzymes, binds the L domain in HIV type 1 Pr55(Gag). Proc Natl Acad Sci USA 2001; 98:7724–7729.

95. Katzmann DJ, Babst M, Emr SD. Ubiquitin-dependent sorting into the multivesicular body pathway requires the function of a conserved endosomal protein sorting complex, ESCRT-I. Cell 2001; 106:145–155.

96. Simon JH, Gaddis NC, Fouchier RA, et al. Evidence for a newly discovered cellular anti-HIV-1 phenotype. Nat Med 1998; 4:1397–1400.

97. Madani N, Kabat D. An endogenous inhibitor of human immunodeficiency virus in human lymphocytes is overcome by the viral Vif protein. J Virol 1998; 72:10251–10255.

98. Sheehy AM, Gaddis NC, Choi JD, et al. Isolation of a human gene that inhibits HIV-1 infection and is suppressed by the viral Vif protein. Nature 2002; 418:646–650.

99. Stopak K, De Noronha C, Yonemoto W, et al. HIV-1 Vif blocks the antiviral activity of APOBEC3G by impairing both its translation and intracellular stability. Mol Cell 2003; 12:591–601.

100. Yu Q, Konig R, Pillai S, et al. Single-strand specificity of APOBEC3G accounts for minus-strand deamination of the HIV genome. Nat Struct Mol Biol 2004; 11:435–442.

101. Mariani R, Chen D, Schrofelbauer B, et al. Species-specific exclusion of APOBEC3G from HIV-1 virions by Vif. Cell 2003; 114:21–31.

102. Marin M, Rose KM, Kozak SL, et al. HIV-1 Vif protein binds the editing enzyme APOBEC3G and induces its degradation. Nat Med 2003; 9:1398–1403.

103. Sheehy AM, Gaddis NC, Malim MH. The antiretroviral enzyme APOBEC3G is degraded by the proteasome in response to HIV-1 Vif. Nat Med 2003; 9:1404–1407.

104. Yu X, Yu Y, Liu B, et al. Induction of APOBEC3G ubiquitination and degradation by an HIV-1 Vif-Cul5-SCF complex. Science 2003; 302:1056–1060.

105. Chiu Y-L, Soros VB, Kreisberg JF, et al. Cellular APOBEC3G restricts HIV-1 infection in resting CD4 T cells. Nature 2005; 435:108–114.

106. Stremlau M, Owens CM, Perron MJ, et al. The cytoplasmic body component TRIM5alpha restricts HIV-1 infection in Old World monkeys. Nature 2004; 427:848–853.

107. Kowalski M, Potz J, Basiripour L, et al. Functional regions of the envelope glycoprotein of human immunodeficiency virus type 1. Science 1987; 237:1351–1355.

108. Westendorp MO, Frank R, Ochsenbauer C, et al. Sensitization of T cells to CD95-mediated apoptosis by HIV-1 Tat and gp120. Nature 1995; 375:497–500.

109. Baur AS, Sawai ET, Dazin P, et al. HIV-1 Nef leads to inhibition or activation of T cells depending on its intracellular localization. Immunity 1994; 1:373–384.

110. Stewart SA, Poon B, Jowett JB, et al. Human immunodeficiency virus type 1 Vpr induces apoptosis following cell cycle arrest. J Virol 1997; 71:5579–5592.

111. Somasundaran M, Robinson HL. Unexpectedly high levels of HIV-1 RNA and protein synthesis in a cytocidal infection. Science 1988; 242:1554–1557.

112. Hanna Z, Kay DG, Rebai N, et al. Nef harbors a major determinant of pathogenicity for an AIDS-like disease induced by HIV-1 in transgenic mice. Cell 1998; 95:163–175.

113. Chao SH, Fujinaga K, Marion JE, et al. Flavopiridol inhibits P-TEFb and blocks HIV-1 replication. J Biol Chem 2000; 275:28345–28348.

114. Wolff B, Sanglier JJ, Wang Y. Leptomycin B is an inhibitor of nuclear export: inhibition of nucleo-cytoplasmic translocation of the human immunodeficiency virus type 1 (HIV-1) Rev protein and Rev-dependent mRNA. Chem Biol 1997; 4:139–147.

CHAPTER 4

The Immune Response to HIV

Clive M. Gray
Bruce Walker

Introduction

Most people in the world live in poverty-stricken conditions where they are continuously confronted with a plethora of pathogenic organisms – some successfully repelled, some resulting in clinically overt disease and others resulting in persistent latent infection. The human immune system has evolved to combat these genetically diverse organisms, including viruses, bacteria and protozoa, through genetically governed responses involving multiple receptors and ligands. Even with clinically overt or persistent infections, most people with an intact immune system ultimately survive most infections.

In marked contrast stands HIV infection. The spread of HIV-1 worldwide represents one of the great challenges to confront host immunity, since the key target is the CD4 lymphocyte, infection and depletion of which severely undermines effective immune responses. As a result, most people who become infected and remain untreated, will ultimately succumb to one or more of the large variety of infectious organisms. The spreading global epidemic has resulted in the infection of over 60 million persons, with over 3 million people having died from AIDS in 2004 alone (www.unaids.org).

The ultimate solution to the HIV epidemic relies on the development of an effective vaccine that can be delivered to those at risk. The ability to achieve this, as yet elusive, goal will be facilitated by a comprehensive understanding of the key immune responses that contribute to protection from infection, or protection from disease progression in those who become infected. In this chapter, we will review the current state of knowledge of what is needed for an AIDS vaccine, first by comparison to effective immune clearance of acute viral infections (such as influenza, rotavirus or respiratory syncytial virus) as well as acute viral infections followed by latent infection (herpes simplex virus or Epstein–Barr virus). This will allow a foundation from which to discuss why successful immune mechanisms are not functional in the majority of HIV-1 infected individuals. Additionally, we will discuss clues as to what may constitute a protective immune response from disease progression in HIV-1 infection that come from investigations of a small proportion of people who are either exposed and uninfected or HIV-1 infected people who do not progress to AIDS and remain clinically healthy. Finally, we will discuss prospects for a vaccine and what aspects may need to be taken into consideration for both prophylactic and therapeutic HIV vaccines, and the considerable challenges that need to be overcome to achieve success.

General Principals of an Antiviral Immune Response

The degree to which pathogenic organisms establish productive infections is determined in part by the integrity of epithelial and mucosal cells: skin, respiratory tract, alimentary tract, urogenital tract and conjunctiva. These regions serve as physical barriers between the exterior and internal environment and any abrasions or lesions will allow potential pathogenic organisms into either the blood or lymphatic circulation. Once these physical barriers have been transcended, there are two major categories of host immune responses, namely innate and acquired immunity.

The innate immune response represents the first line of defence, and serves to rapidly attenuate the impact of most infectious organisms. From an evolutionary perspective, innate immunity shares properties with lower vertebrate mechanisms of engulfment and phagocytosis and the response consists of specialized cells, such as macrophages, natural killer cells, dendritic cells, and polymorphonuclear leukocytes. Infectious organisms that survive the innate immune response, or residues from such a response, are dealt with by the specific acquired immune response.

Acquired immunity has three central tenets: specificity, recognition of protein structures via the interaction of receptors and ligands; diversity, variations in specificity, where multiple receptors interact with different protein structures; and memory, where different T and B cells that have been primed to antigens can be recalled at a subsequent point in time with a more rapid response.

What governs specificity and diversity of the adaptive immune response is the genetic make-up of the host, where genes encoding for the Major Histocompatibility Complex (MHC), T-cell Receptors (TCR) and Immunoglobulins (B-cell receptors) dictate how and which regions of the pathogen are encountered by the immune system. The molecules encoded by these genes are central to specificity, diversity and memory and constitute the internal composition of each individual and is collectively known as 'self.' An acquired immune response that results in the successful clearance of an invading organism can be understood by the exquisite difference in recognition between 'self' and 'non-self.' The ultimate outcome of this process is preservation of 'self' and hence survival.

Acquired Immunity to Viral Infections

The immune system consists of parallel blood and lymphatic circulations, ensuring that different cells participating in an immune response can migrate back and forth between non-lymphoid tissue and the different secondary lymphoid structures (such as the spleen and lymph nodes). Bone marrow is the primary lymphoid organ, where the precursors to all mature immunocompetent cells are derived as pluripotential progenitor cells. B and T cells develop into mature immunocompetent cells in the bone marrow and thymus, respectively. T cells that leave

the thymus are 'naïve' and have yet to encounter invading pathogen.

Lymph nodes are crucial for providing the correct microenvironment and anatomical structures required for initiating an immune response. The micro-anatomical arrangement of the lymph node enables T cells to encounter processed viral proteins presented by specialized antigen presenting cells, which initiates the adaptive immune response. In general terms, if the anatomical arrangement of lymphoid tissue disintegrates due to pathology, the impact will result in disrupted antigen presentation and loss of both B- and T-cell priming and the inability to provide protective immunity.[1]

Movement of T cells from one lymphoid region to another allows both CD4+ and CD8+ T cells to encounter processed antigen in the paracortical region of the lymph node. After engaging and processing antigen in the peripheral tissue, dendritic cells will migrate to lymph nodes, where there is selection of reactive T cells through TcR engagement with viral peptides within the binding groove of the HLA molecules on the surface of the antigen presenting cells. This process results in multiple clones of expanded T cells leading to diversity.

The MHC in humans is known as the Human Leukocyte Antigen (HLA) system and is one of the most polymorphic proteins in the human population.[2] The uniqueness of individuals is partly defined by HLA, where each person has a defined HLA type consisting of pairs of inherited genes. As the sole function of class I and II HLA is to present processed pathogen-derived peptides, or epitopes, to circulating T cells, possible aberrant T-cell function and recognition of self, as in autoimmunity, will thus involve the HLA. Similarly, certain HLA types have been associated with either more rapid course of HIV infection (such as HLA-B*35) or with slow progression (such as HLA-B*57). The manner by which epitopes are processed and bound by the HLA molecule is highly specific and governed by certain rules associated with the binding motif structures of each HLA.

In addition to the TcR, all T cells co-express CD3 on the cell surface and the major subset in humans are CD4+ T cells, important for coordination of the immune response and secretion of multiple cytokines. First identified in murine models, the multitudinous number of cytokines can be placed into a network model of a Th1-type and Th2-type system. A Th1-type response consists of CD4+ T cells liberating a profile of cytokines that direct T-cell immunity and involves IL-1, IL-2, IL-6, IL-12, IL-15, TNFa, and IFNg for example. A Th-2 type response consists of

CD4[+] T cells liberating a profile of cytokines that directs humoral immune responses and are involved in switching on B-cell immunity. These cytokines include, among others, IL-4, IL-5, and IL-10.

In healthy humans, CD8[+] T cells make up the smaller proportion of CD3[+] T cells and are involved in protecting the host from invading pathogens. These cells function by killing virally infected cells, which are marked by the surface expression of HLA class I molecules that present (restrict) virus-derived epitopes that are typically 8–11 amino acids in length. These CD8[+] T cells function with the help of CD4 T-helper cells. The killing potential of CD8[+] T cells is through either perforin/granzyme or Fas-Fas-L interactions. In the case of viral infections, endogenously processed epitopes, derived from the transcription of viral genes, are presented on the surface of the cell by class I HLA molecules. Erupted and effete virally infected cells are engulfed and processed by dendritic cells and virally-derived epitopes are presented via cross-presentation,[3] by class II HLA molecules and drive CD4[+] T-cell responses. Typically, most (99%) expanded viral antigen-specific T-cell effector clones induced in the acute phase of infection will die through apoptosis as the immune response wanes, leaving a small residual population of T-effector memory (TEM) cells that migrate to non-lymphoid tissues or T-central memory (TCM) cells that re-circulate through the lymphatic and blood circulation and can be rapidly reactivated upon secondary exposure to viral antigens.[4]

Immune Response to HIV-1 Infection

The immune response to HIV-1 has been studied extensively, mostly to subtype B infections within the developed world.[5] The course of immunological events from the time of transmission can be divided into the acute, early and chronic phases of infection. The greatest challenges HIV presents to the immune system include the selective infection of CD4[+] T lymphocytes and the extensive viral genetic variability due to mutations.

During acute HIV infection, one of the first immunological responses to occur is the generation of class I MHC restricted CTL.[6] Figure 4.1 shows a composite schema of the possible sequence of immunological responses that occur within the first 12 months of infection. It is believed that robust cellular immune responses in the first few months after viral transmission contribute to the >1000-fold drop in viremia from the typical acute levels of 10 million or more viral RNA copies/mL plasma. Natural history studies in subtype B infections have shown that viral set point achieved within 6 months of infection is prognostic of disease outcome, where high levels of viremia are associated with a more rapid course of infection leading to AIDS.[7] Such natural history studies linking viral load to disease outcome have not yet been performed for clade C, the dominant global clade, or the other non-B clade viruses, and thus it is unclear if there are any clade specific differences in disease progression.

In addition to virus-specific CD8[+] T cells, CD4[+] T cells appear to be critical for immune control.[8] Animal models of chronic viral infections established that virus-specific CD4[+] T cells play an essential role in maintenance of effective immunity,[9] and the immune response to HIV appears to follow these same requirements. The detection of enhanced proliferation of anti-HIV specific CD4[+] T cells in individuals who maintain long-term control of HIV replication[10] and in patients treated for acute infec-

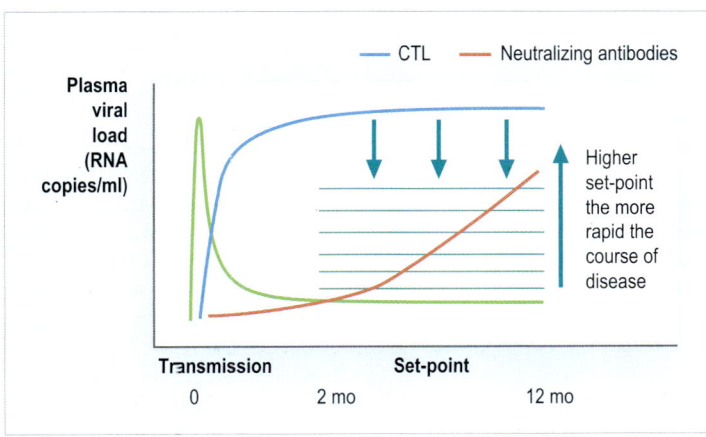

Figure 4.1 Immunological events as they are thought to occur in the first 12 months of HIV-1 infection. There is a rapid CTL response after viral transmission which coincides with the drop in viral load to various levels, or set points. Later, neutralizing antibodies (NaB) emerge and it is thought that the combined effect of both CTL and NaB exert pressure on viral replication: the greater the immune pressure the lower the viral load and set point.

tion with potent antiretroviral therapy[10-12] suggest that the function of these cells is central to influencing viral set point and for controlling virus. It can be speculated that functionally competent anti-HIV CD4[+] T cells can liberate cytokines and influence both CD8[+] T-cell and antibody responses. It has recently been shown that a large number of CD4 cells are infected in the gut and that the bulk of the CD4 pool resides within lymphoid tissue around the gastrointestinal tract. Direct killing of CCR5[+]CD4[+] T cells within the gut[13,14] and memory CD4[+] cells in multiple tissues[15] by AIDS virus has been postulated as the main mechanism for CD4 numbers depletion during SIV infection in monkeys, and extrapolations to HIV-induced depletion of CD4 cells within the human gut have also been made.[16]

Studies in both animal models and humans indicate a dominant role for CD8 T cells in controlling HIV replication. Monkey experiments, where CD8[+] T cells were depleted during acute infection with SIV resulted in persistent high viremia,[17] and when depleted during chronic, or established, infection resulted in a sudden increase in viral load and set point.[17,18] In humans, there is a temporal relationship between the initial drop in viremia in acute infection (Fig. 4.1) and the appearance of class I restricted CTL.[6,19] The antiviral effect of CD8 T cells likely results from two effector mechanisms. *In vitro* studies have shown that CTL can lyse infected cells before new virions are produced, thus inhibiting virus replication,[20-24] and also release soluble factors with anti-HIV properties.[25-27] A critical role for CD8 T-cell responses is also inferred from population data demonstrating evidence of HIV adaptation to HLA class I restricted responses.[28] These data are related to the immune pressure exerted on HIV and its mutation and escape from CTL responses, which in turn have been directed by the HLA of the infected host. To understand the imprint of HLA-restricted CTL responses that can shape the diversity of transmitted HIV strains at a population level is important for developing relevant vaccine candidates on a global level.

In addition to cellular immune responses that emerge rapidly after HIV transmission, active humoral immunity is apparent by the increased titers of anti-Gag antibodies, which are used diagnostically to assess seroconversion. Functional antibodies are those that can block or neutralize HIV entry into CD4-bearing cells and such neutralizing antibodies mainly target the highly variable V3 loop, the CD4 binding domain, and the more conserved gp41 transmembrane protein of HIV-1. Although high titers of neutralizing antibodies can completely prevent infection in animal models, the role of these responses in viral containment following infection remains controversial.[29] During acute infection, these responses appear following the initial drop in viremia,[6] and experimental depletion of B cells in monkeys during acute SIV infection led to delayed emergence of neutralizing antibodies and no change in early viral kinetics.[30] Additionally, passive transfer of neutralizing antibodies in monkeys can protect against intravenous and mucosal challenge of SIV.[31] Thus it is clear that neutralizing antibodies are important for prevention of viral infection, but perhaps less clear once HIV-1 infection has become established. Recent comprehensive longitudinal studies of autologous neutralizing antibody responses following acute infection indicate a significant antiviral effect of these responses, in that the viral inhibitory capacity is of sufficient magnitude to completely replace circulating neutralization sensitive virus with successive populations of neutralization resistant virus.[32,33]

Why the Immune Response Fails to Control HIV

From our discussion so far, HIV infection provokes a burst of immune activity that results in potent targeted CTL responses, CD4 function and the induction of antibodies. These immunological components have been found to be central role-players in effective clearance of many other viral infections, but fail to clear HIV-1 infection without exception. Why is HIV neither eliminated nor effectively contained following infection?

A number of possibilities exist. It is first, important to understand from a virological perspective that HIV-1 establishes persistent infection by infecting CD4-bearing cells and integrates into the host genome as provirus. Both primary and secondary lymphoid tissues are targets for seeding by HIV soon after transmission and the anatomical structures within lymph nodes, spleen and bone marrow are affected by the presence of virus. Consequently, from an immunological perspective, the persistence of antigen directly within the secondary lymphoid structures will influence T- and B-cell clonality and drive cells into a hyperactivated state. As discussed earlier, the high rate of HIV mutability, due to the error prone nature of reverse transcriptase, in response to specific B- and T-cell reactivity leads to immune escape and contributes to viral persistence within the host.

It is also important to understand that 25 years after AIDS was first identified, the critical immune functions that control HIV replication remain to be defined. A simplistic view has been that strong CD8 T-cell responses, together with strong neutralizing antibodies and virus-specific CD4 T cells, would lead to control of viremia. However, attempts to correlate any of these measures with viral load have proven largely unsuccessful. The breadth and magnitude of CD8 T-cell responses do not correlate with control of viremia, at least as measured by IFN gamma responses. Although neutralizing antibodies are detectable, there is again no simple relationship between these and viremia. Even virus-specific CD4 T cells, which seem critical for maintenance of effective cellular and humoral immune responses in animal models of chronic infection, can be found in some persons with progressive infection. Thus, the mechanisms that account for a lack of long-term control of HIV infection are probably complex. The following are some of the factors for which there is now experimental evidence suggesting that they may participate in the ultimate lack of ability to control HIV replication.

Escape from Neutralizing Antibodies

Despite gradual broadening of the neutralizing antibody response following acute infection, it does not become sufficiently broad to neutralize the next population of virus to arise,[32,33] and the neutralizing antibody responses forever lags behind the evolution of the envelope gene. The relevance of neutralization antibody escape in loss of overall control of viremia is open to debate as escape has also been observed in HIV infected individuals who persistently control viremia.[34,35]

Escape from CD8+ T-cell Control

Studies in both acute and chronic HIV infection have shown that mutations in the HIV genome results in viral escape from specific CD8 T-cell recognition. Mutations within targeted epitopes[36,37] can abrogate established CD8 T-cell responses, as can mutations in flanking residues[38,39] that impair normal antigen processing. Both of these lead to loss of recognition by established T-cell responses. The rapid generation of escape mutations within CD8 T-cell epitopes during acute infection,[40] and more recent population data from persons with chronic infection[28,41] support a role for CD8 T-cell selection pressure influencing viral evolution. Thus, as virus evolves with muta-

tions occurring in epitopes, once recognized by CD8+ T cells, the anticipated outcome will be loss of viral control and continued persistence. A major question raised by these findings is whether the result of population selection pressure on HIV will result in the loss of key epitopes through mutation, such that dominant epitopes will be gradually eliminated from the circulating viral population.

CD8+ T-cell Dysfunction

Defects in differentiation and maturation of CTL[42-44] may result in impaired *in vivo* function, and may relate to lack of CD4 help that is critical for maintenance of effective immunity. Most studies to date have defined CD8+ T-cell responses based on the ability to secrete IFN gamma, which based on animal model data may be the last effector response to be lost by CD8+ T cells.[45] Recent data indicate a functional impairment in the ability of CD8+ T cells to proliferate to viral antigen in persons with progressive disease that is maintained in persons with nonprogressing infection,[43] and present in the earliest stages of acute infection when viral load is rapidly declining.[46] Some studies have shown that CTL against HIV-1 may be deficient in perforin production,[27,43] but whether this is due to an intrinsic defect or to recent encounter with antigen is not entirely clear.

Impaired CD4+ T-cell Responses

The composition of functionally distinct subsets of virus-specific CD4 cells, including IL-2- and IL-2/IFN-γ-secreting HIV-1-specific CD4 T cells, may be critical,[47-49] as may cell killing by CD8 cells.[50] Infection of a subset of CD8 T cells that are CD4dim following activation has been demonstrated, suggesting that infection of this population of CD8 T cells may contribute to loss of CD8 T-cell function *in vivo*.[51,52]

Impaired Dendritic Cell Function

There are also recent studies in the SIV model and in a small human clinical trial suggesting impaired induction of immune responses in chronic infection, which may be related to the impaired function of DC during viral infection. These studies,[53] in which adoptive transfer of *in vitro* matured DCs loaded with inactivated virus led to a decrease in set point viremia and increase in virus-specific immune responses, need to be confirmed by additional groups, but suggest that there is impairment in the inductive phase of the immune response.

Lymphoid Structure Degeneration

After infection, HIV-1 resides within the germinal centers of the lymph nodes, spleen, tonsils and thymus and exists, in the main, as whole virus on the surface of follicular dendritic cells (FDC) in the lymph node. As a result, the normal function of FDC in presenting antigen may be overridden. Viral transmission is thought to be cell-associated and productive infection most likely takes place in lymphoid structures in close proximity to the cervix and rectum, where DC from the newly infected individual migrates from the cervical region to lymph nodes elsewhere in the body. Complete virus is most likely carried on dendritic cells by DC-SIGN, which aids in transmission to T cells[54] in the lymph nodes distal to the point of viral transmission. Although there are no clear data relating the dissolution of the lymph node architecture with persistence of virus, and ongoing immune responses, it may be hypothesized that destruction of the platform used to initiate immune responses leads to an overall failure in T-cell priming to new antigens. Evidence from regenerated lymphoid structures after successful antiretroviral treatment supports this notion.[55]

Other Concomitant Infections

The extent to which the ability to control HIV may be impaired by other concomitant infections is a particularly relevant question for those areas where the epidemic is currently most rapidly expanding. In many regions of the world, co-infections with Mycobacterium tuberculosis (mTB)[56] and other co-viral infections are predominant and the impact of co-infections on host immunity to HIV is also relatively unknown. Alternatively, some studies have shown that there may be beneficial protective effects of HIV co-infection with GB virus C (GBV-C),[57] where protection may result from the induction of different chemokines that have anti-HIV properties. However, the mortality rates within cohort studies in populations of mine workers in southern Africa who are co-infected with mTB and HIV suggest that co-bacterial infections are anything but protective.[58,59] Attempting to understand HIV-mediated pathogenesis in an environment where multiple potential co-infections exist represents an added challenge to understand vaccine or treatment mechanisms in the global context of HIV infection.

Evidence for Correlates of Protection to HIV-1 Infection

Even though HIV-1 infection establishes persistence and undermines immunity, there are a small number of people who are infected but are clinically healthy and can control viremia to extraordinarily low levels – less than 50 copies/mL plasma, which is the limit of quantitation by current standard methods. Additionally, there are also individuals who have frequent high-risk sexual encounters and are highly exposed to HIV, but appear to be resistant to infection. These two cohorts of individuals may provide clues to which factors of host immunity correlate with delayed disease or protection from infection.[57] Identity of these immune factors is important for providing clues to protective immunity and for devising successful vaccine strategies. Several cohort studies, including highly exposed persistently seronegative (HEPS) sex workers, occupationally exposed healthcare workers and uninfected babies born to HIV infected mothers, have reported evidence for systemic and mucosal cytotoxic T-cell activity and chemokine receptor mutations as significant associations with seronegative status. Less well-associated factors such as chemokine production, HLA alleles/haplotypes, helper T-cell responses, humoral responses and soluble inhibitory factors have been described, but less uniformly. Evidence for mucosal HIV-specific IgA antibodies in HEPS individuals also provide evidence for possible protective roles of local antibody responses – although these studies often have examined small numbers of individuals.[60]

A caveat when interpreting data derived from HEPS individuals is whether HIV-specific immune responses are protective or reflect HIV-1 antigen exposure. Although this is difficult to address, experiments performed with SCID/beige mice reconstituted with PBMC from HEPS individuals and challenged with R5 using viruses were resistant to infection.[61] When human CD8[+] T cells were depleted in the mice, they became susceptible to HIV infection. Further experiments of this nature have not been repeated and it is unclear what the functional nature of CD8[+] cells were. A more recent exploration of defining which immune factors correlate with protection, or attenuation of disease in HIV infected individuals, has been to identify human genes with polymorphic variants that influence the outcome of HIV-1 exposure or infection. Several aids-restricting genes (ARG) have been identified within the human genome that are related to either resistance or acceleration of disease.[62]

Prospects for Vaccines

A vaccine is of paramount importance to develop and implement as a public health option in many regions of the globe where HIV-1 incidence rates are extremely high. If a preventative vaccine can lower the rate of viral transmission, this will have a significant effect of mitigating the epidemic. Although successful vaccines have been implemented for diseases such as smallpox, polio, measles and hepatitis B, replicating these designs for HIV-1 may not be appropriate.[63] Persistence of HIV leading to chronic infection and the continuous viral evolution in the infected host, to evade antibody and CTL responses, needs to be accounted for. It is known, for example, that chronic persistence of antigen leads to diminished central memory T cells, and the inability of the immune system to mount an effective secondary response.[64] Thus, a vaccine would be required to enhance the pool of central memory, either in a preventative nature or as a therapeutic option. Development of therapeutic vaccines is extremely relevant

for the large numbers of HIV-1 infected individuals, where the aim would be to redirect immunity under the cover of antiretroviral therapy to effectively contain infection. More substantial research is ongoing with preventative vaccine strategies and our discussion will focus on this area.

There is no doubt that a successful preventative vaccine will need to evoke aspects of innate, cellular and humoral immunity.[56] As the major determining factor of disease progression in an individual is viremia and the level of infectiousness is proportional to the magnitude of the viral load in plasma, genital tract secretions and breast-milk, a vaccine capable of controlling viral replication would potentially lower the rate of disease progression and transmission. Although the primary outcome of an efficacious vaccine is prevention from infection, the nature of HIV transmission and its ability to establish infection makes it unlikely that sterilizing immunity will be achieved.

Figure 4.2 shows four potential scenarios of endpoints in HIV efficacy trials. Typically, a phase III vaccine trial measures the efficacy of the candidate

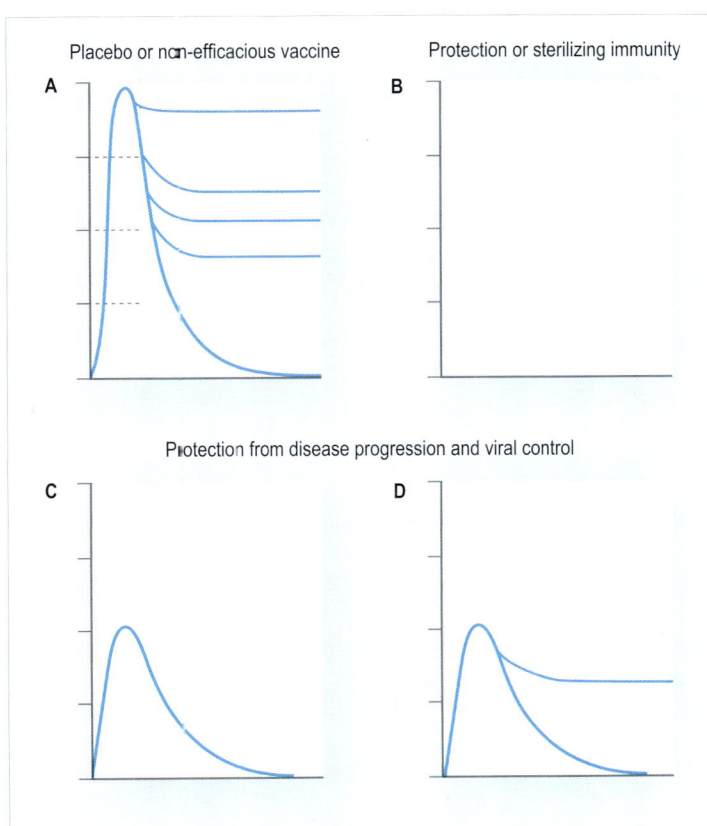

Figure 4.2 Four potential scenarios of measuring vaccine endpoints in efficacy trials: (A) Either the placebo (control) or a non-efficacious vaccine and ineffective at eliciting immune responses that could prevent HIV-1 infection or replication once in the host; (B) a fully efficacious vaccine that can prevent HIV-1 infection by eliciting sterilizing immunity; (C) Attenuation of HIV replication at the time of transmission through a vaccine-induced immune response strong enough to exert pressure on preventing viral replication; (D) Limited attenuation of viral replication, but lower set point and delay of disease progression. (Adapted from UNAIDS).

vaccine, which is compared with a placebo control arm. The primary end-point measurement is lower incidence in the vaccine arm, although it is more likely that a secondary end-point will be levels of viremia and time to set-point.

The immune responses detected in monkeys as well as those detected in HEPS individuals and long-term non-progressors suggest that an effective HIV vaccine will need to elicit neutralizing antibodies, CD4+ T-cell responses and CTL.[56] As the major route of viral transmission is through mucosal barriers, it may be crucial to elicit mucosal vaccine-induced immunity rather than exclusively systemic immunity.[65] One feature of a vaccine-induced response is the elicitation of long-lived memory CD4 and CD8 T cells that can be rapidly recalled in the event of a subsequent exposure or infection with HIV-1. Studies in mice after infection with lymphocytic choriomeningitis virus has shown that CD8+ T cell first differentiate into rapidly dividing and short-lived effector T cells that possess strong CTL activity.[63] After a few weeks, a subset of these cells differentiate into long-lived central memory T cells, which show very little effector function, but proliferate readily after re-encounter with antigen. Extrapolating these studies to humans, the aim of an HIV vaccine response would be to generate pools of vaccine-specific long-lived central memory CD8+ T cells. As discussed above, the persistence of antigen upon HIV infection compromises the development of central memory CD8+ T cells, whereas the transient nature of vaccine-related antigens would create a more favorable environment for induction of central memory.

One of the main challenges of eliciting a relevant vaccine CD8+ T-cell response is matching TcR recognition of epitopes in the vaccine with circulating viral strains in different geographic regions where vaccines are most urgently required. One of the central concepts of HIV vaccine design is to elicit T-cell responses that recognize epitopes that exist in viruses that are transmitted between people. Genetic diversity of HIV-1 has been categorized into multiple clades and numerous circulating recombinant forms (CRF).[66] As a result, individuals infected in West Africa (where CRF02-AG is predominant) may respond to different epitopes that are not present in viral strains infecting individuals in Zimbabwe, China, or India (where subtype C is predominant). In addition to the challenges of viral genetic diversity is the polymorphic nature of HLA and this represents the genetic diversity of peoples in the world that would impact on the specificity of the T-cell response. Figure 4.3 schematically shows the interrelationship between HIV genetic diversity, HLA

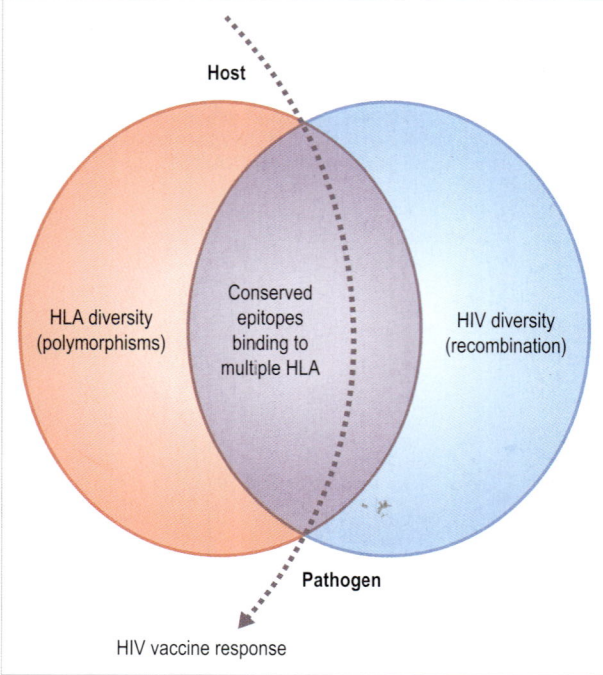

Figure 4.3 The interrelationship between host HLA diversity and HIV diversity. The identity of conserved epitopes that have the ability to bind to multiple HLA backgrounds is the ideal in generating vaccine-induced immunity that is relevant across different HIV-1 subtypes and HLA diversity.

Host

HLA diversity
(polymorphisms)

Conserved
epitopes
binding to
multiple HLA

HIV diversity
(recombination)

Pathogen

HIV vaccine response

diversity and vaccine-induced CTL responses. Where the epitopes converge between viral and human diversity is the point of a globally relevant vaccine response.

There is a multitude of vaccine candidates that are either in early clinical trials or in the pipeline of development (www.iavi.org, www.unaids.org, www.hvtn.org). The most promising candidates are attenuated live vectors containing HIV-1 genes. Such vectors include Sindbis, Adenovirus, Associated adenovirus, Venezuelan Equine Encephalitis Virus, as examples. These vectors have been attenuated so that no infection by the vector can take place after administering of the vaccine formulation. In addition to these vectors, a host of recombinant DNA constructs are available using HIV-1 genes from various clades (www.hvtn.org). It is envisioned that a prime-boost strategy be used where DNA vaccines are used to prime immunity[67] and the vector used to boost specific T-cell immune responses at a later time point, which will serve to focus CD8[+] T cells to recognize an array of epitopes. This heterologous prime-boost approach may cause enough antigen to be transiently processed and presented to T cells to elicit long-lived central memory cells.

Whatever the eventual mechanism of a successful vaccine, immunity will have to be evoked that covers the polymorphism of host genetic diversity, caters for the genetic heterogeneity of HIV-1 across the globe and is durable in its effect. Notwithstanding these challenging scientific issues, uniform access of a stable vaccine to all individuals at an affordable cost is a social and political challenge that needs to be addressed in tandem with scientific development.

Conclusion

HIV infection elicits robust cellular and humoral immune responses, but the vast majority of persons ultimately fail to control viremia and progress to AIDS. Although progress has been made in understanding the reasons for ultimate lack of control, there are critical gaps in our knowledge that need to be resolved to facilitate rational vaccine design, and to guide immunotherapeutic interventions. Among these are the critical ratios of humoral and cellular immune responses, the critical viral antigens to target, the means to induce broadly cross reactive protective immunity to the multiple strains currently fuelling the global epidemics, and vaccine vector systems that are able to elicit potent antiviral immune responses.

Nevertheless, there is reason for optimism. Emerging data suggest that HIV may not be infinitely mutable, but that there are predictable mutations that occur within given residues when they come under immune selection pressure. Whether this knowledge, which is obtainable but not currently fully available, can lead to the generation of a multivalent vaccine that would provide sufficient protection against circulating viruses, when administered with a yet to be identified potent vector, remains to be determined. In the meantime, HIV will remain the most significant infectious disease of our generation, and will continue to extract a disproportionate toll on those most marginalized and disenfranchised in each society.

References

1. van Panhuys N, Perret R, Prout M, et al. Effector lymphoid tissue and its crucial role in protective immunity. Trends Immunol 2005; 26:242–247.
2. Borghans JA, Beltman JB, De Boer RJ. MHC polymorphism under host-pathogen coevolution. Immunogenetics 2004; 55:732–739.
3. Melief CJ. Mini-review: Regulation of cytotoxic T lymphocyte responses by dendritic cells: peaceful coexistence of cross-priming and direct priming? Eur J Immunol 2003; 33:2645–2654.
4. Tough DF. Deciphering the relationship between central and effector memory CD8+ T cells. Trends Immunol 2003; 24:404–407.
5. Korber BTM, Brander C, Haynes BF, et al. HIV Molecular Immunology. Los Alamos, New Mexico: Los Alamos National Laboratory: Theoretical Biology and Biophysics; 2005.
6. Koup RA, Safrit JT, Cao Y, et al. Temporal association of cellular immune responses with the initial control of viremia in primary human immunodeficiency virus type 1 syndrome. J Virol 1994; 68:4650–4655.
7. Lyles CM, Dorrucci M, Vlahov D, et al. Longitudinal human immunodeficiency virus type 1 load in the Italian seroconversion study: correlates and temporal trends of virus load. J Infect Dis 1999; 180:1018–1024.
8. Picker LJ, Maino VC. The CD4(+) T cell response to HIV-1. Curr Opin Immunol 2000; 12:381–386.
9. Day CL, Walker BD. Progress in defining CD4 helper cell responses in chronic viral infections. J Exp Med 2003; 198:1773–1777.
10. Rosenberg ES, Billingsley JM, Caliendo AM, et al. Vigorous HIV-1-specific CD4+ T cell responses associated with control of viremia. Science 1997; 278:1447–1450.
11. Malhotra U, Berrey MM, Huang Y, et al. Effect of combination antiretroviral therapy on T-cell immunity in acute human immunodeficiency virus type 1 infection. J Infect Dis 2000; 181:121–131.
12. Oxenius A, Price DA, Easterbrook PJ, et al. Early highly active antiretroviral therapy for acute HIV-1 infection preserves immune function of CD8+ and CD4+ T lymphocytes. Proc Natl Acad Sci USA 2000; 97:3382–3387.
13. Veazey RS, Lackner AA. HIV swiftly guts the immune system. Nat Med 2005; 11:469–470.
14. Li Q, Duan L, Estes JD, et al. Peak SIV replication in resting memory CD4+ T cells depletes gut lamina propria CD4+ T cells. Nature 2005; 434:1148–1152.

15. Mattapallil JJ, Douek DC, Hill B, et al. Massive infection and loss of memory CD4+ T cells in multiple tissues during acute SIV infection. Nature 2005; 434:1093–1097.

16. Mehandru S, Poles MA, Tenner-Racz K, et al. Primary HIV-1 infection is associated with preferential depletion of CD4+ T lymphocytes from effector sites in the gastrointestinal tract. J Exp Med 2004; 200:761–770.

17. Schmitz JE, Kuroda MJ, Santra S, et al. Control of viremia in simian immunodeficiency virus infection by CD8+ lymphocytes. Science 1999; 283:857–860.

18. Jin X, Bauer DE, Tuttleton SE, et al. Dramatic rise in plasma viremia after CD8(+) T cell depletion in simian immunodeficiency virus-infected macaques. J Exp Med 1999; 189:991–998.

19. Borrow P, Lewicki H, Hahn BH, et al. Virus-specific CD8+ cytotoxic T-lymphocyte activity associated with control of viremia in primary human immunodeficiency virus type 1 infection. J Virol 1994; 68:6103–6110.

20. Tsubota H, Lord CI, Watkins DI, et al. A cytotoxic T lymphocyte inhibits acquired immunodeficiency syndrome virus replication in peripheral blood lymphocytes. J Exp Med 1989; 169:1421–1434.

21. Yang OO, Kalams SA, Rosenzweig M, et al. Efficient lysis of human immunodeficiency virus type 1-infected cells by cytotoxic T lymphocytes. J Virol 1996; 70:5799–5806.

22. Yang OO, Kalams SA, Trocha A, et al. Suppression of human immunodeficiency virus type 1 replication by CD8+ cells: evidence for HLA class I-restricted triggering of cytolytic and noncytolytic mechanisms. J Virol 1997; 71:3120–3128.

23. Van Baalen CA, Schutten M, Huisman RC, et al. Kinetics of antiviral activity by human immunodeficiency virus type 1-specific cytotoxic T lymphocytes (CTL) and rapid selection of CTL escape virus in vitro. J Virol 1998; 72:6851–6857.

24. Yang OO, Sarkis PT, Ali A, et al. Determinant of HIV-1 mutational escape from cytotoxic T lymphocytes. J Exp Med 2003; 197:1365–1375.

25. Cocchi F, DeVico AL, Garzino-Demo A, et al. Identification of RANTES, MIP-1 alpha, and MIP-1 beta as the major HIV-suppressive factors produced by CD8+ T cells. Science 1995; 270:1811–1815.

26. Geiben-Lynn R, Brown N, Walker BD, et al. Purification of a modified form of bovine antithrombin III as an HIV-1 CD8+ T-cell antiviral factor. J Biol Chem 2002; 277:42352–42357.

27. Zhang D, Shankar P, Xu Z, et al. Most antiviral CD8 T cells during chronic viral infection do not express high levels of perforin and are not directly cytotoxic. Blood 2003; 101:226–235.

28. Moore CB, John M, James IR, et al. Evidence of HIV-1 adaptation to HLA-restricted immune responses at a population level. Science 2002; 296:1439–1443.

29. Burton DR, Desrosiers RC, Doms RW, et al. HIV vaccine design and the neutralizing antibody problem. Nat Immunol 2004; 5:233–236.

30. Schmitz JE, Kuroda MJ, Santra S, et al. Effect of humoral immune responses on controlling viremia during primary infection of rhesus monkeys with simian immunodeficiency virus. J Virol 2003; 77:2165–2173.

31. Mascola JR, Stiegler G, VanCott TC, et al. Protection of macaques against vaginal transmission of a pathogenic HIV-1/SIV chimeric virus by passive infusion of neutralizing antibodies. Nat Med 2000; 6:207–210.

32. Richman DD, Wrin T, Little SJ, et al. Rapid evolution of the neutralizing antibody response to HIV type 1 infection. Proc Natl Acad Sci USA 2003; 100:4144–4149.

33. Wei X, Decker JM, Wang S, et al. Antibody neutralization and escape by HIV-1. Nature 2003; 422:307–312.

34. Bradney AP, Scheer S, Crawford JM, et al. Neutralization escape in human immunodeficiency virus type 1-infected long-term nonprogressors. J Infect Dis 1999; 179:1264–1267.

35. Montefiori DC, Altfeld M, Lee PK, et al. Viremia control despite escape from a rapid and potent autologous neutralizing antibody response after therapy cessation in an HIV-1-infected individual. J Immunol 2003; 170:3906–3914.

36. Yokomaku Y, Miura H, Tomiyama H, et al. Impaired processing and presentation of cytotoxic-T-lymphocyte (CTL) epitopes are major escape mechanisms from CTL immune pressure in human immunodeficiency virus type 1 infection. J Virol 2004; 78:1324–1332.

37. Kimura Y, Gushima T, Rawale S, et al. Escape mutations alter proteasome processing of major histocompatibility complex class I-restricted epitopes in persistent hepatitis C virus infection. J Virol 2005; 79:4870–4876.

38. Draenert R, Le Gall S, Pfafferott KJ, et al. Immune selection for altered antigen processing leads to cytotoxic T lymphocyte escape in chronic HIV-1 infection. J Exp Med 2004; 199:905–915.

39. Allen TM, Altfeld M, Yu XG, et al. Selection, transmission, and reversion of an antigen-processing cytotoxic T-lymphocyte escape mutation in human immunodeficiency virus type 1 infection. J Virol 2004; 78:7069–7078.

40. O'Connor DH, Allen TM, Vogel TU, et al. Acute phase cytotoxic T lymphocyte escape is a hallmark of simian immunodeficiency virus infection. Nat Med 2002; 8:493–499.

41. Kiepiela P, Leslie AJ, Honeyborne I, et al. Dominant influence of HLA-B in mediating the potential co-evolution of HIV and HLA. Nature 2004; 432:769–775.

42. Champagne P, Ogg GS, King AS, et al. Skewed maturation of memory HIV-specific CD8 T lymphocytes. Nature 2001; 410:106–111.

43. Migueles SA, Laborico AC, Shupert WL, et al. HIV-specific CD8+ T cell proliferation is coupled to perforin expression and is maintained in nonprogressors. Nat Immunol 2002; 3:1061–1068.

44. Appay V, Dunbar PR, Callan M, et al. Memory CD8+ T cells vary in differentiation phenotype in different persistent virus infections. Nat Med 2002; 8:379–385.

45. Wherry EJ, Blattman JN, Murali-Krishna K, et al. Viral persistence alters CD8 T-cell immunodominance and tissue distribution and results in distinct stages of functional impairment. J Virol 2003; 77:4911–4927.

46. Lichterfeld M, Kaufmann DE, Yu XG, et al. Loss of HIV-1-specific CD8+ T cell proliferation after acute HIV-1 infection and restoration by vaccine-induced HIV-1-specific CD4+ T cells. J Exp Med 2004; 200:701–712.

47. Boaz MJ, Waters A, Murad S, et al. Presence of HIV-1 Gag-specific IFN-gamma+IL-2+ and CD28+IL-2+ CD4 T cell responses is associated with nonprogression in HIV-1 infection. J Immunol 2002; 169:6376–6385.

48. Iyasere C, Tilton JC, Johnson AJ, et al. Diminished proliferation of human immunodeficiency virus-specific CD4+ T cells is associated with diminished interleukin-2 (IL-2) production and is recovered by exogenous IL-2. J Virol 2003; 77:10900–10909.

49. Harari A, Petitpierre S, Vallelian F, et al. Skewed representation of functionally distinct populations of virus-specific CD4 T cells in HIV-1-infected subjects with progressive disease: changes after antiretroviral therapy. Blood 2004; 103:966–972.

50. Boritz E, Palmer BE, Wilson CC. Human immunodeficiency virus type 1 (HIV-1)-specific CD4+ T cells that proliferate in vitro detected in samples from most viremic subjects and inversely associated with plasma HIV-1 levels. J Virol 2004; 78:12638–12646.

51. Cochrane A, Imlach S, Leen C, et al. High levels of human immunodeficiency virus infection of CD8 lymphocytes expressing CD4 in vivo. J Virol 2004; 78:9862–9871.

52. Zloza A, Sullivan YB, Connick E, et al. CD8+ T cells that express CD4 on their surface (CD4dimCD8bright T cells) recognize an antigen-specific target, are detected in vivo, and can be productively infected by T-tropic HIV. Blood 2003; 102:2156–2164.

53. Lu W, Wu X, Lu Y, et al. Therapeutic dendritic-cell vaccine for simian AIDS. Nat Med 2003; 9:27–32.

54. Arrighi JF, Pion M, Garcia E, et al. DC-SIGN-mediated infectious synapse formation enhances X4 HIV-1

transmission from dendritic cells to T cells. J Exp Med 2004; 200:1279–1288

55. Gray CM, Lawrence J, Ranheim EA, et al. Highly active antiretroviral therapy results in HIV type 1 suppression in lymph nodes, increased pools of naive T cells, decreased pools of activated T cells, and diminished frequencies of peripheral activated HIV type 1-specific CD8+ T cells. AIDS Res Hum Retroviruses 2000; 16:1357–1369.

56. Kaufmann SH, McMichael AJ. Annulling a dangerous liaison: vaccination strategies against AIDS and tuberculosis. Nat Med 2005; 11:33–44.

57. Kulkarni PS, Butera ST, Duerr AC. Resistance to HIV-1 infection: lessons learned from studies of highly exposed persistently seronegative (HEPS) individuals. AIDS Rev 2003; 5:87–103.

58. Day JH, Grant AD, Fielding KL, et al. Does tuberculosis increase HIV load? J Infect Dis 2004; 190:1677–1684.

59. Corbett EL, Charalambous S, Moloi VM, et al. Human immunodeficiency virus and the prevalence of undiagnosed tuberculosis in African gold miners. Am J Respir Crit Care Med 2004; 170:673–679.

60. Kaul R, Plummer F, Clerici M, et al. Mucosal IgA in exposed, uninfected subjects: evidence for a role in protection against HIV infection. AIDS 2001; 15:431–432.

61. Zhang C, Cui Y, Houston S, et al. Protective immunity to HIV-1 in SCID/beige mice reconstituted with peripheral blood lymphocytes of exposed but uninfected individuals. Proc Natl Acad Sci USA 1996; 93:14720–14725.

62. O'Brien SJ, Nelson GW. Human genes that limit AIDS. Nat Genet 2004; 36:565–574.

63. Berzofsky JA, Ahlers JD, Janik J, et al. Progress on new vaccine strategies against chronic viral infections. J Clin Invest 2004; 114:450–462.

64. Garber DA, Silvestri G, Feinberg MB. Prospects for an AIDS vaccine: three big questions, no easy answers. Lancet Infect Dis 2004; 4:397–413.

65. Belyakov IM, Berzofsky JA. Immunobiology of mucosal HIV infection and the basis for development of a new generation of mucosal AIDS vaccines. Immunity 2004; 20:247–253.

66. McCutchan FE, Sankale JL, M'Boup S, et al. HIV type 1 circulating recombinant form CRF09_cpx from west Africa combines subtypes A, F, G, and may share ancestors with CRF02_AG and Z321. AIDS Res Hum Retroviruses 2004; 20:819–826.

67. McMichael AJ, Hanke T. HIV vaccines 1983–2003. Nat Med 2003; 9:874–880.

CHAPTER 5

Viral and Host Determinants of HIV-1 Disease Progression

Hanneke Schuitemaker
Angélique B. van't Wout

Introduction

The clinical course of HIV-1 infection can be highly variable, with extremes of disease progression within 12 months after seroconversion or continuous asymptomatic infection for more than 20 years. The loss of CD4[+] T cells is one of the hallmarks of HIV-1 infection and ultimately leads to immunodeficiency. The mechanism by which CD4[+] T cells are lost is still under debate but a component of direct virus mediated killing as well as virus driven chronic immune activation and increased cell turnover is now well accepted. For both mechanisms, HIV-1 load seems to be the driving force. The high variability in the clinical course of HIV-1 infection is therefore determined by the HIV-1 load, which itself is determined by the interplay between viral and host (genetic) factors. In this chapter, we will discuss these factors and their effect on HIV-1 load and disease progression.

Specific (Adaptive) Antiviral Immune Response

Humoral Immune Response

Upon infection with HIV-1, both cellular and humoral immune responses are mounted against the virus. The humoral immune response initially consists mainly of binding antibodies. Only after a few weeks or months, neutralizing antibodies emerge.[1,2] The importance of neutralizing antibodies in controlling infection was shown in SIV infected macaques by B-cell depletion.[3,4] More recently, passive transfer of three broadly neutralizing antibodies resulted in a delay in viral rebound after cessation of antiretroviral therapy in acutely HIV-1 infected individuals.[5] HIV-1 can escape from these neutralizing antibodies using a neutralization resistant phenotype which is associated with changes in the viral envelope. The existence of this escape mechanism was demonstrated in macaques[6] and in a laboratory worker who accidentally got infected with the neutralization sensitive HIV-1 variant IIIB and in whom a neutralization resistant IIIB related variant evolved.[7] A major component of the viral escape mechanism is the repositioning of glycans, the so-called glycan shield. Glycans are strategically positioned and repositioned continuously throughout infection, in a way that affects minimally the interaction of the envelope with the receptor molecules on the cell surface, but hinders maximally the binding of neutralizing antibodies.[2] The neutralizing antibody response is still important however, as escape from humoral immunity is thought to coincide with a loss of viral fitness.[8] This implies that although the humoral immune response may be ineffective due to viral escape, the net effect is a less fit virus, which will give rise to a lower viral load set-point and hence an ameliorated disease course. Recent studies have suggested that early after heterosexual transmission of subtype B virus, the neutralization resistance of HIV-1 may be reduced.[9] This observation would be in line with the hypothesis that in the absence of neutralizing antibodies, rapidly replicating neutralization sensitive variants may be selected. However, after homosexual transmission of subtype B variants this phenomenon was not observed,[10] and also not in heterosexual or vertical transmission of different subtypes.[11] The idea that in the absence of neutralizing antibodies more fit HIV-1 variants are selected is also supported by the observation that late in infection, when HIV-1 specific immunity deteriorates and neutralizing antibodies are declining, HIV-1 load increases reflecting the selection of a more fit viral quasispecies that may be neutralization sensitive again.

Cellular Immune Response: Cytotoxic T Lymphocytes

HIV-1 specific cellular immune responses emerge very rapidly after infection, both in the form of cytotoxic and helper T lymphocytes.[12-14] Several observations indicate that HIV-1 specific CD8[+] cytotoxic T cells (CTLs) contribute to the control of HIV infection. Strong CTL responses are often observed in long term asymptomatic HIV-1 infected individuals but diminish with progression to AIDS.[15] Experimental depletion of CD8[+] T cells in SIV-infected macaques lead to the loss of control of acute infection and to increased viral load in chronic infection.[16,17] The loss of HIV-specific CTL responses with progression of disease was first considered to be due to an actual physical depletion. However, the use of tetrameric human leukocyte antigen (HLA)-peptide complexes in combination with functional assays showed that the loss is merely due to impaired functionality.[18] This loss may be due to the absence of antigenic re-stimulation as a result of disappearance of the epitope as a consequence of viral escape. Escape in even a single epitope may lead to loss of immune control by CTL.[19] Viruses with CTL escape mutations can rapidly overtake the population, in as little as 6 weeks after first emergence.[20] Certain CTL escape mutations have an impact on viral fitness, as is demonstrated by complete reversal of the escape mutation to wild type sequences upon transmission to a new individual.[21] The selective pressure of CTL is such that at a population level, the virus strains circulating in a population have adapted to the most common HLA types in that population.[22] This also results in a protective effect for people with rare HLA types. The complex influence of HLA on HIV-1 disease course will be discussed later in the section on host polymorphisms. Mutations outside CTL epitopes have also been described to influence CTL function, by affecting antigen processing and presentation.[23]

Cellular Immune Response: Helper T Lymphocytes

HIV-1 specific CTL function depends on the presence of functional CD4[+] helper T cells. The presence of CD4[+] helper T cells that proliferate and produce both IL-2 and IFN-γ in response to HIV specific peptide pools early in infection are not predictive for prolonged AIDS free survival.[24] However, the loss of these helper T cells in the course of HIV-1 infection precedes disease progression, suggesting that CD4[+] T cell help may be instrumental in the maintenance of a good CTL response. It was recently demonstrated in mouse models that the presence of CD4[+] T cells during priming of CTLs is essential for the maintenance of memory after the acute infection phase whereas their continuous presence was not required.[25,26] It can thus be envisioned that with the loss of CD4[+] T cells during HIV-1 infection no efficient new CD8[+] T-cell memory is being generated in later phases of the infection.

Mechanisms of CD4 T-cell Loss

Depletion of CD4[+] T cells, which is preceded by a loss of proliferative responses to polyclonal stimuli[27] and recall antigens,[28] is one of the major characteristics of HIV-1 infection.[29] The fact that HIV-1 uses CD4 as a cellular entry receptor together with the observation that CD4[+] T cells are specifically lost in HIV-1 infection led to the logical conclusion that virus-mediated killing of target cells was the main cause for this cell loss. However, the frequency of infected cells in peripheral blood in the chronic phase of infection is too low to account for the ongoing depletion by viral infection.[30,31] Several converging lines of evidence now suggest that hyper-activation of the immune system in response to chronic HIV-1 infection may be the culprit.[32] Hyperactivation is responsible for an increased naive T-cell turnover, leading ultimately to the exhaustion of the naive T-cell compartment, which then cannot compensate for the enhanced death of memory CD4[+] T cells into which the activated CD4[+] T cells mature. Indeed, the level of immune activation was found to be as good, or perhaps even better, a predictor of disease progression than the level of viral replication.[33,34] Additional evidence came from the comparison of SIV infection in Sooty Mangabeys and African Green Monkeys on the one hand and in Asian Macaque species on the other.[35] SIV infection in Asian Macaques generally leads to high virus loads, declining CD4[+] T-cell numbers and disease within 2 years.[36] Sooty Mangabeys and African Green Monkeys can both be infected with SIV and despite overt viral replication these animals have stable CD4 counts and do not progress to disease.[37,38] The stable CD4 counts in the presence of high viral load is in line with the assumption that virus mediated killing has no large effect on total CD4+ T-cell numbers. Despite the high viral load, these animals show no evidence for the hyperactivation of their immune system as observed in SIV infected macaques and HIV-1 infected humans.[38] This implies that although the increased turnover of naive T cells in HIV-1 infected individuals is virus driven, the responsiveness is determined by host factors.

CD4 Depletion in the Gut

In both the SIV macaque model and in HIV-1 infected humans it was demonstrated that already during the phase of primary infection a massive depletion of CD4+ T cells occurs in all tissues, including the gut associated lymphoid tissues (GALT) where more than 80% of T cells reside.[39–42] Although this process occurred within days, the depletion of lymphocytes from the GALT seems to be irreversible.[43] More recently, it was shown that infection and depletion in the acute phase was not restricted to activated memory cells as also a high frequency of infected resting CD4+ T cells could be demonstrated.[44,45] The unique capacity of HIV-1 to replicate in non-dividing cells is in agreement with this observation.[46]

Viral Factors that Influence Viral Load: Biological Phenotype

HIV-1 can vary with respect to biological properties such as replication rate, cell tropism, and neutralization sensitivity. Virus variants with different biological properties dominate in different phases of infection. New infections are generally established by macrophage-tropic HIV-1 variants,[47] which in addition to CD4 use CCR5 as a co-receptor (R5 variants).[48] The early asymptomatic phase is dominated by slowly replicating macrophage-tropic R5 HIV-1 variants.[49] With progression of disease, a shift in the viral quasispecies towards more rapidly replicating T-cell-tropic R5 variants is observed. In about 50% of HIV-1 infected individuals this is associated with the appearance of HIV-1 variants that use CXCR4 as a co-receptor (X4 variants).[50] X4 variants

are associated with an accelerated CD4 T-cell decline and a more rapid disease progression.[51,52] The accelerated loss of CD4+ T cells after appearance of X4 variants can be explained from fact that naive T cells express CXCR4 but not CCR5, while memory cells express both CXCR4 and CCR5.[53] This co-receptor expression pattern makes naive T cells a unique target cell population for X4 variants. Indeed, X4 biological clones were predominantly isolated from naive T cells, whereas both R5 and X4 biological virus clones could be obtained from the memory T cells from the same individuals.[54] It can be envisaged that infection and subsequent virus mediated killing of naive T cells by X4 virus variants directly interferes with T-cell ontogeny as the infected and killed naive T cell will no longer give rise to a daughter cell population.

Evolution of Co-receptor Use

Phylogenetic analyses of HIV-1 envelope sequences have shown that X4 variants directly evolve from R5 variants.[55,56] After the first appearance of X4 variants, both R5 and X4 variants continuously evolve away from the common ancestor and each other. However, this is only evident for the *Env* gene as X4 and R5 virus populations cannot be distinguished on the basis of *Gag* sequences due to frequent recombination events outside the *Env* gene.[57] X4 variants evolve from R5 variants and subsequently, the X4 and R5 viruses co-exist within the same individual. The continued evolution of X4 and R5 variants is also evident from changes in their biological properties over time. Early X4 variants are more sensitive to the inhibitory effect of co-receptor antagonists AMD3100 and T22 than late-stage obtained X4 variants.[58] In analogy, late stage R5 variants from individuals who never developed X4 variants are less sensitive to the inhibition by the natural ligand of CCR5, RANTES,[59] and small-molecule R5 inhibitors.[60] The co-receptor inhibitor resistance of R5 and X4 variants is correlated with the immune status of the host. Although the exact mechanism of resistance remains to be established, the observation is suggestive for selection of HIV-1 variants that use their co-receptor with increasing efficiency as the infection progresses. The fact that this evolution is seen in all study subjects suggests that these high efficiency variants are not transmitted or at least that they do not have an advantage in a newly infected individual. Each infection starts with viral quasispecies that may use its co-receptor less efficiently, but that apparently has other fitness advantage(s) in the new and immuno-competent host.

Viral Accessory Genes

The HIV-1 genome encodes for three structural proteins (Gag, Pol and Env) and six accessory proteins: Vpr, Vpu, Tat, Rev, Nef and Vif. Tat is the transcriptional activator of HIV-1, while Rev functions to shuttle the viral RNAs from the nucleus to the cytoplasm for translation and packaging. Initially, the function of the four other accessory genes was not clear and some were even thought to be dispensable for virus replication based on *in vitro* experiments in permissive cell lines. However, more recent studies *in vitro,* in animal models, and in HIV-1 infected humans have elucidated some of the accessory gene functions, while at the same time providing novel insights into the interactions between the virus and host cell factors that are crucial for virus replication.

Nef

In the SIV macaque model it was demonstrated that inoculation with SIV that lacked the *Nef* gene resulted in infection but not disease progression.[61] Interestingly, animals inoculated with ΔNef viruses were protected against a subsequent SIV challenge.[62] A cohort of individuals in Sydney infected with HIV-1 from the same source and classified as long-term non-progressors, all carried a ΔNef HIV-1 variant.[63] At least three groups of Nef activities are known, which are mostly genetically separable and make use of distinct elements located throughout the Nef molecule.[64] First, Nef is known to deregulate signaling pathways. Second, Nef affects the intracellular trafficking of a number of proteins, including CD4, MHC-I and MHC-II, CD28, DC-SIGN, TNF and HIV-1 Env glycoproteins. Last, Nef has been shown to increase virus infectivity and replication, specifically in primary lymphocytes. Thus, Nef supports viral replication via both direct and indirect mechanisms. While Nef seems to impair antigen-dependent activation of CD4 helper T cells by antigen presenting cells, it simultaneously induces a transcriptional program resembling anti-CD3 T-cell activation.[65] Furthermore, Nef might render CD4[+] T cells more prone to activation by inducing NFAT, NFκB and AP-1 transcription factors.[66] Thus, Nef modulates the function of T-cell cells and APC to uncouple T-cell activation and create an ideal environment for efficient viral propagation, while escaping the specific antiviral immune response. It is also noteworthy that different Nef domains and functions are modulated during disease progression.[67,68]

Vif

The function of the *Vif* gene was established more recently. Vif can counteract the effects of APOBEC3F and APOBEC3G, mediators of a novel mechanism of innate immunity, a potent cellular defense system against retroviral infection.[69,70] APOBEC3F and APOBEC3G are members of the APOBEC superfamily of cytosine deaminases which, in the absence of Vif, are incorporated into the virion by interaction with the viral Gag nucleocapsid protein.[71] During reverse transcription of the viral genome in a new cell, they deaminate cytidine to uracil in newly synthesized minus-strand viral DNA, inducing lethal G-to-A hypermutation in the plus-strand viral DNA.[72,73] Vif can bind both APOBEC3F and APOBEC3G and redirect it by ubiquitination to degradation in the proteasome, thereby preventing incorporation in the virion and protection of the viral DNA from mutation.[74-76] Certain long term non progressors have been identified with HIV-1 variants that lacked a functional *Vif* gene,[77-79] indicating that under these circumstances APOBEC3G may indeed provide the host with an effective defense mechanism. Recent data suggests that APOBEC3G is primarily active in resting T cells and monocytes (but not activated T cells and macrophages), possibly explaining the HIV-1 resistant phenotype of these cells.[80] Polymorphisms in APOBEC3G have also been demonstrated. However, none of the polymorphisms was associated with an altered clinical course of infection in the French Genetics of Resistance to Immunodeficiency Virus (GRIV) cohort.[81] As suggested by the authors, it will be of interest to investigate the other cellular proteins, such as Cullin-5 or Rbx-1, that participate with Vif in APOBEC3G ubiquitination and proteolysis.

Vpr

The viral protein R is reported to have at least two distinct functions.[82] First, Vpr has been shown to interact with host factors involved in cell cycling leading to the G2 arrest observed in infected cells and resulting in higher levels of virus production.[83] Second, Vpr also has a nuclear localization signal and has been proposed to facilitate nuclear localization of the viral pre-integration complex.[84] Monkeys infected with SIV without Vpr function had severely attenuated infections with much lower viral burden and no evidence of disease progression[85] and HIV-1 with a truncated Vpr quickly reverted to wild type in both human and chimpanzee,[86] confirming the role of Vpr in viral pathogenesis. No polymorphisms in the host factors with which Vpr interacts have yet been reported to influence HIV-1 infection.

Vpu

Two distinct functions have been associated with the viral protein U (Vpu), which are associated with distinct functional domains and occur in separate subcellular locations. Vpu interacts with CD4 within the endoplasmic reticulum of infected cells, where it targets CD4 for degradation through interactions with the WD domain protein h-βTrCP.[87] Vpu is also known to enhance HIV-1 particle assembly through an as-yet-undefined mechanism. Curiously, the effect of Vpu on particle release is cell-type-dependent, occurring in most human cells, but not in simian cells. By using human-simian cell heterokaryons, it was shown that inhibition of assembly in human cells is dominant. Vpu overcomes this block to assembly in human cells and in human-simian heterokaryons.[88] The precise mechanism has not been established, but it was speculated that the inhibitor of assembly present in restrictive cells blocks the normal trafficking of Gag through vesicular sorting pathways, and that Vpu releases this block to allow Gag to proceed along this pathway. Vpu is necessary for efficient virus replication on *ex vivo* lymphoid tissue[89] and for pathogenicity in infected macaques.[90]

Host Factors that Influence Viral Load

Several host factors have been identified that directly affect HIV-1 load *in vivo* and consequently the clinical course of infection. The best studied host factors are the major histocompatibility complex and polymorphisms in HIV-1 co-receptors. However, mediators of innate immunity, such as NK-cell receptors and Toll-like receptors and their ligands, and the cellular counterparts of viral proteins are receiving increasing scrutiny. Several host factors associated with resistance to viral entry and replication have been associated with disease progression, with additional factors continuing to be identified.

Human Leukocyte Antigens

Class I alleles from the major histocompatibility complex (MHC) bind viral antigens that are being presented to CTLs. The repertoire of peptides that can be presented depends on the variability of the MHC complex within an individual. Indeed, homozygosity for HLA alleles within an individual has been associated with rapid disease progression.[91-93] For specific groups of class I alleles a profound effect on the outcome of HIV-1 infection has been demonstrated. In multiple studies, HLA-B*27 and *57 have been consistently associated with a favorable prognosis. Both HLA-B*27 and *57 present highly conserved HIV-1 epitopes which may account for the epidemiological association between these HLA types and disease course.[94,95] Viral escape from *HLA-B*27 and *57 restricted CTL by mutations in conserved regions may occur at a high fitness cost, which is supported by the observation that some HLA-B*57 epitopes immediately reverted to wild type sequences upon transmission to a non HLA-B*57 individual.[21] Reduced viral replication of attenuated virus variants will result in lower viral load and delayed disease progression. At the other extreme, *HLA-B*35, and *HLA-B*53 have been associated with an unfavorable prognosis,[91,96-100] but for this association the mechanism is not known. No associations between *HLA-A* or *HLA-C* alleles and disease control have been convincingly documented. Overall, the effect of the HLA-B allele on shaping of the HIV-1 quasispecies and viral load was the strongest.[101] The other interactions between HLA and natural killer cells will be discussed later in the section on natural killer cell receptors.

Chemokine Receptors and Ligands

Two chemokine receptor/ligand families have been found to be most prominent in HIV-1 infection and considerable attention has been given to genetic variation in both ligands and receptors.[102] Members of the C-C chemokine receptor (CCR) family, such as CCR2 and CCR5, are bound by CC-motif chemokine ligands (CCLs), including RANTES, macrophage inflammatory protein (MIP)-1a, MIP-1β, monocyte chemotactic proteins, and others. Members of the C-X-C receptor (CXCR) family, such as CXCR4, are bound by ligands such as CXCL12, which encodes stromal cell-derived factor-1 (SDF-1). The important role of these molecules in HIV-1 infection was recognized more clearly when cells from uninfected persons capable of suppressing replication of macrophage-tropic HIV-1 were found to have increased production levels of RANTES, MIP-1a, and MIP-1β.[103] These chemokines are thought to compete with HIV-1 for its principal co-receptor CCR5 or, less directly, to interfere with replication by down-modulation of co-receptor expression.

CCR5

Variations in both promoter and coding regions of CCR5 have been found to alter the susceptibility for HIV-1/AIDS. Homozygosity for a 32-bp deletion (Δ32) in CCR5 has been associated with almost complete protection from infection,[104] although infection with X4 variants that do not require CCR5 for entry has been reported for several CCR5 Δ32 homozygous individuals.[105] Heterozygosity for the deletion usually confers modest protection against disease progression. The carrier frequency of Δ32 CCR5 is 15–18%, among Caucasians, but the frequencies in other major racial groups are negligible.[106,107] Interestingly, this protection is observed both in individuals harboring only R5 variants and in those also harboring X4 variants.[108] In the latter individuals, the protection is most likely explained by the effect on the co-existing R5 virus populations.

SNPs distributed along the CCR5 promoter sequence appear to be involved in the acquisition of HIV-1 infection and progression to disease. One important set of SNPs has been found in a composite haplotype called 'P1'[109] and in a single subgroup of these SNPs, designated human haplotype E (HHE).[107,100,110,111] In Caucasians, homozygosity for this HHE genotype has been associated with both increased likelihood and an accelerated course of infection.[110] Homozygosity for a haplotype designated 'HHD',[107] which is found more commonly in ethnic African individuals, has been reported to be associated with more rapid progression.[112]

CCR2

Heterozygosity for a valine-to-isoleucine (I) mutation at position 64 in the coding region of CCR2 has been associated with delayed disease progression in HIV-1 infected individuals,[111,113-117] although racial differences have been observed.[100,107,113] The protective effect was even stronger in combination with the CCR5 ?32 allele.[111,114] The delay in disease progression was more pronounced when only R5 variants were present and was not observed after conversion to X4 in CCR2-64I/+ persons. In CCR2-64I/+ subjects, a higher conversion rate to and a higher prevalence of X4 HIV-1 was observed.[117] These findings suggest that the mechanism of action of the CCR2 polymorphism is mediated via R5 HIV-1 variants.

CX3CR1

A deleterious genetic influence of the CX3CR1 M280 genotype on HIV-1 disease progression was reported in the French SEROCO cohort.[118] However, other cohort studies provided no conclusive evidence for an association between this polymorphism in CX3CR1 and the clinical course of HIV-1 infection or virus phenotype evolution.[119-121] Possible explanations for the discrepancy include differences in cohort composition with regards to gender or risk category and the depletion of the rapidly progressing individuals homozygous for the M280 allele among seroprevalent patients.[122] To conclude that this genetic polymorphism indeed influences the clinical course of infection in general, meta-analysis studies are required, as have been performed for several of the other polymorphisms described in this chapter.[114]

CCL5

Recent work suggests that polymorphisms in CCL5, the gene encoding RANTES, alter susceptibility to HIV-1/AIDS.[123,124] Variations at 2 promoter SNPs (at -403 and -28) and at two other downstream sites form haplotypes that differentially modulate RANTES expression and its interference with virus replication. Two haplotypes marked by -403A and -28C or by one of the other shared SNPs have shown some but not complete consistency in their disadvantage to exposed uninfected individuals, as well as to infected individuals.[125,126] Conversely, the -28G variant, which is found much more frequently in Asian individuals, had no effect on susceptibility but was associated with delayed disease progression in HIV-1 infected Japanese populations.[123]

CCL3L1

More recently, the influence of segmental duplications in the CCL3L1 gene, which encodes for the natural ligand of the HIV-1 co-receptor CCR5 (MIP1-alphaP), on HIV-1/AIDS susceptibility was reported. The effect of the number of gene duplications on HIV-1 susceptibility depended on how many copies a person had compared to others of the same ancestry.[127] Individuals with low copy numbers of the gene, relative to their ethnic background, were associated with markedly enhanced HIV-1/AIDS susceptibility. These findings define an important new genetic determinant of HIV-1 susceptibility and further emphasize the importance of the chemokine system, either as elements that inhibit HIV-1 infection or that modulate antiviral immune responses.

CXCL12

Studies of the CXCL12 gene, encoding SDF-1, have focused on a variant 3'A at position 801 in the untranslated region of CXCL12. The effects of either homozygosity or heterozygosity on disease progression have been less consistent than those observed for the CCR and CCL polymorphisms.[114,128,129] Moreover, none of the studies have definitively implicated it as a predisposing or protective factor for susceptibility to infection.

Interleukins

A polymorphism at position -589 in the interleukin 4 (IL-4) promoter region has been described as being associated with both an increased and a delayed acquisition of X4 variants, but did not affect overall disease progression.[130,131] These discrepancies have not been resolved. Individuals carrying the interleukin 10 (IL-10) 5'-592A promoter allele are reported to be at increased risk for HIV-1 infection, and once infected they progress to AIDS more rapidly than homozygotes for the alternative 5'-592 C genotype, particularly in the later stages of HIV-1 infection. An estimated 25–30% of long term non progressors could be attributed to their IL-10 5'-592 C/C promoter genotype.[132]

NK Cell Receptors

Natural killer (NK) cells provide defense in the early stages of the innate immune response against viral infections by producing cytokines and causing cytotoxicity. The killer immunoglobulin-like receptors (KIRs) on NK cells regulate the inhibition and activation of NK-cell responses through recognition of HLA class I molecules on target cells. Associations between KIR epitope combinations expressed by HLA-B/-C haplotypes found in an HIV-1 infected study population may influence NK mediated immune responses.[133] The activating KIR allele KIR3DS1, in combination with HLA-B alleles that encode molecules with isoleucine at position 80 (HLA-B Bw4-80Ile), is associated with delayed progression to AIDS in individuals infected with HIV-1.[134] Interestingly, HLA-B Bw4-80Ile allele was not associated with any of the AIDS outcomes measured, while KIR3DS1 alone was significantly associated with more rapid progression to AIDS, suggesting an epistatic interaction between the two loci. Others reported an effect of the interaction between KIR3DL1 and HLA-B*57 supertype on disease progression.[135]

Toll-like Receptors and Ligands

Rapid immune response to invading microorganisms is facilitated by innate immunity receptor proteins, the Toll-like receptors (TLRs). TLRs are responsible for recognition of conserved pathogen-associated molecular patterns, such as those present in bacterial DNA, lipoglycans and lipoproteins. More recent studies have implicated the TLRs in species-specific dendritic cell (DC) recognition of single stranded RNA from HIV-1,[136] and their ligands modulate enhanced HIV-1-specific T-cell responses through DC interactions.[137] Polymorphisms in TLRs have been reported,[138,139] however, their correlation with HIV-1 disease outcome has not yet been assessed.

Host Cell Factors involved in Cellular Post-entry Restrictions of HIV-1 Replication

Early, post-entry restrictions to retrovirus infection can determine tropism at the species level. HIV-1 encounters a post-entry block in Old World monkeys, whereas SIV of macaques (SIVmac) is blocked in most New World monkey cells. This block occurs prior to or concurrent with reverse transcription in the cytoplasm of the host cell. The viral determinant of susceptibility to the block is the capsid protein and capsid-binding proteins, such as cyclophilin A (CYPA), can modify the degree of the restriction. A tripartite motif (TRIM) protein, TRIM5, was identified as the major factor in rhesus monkey cells restricting HIV-1 infection. Humans express a protein, TRIM5hu, that is 87% identical in amino acid sequence to the rhesus monkey protein, TRIM5rh. Even when expressed at comparable levels, TRIM5hu was less potent at suppressing HIV-1 and SIVmac infection than TRIM5rh. It is conceivable, however, that polymorphisms in TRIM5 itself and/or its expression levels vary among individuals. The host cell protein CYPA, which interacts with primate lentiviral capsid proteins, may also influence how restriction factors such as TRIM5 interact with capsid proteins, thereby dictating the degree of restriction. Other post-entry restriction factors include Murr1, a copper metabolism gene, which is thought to restrict HIV-1 growth in unstimulated $CD4^+$ T cells by inhibiting NFκB function.[140]

Conclusion

As is clear from the above, HIV-1 depends on host cell factors for its replication. In addition, HIV-1 needs to interfere with the innate and adaptive antiviral defenses of the host. In the past few years, a flurry of new papers has reported the identification of novel interactions between viral proteins and host cellular factors. Polymorphisms for several of these factors as described above have been identified and in some cases shown to be associated with disease progression. It is likely that the same will hold true for the other cellular counterparts, such as Murr1, TRIM5a and the as yet unidentified partner of Vpu. Both the identification of the cellular counterparts and the role of any polymorphisms will provide novel insights into HIV-1 replication and new targets for therapeutic intervention. The field of players in the complex battle between HIV-1 and its host is slowly being revealed.

References

1. Richman DD, Wrin T, Little SJ, et al. Rapid evolution of the neutralizing antibody response to HIV type 1 infection. Proc Natl Acad Sci USA 2003; 100:4144–4149.
2. Wei X, Decker JM, Wang S, et al. Antibody neutralization and escape by HIV-1. Nature 2003; 422:307–312.
3. Johnson WE, Lifson JD, Lang SM, et al. Importance of B-cell responses for immunological control of variant strains of simian immunodeficiency virus. J Virol 2003; 77:375–381.
4. Schmitz JE, Kuroda MJ, Santra S, et al. Effect of humoral immune responses on controlling viremia during primary infection of rhesus monkeys with simian immunodeficiency virus. J Virol 2003; 77:2165–2173.
5. Trkola A, Kuster H, Rusert P, et al. Delay of HIV-1 rebound after cessation of antiretroviral therapy through passive transfer of human neutralizing antibodies. Nat Med 2005; 11:615–622.
6. Chackerian B, Rudensey LM, Overbaugh J. Specific N-linked and O-linked glycosylation modifications in the envelope V1 domain of simian immunodeficiency virus variants that evolve in the host alter recognition by neutralizing antibodies. J Virol 1997; 71:7719–7727.
7. Beaumont T, van Nuenen A, Broersen S, et al. Reversal of human immunodeficiency virus type 1 IIIB to a neutralization-resistant phenotype in an accidentally infected laboratory worker with a progressive clinical course. J Virol 2001; 75:2246–2252.
8. Moore JP, Ho DD. HIV-1 neutralization: the consequences of viral adaptation to growth on transformed T cells. AIDS 1995; 9:S117–S136.
9. Derdeyn CA, Decker JM, Bibollet-Ruche F, et al. Envelope-constrained neutralization-sensitive HIV-1 after heterosexual transmission. Science 2004; 303:2019–2022.
10. Frost SD, Liu Y, Pond SL, et al. Characterization of human immunodeficiency virus type 1 (HIV-1) envelope variation and neutralizing antibody responses during transmission of HIV-1 subtype B. J Virol 2005; 79:6523–6527.
11. Chohan B, Lang D, Sagar M, et al. Selection for human immunodeficiency virus type 1 envelope glycosylation variants with shorter V1-V2 loop sequences occurs during transmission of certain genetic subtypes and may impact viral RNA levels. J Virol 2005; 79:6528–6531.
12. Borrow P, Lewicki H, Hahn BH, et al. Virus-specific CD8+ cytotoxic T-lymphocyte activity associated with control of viremia in primary human immunodeficiency virus type 1 infection. J Virol 1994; 68:6103–6110.
13. Harari A, Rizzardi GP, Ellefsen K, et al. Analysis of HIV-1- and CMV-specific memory CD4 T-cell responses during primary and chronic infection. Blood 2002; 100:1381–1387.
14. Koup RA, Safrit JT, Cao Y, et al. Temporal association of cellular immune responses with the initial control of viremia in primary human immunodeficiency virus type 1 syndrome. J Virol 1994; 68:4650–4655.
15. Klein MR, van Baalen CA, Holwerda AM, et al. Kinetics of Gag-specific cytotoxic T lymphocyte responses during the clinical course of HIV-1 infection: a longitudinal analysis of rapid progressors and long-term asymptomatics. J Exp Med 1995; 181:1365–1372.
16. Jin X, Bauer DE, Tuttleton SE, et al. Dramatic rise in plasma viremia after CD8(+) T cell depletion in simian immunodeficiency virus-infected macaques. J Exp Med 1999; 189:991–998.
17. Schmitz JE, Kuroda MJ, Santra S, et al. Control of viremia in simian immunodeficiency virus infection by CD8+ lymphocytes. Science 1999; 283:857–860.
18. Kostense S, Vandenberghe K, Joling J, et al. Persistent numbers of tetramer+ CD8(+) T cells, but loss of interferon-gamma+ HIV-specific T cells during progression to AIDS. Blood 2002; 99:2505–2511.
19. Goulder PJ, Phillips RE, Colbert RA, et al. Late escape from an immunodominant cytotoxic T-lymphocyte response associated with progression to AIDS. Nat Med 1997; 3:212–217.
20. Borrow P, Lewicki H, Wei X, et al. Antiviral pressure exerted by HIV-1-specific cytotoxic T lymphocytes (CTLs) during primary infection demonstrated by rapid selection of CTL escape virus. Nat Med 1997; 3:205–211.
21. Leslie AJ, Pfafferott KJ, Chetty P, et al. HIV evolution: CTL escape mutation and reversion after transmission. Nat Med 2004; 10:282–289.
22. Leslie A, Kavanagh D, Honeyborne I, et al. Transmission and accumulation of CTL escape variants drive negative associations between HIV polymorphisms and HLA. J Exp Med 2005; 201:891–902.
23. Allen TM, Altfeld M, Yu XG, et al. Selection, transmission, and reversion of an antigen-processing cytotoxic T-lymphocyte escape mutation in human immunodeficiency virus type 1 infection. J Virol 2004; 78:7069–7078.
24. Jansen CA, De Cuyper IM, Hooibrink B, et al. Functional HIV-1 specific CD4+ T-cell responses have no prognostic value for progression to AIDS: results from a large, prospective cohort study. Blood 2005; 107:1427–1433.
25. Janssen EM, Lemmens EE, Wolfe T, et al. CD4+ T cells are required for secondary expansion and memory in CD8+ T lymphocytes. Nature 2003; 421:852–856.
26. Sun JC, Williams MA, Bevan MJ. CD4+ T cells are required for the maintenance, not programming, of memory CD8+ T cells after acute infection. Nat Immunol 2004; 5:927–933.
27. Meyaard L, Otto SA, Hooibrink B, et al. Quantitative analysis of CD4+ T cell function in the course of human immunodeficiency virus infection. Gradual decline of both naive and memory alloreactive T cells. J Clin Invest 1994; 94:1947–1952.
28. Wahren B, Morfeldt-Mansson L, Biberfeld G, et al. Characteristics of the specific cell-mediated immune response in human immunodeficiency virus infection. J Virol 1987; 61:2017–2023.
29. Lane HC, Depper JM, Greene WC, et al. Qualitative analysis of immune function in patients with the acquired immunodeficiency syndrome. Evidence for a selective defect in soluble antigen recognition. N Engl J Med 1985; 313:79–84.
30. Douek DC, Brenchley JM, Betts MR, et al. HIV preferentially infects HIV-specific CD4+ T cells. Nature 2002; 417:95–98.
31. Haase AT. Population biology of HIV-1 infection: viral and CD4+ T cell demographics and dynamics in lymphatic tissues. Annu Rev Immunol 1999; 17:625–656.
32. Silvestri G, Feinberg MB. Turnover of lymphocytes and conceptual paradigms in HIV infection. J Clin Invest 2003; 112:821–824.
33. Giorgi JV, Hultin LE, McKeating JA, et al. Shorter survival in advanced human immunodeficiency virus type 1 infection is more closely associated with T lymphocyte activation than with plasma virus burden or virus chemokine coreceptor usage. J Infect Dis 1999; 179:859–870.

34. Hazenberg MD, Otto SA, van Benthem BH, et al. Persistent immune activation in HIV-1 infection is associated with progression to AIDS. AIDS 2003; 17:1881–1888.

35. Silvestri G, Fedanov A, Germon S, et al. Divergent host responses during primary simian immunodeficiency virus SIVsm infection of natural sooty mangabey and nonnatural rhesus macaque hosts. J Virol 2005; 79:4043–4054.

36. Hirsch VM, Fuerst TR, Sutter G, et al. Patterns of viral replication correlate with outcome in simian immunodeficiency virus (SIV)-infected macaques: effect of prior immunization with a trivalent SIV vaccine in modified vaccinia virus prior immunization with a trivalent SIV vaccine in modified vaccinia virus Ankara. J Virol 1996; 70:3741–3752.

37. Broussard SR, Staprans SI, White R, et al. Simian immunodeficiency virus replicates to high levels in naturally infected African green monkeys without inducing immunologic or neurologic disease. J Virol 2001; 75:2262–2275.

38. Silvestri G, Sodora DL, Koup RA, et al. Nonpathogenic SIV infection of sooty mangabeys is characterized by limited bystander immunopathology despite chronic high-level viremia. Immunity 2003; 18:441–452.

39. Brenchley JM, Schacker TW, Ruff LE, et al. CD4+ T cell depletion during all stages of HIV disease occurs predominantly in the gastrointestinal tract. J Exp Med 2004; 200:749–759.

40. Mehandru S, Poles MA, Tenner-Racz K, et al. Primary HIV-1 infection is associated with preferential depletion of CD4+ T lymphocytes from effector sites in the gastrointestinal tract. J Exp Med 2004; 200:761–770.

41. Schneider T, Jahn HU, Schmidt W, et al. Loss of CD4 T lymphocytes in patients infected with human immunodeficiency virus type 1 is more pronounced in the duodenal mucosa than in the peripheral blood. Berl Diarrhea/Wasting Syndr Study Group Gut 1995; 37:524–529.

42. Veazey RS, DeMaria M, Chalifoux LV, et al. Gastrointestinal tract as a major site of CD4+ T cell depletion and viral replication in SIV infection. Science 1998; 280:427–431.

43. Guadalupe M, Reay E, Sankaran S, et al. Severe CD4+ T-cell depletion in gut lymphoid tissue during primary human immunodeficiency virus type 1 infection and substantial delay in restoration following highly active antiretroviral therapy. J Virol 2003; 77:11708–11717.

44. Li Q, Duan L, Estes JD, et al. Peak SIV replication in resting memory CD4+ T cells depletes gut lamina propria CD4+ T cells. Nature 2005; 434:1148–1152.

45. Mattapallil JJ, Douek DC, Hill B, et al. Massive infection and loss of memory CD4+ T cells in multiple tissues during acute SIV infection. Nature 2005; 434:1093–1097.

46. Unutmaz D, KewalRamani VN, Marmon S, et al. Cytokine signals are sufficient for HIV-1 infection of resting human T lymphocytes. J Exp Med 1999; 189:1735–1746.

47. van 't Wout AB, Kootstra NA, Mulder-Kampinga GA, et al. Macrophage-tropic variants initiate human immunodeficiency virus type 1 infection after sexual, parenteral, and vertical transmission. J Clin Invest 1994; 94:2060–2067.

48. Berger EA, Doms RW, Fenyo EM. A new classification for HIV-1. Nature 1998; 391:240.

49. Schuitemaker H, Koot M, Kootstra NA, et al. Biological phenotype of human immunodeficiency virus type 1 clones at different stages of infection: progression of disease is associated with a shift from monocytotropic to T-cell-tropic virus population. J Virol 1992; 66:1354–1360.

50. Koot M, Vos AH, Keet RP, et al. HIV-1 biological phenotype in long-term infected individuals evaluated with an MT-2 cocultivation assay. AIDS 1992; 6:49–54.

51. Bozzette SA, McCutchan JA, Spector SA, et al. A cross-sectional comparison of persons with syncytium- and non-syncytium-inducing human immunodeficiency virus. J Infect Dis 1993; 168:1374–1379.

52. Koot M, Keet IP, Vos AH, et al. Prognostic value of HIV-1 syncytium-inducing phenotype for rate of CD4+ cell depletion and progression to AIDS. Ann Intern Med 1993; 118:681–688.

53. Bleul CC, Wu L, Hoxie JA, et al. The HIV coreceptors CXCR4 and CCR5 are differentially expressed and regulated on human T lymphocytes. Proc Natl Acad Sci USA 1997; 94:1925–1930.

54. Blaak H, van 't Wout AB, Brouwer M, et al. In vivo HIV-1 infection of CD45RA(+)CD4(+) T cells is established primarily by syncytium-inducing variants and correlates with the rate of CD4(+) T cell decline. Proc Natl Acad Sci USA 2000; 97:1269–1274.

55. van Rij RP, Blaak H, Visser JA, et al. Differential coreceptor expression allows for independent evolution of non-syncytium-inducing and syncytium-inducing HIV-1. J Clin Invest 2000; 106:1569.

56. van 't Wout AB, Blaak H, Ran LJ, et al. Evolution of syncytium-inducing and non-syncytium-inducing biological virus clones in relation to replication kinetics during the course of human immunodeficiency virus type 1 infection. J Virol 1998; 72:5099–5107.

57. van Rij RP, Worobey M, Visser JA, et al. Evolution of R5 and X4 human immunodeficiency virus type 1 gag sequences in vivo: evidence for recombination. Virology 2003; 314:451–459.

58. Stalmeijer EH, van Rij RP, Boeser-Nunnink B, et al. In vivo evolution of X4 human immunodeficiency virus type 1 variants in the natural course of infection coincides with decreasing sensitivity to CXCR4 antagonists. J Virol 2004; 78:2722–2728.

59. Koning FA, Kwa D, Boeser-Nunnink B, et al. Decreasing sensitivity to RANTES (regulated on activation, normally T cell-expressed and -secreted) neutralization of CC chemokine receptor 5-using, non-syncytium-inducing virus variants in the course of human immunodeficiency virus type 1 infection. J Infect Dis 2003; 188:864–872.

60. Koning FA, Koevoets C, van der Vorst TJ, et al. Sensitivity of primary R5 HTV-1 to inhibition by RANTES correlates with sensitivity to small-molecule R5 inhibitors. Antivir Ther 2005; 10:231–237.

61. Kestler HW, 3rd DJ, Ringler K, et al. Importance of the nef gene for maintenance of high virus loads and for development of AIDS. Cell 1991; 65:651–662.

62. Daniel MD, Kirchhoff F, Czajak SC, et al. Protective effects of a live attenuated SIV vaccine with a deletion in the Nef gene. Science 1992; 258:1938–1941.

63. Deacon NJ, Tsykin A, Solomon A, et al. Genomic structure of an attenuated quasi species of HIV-1 from a blood transfusion donor and recipients. Science 1995; 270: 988–991.

64. Geyer M, Fackler OT, Peterlin BM. Structure–function relationships in HIV-1 Nef. EMBO Rep 2001; 2:580–585.

65. Simmons A, Aluvihare V, McMichael A. Nef triggers a transcriptional program in T cells imitating single-signal T cell activation and inducing HIV virulence mediators. Immunity 2001; 14:763–777.

66. Fortin JF, Barat C, Beausejour Y, et al. Hyper-responsiveness to stimulation of human immunodeficiency virus-infected CD4+ T cells requires Nef and Tat virus gene products and results from higher NFAT, NF-kappaB, and AP-1 induction. J Biol Chem 2004; 279:39520–39531.

67. Carl S, Greenough TC, Krumbiegel M, et al. Modulation of different human immunodeficiency virus type 1 Nef functions during progression to AIDS. J Virol 2001; 75:3657–3665.

68. Kirchhoff F, Easterbrook PJ, Douglas N, et al. Sequence variations in human immunodeficiency virus type 1 Nef are associated with different stages of disease. J Virol 1999; 73:5497–5508.

69. Sheehy AM, Gaddis NC, Choi JD, et al. Isolation of a human gene that inhibits HIV-1 infection and is suppressed by the viral Vif protein. Nature 2002; 418:646–650.

70. Zheng YH, Irwin D, Kurosu T, et al. Human APOBEC3F is another host factor that blocks human immunodeficiency virus type 1 replication. J Virol 2004; 78:6073–6076.

71. Cen S, Guo F, Niu M, et al. The interaction between HIV-1 Gag and APOBEC3G. J Biol Chem 2004; 279:33177–33184.

72. Mangeat B, Turelli P, Caron G, et al. Broad antiretroviral defence by human APOBEC3G through lethal editing of nascent reverse transcripts. Nature 2003; 424:99–103.

73. Zhang H, Yang B, Pomerantz RJ, et al. The cytidine deaminase CEM15 induces hypermutation in newly synthesized HIV-1 DNA. Nature 2003; 424:94–98.

74. Kobayashi M, Takaori-Kondo A, Miyauchi Y, et al. Ubiquitination of APOBEC3G by an HIV-1 Vif-Cullin5-Elongin B-Elongin C Complex Is Essential for Vif Function. J Biol Chem 2005; 280:18573–18578.

75. Marin M, Rose KM, Kozak SL, et al. HIV-1 Vif protein binds the editing enzyme APOBEC3G and induces its degradation. Nat Med 2003; 9:1398–1403.

76. Sheehy AM, Gaddis NC, Malim MH. The antiretroviral enzyme APOBEC3G is degraded by the proteasome in response to HIV-1 Vif. Nat Med 2003; 9:1404–1407.

77. Alexander L, Aquino-DeJesus MJ, Chan M, et al. Inhibition of human immunodeficiency virus type 1 (HIV-1) replication by a two-amino-acid insertion in HIV-1 Vif from a nonprogressing mother and child. J Virol 2002; 76:10533–10539.

78. Hassaine G, Agostini I, Candotti D, et al. Characterization of human immunodeficiency virus type 1 Vif gene in long-term asymptomatic individuals. Virology 2000; 276:169–180.

79. Sakurai A, Jere A, Yoshida A, et al. Functional analysis of HIV-1 vif genes derived from Japanese long-term nonprogressors and progressors for AIDS. Microbes Infect 2004; 6:799–805.

80. Chiu YL, Soros VB, Kreisberg JF, et al. Cellular APOBEC3G restricts HIV-1 infection in resting CD4+ T cells. Nature 2005; 435:108–114.

81. Do HA, Vasilescu G, Diop T, et al. Exhaustive genotyping of the CEM15 (APOBEC3G) gene and absence of association with AIDS progression in a French cohort. J Infect Dis 2005; 191:159–163.

82. Zhao RY, Bukrinsky M, Elder RT. HIV-1 viral protein R (Vpr) and host cellular responses. Indian J Med Res 2005; 121:270–286.

83. He J, Choe S, Walker R, et al. Human immunodeficiency virus type 1 viral protein R (Vpr) arrests cells in the G2 phase of the cell cycle by inhibiting p34cdc2 activity. J Virol 1995; 69:6705–6711.

84. Heinzinger NK, Bukinsky MI, Haggerty SA, et al. The Vpr protein of human immunodeficiency virus type 1 influences nuclear localization of viral nucleic acids in nondividing host cells. Proc Natl Acad Sci USA 1994; 91:7311–7315.

85. Gibbs JS, Lackner AA, Lang SM, et al. Progression to AIDS in the absence of a gene for vpr or vpx. J Virol 1995; 69:2378–2383.

86. Goh WC, Rogel ME, Kinsey CM, et al. HIV-1 Vpr increases viral expression by manipulation of the cell cycle: a mechanism for selection of Vpr in vivo. Nat Med 1998; 4:65–71.

87. Margottin F, Bour SP, Durand H, et al. A novel human WD protein, h-beta TrCp, that interacts with HIV-1 Vpu connects CD4 to the ER degradation pathway through an F-box motif. Mol Cell 1998; 1:565–574.

88. Varthakavi V, Smith RM, Bour SP, et al. Viral protein U counteracts a human host cell restriction that inhibits HIV-1 particle production. Proc Natl Acad Sci USA 2003; 100:15154–15159.

89. Rucker E, Grivel JC, Munch J, et al. Vpr and Vpu are important for efficient human immunodeficiency virus type 1 replication and CD4+ T-cell depletion in human lymphoid tissue ex vivo. J Virol 2004; 78:12689–12693.

90. Mackay GA, Niu Y, Liu ZQ, et al. Presence of Intact vpu and nef genes in nonpathogenic SHIV is essential for acquisition of pathogenicity of this virus by serial passage in macaques. Virology 2002; 295:133–146.

91. Carrington M, Nelson GW, Martin MP, et al. HLA and HIV-1: heterozygote advantage and B*35-Cw*04 disadvantage. Science 1999; 283:1748–1752.

92. Keet IP, Tang J, Klein MR, et al. Consistent associations of HLA class I and II and transporter gene products with progression of human immunodeficiency virus type 1 infection in homosexual men. J Infect Dis 1999; 180:299–309.

93. Tang J, Costello C, Keet IP, et al. HLA class I homozygosity accelerates disease progression in human immunodeficiency virus type 1 infection. AIDS Res Hum Retroviruses 1999; 15:317–324.

94. Goulder PJ, Edwards A, Phillips RE, et al. Identification of a novel HLA-B*2705-restricted cytotoxic T-lymphocyte epitope within a conserved region of HIV-1 Nef. AIDS 1997; 11:536–538.

95. Migueles SA, Sabbaghian MS, Shupert WL, et al. HLA B*5701 is highly associated with restriction of virus replication in a subgroup of HIV-infected long term nonprogressors. Proc Natl Acad Sci USA 2000; 97:2709–2714.

96. Hendel H, Caillat-Zucman S, Lebuanec H, et al. New class I and II HLA alleles strongly associated with opposite patterns of progression to AIDS. J Immunol 1999; 162:6942–6946.

97. Itescu S, Mathur-Wagh U, Skovron ML, et al. HLA-B35 is associated with accelerated progression to AIDS. J Acquir Immune Defic Syndr 1992; 5:37–45.

98. Kaslow RA, Carrington M, Apple R, et al. Influence of combinations of human major histocompatibility complex genes on the course of HIV-1 infection. Nat Med 1996; 2:405–411.

99. Scorza Smeraldi R, Fabio G, Lazzarin A, et al. HLA-associated susceptibility to AIDS: HLA B35 is a major risk factor for Italian HIV-infected intravenous drug addicts. Hum Immunol 1988; 22:73–79.

100. Tang J, Wilson CM, Meleth S, et al. Host genetic profiles predict virological and immunological control of HIV-1 infection in adolescents. AIDS 2002; 16:2275–2284.

101. Kiepiela P, Leslie AJ, Honeyborne I, et al. Dominant influence of HLA-B in mediating the potential co-evolution of HIV and HLA. Nature 2004; 432:769–775.

102. O'Brien SJ, Moore JP. The effect of genetic variation in chemokines and their receptors on HIV transmission and progression to AIDS. Immunol Rev 2000; 177:99–111.

103. Paxton WA, Martin SR, Tse D, et al. Relative resistance to HIV-1 infection of CD4 lymphocytes from persons who remain uninfected despite multiple high-risk sexual exposure. Nat Med 1996; 2:412–417.

104. Liu R, Paxton WA, Choe S, et al. Homozygous defect in HIV-1 coreceptor accounts for resistance of some multiply-exposed individuals to HIV-1 infection. Cell 1996; 86:367–377.

105. Sheppard HW, Celum C, Michael NL, et al. HIV-1 infection in individuals with the CCR5-Delta32/Delta32 genotype: acquisition of syncytium-inducing virus at seroconversion. J Acquir Immune Defic Syndr 2002; 29:307–313.

106. Dean M, Carrington M, Winkler C, et al. Genetic restriction of HIV-1 infection and progression to AIDS by a deletion allele of the CKR5 structural gene. Hemophilia Growth and Development Study, Multicenter AIDS Cohort Study, Multicenter Hemophilia Cohort Study, San Francisco City Cohort. ALIVE Study Sci 1996; 273:1856–1862.

107. Gonzalez E, Bamshad M, Sato N, et al. Race-specific HIV-1 disease-modifying effects associated with CCR5 haplotypes. Proc Natl Acad Sci USA 1999; 96:12004–12009.

108. de Roda Husman AM, Koot M, Cornelissen M, et al. Association between CCR5 genotype and the clinical course of HIV-1 infection. Ann Intern Med 1997; 127:882–890.

109. Martin MP, Dean M, Smith MW, et al. Genetic acceleration of AIDS progression by a promoter variant of CCR5. Science 1998; 282:1907–1911.

110. Mangano A, Gonzalez E, Dhanda R, et al. Concordance between the CC chemokine receptor 5 genetic determinants that alter risks of transmission and disease progression in

children exposed perinatally to human immunodeficiency virus. J Infect Dis 2001; 183:1574–1585.

111. Tang J, Shelton B, Makhatadze NJ, et al. Distribution of chemokine receptor CCR2 and CCR5 genotypes and their relative contribution to human immunodeficiency virus type 1 (HIV-1) seroconversion, early HIV-1 RNA concentration in plasma, and later disease progression. J Virol 2002; 76:662–672.

112. John GC, Birc T, Overbaugh J, et al. CCR5 promoter polymorphisms in a Kenyan perinatal human immunodeficiency virus type 1 cohort: association with increased 2-year maternal mortality. J Infect Dis 2001; 184:89–92.

113. Anzala AO, Ball TB, Rostron T, et al. CCR2-64I allele and genotype association with delayed AIDS progression in African women. University of Nairobi Collaboration for HIV Research. Lancet 1998; 351:1632–1633.

114. Ioannidis JP, Rosenberg PS, Goedert JJ, et al. Effects of CCR5-Delta32, CCR2-64I, and SDF-1 3'A alleles on HIV-1 disease progression: An international meta-analysis of individual-patient data. Ann Intern Med 2001; 135:782–795.

115. Mangano A, Kopka J, Batalla M, et al. Protective effect of CCR2-64I and not of CCR5-delta32 and SDF1-3'A in pediatric HIV-1 infection. J Acquir Immune Defic Syndr 2000; 23:52–57.

116. Smith MW, Dean M, Carrington M, et al. Contrasting genetic influence of CCR2 and CCR5 variants on HIV-1 infection and disease progression. Hemophilia Growth and Development Study (HGDS), Multicenter AIDS Cohort Study (MACS), Multicenter Hemophilia Cohort Study (MHCS), San Francisco City Cohort (SFCC). ALIVE Study Sci 1997; 277:959–965.

117. van Rij RP, de Roda Husman AM, Brouwer M, et al. Role of CCR2 genotype in the clinical course of syncytium-inducing (SI) or non-SI human immunodeficiency virus type 1 infection and in the time to conversion to SI virus variants. J Infect Dis 1998; 178:1806–1811.

118. Faure S, Meyer L, Costagliola D, et al. Rapid progression to AIDS in HIV+ individuals with a structural variant of the chemokine receptor CX3CR1. Science 2000; 287:2274–2277.

119. Hendel H, Winkler C, An P, et al. Validation of genetic case-control studies in AIDS and application to the CX3CR1 polymorphism. J Acquir Immune Defic Syndr 2001; 26:507–511.

120. Kwa D, Boeser-Nunnink B, Schuitemaker H. Lack of evidence for an association between a polymorphism in CX3CR1 and the clinical course of HIV infection or virus phenotype evolution. AIDS 2003; 17:759–761.

121. McDermott DH, Colla JS, Kleeberger CA, et al. Genetic polymorphism in CX3CR1 and risk of HIV disease. Science 2000; 290:2031.

122. Faure S, Meyer L, Genin E, et al. Deleterious genetic influence of CX3CR1 genotypes on HIV-1 disease progression. J Acquir Immune Defic Syndr 2003; 32:335–337.

123. Liu H, Chao D, Nakayama EE, et al. Polymorphism in RANTES chemokine promoter affects HIV-1 disease progression. Proc Natl Acad Sci USA 1999; 96:4581–4585.

124. McDermott DH, Beecroft MJ, Kleeberger CA, et al. Chemokine RANTES promoter polymorphism affects risk of both HIV infection and disease

progression in the Multicenter AIDS Cohort Study. AIDS 2000; 14:2671–2678.

125. An P, Nelson GW, Wang L, et al. Modulating influence on HIV/AIDS by interacting RANTES gene variants. Proc Natl Acad Sci USA 2002; 99:10002–10007.

126. Gonzalez E, Dhanda R, Bamshad M, et al. Global survey of genetic variation in CCR5, RANTES, and MIP-1alpha: impact on the epidemiology of the HIV-1 pandemic. Proc Natl Acad Sci USA 2001; 98:5199–5204.

127. Gonzalez E, Kulkarni H, Bolivar H, et al. The influence of CCL3L1 gene-containing segmental duplications on HIV-1/AIDS susceptibility. Science 2005; 1:1434–1440.

128. van Rij RP, Broersen S, Goudsmit J, et al. The role of a stromal cell-derived factor-1 chemokine gene variant in the clinical course of HIV-1 infection. AIDS 1998; 12:85–90.

129. Winkler C, Modi W, Smith MW, et al. Genetic restriction of AIDS pathogenesis by an SDF-1 chemokine gene variant. ALIVE Study, Hemophilia Growth and Development Study (HGDS), Multicenter AIDS Cohort Study (MACS), Multicenter Hemophilia Cohort Study (MHCS), San Francisco City Cohort (SFCC). Science 1998; 279:389–393.

130. Kwa D, van Rij RP, Boeser-Nunnink B, et al. Association between an interleukin-4 promoter polymorphism and the acquisition of CXCR4 using HIV-1 variants. AIDS 2003; 17:981–985.

131. Nakayama EE, Hoshino Y, Xin X, et al. Polymorphism in the interleukin-4 promoter affects acquisition of human immunodeficiency virus type 1 syncytium-inducing phenotype. J Virol 2000; 74:5452–5459.

132. Shin HD, Winkler C, Stephens JC, et al. Genetic restriction of HIV-1 pathogenesis to AIDS by promoter alleles of IL10. Proc Natl Acad Sci USA 2000; 97:14467–14472.

133. Gaudieri S, Nolan D, McKinnon E, et al. Associations between KIR epitope combinations expressed by HLA-B/-C haplotypes found in an HIV-1 infected study population may influence NK mediated immune responses. Mol Immunol 2005; 42:557–560.

134. Martin MP, Gao X, Lee JH, et al. Epistatic interaction between KIR3DS1 and HLA-B delays the progression to AIDS. Nat Genet 2002; 31:429–434.

135. Lopez-Vazquez A, Mina-Blanco A, Martinez-Borra J, et al. Interaction between KIR3DL1 and HLA-B*57 supertype alleles influences the progression of HIV-1 infection in a Zambian population. Hum Immunol 2005; 66:285–289.

136. Heil F, Hemmi H, Hochrein H, et al. Species-specific recognition of single-stranded RNA via toll-like receptor 7 and 8. Science 2004; 303:1526–1529.

137. Lore K, Betts MR, Brenchley JM, et al. Toll-like receptor ligands modulate dendritic cells to augment cytomegalovirus- and HIV-1-specific T cell responses. J Immunol 2003; 171:4320–4328.

138. Lazarus R, Klimecki WT, Raby BA, et al. Single-nucleotide polymorphisms in the Toll-like receptor 9 gene (TLR9): frequencies, pairwise linkage disequilibrium, and haplotypes in three U.S. ethnic groups and exploratory case-control disease association studies. Genomics 2003; 81:85–91.

139. Schroder NW, Schumann RR. Single nucleotide polymorphisms of Toll-like receptors and susceptibility to infectious disease. Lancet Infect Dis 2005; 5:156–164.

140. Ganesh L, Burstein E, Guha-Niyogi A, et al. The gene product Murr1 restricts HIV-1 replication in resting CD4+ lymphocytes. Nature 2003; 426:853–857.

CHAPTER 6

Acute HIV Infection

Anthony D. Kelleher
David A. Cooper

Introduction

Although HIV infection is a chronic progressive infection, it is well recognized that the initial stages of the infection are characterized by an acute viral syndrome. Despite this illness often being mild and under-diagnosed, increasing understanding of the links between pathophysiology and clinical manifestations has provided insights into the earliest interactions between host and virus. The virological and immunological events that immediately follow HIV infection are highly dynamic and there is increasing evidence these events impact on long-term outcome of the infection and rates of disease progression. The clinical presentation of initial infection is variously referred to as: acute HIV infection, primary infection illness, acute retroviral syndrome, or seroconversion illness. Although there is variation in the clinical manifestations, there are distinct characteristics associated with this illness. The diagnosis of acute HIV infection is based on a combination of clinical acumen and characteristic findings on a range of laboratory tests. Although there are theoretical arguments supporting the value of therapeutic intervention at this stage of the disease its clinical benefit is yet to be definitively demonstrated. However, the identification of this condition has the potential to impact upon both the care of an individual patient and upon the health of a population by early institution of interventions limiting spread of the infection.

Pathophysiology

By the time a patient presents with clinical manifestations of acute HIV infection, even in those with negative or indeterminate serology, a whole series of virological and immunological events have already occurred (Fig. 6.1). The so-called window period, despite being apparently silent on diagnostic tests, is neither immunologically nor virologically silent. Insight into many of these earliest events has been gained from animal models such as SIV infection of rhesus macaques as these events are impossible to study in humans for a range of practical and ethical reasons.

Most infections occur at mucosal membranes. After crossing epithelial barriers, the initial cells infected by virus are both dendritic cells and CD4+ T cells that populate the mucosal tissues of the genitourinary and/or colonic mucosa. Dendritic cells are capable of harboring and transporting the virus to lymphoid tissue with or without being productively infected.[1] However, whether infected or just transporting the virus, these cells are capable of transferring virus to multiple CD4+ T cells as they fulfil their normal role of antigen presentation to T cells. This interaction simultaneously triggers an immune response consisting of both T-cell (involving activation of both CD4+ and CD8+ T cells) and antibody responses while facilitating infection of responding CD4+ T cells. This process drives preferential infection and subsequent death of HIV-specific CD4+ T

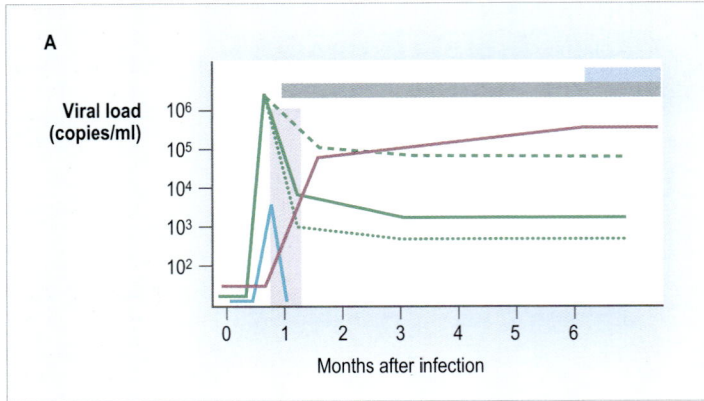

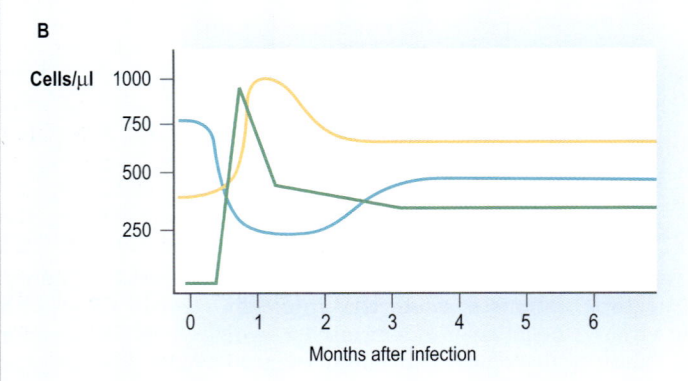

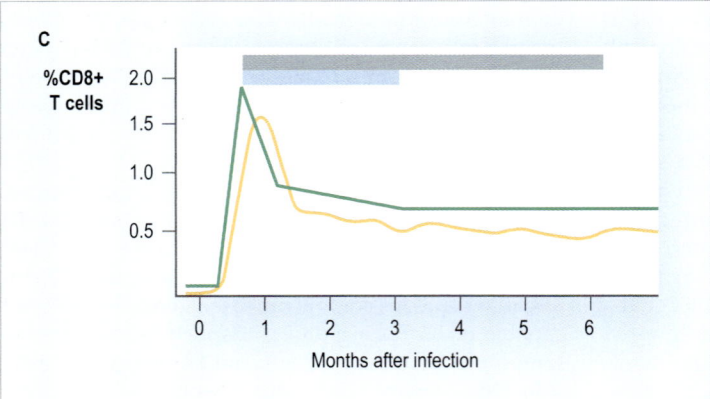

Figure 6.1 Dynamics of virological and immunological events during acute infection and their relationship to diagnostic read outs. (A) Green lines show the changes in plasma viral load measured in RNA copies/mL of plasma. The solid green line shows a typical viral load time course and outcome; the dashed green line shows viral load time course with a likely poor long-term outcome, and the dotted green line shows the time course of the patient likely to have a good prognosis. The blue-gray shaded area indicates the onset and offset of clinical manifestations. The blue line shows the typical time course of p24 antigen detection. The magenta line shows the time course of development of HIV-antibodies. The horizontal gray box shows the period during which a typical EIA will be positive. The purple box shows the timing at which a detuned EIA will become positive. (B) Typical time course of CD4+ and CD8+ T-cell counts in peripheral blood. The blue line is the CD4+ T-cell count; the yellow line is the CD8+T-cell count. A typical viral load curve is shown for reference (green line). (C) The yellow line shows a representative antigen specific CD8+ CTL response as measured by response to a single immuno-dominant epitope. The horizontal boxes show the typical time course of HIV-specific CD4+ T-cell responses and blue horizontal bar shows the presence of CD4+ T cells capable of proliferation and production of IL-2. The gray box shows time course of cells capable of producing IFN-γ.

cells, resulting in the early deletion of these critical cells from the host's immune response to the virus.[2] After infection of lymphoid tissue there is subsequent, rapid dissemination of the virus to multiple tissues including the central nervous system.

CD4+ T-cell Responses

As with any primary immune response, the adaptive immune response takes time to develop. The virus replicates relatively unchecked during this period. Plasma viremia is detectable and viral load increases exponentially (Fig. 6.1). At primary infection in SIV-macaque models there is massive infection and depletion of CD4+ T cells particularly those at tissue sites such as lymphoid tissue, gut, and genitourinary tracts.[3,4] Similar processes appear to be occurring in humans early in HIV-infection.[5,6] This depletion in tissues is reflected in a reduction in CD4+ T-cell count in peripheral blood.

In humans, HIV-specific CD4+ T-cell responses are detectable early in infection.[7,8] Initially, these consist of cells capable of producing both IL-2 and IFN-γ and of proliferating in response to HIV-antigens, but these cells rapidly lose their ability to proliferate and produce IL-2 in the majority of patients (Fig. 6.1C).[8-10] The exception appears to be in those individuals that control virus replication. In the remainder of patients HIV-specific CD4+ T cells are detectable, but consist almost entirely of cells capable of producing IFN-γ without proliferative or IL-2 producing capacity (Fig. 6.1C). This depletion occurs in both peripheral blood and tissues.

T cells homing to peripheral lymphoid tissue such as the gut and genitourinary tracts preferentially express the chemokine receptor CCR5. The preferential depletion of these cells may be due to selective infection and cytolysis due to a heightened susceptibility to infection by the virus strain associated with transmission.[11,12] Preferential infection of CD4+ T cells specifically responding to HIV infection results in loss of these cells and almost certainly accounts for the pathognomic phenomenon of anergy to HIV antigens seen later in HIV infection.[2] Therapy initiated early can preserve this responsiveness and may limit the depletion of these cells from mucosal sites.[5,6]

CD8+ T-cell Responses

In contrast to the decrease in CD4 T-cell numbers, CD8+ T-cell numbers rise dramatically during acute infection (Fig. 6.1B). This increase consists almost entirely of activated T cells.[13] Many of these activated, proliferating and expanding cells are cytotoxic T cells (CTL) specifically targeted to HIV[14-16] (Fig. 6.1C). Their ability to lyse infected targets and prevent infection of new cells is thought to limit viral expansion, halting the exponential increase in plasma viral load that follows initial infection and to at least partially determine the eventual viral set point. While CD8+ CTL are detectable, a second set of CD8+ T cells capable of suppressing viral replication through secretion of a range of soluble factors including MIP1-α, MIP1-β, RANTES and an as yet unidentified cytokine called CAF, is also detectable during acute HIV-infection.[17] Deliberate depletion of CD8+ T cells from SIV-infected macaques at primary infection results in increases of viral load set point and accounts for more rapid disease progression.[18]

In peripheral blood, HIV-specific CD8+ T cells are among the first immune responses detectable, usually during the clinical presentation of acute infection. In macaques, SIV-specific CD8+ T cells can be detected within 8 days of infection.[19] The initial response is usually highly focused on a limited number of high avidity epitopes. The response broadens with time. Responses to a range of HIV proteins, including regulatory and accessory proteins such as Tat and Nef, are present.[20,21]

CD8+ CTL responses place pressure on the virus. Adaptive evolution of the virus to these responses occurs early, allowing selection of immune escape variants capable of evading CTL responses within several weeks of infection.[22,23]

Antibody Responses

Although antibodies to various HIV-proteins, particularly p24 and envelope proteins are detectable soon after infection, most of these antibodies play no clear role in control of infection. The majority of the antibody response is to internal proteins. Of the antibodies directed at the envelope proteins, the overwhelming majority are not neutralizing in nature.[24] Neutralizing antibodies, capable of preventing viral entry and therefore new infection, are slow to arise and are usually detectable not less than 4–8 weeks after infection.[25] When neutralizing antibodies do occur they place pressure on the virus. The virus responds to this pressure rapidly adapting through the generation of escape variants.[26,27] New rounds of neutralizing antibodies are also delayed in their development.

Innate Immune Responses

The role of innate immune responses in primary infection is still not clearly understood. Dendritic cells play a role in transport of virus to lymphoid tissue, and can act as a 'Trojan horse', transmitting captured virus to CD4[+] T cells assisting dissemination of infection. However, dendritic cells play a critical role in the control of infection as they are essential for cross priming and induction of CD8[+] CTL responses as well as CD4[+] T-cell responses.[1] While monocytoid dendritic cell numbers are maintained, plasmacytoid dendritic cell numbers are depleted during primary infection.[28]

Immune and Virological Outcomes at Resolution of Primary Infection

Upon onset of these HIV-specific immune responses viral load declines. CD4[+] T-cell counts partially recover but do not return to normal levels. CD8[+] T-cell numbers drop but remain elevated well above the normal range (Fig. 6.1). These changes maintain a reversed CD4:CD8 T-cell ratio, despite partial normalization of CD4[+] T-cell counts. Markers of immune activation particularly those expressed on the surface of CD8[+] T cells (e.g. CD38) remain substantially increased. Plasma viral load reaches a steady state or set point approximately 3–6 months post-infection.[29] This level reflects a balance between the pathogenicity and replication fitness of the virus and the effectiveness of the host's initial immune response. This level predicts long-term disease outcome (Fig. 6.1).[30]

Virus

Initial infection in the overwhelming majority of cases occurs with the virus using the CCR5 co-receptor. This chemokine receptor is expressed preferentially on monocytes, dendritic cells and memory CD4[+] T cells. Viral tropism for CCR5 is determined by the amino acid sequence of specific regions of Env. The observation of almost exclusive CCR5 co-receptor tropism in viruses isolated early in infection strongly suggests selection of viral strains from within the transmitting host's multiple quasispecies by the process of transmission.

Furthermore, the virus appears highly homogenous, shortly after transmission. Two factors may contribute to homogeneity of transmitted strains. The first is the concept of a molecular sieve, where the process of transmission selects for the variants most capable of transmission from among the swarm of quasispecies in the transmitting host. Certain envelope variants appear to have an advantage during the transmission process. The selection of CCR5 tropic variants is the clearest example. More recently, in subtype C virus, variants carrying *Env* sequences with shorter V1–V4 intervals and reduced numbers of glycosylation sites appear to be preferentially transmitted.[31] Additionally, homogeneity of transmitted strains may be contributed to by rapid viral adaptation to its new host post-transmission. Post-transmission, the virus tends to revert from mutations that were advantageous in the original host towards wild type. This process of reversion affects both drug resistance and immune escape mutations.[32,33] The rate of reversion inversely correlates with the fitness cost to the virus in its new host with reversion of non-advantageous mutations in the new host occurring very quickly.

Despite these processes, a range of adaptive mutations within the transmitted virus may be maintained. Horizontal and vertical transmission of both drug resistance mutations and immune escape mutations are well documented.[34,35] However, thereafter, mutations reflecting adaptation to the new host also occur rapidly with mutations allowing escape from both CTL and neutralizing antibody pressure arising rapidly.[22,23,27] The virus adapts to the altered pressures placed upon it, with selection of the most replication-competent variants occurring rapidly. Variation can occur in all genes. The reasons for differences in the rate of variation relate to varying levels of gene product plasticity and differences in the pressures applied.

Co-infection and Superinfection

Although co-infection with two viruses at primary infection is rare, superinfection with a second virus within the first two years post initial infection has been reported with increasing frequency, at least in non-B subtype infections. Super-infection, in B subtype infections appears rare or at least uncommon,[36–39] however, in areas where micro-epidemics of different subtypes intersect superinfection appears more common.[40,41]

Clinical Manifestations

The rate of recognition of the clinical manifestations of primary infection varies markedly. An acute illness associated with recent infection with HIV-1 can be identified in the majority of individuals with reported rates ranging from 50–90%.[42–47] Initial descriptions described the illness as resembling infectious mononucleosis, with the major manifestations being fever, pharyngitis and adenopathy,[42] but further studies have demonstrated that using this triad alone to describe the clinical manifestations is restrictive.[43] Symptoms associated with initial infection and subsequent seroconversion can vary from completely absent through to an acute debilitating illness requiring hospitalization. The rate of identification is dependent on high levels of clinical suspicion, experience with making the diagnosis, the availability of medical resources, as well as suspicion on the part of the patient. Although the overwhelming majority of reports of this illness have been in the context of the developed world with subtype B infections, similar manifestations have been reported with other viral subtypes in developing world settings. Similarly, although most reported series also arise from cohorts where the major mode of transmission is sexual, similar prevalence of symptomatic illness and similar clinical manifestations have been reported in intravenous drug users.[10,48] In adults, clinical manifestations and severity are not dependent on age, sex, race, or geographical factors. Although no concurrent studies have been performed, a study in a US population showed that 49% sought medical attention for symptoms,[49] while up to 44% of African women took some time off work due to primary infection symptoms.[50] Although published reports are sparse, similar manifestations are seen in adolescents.[51]

The time from exposure to illness is typically 2–4 weeks (range: 6–42 days),[42–47] but there are rare, isolated reports of delayed seroconversion of up to 12 months post-exposure. The acute illness typically lasts approximately 3 weeks and is of rapid onset. In the main, the symptoms are self-limiting. However, up to 20% of cases can require hospitalization or be associated with the presence of opportunistic infections like candidiasis, herpes zoster, cryptococcosis and *Pneumocystis jirovecii* pneumonia. The likelihood of primary infection being complicated by an opportunistic infection is related to the extent of CD4+ T-cell depression.[52]

The main clinical manifestations are fever, pharyngitis, adenopathy, rash, myalgia or arthralgia, headaches, and fatigue or asthenia. The pharyngitis is non-exudative and the tonsils are not coated. The rash is classically maculopapular, symmetrical with lesions 0.5–1 cm in diameter affecting face and or trunk, but may also affect the hands including the palms. Other manifestations include mouth ulcers and gastrointestinal upset including diarrhea, odynophagia, anorexia, abdominal pain, vomiting. Headaches can be associated with retro-orbital pain exacerbated by movement of the eyes and meningitic or encephalitic symptoms and signs. Lymphadenopathy tends to be more common in the cervical region but can affect axillary and inguinal regions.[42–47,52]

The originally described triad of dominant manifestations, fever, pharyngitis and lymphadenopathy occurs in a significant minority of patients. Although fever is the most common manifestation, it occurs in less than three-quarters of patients. In the absence of a typical mononucleosis like presentation, fever is most commonly associated with headache, oral ulceration and/or abdominal pain. In the absence of fever the most common manifestations are pharyngitis, lethargy, myalgia, rash, headache and adenopathy.[43] Lymphadenopathy may be slow to resolve, persisting well after the resolution of other manifestations.

Clinical presentations are reasonably non-specific and not easily distinguishable from other viral illnesses on clinical grounds alone. However, this constellation of symptoms in those at risk should trigger consideration of primary infection illness in the differential diagnosis and should initiate laboratory investigation including HIV serology.

The severity of the illness appears to impact on long-term outcome, with greater severity predicting more rapid progression to disease. More rapid CD4+ T-cell count declines have been documented in those who present to a physician.[53] The presence of candidiasis, neurological involvement or a prolonged illness lasting more than 14 days is associated with a worse prognosis.[43]

Co-infection with other viruses, such as cytomegalovirus (CMV), or other sexually transmitted infections (STIs) occur. These co-infections can make the clinical presentation more complicated.[54] Co-infection with other viruses such as herpes viruses, hepatitis B or C viruses or other STIs such as chlamydia or syphilis must be considered in the diagnostic work-up.

As stated, race, mode of acquisition, or viral subtype do not appear to impact upon the severity of the illness. Pre-existing impaired immune responses as demonstrated by low pre-existing CD4+ T-cell count, low CD4:CD8 T-cell ratios or impaired delayed type-hypersensitivity reactions are associated with increased risk of a symptomatic illness, as is transmission from an index case with advanced HIV disease.[55,56]

Diagnosis

Clinical suspicion, based upon recognition of the constellation of clinical signs detailed in the previous section, combined with knowledge of possible exposure to the virus in the previous 2–8 weeks, plus laboratory confirmation of recent HIV infection, are the corner stones of diagnosis. For these reasons, the diagnosis should always be considered in individuals presenting with apparently non-specific symptoms if they belong to a risk group for HIV-infection. The differential diagnosis of primary HIV-1 infection includes other viral infections, particularly with herpes viruses, such as Epstein-Barr virus (EBV) and CMV, but also includes other viral illnesses and STIs, particularly syphilis. Usually, the confirmation or exclusion of the diagnosis of acute HIV-infection in the laboratory is straightforward. Therefore, the critical step in the process is the consideration of the diagnosis as a possibility.

Early diagnosis has advantages for both the individual and the population. It allows institution of therapies in the context of a relatively intact immune system. Furthermore, effective therapy reduces viral load and therefore viral turnover, markedly limiting the rate at which virus mutants arise, allowing adaptation to either drug pressure or immune responses. As the severity of the illness has implications for long-term outcome, it may influence decisions regarding timing of institution of therapy. Early initiation of risk-modification counselling limits the potential for transmission, particularly as transmission probability increases with high viral loads such as those that characterize primary infection.[57–60] However, the effectiveness of this intervention will depend upon the stage of the epidemic and the extent to which transmission is to casual partners.[61]

Laboratory Testing and Diagnosis

Although nucleic acid testing is playing a greater role in the diagnosis and management of acute HIV-infection, serology is still the mainstay of diagnosis. The relative susceptibility of nucleic acid testing to false-negative results as a result of sequence variation, particularly across different viral subtypes, still prevents these tests becoming the mainstay of diagnosis.

The routine detection of primary infection relies on the generation of antibodies to the virus. As these take a finite period to develop, there is an unavoidable window period after infection when these tests will be negative, even in the presence of established infection (Fig. 6.1). The length of this period is, to some extent, dependent upon the sensitivity of the test used. In general, those assays where the viral proteins are derived from viral lysates alone are less sensitive than those in which lysates are supplemented by recombinant proteins or peptides. The window period can be further shortened by detection of virus directly, either through protein based assays for the detection of p24 protein or nucleic acid testing based on either the detection of pro-viral DNA or viral RNA (Fig. 6.1). However, even these tests will be negative for up to 2 weeks following infection.[62]

Criteria for diagnosis of HIV-1 infection vary from country to country but the diagnosis in the laboratory of acute HIV infection is dependent upon either an evolving pattern of antibody production or a new positive test in the presence of a documented recent negative test.

Serology

A range of tests are available for detection of antibodies that will make the diagnosis of HIV infection. These include a variety of enzyme immunoassay (EIA) type technologies and immunoblotting. These now include a variety of 'point of care' testing platforms that in general have lower specificity and sensitivity than the standard laboratory based tests. This type of test may have a role in diagnosis particularly in the absence of formal laboratory support in resource poor settings.[63]

As is typical of immune responses to infection anti-HIV IgM antibodies precede the development of IgG antibodies. However, detection of IgM antibodies alone is not routinely used in the diagnosis of recent HIV infection because of unacceptable rates of false-positive results. Antibodies are usually detectable by EIA or western blot within 2 weeks of infection, however the length of this window period varies depending on the diagnostic kit used (Fig. 6.1).

Immunoblotting demonstrates that antibodies develop in typical and predictable patterns (Fig. 6.2). This knowledge can be used for early identification of likely seroconverters triggering other testing to support the diagnosis of early or acute HIV infection. These tests include direct detection of virus (see below). Antibodies to p24 or Env are typically the earliest antibodies detectable with virtually all sera being positive 2 weeks or more after the onset of the acute illness. Antibodies to other proteins develop

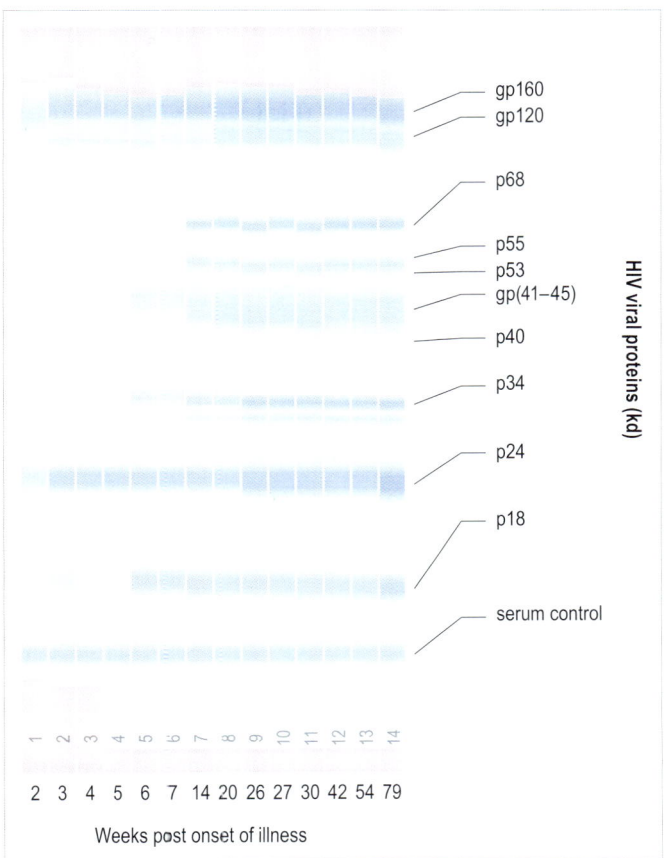

Figure 6.2 Development of HIV-antibodies over time, following infection. Sequential immunoblots performed on serum samples from a typical seroconverter showing characteristic pattern of antibodies to various HIV-proteins at acute infection.

sequentially with a fully positive western blot present by 3 months after infection. However, individuals identified soon after exposure may have negative EIA and negative or indeterminate immunoblot results at the time of their first blood draw. Definitive serological diagnosis then depends on tracking responses over time until diagnostic criteria are fulfilled. Laboratories interested in studying acute infection have developed algorithms for the rapid detection and confirmation of these cases (Fig. 6.3).

Importantly, highly suppressive antiretroviral therapy commenced early in the course of acute HIV-infection can change the pattern of antibody development resulting in freezing antibody development at the stage at which therapy was commenced.[64] This can cause diagnostic difficulties, however upon interruption of therapy and subsequent increases in viral load, antibody responses develop rapidly to a fully positive immunoblot pattern.

Detuned Serology and other Testing to Detect Recent Infection

In the absence of a developing antibody pattern, diagnosis of early infection is usually dependent upon the availability of recently negative serology. However, a range of serological techniques are becoming available that can indicate recent infection. These techniques are based on the observation that both the intensity and the affinity of the antibodies increase over time. The best known of these techniques is the 'detuned' EIA. In these assays, the sensitivity of a standard EIA is deliberately compromised through increasing the dilution of the sera tested and reducing incubation times. In these compromised EIA, sera from individuals with fully established infection still produce a positive response, but sera from those with recent infection will give a negative response and therefore 'detune'. The period over which recent infection can be detected by

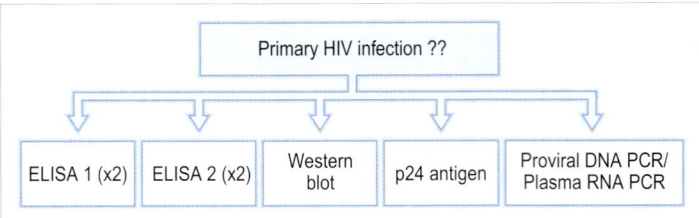

Figure 6.3 An example of a 'flat' diagnostic algorithm for rapid identification of true acute infection cases. A barrage of diagnostic tests is set up in parallel, allowing for faster turnaround times, but this is a more expensive strategy and is usually only adopted in reference laboratories with an interest in primary infection.

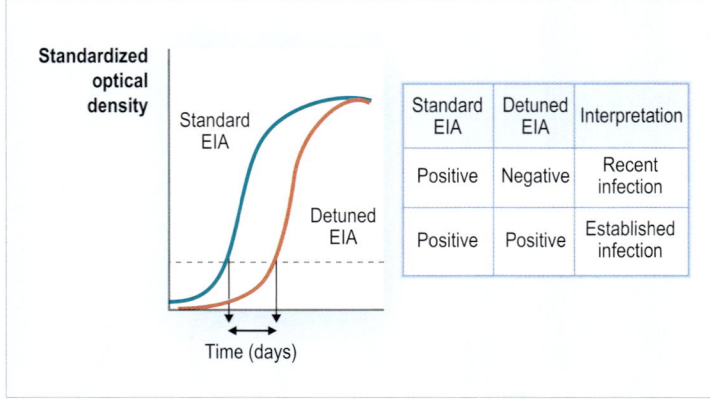

Figure 6.4 Relative performance of a standard diagnostic EIA and a detuned EIA. The detuned EIA will become positive several months later than the standard highly optimized and sensitive diagnostic EIA. In the interval shown by the double-headed arrow, the diagnosis of a recent infection can be made by the discrepant results between the two tests.

detuned EIAs varies from test to test, but in general these assays detect infections within the last 6 months (Figs. 6.1, 6.4).[63]

However, this assay performs with quite different characteristics in non-B subtype viruses, limiting its utility outside the developed world.[65] More recent developments with IgG capture EIAs may have overcome some of these problems.[66,67] Other methodologies for detecting recent infection depend on the affinity maturation of antibodies to particular epitopes or detection of development of p24 antibodies of a particular isotype.[68] However, the performance of these tests on non-B subtypes has not been assessed. Another mechanism of diagnosing early infection employs an algorithm that takes into account the characteristic patterns in development of individual bands and intensities of bands upon western blot. This simple algorithm appears to have greater specificity for recent infection than detuned testing. The further development of this type of test will aid with collection of epidemiologic data on rates of new infections, rates of disease progression and early diagnosis for individuals.

Detection of Virus

The main role of direct viral detection in the diagnosis of primary infection is in reducing the window period in those with negative or indeterminate serological testing. The ability to directly detect viral components, p24 or nucleic acid (plasma RNA or proviral DNA) supports the likely diagnosis of HIV infection.

p24 Antigen Detection

This test employs EIA technology. The test is highly specific and, although not sensitive in chronic disease, is characteristically transiently positive early in acute infection in those with negative or very early antibody responses. The test is usually positive 3–6 days prior to a sensitive antibody EIA (Fig. 6.1).[62]

Many commercially available tests now combine antibody and antigen detection in a single EIA. These kits offer significant advantages in screening for positive diagnoses especially at primary infection. Subsequent testing will reveal whether the positive result is driven by the presence of antigen or antibody. The majority of the latest generation of p24 antigen tests ('4th generation kits') perform well with non-B clade isolates.[69]

Nucleic Acid Testing

Detection of proviral DNA by PCR techniques is a sensitive and specific way of diagnosing HIV infection and is a very useful adjunct test in the context of primary infection in those with negative or indeterminate serology. The test is often positive up to 2 days prior to the p24 antibody test (Fig. 6.1), however, it works less efficiently in non-subtype B infections. Viral RNA can be used as an alternative, but this test has a low but problematical false-positive rate in true seronegatives. Therefore, the viral load detected must be >5000 copies/mL on two separate occasions before the diagnosis can be made with certainty. Used in this way, the test usually first becomes positive about the same time as the p24 antigen. Alternative qualitative RNA detection kits have been developed for screening of blood donations can be used to screen pooled samples. These give positive read outs at lower RNA levels and therefore reduce the window period further but are not currently approved for use in routine diagnosis.[62] As with the proviral DNA test, RNA tests are susceptible to false-negative results in variant strains.

Viral Load During Primary Infection

Following diagnosis, the patient is usually monitored using standard surrogate markers of disease progression, viral load and CD4+ T-cell count. A low nadir CD4+ cells count and higher viral load at 2–4 months, but not peak viral load, is associated with a poorer prognosis,[53,70] while rapid falls in viral load are associated with a better prognosis. Set point viral load is attained between 3–6 months post-infection,[29] and the higher this level, the worse the prognosis.

Drug Resistance Testing

Drug resistance can be determined either phenotypically or genotypically. The determination of drug resistance at primary infection is generally recommended by expert panels and can serve two purposes. First, it can serve as a public health surveillance mechanism providing information regarding population rates of transmission of drug resistant variants. Second, it provides important information for the individual if therapeutic intervention is being considered. Rates of transmitted resistance vary markedly between populations.[71] In the absence of drug pressure, some of these mutations revert over time, while some, particularly those that are compensated by secondary mutations or those that do not significantly impact on viral fitness, tend to be maintained. The impact of these transmitted mutations on long-term outcome is still to be determined,

but theoretically, they will compromise response to antiretroviral therapy (ART).

Transmitted resistance mutations may behave differently from those in an individual stopping therapy where there is often rapid outgrowth of wild type or reversion variants. Mutations may be maintained post-transmission for much longer periods than after withdrawal of therapy. While the M184V 3TC mutation often reverts rapidly and the T215Y AZT mutation partially reverts to 215S/C/D, others, particularly the K103N mutation may be maintained for long periods of time.[72]

Management

Once the definitive diagnosis is made, it must be communicated with the patient in a clear and supportive manner. The diagnosis must be fully understood by the patient who must also understand the need to adopt safe practices that minimize further spread of the infection. There is evidence that earlier diagnosis if linked to effective counselling services can modify behavior and reduce transmission at a time of high viral load and therefore the likely probability of transmission per unsafe event.[73] Therapy of primary infection is supportive. The initiation of highly active antiretroviral therapy (HAART) during acute infection is suggested by a range of treatment guidelines, but usually only in the context of clinical trial. Although there are theoretical reasons to support this approach, there are still no definitive data from controlled clinical trials which demonstrate that combination antiretroviral chemotherapy has a positive effect on long term clinical outcome.[74] Although the first randomized trial of zidovudine monotherapy at primary infection suggested a therapeutic benefit in the short term, longer-term follow-up suggested this effect was diluted with time.[75,76] Placebo controlled studies have not been conducted in the HAART era. Combination antiretroviral therapy is definitely effective in improving both CD4+ T-cell count and viral load, compared with untreated historical controls, while those patients are on treatment. However, the long-term advantage of these regimens has not been demonstrated and in general CD4+ T-cell counts and viral load return to similar set points as those untreated individuals upon cessation of therapy.[74] Other therapeutic approaches such as structured treatment interruptions and short course therapy lasting up to 12 months have been advocated after apparent success in selected individuals. Definitive evidence of the clinical superiority of these strategies awaits the results of properly conducted randomized clinical trials. There are significant amounts of data suggesting improvements or maintenance of various functional HIV-specific immune responses mediated by both CD4[+] and CD8[+] T cells however, the impact of these changes on long term outcome are unclear at this time.[7,8]

The presumed benefits of early intervention with suppressive HAART include reduction in viral load resulting in reduction of transmission and preservation of the immune system preventing depletion of CD4[+] T cells. Although there has been fairly universal acceptance of initiation of therapy for those diagnosed during acute infection, attitudes of physicians are becoming more conservative driven by the lack of efficacy data and the cumulative toxicities of HAART regimens. Recent data suggest that adverse events, including gastrointestinal upsets, lipodystrophy and mood disorders, are recorded in 51% of individuals treated with only 75% achieving good viral load control.[77] Currently, there are at least two randomized studies exploring the effects various forms of ART initiated during acute or early primary infection against no therapy. Hopefully, these will give some definitive guidance on therapeutic intervention during primary infection.

Conclusion

Primary infection is a dynamic process. To a significant degree, long-term outcomes of the natural history of HIV-infection are determined by the pathophysiological events occurring during this period. Clearer understanding of the correlates of these outcomes will aid in identification of those most likely to benefit from early therapeutic intervention. Identification of patients during acute infection allows for ideal management of the infection from its earliest stages and has the potential to significantly impact further spread of the epidemic through early institution of risk reduction strategies.

References

1. Rinaldo CR Jr, Piazza P. Virus infection of dendritic cells: portal for host invasion and host defense. Trends Microbiol 2004; 12:337–345.
2. Douek DC , Brenchley JM, Betts MR, et al. HIV preferentially infects HIV-specific CD4[+] T cells. Nature 2002; 417:95–98.
3. Couedel-Courteille A, Pretet JL, Barget N, et al. Delayed viral replication and CD4(+) T cell depletion in the rectosigmoid mucosa of macaques during primary rectal SIV infection. Virology 2003; 316:290–301.
4. Veazey RS, DeMaria M, Chalifoux LV, et al. Gastrointestinal tract as a major site of CD4+ T cell depletion and viral replication in SIV infection. Science 1998; 280:427–431.
5. Guadalupe M, Reay E, Sankaran S, et al. Severe CD4+ T-cell depletion in gut lymphoid tissue during primary human immunodeficiency virus type 1 infection and substantial delay in restoration following highly active antiretroviral therapy. J Virol 2003; 77:11708–11717.
6. Mehandru S, Poles MA, Tenner-Racz K, et al. Primary HIV-1 infection is associated with preferential depletion of CD4+ T lymphocytes from effector sites in the gastrointestinal tract. J Exp Med 2004; 200:761–770.
7. Rosenberg ES, Billingsley JM, Caliendo AM, et al. Vigorous HIV-1-specific CD4+T cell responses associated with control of viremia. Science 1997; 278:1447–1450.
8. Oxenius A, Price DA, Easterbrook PJ, et al. Early highly active antiretroviral therapy for acute HIV-1 infection preserves immune function of CD8+ and CD4+ T lymphocytes. Proc Natl Acad Sci USA 2000; 97:3382–3387.
9. Younes SA, Yassine-Diab B, Dumont AR, et al. HIV-1 viremia prevents the establishment of interleukin 2-producing HIV-specific memory CD4+ T cells endowed with proliferative capacity. J Exp Med 2003; 198:1909–1922.
10. Routy JP, Vanhems P, Rouleau D, et al. Comparison of the clinical features of acute HIV-1 infection in patients infected sexually or through injection drug use. J Acquir Immune Defic Syndr 2000; 24:425–432.
11. Zaunders JJ, Kaufmann GR, Cunningham PH, et al. Increased turnover of CCR5+ and redistribution of CCR5-CD4 T lymphocytes during primary human immunodeficiency virus type 1 infection. J Infect Dis 2001; 183:736–743.
12. Zaunders JJ, Moutouh-de Parseval L, et al. Polyclonal proliferation and apoptosis of CCR5+ T lymphocytes during primary human immunodeficiency virus type 1 infection: regulation by interleukin (IL)-2, IL-15, and Bcl-2. J Infect Dis 2003; 187:1735–1747.
13. Zaunders J, Carr A, McNally L, et al. Effects of primary HIV-1 infection on subsets of CD4+ and CD8+ T lymphocytes. AIDS 1995; 9:561–566.
14. Pantaleo G, Demarest JF, Soudeyns H, et al. Major expansion of CD8+ T cells with a predominant VB usage during the primary immune response to HIV. Nature 1994; 370:463–467.
15. Koup RA, Safrit JT, Cao Y, et al. Temporal association of cellular immune responses with initial control of viraemia in primary human immunodeficiency type 1 syndrome. J Virol 1994; 68:4650–4655.
16. Wilson JD, Ogg GS, Allen RL, et al. Direct visualization of the HIV-1-specific cytotoxic T lymphocyte (CTL) response during primary HIV infection. AIDS 2000; 14:225–233.
17. Mackewicz CE, Yang LC, Lifson JD, et al. Non-cytolytic CD8 T-cell anti-HIV responses in primary HIV-1 infection. Lancet 1994; 344:1671–1673.
18. Jin X, Bauer DE, Tuttleton SE, et al. Dramatic rise in plasma viremia after CD8+ T cell depletion in Simian immunodeficiency virus-infected macaques. J Exp Med 1999; 189:991–998.
19. Reimann KA, Tenner-Racz K, Racz P, et al. Immunopathogenic events in acute infection of Rhesus monkeys with simian immunodeficiency virus of Macaques. J Virol 1994; 68:2362–2370.
20. Cao J, McNevin J, Holte S, et al. Comprehensive analysis of human immunodeficiency virus type 1 (HIV-1)-specific gamma interferon-secreting CD8+ T cells in primary HIV-1 infection. J Virol 2003; 77:6867–6878.
21. Lichterfeld M, Yu XG, Cohen D, et al. HIV-1 nef is preferentially recognized by CD T cells in primary HIV-1 infection despite a relatively high degree of genetic diversity. AIDS 2004; 18:1383–1392.
22. Price DA, Goulder PJ, Klenerman P, et al. Positive selection of cytotoxic T lymphocyte escape variants during primary infection. Proc Natl Acad Sci USA 1997; 94:1890–1895.

23. Borrow P, Lewicki H, Wei X, et al. Antiviral pressure exerted by HIV-1 specific cytotoxic T lymphocytes (CTLs) during primary infection demonstrated by rapid selection of CTL escape virus. Nat Med 1997; 3:205–211.

24. Burton DR. A vaccine for HIV type 1: the antibody perspective. Proc Natl Acad Sci USA 1997; 94: 10018–10023.

25. Richman DD, Wrin T, Little SJ, et al. Rapid evolution of the neutralizing antibody response to HIV type 1 infection. Proc Natl Acad Sci USA 2003; 100:4144–4149.

26. Arendrup M, Nielsen C, Hansen JE, et al. Autologous HIV-1 neutralizing antibodies: Emergence of neutralizing resistant escape virus and subsequent development of escape virus neutralizing antibodies. J Acquir Immune Defic Syndr 1992; 5:303–307.

27. Desrosiers RC. Escape from neutralizing antibody responses by sequence variation in the SIV envelope. 7th Annual Conference of the Australian Society for HIV Medicine; 1995.

28. Pacanowski J, Kahi S, Baillet M, et al. Reduced blood CD123+ (lymphoid) and CD11c+ (myeloid) dendritic cell numbers in primary HIV-1 infection. Blood 2001; 98:3016–3021.

29. Kaufmann GR, Cunningham P, Kelleher AD, et al. Patterns of viral dynamics during primary human immunodeficiency virus type 1 infection. Syd Primary HIV Infect Study Group J Infect Dis 1998; 178:1812–1815.

30. Mellors JW, Kingsley LA, Rinaldo CR Jr, et al. Quantitation of HIV-1 RNA in plasma predicts outcome after seroconversion. Ann Intern Med 1995; 122:573–579.

31. Derdeyn CA, Decker JM, Bibollet-Ruche F, et al. Envelope-constrained neutralization-sensitive HIV-1 after heterosexual transmission. Science 2004; 303:2019–2022.

32. Allen TM, Altfeld M, Yu XG, et al. Selection, transmission, and reversion of an antigen-processing cytotoxic T-lymphocyte escape mutation in human immunodeficiency virus type 1 infection. J Virol 2004; 78:7069–7078.

33. Friedrich TC, Dodds EJ, Yant LJ, et al. Reversion of CTL escape-variant immunodeficiency viruses in vivo. Nat Med 2004; 10:275–281.

34. Leslie AJ, Pfafferott KJ, Chetty P, et al. HIV evolution: CTL escape mutation and reversion after transmission. Nat Med 2004; 10:282–289.

35. Goulder PJ, Brander C, Tang Y, et al. Evolution and transmission of stable CTL escape mutations in HIV infection. Nature 2001; 412:334–338.

36. Koelsch KK, Smith DM, Little SJ, et al. Clade B HIV-1 superinfection with wild-type virus after primary infection with drug-resistant clade B virus. AIDS 2003; 17:11–16.

37. Altfeld M, Allen TM, Yu XG, et al. HIV-1 superinfection despite broad CD8+ T-cell responses containing replication of the primary virus. Nature 2002; 420:434–439.

38. Yerly S, Jost S, Monnat M, et al. HIV-1 co/super-infection in intravenous drug users. AIDS 2004; 18:1413–1421.

39. Smith DM, Wong JK, Hightower GK, et al. Incidence of HIV superinfection following primary infection. JAMA 2004; 292:1177–1178.

40. Sagar M, Lavreys L, Baeten JM, et al. Infection with multiple human immunodeficiency virus type 1 variants is associated with faster disease progression. J Virol 2003; 77:12921–12926.

41. Ritola K, Pilcher CD, Fiscus SA, et al. Multiple V1/V2 env variants are frequently present during primary infection with human immunodeficiency virus type 1. J Virol 2004; 78:11208–11218.

42. Cooper DA, Gold J, MacLean P, et al. Acute AIDS retrovirus infection. Lancet 1985; 1:537–540.

43. Vanhems P, Allard R, Cooper DA, et al. Acute Human Immunodeficiency virus type 1 disease as a mononucleosis-like illness: Is the Diagnosis too restrictive. Clin Infect Dis 1997; 24:965–970.

44. Pedersen C, Lindhardt BO, Jensen BL, et al. Clinical course of primary HIV infection: Consequences for subsequent course of infection. BMJ 1989; 299:965.

45. Ho DD, Sarngadharan MG, Resnick L, et al. Primary T-lymphotropic virus type III infection. Ann Intern Med 1985; 103:880–883.

46. Wolf F de, Lange JMA, Bakker M, et al. Influenza syndrome in homosexual men: A prospective diagnostic study. J R Coll Gen Pr 1988; 38:443.

47. Tindall B, Barker S, Donovan B, et al. Characterization of the acute clinical illness associated with human immunodeficiency virus infection. Arch Intern Med 1988; 148:945.

48. Montessori V, Rouleau D, Raboud J, et al. Clinical Characteristics of Primary HIV infection in intravenous drug users. AIDS 2000; 14:1868–1870.

49. Celum CL, Buchbinder SP, Donnell D, et al. Early Human Immunodeficiency virus (HIV) infection in the HIV Network for Prevention Trials Vaccine Preparedness Cohort: risk behaviors, symptoms and early plasma and genital track virus load. J Infect Dis 2001; 183:23–25.

50. Lavreys L, Thompson ML, Martin HL, et al. Primary Immunodeficiency virus Type 1 infection: clinical manifestations among women in Mombasa, Kenya. Clin Infect Dis 2000; 30:486–490.

51. Aggarwal M, Rein J. Acute human immunodeficiency virus syndrome in an adolescent. Pediatrics 2003; 112:e323.

52. Carr A, Cooper DA. Primary HIV infection. In: Sande MA, Volberding PA, eds. The medical management of AIDS. Philadelphia: WB Saunders; 1999:67–78.

53. Schacker T, Hughes J, Shea T, et al. Biological and virological characteristics of Primary HIV infection. Ann Intern Med 1998; 128:613–620.

54. Bonetti A, Weber R, Vogt MW, et al. Acute co-infection with human immunodeficiency virus (HIV) and cytomegalovirus. Ann Intern Med 1990; 111:293.

55. Ward JW, Bush TJ, Perkins HA, et al. The natural history of transfusion-associated HIV infection: factors influencing progression to disease. N Engl J Med 1989; 321:947.

56. Marion SA, Schecter MT, Weaver MS, et al. Evidence that prior immune dysfunction pre-disposes to human immunodeficiency virus infection in homosexual men. J Acquir Immune Defic Syndr 1989; 2:178.

57. Quinn TC, Wawer MJ, Sewankambo N, et al. Viral load and Heterosexual transmission of human immunodeficiency virus type 1. N Engl J Med 2000; 342:921–929.

58. Gray RH, Wawer MJ, Brookmeyer R, et al. Probability of HIV-1 transmission per coital act in monogamous heterosexual, HIV-1 discordant couples in Rakai, Uganda. Lancet 2001; 357:1149–1153.

59. Chakraborty H, Sen PK, Helms RW, et al. Viral burden in genital secretions determines male to female sexual transmission of HIV-1: A probabilistic empirical model. AIDS 2001; 15:621–627.

60. O'Brien TR, Busch MP, Donegan E, et al. Heterosexual transmission of human immunodeficiency virus type 1from transfusion recipients to their sex partners. J Acquir Immune Defic Syndr 1994; 7:705–710.

61. Xiridou M, Geskus R, de Wit J, et al. Primary HIV infection as source of HIV transmission within steady and casual partnerships among homosexual men. AIDS 2004; 18:1311–1320.

62. Fiebig EW, Wright DJ, Rawal BD, et al. Dynamics of HIV viremia and antibody seroconversion in plasma donors: implications for diagnosis and staging of primary HIV infection. AIDS 2003; 17:1871–1879.

63. Respess RA, Rayfield MA, Dondero TJ. Laboratory testing and rapid HIV assays: applications for HIV surveillance in hard-to-reach populations. AIDS Suppl 2001; 3:49–59.

64. Zaunders JJ, Cunningham PH, Kelleher AD, et al. Potent antiretroviral therapy of primary HIV-1 infection: partial normalization of T lymphocyte subsets and limited reduction of proviral DNA despite clearance of plasma viremia. J Infect Dis 1999; 180:320–329.

65. Young CL, Hu DJ, Byers R, et al. Evaluation of a sensitive/less sensitive testing algorithm using the bioMérieux Vironostika-LS assay for detecting recent HIV-1 subtype B9

or E infection in Thailand. AIDS Res Hum Retroviruses 2003; 19:481–486.

66. Hu DJ, Vanichseni S, Mock PA, et al. HIV type 1 incidence estimates by detection of recent infection from a cross-sectional sampling of injection drug users in Bangkok: Use of the IgG capture BED enzyme immunoassay. AIDS Res Hum Retroviruses 2003; 19:727–730.

67. Dobbs T, Kennedy S, Pau CP, et al. Performance characteristics of the immunoglobulin G-capture BED-enzyme immunoassay, an assay to detect recent human immunodeficiency virus type 1 seroconversion. J Clin Microbiol 2004; 42:2623–2638.

68. Wilson KM, Johnson EI, Croom HA, et al. Incidence immunoassay for distinguishing recent from established HIV-1 infection in therapy-naive populations. AIDS 2004; 18:2253–2259.

69. Weber B, Thorstensson R, Tanprasert S, et al. Reduction of the diagnostic window in three cases of human immunodeficiency-1 subtype E primary infection with fourth-generation HIV screening assays. Vox Sang 2003; 85:73–79.

70. Kaufmann GR, Cunningham P, Zaunders J, et al. Impact of early HIV-1 RNA and T-lymphocyte dynamics during primary HIV-1 infection on the subsequent course of HIV-1 RNA levels and CD4+ T-lymphocyte counts in the first year of HIV-1 infection. Syd Primary HIV Infect Study Group. J Acquir Immune Defic Syndr 1999; 22:437–444.

71. Ammaranond P, Cunningham P, Oelrichs R, et al. Rates of transmission of antiretroviral drug resistant strains of HIV-1. J Clin Virol 2003; 26:153–161.

72. Barbour JD, Hecht FM, Wrin T, et al. Persistence of primary drug resistance among recently HIV-1 Infected adults. AIDS 2004; 18:1863–1689.

73. Pilcher CD, Fiscus SA, Nguyen TQ, et al. Detection of Acute Infections during HIV Testing in North Carolina. N Eng J Med 2005; 352:1873–1883.

74. Smith DE, Walker BD, Cooper DA, et al. Is antiretroviral treatment of primary HIV infection clinically justified on the basis of current evidence? AIDS 2004; 18:709–718.

75. Kinloch-De Loes S, Hirschel BJ, Hoen B, et al. A controlled trial of zidovudine in primary human immunodeficiency virus infection. N Engl J Med 1995; 333:408–413.

76. Lindback S, Vizzard J, Cooper DA, et al. Long term prognosis following zidovudine monotherapy in primary human immunodeficiency virus type 1 infection. J Infect Dis 1999; 179:1549–1552.

77. Schiffer V, Deveau C, Meyer L, et al. Recent changes in the management of primary HIV-1 infection: results from the French PRIMO cohort. HIV Med 2004; 5:326–333.

CHAPTER 7

Biology of HIV-1 Transmission

Julie Overbaugh

Introduction

HIV-1 has spread rapidly around the globe, and in some parts of sub-Saharan Africa infects up to one-third of adults aged 15–49. Indeed, the effects of HIV-1 have been most devastating in the developing world: of the estimated 5 million new infections occurring each year, nearly 95% take place there (www.unaids.org).

HIV-1 can be transmitted sexually, from mothers to their infants, and via contaminated blood. Globally, heterosexual transmission accounts for the vast majority of new cases of HIV-1 infection, and the epidemic has had similar impact on men and women, with cases in women on the rise.[1] Since sexually infected women who become pregnant can in turn transmit the virus to their infants (called vertical transmission), preventing sexual transmission is viewed as key to slowing the HIV-1 pandemic.

Despite the virus's remarkable spread, the risk of transmission per exposure is low; estimates are on the order of 0.1% per contact for heterosexual transmission; The per-contact risk is higher (~1%) for male-to-male sexual transmission, and for blood exposures via contaminated needles (called parenteral transmission).[2] These numbers may underestimate the risk for persons who have other endogenous or exogenous risk factors that increase their susceptibility, as host factors of the source partner as well as those of the exposed individual are known to alter transmission risk. Certain features of the virus may also influence its fitness for transmission. Thus, the per-contact risk should be considered an average estimate that may be much higher (or lower) under certain circumstances, as discussed below.

HIV-1 can be transmitted from an infected mother to her infant *in utero*, during delivery, or through breast-feeding.[3,4] In the absence of any interventions to reduce transmission, approximately one-third of infants born to HIV-1-infected mothers will become infected. In breast-feeding populations, the risk of HIV-1 infection is almost double the risk in non-breast-feeding populations. While it may seem reasonable to therefore recommend against breast-feeding for all HIV-1-infected mothers, this must be balanced with the potential for increased mortality due to other infectious diseases, which can often occur in regions where access to clean water is limited. Fortunately, mother-to-child transmission of HIV-1 can be lowered considerably by antiviral treatment. In developed countries where state-of-the-art treatment is available, and HIV-1 infected mothers do not breast-feed, transmission is as low as 1–2%.

Factors in the Infecting Partner that Determine the Likelihood of Transmission

Higher virus levels in the infecting host (also called index case or source partner) are highly correlated with infection.[2] This is perhaps unsurprising, as one might expect that exposure to a higher dose of virus would increase the likelihood of transmission. In most studies, viral levels have been defined by measuring systemic HIV-1 RNA in plasma, even though plasma may not be the major bodily fluid to which the person is exposed to during sexual contact. However, the levels of virus in blood plasma are highly correlated with the viral levels in other body fluids, such as genital secretions, and it is likely these genital virus levels would similarly correlate to risk of sexual transmission. The presence of sexually transmitted diseases (STDs) has been shown to increase risk of transmission. Many STDs increase genital HIV-1 levels, which could in turn increase risk by increasing HIV-1 exposure. However, a direct link between genital virus levels and increased risk of sexual transmission has not yet been established.

Virus levels are highest during acute (primary) HIV-1 infection, before the virus is contained by the host, and this is thought to be the time when a person is most infectious.[2] Viral levels drop after primary infection resolves, and then slowly and steadily increase over time. Thus, the advanced stage of HIV-1 infection, when CD4$^+$ T-lymphocyte counts are low, is also a time when a person is potentially highly infectious, although probably less so than during primary infection.

There are several risk factors common to both vertical transmission and sexual transmission, including the levels of plasma virus in the index case.[2,4] In the case of vertical transmission, it has been shown that the levels of maternal breast-milk virus and genital virus correlate with the risk of infant infection. Poor breast health in a breast-feeding mother, particularly mastitis, increases infant risk of infection.

Premature birth has been associated with increased infant HIV-1 infection, which could reflect an increased risk of premature birth for infants infected *in utero*, rather than prematurity leading to a greater chance of HIV-1 infection. A prolonged duration of ruptured membranes is associated with increased transmission, whereas cesarean-section birth is associated with decreased risk. Presumably, these associations reflect the fact that during transit through the birth canal, the infant may be exposed to HIV-1 in both blood and genital secretions.

Factors in Viral Selection

HIV-1 is highly genetically variable and it continually evolves and adapts in the infected host.[5] HIV-1 seems to undergo a selective bottleneck during transmission because very few viruses are apparently transmitted from one host to another. It is possible that this bottleneck is at least partially a result of stochastic events that reflect the low frequency at which HIV-1 is transmitted. But it may also indicate that there is selection for particular variants with certain properties. The major lines of evidence to

support selective transmission include the observations that (1) the early virus population is often genetically less diverse than the source-virus population; and (2) viruses present early in infection tend to infect cells using one particular co-receptor (CCR5).

Several studies have shown that the virus population early in infection, which is presumably very similar to the virus that was transmitted, is genetically more homogeneous than the virus population that is present during chronic infection. The viral sequences present during the early stages of infection are often remarkably homogeneous, particularly in some studies of men and infants. However, in women there is evidence that multiple viral sequences are sometimes transmitted, and this has been observed at low frequency in men as well. Even in cases where the virus is heterogeneous early in infection, it appears to be less diverse than what would be expected during chronic infection, suggesting that only a subset of variants are successfully transmitted. However, it is also possible that the limited diversity of transmitted strains in some cases indicates that the source partners harbored a virus population of limited diversity, perhaps because they transmitted during their primary infection. Detailed studies of viruses in both the index case and their newly infected partner (transmission pairs) near the time of HIV-1 acquisition will be needed to better address these questions.

No matter what the complexity of the viral genotype, the viruses present within the first few months after infection almost invariably require the CCR5 co-receptor for entry (these are called R5 viruses).[5-7] CCR5 is one of two major HIV-1 co-receptors (the other being CXCR4), and the co-receptor, along with the CD4 receptor, is critical for HIV-1 entry into cells. The observation that most recently transmitted viruses are R5 viruses suggests that CCR5 variants are favored for transmission. This apparent selection for R5 viruses occurs during all routes of transmission, including sexual, vertical, and parenteral routes. In support of this model, it has been shown that individuals who do not express cell surface CCR5 due to a specific genetic polymorphism are less susceptible to HIV infection (see also below).

Despite the fact that transmitted viruses share a common co-receptor requirement, the viruses transmitted from different individuals are quite genetically distinct. This diversity has made vaccine development a daunting prospect. Thus, there has been considerable interest in defining common features among transmitted viral strains. Recently, signature sequence characteristics have been noted among viruses present early in infection, at least in some populations. In two studies of recently infected African individuals, the early viruses were found to have envelope proteins with short loop sequences that had relatively few glycosylation sites compared to viruses present in the index case, or in the circulating viruses. Vertically transmitted viruses also tend to be less glycosylated than those in the mother (the index case).[8] However, this sequence pattern was not observed in recently transmitted viruses characterized from US individuals who acquired HIV-1 through sexual contact. Thus, the sequence characteristics of transmitted viruses may not be the same in different risk groups, or in strains circulating in different regions (the African populations were infected with subtype A and C, all through heterosexual contact, whereas the US population was infected with subtype B, primarily via male-to-male transmission).[9–41] However, even if the sequence signatures of transmitted viruses are not generalizable across all virus subtypes, they may nonetheless provide insights into which biological properties of viruses increase their fitness for transmission.

Endogenous Host Factors

Host Genetics

Multiple host genetic polymorphisms have been linked to HIV-1 susceptibility.[12,13] The mutations that have been identified derive largely from targeted studies focused on genes that code for host factors known to be critical for HIV-1 replication. For example, many studies have focused on allelic variation within co-receptor genes, or genes coding for ligands that bind the HIV-1 co-receptors (e.g. CCL5/RANTES for CCR5 and CXCL12/SDF1 for CXCR4) and thus potentially compete for HIV-1 entry. Therefore, alterations in the expression or function of the proteins encoded by these genes could impact HIV-1 replication at the cellular level. Overall, studies of host genetic factors have provided a somewhat complex view of the effects of host genetics on HIV-1 transmission, as consistent results have not always been found across studies. This may partially be due to the complexity of the interactions between the different alleles, as well as differences in allele frequency and other factors in the populations examined. Moreover, with many of the mutations it is unclear whether they actually affect protein levels or function, or whether they were detected because they are genetically linked to other mutations in nearby genes, which play a more direct role in transmission.

Some studies have found clear and consistent evidence for a direct association between host genetics and HIV-1 susceptibility. This is the case with CCR5, where an inactivating genetic mutation ($\Delta 32$), which is present in a small fraction of Caucasians, has been associated with reduced susceptibility to HIV-1 infection in high-risk individuals with the homozygous $\Delta 32$ CCR5 allele. Lymphocytes and macrophages from these individuals are not permissive to replication of R5 viruses, providing biological support for the observed associations. However, this mutation is not found in Africans, and therefore is not a modulating risk factor for the African epidemic. Thus, although the $\Delta 32$ CCR5 mutation can have pronounced effects on HIV-1 susceptibility for an exposed individual, it has had limited global impact on HIV-1 spread.

A variety of other mutations in CCR5, found particularly in the promoter region, also appear to affect HIV-1 susceptibility. In addition, single nucleotide polymorphisms (SNPs) in several genes that encode chemokines or cytokines have been linked to HIV-1 susceptibility. In some cases, a particular haplotype, one that includes several SNPs, has been associated with susceptibility. The biological mechanism of action of most of these mutations, alone or in combination, remains to be elucidated.

Genetic variations in loci encoding molecules that play a role in acquired immunity have also been associated with HIV-1 transmission risk. Several studies suggest that human leukocyte antigen (HLA) allele concordance between the index case and the uninfected partner may increase the risk of transmission. HLA proteins are acquired on the virus as it buds from the host cell, and it has been postulated that discordance of HLA may mark the infectious virus as more immunologically foreign, and thus decrease transmission.

It is likely that other host genetic factors that affect HIV-1 transmission will be uncovered as we identify additional host cell proteins involved in HIV-1 replication. Indeed, a plethora of such proteins have been discovered recently (e.g. APOBEC3G, TRIM5a, APCE1, etc.), and the corresponding genes are being closely scrutinized for SNPs associated with HIV-1 susceptibility. Such candidate gene approaches have been fruitful, but are dependent on the initial identification of a host factor involved in HIV-1 replication. It seems likely that a more global genomic approach, which would sample a larger number of genes independently of whether they have an established link to HIV-1 replication, may yield a much longer list of polymorphisms involved in HIV-1 susceptibility. Unfortunately, such approaches are technically daunting at present. Until this becomes more feasible, there remain plenty of puzzles to resolve regarding the mechanisms that underlie some of the associations already observed.

Exogenous Host Factors

STDs, Female Hormones, Male Circumcision

Sexually transmitted diseases are a major risk factor for HIV-1 infection, and both ulcerative and non-ulcerative STDs have been shown to increase susceptibility to HIV-1.[2,14,15] These include a variety of specific sexually acquired infections, both viral (e.g. herpes simplex virus type 2, HSV-2) and bacterial (e.g. *Neisseria gonorrhoeae* and *Treponema pallidum*). It is likely that these STDs enhance susceptibility in part by increasing the number of activated T lymphocytes, which are targets for HIV-1 infection, at mucosal surfaces. In addition, some may disrupt mucosal integrity, providing access to T lymphocytes and other potential target cells in the submucosa.

The estimates of the effect of STDs on the risk of HIV-1 infection vary from study to study, but are likely to be in the range of 2–5-fold. Given the high prevalence of STDs in many parts of the world, the overall impact of STDs on HIV-1 spread is therefore likely to be significant. A recent clinical trial suggested that syndromic treatment of bacterial STDs may reduce HIV-1 infection, and thus provides a promising intervention to reduce both STD and HIV-1 infections. However, a subsequent mass-treatment trial for STDs did not show any benefit in reducing HIV-1 transmission rates. Thus, the benefit of broad STD treatment may be limited to certain populations, or to specific approaches to treatment. The impact of treatment for HSV-2 on HIV-1 acquisition is currently being evaluated.

In men, lack of circumcision increases their risk of HIV-1 acquisition, whereas for women, the use of hormonal contraceptives increases their risk of acquiring the virus. The results of recent clinical trials of male circumcision support a role for circumcision in reducing the risk of HIV-1 infection in men. The association between use of hormonal contraceptives and HIV-1 susceptibility has not been observed in all studies, particularly those in which there is not frequent monitoring to permit good estimates of the time of infection. However, this association has been observed in cases where information was available on hormonal contraceptive use very close to the time of HIV-1 acquisition. Importantly, it was observed after controlling for such confounding variables as condom use and sexual frequency. The findings in humans are supported by studies in the macaque model showing that progesterone increased the risk of SIV infection in the monkeys.

The mechanism by which exogenous female hormones influence HIV-1 susceptibility is not known. Several hypotheses have been suggested, including: (1) vaginal thinning leading to easier HIV-1 penetration; (2) changes in the resident mucosal cell population, potentially resulting in an influx of HIV-1-susceptible cells; and (3) alterations in cell susceptibility that result from changes in expression of host-cell proteins that are critical for HIV-1 replication. If such changes occur in response to exogenous hormones, it is possible that they may also occur during the normal hormonal fluctuations that regulate the menstrual cycle. However, there is currently no data to support this hypothesis.

Early Target Cells and Initial Virus-Host Dynamics

At least two molecules are required for HIV-1 entry into cells: CD4, plus a multiple-membrane-spanning chemokine receptor, such as CCR5 or CXCR4.[5,15] Because CD4 is required for virus binding, the host range of HIV-1 is largely restricted to CD4-positive cells, which include a subset of T lymphocytes (T-helper cells), cells of the monocyte lineage, and dendritic cells. Each of these cells is therefore a potential target for initial HIV-1 infection, and there is some evidence to support a role for each in early infection. However, as much of this information derives from either animal or culture model systems, each of which has limitations; the initial target cell for HIV-1 infection in a new host is not known.

In vitro studies suggest that CD4+ T lymphocytes must be activated to become productively infected by HIV-1, although CD4+ T lymphocytes that have the phenotype of resting cells have been shown to harbor HIV-1 *in vivo*. Certainly, CD4+ T lymphocytes are important either in the initial infection event and/or in subsequent dissemination of the virus from the mucosal site of entry. One currently favored model is that initial infection of CD4+ T lymphocytes is facilitated by dendritic cells (DCs).[16] DCs express CD4 and, depending on their maturation state, may express HIV-1 co-receptor(s). Immature DCs express CCR5 and can be infected by HIV-1 *in vitro*, whereas mature DCs cannot. More importantly, both immature and mature DCs have been shown to capture HIV-1 via a C-type lectin receptor (e.g. DC-SIGN) and transfer it to CD4+ T lymphocytes *in vitro*. Thus, one plausible model of HIV-1 transmission is that DCs positioned just below the mucosal epithelium capture HIV-1 and facilitate its transfer to lymphocytes, where the virus rapidly replicates and amplifies. Indeed, in animal model studies, virus dissemination to the draining lymph node has been shown to occur within 1 to 2 days after vaginal inoculation, and DCs have been implicated.

There is uncertainty over whether any of these models reflect reality which stems from our inability to study the earliest events in HIV-1 infection. Generally, infection cannot be detected, at least using non-invasive methods, for several weeks after the initial transmission, at which time the virus has become well established throughout the host tissues. Thus, the earliest events that lead to successful HIV-1 transmission have simply not been studied. Some studies have been conducted in animal model systems, but these have employed a very high inoculum, and viruses that are unlikely to represent the ones typically transmitted between humans. Thus, it is hard to know how well these models mimic HIV-1 transmission. Remarkably, it is not even clear if the virus that is transmitted is cell-free (extracellular, free virus) or cell-associated. Without good knowledge of the precise molecular interactions that govern initial infection, the design of interventions to target them is particularly challenging.

Superinfection

Re-infection by HIV-1 from another Source Partner

More and more data have been accumulating to suggest that transmission of HIV-1 occurs in the face of pre-existing HIV-1 infection.[17-20] Over the years, numerous studies have reported dual infection by two HIV-1 strains that were so unrelated as to be unlikely to have come from a single source. Dual infection has been identified in cases where there were viruses from two different HIV-1 subtypes, which typically differ by ~30% in their envelope proteins. Such variation extends well beyond what is typical *de novo* variation of the virus within a subject (up to 1% per year and usually not much more than ~5% overall during the course of a single infection). Because dual infections were identified in cross-sectional studies, it was not possible to establish exactly

when the second transmission event occurred, and indeed, whether it occurred in the person under study or in their source partner. Notably, HIV-1 intersubtype recombinants are common in many parts of the world where HIV-1 subtypes co-exist; these most certainly reflect dual or sequential infections, as they arise only after a cell becomes dually infected.

More definitive evidence for superinfection has come from some intensively monitored subjects who were part of various trials or studies. In these cases, one virus was detected over several visits, and then a second virus, which differed more than would be expected by *de novo* variation, emerged in the virus population. One case presented particularly compelling evidence for superinfection: after the person had engaged in high-risk behavior on holiday, a second strain was detected that was characteristic of those circulating in the region where the subject had vacationed.[21] However, many of these cases were somewhat unusual because the subjects had had treatment interruptions, or showed evidence of a less virulent initial virus, in some cases because it had acquired drug-resistance mutations, presumably in a treated source partner prior to transmission.

Several recent studies suggest that re-infections could be almost as common as initial infections, and that they occur in the face of high levels of replication of the first virus. This suggests that re-infection can occur even when the host already harbors a virus that is highly fit and well established. Of concern is the fact that re-infections appear to be occurring in some cases at a time when immune responses have had adequate time to develop to the first infection, but before immune function is completely compromised later in infection. These findings suggest that the immune responses that are generated to counteract one strain of HIV-1 do little to block transmission of a second strain.

Preventing HIV-1 Transmission

An HIV-1 vaccine is the best method to significantly impact HIV-1 spread and thus is the holy grail of HIV-1 prevention efforts. However, an effective HIV-1 vaccine is not likely to become available any time in the near future. In the meantime, much of HIV-1 prevention has focused on educational efforts to reduce risk behaviors and consequent exposure. In addition, the use of antiretrovirals to treat infected individuals may help reduce virus spread, because these treatments reduce source virus levels. Indeed, treatment of infected mothers has been repeatedly shown to reduce transmission to their infants, and similar effects are likely in cases of sexual and parenteral transmission. Thus, treatment may not only benefit the infected individual, but it can also have an effect at the population level.

Other methods for blocking transmission show promise, at least in model systems. For example, passive administration of antibodies has been shown to block transmission in macaque models. Such interventions are being considered to prevent mother-to-infant transmission in humans, particularly during breast-feeding. However, the passive immunization approach is currently limited because it requires too much of the antibody needed to block infection. In addition, the antigenic diversity of HIV-1 strains presents major challenges for all immune-based approaches to prevention. Thus, highly potent and broadly neutralizing antibodies or antibody cocktails are likely to be needed to make passive immunization efficacious. Similarly, compounds that competitively block HIV-1 binding to the CCR5 co-receptor have been shown to block infection in animal models. Such compounds, which are most effective when applied topically at the site of exposure just prior to sexual intercourse (as a microbicide),[22] currently appear to be one of the more promising means to prevent HIV-1 spread. Other broad spectrum microbicides, such as polyanion molecules, are also being considered. However, clinical trials of such compounds are just beginning, and thus their acceptability, tolerability, and efficacy in humans remains to be determined.

Prevention efforts have certainly been more challenging given our rather limited understanding of the initial events in HIV-1 transmission. Critical aspects of transmission, such as the precise source of the virus and initial target cells for infection are not known. Without a better understanding of the factors that encourage or discourage transmission of HIV-1, we have little hope of stopping its spread.

References

1. Quinn TC, Overbaugh J. HIV/AIDS in women: an expanding epidemic. Science 2005; 308:1582–1583.

2. Baeten JM, Overbaugh J. Measuring the infectiousness of persons with HIV-1: Opportunities for preventing sexual HIV-1 transmission. Curr HIV Res 2003; 1:69–86.

3. John GC, Kreiss J. Mother-to-child transmission of human immunodeficiency virus type 1. Epidemiol Rev 1996; 18:149–157.

4. John-Stewart G, Mbori-Ngacha D, Ekpini R, et al. Breastfeeding and transmission of HIV-1. J Acquir Immune Defic Syndr 2004; 35:196–202.

5. Overbaugh J, Bangham CR. Selection forces and constraints on retroviral sequence variation. Science 2001; 292:1106–1109.

6. Berger EA, Murphy PM, Farber JM. Chemokine receptors as HIV-1 coreceptors: roles in viral entry, tropism, and disease. Annu Rev Immunol 1999; 17:657–700.

7. Hoffman TL, Doms RW. Chemokines and coreceptors in HIV/SIV-host interactions. AIDS 1998; 12:17–26.

8. Wu X, Parast AB, Richardson BA, et al. Neutralization escape variants of human immunodeficiency virus type 1 are transmitted from mother to infant. J Virol 2006; 80:835–844.

9. Chohan B, Lang D, Sagar M, et al. Selection for human immunodeficiency virus type 1 envelope glycosylation variants with shorter V1-V2 loop sequences occurs during transmission of certain genetic subtypes and may impact viral RNA levels. J Virol 2005; 79:6528–6531.

10. Derdeyn CA, Decker JM, Bibollet-Ruche F, et al. Envelope-constrained neutralization-sensitive HIV-1 after heterosexual transmission. Science 2004; 303:2019–2022.

11. Frost SD, Liu Y, Pond SL, et al. Characterization of human immunodeficiency virus type 1 (HIV-1) envelope variation and neutralizing antibody responses during transmission of HIV-1 subtype B. J Virol 2005; 79:6523–6527.

12. Kaslow RA, Dorak T, Tang JJ. Influence of host genetic variation on susceptibility to HIV Type 1 infection. J Infect Dis 2005; 191:68–77.

13. O'Brien SJ, Nelson GW. Human genes that limit AIDS. Nat Genet 2004; 36:565–574.

14. Benki S, McClelland RS, Overbaugh J. Risk factors for human immunodeficiency virus type-1 acquisition in women in Africa. J Neurovirol 2005; 11:S58–S65.

15. Fleming DT, Wasserheit JN. From epidemiological synergy to public health policy and practice: the contribution of other sexually transmitted diseases to sexual transmission of HIV infection. Sex Transm Infect 1999; 75:3–17.

16. Pope M, Haase AT. Transmission, acute HIV-1 infection and the quest for strategies to prevent infection. Nat Med 2003; 9:847–852.

17. Allen TM, Altfeld M. HIV-1 superinfection. J Allergy Clin Immunol 2003; 112:829–836.

18. Blackard JT, Mayer KH. HIV superinfection in the era of increased sexual risk-taking. Sex Transm Dis 2004; 31:201–204.

19. Chan DJ. HIV-1 superinfection: evidence and impact. Curr HIV Res 2004; 2:271–274.

20. Smith DM, Richman DD, Little SJ. HIV superinfection. J Infect Dis 2005; 192:438–444.

21. Jost S, Bernard MC, Kaiser L, et al. A patient with HIV-1 superinfection. N Engl J Med 2002; 347:731–736.

22. Shattock RJ, Moore JP. Inhibiting sexual transmission of HIV-1 infection. Nat Rev Microbiol 2003; 1:25–34.

CHAPTER 8

The Design of a Global AIDS Vaccine

John R. Mascola
Richard A. Koup

Introduction

The enormous human toll of the global human immunodeficiency virus type 1 (HIV-1)/acquired immunodeficiency syndrome (AIDS) pandemic has appropriately focused scientific resources on the development of an effective AIDS vaccine. Despite a remarkable expansion of scientific knowledge about HIV-1, the conduct of numerous phase I vaccine studies and the successful completion of a phase III efficacy trail, there are still many hurdles to overcome before successful AIDS vaccine development. Among these challenges are the incomplete knowledge regarding protective immunity, the extensive genetic diversity of the virus, and viral immune evasion mechanisms. Despite considerable progress we are still learning how best to optimize immunogens and vaccination strategies to elicit protective HIV-1 specific immune responses in humans. Numerous vaccine prototypes have now been studied in pre-clinical and early phase I testing, most based on reasonable assumptions about the need to induce HIV-1 specific CD8 T-cell immunity or antiviral neutralizing antibodies, yet we still lack a vaccine.

The choice of antigens for HIV vaccine design begins with the 12 or so gene products normally expressed by the virus. Among these viral gene products are the major structural proteins, as well as the potent viral regulatory genes, that control the expression of HIV during infection. The structural proteins, Gag, Pol and Env, have long been considered the major targets relevant to HIV vaccine design, because exposure of Env on the surface of the virus particle is the most accessible target to antibody neu-

tralization and because the internal proteins, Gag and Pol, are relatively abundant proteins and are therefore logical targets for recognition by the cellular arm of the immune system.

While the Env and Gag proteins are the most abundant viral proteins, and likely to be readily exposed to the immune system during natural infection, there are reasons to consider additional viral proteins as components of HIV vaccines. The expression of HIV gene products within infected cells begins with the synthesis of the early, highly spliced RNA species that give rise to the Tat, Rev and Nef gene products. These regulatory proteins are synthesized at lower levels within the cell; however, they regulate the expression of the viral structural proteins made from the unspliced messages at later points in the virus replication cycle. Therefore, these proteins would appear to offer reasonable 'early' targets. For this reason, the Tat, Rev and Nef proteins have been proposed as components of vaccines. However, we do not have a known correlate of immune protection in HIV infection. Therefore, choosing the appropriate antigens to include in a vaccine will have to be made based upon consideration of antigen size, variability, expression levels, expression timing, and immunogenicity.[1]

In addition to the specific gene products that can serve as components of a vaccine, the character of the immune response generated to these gene products is of paramount importance to HIV vaccine design strategies. It is likely that the containment of HIV will be more effective when multiple epitopes can be presented to the immune system, providing greater negative pressure on viral replication. Theoretically, it is desirable to generate T-cell immunity to multiple conserved and sequence-constrained regions encompassing a large percentage of the viral open reading frames. Although antibody responses can be generated to nearly all of the viral proteins, the ability to generate relevant broadly neutralizing antibodies to the viral envelope is perhaps the most important challenge in HIV vaccine research. The ability to develop these antibodies to any specific HIV strain, as well as to deal with the enormous clade and strain diversity of the HIV envelope, poses a major challenge to effective AIDS vaccine development. This chapter will provide an overview of the rationale for some of these vaccine strategies and the choice of immunogens to include in a candidate vaccine.

Vaccines Designed to Elicit HIV-1 Specific Cd8 T-cell Responses

Many current HIV-1 vaccine strategies are aimed at inducing HIV-specific CD8 T-cell immunity. CD8 T cells can inhibit HIV-1 replication *in vitro* and their emergence in primary HIV-1 infection precedes the initial drop in plasma viremia.[2,3] Such cells are also readily detected in long-term non-progressing patients. These data suggest that HIV-1 specific CD8 T cells play an important role in controlling HIV-1 replication. More direct proof comes from the simian immunodeficiency virus (SIV) macaque model where depletion of CD8 T cells by anti-CD8 antibody infusion was directly correlated with a rise in SIV plasma viremia.[4,5] Similarly, animals depleted of CD8 T cells prior to SIV infection were unable to control initial viral replication.[6] Initial data from vaccine experiments in non-human primates has confirmed the importance of T-cell immunity. In the SIV and SHIV challenge models, the level of vaccine induced and anamnestic T-cell responses generally correlates with the level of protection mediated by immunization.[7-9] After viral challenge, vaccinated animals can experience long-term reductions in plasma viremia and preservation of CD4 T cells. Based on these types of data, a major goal of many HIV-1 vaccine strategies is the generation of cellular immunity, particularly HIV-1 specific CD8 T cells. These types of vaccines are often referred to as cytotoxic T-cell (CTL)-based vaccines.

Gene-based Vaccine Strategies

The safety concerns inherent in the traditional approaches of live attenuated and whole-inactivated virus vaccination have made these modalities impractical for human HIV/AIDS vaccine development. This has led to a plethora of novel vaccine strategies aimed at generating potent cellular immunity. These newer gene-based vaccines include DNA plasmids and recombinant viral vectors each encoding viral immunogens under the control of potent eukaryotic promoters. DNA plasmid immunization can induce detectable immune responses in non-human primates,[8] but more robust responses are generated after boosting with a viral vector. This bimodal strategy of DNA prime followed by viral vector boost, has become a common approach for eliciting cellular immune responses.[7,9] However, viral vectors alone or in sequential combinations may also produce robust immunity.[9]

Vectors of the pox family of viruses have been the most extensively studied as SIV and HIV vaccine products. Initial studies were performed with the prototype replication competent vaccinia virus; more recent studies have used less pathogenic poxviruses such as modified vaccinia Ankara (MVA), NYVAC (New York vaccinia virus attenuated by gene deletions) and canarypox (ALVAC). Other replication competent viral vectors include attenuated serotypes 4 and 7 adenovirus, vesicular stomatitis virus (VSV) and poliovirus. Each of these can induce cellular immune responses in non-human primates. Viral vectors engineered to produce a single cycle of infection and gene delivery have some inherent safety advantages and may have a more direct road to human phase I studies. These include vectors of the alphavirus family (such as Venezuelan equine encephalitis virus, Semliki forest virus and Sindbis), recombinant serotype-5 adenovirus (ADV), adeno-associated virus (AAV) and herpes simplex virus (HSV). The details of these gene-based vectors are reviewed in greater detail elsewhere.[1,6,10] Among these replication defective viral vectors, the largest body of human clinical data exists for serotype 5 ADV, as these constructs have been used as vectors for gene therapy. Immunization data from non-human primate studies with ADV vectors are promising[9,11] and such vectors are in phase I human trials. Due to the potential for decreased immunogenicity in people with pre-existing ADV-5 immunity, novel ADV serotypes and other strategies are being considered to circumvent the problem of pre-existing immunity.

Choice of Immunogens

HIV-1 encodes more than 12 gene products, but vaccine design is complicated by the considerable genetic diversity of the virus. Some viral proteins show greater diversity than others, with the Env and Gag regions showing 70–85% identity among isolates, while Pol shows a much higher degree of conservation. For vaccine design, it is important to consider ways to induce coverage against this diversity, whether through the inclusion of immunogens from various representative strains or through the presentation of consensus or ancestral sequences. The optimal approach to this problem is not yet known and will be an important subject of future investigation. In addition to antigenic complexity, the variability of the major histocompatibility complex in humans adds to the unpredictable nature of immune responsiveness to any given epitope. Since gene-based vectors can be readily manipulated, investigators can make rational choices about the immunogens to include in a vaccine, and these can be empirically tested in clinical trials (Table 8.1).[12-22] While knowledge of HLA-restricted epitopes in natural infection and data from non-human primate animal models provide some insights about possible immunogens, there is little direct scientific evidence to guide the choice of immunogen selection for an HIV-1 vaccine. In addition, the genetic diversity of HIV-1 does not necessarily reflect differences in immunogenicity between viral isolates. So how genetic variability of the virus will affect the breadth of protective immune mechanisms remains unknown. These uncertainties result in numerous empirical choices for candidate vaccines. Eventually, decisions about advancement into clinical trials will need to come from carefully derived data on the type and potency of immune responses generated. Currently, there are various vaccine approaches under development, which include those containing single conserved genes, genes genetically matched to geographic region, multiple genes representing diverse HIV-1 strains and consensus gene sequences.[1,6,10]

Because CTLs are more likely than antibodies to be effective against internal viral proteins, much attention has focused on the use of Gag and Pol proteins as immunogens. While HIV-1 strains belonging to the same genetic subtype can differ by up to 20% in the amino acid sequence of their envelope proteins, and by up to 35% between genetic subtypes, inter-subtype diversity for Gag is about 15% and for Pol about 10%.[23] Thus, one approach toward CTL-based vaccines is to target proteins that are 85–90% conserved among diverse HIV-1 strains. If the immune responses to Gag and Pol were to be protective, a candidate vaccine may not need to be multivalent. There are limited data to support or refute this approach.[24] Non-human primate studies

indicate that DNA and/or viral vector immunization with Gag or Gag-Pol constructs induces partial protection against a homologous SIV challenge.[25,26] These studies confirm a likely role for these internal proteins in a vaccine, but do not address the breadth of protective immunity in the setting of heterologous virus challenge. Recombinant adenovirus (ADV) type 5 expressing SIV Gag has also been shown to provide partial protection against homologous SHIV-challenge, and this product has advanced to phase I human studies.[9]

One potential obstacle to CTL-based vaccines is the documented emergence of CTL escape. In the SHIV-macaque model, the partial protection afforded by SIV Gag-specific CD8 T-cell responses can be overcome by a single mutation in the immunodominant Gag CTL epitope. This resulted in increased plasma viremia and disease progression in several Gag vaccinated animals.[27] In humans, CTL escape from a conserved HLA B27-resrticted Gag CTL epitope leads to loss of recognition and disease progression.[28] These data provide a conceptual rationale for the inclusion of multiple genes in a vaccine construct; i.e. pre-existing immune responses to a diverse array of epitopes may prevent or limit viral escape from vaccine-induced responses. Indeed, many groups of investigators have developed gene-based constructs that express multiple proteins, such as those that express Gag, Pol and Env.[7,8] In addition to Gag, Pol and Env proteins, there has been interest in the inclusion of regulatory genes such as Tat, Rev and Nef. Among these, Tat has received the most attention because it is expressed early after viral infection and therefore may be an initial target for pre-existing vaccine induced responses.[29] While macaque challenge studies have yielded conflicting data about the effect of a Tat vaccination,[30,31] there remains interest in both protein and gene-based immunization strategies for Tat, and there are plans for a phase I human study of a recombinant Tat protein.

The identification of optimal antigens to include in an HIV vaccine designed to elicit a cellular immune response also requires careful consideration of protein length, variability, and immunogenicity. By studying the immune responses to HIV proteins in infected individuals, some fundamental characteristics of the antigens, and their appropriateness for inclusion in a vaccine, have been delineated. While the vast majority of defined epitopes are found in HIV Gag, Pol, Env, and Nef,[32] recent evidence indicates that the accessory proteins Tat, Rev, Vif, Vpu, and Vpr are also commonly recognized,[33,34] albeit at a considerably lower magnitude in most individuals.

Table 8.1 Advanced clinical trials of HIV preventive vaccines[12-14]

Producer/ trials group	HIV genes represented	HIV subtypes	Vaccine type	Expected immunity	Country/ region	Size	Outcome
Efficacy trials (Phase IIb or III) completed or ongoing as of January 2006							
VaxGen	Env	B	protein	Ab	US, Canada, Netherlands	5403	No efficacy[15]
VaxGen	Env	B,E	protein	Ab	Thailand	2546	No efficacy[16]
Sanofi-Pasteur + VaxGen/USMHRP/TAVEG	Gag, Pol, Env	B,E	canarypox + protein	T-cell + Ab	Thailand	16,000	In progress[17]
Merck/HVTN	Gag, Pol, Nef	B	type 5 adenovector	T-cell	US, Canada, Peru, Australia, Haiti, DR	3000	In progress
Confirmatory immunogenicity trials (Phase II or Large Phase I/II) 2002–2006[a]							
Sanofi-Pasteur + VaxGen/HVTN	Gag, Pro, RT, Nef, Env	B,B	canarypox + protein	T-cell + Ab	US	330	Low cellular responses[b]
MRC Oxford/IAVI/KAVI	Gag, Pol, Nef, Env	A,A	DNA + MVA	T-cell	UK, Kenya	111	Low cellular responses[b]
Merck/HVTN	Gag	B	type 5 adenovector	T-cell	US, Caribbean, Southern Africa, South America, Thailand	435	In progress
Sanofi-Pasteur + ANRS	Gag, Pol, Nef	B	lipopeptides	T-cell	France	132	In progress
Sanofi-Pasteur + ANRS/HVTN	Gag, Pol, Nef	B	lipopeptides	T-cell	US	174	In progress
Vaccine Research Center, NIAID, NIH/HVTN/IAVI/USMHRP	Gag, Pol, Nef, Env	B,A,B,C	DNA + type 5 adenovector	T-cell	US, Caribbean, East Africa, South Africa, S. America	916	In progress
Targeted Genetics/IAVI	Gag, Pro, RT	C	AAV	T-cell+ Ab	South Africa	78	In progress

Note: Approximately 30 additional products, including DNA plasmids, viral vectors, peptides, and proteins, alone or in combination, are currently in Phase I or Phase I/II trials to assess safety and preliminary immunogenicity. For regularly updated listings of HIV vaccine trials, see references [12-14]. [a]Earlier confirmatory immunogenicity trials included envelope subunits[18-20] and a canarypox vector[19] that did not progress to efficacy testing; the envelope subunits later tested for efficacy by VaxGen[18,21], and the canarypox vector/envelope subunit combination currently being tested for efficacy in Thailand.[22] [b]Cellular responses as detected by interferon-gamma ELIspot assay. The correlation between ELIspot responses and protective immunity against HIV has not been established. Ab, antibody; AAV, adeno-associated virus; ANRS, Agence Nationale de Recherches sur le SIDA (France); HVTN, HIV Vaccine Trials Network; IAVI, International AIDS Vaccine Initiative; KAVI, Kenya AIDS Vaccine Initiative; NIAID, National Institute of Allergy and Infectious Disease (US); NIH, National Institutes of Health (US); MRC, Medical Research Council (UK); TAVEG, Thailand AIDS Vaccine Evaluation Group; USMHRP, United States Military HIV Research Program. (*Source:* Laurence Peiperl.)

One could argue that HIV Gag and Pol, being the most highly conserved HIV proteins that contains the largest number of defined epitopes,[32] should be the best candidate antigens to employ in an HIV vaccine. However, responses to the more variable accessory proteins are quite substantial in many HIV-infected patients,[33,34] yet their high sequence variability may make them poor candidates to include in a vaccine[35] even taking into consideration their early expression within the viral life cycle. Normalizing the T-cell response to take into account the protein length, it has been found that HIV Gag and Nef are the most frequently recognized antigens by CD8 T cells, on a response per amino acid basis.[35] Interestingly, the accessory protein Nef, despite its relatively high variability, elicits an extremely strong CD8+ T-cell response, targeted primarily to the more conserved regions of the protein. Overall, on the basis of length, variability, and immunogenicity, most investigators agree that one or more of the HIV antigens Gag, Pol, Env, and Nef should be included in a vaccine.[35]

To further address the issue of HIV-1 diversity and vaccine development, the Vaccine Research Center (VRC) of the National Institutes of Allergy and Infectious Disease, National Institutes of Health sponsored a meeting in collaboration with the World Health Organization and the Joint United Nations Programme on HIV/AIDS. The meeting led to consensus recommendations on how best to address this scientific issue in the context of current vaccine efforts.[36] There was general agreement that HIV-1 genetic diversity may be an obstacle to vaccine development, but that there is little scientific rationale for matching vaccine clades to the particular country from which they emanate. Testing of multiclade vaccines was suggested, but practical limitations on manufacturing and testing dictate that vaccine candidates should be representative of clades rather than be country-specific. As a result of this meeting in July 2001, the VRC undertook plans to develop a multivalent, multiclade immunogen, based on DNA plasmids and recombinant ADV vectors. This candidate vaccine contains six DNA plasmid constructs. One plasmid each encodes a Gag, Pol, and Nef protein based on the clade B HxB2 viral sequence. The other three plasmids encode the gp145 envelope sequence from a clade A, B, and C virus strain, respectively. Three recombinant ADV constructs, expressing the same Env proteins with slight modifications, and a fourth ADV construct encoding a Gag-Pol fusion protein will be used to boost the DNA immunization. The components of this vaccine strategy have been tested in non-human primates[37]

and are currently being evaluated in human phase I and II studies.

An additional approach to viral diversity is to match the immunogen to the predominant clade present in the region where the vaccine will be tested. One such DNA/MVA prime boost approach includes a consensus clade A Gag protein fused to a string of partially overlapping clade A-derived CTL epitopes.[38] The Gag protein includes both HLA class I and II restricted epitopes to induce T-cell help thought to be important in induction of potent immune responses. This candidate vaccine has been through pre-clinical testing and is currently in phase I trails in the UK and Kenya (where clade A viruses predominate). As an alternative to clade specific vaccine constructs, some have suggested that evolutionary relationships may be more useful than regional considerations.[23] They propose the use of consensus or ancestral sequences that would be used to minimize the genetic differences between vaccine strains and contemporary isolates. This is an intriguing approach to CTL-based immunization. Rather than the arbitrary choice of a gene based on one circulating HIV-1 strain, it is hoped that a consensus or ancestral sequence would induce an immune response that is reactive with a greater proportion of circulating viruses than any one existing virus sequence. Immunogens incorporating these types of designs are progressing through pre-clinical evaluation, and such studies should indicate if the breadth of immunity against present day circulating strains is increased by this approach.

Vaccines Designed to Elicit Neutralizing Antibodies

Traditional viral vaccines, such as those for polio, influenza and hepatitis B, elicit neutralizing antibodies that play a major role in conferring protective immunity. The success of the hepatitis B vaccine, based on recombinant protein expression of the viral surface antigen, led to optimism that the surface glycoprotein of HIV-1 could also be expressed and used as an effective vaccine. However, phase I studies of monomeric gp120 and gp160 vaccine products demonstrated that the neutralizing antibodies elicited were active only against laboratory-adapted rather than primary HIV-1 isolates.[39] While the implications of these *in vitro* data were initially not entirely clear, the successful completion of a phase III trial of a bivalent gp120 recombinant protein vaccine has provided evidence that the antibody response elicited was not protective.[40] We now appreciate that HIV-1 employs a complex array of immune evasion mechanisms to avoid antibody-mediated neutralization.[41-45] The genetic diversity among HIV-1 strains translates into an extraordinary level of antigenic diversity, particularly in Env. The potentially vulnerable regions of the Env, such as receptor binding sites or fusion domains appear to be either poorly immunogenic or shielded from antibody reactivity. In addition, the HIV-1 Env is heavily glycosylated and such sugar moieties impede antibody binding to Env. Finally, the trimeric nature of the gp120/gp41 complex, together with the variable loop regions, appears to form a structure that shields key epitopes for neutralizing antibodies.[46] With regard to fist generation monomeric gp120 vaccines, the gp120 antibodies elicited did not effectively bind to the native trimeric gp120/gp41 complex on virions, and thus did not neutralize most primary HIV-1 strains.[39,47] In contrast to these vaccine sera, antibodies elicited during natural HIV-1 infection can sometimes neutralize primary HIV-1 stains.[39,48,49] Assays of HIV-1 positive sera and isolation of neutralizing mAbs suggest that such neutralizing antibodies are a minor subset of the Env reactive antibodies elicited during natural infection.[42,47] Nonetheless, this provides evidence that the humoral immune system does find ways to overcome the barriers to HIV-1 neutralization. Evidence that appropriately potent neutralizing antibodies can protect comes from studies of passive antibody immunization followed by SHIV-challenge. In these studies, neutralizing monoclonal antibodies could prevent the establishment of infection or mediate long-term reductions in plasma viremia.[50] Thus, newer antibody-based vaccines approaches are aimed at the development of immunogens that improve the potency of antibodies generated, and their breadth of reactivity.

Design of Improved Antibody-Based Immunogens

One approach to improving antibody responses is based on the hypothesis that a protein immunogen should closely mimic the native HIV-1 envelope glycoprotein structure. Antibody mapping studies, and the more recent HIV-1 gp120 atomic structure, suggest that many epitopes on monomeric gp120 are unavailable within the context of the native trimeric Env.[45,46] This suggests that a trimeric envelope protein might elicit antibodies to epitopes that are exposed on the native envelope glycoprotein and therefore

neutralize HIV-1. Several groups are pursuing this strategy,[51,52] and emerging data suggest that these oligomeric protein immunogens elicit more potent neutralizing antibody responses than monomeric gp120.[53] While such immunogens do appear to be qualitatively different than prior gp120 immunogens, the antibody specificities elicited are still not well characterized and additional research will be required to achieve the ultimate goal of inducing antibodies similar to the well characterized neutralizing IgG monoclonal antibodies (mAbs) such as b12, 2G12, 2F5 and 4E10. Thus, a related approach attempts to use the specific epitopes of the well-known neutralizing mAbs as immunogens. These immunogens can be linear peptides, peptide mimetics, or modified Env structures designed to optimize the immunogenicity of a known epitope.[46] For several reasons, the membrane proximal region of gp41 has engendered particular interest for vaccine design. Two broadly neutralizing mAbs are directed against this fairly conserved region of gp41 and epitope mapping of mAbs 2F5 and 4E10 initially suggested that the epitopes had a linear conformation. However, attempt to elicit 2F5- or 4E10-like antibodies using linear peptides have been unsuccessful and recent structural data demonstrates a more complex non-linear conformation of this ectodomain region of gp41.[46] Thus, more recent work has focused on an understanding of the structural basis of gp41-mediated viral neutralization, in hopes that this will lead to novel strategies for immunogen design.[54,55]

A complementary approach to the design of antibody-based vaccines is to introduce specific modifications to the HIV-1 envelope structure in order to better expose or stabilize key epitopes. Since HIV-1 is a chronically replicating lentivirus, it must continually evade the host's antibody response.[43,44] Our understanding of these immune evasion mechanisms has increased dramatically over the past few years and there is optimism that this will lead to novel immunogen strategies.[46,56] As noted above, HIV-1 uses variable loop structures, sugar moieties and the tertiary conformation of the trimeric envelope structure to shield neutralization epitopes.[45] Thus, it may be possible to modify the envelope structure to highlight neutralization epitopes that are otherwise cryptic or sub-optimally immunogenic. The removal of specific glycosylation sites, or of variable loop regions, can lead to better exposure of neutralization epitopes, making the virus highly sensitive to neutralizing antibodies. Immunogens based on these modifications may generate better neutralizing antibody responses,[57-59] but it is not yet clear if the antibodies elicited will be able to bind the native envelope glycoprotein present on most primary viruses.[46,50] Our group at the VRC has designed a gene-based Env immunogen with deletions in the gp120/41 cleavage site, the fusion domain and the gp41 heptad repeats. These mutations appear to stabilize the Env conformation and improve antibody responses in immunized animals.[61] More recently, we have shown that removal of the V12 region, and selective modifications to stabilize the V3 loop, can improve the neutralization potency of V3 loop antibodies elicited by Env immunization.[62] While the breadth of neutralization by V3 antibodies is limited,[63] this proof of concept suggests that the immunogenicity of other neutralizing antibody epitopes may be improved by structural modifications to Env. Another recent approach uses a hyperglycosylated envelope glycoprotein that shields most non-neutralizing epitopes. This type of modified envelope is designed to preferentially bind antibodies directed against the CD4 binding site of gp120, particularly the potently neutralizing IgG1b12.[64]

Other investigators have tried to stabilize envelope glycoprotein intermediates that arise during the process of virus-cell fusion. HIV-1 Env fusion is triggered by sequential binding to CD4 and to the CCR5 or CXCR4 co-receptor. Since the fusion machinery of HIV-1 is highly conserved, such fusion intermediate epitopes are potential targets for neutralizing antibodies. These include epitopes on the chemokine binding domain that are induced after CD4 binding[65] and on the pre-hairpin intermediate that forms prior to the final steps of fusion.[66] While we have an improved understanding of the structure and function of these epitopes, they have so far been difficult targets for vaccine design. For example, several mAbs directed against the conserved co-receptor binding domain of Env have been described. The mAbs, such as mAb 17b, neutralize HIV-1 only if the epitope has been exposed by prior Env binding to CD4; i.e. by itself, mAb 17b does not neutralize HIV-1. This lack of neutralization appears to be the result of both kinetic and spatial constraints. During HIV-1 fusion, the CD4 induced co-receptor binding domain may only briefly be accessible to antibody. Recent evidence demonstrates that mAb 17b can neutralize HIV-1 as a single chain or Fab fragment, but not as an IgG. These constraints on IgG molecules suggest that it may be difficult to target HIV-1 via this region, unless a strategy can be designed to expose the epitope, perhaps with an antibody that mimics binding to CD4. Similarly, antibodies to epitopes on the pre-hairpin fusion intermediates of gp41 do not neutralize the virus. This region may be only transiently exposed during fusion and may be spatially constrained by close proximity to the cell membrane. Fortunately, there are regions on the ectodomain of gp41, such as those bound by mAbs 2F5 and 4E10 mentioned above, that do present vulnerable epitopes on gp41. This has focused vaccine design efforts on the membrane proximal region of gp41.[46]

Breadth of the Neutralizing Antibody Response

Numerous studies of antibody reactivity have demonstrated that HIV-1 displays a remarkable amount of antigenic diversity. While genetic subtype may not strictly correspond to a neutralization serotype, there is ample evidence that the antibody response in natural infection is not broadly neutralizing. Sera or mAbs from most clade B HIV-1 infected patients have a limited breadth of activity against clade B viruses and even less activity against viruses from other clades.[49,63] A few sera appear to be broadly neutralizing, yet the specificities of antibodies that combine to create this broad neutralizing activity have not been well defined. Additionally, even potent neutralizing mAbs such as 2F5 and b12 neutralize only 70–90% of clade B viruses and an even lower percentage of non-clade B viruses.[63] Since most current immunogens induce neutralizing antibodies of modest potency and breadth, the antigenic diversity of HIV-1 is viewed as a major obstacle for antibody-based vaccines.

To address the problem of breadth of immunity, some groups are constructing envelope immunogens from non-clade B subtypes[37,38,67] Given the genetic diversity among HIV-1 clades, it is possible that the antibody response induced by a vaccine immunogen will react more potently with closely related viruses. However, little is know about the specificities of antibodies elicited by most vaccines, or their breadth of reactivity. If a vaccine elicits antibodies to an immunogenic but variable region of the HIV-1 envelope, such as the V3 loop, it may be necessary to produce a multivalent immunogen to broaden the antibody response. There have been few studies evaluating multivalent antibody-based immunogens,[68] but several groups of investigators are pursing this approach. The gene-based immunization platforms discussed above, such as DNA and ADV, allow fairly rapid construction of gene constructs which facilitate the testing of multivalent multiclade immunogens.

To most effectively assess and compare the neutralizing antibody response elicited by various vaccine immunogens, standard panels of diverse HIV-1 isolates should be used. This would allow systematic comparisons of novel immunogens based on the magnitude and breadth of the neutralizing antibody response against the same sets of well-characterized viruses. A consensus working group has recently recommended the use of clonal Env-pseudoviruses for this purpose.[69] Such recombinant Env-pseudoviruses are commonly made by co-transfection of an Env-defective HIV-1 molecular clone together with an expression plasmid encoding the Env of interest. The resulting Env-pseudotyped virions produce a single round of infection that can be monitored by reporter genes encoded in the virus or in an engineered cell line. The recent study by Binley and co-workers, in which over 90 Env-pseudoviruses were studies with well known antibody reagents, is a clear example of the utility of this proposed assay.[63] There are several advantages to this assay format. The glycoprotein amino acid sequence of these Env-pseudoviruses is precisely known and exists in a stable plasmid form. This facilies reagent transfer and standardization across laboratories and adds to the precision of the assay. In addition, molecularly cloned pseudoviruses enhance the scientific value of the assay by permitting antibody specificities to be mapped in relation to a precisely known Env sequence. Mapping the NAb response generated by different vaccines should provide valuable information for future immunogen design. The first standard virus panel, based on clade B viruses, has been constructed.[70] Similar virus panels for non-clade B viruses are currently being constructed and evaluated. In summary, the ultimate success of our efforts to elicit anti-HIV-1 neutralizing antibodies will likely require a combination of systematic approaches. These include rational antigen design based on structural knowledge, empirical testing of immunogens, standardized virus panels to assess and the antibody response and mapping of immune responses to understand the type of antibody responses elicited by specific immunogens.

References

1. Nabel GJ. Challenges and opportunities for development of an AIDS vaccine. Nature 2001; 410:1002–1007.
2. Borrow P, Lewicki H, Hahn BH, et al. Virus-specific CD8+ cytotoxic T-lymphocyte activity associated with control of viremia in primary human immunodeficiency virus type 1 infection. J Virol 1994; 68:6103–6110.
3. Koup RA, Safrit JT, Cao Y, et al. Temporal association of cellular immune responses with the initial control of viremia in primary human immunodeficiency virus type 1 syndrome. J Virol 1994; 68:4650–4655.
4. Jin X, Bauer DE, Tuttleton SE, et al. Dramatic rise in plasma viremia after CD8(+) T cell depletion in simian immunodeficiency virus-infected macaques. J Exp Med 1999; 189:991–998.
5. Schmitz JE, Kuroda MJ, Santra S, et al. Control of viremia in simian immunodeficiency virus infection by CD8+ lymphocytes. Science 1999; 283:857–860.
6. Letvin NL, Barouch DH, Montefiori DC. Prospects for vaccine protection against HIV-1 infection and AIDS. Annu Rev Immunol 2002; 20:73–99.
7. Amara RR, Villinger F, Altman JD, et al. Control of a mucosal challenge and prevention of AIDS by a multiprotein DNA/MVA vaccine. Science 2001; 292:69–74.
8. Barouch DH, Santra S, Schmitz JE, et al. Control of viremia and prevention of clinical AIDS in rhesus monkeys by cytokine-augmented DNA vaccination. Science 2000; 290:486–492.
9. Shiver JW, Fu TM, Chen L, et al. Replication-incompetent adenoviral vaccine vector elicits effective anti-immunodeficiency-virus immunity. Nature 2002; 415:331–335.
10. Mascola JR, Nabel GJ. Vaccines for the prevention of HIV-1 disease. Curr Opin Immunol 2001; 13:489–495.
11. Letvin NL, Huang Y, Chakrabarti BK, et al. Heterologous envelope immunogens contribute to AIDS vaccine protection in rhesus monkeys. J Virol 2004; 78:7490–7497.
12. International AIDS Vaccine Initiative (IAVI). Vaccine trials database. Online. Available: www.iavireport.org/trialsdb
13. NIH. ClinicalTrials.gov Database. Online. Available: www.clinicaltrials.gov
14. HIV Vaccine Trials Network (HVTN). Pipeline Project. Online. Available: http://chi.ucsf.edu/vaccines
15. Flynn NM, Forthal DN, Harro CD, et al. Placebo-controlled phase 3 trial of a recombinant glycoprotein 120 vaccine to prevent HIV-1 infection. J Infect Dis 2005; 191:654–665.
16. Pitisutithum P. Efficacy of AIDSVAX B/E vaccines in injection drug use. Paper presented at the 11th Conference on Retroviruses and Opportunistic Infections, San Francisco, 2004.
17. Rerks-Ngam S. An update of progress in the Thai HIV prime boost vaccine trial: vCP1521 (ALVAC-HIV) + gp120 B/E (AIDSVAX B/E). AIDS Vaccine Conference, Montreal, 2005.
18. McElrath MJ, Corey L, Montefiori D, et al. A phase II study of two HIV type 1 envelope vaccines, comparing their immunogenicity in populations at risk for acquiring HIV type 1 infection. AIDS Vaccine Evaluation Group. AIDS Res Hum Retroviruses 2000; 16:907–919.
19. Belshe RB, Stevens C, Gorse GJ, et al. Safety and immunogenicity of a canarypox-vectored human immunodeficiency virus Type 1 vaccine with or without gp120: a phase 2 study in higher- and lower-risk volunteers. J Infect Dis 2001; 183:1343–1352.
20. Pitisuttithum P, Nitayaphan S, Thongcharoen P, et al. Safety and immunogenicity of combinations of recombinant subtype E and B human immunodeficiency virus type 1 envelope glycoprotein 120 vaccines in healthy Thai adults. J Infect Dis 2003; 188:219–227.
21. Pitisuttithum P, Berman PW, Phonrat B, et al. Phase I/II study of a candidate vaccine designed against the B and E subtypes of HIV-1. J Acquir Immune Defic Syndr 2004; 37:1160–1165.
22. Nitayaphan S, Pitisuttithum P, Karnasuta C, et al. Safety and immunogenicity of an HIV subtype B and E prime-boost vaccine combination in HIV-negative Thai adults. J Infect Dis 2004; 190:702–706.
23. Gaschen B, Taylor J, Yusim K, et al. Diversity considerations in HIV-1 vaccine selection. Science 2002; 296:2354–2360.
24. McMichael A, Hanke T. The quest for an AIDS vaccine: is the CD8+ T-cell approach feasible? Nat Rev Immunol 2002; 2:283–291.
25. Amara RR, Smith JM, Staprans SI, et al. Critical role for Env as well as Gag-Pol in control of a simian-human

immunodeficiency virus 89.6P challenge by a DNA prime/recombinant modified vaccinia virus Ankara vaccine. J Virol 2002; 76:6138–6146.

26. Ourmanov I, Brown CR, Moss B, et al. Comparative efficacy of recombinant modified vaccinia virus Ankara expressing simian immunodeficiency virus (SIV) Gag-Pol and/or Env in macaques challenged with pathogenic SIV. J Virol 2000; 74:2740–2751.

27. Barouch DH, Kunstman J, Kuroda MJ, et al. Eventual AIDS vaccine failure in a rhesus monkey by viral escape from cytotoxic T lymphocytes. Nature 2002; 415:335–339.

28. Goulder PJ, Brander C, Tang Y, et al. Evolution and transmission of stable CTL escape mutations in HIV infection. Nature 2001; 412:334–338.

29. Allen TM, O'Connor DH, Jing P, et al. Tat-specific cytotoxic T lymphocytes select for SIV escape variants during resolution of primary viraemia. Nature 2000; 407:386–390.

30. Allen TM, Mortara L, Mothe BR, et al. Tat-vaccinated macaques do not control simian immunodeficiency virus SIVmac239 replication. J Virol 2002; 76:4108–4112.

31. Cafaro A, Caputo A, Fracasso C, et al. Control of SHIV-89.6P-infection of cynomolgus monkeys by HIV-1 Tat protein vaccine. Nat Med 1999; 5:643–650.

32. HIV Immunology and HIV/SIV Vaccine Databases. Theoretical biology and biophysics. Los Alamos, New Mexico: Los Alamos National Laboratory.

33. Addo MM, Yu XG, Rathod A, et al. Comprehensive epitope analysis of human immunodeficiency virus type 1 (HIV-1)-specific T-cell responses directed against the entire expressed HIV-1 genome demonstrate broadly directed responses, but no correlation to viral load. J Virol 2003; 77:2081–2092.

34. Betts MR, Ambrozak DR, Douek DC, et al. Analysis of total human immunodeficiency virus (HIV)-specific CD4(+) and CD8(+) T-cell responses: relationship to viral load in untreated HIV infection. J Virol 2001; 75:11983–11991.

35. Betts MR, Yusim K, Koup RA. Optimal antigens for HIV vaccines based on CD8+ T response, protein length, and sequence variability. DNA Cell Biol 2002; 21:665–670.

36. Nabel G, Makgoba W, Esparza J. HIV-1 diversity and vaccine development. Science 2002; 296:2335.

37. Seaman MS, Xu L, Beaudry K, et al. Multiclade human immunodeficiency virus type 1 envelope immunogens elicit broad cellular and humoral immunity in rhesus monkeys. J Virol 2005; 79:2956–2963.

38. Hanke T, McMichael AJ. Design and construction of an experimental HIV-1 vaccine for a year-2000 clinical trial in Kenya. Nat Med 2000; 6:951–955.

39. Mascola JR, Snyder SW, Weislow OS, et al. Immunization with envelope subunit vaccine products elicits neutralizing antibodies against laboratory-adapted but not primary isolates of human immunodeficiency virus type 1. The National Institute of Allergy and Infectious Diseases AIDS Vaccine Evaluation Group. J Infect Dis 1996; 173:340–348.

40. Graham BS, Mascola JR. Lessons from Failure–Preparing for Future HIV-1 Vaccine Efficacy Trials. J Infect Dis 2005; 191:647–649.

41. Kwong PD, Wyatt R, Robinson J, et al. Structure of an HIV gp120 envelope glycoprotein in complex with the CD4 receptor and a neutralizing human antibody. Nature 1998; 393:648–659.

42. Parren PW, Moore JP, Burton DR, et al. The neutralizing antibody response to HIV-1: viral evasion and escape from humoral immunity. AIDS 1999; 13:137–162.

43. Richman DD, Wrin T, Little SJ, et al. Rapid evolution of the neutralizing antibody response to HIV type 1 infection. Proc Natl Acad Sci USA 2003; 100:4144–4149.

44. Wei X, Decker JM, Wang S, et al. Antibody neutralization and escape by HIV-1. Nature 2003; 422:307–312.

45. Wyatt R, Sodroski J. The HIV-1 envelope glycoproteins: fusogens, antigens, and immunogens. Science 1998; 280:1884–1888.

46. Burton DR, Desrosiers RC, Doms RW, et al. HIV vaccine design and the neutralizing antibody problem. Nat Immunol 2004; 5:233–236.

47. Moore JP, Cao Y, Qing L, et al. Primary isolates of human immunodeficiency virus type 1 are relatively resistant to neutralization by monoclonal antibodies to gp120, and their neutralization is not predicted by studies with monomeric gp120. J Virol 1995; 69:101–109.

48. Bradney AP, Scheer S, Crawford JM, et al. Neutralization escape in human immunodeficiency virus type 1-infected long-term nonprogressors. J Infect Dis 1999; 179:1264–1267.

49. Bures R, Morris L, Williamson C, et al. Regional clustering of shared neutralization determinants on primary isolates of clade C human immunodeficiency virus type 1 from South Africa. J Virol 2002; 76:2233–2244.

50. Mascola JR. Defining the protective antibody response for HIV-1. Curr Mol Med 2003; 3:209–216.

51. Binley JM, Sanders RW, Clas B, et al. A recombinant human immunodeficiency virus type 1 envelope glycoprotein complex stabilized by an intermolecular disulfide bond between the gp120 and gp41 subunits is an antigenic mimic of the trimeric virion-associated structure. J Virol 2000; 74:627–643.

52. Farzan M, Choe H, Desjardins E, et al. Stabilization of human immunodeficiency virus type 1 envelope glycoprotein trimers by disulfide bonds introduced into the gp41 glycoprotein ectodomain. J Virol 1998; 72:7620–7625.

53. Yang X, Wyatt R, Sodroski J. Improved elicitation of neutralizing antibodies against primary human immunodeficiency viruses by soluble stabilized envelope glycoprotein trimers. J Virol 2001; 75:1165–1171.

54. Cardoso RM, Zwick MB, Stanfield RL, et al. Broadly neutralizing anti-HIV antibody 4E10 recognizes a helical conformation of a highly conserved fusion-associated motif in gp41. Immunity 2005; 22:163–173.

55. Ofek G, Tang M, Sambor A, et al. Structure and mechanistic analysis of the anti-human immunodeficiency virus type 1 antibody 2F5 in complex with its gp41 epitope. J Virol 2004; 78:10724–10737.

56. Kwong PD, Doyle ML, Casper DJ, et al. HIV-1 evades antibody-mediated neutralization through conformational masking of receptor-binding sites. Nature 2002; 420:678–682.

57. Barnett SW, Lu S, Srivastava I, et al. The ability of an oligomeric human immunodeficiency virus type 1 (HIV-1) envelope antigen to elicit neutralizing antibodies against primary HIV-1 isolates is improved following partial deletion of the second hypervariable region. J Virol 2001; 75:5526–5540.

58. Kolchinsky P, Kiprilov E, Sodroski J. Increased neutralization sensitivity of CD4-independent human immunodeficiency virus variants. J Virol 2001; 75:2041–2050.

59. Ly A, Stamatatos L. V2 loop glycosylation of the human immunodeficiency virus type 1 SF162 envelope facilitates interaction of this protein with CD4 and CCR5 receptors and protects the virus from neutralization by anti-V3 loop and anti-CD4 binding site antibodies. J Virol 2000; 74:6769–6776.

60. Kim YB, Han DP, Cao C, et al. Immunogenicity and ability of variable loop-deleted human immunodeficiency virus type 1 envelope glycoproteins to elicit neutralizing antibodies. Virology 2003; 305:124–137.

61. Chakrabarti BK, Kong WP, Wu BY, et al. Modifications of the human immunodeficiency virus envelope glycoprotein enhance immunogenicity for genetic immunization. J Virol 2002; 76:5357–5368.

62. Yang ZY, Chakrabarti BK, Xu L, et al. Selective modifications of variable loops alters tropism and enhances immunogenicity of HIV-1 envelope. J Virol 2004; 78:4029–4036.

63. Binley JM, Wrin T, Korber B, et al. Comprehensive cross-clade neutralization analysis of a panel of anti-human immunodeficiency virus type 1 monoclonal antibodies. J Virol 2004; 78:13232–13252.

64. Pantophlet R, Wilson IA, Burton DR. Hyperglycosylated mutants of human immunodeficiency virus (HIV) type 1 monomeric gp120 as novel antigens for HIV vaccine design. J Virol 2003; 77:5889–5901.

65. Fouts TR, Tuskan R, Godfrey K, et al. Expression and characterization of a single-chain polypeptide analogue of the human immunodeficiency virus type 1 gp120-CD4 receptor complex. J Virol 2000; 74:11427–11436.

66. He Y, Vassell R, Zaitseva M, et al. Peptides trap the human immunodeficiency virus type 1 envelope glycoprotein fusion intermediate at two sites. J Virol 2003; 77:1666–1671.

67. Williamson C, Morris L, Maughan MF, et al. Characterization and selection of HIV-1 subtype C isolates for use in vaccine development. AIDS Res Hum Retroviruses 2003; 19:133–144.

68. Cho MW, Kim YB, Lee MK, et al. Polyvalent Envelope Glycoprotein Vaccine Elicits a Broader Neutralizing Antibody Response but Is Unable To Provide Sterilizing Protection against Heterologous Simian/Human Immunodeficiency Virus Infection in Pigtailed Macaques. J Virol 2001; 75:2224–2234.

69. Mascola JR, D'Souza PD, Gilbert P, et al. Recommendations for the Design and Use of Standard Virus Panels to Assess Neutralizing Antibody Responses Elicited by Candidate HIV-1 Vaccines. J Virol Press 2005; 79:10103–10107.

70. Li M, Gao F, Mascola JR, et al. Human immunodeficiency virus type 1 env clones from acute and early subtype B infections for standardized assessments of vaccine-elicited neutralizing antibodies. J Virol 2005; 79: 10108–10125.

CHAPTER 9

HIV Prevention

Helene D. Gayle

Introduction

Curbing the expansion of HIV/AIDS represents one of the world's most pressing priorities. Since HIV/AIDS was first recognized more than 25 years ago, a substantial body of data has developed on effective strategies for preventing the transmission of HIV.

This chapter summarizes the evidence base for HIV prevention. After briefly describing the epidemiology of HIV to put in context the modes of transmission upon which prevention strategies are based, the chapter identifies the prevention strategies that have been proven to be effective. The chapter also notes additional prevention options that may hold promise but have yet to be proven effective.

Epidemiology of HIV/AIDS

Since AIDS was first identified in 1981, the disease has rapidly become the world's most serious health threat. Through the end of 2006, nearly 60 million infections had occurred, and more than 20 million people worldwide had died. As Figure 9.1 indicates, by the end of 2006, an estimated 39.5 million people worldwide were living with HIV.[1]

Sub-Saharan Africa remains the hardest-hit region, accounting for 29.7 million people living with HIV and for 2.8 million new HIV infections in 2006. Asia had 7.8 million people living with HIV by the end of 2006. HIV is spreading fastest in Eastern Europe and Central Asia. The Caribbean basin has the second highest rate of infection after Africa.[1]

The epidemic shows little sign of slowing. There were more new HIV infections and more AIDS deaths in 2006 than in any previous year. The risk of a major expansion of HIV/AIDS is most apparent in some of the world's most populous countries, including China and India.

Although AIDS in its early years was predominantly a disease of men, women now represent one in two people living with HIV worldwide, including a majority of prevalent and incident infections in Africa. Young people are also especially vulnerable to infection; 15–24-year-olds account for half of all new infections.[1]

HIV is transmitted in one of three ways: through sexual contact, blood-borne transmission, or transmission from mother-to-child. Globally, the most common route of transmission is sexual, accounting for approximately 80% of infections worldwide and more than 90% of infections in sub-Saharan Africa.[2] Receptive anal intercourse is the most efficient means of sexual transmission of HIV, with a per-contact likelihood of infection that is four times higher than for receptive vaginal intercourse and nearly 27 times higher than for insertive anal or vaginal intercourse.[3] As these figures indicate, male-to-female transmission is significantly more efficient than female-to-male transmission. Worldwide, heterosexual intercourse is the leading route of sexual transmission, although men who have sex with men (MSM) account for an estimated 5–10% of infections,[4] including the largest share of infections in Latin America and in many high-income countries.[1]

The second route of HIV transmission – and the most efficient – is blood-borne exposure to the virus. The most common source of blood-borne transmission is injecting-drug use, which accounts for the largest share of cases in Eastern Europe, parts of Asia, and the southern cone of Latin America. Receipt of an HIV-infected blood transfusion also readily

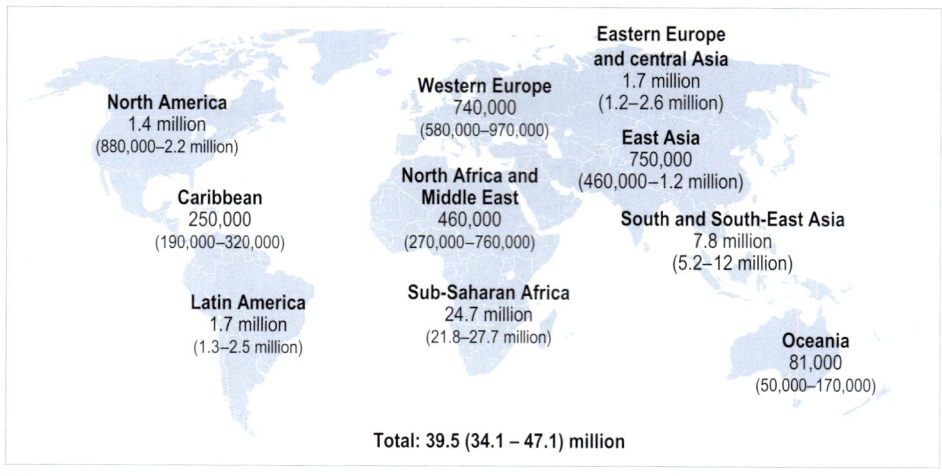

Figure 9.1 Adults and children estimated to be living with HIV as of end-2006.[1]

transmits HIV, leading to HIV infection 89% of the time.[5] Although blood transfusions account for an estimated 5–10% of cumulative infections worldwide,[6] incidence of such cases has declined in recent years as more countries have implemented standard blood control procedures. Re-use of injecting equipment in health care settings resulted in approximately 5% of new HIV infections in 2000.[7]

Third, more than 600,000 newborns contract HIV each year before birth, during delivery, or as a result of breast-feeding.[1] In the absence of any preventive intervention, an infant born to an HIV-infected, breast-feeding mother faces around a 30% chance of contracting HIV.

While it is common to speak of a single global epidemic, the reality is that HIV/AIDS is highly diverse in all regions. In the Latin America and Caribbean region, for example, MSM represent the largest share of cases overall, but injection drug use predominates in parts of South America and heterosexual intercourse is the primary source of transmission in the Caribbean. The broad variation of the epidemic has important implications for HIV prevention, requiring that national programs pursue a range of evidence-based prevention strategies tailored to local circumstances and to the populations at highest risk.

The Evidence Base for HIV Prevention

Despite a wealth of effective prevention strategies, the global epidemic continues to expand. While

some question whether existing prevention methods are capable of slowing the spread of the epidemic, the limited impact of prevention efforts stems in large measure from low levels of prevention coverage. In 2003, a panel of leading prevention experts reported that fewer than one in five people at high risk of infection had access to the most basic prevention services.[8] Extrapolating from available data on the effectiveness of existing prevention strategies, Stover and co-workers determined that a scaling-up of a limited number of existing interventions could prevent 63% of all infections projected to occur between 2002 and 2010.[9]

Although globally, the epidemic continues to grow, numerous countries have reversed their national epidemics by implementing strong prevention programs. In high-income countries, risk behaviors and HIV incidence among MSM and injecting-drugs users (IDUs) declined sharply in the 1980s and 1990s, respectively, following initiation of prevention programs targeting these groups. Among middle- and low-income countries, Senegal averted a major epidemic, and Thailand and Uganda reversed serious national epidemics, by undertaking prevention efforts that were strongly supported by national political leaders.[10]

The discussion below examines what is currently known – and what remains to be clarified – regarding effective prevention strategies for each of the three main routes of HIV transmission. As Box 9.1 illustrates, a broad range of prevention strategies have proven effective in reducing the risk of HIV transmission. Because developing countries account for approximately 95% of the world's HIV infections, this chapter primarily focuses on prevention measures in resource-limited settings.

Preventing Sexual Transmission

A wide range of interventions has proven effective to prevent sexual transmission, the single greatest contributor to the global epidemic.

Behavior Change Programs

Behavioral interventions to prevent HIV transmission may seek to encourage abstinence and delayed initiation of sexual behavior, promote monogamy and reduce the number of sexual partners, increase condom use, and forge new social norms that discourage risky behavior. Behavior change programs typically include one or more of the following components that have proven effective in prevention trials:

Targeted Counseling and Behavior Change Communication

Prevention counseling helps reduce HIV-related risk behaviors.[11] Counseling may be provided in connection with HIV testing or as a stand-alone intervention in community-based settings. While it is optimally effective for individuals at risk to be exposed to multiple counseling sessions, studies indicate that a single session of client-centered counseling results in significant reductions in acquisition of sexually transmitted disease.[11]

Community Interventions

Interventions that seek to affect the norms of entire communities or discrete social networks have also been shown to reduce the behaviors that can transmit HIV.[12]

Condom Promotion

Studies overwhelmingly demonstrate that condoms are highly effective in preventing HIV transmission. A 2001 report by the US National Institutes of Health analyzed several studies on condom effectiveness, and concluded that consistent use of condoms can reduce an individual's risk of HIV transmission by 85%.[13] Among sexually active people in developing countries, including hard-hit sub-Saharan Africa, condom use is rare.[14] Accordingly, substantial effort has been directed toward the implementation and evaluation of interventions to encourage condom use. Initiatives that increase the accessibility of condoms have been shown to lead to significant increases in condom use.[15] Social marketing strategies have also proven effective in promoting increased condom use.[16]

Peer-based Programs

Youth-oriented prevention programs have proven especially effective when peers have been used to deliver the intervention.[17] Excluding interventions to prevent mother-to-child HIV transmission, peer-based prevention programs for sex workers produce the largest single reduction in disability-adjusted life years lost of any category of HIV prevention intervention in Africa.[18]

School-based Sex Education

School-based programs provide health information to young people and reinforce healthy norms. A school-based education intervention in Namibia resulted in positive changes in HIV-related behaviors, intention to use condom, and perceptions of the efficacy of condoms.[19] Some studies suggest that sex education alone is often insufficient to generate long-term behavior change and should be supplemented with other youth-targeted interventions.[20] By definition, school-based programs do not reach out-of-school youth, who are often at high risk of transmission and require targeted prevention interventions.

Voluntary Counseling and Testing (VCT)

Knowledge of HIV serostatus normally leads individuals to avoid engaging in behaviors that could expose others to HIV. A study involving more than 4000 people in Kenya, Tanzania and Trinidad found that VCT was more effective in reducing reported risk behaviors than simple provision of health information.[21]

STD Screening and Treatment

Untreated STDs increase, by several orders of magnitude, the risk of sexual HIV transmission.[22] A study in Tanzania found that enhanced provision of STD treatment by trained health care providers reduced HIV incidence in six intervention sites by 38%.[23] As noted below, clarity does not currently exist regarding optimal strategies for maximizing the HIV prevention impact of STD control in some settings. Clinical trials are underway to produce needed insight to facilitate implementation of STD control strategies that have maximum impact on the rate of HIV transmission.

Preventing Blood-borne Transmission

Research has documented the effectiveness of several measures to prevent blood-borne transmission of HIV.

Harm Reduction Programs

Harm reduction involves a combination of health promotion strategies for IDUs, including needle and syringe exchange programs, ready access to effective drug treatment, and provision of counseling and condoms. Strong evidence demonstrates the effectiveness of each element of the harm reduction approach.

Needle and Syringe Exchange

Studies indicate that needle exchange projects reduce the risk of HIV transmission without encouraging increased drug use.[24] For individuals who have yet to achieve recovery from their substance addiction, such projects reduce the harm from drug use by providing access to clean injection equipment, client-centered counseling, and assistance in entering drug

treatment. International experience reveals that early initiation of needle exchange programs is often critical to the ability of large cities to avoid major HIV outbreaks in their IDU populations.[25]

Drug Substitution Programs

Methadone maintenance is both safe and effective as treatment for drug addiction.[26] In 2002, the US Food and Drug Administration gave approval to two formulations of buprenorphine (Subutex/Suboxone) for physician-administered opioid addiction treatment, providing an office-based alternative to methadone. Methadone maintenance and other forms of substance abuse treatment reduce the risk of HIV transmission by helping individuals avoid the drug-using behaviors that can lead to HIV infection. The impact of drug treatment modalities on the rate of HIV transmission is currently limited by laws in some countries that prohibit or restrict the use of methadone maintenance of other drug substitution strategies. For all substance abuse treatment modalities, relapse is common, requiring both strong individual commitment on the part of the client and flexible, accessible service systems.

Counseling and Condom Provision

Small group interventions, individual counseling, and other psychosocial interventions have been demonstrated to help IDUs reduce the frequency of drug injection or unprotected sex.[27] Behavioral interventions for IDUs appear more successful in altering drug injecting practices than in promoting safer sex.

Implementation of Blood Safety Practices

Studies in North America indicate that screening of blood reduces the risk of HIV transmission to approximately one in every 500 000 transfusions.[28] Standard blood safety practices include use of low-risk blood donors and promotion of appropriate clinical use of blood.

Proper Infection Control in Health Care Settings

To prevent blood-borne transmission of HIV and other diseases, health care workers, emergency personnel, and others who might experience occupational exposure to blood or body fluids are advised to take 'universal precautions.' This approach, which treats all blood as potentially infectious, includes gloves, gowns, goggles, proper disposal of waste and other infection control practices.[29] A critical component of universal precautions is the prohibition on re-use of needles and syringes. In Romania, the risk of injection-related transmission in health care settings was eliminated after national authorities mandated the use of single-injection devices.[30]

Post-exposure Prophylaxis

Initiation of a 4-week antiretroviral regimen within hours of an occupational blood exposure has been shown to reduce the risk of HIV transmission to the health care worker.[31]

Preventing Mother-to-child Transmission

Effective prevention of mother-to-child transmission (PMTCT) ideally encompasses a package of prevention elements, including primary prevention services for women of childbearing age, reproductive health services, VCT in the context of comprehensive prenatal care, administration to mother and newborn of nevirapine (Viramune) or short-course zidovudine (Retrovir), and counseling and assistance to facilitate alternatives to breast-feeding. Unfortunately, prevailing realities in low-income countries often make it challenging to obtain meaningful PMTCT coverage. Many women do not obtain reproductive health services or prenatal care, many do not know their serostatus and also lack meaningful access to VCT, many first present late in the course of pregnancy, PMTCT projects that deliver nevirapine or zidovudine are not accessible in many parts of the world, and effective alternatives to breast-feeding often do not exist. It was estimated that PMTCT coverage in low- and middle-income countries in 2001 was approximately 5%, with coverage of only 1% in sub-Saharan Africa, which accounts for 90% of all cases of mother-to-child transmission.[8] Substantial operational research and analysis is presently focused on strategies to bring PMTCT to broad scale. Proven approaches include:

Antiretroviral Therapy

Research has identified three effective strategies to reduce the risk of mother-to-child transmission through the administration to mother and newborn of antiretroviral drugs. The most effective, but more costly, regimen involves a three-part regimen of zidovudine that is initiated prior to delivery. This three-part zidovudine regimen reduces transmission risk by two-thirds.[32] The second strategy – a shorter, less expensive course of zidovudine – reduces the risk of transmission by 50% among non-breast-feeding women and by 37–38% for women who breast-feed.[33] The third, simplest and most inexpensive strategy involves the intrapartum and neonatal single-dose administration of nevirapine. This strategy lowers the risk of transmission by 50% among women who breast-feed and appears to be more effective than short-course zidovudine.[34]

As noted, limited health care access and knowledge of serostatus diminish the reach of PMTCT programs, leading clinicians, program planners, and researchers to consider additional strategies to expand the access of pregnant women to preventive services. Where circumstances do not permit administration of nevirapine to the mother prior to delivery, evidence indicates that administration of post-exposure prophylaxis to the newborn reduces the risk of transmission, with a combination regimen of nevirapine and zidovudine appearing to be superior to nevirapine alone.[35]

Cesarean Delivery

Cesarean delivery prior to labor and membrane rupture lowers the risk of mother-to-child transmission.[36] The applicability of this finding in resource-poor settings remains unclear due to the increased likelihood of post-operative complications and limited access to hospital birthing facilities.

Breast-feeding Alternatives

Prolonged breast-feeding more than doubles the likelihood of mother-to-child transmission of HIV.[37] While avoiding breast-feeding represents an obvious HIV prevention strategy, it is sometimes not feasible in resource-limited settings. Because evidence indicates that mixed feeding (breast milk and formula or other substance) has a higher risk of transmission than exclusive breast-feeding,[38] mothers should be counseled on the superiority of early weaning over mixed feeding.

Reproductive Health Services

In addition to contributing to the reduction of sexual transmission through the provision of health education and treatment for STDs, reproductive health services help counsel women who are either HIV-positive or at risk of infection on strategies for avoiding unwanted pregnancies.[2]

Implementing Effective Prevention Programs

While studies have documented the efficacy of numerous HIV prevention strategies, these measures must be effectively implemented in developing countries and reach optimal coverage levels to have an impact on the epidemic. Accumulated learning has identified certain key principles for implementation of effective prevention strategies at the country level:

Combination Prevention

Because HIV epidemics and the social and cultural environments that increase vulnerability to transmission are inherently complex, no single prevention approach is likely to achieve optimal success in reducing infection rates. Rather, it is now widely recognized that effective prevention requires the simultaneous implementation of a combination of proven prevention strategies. Combination prevention targets multiple populations and routes of transmission and affects the behavioral, biological and environmental factors that influence individual risk.

Funding

An analysis by an expert panel in 2003 found that spending on HIV prevention is roughly one-third of what is needed to mount a comprehensive response.[8] To reach the resource levels needed to mount an effective prevention effort, greater investments in prevention efforts are needed from all sources, including international donors and developing country governments.

Adequate Coverage Levels

Proven prevention strategies can have an impact on national epidemics only when they reach a sufficient percentage of the target population. At publication, critical prevention interventions were reaching only a fraction of those at risk – a factor not only of inadequate funding but of prevailing capacity limitations in developing countries.[39] To reach the coverage levels needed to halt the epidemic, international donors and technical agencies should work with countries to develop and implement strategic plans to preserve, build and sustain the national capacity needed to ensure a robust prevention effort.

Targeting Populations at Risk

Prevention programs must be effectively directed toward those at highest risk. This is especially important in low-level or concentrated epidemics, when the potential exists to prevent a major outbreak of infection into other populations. A 2004 analysis by UNAIDS, however, found that many countries appear to be allocating disproportionate amounts of prevention resources to the general population or groups at limited risk, potentially neglecting the populations at highest risk of infection.[40]

Political Support

In every country that has achieved major, sustained progress against HIV, senior political and cultural leaders have exhibited strong support for the fight against HIV/AIDS.[10]

Supportive Policies

Because social and economic conditions can increase the likelihood of risk behavior, policy reforms are often needed to address the factors that increase vulnerability to HIV. A climate of stigma and discrimination impedes open discussion of HIV and deters individuals from being tested or from seeking voluntary counseling and testing; to create an attitudinal environment that is more conducive to risk reduction, countries should enact and enforce laws protecting individuals from HIV-related discrimination and provide financial and political support for organizations of people living with HIV. Measures are also required to reduce women's economic and social dependence on men, such as enactment of laws that provide women with the right of inheritance, micro-finance initiatives that help women earn a living, and girls' education initiatives.

Capitalizing on Treatment Access

Following sharp declines in the prices of antiretroviral drugs in developing countries, the global community embarked on an unprecedented effort to expand HIV treatment access in resource-limited settings.[41] Greater treatment access will strengthen HIV prevention efforts, encouraging knowledge of serostatus, reducing the infectivity of people living with HIV, and attracting individuals to health care settings, where condoms can be provided and prevention methods reinforced. Experience in high-income countries, however, indicates that introduction of improved therapies may cause individuals to increase their risk behavior, potentially offsetting the prevention benefits of treatment access.[42] To capitalize on the prevention potential of treatment access and to avert detrimental behavioral responses, donors and national programs should work together to integrate HIV prevention services in clinical settings, deliver prevention services to people living with HIV, and adapt prevention messages for HIV-negative and untested individuals to respond to potential changes in perception as a result of treatment.[43]

Unanswered Questions and Key Research Priorities

While working to implement existing strategies that are known to be effective, the global community should work to improve these strategies and prepare for the rapid introduction of new prevention technologies and expanded prevention options that are likely to emerge in the coming years as a result of current research:

HIV Vaccines

Although research suggests that it will likely be several years before the emergence of a safe and effective preventive vaccine, the global need for an HIV vaccine mandates significant public and private sector support for vaccine-related research and development. The International AIDS Vaccine Initiative estimated that spending on HIV/AIDS vaccine research and development in 2003 from all sources (including both public and private sectors) was roughly half of the amount required needed to underwrite a robust global research effort. To accelerate the search for an HIV vaccine, key stakeholders in the HIV/AIDS field united in 2004 to establish the Global HIV Vaccine Enterprise, an alliance of independent agencies that seeks to promote greater collaboration and improved strategic focus among vaccine researchers.[44]

Female-controlled Prevention

New Chemical or Barrier Methods

A major weakness of current prevention efforts is the shortage of effective prevention methods that can be controlled by women, who often lack the ability to negotiate condom use with their male partners. In recent years, research attention has increas-

ingly focused on the development of one or more microbicides, substances that women could apply vaginally to prevent infection or thwart the virus from replicating following sexual exposure. At publication, more than 50 candidate microbicides were in various stages of development, with six having entered large-scale human efficacy trials.[45] (Limited research attention has focused on the development of a rectal microbicide to reduce the risk of transmission during anal intercourse.) In addition, researchers are investigating use of the female diaphragm to prevent male-to-female sexual transmission.[46] The first generation of the female (or vaginal) condom has proven effective in reducing the risk of HIV transmission,[47] and research is now seeking to identify even more efficacious versions of this prevention tool.

STD Control

Although STDs are strongly correlated with HIV transmission, implementation of enhanced STD treatment in Uganda did not reduce HIV incidence,[48] a finding that conflicted with the above-noted research results from Tanzania. Subsequent analysis indicates that the lower levels of risk behavior in Uganda, resulting from the success of longstanding HIV prevention efforts in that country, likely explain the contrasting results of the Tanzania and Uganda trials.[49] This analysis suggests that STD control may be most effective as an HIV prevention strategy when initiated earlier in the course of national epidemics and when sexual risk behaviors are high. Additional research is needed to clarify optimal STD control strategies under different circumstances. In particular, study is needed to examine strategies to minimize the role of herpes simplex virus 2 (HSV-2) in facilitating the transmission of HIV.[50] A multi-country trial in Africa, India and Latin America, underway at publication, seeks to determine whether daily administration of acyclovir (Zovirax), an off-patent treatment for HSV-2, reduces the risk of HIV transmission.[51]

Circumcision

Observational studies have long noted that countries with high rates of circumcised men tend to have lower HIV infection levels than countries where circumcision is less common.[52] In 2005, the first randomized clinical trial of male circumcision as an HIV prevention method found that the intervention reduced the risk of female-to-male HIV transmission by approximately 60%.[53] In an effort to confirm these findings and assess their applicability in other settings, efficacy trials for male circumcision were ongoing in 2006 in Kenya and Uganda.

Antiretroviral Therapy

The risk of sexual transmission is strongly correlated with the plasma level of virus in the infected individual.[54] Antiretroviral therapy (ART) significantly reduces the level of virus, often to the point that HIV cannot be detected in the patient's blood by standard tests.[55] As a result, it is possible that widespread use of ART for treatment may also have a preventive impact. More specifically, use of ART as either pre or post exposure is being more closely evaluated. On the basis of evidence demonstrating the effectiveness of ART/PEP following percutaneous exposure (see above), it is suggested that a 4-week course of ART should uniformly be initiated following a sexual assault or after a consensual episode of unprotected sex. Observational studies suggest that PEP may reduce the risk of HIV acquisition following sexual exposure,[56] and in 2005 the US Centers for Disease Control published recommendations endorsing PEP as a recognized HIV prevention method following non-occupational exposure.[57] In addition, trials are either planned or enrolling participants in industrialized and developing countries to determine whether daily administration to HIV negative persons of tenofovir (Viread), an antiretroviral with an especially attractive resistance profile and few side effects, might reduce the risk of HIV acquisition.[58]

Prevention Programs for People with HIV

Historically, prevention programs in both developing and industrialized countries have primarily focused on individuals who are either uninfected or unaware of their serostatus. In recent years, a growing number of public health experts have argued for the implementation of prevention interventions that specifically target people with HIV. At present, evidence is lacking on the most effective strategies to encourage safer behavior among people with HIV.

PMTCT Resistance

The most economically feasible approach to preventing mother-to-child transmission – single-dose nevi-

rapine to mother and child – has been shown to cause drug resistance in a substantial portion of HIV-infected mothers.[33] While the risk of resistance does not currently justify withdrawal of nevirapine to prevent mother-to-child transmission, it is clear that alternative interventions are needed.

Breast-feeding

Greater clarity is required on the factors that increase the risk of HIV transmission through breast-feeding and on prevention strategies that can be feasibly implement to minimize the HIV-related risk associated with infant feeding. Consensus is needed on when mothers who initiate breast-feeding should switch to replacement feeding.

Conclusion

The HIV epidemic constitutes the world's most pressing public health threat. To respond effectively, the world must adopt a comprehensive response that provides treatment to those who are infected, while greatly expanding access to evidence-based prevention programs appropriate to at-risk populations. It is essential that prevention interventions achieve sufficient coverage levels to have an impact, and that future biomedical approaches be closely integrated with existing behavioral prevention interventions. Not only are prevention efforts essential to saving millions of lives, but they are also critical to ensuring the long-term financial and logistical viability of HIV/AIDS treatment initiatives.

References

1. UNAIDS. Report on the global AIDS epidemic. UNAIDS; 2006.
2. Askew I, Berer M. The contribution of sexual and reproductive health services to the fight against HIV/AIDS: A review. Repro Health Matters 2003; 11:51–73.
3. Royce R, et al. Sexual transmission of HIV. N Engl J Med 1997; 336:1072–1078.
4. UNAIDS. Men who have sex with men. Technical update. UNAIDS; 2001.
5. Busch M, Operskalski EA, Mosley JW et al. Factors influencing human immunodeficiency virus type 1 transmission by blood transfusion. J Infect Dis 1996; 174:26–33.
6. UNAIDS. Blood safety and HIV. UNAIDS best practice collection. UNAIDS; 1997.
7. Hauri AM, Armstrong GL, Hutin YJ. The global burden of disease attributable to contaminated injections given in health care settings. Int J STD AIDS 2004; 15:7–16.
8. Global HIV Prevention Working Group. Access to HIV prevention: Closing the gap. Global HIV Prevention Working Group; 2003.

9. Stover J, Walker N, Garnett GP, et al. Can we reverse the HIV/AIDS pandemic with an expanded response? Lancet 2002; 360:73–77.

10. UNAIDS. HIV prevention needs and successes – an update on HIV prevention success in Senegal, Thailand and Uganda. UNAIDS; 2001.

11. Kamb M, Fishbein M, Douglas JM, et al. Efficacy of risk-reduction counseling to prevent human immunodeficiency virus and sexually transmitted diseases: A randomized controlled trial. JAMA 1998; 280:1161–1167.

12. Kegeles SM, Hays RB, Coates TJ. The Mpowerment Project: a community–level HIV prevention intervention for young gay men. Am J Pub Health 1996; 86:1129–1136.

13. National Institute of Allergy and Infectious Diseases, National Institutes of Health. Workshop Summary: Scientific evidence on condom effectiveness for sexually transmitted disease (STD) prevention. National Institute of Allergy and Infectious Diseases, National Institutes of Health; 2001.

14. Norman L. Predictors of consistent condom use: a hierarchical analysis of adults from Kenya, Tanzania and Trinidad. Int J STD AIDS 2003; 14:584–590.

15. Celentano D, Bond KC, Lules CM, et al. Preventive intervention to reduce sexually transmitted infections: a field trial in the Royal Thai Army. Arch Intern Med 2000; 160:535–540.

16. Meekers D. Going underground and going after women: trends in sexual risk behaviors among gold miners in South Africa. Int J STD AIDS 2000; 11:21–26.

17. Bianco M, Pagani LI. Evaluation of an intervention in training adolescents as peer educators in Argentina. Abstract 33539. XII International Conference on AIDS, Geneva, 1998.

18. Creese A, Floyd K, Alban A, et al. Cost-effectiveness of HIV/AIDS interventions in Africa: a systematic review of the evidence. Lancet 2002; 359:1635–1643.

19. Stanton BF, Li X, Kanihuata J, et al. Increased protected sex and abstinence among Namibian youth following a HIV risk-reduction intervention: a randomized, longitudinal study. AIDS 1998; 12:2473–2480.

20. Betts SC, Peterson DJ, Huebner AJ, et al. Zimbabwean adolescents' condom use: what makes a difference? Implications for intervention. J Adolesc Health 2003; 33:165–171.

21. Voluntary HIV-1 Counseling and Testing Efficacy Study Group. Efficacy of voluntary HIV-1 counseling and testing in individuals and couples in Kenya, Tanzania, and Trinidad: a randomized trial. Lancet 2000; 356:103–112.

22. US Centers for Disease Control and Prevention. HIV prevention through early detection and treatment of other sexually transmitted diseases – United States. Recommendations of the Advisory Committee for HIV and STD Prevention. MMWR 1998; 47:1–24.

23. Grosskurth H, Mosha F, Todd J, et al. Impact of improved treatment of sexually transmitted diseases on HIV infection in rural Tanzania: randomized controlled trial. Lancet 1995; 346:530–536.

24. Vlahov D, Junge B. The role of needle exchange programs in HIV prevention. Public Health Rep 1998; (Suppl 1):75–80.

25. Hurley S, Jolley DJ, Kaldor JM, et al. Effectiveness of needle exchange programmes for prevention of HIV infection. Lancet 1997; 349:1797–1800.

26. National Consensus Development Panel on Effective Medical Treatment of Opiate Addiction. Effective medical treatment of opiate addiction. JAMA 1998; 280:1936–1943.

27. Gibson DR, McCusker J, Chesney M, et al. Effectiveness of psychosocial interventions in preventing HIV risk behavior in injecting drug users. AIDS 1998; 12:919–929.

28. Sloand E, Pitt E, Klein HG. Safety of the Blood Supply. JAMA 1995; 274:1368–1373.

29. US Centers for Disease Control and Prevention. Guidelines for prevention of transmission of human immunodeficiency virus and hepatitis B virus to health-care and public-safety workers. MMWR 1989; 38(Suppl 6):1–36.

30. US Centers for Disease Control and Prevention. Injection practices among nurses – Valcea, Romania, 1998. MMWR 2001; 50:59–61.

31. Cardo D, Culver DH, Ciesielski CA, et al. A Case-control study of HIV seroconversion in health care workers after percutaneous exposure. N Engl J Med 1997; 337:1485–1490.

32. Connor EM, Sperling RS, Gelber R, et al. Reduction of maternal-infant transmission of human immunodeficiency virus type 1 with Zidovudine treatment. N Engl J Med 1994; 331:1173–1180.

33. Shaffer N, Chuachoowong R, Mock PA, et al. Short-course zidovudine for perinatal HIV-1 transmission in Bangkok, Thailand: a randomized controlled trial. Lancet 1999; 353:773–780.

34. Guay L, Musoke P, Fleming T, et al. Intrapartum and neonatal single-dose nevirapine compared with zidovudine for prevention of mother-to-child transmission of HIV-1 in Kampala. Uganda: HIVNET 012 randomized trial. Lancet 1999; 354:795–802.

35. Taha TE, Kumwenda NI, Gibbons A, et al. Short postexposure prophylaxis in newborn babies to reduce mother-to-child transmission of HIV-1: NVAZ randomized clinical trial. Lancet 2003; 362:1171–1177.

36. International Perinatal HIV Group. The mode of delivery and the risk of vertical transmission of human immunodeficiency virus type 1. A meta-analysis of 15 prospective cohort studies. N Engl J Med 1999; 340:977–987.

37. Nduati R, John G, Mbori-Ngacha D, et al. Effect of breastfeeding and formula feeding on transmission of HIV-1: a randomized clinical trial. JAMA 2000; 283:1167–1174.

38. Coutsoudis A, Pillay K, Spooner E, et al. Influence of infant-feeding patterns on early mother-to-child transmission of HIV-1 in Durban, South Africa: a prospective cohort study. Lancet 1999; 354:471–476.

39. UNAIDS. Resource needs for an expanded response to AIDS in low- and middle-income countries. UNAIDS; 2005.

40. UNAIDS. National spending for AIDS. UNAIDS; 2004.

41. World Health Organization. Treating 3 million by 2005: making it happen. Geneva: World Health Organization; 2003.

42. Kelly JA, Hoffman RG, Rompa D, et al. Protease inhibitor combination therapies and perceptions of gay men regarding AIDS severity and the need to maintain safer sex. AIDS 1998; 12:91–95.

43. Global HIV Prevention Working Group. HIV prevention in the era of expanded treatment access. Global HIV Prevention Working Group; 2004.

44. Coordinating Committee of Global HIV/AIDS Vaccine Enterprise of The Global HIV/AIDS Vaccine Enterprise. Scientific strategic plan. PLoS Med 2005; 2:e25.

45. Rosenberg Z. State of the art report on development and use of microbicides. Plenary address, XV International Conference on HIV/AIDS, July 2004, Bangkok; 2005.

46. Moench TR, Chipato T, Padian NS. Preventing disease by protecting the cervix: the unexplored promise of internal vaginal barrier devices. AIDS 2001; 15:1595–1602.

47. Trussell J, Sturgen K, Strickler J, et al. Comparative contraceptive efficacy of the female condom and other barrier methods. Fam Plann Perspect 1994; 26:66–72.

48. Wawer M, et al. Control of sexually transmitted diseases for AIDS prevention in Uganda: a randomized community trial. Lancet 1999; 353:525–535.

49. Orroth K, Korenromp EL, White RG, et al. Higher risk behaviour and rates of sexually transmitted diseases in Mwanza compared to Uganda may help explain HIV prevention trial outcomes. AIDS 2003; 17:2653–2660.

50. Renzi C, Douglas JM Jr, Foster M, et al. Herpes simplex virus type 2 infection as a risk factor for human immunodeficiency virus acquisition among men who have sex with men. J Infect Dis 2003; 187:19–25.

51. Corey L, Wald A, Celum CL, et al. The effects of herpes simplex virus-2 on HIV-1 acquisition and transmission: A review of two overlapping epidemics. J Acquir Immune Defic Syndr 2004; 35:435–445.

52. Weiss HA, Quigley MA, Hayes RJ et al. Male circumcision and risk of HIV infection in sub-Saharan Africa: a systematic review and meta-analysis. AIDS 2000; 14:2361–2370.

53. Auvert B, Taljaard D, Lagarde E, et al. Randomized, controlled intervention trial of male circumcision for reduction of HIV infection risk: the ANRS 1265 trial. PLoS Med 2005; 2:e298.

54. Quinn T, Wawer MJ, Brookmeyer R, et al. Viral load and heterosexual transmission of human immunodeficiency virus type 1. N Engl J Med 2001; 342:921–929.

55. Palella FJ Jr, Delaney KM, Moorman AC, et al. Declining morbidity and mortality among patients with advanced human immunodeficiency virus infections. N Engl J Med 1998; 338:853–860.

56. Schechter M, do Lago RF, Mendelsohn AB, et al. Behavioral impact, acceptability and HIV incidence among homosexual men with access to postexposure chemoprophylaxis for HIV. J Acquir Immune Defic Syndr 2004; 35:519–525.

57. Centers for Disease Control and Prevention (CDC). Antiretroviral postexposure prophylaxis after sexual, injecting-drug use, or other nonoccupational exposure to HIV in the United States: Recommendations from the US Department of Health and Human Services. MMWR 2005; 54:1–20.

58. Van Rompay KK, Berardi CJ, Aguirre NL, et al. Two doses of PMPA protect newborn macaques against oral simian immunodeficiency virus infection. AIDS 1998; 12:79–83.

CHAPTER 10

Laboratory Testing for HIV Infection

James C. Shepherd
Oliver Laeyendecker
Thomas C. Quinn

Introduction

In the 20 years since HIV infection was first recognized it has spurred the development of a number of laboratory tests to aid in the diagnosis and management of the disease. The use of these tests has become well established in America and Europe and there are a number of up-to-date reviews of HIV laboratory testing available for these areas.[1] There is less experience with using laboratory testing in the developing world where HIV subtypes may be different, host responses to the virus may vary and technical and financial resources may be limited. There is a recent comprehensive review of laboratory services for antiretroviral therapy monitoring in resource-limited settings published on the web by WHO (www.who.int/hiv/). In this chapter, laboratory tests for the diagnosis and management of HIV infection are described with an emphasis on those in use or applicable to resource limited settings.

Initially, tests for the diagnosis of HIV infection, including tests of body fluids other than blood, and tests for incident versus prevalent infections are described. Next, tests that measure the robustness of the immune system, including relatively simple tests for measuring CD4+ T cells are described. Tests that measure the amount of virus present in an individual, both for diagnosis, prognosis and monitoring of therapy are then presented. Finally, an overview of tests that detect drug resistance mutations in HIV are described. None of these tests are valuable without accurate quality control procedures to validate the results being generated. Pricing* for each of the tests kits are shown when possible but do not reflect technician costs which vary greatly by country and by region. Significant price reductions for some reagents have been negotiated by WHO and the Clinton Foundation (www.clintonfoundation.org) in order to make these tests more affordable.

Diagnostic Testing

During, or shortly after, the clinical presentation of acute retroviral infection, IgM antibodies to Gag (p17,p24,p55) and Env (gp41,120,160) first appear.[2] This response seems similar throughout the world, regardless of HIV subtype or host population.[3] The appearance of the IgM response is followed weeks to months later by IgG antibodies to *Gag* and *Env* epitopes and later still to viral enzymes and regulatory proteins. The time to first detectable IgG seroconversion by enzyme immunoassay in most studies in Europe and America is 2 weeks with a median of 3–4 weeks.[2] Almost all newly HIV-infected individuals will have detectable IgG by 6 months.

Currently the most established tests for detecting HIV infection rely on an enzyme-linked immunoabsorbent assay (ELISA) as an initial screening test

---

*Prices are quoted from UNAIDS, UNICEF, WHO, MSF – Sources and prices of selected drugs and diagnostics for people living with HIV/AIDS; www.unaids.org/en/in+focus June 2004.

(cost US$1–1.50 per test). This method involves coating a solid surface such as the plastic of a 96 well plate with antigen and using this as an affinity matrix for IgG present in a serum sample 1st generation ELISA used crude lysates of HIV as antigen, followed by 2nd and 3rd generation tests using increasingly refined recombinant preparations of HIV proteins to coat the plastic. Current 4th generation tests use a combination of IgG antibody capture by the immobilized recombinant antigen and HIV antigen capture by immobilized antibody simultaneously in the same reaction to increase sensitivity.[4] The consequent reduction in the 'window period', particularly in developing world areas where incident infection is frequent, is important to reduce the number of false-negative results.

The mechanics of ELISA lend themselves to high throughput, rapid testing with automation and this is the preferred screening test in the developed world. The US FDA and the WHO have validated a number of these assays for use worldwide (see www.fda.gov/cber/products/testkits/htm; www.who.int/diagnostics_laboratory/evaluations/hiv/en). The ELISA has also been evaluated in less developed countries with a variety of HIV subtypes and similar results for accuracy have been obtained.[3,5] The cost-benefit analysis of frequency of HIV testing will depend on the background risk of the population and the background incidence in the population but in developed countries testing is rarely recommended more frequently than annually.

Despite high specificity, the use of ELISA in populations where the prevalence of disease is low will lead to a high proportion of positive results being false. Thus, the preferred testing strategy in the developed world is to confirm positive or indeterminate (an intermediate colorimetric reaction) results in the ELISA with a second test, Western blot. This uses a similar concept to ELISA but the immobilized antigens are first separated by size through SDS-PAGE electrophoresis and then bound to a solid medium. Antibody reactivity to different sized proteins of HIV can be determined. The criteria for a Western blot positive test vary depending on the manufacturer of the test kit and the fluid being tested. In general, sera with antibodies reactive to gp120 and gp160 plus either gp41 or p24 must be present to confirm a positive ELISA.[2] Western blots require significant time and resources and are costly (US$11 per test), and therefore are not suited to many parts of the world where the prevalence of HIV is high.

A test that has worked well in resource-poor areas is the rapid HIV test. There are several of these

approved for use both by the FDA and the WHO. The basic method requires spotting of whole blood or serum/plasma on a test strip with HIV antigen prebound (www.cdc.gov/hiv/rapid_testing). Lateral chromatography of the antibodies within the test strip and reaction with the immobilized HIV proteins is revealed colorimetrically in a 'pregnancy test' fashion within minutes. These tests have higher than 99% sensitivity and specificity when combined with a confirmatory test such as Western blot in the developed world or a second rapid test in the developing world.[6] The lack of sample preparation, ease of storage, simple visual readout, speed and cost (US$0.47–1.30) make these tests attractive for use all over the world and they have been evaluated in a number of African countries where their sensitivity and specificity profiles have been comparable with results in Europe and America.[5,7,8] A number of algorithms (Fig. 10.1) have been developed for confirmation of rapid testing results without resort to ELISA or Western blotting and these have been validated in different resource poor settings.[9]

Other screening strategies for HIV infection have tested for the presence of antibodies in fluids other than blood. Levels of IgG are much lower in urine than in plasma but a highly sensitive screening test for urine, similar to ELISA, has a reported sensitivity of 99% and a specificity of 94% and is FDA approved.[10] A positive result should be confirmed with a standard serological ELISA. Saliva contains much higher concentrations of IgA and IgG than blood and there is an FDA approved collection method involving soaking a pad in the mouth and then testing the adsorbed antibodies in a standard ELISA/western blot system, which is extremely sensitive and specific.[11] An ELISA test for IgG in cervico-vaginal secretions is available. The principle benefit of these approaches lie in their convenience for the patient and the lessened risk of needlestick injury to the tester but their reliance on ELISA for screening or confirmation make them less adaptable to the developing world.

Vertical transmission of HIV presents a particular diagnostic challenge as placentally transfered maternal antibodies can persist in the neonate for as long as 18 months post-partum.[12] Nucleic acid testing (DNA or RNA) provides the most sensitive method for diagnosing HIV in an infant.[13] At four to six weeks of age most infants can be diagnosed using these methods.

For epidemiological purposes, it is important to measure the incidence of HIV infection in populations. Recently and chronically infected individuals can be differentiated by biological changes that

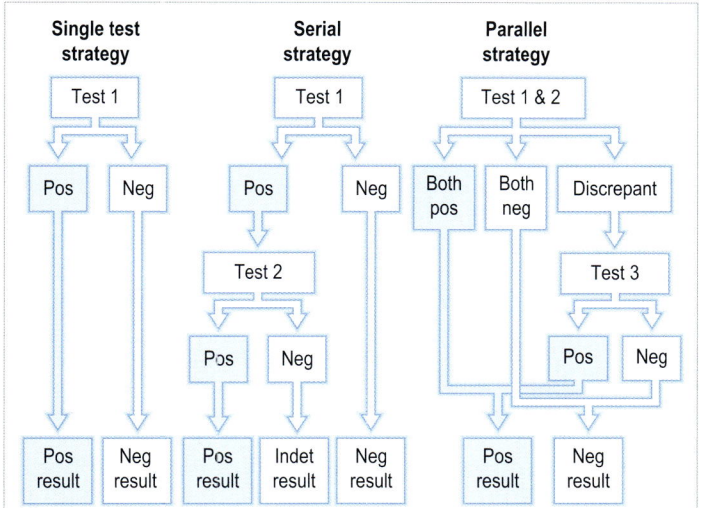

Figure 10.1 Testing algorithm for use with rapid testing. Pos, positive; Neg, negative; Indet, indeterminate.

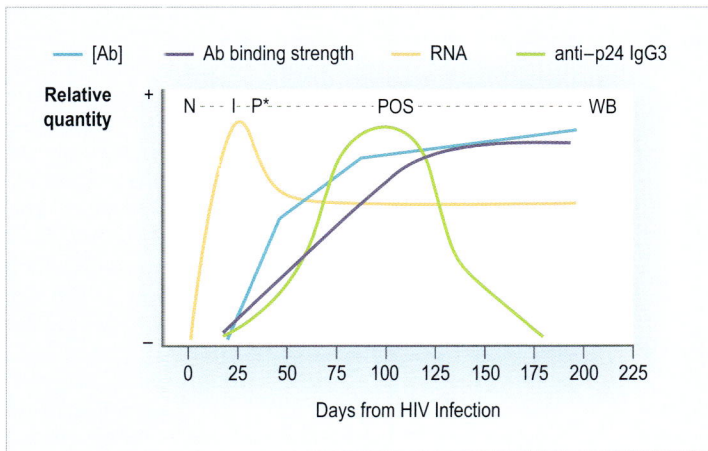

Figure 10.2 Biological changes that occur early in HIV infection. HIV virus in blood increases and falls to a viral set point (RNA, orange line); concentration of antibody specific to HIV increases (Ab, light blue line). The binding strength of antibody specific to HIV antigen increases and plateaus (Ab binding strength, dark blue line); switching of antibody isotype occurs with the temporal appearance of IgG3 specific to HIV (anti-p24 IgG$_3$, green line).

occur as the immune system matures its response to the infection. The evolution of the immune response is shown in Figure 10.2. There is a window period of approximately 3 weeks, where HIV RNA can be detected but an antibody response to the virus is not detectable. During the initial development of the humoral response, the strength of binding and concentration of antibody specific for HIV increases with time. There is also a switching of the class of antibody to the virus. An epidemiological tool for determining incidence rates from cross-sectional population sampling exploit these biologic differences between incident and chronically infected individuals. The most commonly used protocol is STARHS (Serological Testing Algorithm for Recent HIV Seroconversion).[14] This is a sensitive, standard ELISA for blood IgG that is followed by a 'detuned' ELISA using more dilute sample and reduced reaction incubation times. Evaluation of this test has demonstrated that it is an accurate method to detect individuals who have become infected within a 'window period' of approximately 170 days and is therefore a good screening tool for incident infection. It has been used with success in the USA but requires adaptation to non-US populations and non-subtype B infections. Polymerase chain reaction (PCR) of pooled blood samples to detect viral RNA positive samples before antibody has developed has been pioneered in North Carolina, USA and may be the most sensitive and specific method for detecting incident infection in at risk populations.[15] It has not been tested in resource-poor areas but may be rapidly adaptable to Eastern Europe or China where PCR technology is already available.

Laboratory diagnosis of HIV-2 is frequently necessary depending on geographical area, travel and exposure history. Infection with HIV-2 is prevalent in West Africa and in many cases, HIV-1 infected people are also infected with HIV-2, although it is rare in the rest of the world. The virus is less transmissible, replicates more slowly and causes a slower rate of T-cell decline and there are few standardized tests useful for management. The diagnostic testing methodology for HIV-2 is identical to HIV-1 except that the serological tests are specific for antibodies against HIV-2 proteins. Currently there are no commercially available assays for HIV-2 viral load or Western blot testing. However, HIV-2 viral load data can be generated by real time RT-PCR using primers specific for HIV-2.[16] Western blot testing for HIV-2 has been previously described[17] and is performed by a number of groups as a 'home brew' assay. There are diagnostic ELISA tests available specifically for HIV-2 and one test available for diagnosis of both HIV-1 and HIV-2 simultaneously,[18] although 20–30% of HIV-1 ELISA tests do not detect antibodies to HIV-2.[1]

Monitoring Patient Health

Tests for Estimating T lymphocytes

Monitoring of the health of the immune system is accomplished with estimates of the number of $CD4^+$ T cells circulating in a person's bloodstream. This is the most reliable prognostic test available[19] and is the primary means of deciding need for anti-viral treatment. Tests of $CD8^+$ T cells are valuable to measure anti-HIV cytolytic activity as a research tool but their number has not been found to correlate with clinical outcome.

The value of a $CD4^+$ determination at any particular time point is approximate, with wide confidence intervals. Thus, the utility of testing is mainly in observing trends. The recommended interval of testing is 3–6 months (see DHHS, WHO guidelines). A result markedly different from prior results should be repeated. In addition, many factors other than HIV-1 influence the CD4 T-cell count, including diurnal variation, intercurrent illness, corticosteroid use, idiopathic lymphocytopenia and splenectomy.[1] Of significance in some parts of the world, most notably Brazil and Haiti, is the interaction between HIV-1 and HTLV-1 co-infection. In these patients the

true level of immunosuppression is more accurately represented by a $CD4^+$ T-cell value half as high as that actually measured.[20] The $CD4^+$ T-cell fraction of total lymphocytes, expressed as a $CD4^+$ percentage, is sometimes used to account for variation in the total number of T cells but this has not been found to correlate as accurately with risk for opportunistic infection as the absolute count.[21] The total lymphocyte count has been used with some success in resource-poor areas as a surrogate for T-cell counting although the sensitivity of this strategy was found to be low in a cohort in Uganda.[22]

The standard method in America and Europe for measurement of $CD4^+$ T cells is by flow cytometry. This requires a fresh blood sample and antibody reagents specific for CD4 and CD8 that are labeled with fluorescent molecules. The number of labeled cells present is counted by flow of individual cells past a fluorescence detector. This is expensive, both in equipment and reagents (US$6–20 per test), and requires frequent calibration of the machine. A variation on standard flow cytometry for CD4 counting is leukogating. The primary advantage of leukogating is the ability to do the analysis in a single reaction with a lowered cost of reagents (<US$4 per test) but still requires an expensive flow cytometer for detection. For medium throughput applications, a microflow method that is more portable and uses smaller volumes has been developed (Guava Technologies). Lower throughput methods such as FACSCount (Becton-Dickinson) and PointCare (Beckman Coulter) give automated, absolute or absolute plus percentage CD4 counts, respectively, making the PointCare machine more useful for pediatric monitoring. Alternative, low throughput (<10 samples per day) methods that have been developed specifically for resource-limited laboratories are Cyto-Spheres (Beckman Coulter) (US$4–8 per test) and Dynabeads (Dynal Biotech) (US$3–5 per test). The former uses latex beads coated with anti-CD4 monoclonal antibody to 'rosette' CD4 lymphocytes that can then be counted in a hematocytometer by light microscopy. The latter uses magnetic beads that are coated with anti-CD4 antibody to purify CD4 lymphocytes from whole blood using a magnet. Both of these 'low-tech' methods correlate well with flow cytometry both in Europe and the developing world.[23]

Routine Laboratory Testing

Most of this chapter describes in detail the laboratory testing that is unique to the diagnosis and management of HIV. However, there are a number of routine screening tests that should be repeated at intervals during the management of HIV infection and these are summarized in Table 10.1. It should be remembered that the normal parameters for most of these tests have been developed in North American and European populations and will need to be adjusted to local population norms.

Monitoring Viral Replication

Viral Load Testing

Assays that detect the virus itself have been developed for two purposes – to detect incident infection earlier than possible with antibody testing and, more frequently, to monitor antiretroviral therapy. Antigen capture assays that detect p24, an early viral antigen, have been evaluated for early diagnosis and monitoring of therapy and have been incorporated into the strategy of antibody/antigen detection in the 4th generation ELISA.[4] As a screening tool in developed countries for early infection it has not been as popular as the STARHS technique or more sensitive nucleic acid detection methods. Limited evidence has suggested that p24 quantification (US$10 per test) may potentially replace nucleic acid quantification as a measure of viral load.[24] In the developing world the reliance of p24 detection on ELISA type technology has hampered its widespread use for monitoring of therapy, although it has been successfully used to reduce the 'window period' in subtype E infections in a research study.[25] There is evidence that although the specificity of p24 testing is close to 100% the sensitivity in non-subtype B infections can be quite low.[26]

Much more widely used are tests that detect and measure viral nucleic acid in blood and other body fluids. The most commonly used of these in the developed world is Reverse-Transcriptase Polymerase Chain Reaction (RT-PCR) of viral RNA isolated from plasma (US$20–100 per test). Viral RNA is extracted and transcribed to single stranded DNA and amplified by PCR. There is an ultrasensitive version of this test that can reliably measure virus as low as 50 RNA copies/mL in plasma as well as a standard version with sensitivity to 400 RNA copies/mL. There are tests in development which can measure virus at levels as low as 20 copies/mL. Sensitivity for diagnosis is excellent but specificity is significantly lower than serology and therefore these tests are not routinely recommended for primary

screening, except for acute HIV infection.[27] The level of viral replication is very high during acute HIV infection and can be used for diagnosis of early HIV infection, particularly if the assay consistently reports an elevated viral load of at least 100 000 copies/mL. Values below 10 000 copies/mL are to be viewed with suspicion in the diagnosis of acute HIV[28] Another proven technology frequently used for the quantification of HIV viral loads is branched DNA (bDNA). In this method, HIV RNA is captured by one set of immobilized oligonucleotides and detected by a second set. Amplification of the target is achieved by hybridizing with a successive set of probes attached to a signaling enzyme.

The principal use of viral load monitoring is in prognostication and monitoring of therapy. It is well established in Europe and America that those individuals with higher viral loads progress to AIDS more rapidly than those with lower viral loads.[19] It is also well established in developing world practice that the most sensitive test for detecting failure of antiretroviral therapy is viral load. Thus, the very first sign that the virus is no longer completely susceptible to the antiretroviral drugs administered is a rising viral load rather than a falling CD4 T-cell count. Initial therapy should result in a 10-fold decrease in viral load within 1 week of initiating therapy and a 100-fold decline by 4 weeks.[1] Successfully treated patients should have a viral load below the limit of detection by an ultrasensitive test at 3 months. Reasons for declines in viral loads less dramatic than these after initiation of HAART are most commonly poor compliance with therapy or viral resistance to drugs. The standard error of viral load measurement is approximately 0.3 log copies/mL so any change in viral load less than this is not considered significant.

Current practice guidelines (Department of Health and Social Services, USA, www.aidsinfo.nih.gov) recommend a baseline viral load followed by regular measurements every 3 months, regardless of whether the patient is on therapy or not. This allows a rapid response to the emergence of resistant virus in individuals already on drug therapy, and initiation of therapy in those with a rising viral load and a falling CD4 T-cell count. It has been observed that viral RNA detection by PCR behaves slightly differently to RNA detection by branched-chain DNA methods. The low cut-off for sensitivity is 50 copies/mL with PCR-based methods and 75 copies/mL with bDNA methods. Often a persistently positive result at the very low range of PCR will be below detection by bDNA. The clinical significance of these differences is unclear as patients with a persistent but very

Table 10.1 Pocket guide to adult HIV/AIDS treatment, January 2005

Test	Comment

HIV serology	Sensitivity and specificity standard serology is >99%
	   False positives: human error
	   False negatives: usually 'window period'
	Acute HIV: HIV RNA level >10 000 copies/mL; confirm seroconversion
	Rapid tests: confirm positives

CD4	Reproducibility: 95% CI = 30% False high levels – splenectomy (use CD4%) concurrent HTLV-1 Repeat every 3–6 months % – CD4 >500 = >29%, 200–500 = 14–28%, <200 = <14%
HIV viral load	Reproducibility: 95% CI = 0.3 log 10 copies/mL or 50% Repeat every 3–4 months
CBC	Repeat every 3–6 months; more frequently as indicated Macrocytosis with AZT and d4T
Chemical profile	Include LFT and renal function Repeat LFT with all Pls and NNRTIs, ETOH and hepatitis Repeat renal function with IDV and TDF
Hepatitis screen	Anti-HCV, anti-HAV anti-HbsAg (if prior vaccine) or anti-HBcAg Abnormal LFT: get anti-HCV and HBsAg Positive anti-HCV: get quantitative HCV Neg anti-HBs: vaccinate for HBV Pos HBsAg or anti-HCV: get LFTs Neg anti-HAV: HAV vaccine routine
Fasting lipid profile and glucose	Patient at risk Baseline for HAART; repeat at 3–4 months and then yearly
Toxoplasma IgG	10–15% positive in US
PPD	Indicated if no history of TB or prior pos. PPD Induration >5 mm is indication for INH × 9 months
PAP smear	Baseline, at 6 months and then annual; if 'inadequate' – repeat; if atypia – refer to gynecologist
Chest X-ray	Indicated with pulmonary sx, positive PPD or history of chest disease; some do baseline X-ray routinely
Urinary NAAT for gonorrhea and chlamydia	'Consider' in sexually active patients Repeat at 6–12 month intervals depending on risk
VDRL	Baseline and repeat annually in sexually active patients Confirm positives with FTA-ABS
Renal screen	Urinalysis and creatinine
	If ≥1+ proteinuria or elevated creatinine: quantify urine protein and do renal ultrasound.

Reprinted with permission of Bartlett and Gallant[1]; ©2004 John G. Bartlett.

low level of viremia do not appear to collect resistance mutations.[29]

Evidence that the RT-PCR and bDNA based measurements are adaptable to non-subtype B HIV-1 is limited but current studies suggest that bDNA-based measurements may be the most reliable with subtypes A through G.[30] Of the PCR based tests the Roche Amplicor version 1.5 demonstrated good reproducibility with non-subtype B HIV-1 although an earlier version, 1.0, was not adequate for non-B subtypes. Nevertheless, the requirements for an antiseptic, dust-free environment, constant electricity, pure water and significant equipment expenditure make viral nucleic acid detection one of the hardest tests to introduce into resource-poor laboratories. RNA is a notoriously unstable molecule and difficult to work with and the technique of PCR exquisitely sensitive to contaminants. There is an urgent need for development of viral detection methods that are useful clinically but do not require delicate equipment or distilled water. Detection of viral DNA is extremely sensitive and DNA is a more stable molecule than RNA but there is limited data on the correlation between circulating pro-viral DNA and viral replication.[31]

Monitoring Drug Resistance Mutations

The final cornerstone of laboratory monitoring of HIV is drug resistance testing. The importance of this is growing as the prevalence of HIV strains resistant to ART grows and the transmission of drug-resistant strains increases. Current estimates in the USA put the frequency of new infections caused by viruses with at least one major drug resistance mutation at around 10–25%.[32] This figure is likely to be reached in the developing world as antiretrovirals are increasingly used. The indications for resistance testing are growing from the original FDA-approved indications for rational drug selection in a patient on antiretroviral therapy that has either had a less than satisfactory response to a new regimen or a rising viral load on an established regimen.[33] It is now recommended by many authorities for patients with new or chronic infections prior to selection of their first ART regimen (DHHS, www.aidsinfo.nih.gov/guidelines; IAS-USA, www.iasusa.org). It is proposed by WHO to monitor treatment of naïve individuals by country and regional sampling to detect the rate of drug-resistant viral transmission in different geographical areas of the developing world and respond accordingly (www.who.int/hiv/).

The most commonly used and cheaper test of resistant mutations is genotypic (US$300–500 per test), as opposed to the more time consuming and laborious phenotypic testing (US$800–1000 per test). Genotyping involves amplification of the reverse transcriptase and protease genes by RT-PCR from the circulating swarm of viral RNA and DNA sequencing of the major products of the amplification. Currently there are two FDA approved assays for the genotypic assessment for resistant virus, (Trugene by Visible Genetics and ViroSeq by Applied Biosystems).[34,35] The mutations are reported as amino-acid substitutions at specific numbered codons and the interpretation of drug susceptibility is aided by computer algorithms using rules generated from past data, most of which have been generated from sequencing of subtype B.[33] The test requires a viral load of at least 500 copies/mL and in most cases unless the selecting drug is present or recently withdrawn, the predominant species detected will be wild-type virus, which tends to outgrow mutated virus. Indeed, recent evidence suggests that transmitted drug-resistant virus may revert to wild type over time in the absence of drug selection pressure.[36] The extraction of viral RNA, amplification by RT-PCR, and sequencing of amplified products and their analysis requires a laboratory with stable electricity, clean water, a highly trained staff, a dedicated laboratory manager and initial investment in instrumentation of well over US$100 000.

The phenotyping, assay also involves an initial amplification of the reverse transcriptase and protease genes which are then cloned into an HIV pseudotyping vector which is then grown in the presence of permissive tissue culture cells and drug. The results are easier to interpret for single agents – the virus either grows efficiently in the drug's presence or not, but combinations of drugs in a phenotypic assay are still being evaluated.[37] The reliance on tissue culture imposes the rigors of sterility upon a laboratory and this may limit its attractiveness to resource limited sites.

There is a pressing need for more information on mutations and mutational pathways in HIV-1 subtypes other than B and correlations between codon substitutions and phenotypic changes in drug susceptibility.[38] As more HIV infected people are treated all over the world this data will become invaluable for guiding therapeutic decisions.

Quality Assurance and Quality Control

As with all clinically useful tests QA/QC is crucial. The accuracy of the results of all the tests described here are highly dependent upon the level of training of the technical staff and the maintenance and calibration of the equipment. In addition, the reproducibility of testing must be assured. Thus all labs performing laboratory monitoring for HIV diagnosis and management should be part of a network where each site can check their results against a panel of standards validated at other sites. In addition, there should be a mechanism whereby 'low-tech' tests can be compared with 'high-tech' gold standard tests at suitable intervals. Biological standards can be purchased commercially. Standards for testing in the USA are determined by the College of American

Pathology (www.cap.org). The WHO is facilitating the establishment of an electronic data monitoring system for QA/QC of resource-poor laboratories.

References

1. Bartlett JG, Gallant JE. Medical management of HIV infection. Baltimore, MD: Johns Hopkins Medicine Health Publishing Business Group; 2004.

2. Mylonakis E, Paliou M, Lally M, et al. Laboratory testing for infection with the human immunodeficiency virus: established and novel approaches. Am J Med 2000; 109:568–576.

3. Beelaert G, Vercauteren G, Fransen K, et al. Comparative evaluation of eight commercial enzyme linked immunosorbent assays and 14 simple assays for detection of antibodies to HIV. J Virol Methods 2002; 105:197–206.

4. Weber B, Meier T, Enders G. Fourth generation human immunodeficiency virus (HIV) screening assays with an improved sensitivity for p24 antigen close the second diagnostic window in primary HIV infection. J Clin Virol 2002; 25:357–359.

5. Makuwa M, Souquiere S, Niangui MT, et al. Reliability of rapid diagnostic tests for HIV variant infection. J Virol Methods 2002; 103:183–190.

6. Urassa W, Nozohoor S, Jaffer S, et al. Evaluation of an alternative confirmatory strategy for the diagnosis of HIV infection in Dar Es Salaam, Tanzania, based on simple rapid assays. J Virol Methods 2002; 100:115–120.

7. Solomon SS, Pulimi S, Rodriguez II, et al. Dried blood spots are an acceptable and useful HIV surveillance tool in a remote developing world setting. Int J STD AIDS 2004; 15:658–661.

8. Phili R, Vardas E. Evaluation of a rapid human immunodeficiency virus test at two community clinics in Kwazulu-Natal. S Afr Med J 2002; 92:818–821.

9. Wright RJ, Stringer JS. Rapid testing strategies for HIV-1 serodiagnosis in high-prevalence African settings. Am J Prev Med 2004; 27:42–48.

10. Urnovitz HB, Sturge JC, Gottfried TD, et al. Urine antibody tests: new insights into the dynamics of HIV-1 infection. Clin Chem 1999; 45:1602–1613.

11. de Morgado Moura Machedo JE, Kayita J, Bakaki P, et al. IgA antibodies to human immunodeficiency virus in serum, saliva and urine for early diagnosis of immunodeficiency virus infection in Ugandan infants. Pediatr Infect Dis J 2003; 22:193–195.

12. Committee on Pediatric AIDS. Identification and care of HIV-exposed and HIV-infected infants, children and adolescents in faster care. Pediatrics 2000; 106:149–153.

13. Steketee RW, Abrams EJ, Thea DM, et al. Early detection of perinatal human immunodeficiency virus (HIV) type 1 infection using HIV RNA amplification and detection. N Y City Perinatal HIV Transm Collab Study J Infect Dis 1997; 175:707–711.

14. Janssen RS, Satten GA, Stramer SL, et al. New testing strategy to detect early HIV-1 infection for use in incidence estimates and for clinical and prevention purposes. JAMA 1998; 280:42–48.

15. Pilcher CD, Fiscus SA, Nguyen TQ, et al. Detection of acute infections during HIV testing in North Carolina. N Engl J Med 2005; 352:1873–1883.

16. Ruelle J, Mukadi BK, Schutten M, et al. Quantitative real-time PCR on Lightcycler for the detection of human immunodeficiency virus type 2 (HIV-2). J Virol Methods 2004; 117:67–74.

17. Parekh BS, Pau CP, Granade TC, et al. Oligomeric nature of transmembrane glycoproteins of HIV-2: procedures for their efficient dissociation and preparation of Western blots for diagnosis. AIDS 1991; 5:1009–1013.

18. Holguin A. Evaluation of three rapid tests for detection of antibodies to HIV-1 non-B subtypes. J Virol Methods 2004; 115:105–107.

19. Mellors JW, Munoz A, Giorgi JV, et al. Plasma viral load and CD4+ lymphocytes as prognostic markers of HIV-1 infection. Ann Intern Med 1997; 126:946–954.

20. Schechter M, Harrison LH, Halsey NA, et al. Coinfection with human T-cell lymphotropic virus type I and HIV in Brazil. Impact on markers of HIV disease progression. JAMA 1994; 271:353–357.

21. Gebo KA, Gallant JE, Keruly JC, et al. Absolute CD4 vs. CD4 percentage for predicting the risk of opportunistic illness in HIV infection. J Acquir Immune Defic Syndr 2004; 36:1028–1033.

22. Kamya MR, Semitala FC, Quinn TC, et al. Total lymphocyte count of 1200 is not a sensitive predictor of CD4 lymphocyte count among patients with HIV disease in Kampala, Uganda. Afr Health Sci 2004; 4:94–101.

23. Didier JM, Kazatchkine MD, Demouchy C, et al. Comparative assessment of five alternative methods for CD4+ T-lymphocyte enumeration for implementation in developing countries. J Acquir Immune Defic Syndr 2001; 26:193–195.

24. Sterling TR, Hoover DR, Astemborski J, et al. Heat-denatured human immunodeficiency virus type 1 protein 24 antigen: prognostic value in adults with early-stage disease. J Infect Dis 2002; 186:1181–1185.

25. Weber B, Thorstensson R, Tanprasert S, et al. Reduction of the diagnostic window in three cases of human immunodeficiency-1 subtype E primary infection with fourth-generation HIV screening assays. Vox Sang 2003; 85:73–79.

26. Burgisser P, Vernazza P, Flepp M, et al. Performance of five different assays for the quantification of viral load in persons infected with various subtypes of HIV-1. Swiss HIV Cohort Study. J Acquir Immune Defic Syndr 2000; 23:138–144.

27. Daar ES, Little S, Pitt J, et al. Diagnosis of primary HIV-1 infection. Angeles Cty Primary HIV Infect Recruitment Network Ann Intern Med 2001; 134:25–29.

28. Rich JD, Merriman NA, Mylonakis E, et al. Misdiagnosis of HIV infection by HIV-1 plasma viral load testing: a case series. Ann Intern Med 1999; 130:37–39.

29. Kieffer TL, Finucane MM, Nettles RE, et al. Genotypic analysis of HIV-1 drug resistance at the limit of detection: virus production without evolution in treated adults with undetectable HIV loads. J Infect Dis 2004; 189:1452–1465.

30. Elbeik T, Alvord WG, Trichavaroj R, et al. Comparative analysis of HIV-1 viral load assays on subtype quantification: Bayer Versant HIV-1 RNA 3.0 versus Roche Amplicor HIV-1 Monitor version 1.5. J Acquir Immune Defic Syndr 2002; 29:330–339.

31. Hatzakis AE, Touloumi G, Pantazis N, et al. Cellular HIV-1 DNA load predicts HIV-RNA rebound and the outcome of highly active antiretroviral therapy. AIDS 2004; 18:2261–2267.

32. Little SJ, Holte S, Routy JP, et al. Antiretroviral-drug resistance among patients recently infected with HIV. N Engl J Med 2002; 347:385–394.

33. Hirsch MS, Brun-Vezinet F, Clotet B, et al. Antiretroviral drug resistance testing in adults infected with human immunodeficiency virus type 1: 2003 recommendations of an International AIDS Society-USA Panel. Clin Infect Dis 2003; 37:113–128.

34. Eshleman SH, Hoover DR, Chen S, et al. Resistance after single-dose nevirapine prophylaxis emerges in a high proportion of Malawian newborns. AIDS 2005; 19:2167–2169.

35. Tong CY, Mullen J, Kulasegaram R, et al. Genotyping of B and non-B subtypes of human immunodeficiency virus type 1. J Clin Microbiol 2005; 43:4623–4627.

36. Gandhi RT, Wurcel A, Rosenberg ES, et al. Progressive reversion of human immunodeficiency virus type 1 resistance mutations in vivo after transmission of a

multiply drug-resistant virus. Clin Infect Dis 2003; 37:1693–1698.

37. Hachiya A, Matsuoka-Aizawa S, Tsuchiya K, et al. All-in-One assay, a direct phenotypic anti-human immunodeficiency virus type 1 drug resistance assay for three-drug combination therapies that takes into consideration in vivo drug concentrations. J Virol Methods 2003; 111:43–53.

38. Visco-Comandini U, Balotta C. Genotypic resistance tests for the management of the HIV-infected patient with non-B viral isolates. Scand J Infect Dis 2003; 106:S75–S79.

CHAPTER 11

Testing and Counseling

Rhoda Wanyenze
Primo Madra
Allan Ronald

Introduction

Information, education and counseling have been the foundation of HIV prevention strategies since the behavioral determinants of the epidemic were first understood in the early 1980s. Counseling can be defined as an interactive participatory discussion directed at least in part by the client and with the clients consent. and relevant to and respectful of the clients' culture, beliefs, traditions, gender, age, and sexual orientation. Counseling evolved historically as a discipline within the field of psychology and found its scientific boundaries within the several theories that have been offered to explain human behavior. Over the past 25 years, HIV counseling has developed as a separate field of care and inquiry with increasing sophistication and scientific evidence and a body of knowledge with over 500 articles in the health literature. This chapter will review counseling from the perspective of 'learning' about one's HIV status in both industrialized and developing countries. Issues around client education and counseling to ensure adherence to care and antiretroviral regimens are discussed in Chapter 19. HIV counseling associated with an HIV test has usually been divided into pretest counseling to inform an individual about the benefits and risks followed by a post-test experience with one or several sessions to enable the client to assimilate and cope with the information, reduce risks of acquiring or transmitting the virus, and make good decisions about the future.

Early and throughout the HIV epidemic, human rights have frequently been seen to conflict with the 'greater good' of public health and widespread even mandatory testing with labeling of positives has been promoted as a strategy to control the epidemic. This led to abuse of testing which in turn encouraged fear of testing with the stigmatization of individuals and populations. Testing was avoided, denial ensued, and ultimately prevention and care programs were compromised. As a result, in many countries, fewer than 10% of HIV-infected individuals particularly in resource constrained societies have learned their HIV serostatus. Consent, confidentiality and compassionate counseling are the prerequisites for ethical testing processes to ensure that human rights are upheld in the implementation and scale-up of programs for diagnosing HIV infection. Counseling should be personalized to the individuals' risk behaviors and should enable the individual to both reduce transmission possibilities and access care and support services.

Historically, health care providers have been successful at delivering brief counseling messages, such as smoking cessation and nutrition during routine care.[1] However, most routine HIV care interactions are not accompanied by these focused messages; adequate risk assessments do not occur and tests or 'counseling sessions' are not offered to at-risk individuals.[2] A recent study among HIV-positive individuals found that a message framed to emphasize consequences of unsafe sex was effective and reduced unprotected intercourse by 38%.[1] The study also found that a negative 'loss framed' message was more effective in this setting than a 'gain framed' message about the consequences of unsafe sex. Strategies to take advantage of care opportunities through training health care providers with some counseling techniques have been largely overlooked and require further development as a means to reduce HIV transmission.

General HIV Screening Recommendations

The United States Preventative Services Task Force (USPSTF) has recently released guidelines for HIV screening.[2] They are updated from those previously suggested by the United States Centers for Disease Control in 1993 and revised in 2001.[3,4] They recommend that all adolescents and adults with at least one risk factor or residing in high prevalence settings (defined as >1%) or high-risk settings (such as STD clinics, correctional facilities, homeless shelters) be offered screening. This implies that all hospitalized adults be routinely offered screening in settings in which the prevalence is >1%.[2] It is also recommended that all pregnant women should be screened with an opt-out provision, regardless of risk factors or presumed background setting. These are wide-ranging recommendations and although they are now being discussed and generally accepted in many industrialized countries, they may be associated with negative outcomes in societies where an HIV positive serostatus leads to stigma and loss of rights. However, as care programs become widely available it is hoped that knowledge, counseling, and support will lead to action with care including access to antiretroviral treatment (ART) and reduced transmission as the outcomes. Testing strategies including HIV screening and confirmation procedures are further presented in Chapter 10.

Behavioral Theories

Behaviors that are critical to HIV/AIDS prevention and care are determined by a complex set of individual and environmental factors that behavioral theories try to explain. Understanding behavioral models enables critical analysis of the situation of the individual, group or the environment in order to identify appropriate prevention and care interventions.

The main outcomes of HIV counseling and testing are risk reduction for both positive and negative individuals, and linkage to care. All these aspects involve a series of decision making processes, beginning with the decision to test, and leading to decisions to reduce risk, to disclose status after testing, to seek HIV/AIDS care and even to take medications

as prescribed. Adopting and maintaining of positive behaviors is determined by several factors as outlined in the behavioral theories.

The following are the commonly used theories in HIV/AIDS prevention and care.

The Health Belief Model

This theory was developed by Rosenstock in the 1950s.[5] It stipulates that all health-related behaviors depend on four key beliefs about perceptions regarding the condition: *susceptibility* to the condition, its *severity*, the *benefits* of adopting a new behavior and the *barriers* to implementing that behavior. For an HIV prevention initiative, these might include the beliefs that a person is at risk of HIV infection, the consequences of acquiring HIV, the benefit of adopting risk reduction behaviors such as condom use or limiting number of sexual partners, and the barriers to adopting risk reduction behavior. An example of the latter might be the belief that condoms do not work. The decisions to go for a test, access care, and disclose results to sexual partners can be similarly evaluated.

Theory of Reasoned Action

In order for behavior change to occur, there must be an intention to change.[6] Intentions in turn are influenced by two factors: personal attitudes towards the behavior and subjective group norms regarding that behavior. The subjective norms are defined for the individual by the opinion of peers and influenced by the social environment. Several HIV/AIDS interventions have used this model, for example use of peer counselors among youth and commercial sex workers.

Social Learning (Cognitive) Theory

This theory recognizes three factors: behavior, social environment and physical environment as influencing each other. It proposes that social and physical environments are critical in reinforcing and shaping the beliefs that determine health-related behavior.[7] The key components of this theory are: self-efficacy (a person's belief about his/her ability and confidence in performing the new behavior), outcome expectation (the extent to which a person values the expected outcome) and skill acquisition (obtaining and/or increasing skills either through direct experience or by modeling others).

Stages of Change (Transtheoretical) Model

This theory was developed in the 1990s by Prochaska and co-workers, to help people stop smoking.[8] It postulates that behavior change occurs in a series of five stages that starts from not being aware of the negative effects of a behavior to a stage of maintaining safer behavior. The process is however not linear and often involves relapses. The stages are: *pre-contemplation* (not aware of risk), *contemplation* (recognizes that the behavior puts them at risk but not committed to changing behavior), *preparation* (taking steps to change behavior), *action* (person has changed behavior recently), and *maintenance* (person has maintained behavior change for a long time and has adapted to the change). This theory applies to many aspects of HIV/AIDS care and prevention practices, for example, the decision to reduce the number of sexual partners or to use condoms and the decision to access care and adhere to medications. The theory emphasizes the need for ongoing support in critical issues in order to sustain the new behavior. It helps us recognize relapses and address them when they occur.

Diffusion of Innovation

This theory explains how new ideas or behaviors are introduced and become accepted by a community. People in the same community adopt new behaviors at different rates and respond to different methods of intervention.[9] The key components of this theory are: communication channels, opinion leaders, time and process. When introducing a new HIV/AIDS intervention, care should be taken to determine appropriate timing, approaches, and communication channels. Public HIV testing of prominent people in the society in order to increase acceptability of testing is one such example.

Harm Reduction

This theory recognizes that harmful behaviors exist and counseling aims at reducing the negative effects.[10] Practices like commercial sex work and injection drug use (IDU) presumably cannot be eliminated from communities. Under these circumstances, the main strategy is to ensure that people do not acquire infections like HIV/AIDS when they engage in these practices. Commonly used interventions here include promoting condom use for all clients among commercial sex workers

(CSWs) or needle exchange programs among IDUs. This does not imply that CSW and IDU are acceptable practices in all communities but rather that these individuals and their contacts should be protected from infections with their active participation. Sometimes these harm reduction programs are offered within the context of complementary programs that seek to offer options to abandon risky practices.

AIDS Risk Reduction Model

This theory was developed by Catania.[11] It suggests that in order to change behavior, one must first label the behavior as risky, then make a commitment to reduce the behavior and finally take action to perform the desired change. The theory combines aspects of the Health Belief model, Diffusion of Information model and the Social Learning (cognitive) theory. In order for one to label a behavior as a risk for HIV infection, one must have knowledge of how HIV is prevented and transmitted, perceive that one is at risk of infection, and believe that HIV is undesirable.

The theories outlined above reinforce each other but broadly cover the individual beliefs and environmental influences including community beliefs and norms, peer pressure and the process of changing and maintaining behaviors. In practice, HIV/AIDS programs may use these theories by adopting best practices without a critical analysis of the behavioral theories. This often is effective if the program has been adopted from a society with similar cultures and circumstances. Ideally, programs should be evaluated before transfer of counseling strategies and technologies to different cultural groups. Also, a program that has been running well can reach a point in time when it has to be redesigned as the circumstances change. At this point in time, it may be important to refer to behavioral theories to guide situation analysis and strategy change.

Benefits of HIV Counseling and Testing

The benefits that arise from HIV counseling and testing are due to the information that is usually provided and discussed before and after testing, and the specific knowledge acquired of ones' HIV status. Counseling and testing has benefits for HIV positive and negative individuals, their families, and communities.

Benefits to the Individual

Knowledge of HIV status assists an individual to make better choices for themselves, plan for their future and facilitate access to care. This is more beneficial when specific care is begun early in the course of infection, delaying and even avoiding progression to clinical AIDS with life-threatening opportunistic complications.[12] Costly hospitalizations and erroneous diagnosis can be avoided. Patients can prepare for initiation of ART and ensure that progress can be monitored and drug access is possible when required.[13] Also after knowing their HIV status, HIV positive individuals can avoid HIV re-infection and other STIs, and prevent HIV transmission to sexual partners through safer sex practices. Counseling and testing encourages disclosure of HIV status to sexual partners, especially when offered to couples.[14] HIV positive individuals or couples can decide whether or not to have children and if they chose to have children, to avail themselves of 'prevention of mother-to-child' transmission services.

The efficacy of HIV counseling and testing as a risk reduction strategy has been demonstrated in several studies.[15,16] Although some literature indicates that risk reduction among HIV negative individuals may be less evident, some interventions have shown significant risk reduction especially when people are tested as couples.[17] Testing for HIV can also alleviate anxiety and fear for individuals who have concerns. Individuals may have an underlying illness that leads them to seek an HIV test. Access to care for this illness especially for tuberculosis in countries with high endemicity, should be offered during the post-test counseling sessions.

Benefits to the Couple

HIV negative individuals in discordant relationships are at very high risk of acquiring HIV infection. Testing for couples is the most efficient way of identifying and preventing infection among couples.[17,18] Testing for couples also allows for joint risk reduction planning and decision-making for critical interventions including PMTCT and care for the infected individuals. Risk reduction is more prominent when people are tested as couples.[19]

Benefits to the Family and Community

HIV counseling and testing benefits families when HIV/AIDS information has been provided to entire families or households as in family-based or home-based HIV counseling and testing. Even when provided to individuals, disclosure of HIV status and discussion of HIV/AIDS with family members offers an opportunity for enhancing prevention and care for positive individuals. When many people in a community under go counseling and testing and receive information on HIV care and prevention it ultimately impacts on general community beliefs, norms and behavior and may reduce HIV-related stigma.

Disclosure of HIV status publicly allows for interaction and formation of groups of people living with HIV/AIDS. These groups support each other and advocate for rights and needs for people living with HIV including care and non-discrimination. This may serve as a catalyst for the implementation of care and support services. These groups have also played a significant role in dissemination of HIV prevention information.

In addition to the benefits highlighted above, HIV counseling and testing is a cost-effective intervention.[20,21] The cost-effectiveness is increased in settings where HIV prevalence is higher, when counseling is offered to couples and when utilization rates are high.[20] Studies have also compared cost-effectiveness of various HIV testing approaches. It has been demonstrated that routine offer of HIV testing to all patients attending STD and emergency units is more cost-effective than an offer of testing based on risk assessment.[22,23]

Negative Outcomes of HIV Counseling and Testing

Coercion, which may be subtle or obvious, is a risk of all types of HIV testing. Except in mandatory testing counseling sessions, the counselor should offer the client the opportunity to opt out (right of refusal) once the 'facts' are shared and the client clearly understands the possible risks and benefits. Clients also need the alternative of requesting delays in making a decision or asking for another counselor or further support from family or friends. In particular with group counseling, 'herd mentality' may propel the client to a decision that might not have other wise been made.

Studies have identified increased risks of physical abuse, usually by the 'intimate partner' both among women who are HIV positive and following disclosure of status.[24,25] Commonly documented negative outcomes of HIV testing and disclosure of HIV status include domestic violence, abandonment, stigma and discrimination.[24] However, with adequate counseling and support, these negative outcomes can be minimized.[26] Counselors need to recognize the possibility of violence occurring and provide support and other options for women including access, if necessary, to a 'safe house' should be offered. Couples counseling may reduce these tragic outcomes. Gender sensitivity training and skills at eliciting abuse are essential for HIV counseling.

Models of HIV Counseling and Testing

The first HIV counseling and testing model described and scaled up globally was referred to as 'voluntary counseling and testing' (VCT) and it remains the most commonly used model throughout the world. However, due to the need to expand access to HIV counseling and testing, other models or approaches to HIV counseling and testing have evolved over time. These models still hinge on consent, confidentiality and counseling; the three 'Cs' as described by UNAIDS.[22] Informed consent implies that individuals are given adequate information about HIV/AIDS including the risks and benefits and the process of testing, to guide the decision to test or not to test. Counseling or information accompanying HIV testing and disclosure of results ensures that the individual receives adequate information to make decisions about risk reduction and access to support and care for those who are HIV positive. Also, an ill HIV negative individual who may seek VCT due to symptoms should be provided with referrals for relevant care such as tuberculosis and/or sexually

transmitted infection management. To ensure confidentiality, HIV results should be disclosed only to the client. Disclosure of results to a third party should be done by the client or with their permission. However, when it is deemed that the individual poses a risk to others, the provider may disclose the status to those who are at risk although the legal basis for this may vary from one country to another.

Counselors need to anticipate, clearly explain and address beliefs and misinformation that may affect prevention, and adherence to care interventions. Some examples are beliefs in spiritual cure, traditional or herbal medications and other forms of treatment that are not scientifically proven. The window period when an individual who has recently acquired HIV infection may not have developed detectable antibodies needs to be explained. Individuals who have tested HIV negative may be offered a repeat test in 3 months in case they were initially tested within the window period; not all individuals testing negative need to be tested again in the absence of recent exposure.

Voluntary HIV Counseling and Testing (VCT)

VCT is an approach where HIV counseling and testing is initiated by a client who desires, for whatever reason, to determine his/her HIV status. It has structured components including pre-test counseling, consent, post-test counseling, disclosure of results to clients, and referral of HIV positive individuals for ongoing care. The VCT model emphasizes prevention through risk assessment and risk reduction counseling. Typically, counseling pre- and post-test is provided on one-to-one basis. However, there have been several variations in this model including group pre-test counseling due to resource limitations (time, space, and personnel). Group pre-test counseling has been commonly used in busy settings such as ANC/PMTCT and high volume VCT centers. VCT is offered in different settings including freestanding sites, health facilities, in the workplace, and as outreach services. A freestanding VCT site is usually an HIV testing site that does not provide other HIV care services. Freestanding facilities should have adequate referral linkages for clients who test HIV positive. Because of the need to ensure that HIV positive clients are adequately linked to care, some freestanding sites have integrated other related services such as TB screening, STD screening and treatment, OI treatment and prophylaxis.

Box 11.1

Minimum information for HIV counseling and testing

Irrespective of the model of HIV counseling and testing, all individuals should receive the following information:

- Understand the clinical and prevention benefits of testing
- Be aware of the right to opt out
- Learn of the follow-up services that will be offered
- Realize the importance of partner notification and testing
- Realize the need for HIV risk reduction when necessary

Routine HIV Testing and Counseling (RTC)

Routine HIV Testing and Counseling (RTC) is a provider-initiated approach where testing is offered to all patients or clients presenting to a facility, irrespective of the presenting complaint.[27,28] RTC is frequently referred to as the 'opt out' approach because the patients have the right to decline testing. Several other terminologies have been used to describe routine HIV testing including 'routine HIV counseling and testing' (RCT) and 'routine offer of HIV testing' (ROT). The aim of RTC is to provide comprehensive care for HIV infected patients. In RTC brief pre-test information is provided to ensure informed consent. Risk reduction information is delivered post-test and the messages are tailored to the outcome of the test; positive or negative. The post-test information includes disclosure of HIV status to sexual partners and partner testing, and other options of reducing risk of transmission or acquisition of HIV infection. Care for HIV positive patients is initiated on diagnosis and referral provided for additional or follow-up care and treatment. Confidentiality should be ensured for all patient information including the HIV results; results should only be accessed by health care providers who are involved in managing the patient.

The arguments for adoption of the RTC model in the health care setting include concern that testing is rarely requested by patients because the usual practice is for health care providers to propose all investigations required by patients.[29]

HIV testing based on risk assessment is inaccurate due to difficulties in eliciting risk information because individuals may either not volunteer risk information or may not perceive themselves as at risk[30] and that the offer of testing based on symptoms is inaccurate and misses many HIV infected individuals leading to an HIV diagnosis at a late stage of the illness.[31] The Public Health approach to prevention of infections requires improved case identification and notification.[32] Studies and pilot programs have shown that RTC is efficient in identifying previously undiagnosed HIV infections in the health care setting.[33,34] As a result of these arguments and experiences, policies worldwide are changing to adopt RTC in health care setting.[4,27] RTC is now the standard of care for pregnant mothers in the developed world in an effort to reduce mother-to-child HIV transmission.[35] RTC has also been offered in other facilities that serve high-risk groups including alcohol and drug rehabilitation centers.

Diagnostic HIV Testing

Diagnostic HIV testing is also a health care provider initiated approach but testing under this model is offered when a patient has clinical signs and symptoms that are suggestive of HIV infection. Patients should be given sufficient information to make an informed decision, and still retain the right to opt-out of testing. However, in circumstances where the patient is not in a position to consent, for example an unconscious patient or those with psychiatric illness, the test can be obtained in most countries if the results are deemed essential for patient management.[27] If this happens, attempts should be made to communicate to the patient and disclose the results with adequate post-test information/counseling and linkage to care for those who are HIV positive.

Home Based HIV Counseling and Testing (HBHCT)

HIV counseling and testing can be provided by outreach teams within the home setting. This can occur for entire communities using a door-to-door approach. A variation of this is the family based approach where HIV counseling and testing is offered to households with an index HIV positive patient as opposed to entire communities. With the family based approach there is increased likelihood of identifying HIV positive individuals in these households (children and sexual partners of index positive patients) and allow reduced transmission to HIV negative partners if couples are discordant. In circumstances where it is not possible to provide family-based testing within the homes, family members can be encouraged to be tested in health units or other testing facilities. In HBHCT, the aim is to provide counseling and testing to the entire household. Pre-test information is usually given in groups but disclosure of results and post-test counseling are individualized. Several pilot programs have offered testing in the home setting with high acceptability and have identified a number of HIV infected individuals with substantial discordance rates among couples.[36-38] HBHCT has the added advantage of increasing access to HIV testing; lack of money for transport to testing sites has been documented as a barrier to testing. It has also been observed that HBHCT facilitates disclosure of results to sexual partners and minimizes negative outcomes.[34] HIV testing in the home setting requires provision of information, and linkage to care for identified HIV positive clients.

Mandatory Testing

Mandatory HIV testing of donors is required prior to all procedures involving transfer of body fluids or parts. This most commonly occurs in screening prior to blood transfusion. Counseling in these situations may require special care as the client may be especially unsuspecting and vulnerable. Outside these circumstances, mandatory HIV testing has been practiced in pre-employment screening, for example recruitment into certain employment areas such as the military or immigration. However, mandatory testing in these situations is usually coercive and should be resisted with legal or other human rights strategies. Wherever mandatory testing has been done, results should be disclosed with adequate support and information with linkage to care for those who are HIV positive.

Counseling for Special Groups

Peer Counseling

In peer counseling, the services are provided by individuals with common characteristics or experiences. Examples include youth and commercial sex workers. Peer counseling is based on the theory of reasoned action that recognizes that peers have a strong influence on behavior of an individual. In this model, individuals are trained to provide services to their peers. Its intent is to help shape the 'norms' of groups as well as assist the individual to become accepted within the group and be compliant with those 'norms'.

HIV Counseling and Testing for Children

The majority of children at risk of HIV infection have not benefited from VCT or other counseling activities largely due to lack of clarity on policy regarding consent procedures and disclosure of HIV results. This is now becoming a specialized area with active involvement of parents or guardians for legal minors. Issues of sexual abuse may arise with children; testing may be required for molestation or rape. This requires perceptive skilled counselors usually with special training. Another challenge with HIV testing for children is the limited access to technologies required for HIV diagnosis among children below 18 months; these are costly and often unavailable especially in resource limited setting.

Counseling for adolescents has special challenges. Many young people begin sexual activity or are pressured to become sexually active during teen years and need support to make healthy choices. The female genital tract is generally more susceptible to acquiring HIV during adolescence. Many young people accept information and counseling more readily from peers than from older adults. Legal minors who cannot consent for HIV counseling and testing are often sexually active and require to access HIV prevention and care services. The need for parental consent may prevent them from accessing HIV testing. In HIV counseling and testing of adolescents, it is critical to balance the requirements for protection and involvement of parents/guardians and the need to diagnose HIV infection and access prevention and care interventions.

Couples Counseling

Mutually sexually-faithful couples were not initially recognized to be at significant risk of HIV. However we now know that the HIV discordance rate among currently monogamous couples in many countries is high, yet messages like the ABC model (Abstinence, Be faithful and Condom use) often emphasize faithfulness without encouraging testing.[39] Disclosure of HIV results to sexual partners when people have tested as individuals is known to be low for various reasons including stigma and fear of negative outcomes, such as abandonment and domestic violence. The negative outcomes of disclosure are less common when people test as couples.[22]

Counseling discordant couples requires insight into the ongoing difficulties of routinely using condoms, maintaining sexual interest, understanding the desire for parenting, and keeping couples together. Studies from Africa have found that couples counseling can reduce transmission by about 50% and over 80% of established couples remain in the relationship.[26]

Prisoners

Most prisons do not have comprehensive HIV/AIDS programs including testing for HIV and programs that target the general population may not be accessed by prisoners. Prisoners because of their vulnerability end up engaging in risky sexual behaviors including unprotected sex. Lack of access to HIV prevention and care by prisoners may ultimately lead to increased transmission in the general population because prisoners move in and out of prisons and mix with the communities.

Sex Workers

Commercial sex work (CSW) or prostitution is a global phenomenon complicated by stigmatization, slavery, abuse, extreme deprivation of human rights, drug addiction and denigration of the individual providing these services. Unfortunately, the demand for purchased sex is growing and as result in many societies, the number of sex workers is increasing even though illegal in many countries. The contribution of CSW to HIV incidence has been estimated in Benin and Ghana and in both countries, it accounts for 25% or more of incident cases.[40] The University of Nairobi HIV study group has pioneered peer counseling and support initiatives in Kenya for over two decades with over 10 000 prostitutes. In these studies, effective counseling and support with or without testing reduces HIV incidence by 50% or more.[41]

Because of the restrictions to commercial sex work, prostitutes may not access social services including HIV/AIDS care and prevention. In addition, they are highly mobile and operate at times of the day when services are not available. Because of this, HIV counseling and testing programs directed at the general population may not reach the commercial sex workers. Yet, the CSWs are a high risk for acquisition of STIs and HIV and an important group for transmission on account of their high rate of partner change. HIV testing services targeting commercial sex workers must take into account these special circumstances and be responsive to the needs of the commercial sex workers. In 407 drug involved prostitutes in Miami Florida, a VCT program resulted in increased access to care for their addiction (2.4×), reduced overall sex work (2.2×) and reduced unprotected sex (1.9×) more frequently among HIV positive compared with HIV negative women.[42]

Individuals at Risk from Same Sex Practices

Men having Sex with Men (MSM) like CSWs are often stigmatized and in many societies they may not disclose their sexual orientation. The nature of their sexual practice particularly anal insertive sex puts them at a higher risk of infection and hence need special attention. Similarly, the spouses of bisexual men who also engage in MSM practices may be at an increased risk of HIV acquisition.

Opportunities need to be provided during counseling for men and women to discuss their sexual orientation, practices and concerns in a non judgmental safe setting in which the counselor supports the person with harm reduction information. Peer counseling may be particularly important for individuals who have same sex relationships.

Injection Drug Users (IDUs)

IDUs like some of the earlier groups are also stigmatized and criminalized and are often not readily accessible for HIV testing. Their risk of HIV acquisition is substantially higher than most other at risk groups and harm reduction initiatives can be particularly effective if offered through appropriately designed counseling and support programs. Many IDUs are young, sexually active and a potential bridge for HIV transmission to move from parenteral to sexual transmission and infect new at risk populations. Some IDUs engage in sex work to support their addiction. Many IDUs are at risk of other agents transmissible from shared needles particularly Hepatitis B and C. Counselors must be informed and provide information on these potential infections as well as HIV.

Ongoing Counseling Support and Prevention Interventions for HIV-infected Individuals

One session of counseling during HIV testing may not be sufficient to sustain behavior change and enable the client to cope with their HIV status. Additional counseling may be provided by health providers at the HIV care outlets or by peers, for example in post-test groups. These additional counseling sessions should address psychosocial issues, actual and anticipated care needs and prevention of HIV transmission.

Most HIV positive individuals may have one or more uninfected sexual partners and studies have shown that risk reduction following HIV testing can be more effective among HIV positive individuals than in HIV negative ones.[19] This has led to the development of the 'prevention with positives' strategy.[43,44] 'Prevention with positives' counseling refers to interventions directed towards HIV positive individuals to enable them to reduce the risk of transmitting HIV infection to others.

Prevention with positives interventions include identification of HIV-infected individuals through routine testing of patients in the health care setting and other HIV counseling and testing innovations. Other components include risk reduction counseling, screening and treatment of sexually transmitted infections, disclosure of HIV status and testing of sexual partners, and prevention of mother to child transmission.[44] Barriers to access of 'prevention with positives' counseling include limited skills and knowledge for prevention counseling among clinicians, poor communication between patients and providers, and the additional time required for counseling in the setting of busy care centers.[45–47]

Counseling with prevention interventions at the time of primary infection has been shown to be a remarkably effective strategy in a US study.[48] With special serological assays, recent seroconversions can be identified. These individuals characteristically have a very high viral load, may have risky sexual behaviors with multiple partners, and frequently have sexual partners who are HIV negative. If identified either through clinical recognition of the primary illness or through screening, behavior change may be encouraged early in the course of HIV infection.

Quality Assurance in HIV Counseling and Testing

While there is need to quickly expand HIV counseling and testing services to reach as many people as possible, it is necessary to ensure quality services. Quality can be looked at from the perspectives of the provider and the client.[49] From the perspective of the client, it is important to ensure that the services meet their needs, are acceptable and appropriate. Infrastructure (e.g. space), supplies and skilled providers are essential requirements for provision of quality HIV counseling and testing services. All these aspects ultimately affect client satisfaction and service utilization and should be in place before accreditation of counseling and testing programs.

To ensure high quality services and that all these aspects are maintained, it is important to have a monitoring and evaluation system in place for early and appropriate corrective measures.[50] There should be checks and balances with continuous feedback into program implementation. Guidelines and standards of what must be in place to have an approved counseling and testing program should be available, and providers of counseling and testing services should be conversant with these procedures. Specific areas that need to be monitored in HIV counseling and testing include:

- Counseling: It is important to ensure that adequate information is provided (with proper informed consent), culturally sensitive approaches and messages. It is also necessary to provide appropriate risk reduction and linkage to care information for HIV positive individuals.
- HIV testing: HIV test results should be accurate. The entire process of handling and storage of laboratory supplies should be appropriate (e.g. some rapid test kits may require cold storage). Usually, for testing programs, a proportion of tested samples are retested in a reference laboratory to substantiate the quality of the testing process and outcome.
- Outcomes of HIV counseling and testing: There are several outcomes that have been demonstrated through studies and programs (e.g. risk reduction, reduction in seroconversion, STD and pregnancy rates post-test). However, at programmatic level, it may not be possible to evaluate the entire range of outcomes. HIV counseling and testing programs should document the number of individuals tested, number of individuals receiving results, number of HIV infections identified and number of infected individuals linked to care.
- Infrastructure and skilled personnel for counseling and testing.
- Tracking of supplies is necessary to avoid stock out of testing supplies.

Human Resource Priorities

No study of the global human resources required for HIV counseling has been compiled so any estimates should be seen as a 'best guess'. No international guidelines have been developed for accrediting and approving HIV counseling programs. In many countries, counselor or psychological professional bodies have been established but these are often 'generalist' groups and not usually organized for HIV focused activities. However, professional bodies and academic units need to be established to create standards, advocate for formal recognition, facilitate research and enable self regulation. HIV counselor training currently varies from a very short 2-week beginner course offered by many institutions, to an academic PhD program with additional postdoctoral clinical and research experience. Trainees acquire very different skills and professional attributes with these widely varying educational programs. Research is needed to determine requirements to provide an 'acceptable' level of competence for

HIV counseling activities. This should include antecedent preparation, curriculum content, practical experience, and instructional methods. In particular it is uncertain whether a background in health as a caregiver enables counselors to be more capable and understanding as well as able to be available for 'multitasking' as a member of the care team as well as a counselor.

The size of a counselor's case portfolio depends on the acuity of client illness and the expectations of longitudinal client support particularly if antiretroviral drug education and adherence counseling are included. Ideally, most clients should be offered about one hour at the initial visit and 15–30 min every 4–12 weeks. Using these numbers, a counselor should have a maximum of 300 HIV positive clients and a country such as Uganda with about 1 million presumed infected individuals would require about 2500 full time counselors if two-thirds of HIV positive individuals were identified and were receiving ongoing support. Group counseling may enable some efficiency in counselor utilization to occur but it requires additional research to prove 'equivalency' in outcomes. Also in most testing paradigms, large numbers of tested individuals are found to be HIV negative and these individuals still require post-test counseling and some support.

Counseling supervisors may be more experienced counselors or senior health care personnel. Supervisory challenges include allocating work load fairly, maintaining counselor motivation, ensuring that most clients are satisfied with individual counselors, and acknowledging and supporting their role in the care team. Counselors have their own beliefs and prejudices from their faith, culture, traditions, and experience. These need to be recognized and openly discussed with fellow counselors and supervisors. They must not be allowed to create a condemning atmosphere during the counseling process. Occasionally a counselor may wish to be excused from counseling a client when these beliefs or attitudes interfere with the clients perceived needs.

Counselors must have opportunity for ongoing education. HIV/AIDS is a rapidly changing area and the 'knowledge base' grows at least 20–30% per year. Prevention and care activities are constantly evolving. The content, and approaches to counseling need to be updated in order to ensure that they remain relevant to the prevailing circumstances. It is also important to tailor the counseling content and approaches to the social cultural and economic circumstances. Courses, more advanced academic degrees and learning 'at work' all need to be available options. Counselors are also at risk of burn out

from the ongoing efforts to address difficult often refractory problems. Support for individuals from peers and supervisors is essential.

Counseling research should also be a priority. Operational research to address questions of how and why; systems research to create further efficiencies; randomized controlled trials to test hypotheses and outcomes research to validate various counseling theories are all necessary to build the case for counseling.

References

1. Richardson JL, Milam J, McCutchan A, et al. Effect of brief safer sex counseling by medical providers to HIV-1 seropositive patients: a multicentre assessment. AIDS 2004; 18:1179–1186.
2. Chou R, Smits AK, Huffman LH, et al. Prenatal screening for HIV: A review of the evidence for the US. Preventive Services Task Force. Ann Intern Med 2005; 143:55–73.
3. CDC. Technical guidance on HIV counseling. MMWR 1993; 42:5–9.
4. CDC. Revised guidelines for HIV counseling, testing, and referral. MMWR Recomm Rep 2001; 50:1–57.
5. Rosenstock IM, Strecher VJ, Becker MH. The health belief model and HIV risk behavior change. In: DiClemente RJ, ed. Preventing AIDS: theories and methods of behavioral interventions. New York: Plenum Press; 1994.
6. Fishbein M, Middlestadt SE. Using the theory of reasoned action as a framework for understanding and changing AIDS-related behaviors. In: Wasserheit JN, ed. Primary prevention of AIDS: Psychological approaches. New York, NY: Sage; 1989.
7. Bandura A. Social cognitive theory and exercise of control over HIV infection. In: DiClemente RJ, ed. Preventing AIDS: Theories and methods of behavioral interventions. New York: Plenum Press; 1994.
8. Prochaska JO, DiClemente CC, Norcross JC. In search of how people change. Am Psychol 1992; 47:1102–1114.
9. Rogers EM. Diffusion of innovations. 3rd edn. New York, NY: Free Press; 1983.
10. Brettle RP. HIV and harm reduction for injection drug users. AIDS 1991; 5:125–136.
11. Catania JA, Kegeles SM, Coates TJ. Toward an understanding of risk behavior: An AIDS risk reduction model. Health Educ Q 1990; 17:53–72.
12. Mermin J, Lule J, Ekwaru JP, et al. Effect of co-trimoxazole prophylaxis on morbidity, mortality, CD4-cell count, and viral load in HIV infection in rural Uganda. Lancet 2004; 364:1428–1434.
13. UNAIDS/WHO. Emergency scale-up of antiretroviral therapy in resource-limited settings: technical and operational recommendations to achieve 3 by 5. Lusaka Zambia: UNAIDS/WHO; 2003.
14. WHO. Increasing access to HIV testing and counselling: Report of WHO consultation 19–21 November 2002. Geneva, Switzerland: WHO; 2002.
15. Gresenguet G, Sehonou J, Bassirou B, et al. Voluntary HIV counseling and testing: experience among the sexually active population in Bangui, Central African Republic. J Acquir Immune Defic Syndr 2002; 31:106–114.
16. Allen S, Tice J, Perre P Van de, et al. Effect of serotesting with counselling on condom use and seroconversion among HIV discordant couples in Africa. Br Med J 1992; 304:1605–1609.
17. The Voluntary HIV-1 Counseling and Testing Efficacy Study Group. Efficacy of voluntary HIV-1 counseling and testing in individuals and couples in Kenya, Tanzania, and Trinidad: a randomized trial. Lancet 2000; 356:103–112.

18. Painter TM. Voluntary counseling and testing for couples: a high-leverage intervention for HIV/AIDS prevention in sub-Saharan Africa. Soc Sci Med 2001; 53:1397–1411.
19. UNAIDS. The impact of voluntary counseling and testing: A global review of the benefits and challenges. Geneva Switzerland UNAIDS; 2001.
20. Sweat M, Gregoric S, Sangiwa G, et al. Cost-effectiveness of VCT in reducing sexual transmission of HIV-1 in Kenya and Tanzania. Lancet 2000; 356:113–121.
21. Creese A, Floyd K, Alban A, et al. Cost-effectiveness of HIV/AIDS interventions in Africa: A systematic review of the evidence. Lancet 2002; 359:1635–1642.
22. Philips KA, Fernyak S. The cost-effectiveness of expanded HIV counseling and testing in primary care settings: A first look. AIDS 2000; 14:2159–2169.
23. Bos JM, van der Meijden WI, Swart W, et al. Postma Routine HIV screening of sexually transmitted disease clinic attenders has favorable cost-effectiveness ratio in low HIV prevalence settings. AIDS 2002; 16:1185–1187.
24. Semrau K, Kuhn L, Vwalika C, et al. Women in couples antenatal HIV counseling and testing are not more likely to report adverse social events. AIDS 2005; 19:603–609.
25. Medley A, Garcia-Moreno C, McGill S, et al. Rates, barriers and outcomes of HIV serostatus disclosure among women in developing countries: implications for prevention of mother-to-child transmission programmes. Bull World Health Organ 2004; 82:299–307.
26. Fonck K, Els L, Kidula N, et al. Increased Risk of HIV in Women Experiencing Physical Partner Violence in Nairobi, Kenya. AIDS Behav 2005; 9:335–339.
27. UNAIDS/WHO. Policy statement on HIV testing. Geneva, Switzerland: UNAIDS/WHO; June 2004.
28. WHO. The right to know: new approaches to HIV testing and counseling. Geneva, Switzerland: WHO; 2003.
29. Wanyenze R, Kamya M, Liechty C, et al. Inpatient HIV counseling and testing practices at an urban teaching and national referral hospital in Kampala, Uganda. AIDS and Behavior.
30. Beckwith CG, Flanigan TP, Carlos del Rio, et al. It is time to implement routine, not risk-based HIV testing. Clin Infect Dis 2005; 40:1037–1040.
31. Kwesigabo G, Killewo JZ, Sandstrom A, et al. Prevalence of HIV infection among hospital patients in North West Tanzania. AIDS Care 1999; 11:87–93.
32. De Cock KM. Mbori-Ngacha and Marum E. Shadow on the continent: public health and HIV/AIDS in Africa in the 21st century. Lancet 2002; 360:67–72.
33. Center for Disease Control (CDC). Routinely recommended HIV testing at an urban urgent-care clinic, Atlanta, Georgia, 2000. MMWR 2001; 50:538–541.
34. CDC. Voluntary HIV testing as part of routine medical care, Massachusetts, 2002. MMWR 2002; 53:523–526.
35. CDC. Revised recommendations for HIV screening of pregnant women. MMWR Recomm Rep 2001; 50:63–85.
36. AIDS Information Center (AIC). Annual report, 2004. Kampala, Uganda: AIDS Information Center; 2005.
37. Wolff B, Nyanzi B, Katongole G, et al. Evaluation of a home-based voluntary counselling and testing intervention in rural Uganda. Health Policy Plan 2005; 20:109–116.
38. Matovu JK, Kigozi G, Nalugoda F, et al. The Rakai Project counselling programme experience. Trop Med Int Health 2002; 7:1064–1067.
39. Malamba SS, Mermin JH, Bunnel R, et al. Couples at risk: HIV-1 concordance and discordance among sexual partners receiving voluntary counseling and testing in Uganda. J Acquir Immune Defic Syndr 2005; 39:576–580.
40. Alary M, Lowndes CM. The central role of the clients of female sexworkers in the dynamics of heterosexual HIV transmission in sub-Saharan Africa. AIDS 2004; 18:917–925.
41. Kaul R, Kimani J, Nagelkerke NJ, et al. Kibera HIV Study Group. Monthly antibiotic chemoprophylaxis and incidence of sexually transmitted infections and HIV-1 infection in Kenyan sex workers: a randomized controlled trial. JAMA 2004; 291:2555–2562.
42. Inciardi JA, Surratt HL, Kurtz SP, et al. The effect of serostatus on HIV risk behavior change among women sex workers in Miami, FL. AIDS Care 2005; 17(Suppl):88–101.
43. Jansen RS, Holtgrave DR, Valdiserri RO, et al. The serostatus approach to fighting the HIV epidemic: prevention strategies for infected individuals. Am J Pub Health 2001; 91:1016–1020.
44. CDC. Advancing HIV prevention: New strategies for a changing epidemic. MMWR 2003; 52:329–332.
45. Morin SF, Koester KA, Steward WT, et al. Missed opportunities: prevention with HIV-infected patients in clinical care settings. J Acquir Immune Defic Syndr 2004; 36:960–966.
46. Myers JJ, Steward WT, Charlebois E, et al. Written clinic procedures enhance delivery of HIV prevention with positive counseling in primary health care settings. J Acquir Immune Defic Syndr 2004; 1:95–100.
47. Marks G, Richardson JL, Crepaz N, et al. Are HIV care providers talking with patients about safer sex and disclosure?: A multi-clinic assessment. AIDS 2002; 16:1953–1957.
48. Pilcher CD, Fiscus SA, Nguyen TQ, et al. Detection of acute infections during HIV testing in North Carolina. N Engl J Med 2005; 352:1873–1883.
49. Brown LD, Franco LM, Rafeh N, et al. Quality assurance of health care in developing countries. Quality Assurance Project. Bethesda, MD USA: Quality Assurance Project; 1995.
50. UNAIDS 2000. Tools for evaluating HIV voluntary counseling and testing. Geneva, Switzerland: UNAIDS; 2000.

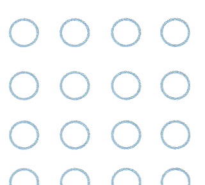

CHAPTER 12

New HIV Drug Development

Ferdinand W. N. M. Wit

Joep M. A. Lange

Paul A. Volberding

The Need for New Antiretroviral Agents

This chapter will review important trends in the development programs of several new and experimental antiretroviral targets. These new agents will be discussed in the order of the point in the viral life cycle that they target (see also Ch. 3).

The introduction of highly active antiretroviral therapy (HAART) in the mid-1990s has been hailed as one of the greatest achievements of modern medicine. Currently, 25 antiretroviral agents and combination-tablets are licensed for the treatment of HIV-1 infection. However, there is still an urgent need for new antiretroviral agents because of several problems with the currently available antiretroviral agents.

First, HAART does not completely block the ability of HIV-1 to infect new cells. In patients using apparently fully suppressive HAART there is evidence of ongoing low-level HIV-1 replication and viral evolution, and replication-competent proviral HIV-1 DNA is found in long-lived resting CD4 T lymphocytes. Therefore, it seems unrealistic to assume that present-day HAART alone will eradicate HIV-1 from an infected individual within a reasonable period of time, so antiretroviral treatment with the currently available agents will likely need to be continued indefinitely.

Second, the long-term use of HAART is associated with considerable toxicity. The pressing need for antiretroviral agents led to the accelerated approval of new compounds by the regulatory authorities. Therefore, little was known about the mid- and long-term adverse effects of these agents. In certain studies, up to half the patients had changed their initial HAART regimen within 48 weeks after initiating HAART, mostly because of drug related adverse effects.

Third, for HAART to be virologically successful, near-perfect (>95%) adherence is necessary. High pill-burdens, food-restrictions, very strict dosing schedules, and the frequent occurrence of antiretroviral drug-related toxicities make it more difficult for patients to stay fully compliant with the prescribed antiretroviral regimen.

Because of these problems, high rates of virological treatment failure of HAART have been reported in several cohort studies. Once resistance to certain drugs has developed, the resistant viral strains will not disappear from the viral pool in an individual patient. Unfortunately, there is considerable cross-resistance between members of the same drug class, and at the moment antiretroviral agents from only four classes are available limiting the number of truly 'highly active' regimens that can be used sequentially. Virological treatment failure occurs even more often with second-line and salvage regimens then with first-line HAART. This is mainly because of (1) (partial) cross-resistance between agents in the first and second regimen, (2) the reluctance of patients and physicians[1,2] to use the only available fusion-inhibitor enfuvirtide in a timely manner because enfuvirtide needs to be administered subcutaneously, and (3) most patients who are non-adherent to their first regimen often also have difficulties to be fully compliant with the second-line regimen. The fact that enfuvirtide is almost exclusively used in so-called deep-salvage regimens where enfuvirtide is more often than not the only truly new drug (i.e. not previously been used) combined with recycled agents, is especially worrying in light of the favorable treatment results reported when enfuvirtide is combined with another 'new' drug in the TORO, POWER, and RESIST studies.[3-6] Currently, there are a great many patients who have already been treated unsuccessfully with all available antiretroviral agents, and desperately need new antiretroviral agents. But also the patients that are currently successfully treated would greatly benefit if new and better agents would become available, because the old maxim 'don't fix what ain't broke' certainly does not apply to antiretroviral therapy. A good example of this is what happened when tenofovir and atazanavir were licensed. These agents were substituted for other antiretroviral agents by a large number of patients who were successfully treated with regimens that were however more toxic and less convenient to use than these newer agents. Finally, transmission of drug-resistant viral strains is on the rise, occurring in between 5% and 20% of newly infected individuals, limiting the treatment options of these individuals before they have ever taken a single antiretroviral drug.

Because of these shortcomings of currently available antiretroviral agents, there is still a pressing need for the speedy development of new and better antiretroviral agents. The ideal new antiretroviral agent should have no cross-resistance with currently available drugs, but instead should preferably be from an entirely different drug class, e.g. integrase inhibitors or CCR5 inhibitors. Furthermore, these new agents should also improve upon the available drugs with regard to antiretroviral potency, genetic barrier for the development of resistance, pharmacokinetic properties, both short- and long-term tolerability, ease of use, and pill burden. And finally, if a new agent is easy and cheap to produce, this would increase the probability that this agent would also become available for patients in resource-poor settings where the vast majority of HIV-1 infected patients live and better drugs are so desperately needed.

HIV Attachment and Entry Inhibitors

Attachment Inhibitors

These compounds block the gp120-CD4 interaction, thereby preventing further interaction of Env with the co-receptors CCR5 or CXCR4, effectively preventing fusion of the viral and cellular membranes from taking pace. Unlike the chemokine receptor inhibitors, the attachment inhibitors are active against both CCR5- and CXCR4-tropic strains.

PRO542

PRO542, a tetravalent fusion protein containing the D1 and D2 domains of human CD4 and the heavy- and light-chain constant regions of human IgG2, has shown promise as an attachment inhibitor in phase I and phase II testing. However, this protein-based attachment inhibitor requires parenteral administration, but fortunately has a long half-life of 3–4 days.[7,8]

TNX-355

Binding of the gp120 to the CD4 receptor induces a conformational change in the D2 domain of the CD4 molecule. TNX-355 is a humanized anti-CD4 IgG4 monoclonal antibody that specifically binds to this epitope in the D2 domain of CD4, preventing further interactions of gp120 with the chemokine co-receptors CCR5 or CXCR4.[9] This protein-based attachment inhibitor requires parenteral administration. TNX-355 has antiretroviral activity against viral strains that use the CCR5 and/or the CXCR4 chemokine receptor, and works synergistically with the fusion inhibitor enfuvirtide.[10]

In a phase II, placebo-controlled study 82 triple-class treatment-experienced subjects were treated for 24 weeks with optimized background therapy with or without the addition of TNX-355. TNX-355 was dosed 15 mg/kg infused every 2 weeks, or 10 mg/kg infused weekly for 8 weeks, followed by 10 mg/kg infused every 2 weeks. In the placebo arm of the study, the mean decrease of plasma HIV-1 RNA levels was -0.20 $\log_{10}$ copies/mL, compared with -0.95 and -1.16 $\log_{10}$ copies/mL in the TNX-355 arms.[11] Five subjects experienced a serious adverse event in this study, but none of these events were considered to be related to the use of study drug by the investigators. There appeared to be no major detrimental effects of the blocking of the CD4 receptor on the CD4+ T-cell counts, as the CD4 cell increase was comparable in all study arms.

BMS488043

BMS488043 represents a promising second-generation attachment inhibitor that blocks the interaction of CD4 with gp120. Monotherapy with BMS488043 dose 800 or 1800 mg b.i.d. for 8 days in HIV-1 infected subjects resulted in a average decrease in plasma HIV-1 RNA levels of 1.01 and 1.23 $\log_{10}$ copies/mL, respectively.[12] BMS488043 was generally well tolerated. Resistance has been demonstrated to develop *in vitro*, with the signature mutations V68A, S375W, M426L, M434I, S440R, and M475I in gp120.[13] Unfortunately, as of August 2004, further development of this agent has been halted by its manufacturer.

Chemokine Receptor Inhibitors

A dozen chemokine receptors can function as HIV-1 co-receptors, but only CCR5 and CXCR4 are relevant for the pathogenesis of HIV-1 disease *in vivo*.[14] CCR5 is used by macrophage-tropic, non-syncytium-inducing (R5-tropic) viruses. The R5-tropic viruses are virtually the only strains that establish new infections after mucosal or intravenous transmission. CXCR4 is used by T-cell-tropic, syncytium-inducing (X4) viruses. X4-tropic viruses are rarely present in the early phases of HIV-1 infection. During the natural course of HIV-1 infection, they generally emerge only after many years, but only in about half the patients. The switch from R5- to X4- or dual-tropic strains is associated with more rapid disease progression.[15] Individuals homozygous for the CCR5 Δ32 mutation are almost completely resistant to HIV infection.[16] Individuals with the CCR5 Δ32/Δ32 genotype are healthy and have no apparent immunologic or other diseases. This has resulted in much research into compounds that can block HIV-1 replication by interfering with the interaction of the viral envelope with CCR5. A major concern is the possible rapid emergence of CXCR4-using variants during treatment with CCR5 antagonists, which result in a more rapid disease course. CCR5 inhibitors might also be used as vaginal microbicides to prevent HIV-1 infection.[17]

Researchers are generally somewhat more cautious about the prospects of developing a novel CXCR4 antagonist, because SDF1-knockout (stromal-derived factor-1), the only known natural ligand for CXCR4, is lethal in mice, raising concerns about the potential toxicities of this approach.

Vicriviroc (Schering D, SCH-D,)

Schering D is the successor of SCH-C (development of SCH-C was halted because of prolongation of QT intervals) with increased antiretroviral potency. It can be dosed orally twice-daily, and has a half-life of about 24 h. In contrast to the PIs and NNRTIs, it appears that for vicriviroc and all other CCR5 inhibi-

tors, the most import pharmacokinetic parameter is not the C_{min}, but the area under the curve.[18]

A 14-day randomized, double-blinded placebo-controlled, dose-finding study with 48 treatment-naive subjects treated with 10, 25, or 50 mg b.i.d. found that of the subjects in the highest dose group, 81% experienced a decline in the plasma HIV-1 RNA levels of at least 1 $\log_{10}$ copies/mL, and 45% of at least 1.5 $\log_{10}$ copies/mL.[19] One subject had dual-tropic virus at baseline and experienced a decrease in the plasma HIV-1 RNA levels of only 0.5 $\log_{10}$ copies/mL. SCH-D was generally well tolerated, and no electrocardiographic abnormalities were observed.

Clinical studies of SCH-D in treatment-naive patients have been halted because of inferior results of SCH-D compared with efavirenz both in combination with Combivir. The development of SCH-D for treatment-experienced patients continues.

Maraviroc (UK427-857)

Maraviroc is a small molecule antagonist of the CCR5 receptor with potent *in vitro* antiviral activity (IC90 of ~2 nmol/L). In animal studies there were no signs of immunotoxicity with doses up to 300 mg/kg per day.[20] It is safe and well tolerated in healthy volunteers. There is no evidence of QT prolongation following single doses up to 900 mg or multiple doses up to 300 mg b.i.d. Postural hypotension was seen primarily at doses of 600 mg and more. There is no significant impact of food on short-term efficacy, but there are significant PK interactions with commonly used antiretrovirals (NNRTI and PI). Maraviroc is potentially a substrate for the P-glycoprotein, so clinically significant interactions with protease inhibitors like ritonavir might occur.[21] No *in vitro* evidence of antagonism with any members of the other four classes of antiretroviral agents. There is evidence of some synergy with enfuvirtide. *In vitro* resistance has been very slow to develop. In serial passage experiments three out of six viruses developed resistance to maraviroc over 14 weeks; two strains continued to use CCR5 as a co-receptor, and one strain showed a switch to CXCR4 use in cultures passaged in the presence or absence of maraviroc. Some strains that were resistant to maraviroc were found to retain sensitivity for other CCR5 inhibitors.[22-24] A possible reason that viral strains that are resistant to (any) CCR5 inhibitors do not always switch to the use of the CXCR4 receptor might be that the mutant virus now utilizes the receptor-inhibitor complex for viral entry.[25] There are comparable reductions of the plasma HIV-1 RNA levels at total daily doses of 100 mg or more of about 1.5 $\log_{10}$ copies/mL.[26]

Antiviral activity against primary isolates from different clades appears to be similar.[27] In one of the phase II studies, the 1007 study, there was one patient with dual-tropic virus at baseline that was inadvertently enrolled and treated with maraviroc 100 mg b.i.d. for 10 days. There were no changes in plasma HIV-1 RNA levels. The CCR5-tropic variants declined during treatment and returned to baseline levels after cessation of treatment.[28] In another phase II study, the 1015 study, there were two patients with emergence of CXCR4-tropic variants during treatment with maraviroc 100 mg q.d. for 10 days. In patient 1, the plasma HIV-1 RNA decline was −0.71 $\log_{10}$ copies/mL with transient emergence of dual-tropic virus at day 11 which reverted to CCR5-tropic at day 40. In patient 2, the plasma HIV-1 RNA decline was −1.26 $\log_{10}$ copies/mL and dual-tropic virus was detected from day 11 onwards.[29] Phylogenetic analysis suggested that the R5/X4 variants which emerged post-treatment in each patient most likely expanded from a pre-treatment R5/X4 virus reservoir, rather than co-receptor switching of an R5 clone. R5 variants remained the predominant virus species post-treatment. Patient 1 reverted to an R5 phenotype and in patient 2, the R5 variant constituted more than 80% of the circulating virus after 1 year of follow-up. Clonal analysis of pre-treatment samples did not predict emergence and persistence of a dual-tropic phenotype. These cases underscore the need for very sensitive screening assay before any patient is being treated with any CCR5 inhibitor.

Recently, it was reported that a subject from one of the studies with maraviroc had developed serious hepatotoxicity. Even though this subject had several other risk factors for developing liver toxicity, this event is particularly worrisome in light of the hepatotoxicity problems seen with aplaviroc.

Aplaviroc (GSK873140, AK602)

Aplaviroc is a spirodiketopiperazine CCR5 antagonist and has prolonged receptor occupancy. Its half-life is more than 100 h, and it has a prolonged receptor occupancy.[30] Aplaviroc is specific for CCR5 and has no activity against CXCR4. Aplaviroc prevents the natural ligands MIP-1a and MIP-1b, but not RANTES, from interacting with the CCR5 receptor.[31]

In a double-blind, randomized, placebo-controlled phase Ib/IIa study, aplaviroc monotherapy for 10 days was found to have potent antiretroviral activity against R5-tropic HIV-1 in both treatment-naive and -experienced subjects.[32] A total of 40 subjects were randomized to aplaviroc 200 mg q.d., 200 mg b.i.d., 400 mg q.d., 600 mg b.i.d., or placebo. All patients

had CCR5-tropic virus at baseline. The decreases in plasma HIV-1 RNA levels were dose dependent, ranging from −0.51 in the 200 mg q.d. to −1.49 $\log_{10}$ copies/mL in the 600 mg b.i.d. arm. The nadir of the plasma HIV-1 RNA levels occurred most often at day 12, 2 days after discontinuation of the drug, probably because of the prolonged receptor occupancy. The antiretroviral effect was similar for the treatment-naive and -experienced subjects. In one subject, dual-tropic virus was detected after 10 days of treatment, but not on day 1, 5, and day 24. More sensitive analyses revealed that this subject already had dual-tropic viruses at baseline but below the detection limit of the used assay. In this study, aplaviroc was generally well tolerated, with the most frequent side-effects being diarrhea, nausea, and abdominal pain, but these gastrointestinal adverse events usually disappeared after a few days of continued treatment. No electrocardiography abnormalities were observed.

However, currently, the development of aplaviroc is put on hold because of several cases of hepatotoxicity in phase II and III studies.[33] In light of the problems with aplaviroc and maraviroc, it is interesting to note that CCR5 deficiency exacerbates experimental T-cell mediated hepatitis in mice.[34] If *in vivo* CCR5 indeed acts as a brake to the immune response to limit liver inflammation, severe hepatotoxicity might turn out to be a problem associated with the whole class of CCR5 inhibitors.

AMD3100 (JM3100)

AMD3100 is a CXCR4 antagonist. It can block HIV-1 replication in mouse models and *in vitro*.[35] Clinical development of AMD3100 has been halted since May 2001 because of disappointing antiretroviral activity and possible cardiac toxicity.

AMD070

AMD070 is also a CXCR4 antagonist and has additive or synergistic effects *in vitro* in combination with other antiretroviral agents.[36] AMD070 has good oral bioavailability without a food effect in healthy volunteers and transient leukocytosis after a single oral dose between 50 and 400 mg.[37] Phase Ib/IIa studies in HIV-1 infected subjects are currently ongoing.

Fusion Inhibitors

There is currently one licensed drug is this class, enfuvirtide (Fuzeon, T-20). This drug, a subcutaneously injected 36 amino acid polypeptide, binds to the tethered uncoiled gp41 and prevents its recoiling and thus blocks viral-cell fusion. *In vitro* data suggests that enfuvirtide acts synergistically with chemokine receptor inhibitors, and it appears there is no cross-resistance between enfuvirtide and the CCR5 inhibitors.[38,39]

T-1249

T-1249 is, like T-20, an amino acid polypeptide, targeted at the viral p41, and needs to be administered subcutaneously. Early clinical trials reported average declines in the plasma HIV-1 RNA levels of 1.96 log10 copies/mL after 14 days of monotherapy with T-1249 dosed 200 mg q.d.[40] T-1249 appears to retain antiretroviral activity in 67% of patients resistant to T-20.[41-43] Clinical development of T-1249 was permanently discontinued in January 2004. The reason that was reported by its manufacturer Trimeris, were problems with the formulation of T-1249.

Reverse Transcriptase Inhibitors

Nucleos/tide-analogue Reverse Transcriptase Inhibitors

Elvucitabine (β-L-Fd4C)

Elvucitabine is a nucleoside-analogue RT inhibitor (NRTI) that is remarkable in the sense that it has a half-life of 4 days. It pharmacokinetic profile supports once-daily dosing. It retains antiretroviral activity against NRTI-resistant viruses. The major toxicity of this agent is bone marrow suppression, especially at higher doses. It does not inhibit DNA polymerase gamma. In a phase IIa study elvucitabine was dosed 5 or 10 mg once daily or 20 mg every other day. All 24 patients were also treated with lopinavir/ritonavir BID. After 21 days of treatment, the median decrease of plasma HIV-1 RNA levels was −1.8, −1.9, and −2.0 $\log_{10}$ copies/mL, respectively.[44]

Dexelvucitabine (Reverset, d-d4FC)

Reverset retains antiretroviral activity against NRTI-resistant viruses, but its activity is decreased when the Q151M or K65R mutations are present. Reverset is generally well tolerated. After 10 days of monotherapy in 30 treatment-naive subjects with doses of 50, 100, or 200 mg q.d. the decrease in plasma HIV-1 RNA levels were −1.67, −1.74, and −1.77 $\log_{10}$ copies/mL.[45]

The virologic treatment responses in treatment-experienced subjects were found to be somewhat lower with an average decline of the plasma HIV-1 RNA levels of −0.8 $\log_{10}$ copies/mL after 10 days of treatment with elvucitabine added to a failing regimen.[46]

In a randomized, double-blind, placebo-controlled, phase IIb study Reverset dosed 50, 100, or 200 mg q.d. and added to the failing regimen of treatment-experienced patients, the mean decrease in plasma HIV-1 RNA levels after 2 weeks was −0.5, −0.3, and −0.7 $\log_{10}$ copies/mL, respectively.[47] The most frequently reported adverse events were fatigue, gastrointestinal complaints, and headache. Several severe adverse events occurred in patients who were also treated concomitantly with didanosine (Videx).

SPD754 (-dOTC, BCH-10618, AVX754)

Although SPD754 is similar in structure to lamivudine, it retains antiretroviral activity against lamivudine-resistant viral strains. SPD754 is antagonistic with lamivudine because of lower intracellular triphosphate levels.[48] It can be dosed orally, twice daily. It was found to have only limited inhibitory activity against the DNA polymerase gamma in tissue culture model.[49] Monotherapy with SPD754 for 10 days in treatment-naive subjects in a randomized, double-blind, placebo-controlled dose-finding study, with dose levels between 400 and 1600 mg daily, resulted in a average decrease in the plasma HIV-1 RNA levels between 1.18 and 1.65 $\log_{10}$ copies/mL.[50] SPD764 was generally well tolerated.

DAPD (amdoxovir)

DAPD is a NRTI with potent antiretroviral activity against HIV-1 and HBV. In phase I and II studies, the compound appeared to be useful in salvage settings, although it has limited antiretroviral activity against viral strains harboring the K65R or L74V mutations. DAPD, dosed 500 mg b.i.d., added to the regimens of six highly treatment-experienced subjects resulted in a decrease of the plasma HIV-1 RNA levels of almost 2 $\log_{10}$ copies/mL.[51] Unexpectedly, there were problems with lens opacities in an animal model. Gilead Sciences halted further development of this compound in January 2004, although several clinical studies with DAPD continued. The ACTG 5118 study was a randomized, placebo-controlled pilot study in which treatment-experienced subjects received DAPD or placebo both in combination with enfuvirtide plus optimized background therapy.[52] An interim analysis after 24 weeks of treatment of 18 subjects revealed that the use of DAPD was safe (no cataract formation was observed), but there was only a tiny 0.3 $\log_{10}$ greater decrease in the plasma HIV-1 RNA levels compared to the placebo arm. Another study, also sponsored by the ACTG, in which DAPD is combined with immunomodulatory agent mycophenolic acid, is still ongoing. It is hoped that the mycophenolic acid enhances the antiretroviral activity of DAPD.

Non-nucleoside Reverse Transcriptase Inhibitors

One of the major drawbacks of the currently licensed non-nucleoside reverse transcriptase inhibitors (NNRTI) is their low genetic barrier for the development of resistance and high level cross-resistance between these agents.

Etravirine (TMC125)

The molecular structure TMC125 is optimized for strong binding in the apolar pocket of the HIV-1 reverse transcriptase. It is a flexible molecule and this property enables it to retain this strong binding capacity even when the binding site has mutated. TMC125 is an NNRTI that retains potent *in vitro* antiviral activity against HIV-1 strains resistant for currently licensed NNRTI. TMC125 has a more than fourfold higher exposure in the lymph nodes than in plasma.

TMC125 has demonstrated remarkable antiviral potency in treatment-naive patients. TMC125 monotherapy for 7 days was found to exert similar initial antiviral potency as a five-drug, triple-class antiretroviral regimen in treatment-naive subjects. The median decline in plasma HIV-1 RNA after 7 days was 1.92 and 1.76 $\log_{10}$ copies/mL, respectively.[53]

In the TMC125-C207 study 16 highly NNRTI-resistant patients were treated with TMC125 monotherapy for 1 week, during which the plasma viral load dropped 0.9 $\log_{10}$ copies/mL.[54]

The TMC125-C223 was a partially-blinded, randomized, dose-finding study in which 199 patients with resistance to NNRTI and PI were treated for 48 weeks with an optimized background with or without the addition of TMC125.[55,56] The subjects had NNRTI resistance and at least three primary PI resistance mutations. TMC125 was dosed 400 or 800 mg b.i.d. A planned interim-analysis after 24 weeks of treatment found that in the control-arm with optimized background therapy only, plasma HIV-1 RNA levels declined on average with −0.19 $\log_{10}$ copies/mL, whereas the subjects treated with the highest dose of TMC125 experienced a decline of −1.18 $\log_{10}$

copies/mL. Only 8% of subjects in the control arm reached plasma HIV-1 RNA levels below 400 copies/mL compared with 38% in the highest TMC125 dose group. It was observed that the use of enfuvirtide significantly increased the virological treatment response rates in enfuvirtide-naive subjects. TMC125 was generally well tolerated, with the most frequently occurring adverse events being diarrhea, rash, fatigue, nausea, pyrexia, and insomnia. However, one death due to myocardial infarction with cardiac failure was possibly attributable to the use of TMC125. Grade 3/4 TMC125-related skin rash occurred in 2% of subjects using TMC125. All grade skin rashes occurred in 20% of subjects using TMC125 and 8% of controls. The median duration to the onset of rash was 13 days, and there was no correlation with the baseline CD4 cell counts. Pancreatitis developed in 2% of patients, grade 3/4 hyperamylasemia occurred in 8% of subjects. The 800 mg b.i.d. dose of TMC125 has been selected for further testing in phase III studies.

TMC125 is currently being tested in two phase III studies with heavily treatment-experienced subjects (DUET-1 and -2, also called TMC125-C206 and TMC125-C216). In these studies, TMC125 will be combined with TMC114. Furthermore, a new formulation of TMC125 is being evaluated. This new formulation will allow for a much lower dose of 200 mg b.i.d.

Recently, the phase II TMC125-C227 study, which compared the use of TMC125 with PI, both in combination with 2 NRTI, in NNRTI-experienced but PI-naive subjects, was stopped early because the virological treatment response was inferior in the TMC125 arm compared with the PI arm. This decision has so far not had an impact on the further developmental program of TMC125, with both DUET studies in which different patient populations are enrolled than in the TMC125-C227 study, continuing as planned.

TMC278

TMC278 is a potent NNRTI with a high genetic barrier to resistance development. It retains good antiviral activity against HIV-strains resistant to currently licensed NNRTI. It has favorable pharmacokinetics, with a half-life of 38 h, making possible q.d. dosing. It can potentially be co-formulated with other ARVs.[57]

The TMC278-C201 study was a randomized, double-blind, placebo-controlled dose-escalating (25, 50, 100, or 150 mg q.d.) phase IIa trial in 47 antiretroviral-naive, HIV-1 infected subjects. TMC278 oral solution was given once daily as monotherapy for 7 days. The median change in plasma HIV-1 RNA levels across all TMC278 groups was around −1.2 $\log_{10}$ copies/mL.[58] TMC278 was generally well tolerated, with headache, fatigue, nausea, and insomnia being most often reported. There was only one grade 1 rash on day 3 that had resolved by day 7, despite continued dosing.

Capravirine (AG1549)

Capravirine retains potent antiretroviral activity against viral strains harboring the K103N NNRTI-resistance mutation, but its activity is lessened by the Y181C mutation. Capravirine monotherapy with 700–2100 mg b.i.d. for 10 days in treatment-naive subjects resulted in a decrease in the plasma HIV-1 RNA levels of between 1.23 and 1.69 $\log_{10}$ copies/mL.[59] Around 50% of 179 NNRTI-experienced subjects obtained plasma HIV-1 RNA levels below 400 copies/mL after 12 weeks of treatment with capravirine, dosed 700 or 1400 mg b.i.d., plus nelfinavir plus two new NRTI, however, this was not significantly better than the 46% in the placebo arm of the study.[60] The mean decrease in plasma HIV-1 RNA levels were −2.1, −2.3, and −2.4 $\log_{10}$ copies/mL for placebo, capravirine 700 mg b.i.d., and capravirine 1400 mg b.i.d., respectively. The most frequent side-effects were diarrhea, nausea, and vomiting.

GW695634

GW695634 is a prodrug of the previously tested compound GW678248. GW695634 has a half-life of 10–18 h and can be taken orally twice daily.[61] GW695634 is active against 80% of NNRTI-resistant strains.[62] Multiple doses of 100–400 mg b.i.d. are generally well tolerated.[63] After 7 days of monotherapy with GW695634 dosed 100, 200, 300, or 400 mg b.i.d. in 46 treatment-experienced subjects, the mean decrease in plasma HIV-1 RNA levels were between 1.1 and 1.7 $\log_{10}$ copies/mL.[64] GW695634 was generally well tolerated. The most frequently occurring adverse events were rash, nausea, and diarrhea.

BILR 355 BS

BILR 355 BS is a new NNRTI with potent antiretroviral activity against viral strains with multiple NNRTI-resistance mutations.[65,66] It is also active against many different HIV-1 subtypes. The pharmacokinetic profile of BILR 355 BS is enhanced by the co-administration of ritonavir. BILR 355 BS is currently undergoing testing in phase II studies.

Nucleotide-competing Reverse Transcriptase Inhibitors

Nucleotide-competing RT inhibitors (NcRTI) resemble the classic non-nucleoside RT inhibitors in that they are also not analogues of nucleosides, so they need not to be triphosphorylated intracellularly to become active. The NNRTI inhibit the RT by binding into a pocket not part of the active site of the enzyme, thereby inducing a conformational state of the RT that is enzymatically inactive. However, the NcRTI strongly bind to the active site of the RT thereby directly competing with the natural substrates of the RT, the natural nucleotides. Several candidate compounds have been synthesized, but none of them have yet entered human trials. It appears these compounds are less active against HIV-2. NcRTI retain full antiretroviral activity against NNRTI-resistant strains.

Compound-1 (compound-X)

Compound-1 is the prototype of this new class of antiretroviral agents.[67] It has an IC_{50} of 16 nM in the presence of physiologic concentrations of ATP.[68,69] No *in vivo* studies have thus far been performed.

RNase H Inhibitors

The HIV-1 reverse transcriptase has two enzymatic activities: (1) reverse transcriptase, and (2) RNase H. RNase H destroys the HIV-1 RNA-strand after the minus-strand HIV-1 DNA has been synthesized, it removes the tRNA, and generates the primer that initiates the synthesis of the plus-strand HIV-1 DNA.

KMMP05

KMMP05 is a N-acyl hydrazone RNase H inhibitor.[70] So far only *in vitro* data are available on this compound. It specifically inhibits the RNase H activity of the HIV-1 RT but not the polymerase activity. Its IC_{50} is 0.5 µmol/l. The binding site on the HIV-1 RT partially overlaps the NNRTI-binding pocket, suggesting it might be possible that derivatives of KMMP05 also have an inhibitory effect on the polymerase function of the HIV-1 RT. The mechanism by which KMMP05 inhibits the RNase H activity might be by altering the trajectory of the nucleic acid or enzyme processivity. RNase H inhibitors probably do not have cross-resistance with the other classes of RT inhibitors.

Integrase Inhibitors

The HIV-1 integrase is an enzyme that is necessary for the integration of the provirus into the host genome. By inhibiting the HIV-1 integrase a permanent infection of the host cell can be prevented. Many groups have been working on developing an integrase inhibitor for many years, but progress has proved to be very slow.

L-870810

It appears that resistance is very slow to develop against L-870810, *in vitro* this process takes several months. A small double-blind, placebo-controlled proof-of-concept study has been performed. Thirty subjects received 10-day monotherapy with L-870810 dosed either 400 mg or 200 mg twice daily. The median decrease in plasma HIV-1 RNA levels was 1.77 and 1.73 $\log_{10}$ copies/mL, respectively. The compound was generally well tolerated.[71] Unfortunately, its development program has been put on hold because of liver and kidney toxicities observed in dog studies.

MK-0518

MK-0518 is a candidate integrase inhibitor that has potent antiretroviral activity *in vitro*. Animal studies of up to 12 months duration have not demonstrated any significant toxicity. MK-0518 has shown potent suppression of HIV-1 replication and good tolerability in a randomized, double-blind, placebo-controlled, phase 2, dose-ranging study.[72] A total of 35 treatment-naive subjects were treated with doses of MK-0518 ranging from 100 mg b.i.d. to 600 mg b.i.d. After 10 days of treatment, the mean decrease in plasma HIV-1 RNA levels was −1.7 to −2.2 $\log_{10}$ copies/mL across MK-0518 dose groups, but no dose effect was observed. No serious adverse events occurred, with the most common mild adverse events being dizziness, headache, and fatigue. A study in which MK-0518 is compared with efavirenz is ongoing.

GS9137 (JTK-303)

GS9137 is a low-molecular weight compound that is orally bioavailable and can be dosed once-daily. It has potent antiretroviral activity *in vitro*. It is well tolerated in single doses up to 800 mg in healthy subjects. A 10-day double-blind, randomized, placebo-controlled phase I/II dose-escalation study in treatment-naive HIV-positive subjects has recently been completed. Development will continue further with a phase IIb study in which GS9137 is dosed at 20, 50, and 125 mg q.d., in combination with ritonavir.

Maturation Inhibitors

PA-457

The compound PA-457 is the first representative of a new class of antiretroviral agents called maturation inhibitors. Maturation inhibitors inhibit viral replication by interfering with the cleavage of the HIV-1 capsid precursor (p25) into mature capsid (p24). This results in defective core formation and renders the produced viral particles non-infective.[73] PA-457 can be administered orally, has a long half-life of approximately 60 h, and can be administered once daily. It does not inhibit cytochrome p450, and likely has no significant interactions with currently available antiretroviral agents.

A randomized, double-blind, placebo-controlled dose-ranging study investigated monotherapy with four doses of PA-457 in 32 treatment-naive and experienced subjects.[74] Subjects were randomized to receive 25, 50, 100, or 200 mg q.d. PK analyses revealed that the steady state was reached only after 7 days of dosing. After 10 days of treatment with PA-457 the plasma HIV-1 RNA levels declined an average of −1.03 $\log_{10}$ copies/mL with the highest dose tested of 200 mg. The virological treatment response was comparable in treatment-naive and -experienced subjects. No p25-cleavage site mutations were observed in any of the subjects. PA-457 was generally well tolerated, with the most frequent side-effect being gastrointestinal discomfort. No hepatic or renal laboratory abnormalities were observed. No significant lipid changes occurred, only transient triglyceride elevations were observed in a single subject.

Protease Inhibitors

Tipranavir (Aptivus)

The two pivotal phase III studies for the developmental program of tipranavir were the parallel RESIST-1 and -2 studies. RESIST-1 enrolled patients from North America and Australia, RESIST-2 enrolled patients from Europe and Latin America. Both studies were open-label, randomized comparisons of 48 weeks of treatment with tipranavir/ritonavir or comparator boosted-PI both with optimized background treatment in triple-class treatment-experienced subjects. In a pooled analysis of the RESIST-1 and -2 studies, containing data on 1483 subjects, the subjects treated with tipranavir had a significant reduced risk of treatment failure (hazard ratio 0.63), greater decreases in plasma HIV-1 RNA levels (−1.14 vs −0.54, respectively), greater percentage of patients with plasma HIV-1 RNA levels below 50 copies/mL (22.8% vs 10.2%, respectively), and a greater increase in the CD4 cell counts (+45 vs +21 cells/mm^3, respectively).[6] In enfuvirtide-naive subjects, concomitant treatment with enfuvirtide further increased the response rate to 35.8% in the tipranavir group and 14.4% in the control group. The overall safety and tolerability in the tipranavir group was comparable to the control group. Grade 3/4 elevations of liver enzymes (ALT 9.7% vs 4.2%, respectively), total cholesterol (2.1% vs 0.4%, respectively), and triglycerides (24.9% vs 13.0%, respectively) occurred more often in the tipranavir group compared with the control group. In a substudy of the RESIST-1 and -2 studies, tipranavir/ritonavir was also found to be virologically superior to treatment with lopinavir/ritonavir after 24 weeks of follow-up.[75]

Tipranavir appears to significantly decrease the concentrations of concomitantly administered amprenavir (−51%), lopinavir (−45%), and saquinavir (−84%).[76] Tipranavir has recently been licensed in the USA and Europe for the treatment of HIV-1 infection in treatment-experienced patients. It is dosed 500 mg b.i.d. and must be boosted with ritonavir 200 mg b.i.d.

Darunavir (TMC114)

Darunavir, better known as TMC114, has potent antiviral activity against HIV-1 strains that is resistant to currently licensed protease inhibitors (PIs). Its poor bioavailability makes boosting with low-dose ritonavir necessary. The parallel POWER-1 and -2 dose-ranging studies identified a TMC114 dose of 600 mg b.i.d. plus ritonavir 100 mg b.i.d. as the optimal dose in treatment-experienced patients.[5] In both the POWER-1 and -2 study, 278 triple-class experienced subjects were treated for 24 weeks with optimized backbone plus TMC114/r (600/100 b.i.d.) and were found to have better virologic and immunologic outcomes than subjects treated with optimized backbone plus investigator-selected comparator PIs. In the planned interim analysis of the combined datasets of the POWER-1 and -2 studies (TMC114-C213/C202) at 24 weeks of treatment, the mean reduction of plasma HIV-1 RNA levels was −1.85 and −0.27 log$_{10}$ copies/mL for TMC114/r 600/100

b.i.d. and placebo, respectively. The percentage of patients with plasma HIV-1 RNA levels below 50 copies/mL was 47% and 9%, respectively, but these numbers increased markedly when enfuvirtide-naive subjects were concomitantly treated with enfuvirtide: 67% and 16%, respectively. The mean increase of the CD4 cell count was +75 and +15 cells/mm^3, respectively. The most frequently occurring side-effects with TMC114/r are headache, nausea, diarrhea, insomnia, and fatigue. No serious liver-related adverse events were reported. Patients co-infected with hepatitis B or C virus had similar safety profiles compared with the overall study population.

Brecanavir (GW640385, VX-385)

Brecanavir has *in vitro* potent antiretroviral activity against viral strains harboring multiple PI resistance mutations. It has good bioavailability after pharmacologic boosting with ritonavir. It has good tolerability in healthy volunteers, and no cardiac arrhythmias have been noted.

In the HPR10006 trial, an open-label, single-arm, exploratory phase II study, 31 treatment-naive and -experienced subjects were treated with brecanavir for 48 weeks.[77] Subjects were treated with brecanavir/ritonavir plus 2 NRTI. Brecanavir/ritonavir was dosed 300/100 mg b.i.d. Six patients harbored viruses with PI resistance mutations. A planned interim-analyses after 24 weeks of treatment found that 77% of the subjects had plasma HIV-1 RNA levels below 50 copies/mL, with a median increase of the CD4 cell count of 84 cells/mm^3. Plasma HIV-1 RNA levels decreased in both treatment-naive and -experienced subjects. The most frequent clinical adverse events were fatigue, nausea, and dyspepsia. The most frequent grade 3/4 laboratory abnormalities were CK elevations (10%) and hypertriglyceridemia (6%). Total cholesterol increased on average with 30.9 mg/dL, and triglycerides with 62.3 mg/dL. Currently, a dose-ranging study with PI-experienced subjects is ongoing.

References

1. Youle M, Arastéh K, Clotet B, et al. Potential barriers and motivators to enfuvirtide use: Physician and patient perspectives of injectable antiretrovirals (ARVs). Program and abstracts of the European AIDS Clinical Society, 10th European AIDS Conference, Dublin, Ireland: 17–20 November 2005; Poster PE7.3/24.
2. Horne R, Clotet R, Cohen C, et al. Treatment-experienced patient perceptions of self-injectable therapy. Program and abstracts of the European AIDS Clinical Society, 10th European AIDS Conference, Dublin, Ireland: 17–20 November 2005; Poster PE7.3/25.

3. Lazzarin A, Clotet B, Cooper D, et al. TORO 2 Study Group. Efficacy of enfuvirtide in patients infected with drug-resistant HIV-1 in Europe and Australia. N Engl J Med 2003; 348:2186–2195.

4. Lalezari JP, Henry K, O'Hearn M, et al. TORO 1 Study Group. Enfuvirtide, an HIV-1 fusion inhibitor, for drug-resistant HIV infection in North and South America. N Engl J Med 2003; 348:2175–2185. [Erratum in: N Engl J Med 2003; 349:1100].

5. Katlama C, Berger D, Bellos N, et al. Efficacy of TMC114/r in 3-class experienced patients with limited treatment options: 24-week planned interim analysis of 2 96-week multinational dose-finding trials. Program and abstracts of the 12th Conference on Retroviruses and Opportunistic Infections, Boston, MA: 22–25 February 2005; Abstract 164LB.

6. Cahn P, Hicks C. 48 Week meta-analyses demonstrate superiority of protease inhibitor (PI) Tipranavir + Ritonavir (TPV/r) over an optimized PI (CPI/r) regimen in antiretroviral (ARV) experienced patients. 10th European AIDS Conference, Dublin, Ireland: 17–20 November 2005; Abstract No. PS 3/8.

7. Jacobson JM, Lowy I, Fletcher CV, et al. Single-dose safety, pharmacology, and antiviral activity of the human immunodeficiency virus (HIV) type 1 entry inhibitor PRO 542 in HIV-infected adults. J Infect Dis 2000; 182:326–329

8. Jacobson JM, Israel RJ, Lowy I, et al. Treatment of advanced human immunodeficiency virus type 1 disease with the viral entry inhibitor PRO 542. Antimicrob Agents Chemother 2004; 48:423–429.

9. Kuritzkes DR, Jacobson J, Powderly WG, et al. Antiretroviral activity of the anti-CD4 monoclonal antibody TNX-355 in patients infected with HIV type 1. J Infect Dis 2004; 189:286–291.

10. Godofsky E, Zhang X, Sorenson M, et al. In vitro antiretroviral activity of the humanized anti-CD4 monoclonal antibody, TNX-355, against CCR5, CXCR4, and dual-tropic isolates and synergy with enfuvirtide. 45th Interscience Conference on Antimicrobial Agents and Chemotherapy, Washington, DC: 16–29 December 2005; Abstract LB-26.

11. Norris, D, Morales J, Gathe J, et al. TNX-355 in combination with optimized background regimen (OBR) exhibits greater antiviral activity than OBR alone in HIV treatment experienced patients. Program and abstracts of the 45th Interscience Conference of Antimicrobial Agents and Chemotherapy Washington, DC: 16–19 December 2005, Abstract LB 2–26.

12. Hanna G, Lalezari J, Hellinger J, et al. Antiviral activity, safety and tolerability of a novel oral small molecule HIV-1 attachment inhibitor BMS-488043 in HIV-1 infected subjects. 11th Conference on Retroviruses and Opportunistic Infections, San Francisco, CA: 2004; Abstract 141.

13. Lin PF, Ho HT, Gong YF, et al. Characterization of a small molecule HIV-1 attachment inhibitor BMS-488043: virology, resistance and mechanism of action. 11th Conference on Retroviruses and Opportunistic Infections, San Francisco, CA: 2004; Abstract 534.

14. Doms RW, Trono D. The plasma membrane as a combat zone in the HIV battlefield. Genes Dev 2000; 14:2677–2688.

15. Scarlatti G, Tresoldi E, Bjorndal A, et al. In vivo evolution of HIV-1 co-receptor usage and sensitivity to chemokine-mediated suppression. Nat Med 1997; 3:1259–1265.

16. Liu R, Paxton WA, Choe S, et al. Homozygous defect in HIV-1 coreceptor accounts for resistance of some multiply-exposed individuals to HIV-1 infection. Cell 1996; 86:367–377.

17. Lederman MM, Veazey RS, Offord R, et al. Prevention of vaginal SHIV transmission in rhesus macaques through inhibition of CCR5. Science 2004; 306:485–487.

18. Hendrix CW. Clinical pharmacokinetics and pharmacodynamics of chemokine inhibitors: implications for rational dosing. Program and abstracts of the 12th Conference on Retroviruses and Opportunistic Infections, Boston, MA: 22–25 February 2005; Abstract 58.

19. Schurmann D, Rouzier R, Nougarede R, et al. SCH-D: Antiviral activity of a CCR5 receptor antagonist. 11th Conference on Retroviruses and Opportunistic Infections, San Francisco, CA: 2004; Abstract 140LB.

20. Peters C, Kawabata T, Syntin P. Assessment of immunotoxic potential of maraviroc (UK-427857) in cynomolgus monkeys. Program and abstracts of the 45th Interscience Conference of Antimicrobial Agents and Chemotherapy, Washington, DC: 16–19 December 2005; Abstract H-1100.

21. Walker DK, Abel S, Comby P, et al. Species differences in the disposition of the CCR5 antagonist, UK-427857, a new potential treatment for HIV. Drug Metab Dispos 2005; 33:587–595.

22. Dorr P, Macartney M, Rickett G et al. UK-427857. A novel small molecule HIV entry inhibitor is a specific antagonist of the chemokine receptor CCR5. Program and abstracts of the 10th Conference on Retroviruses and Opportunistic Infections, Boston, MA: 10–14 February 2003; Oral Presentation 12.

23. Westby M, Smith-Burchnell C, Hamilton D, et al. Structurally related HIV co-receptor antagonists bind to similar regions of CCR5 but have differential activities against UK-427857-resistant primary isolates. Program and abstracts of the 12th Conference on Retroviruses and Opportunistic Infections, Boston, MA: 22–25 February 2005; Abstract 96.

24. Westby M, Mori J, Smith-Burchnell C, et al. Maraviroc (UK-427857)-resistant HIV-1 variants, selected by serial passage, are sensitive to CCR5 antagonists and T-20. Antivir Ther 2005; 10:S72.

25. Petropoulos CJ, Huang W, Toma J, et al. Resistance to HIV chemokine receptor antagonists. Program and abstracts of the 12th Conference on Retroviruses and Opportunistic Infections, Boston, MA: 22–25 February 2005; Abstract 59.

26. Fätkenheuer G, Pozniak A, Johnson M, et al. Evaluation of dosing frequency and food effect on viral load reduction during short-term monotherapy with UK-427857 a novel CCR5 antagonist. Program and abstracts of the XV International AIDS Conference, Bangkok, Thailand: 11–16 July 2004; Abstract TuPeB4489.

27. Macartney MJ, Dorr PK, Smith-Burchnell C, et al. In vitro antiviral profile of UK-427857, a novel CCR5 antagonist. Abstracts of the 43rd Annual Interscience Conference on Antimicrobial Agents and Chemotherapy (43rd ICAAC), Chicago, IL: 14–17 September 2003. Abstract H-875.

28. Westby M, Whitcomb J, Huang W, et al. Reversible predominance of CXCR4. Utilising variants in a non-responsive dual tropic patient receiving the CCR5 antagonist UK-427857. 11th Conference on Retroviruses and Opportunistic Infection, San Francisco CA: 8–11 February 2004; Abstract 538.

29. Lewis ME, Van der Ryst E, Youle M, et al. Phylogenetic analysis and co-receptor tropism of HIV-1 envelope sequences from two patients with emergence of CXCR4 using virus following treatment with the CCR5 antagonist UK-427857. Program and abstracts of the 44th Annual ICAAC Meeting, Washington, DC: 30 October–2 November, 2004; Abstract H-584b.

30. Sparks S, Adkison K, Shachoy-Clark A, et al. Prolonged duration of CCR5 occupancy by 873140 in HIV-positive subjects. Program and abstracts of the 12th Conference on Retroviruses and Opportunistic Infections, Boston, MA: 22–25 February 2005; Abstract 77.

31. Demarest J, Sparks S, Watson C, et al. Prolonged and unique binding of a novel CCR5 antagonist, 873140. Program and abstracts of the 44th Interscience Conference of Antimicrobial Agents and Chemotherapy, Washington, DC: 30 October–2 November 2004; Abstract H-211.

32. Lalezari J, Thompson M, Kumar P, et al. Antiviral activity and safety of 873140, a novel CCR5 antagonist, during short-term monotherapy in HIV-infected adults AIDS. 2005; 19:1443–1448.

33. Steel HM. Special presentation on aplaviroc-related hepatotoxicity. Program and abstracts of the European AIDS Clinical Society 10th European AIDS Conference, Dublin, Ireland: 17–20 November 2005; Special presentation.

34. Moreno C, Gustot T, Nicaise C, et al. CCR deficiency exacerbates T-cell medicated hepatitis in mice. Hepatology 2005; 42:854–862

35. Schols D, Claes S, De Clercq E, et al. AMD-3100, a CXCR4 antagonist, reduced HIV viral load and X4 virus levels in humans. Program and abstracts of the 9th Conference on Retroviruses and Opportunistic Infections, Seattle, Washington: 24–28 February 2002; Abstract 2.

36. Schols D, Claes S, Hatse S, et al. Anti-HIV activity profile of AMD070, an orally bioavailable CXCR4 antagonist H. 10th Conference on Retroviruses and Opportunistic Infections, Boston, MA: 2003; Abstract 563.

37. Stone N, Dunaway S, Flexner C, et al. Biologic activity of an orally bioavailable CXCR4 antagonist in human subjects. Program and abstracts of the 5th International Workshop on Clinical Pharmacology of HIV Therapy, Rome, Italy: 1–3 April 2004; Abstract 5.3.

38. Strizki J, Wojcik L, Marozsan A, et al. Properties of in vitro generated HIV-1 variants resistant to the CCR5 antagonists SCH 351125 and SCH 417690. Antivir Ther 2005; 10:S66.

39. LaBranche C, Davison D, Ferris R, et al. Studies with 873140, a novel CCR5 antagonist, demonstrate synergy with enfuvirtide and potent inhibition of enfuvirtide-resistant R5-tropic HIV-1. Antivir Ther 2005; 10:S73.

40. Gulick R, Eron J, Bartlett JA, et al. Complete analysis of T-1249-101: safety, pharmacokinetics and antiviral activity of T-1249, a peptide inhibitor of HIV membrane fusion. 42nd Interscience Conference on Antimicrobial Agents and Chemotherapy, San Diego, CA: 2002; Abstract H-1075.

41. Miralles GD, DeMasi R, Sista P, et al. Baseline genotype and prior antiretroviral history do not affect virological response to T-1249. Antivir Ther 2002; 6:S4

42. Miralles GD, Lalezari JP, Bellos N, et al. T-1249 demonstrates potent antiviral activity over 10 day dosing in most patients who have failed a regimen containing enfuvirtide (ENF): planned interim analysis of T1249-102, a phase I/II study. 10th Conference on Retroviruses and Opportunistic Infections, Boston, MA: 10–14 February 2003; Abstract 14LB.

43. Sista P, Melby T, Dhingra U, et al. The fusion inhibitors T-20 and T-1249 demonstrate potent in vitro antiviral activity against clade E HIV-1 isolates resistant to reverse transcriptase and protease inhibitors and non-B clades. Antivir Ther 2001; 6:S3

44. Colucci P, Pottage J, Robison H, et al. Program and abstracts of the 45th Interscience Conference on Antimicrobial Agents and Chemotherapy, Washington, DC: 16–19 December 2005; Abstract LB-27.

45. Murphy RL, Schürmann D, Beard A, et al. Tolerance and potent anti-HIV-1 activity of Reverset following 10 days of mono-therapy in treatment-naive individuals. Program and abstracts of the 11th Conference on Retroviruses and Opportunistic Infections, San Francisco, CA: 8–11 February 2004; Abstract 137.

46. Murphy RL, Schürmann D, Beard A, et al. Potent anti-HIV-1 activity of Reverset™ following 10 days of monotherapy in treatment-naive individuals. Program and abstracts of the XV International AIDS Conference, Bangkok, Thailand. 11–16 July 2004; Abstract MoOrB1056.

47. Cohen C, Katlama C, Murphy R, et al. Antiretroviral activity and tolerability of Reverset (Dd4FC), a new fluoro-cytidine nucleoside analog when used in combination therapy in treatment-experienced patients: results of phase IIb study RVT-203. Program and abstracts of the 3rd International AIDS Society Conference on the HIV Pathogenesis and Treatment, Rio de Janeiro, Brazil: 24–27 July 2005; Abstract WeOaLB0103.

48. Bethell R, Adams J, De Muys J, et al. Pharmacological evaluation of a dual deoxycytidine analogue combination: 3TC and SPD754. Program and abstracts of the 11th Conference on Retroviruses and Opportunistic Infections, San Francisco, CA: 8–11 February 2004; Abstract 138.

49. Bethell R, De Rooj E, Smolders K, et al. Comparison of the in vitro mitochondrial toxicity of SPD754 in HepG2 cells with nine other nucleoside reverse transcriptase inhibitors. Program and abstracts of the 44th Interscience Conference of Antimicrobial Agents and Chemotherapy, Washington, DC. 30 October–2 November 2004; Abstract H-207.

50. Cahn P, Lange J, Cassetti I, et al. Anti HIV-1 activity of SPD754, a new NRTI: results of a 10-day monotherapy study in treatment-naive HIV patients. Program and abstracts of the 2nd IAS Conference on HIV Pathogenesis and Treatment, Paris, France: 13–16 July 2003; Abstract LB15.

51. Eron J, Merigan T, Kilby M, et al. Clinical HIV suppression after short-term monotherapy with DAPD. 40th Interscience Conference on Antimicrobial Agents and Chemotherapy, Toronto: 2000; Abstract 690.

52. Gripshover B, Santana J, Ribaudo H, et al. A randomized, placebo-controlled trial of amdoxovir vs placebo with enfuvirtide plus optimized background therapy for HIV-infected subjects failing current therapy (AACTG 5118). Program and abstracts of the 12th Conference on Retroviruses and Opportunistic Infections; 22–25 February 2005; Boston, MA. Abstract 553.

53. Sankatsing SU, Weverling GJ, Peeters M, et al. TMC125 exerts similar initial antiviral potency as a five-drug, triple class antiretroviral regimen. AIDS 2003; 17:2623–2627.

54. Gazzard B, Pozniak A, Rosenbaum W, et al. An open-label assessment of TMC 125-a new, next-generation NNRTI, for 7 days in HIV-1 infected individuals with NNRTI resistance. AIDS 2003; 17:49–54.

55. Nadler JP, Grossman HA, Hicks C, et al. Efficacy and tolerability of TMC125 in HIV patients with NNRTI and PI resistance at 24 weeks: TMC125-C223. 10th European AIDS Conference/European AIDS Clinical Society, Dublin, Ireland: 2005; Abstract LBPS3/7A.

56. Grossman HA, Hicks C, Nadler, et al. Efficacy and tolerability of TMC125 in HIV patients with NNRTI and PI resistance at 24 weeks: tmc-c223. Program and abstracts of the 45th Interscience Conference of Antimicrobial Agents and Chemotherapy, Washington DC: 16–19 December 2005; Abstract H-416C.

57. de Béthune MP, Andries K, Azijn H. TMC278, a new potent NNRTI, with an increased barrier to resistance and good pharmacokinetic Profile. Program and abstracts of the 12th Conference on Retroviruses and Opportunistic Infections, Boston, MA: 22–25 February 2005; Abstract 556.

58. Goebel F, Yakovlev A, Pozniak A, et al. TMC278: potent anti-HIV activity in antiretroviral therapy-naive patients. Program and abstracts of the 12th Conference on Retroviruses and Opportunistic Infections, Boston, MA: 22–25 February 2005; Abstract 160.

59. Hernandez J, Amador L, Amantea M, et al. Short-course monotherapy with AG1549, a novel nonnucleoside reverse transcriptase inhibitor (NNRTI), in antiretroviral naive patients. Program and abstracts of the 7th Conference on Retroviruses and Opportunistic Infections: 30 January–2 February 2000; Abstract 669.

60. Pesano R, Piraino S, Hawley P, et al. 24 week safety, tolerability, and efficacy of capravirine as add-on therapy to nelfinavir and 2 nucleoside reverse transcriptase inhibitors in patients failing a non-nucleoside reverse transcriptase inhibitor-based regimen. Program and abstracts of the 12th Conference on Retroviruses and Opportunistic Infections, Boston, MA: 22–25 February 2005; Abstract 555.

61. Denning J, Kim J, Sanderson B, et al. A double-blind, parallel, randomized, placebo-controlled, single ascending dose study to investigate 695634X and 678248X safety, tolerability and pharmacokinetics following oral administration of 695634G to healthy male subjects (NN210001). Program and abstracts of the XV International AIDS Conference, Bangkok, Thailand: 11–16 July 2004; Abstract TuPeB4480.

62. Romines K, St. Clair M, Hazen R, et al. Antiviral characterization of GW8248, a novel benzophenone non-nucleoside reverse transcriptase inhibitor. Program and abstracts of the 2nd International AIDS Society Conference on HIV Pathogenesis and Treatment, Paris, France: 13–16 July 2003; Abstract 535.

63. Kim Y, Symonds W, Steel H, et al. Safety and pharmacokinetics (PK) of 695634 following repeat oral dose administration to healthy subjects. Program and abstracts of the 44th Interscience Conference on Antimicrobial Agents and Chemotherapy, Washington, DC: 30 October –2 November 2004; Abstract A23.

64. Becker S, Lalezari J, Walworth C, et al. Antiviral activity and safety of GW695634, a novel next generation NNRTI, in NNRTI-resistant HIV-1 infected patients. Program and abstracts of the 3rd International AIDS Society Conference on the HIV Pathogenesis and Treatment, Rio de Janeiro, Brazil: 24–27 July 2005; Abstract WePe62C03.

65. Bonneau P, Robinson P, Duan J, et al. Antiviral characterization and human experience with BILR 355 BS, a novel next-generation non-nucleoside reverse transcriptase inhibitor with a broad anti HIV-1 profile. Program and abstracts of the 12th Conference on Retroviruses and Opportunistic Infections, Boston, MA: 22–25 February 2005; Abstract 558.

66. Coulombe R, Fink D, Landry S, et al. Crystallographic study with BILR 355 BS, a novel nonnucleoside reverse transcriptase inhibitor (NNRTI) with a broad anti HIV-1 profile. Program and abstracts of the 3rd International AIDS Society Conference on the HIV Pathogenesis and Treatment, Rio de Janeiro, Brazil: 24–27 July 2005; Abstract WePp0105.

67. Jochmans D, Kestelyn B, Marchand B, et al. Identification and biochemical characterization of a new class of HIV inhibitors: nucleotide-competing reverse transcriptase inhibitors. Program and abstracts of the 12th Conference on Retroviruses and Opportunistic Infections, Boston, MA: 22–25 February 2005; Abstract 156.

68. Jochmans D, Van Schoubroeck B, Ivens T, et al. ATP enhances the inhibitory effect of NcRTIs (nucleotide-competing RT inhibitors). Antivir Ther 2005; 10:S93.

69. Deval J, Jochmans D, Hertogs K, et al. Mechanistic differences between novel nucleotide-competing reverse transcriptase inhibitors (NcRTIs) and classical chain-terminators. Antivir Ther 2005; 10:S94

70. Himmel D, Sarafianos S, Clark A, et al. Crystal structure of a complex of HIV-1 reverse transcriptase with an RNase H inhibitor bound at a novel site on the enzyme. Program and abstracts of the 12th Conference on Retroviruses and Opportunistic Infections, Boston, MA: 22–25 February 2005; Abstract 157.

71. Little S, Drusano G, Schooley R, et al. Antiretroviral effect of L-000870810, a novel HIV-1 integrase inhibitor, in HIV-1-infected patients. Program and abstracts of the 12th Conference on Retroviruses and Opportunistic Infections, Boston, MA: 22–25 February 2005; Abstract 161.

72. Morales-Ramirez JO, Teppler H, Kovacs C, et al. Antiretroviral effect of MK-0518, a novel HIV-1 integrase inhibitor, in ART-naive HIV-1 infected patients. Program and abstracts of the European AIDS Clinical Society 10th European AIDS Conference, Dublin, Ireland: 17–20 November 2005; Abstract LBPS1/6.

73. Li F, Goila-Gaur R, Salzwedel K, et al. PA-457: a potent HIV inhibitor that disrupts core condensation by targeting a late step in Gag processing. Proc Natl Acad Sci USA 2003; 100:13555–13560.

74. Beatty G, Lalezari J, Eron J, et al. Safety and antiviral activity of PA-457, the first-in-class maturation inhibitor, in a 10-Day monotherapy study in HIV-1 infected patients. Program and abstracts of the 45th Interscience Conference of Antimicrobial Agents and Chemotherapy, Washington, DC: 16–19 December 2005; Abstract H-416D.

75. Cooper D, Hicks C, Lazzarin A, et al. 24-week RESIST study analyses: the efficacy of tipranavir/ritonavir (TPV/r) is superior to lopinavir/ritonavir LPV/r), and the TPV/r treatment response is enhanced by inclusion of genotypically active antiretrovirals in the optimized background regimen (OBR). Program and abstracts of the 12th Conference on Retroviruses and Opportunistic Infections, Boston, MA: 22–25 February 2005; Abstract 560.

76. Walmsley S, Leith J, Katlama C, et al. Pharmacokinetics and safety of tipranavir/ritonavir (TPV/r) alone or in combination with saquinavir (SQV), amprenavir (APV), or lopinavir (LPV): interim analysis of BI1182.51. Program and abstracts of the XV International AIDS Conference, Bangkok, Thailand: 11–16 July 2004; Abstract WeOrB1236.

77. Ward D, Lalezari J, Thompson M et al. Preliminary antiviral activity and safety of 640385/ritonavir in HIV-infected patients (Study HPR10006): an 8-week interim analysis. 45th Annual Interscience Conference on Antimicrobial Agents and Chemotherapy, Washington, DC: 16–19 December 2005; Abstract H-412 (oral).

CHAPTER 13

Overview of Antiretroviral Therapy

Paul A. Volberding

Introduction

Antiretroviral (ARV) therapy is one of the most dramatic examples of successful drug development in the history of medicine. ARV therapy, when used appropriately, can reduce HIV replication to extremely low levels. It can allow the restoration of even advanced immune deficiency to safe levels in the vast majority of treated persons and the recovery and maintenance of health in a previously progressive and uniformly fatal syndrome. ARV can, furthermore, reduce HIV transmission and even prevent initial infection. The obvious benefits of ARV therapy realized in wealthy economies are leading to efforts to make treatment available as well in some of the world's poorest economies being devastated by the HIV epidemic.

Success in ARV therapy is not difficult, but does require substantial resources and the careful application of principles learned from clinical trials and experience from treatment program development. Drugs that form potent multi-agent regimens must be continuously available and affordable. Laboratory assays must be available to diagnose HIV infection and, ideally, to stage the illness and monitor treatment response and toxicity. Also desirable are assays used to detect ARV resistance both to improve initial response and to adjust regimens that have lost some effectiveness. Effective ARV therapy also requires access to health care providers – physicians and others – sufficiently trained to diagnose infection, to select effective drug combinations and to initiate them at the appropriate stage in HIV disease. Providers must be expert in educating patients in medica-tion adherence and in managing ARV toxicity and drug interactions. They must also be able to adjust regimens to maintain clinical benefits despite drug resistance.

This chapter will provide a brief review of the biology of HIV therapy and the essential questions of ARV management including the design and timing of initial combination regimens and of secondary or salvage therapy. It will summarize current ARV drugs with respect to common toxicities, resistance patterns, and drug interactions, but will defer to other chapters that deal with many of these topics in much more detail.

The central goal of HIV therapy is suppression of viral replication sufficient to prevent the selection of drug resistance mutations.[1-4] Potent ARV regimens, however, allow some very low-level HIV replication, but not enough to result in resistance.[5,6] Successful ARV therapy must durably restore or maintain immune competence and the control of infections and malignancies that defined the AIDS syndrome. In patients infected with HIV resistant to multiple ARV agents and even entire drug classes, therapy may not fully suppress viremia, but can still dra-matically slow disease progression.[7,8] The goal of all HIV therapy is, therefore, prolonged high quality survival making this another treatable, if not curable, chronic disease.

The Natural History of HIV Infection

Untreated HIV infection results in persisting and relatively constant levels of viremia and a progressive immune attrition reflected most obviously, but only in part, by a decline in the numbers of circulating CD4 positive T lymphocytes.[9] The rate of CD4 cell loss varies widely among infected individuals but averages 60–80 cells/mm^3 annually.[10,11] Constitutional symptoms and serious infections and malignancies arise with immune attrition, particularly when the peripheral CD4 cell count falls below 200 cells/mm^3. Many with initial, or acute, primary HIV infection have a one to two week clinical illness.[12,13] Following recovery from any symptoms of this acute phase of HIV infection, most are asymptomatic until much later in the disease course, often ten or more years following infection.[14] With progressing disease, some experience constitutional signs and symptoms – chronic or recurring fevers, malaise, weight loss or other evidence of chronic inflammation. Advanced HIV disease, also termed AIDS, when the CD4 cell count is below 200/mm^3, is punctuated by opportunistic infections and malignancies that range from treatable inconveniences to rapidly fatal and irreversible acute illnesses. While some progress from initial infection to death in as little as 12 months, others have survived infection for more than 20 years with no apparent ill health.[15,16]

HIV disease is staged by the CD4 cell count, with numbers above 500/mm^3 considered in the normal range, while those below 200/mm^3 indicate advanced disease or AIDS. As the risk of specific opportunistic diseases correlates closely with the CD4 cell count, this test is of particular value in patient management. By contrast, levels of HIV viremia are less predictive of disease stage, but may correlate with the rate of disease progression.

The HIV Life Cycle

Reviewed in detail elsewhere, a brief summary of the HIV life cycle focused on targets of existing drugs, can help in considering ARV regimen design. These targets will be considered early, middle or late in the life cycle, corresponding to currently approved ARV drugs blocking cell entry, reverse transcription or HIV protease processing.

Early Targets in the HIV Life Cycle

After the viral surface glycoprotein , gp120, and the cell surface protein, CD4, interact in attachment,[17] the CD4 changes its conformation to allow the engagement into this complex of a second cell surface protein, the co-receptor, whose natural function is to act as a chemokine receptor, either CCR5 or CXCR4.[18-20] The CD4-gp120-chemokine receptor complex in turn activates the viral gp41 which uncoils its triple helical structure, elongates, and inserts a fusion protein into the cell surface membrane. The gp41 then returns to its tight configuration and the recoiling of gp41, now tethered to the cell, approximates the viral and cell membranes resulting in their fusion.[21] Active drug development efforts are designing drugs to interfere with one or more points in this early life cycle phase and one, enfuvirtide, is already approved.[22] This drug, a subcutaneously injected 36 amino acid polypeptide, binds to the tethered uncoiled gp41 and prevents its recoiling and thus blocks viral-cell fusion. These 'early' acting drugs can actually prevent cellular HIV infection, in contrast to other available ARV drugs.

Middle Targets in the HIV Life Cycle

Following membrane fusion, the viral core enters and uncoats in the target cell cytoplasm where the viral genes encoded on the single-strand HIV RNA genome are reverse transcribed into a dual-strand DNA copy.[23] The enzyme that facilitates this, reverse transcriptase, is the target of many ARV drugs, some structural analogs of normal nucleosides or nucleotides.[24,25] Other drugs that block this enzyme, the non-nucleosides, bind to the enzyme's active site, but have a chemical structure that does not resemble nucleosides.[26-28] Reverse transcriptase inhibitors of both types only act following cellular infection by HIV. By convention, the nucleoside (or nucleotide) – like reverse transcriptase drugs are called the NRTIs while the non-nucleoside agents are called the NNRTIs.

Other targets in the middle phase of replication are being explored. The most active area in this focuses on HIV integrase, the enzyme that enables the incorporation of the viral genome into that of the host cell. Several HIV integrase inhibitors are in development and show real promise, but are not yet approved for use.[29]

Late Targets in the HIV Life Cycle

As the new HIV virion forms inside the cell membrane and then buds into the extracellular environment, trimming of the structural or gag-related proteins by HIV protease is necessary for full infectivity. HIV protease inhibitors are potent ARV drugs.[30] Several are in use and more are being developed. Co-administration of certain HIV protease inhibitors with a low dose of ritonavir, another drug from this class, is used to block protease inhibitor catabolism. This increases plasma drug levels and allows added potency and convenience.[31] By convention, HIV protease inhibitors are called PIs. The co-administration of low-dose ritonavir is commonly called 'boosting.' A ritonavir boosted PI is counted as a single drug as the ritonavir dose, by itself, is sub-therapeutic Newer drug development in the late life cycle events is targeting Gag protein maturation[32] or blocking the activity of the viral gene Vif,[33] which appears to act by inhibiting innate cellular antiretroviral factors.

Elements in the Design of ARV Regimens

Achieving treatment goals, suppressing HIV replication to the lowest possible levels, currently requires the simultaneous use of multiple ARV drugs. Typically, one drug is either an NNRTI or a PI (often a boosted one). These 'cornerstone' or 'third agent' drugs are almost always combined with two NRTIs. As a boosted PI is counted as only one active drug, such regimens are often termed triple-agent ARV therapy. The use of an NRTI as a 'third drug' (thus forming a three drug NRTI combination) has been attempted but is less potent and is not a preferred option in most settings.[34] The choice of the two drug NRTI 'backbone' of the regimen is as important as the 'cornerstone' drug. Each drug in a typical triple drug combination must be considered on its own in terms of potency, convenience and toxicity, but the entire regimen must be similarly considered. Designing an optimum regimen must be individualized for each patient. The regimen must be compatible in terms of ease of use and tolerability for that person as its administration needs to be convenient to allow long-term medication adherence. Adverse drug interactions must be avoided and any baseline resistance mutations of each drug must be reviewed, to avoid compromised potency which can limit long-term clinical benefit.

Summarizing each ARV drug and all possible regimens of choice is beyond the scope of this review, although Table 13.1 offers a brief overview of commonly used agents. Excellent summaries of this information are included in guidelines published by national and international organizations. In the USA, both the DHHS[4] and the IAS-USA guidelines[2] are frequently updated. The DHHS guidelines serve as an especially extensive information resource for many aspects of drug toxicity, potency and drug interactions. The IAS-USA also publishes updated guidelines of ARV resistance testing,[35] which are extremely useful for clinical treatment planning. Other chapters in this book address HIV biology and important ARV treatment issues including drug toxicity, drug resistance, adherence, and drug interactions. These chapters should be consulted for this crucial information.

An Overview of Common ARV Regimens

Most effective ARV regimens consist of a dual NRTI 'backbone' and a third or 'cornerstone' drug.[2,4]

Dual NRTI Backbone

Of all possible two-drug NRTI combinations, several are commonly prescribed, while others are to be avoided and yet others can be useful in specific situations affected by prior toxicity or drug resistance. Preferred combinations increasingly are co-formulations of two drugs in a single pill, increasing convenience and potentially improving medication adherence.[36,37]

Zidovudine (ZDV) and Lamivudine (3TC)

This combination was the first to be co-formulated and, as it contains two of the first ARVs approved, has had extensive use. The main disadvantage is that it must be used twice daily. Zidovudine also can cause anemia,[38,39] although not typically of severe grade. This combination has minimal drug interactions with other ARV drugs. The resistance barrier with zidovudine is broad, while a single mutation, M184V, confers high level lamivudine resistance. Lamivudine is also active against hepatitis B virus (HBV), but which, as a single active drug can lead to HBV resistance.[40,41] This should be considered in designing ARV regimens for those with HBV co-infection.

Tenofovir (TDF) and Emtricitabine (FTC)

This is a newer co-formulation with less extensive clinical use. This is a potent and convenient one pill, once daily backbone. Both agents are well tolerated in short-term use. Questions of potential long-term renal or bone toxicity with tenofovir remain under investigation.[42] Tenofovir has interactions, especially with didanosine (ddI levels increase)[43,44] and atazanavir (ATZ levels decrease)[45] and its own levels are somewhat elevated by boosted PIs. The resistance pattern of emtricitabine is the same as lamivudine. Both drugs in this co-formulation are active against HBV although not approved for this indication. The HIV resistance pattern of tenofovir includes a K65R

Table 13.1 Antiretroviral drugs in common use

Drug class	Generic drug name	Common abbreviation	Dose in common formulation	Dosing in adults*	Comments
Nucleoside/ nucleotide Reverse Transcriptase Inhibitors (NRTI)	Zidovudine	ZDV	100 caps, 300 mg tabs (also available in two fixed dose combinations; one with lamivudine, another with both lamivudine and abacavir)	300 mg b.i.d.	Common side-effects, anemia, macrocytosis. Must be used b.i.d. Should not be used with d4T.
	Stavudine	d4T	15, 20, 30 40 mg caps	40 mg b.i.d. if >60 kg; 30 mg b.i.d. if <60 kg	Commonly causes peripheral neuropathy lipoatrophy. Lactic acidosis, pancreatitis more common when used with ddl.
	Didanosine	ddl	125, 200, 250, 400 mg EC caps	400 mg q.d. if >60 kg; 250 mg q.d. if <60 kg or if <60 kg or if used with TDF	See caution with d4T. Reduce dose when used with tenofovir.
	Lamivudine	3TC	150, 300 mg tabs	150 mg b.i.d. or 300 mg q.d.	Well tolerated.
	Abacavir	ABC	300 mg tabs (also available in two fixed dose combinations, one with lamivudine, and one with both lamivudine and zidovudine)	300 mg b.i.d. or 600 mg q.d.	Can cause rash and systemic hypersensitivity reaction that can be fatal if drug not stopped or if it is reinitiated after initial reaction.
	Tenofovir	TDF	300 mg tabs (also available in a fixed dose combination with emtricitabine)	300 mg q.d.	Combination of TDF with ddl may have reduced potency.
	Emtricitabine	FTC	200 mg caps	200 mg q.d.	Well tolerated.
Non-nucleoside Reverse Transcriptase Inhibitors (NNRTI)	Efavirenz	EFV	50, 100, 200 mg caps or 600 mg tabs	600 mg q.d.	Can cause rash, CNS side-effects. Both usually transient. Can cause severe teratogenicity. Take on empty stomach, usually at bedtime.
	Nevirapine	NVP	200 mg tabs	200 mg q.d. for first 14 days, then 200 mg b.i.d.	Can cause rash, hypersensitivity with hepatotoxicity; occasionally fatal.

Class	Drug	Abbrev.	Formulation	Dosing	Comments
Protease Inhibitor (PI)	Indinavir	IDV	200, 333, 400 mg caps	800 mg b.i.d. with RTV boosting dose of 100–200 mg	Hyperbilirubinemia, retinoid-like effects, renal stones, GI disorders. Should be taken with extra hydration.
	Ritonavir	RTV	100 mg caps	600 mg b.i.d. as sole PI. 100–200 mg b.i.d. or q.d. as boost for other PI.	Rarely used as sole PI as GI disorders, hyperlipidemia common.
	Saquinavir hard gel	SQV-hgc	500 mg tabs	1000 mg b.i.d. with RTV boosting dose of 100 mg b.i.d. or 400 mg b.i.d. with RTV 400 mg b.i.d.	Only approved for b.i.d. use. Must be used in combination with RTV. Causes GI disorders, hyperlipidemias.
	Lopinavir/r	LPV/r	133.3 mg LPV+ 33.3 mg RTV caps	3 caps b.i.d. or 6 caps q.d. (if treatment naive)	Can cause GI disorders, hyperlipidemia. Increase to 4 caps b.i.d. if combined with EFV or NVP.
	Atazanavir	ATV	100, 150, 200 mg caps	400 mg q.d.;300 mg q.d. if boosted with 100 mg RTV	Causes elevated indirect bilirubin levels. Little lipid or GI effects. Must be ritonavir boosted when used with tenofovir.
	Fos-Amprenavir	f-APV	700 mg tabs	1400 mg q.d. with 200 mg RTV or 700 mg b.i.d. with 100 mg RTV	Can cause rash, GI disorders, hyperlipidemia.
	Tipranavir	TPV	250 mg caps	500 mg q.d. with 200 mg RTV	Approved only in salvage therapy. Must be ritonavir boosted. Can cause hepatotoxicity GI disorders, hyperlipidemia. Not for use in patients with moderate/severe hepatic insufficiency.
	Darunavir	DRV	300 mg tabs	600 mg b.i.d. with 100 mg ritonavir boosting	Refines potency in HIV moderately resistant to other drugs in PI class.
Fusion Inhibitor	Enfuvirtide	T20	Vial of 108 mg lyophilized powder reconstituted with 1.1 mL sterile water.	90 mg s.q. b.i.d.	Commonly causes injection site reactions.

mutation that can lead to cross-resistance with some other drugs in this class. This mutation is rare if either a thymidine analog, or a potent 'cornerstone' drug is co-administered. Triple nucleoside regimens including tenofovir without either a thymidine NRTI or a potent third drug have led to a high viral break-through, frequently with the K65R mutation.[46,47]

Abacavir (ABC) and Lamivudine (3TC)

The third NRTI co-formulation, also one pill, once daily, has had extensive clinical application.[48] Abacavir is a potent non-thymidine NRTI with no significant drug interactions. It, along with lamivudine, is well tolerated in long-term use. It, however, has an uncommon, but occasionally severe hypersensitivity reaction in early use characterized by fever, rash, malaise, and, in extreme cases where the drug is continued or reintroduced, circulatory collapse and death.[49,50] The rate of this reaction may be reduced with genetic screening. Drug interactions with this combination are uncommon. Drug resistance patterns with abacavir are similar to tenofovir with a K65R mutation, but also seen is the L74V mutation.

Comments on Other NRTIs

Didanosine (ddI) is a drug used daily in an enteric coated formulation. It is well tolerated in the short term, although some note a mild gastrointestinal (GI) reaction. It has been associated with pancreatitis, usually in longer-term use, especially if combined with stavudine, a combination contraindicated in women and relatively contraindicated in all patients.[51] Didanosine is often used with lamivudine, zidovudine or tenofovir. As tenofovir increases didanosine levels, dose adjustment is needed. An attenuated CD4 response to ARV therapy has been reported with tenofovir and didanosine, especially if the ddI dose is not appropriately reduced,[52,53] and some trials have suggested a lower potency with the tenofovir combination when used with an NNRTI-based regimen.[54,55]

Stavudine

This thymidine analog has been used extensively but is strongly associated with peripheral lipotrophy.[56] It can also cause peripheral neuropathy[57] when used with didanosine, pancreatitis and lactic acidosis.[51] While well tolerated in short-term use, long-term toxicities limit its current application. Stavudine has also been used in generic formulations in resource constrained settings due to low cost. Even there, alternatives should be sought, if possible.

Cornerstone agents

Non-nucleoside RTIs

Efavirenz (EFV) Efavirenz is a potent, once daily NNRTI and the preferred 'third agent' in many initial ARV triple drug regimens.[2,4] It is well tolerated in the long term. Short-term toxicity is usually temporary and does not require treatment interruption. Most common is a rash and/or central nervous system symptoms including vivid dreams.[58] The resistance pattern of efavirenz overlaps that of other drugs in this class. Even single mutations, especially K103N and Y181 C or I can lead to high level resistance. The long serum half-life of efavirenz, on the other hand, may allow durable activity and limited resistance selection even with compromised adherence.[59] One important aspect of efavirenz is its fetal toxicity.[60] Seen both in primate trials and in human use, efavirenz can cause CNS defects exposed in infants, especially in the first trimester. Efavirenz should be used extremely cautiously in women who may become pregnant while taking the drug. Other drugs should be used when possible. If efavirenz is used, women should be fully informed about the need for effective contraception.

Nevirapine Nevirapine is similar in many respects to efavirenz, but may be somewhat less potent. Its short-term toxicity also includes a rash[61,62] but not the CNS side-effects of efavirenz. Nevirapine, however, has been associated with an uncommon but occasionally severe or even fatal hepatic hypersensitivity reaction.[63] This is more common in women and in those with more preserved CD4 cell counts. Its resistance overlaps that of efavirenz. Nevirapine has been widely used during pregnancy where it reduces HIV transmission to the infant.

Protease Inhibitors (PIs)

As a class, PIs have been associated with both short term and persisting GI distress and hyperlipidemia. One PI, indinavir, has a unique renal toxicity, as well as a retinoid-like constellation of cutaneous effects. One of the newer PIs, atazanavir, has no lipid effects, and less GI toxicity, but does commonly cause an elevated indirect hyperbilirubinemia, not infrequently with visible icterus or jaundice.

With the exception of nelfinavir, all PIs are pharmacologically boosted with the co-administration of low-dose ritonavir. This typically adds both potency and convenience, enabling less frequent administration and fewer pills per dose. As a class, PIs have a broad genetic resistance barrier. Each has a characteristic set of induced mutations, described more fully in the chapter on ARV drug resistance.

Lopinavir (LPV)/Ritonavir (RTV) This co-formulated PI (the only one in this class) can be used once or twice daily.[30] It is potent but is associated with moderate GI complaints and can increase adverse lipid profiles.[64,65] LPV/RTV has modest interactions with other ARV drugs, most notably with efavirenz. The potency and broad resistance barrier of this boosted PI and the unique convenience of the co-formulation have made it popular both as an initial 'cornerstone' agent and in salvage regimens. A newly released formulation may have less GI toxicity and does not require refrigeration.

Atazanavir (ATZ)/Ritonavir (RTV) Atazanavir is a newer PI and the first developed and approved for once daily administration.[66] Ritonavir boosting improves drug levels without apparently increased toxicity in shorter-term studies.[67] This combination is typically well tolerated with less GI and possibly by lipid effects than other PIs.[68] Indirect hyperbilirubinemia is common. While not a true hepatotoxicity, resulting sclera icterus or jaundice may be of concern to the treated patients who should be appropriately informed. Ritonavir boosted atazanavir has been most thoroughly tested in salvage regimens where it is approved in the USA. While widely used in initial therapy, studies for this indication are in progress. Atazanavir should not be used unboosted with tenofovir as its levels are reduced by that NRTI, and levels are reduced by the concurrent use of proton pump inhibitors.[45]

Darunavir (DRV) Darunavir is a recently approved protease inhibitor. Its primary attraction is its potency against HIV with moderate resistance to other PI agents. It should be ritonavir boosted and its main use is in salvage regimens. It has typical PI side effects, including GI disturbance and hyper-lipidemias.

Other Boosted PIs

In order of their development, indinavir (IDV), saquinavir (SQV) – in its two formulations as Inverase (INV) or Fortovase (FTV), and fos-amprenavir (fos-APV) are all boosted by low dose ritonavir. Though in somewhat less common current use than the other boosted PIs above, each is potent and can have a place in individualized ARV regimens. Indinavir is declining in use due to more common toxicities and dose inconvenience. Indinavir can cause hyperglycemia and uncommonly, renal disease.[69] More common side-effects include renal stones due to precipitated excreted drug and retinoid-like cutaneous reactions.[70] Even boosted indinavir must be used twice daily, further limiting its use. Saquinavir (as the hard gel Inverase formulation[71] – the soft gel having been removed from sales) and fos-amprenavir,[72,73] by contrast are better tolerated, although like most other PIs can cause GI distress and hyperlipidemia. As with all boosted PI's, these agents have a broad genetic resistance barrier.

Nelfinavir (NFV) Unique among the PIs, nelfinavir is not ritonavir-boosted and is thus used alone. This, and the need for twice daily dosing, has limited its use except in ritonavir intolerant patients. It is a relatively potent drug, although probably less so than boosted PIs.[30] Nelfinavir commonly causes GI distress, especially diarrhea, and can raise serum lipid levels. It has been widely used during pregnancy where it is considered quite safe.[74]

Fusion Inhibitors

Enfuvirtide (or T-20) is a polypeptide that blocks the entry of HIV into cells.[22] It is given subcutaneously twice daily and is well tolerated apart from the need for injection and for nearly universal reactions at the injection site. When used along with other active drugs, enfuvirtide has been a potent antiviral drug.[75,76] It is usually used against HIV with accumulated resistance to two or even all three of the other classes of antiretroviral medications.

Clinical Application of ARV Regimens

Successful management of HIV infection requires the prescription of a potent ARV drug combination at an appropriate point in the disease course. This regimen must be taken correctly and continuously during what is now a chronic and non-curable infection. Decisions are relatively straightforward with initial ARV therapy, but become much more complex later in the face of increasing drug resistance, seen over time in most patients, or with unexpected or severe side-effects or drug interactions.

ARV Regimen Design

The choice of a specific ARV regimen is an absolutely crucial one as a good choice, individualized for that person's needs and concerns can result in extremely gratifying disease recovery and durable benefit (Table 13.2). This choice should consider the patient's wishes for once or twice daily treatment, the need

Table 13.2 Common antiretroviral regimens using FDC backbones

Regimen	Advantages	Disadvantages
[ZDV+3TC]+EFV		ZDV+3TC is b.i.d., EFV is q.d., two drugs with low resistance barrier.
[ZDV+3TC]+NVP	All b.i.d. after first 2 weeks	Two drugs with low resistance barrier, no q.d. option.
[ZDV+3TC]+[LPV/rtv*]	All b.i.d. (although PI can be q.d.)	No q.d. option.
[ZDV+3TC]+SQV-hgc/rtv	All b.i.d. (although PI can be q.d.)	No q.d. option.
[ZDV+3TC]+f-APV/rtv	All b.i.d. (although PI can be q.d.)	No q.d. option.
[ZDV+3TC]+ATV/rtv		ZDV+3TC is b.i.d., ATV/rtv is q.d.
[ZDV+3TC]+IDV/rtv	All b.i.d.	No q.d. option.
[ZDV+3TC]+NFV	All b.i.d.	No q.d. option.
[TDF+FTC]+EFV	All q.d. in two pills	Two drugs with low resistance barrier.
[TDF+FTC]+NVP		Two drugs with low resistance barrier, NVP usually b.i.d.
[TDF+FTC]+[LPV/rtv]	Can be q.d.	
[TDF+FTC]+SQV-hgc/rtv	Can be q.d.	
[TDF+FTC]+f-APV/rtv	Can be q.d.	
[TDF+FTC]+ATV/rtv	All q.d.	
[TDF+FTC]+IDV/rtv		No q.d. option.
[TDF+FTC]+NFV		No q.d. option.
[ABC+3TC]+EFV	All q.d.	ABC and EFV can both cause rash, two drugs with low resistance barrier.
[ABC+3TC]+NVP		ABC and NVP can both cause rash, two drugs with low resistance barrier, NVP usually b.i.d.
[ABC+3TC]+[LPV/rtv]	Can be q.d.	
[ABC+3TC]+SQV-hgc/rtv	Can be q.d.	
[ABC+3TC]+f-APV/rtv	Can be q.d.	ABC and f-APV can each cause rash.
[ABC+3TC]+ATV/rtv	All q.d.	
[ABC+3TC]+IDV/rtv		No q.d. option.
[ABC+3TC]+NFV		No q.d. option.
[ZDV+3TC+ABC]	All one pill b.i.d.	Less potent than regimens with NNRTI or PI component.

for other medications that might cause adverse interactions, and other health conditions, such as hyperlipidemia that may increase long term complications with certain drugs. Also, the patient's concern for specific side-effects should be elicited. For example, some patients are less willing to tolerate ongoing diarrhea, even if mild, which can complicate some ARV drugs. Some patients find the vivid dreams, sometimes associated with efavirenz, disturbing, while others do not.

Ideally, all ARV agents can be used simultaneously without complicating restrictions on food or fluid intake. All possible drug interactions, both within the ARV regimen and with any other prescribed or non-prescribed drugs, must also be considered and, when possible, avoided. The presence of pre-existing genetic ARV resistance mutations should be tested. While not yet in common use, host genomic testing might identify variations in drug toxicity or metabolism, enabling even more rational regimen design. Certain HLA types, for example, are associated with a higher risk for abacavir hypersensitivity[77] and, if detected, may lead to the choice of alternative agents.

Optimal Timing of Initial ARV Therapy

ARV therapy of very recently acquired HIV infection is of uncertain benefit, and the appropriate subject of ongoing clinical trials.[78,79] Chronic HIV infection – generally defined as beginning about 12 months after exposure – should be treated before the onset of opportunistic infections or malignancies. Where available, treatment is guided by CD4+ T-lymphocyte counts and, to a lesser degree, plasma viral loads. Specific drug regimens are selected based on existing ARV drug resistance and by the patient's specific circumstances. Absent resource constraints, US and most European guidelines suggest ARV initiation after the CD4 cell count falls below 350 cells/mm^3 but before it falls below 200/mm^3.[2,4] When resources are very limited, ARV is recommended at the onset of clinical disease or when the CD4 count falls below 200/mm^3.[80] Immunologic and clinical recovery is expected even when ARV use is delayed until late disease stages, but immune restoration may be less robust in those cases.[81,82] Experimental data suggest even earlier ARV initiation – before the CD4 count falls to 350/mm^3 for example – may prove superior, but this is still the subject of ongoing clinical investigation.[83] As a treatment strategy, such very early treatment may allow later prolonged periods of intentional drug interruption to limit drug exposure before reinitiation prompted by a decline in CD4 cell counts, but this remains controversial given recent failures of trials using this approach.[84]

Before ARV is first prescribed, co-incident illness should be considered as it may affect ARV choice. In advanced stage HIV disease, opportunistic infections or cancers may require immediate management. Whether ARV drugs should be used while acute opportunistic infections are being controlled, or deferred for some time is unknown. Patients may also have infections related to their HIV exposure history such as sexually transmitted infections or those related to parental or maternal exposure including hepatitis viruses B or C. Pregnancy should also be considered as it can affect the choice of ARV drugs. Most notably, efavirenz should be avoided in pregnancy.[60] Chronic health problems that may be exacerbated during ARV therapy such as hyperlipidemia or hyperglycemia should be diagnosed and appropriately managed. Also, a thorough medication history is required as ARV drugs may lead to adverse interactions. The drug history should include non-prescription and illicit agents, and herbal remedies. Proton-pump inhibitors and H2 blockers, in common over-the-counter use, should be specifically assessed as they can decrease the absorption of ARV drugs –

notably atazanavir.[85] Finally, underlying factors that might affect drug absorption or metabolism should be assessed at baseline, especially renal function. Guidelines for ARV use in the setting of chronic kidney disease are currently being published.[86]

The patient should be fully informed before ARV drugs are first prescribed. Patient counseling should include information on potential drug side-effects, the importance of excellent and continuous medication adherence, and the need for on-going safe transmission behavior. The patient initiating ARV should have access to sources knowledgeable in ARV use should questions or concerns arise.

Baseline laboratory testing should ideally include CD4 cell counts and plasma viral load and, increasingly, drug resistance genotyping. In resource constrained settings, laboratory tests may not be available, and clinical recovery used to guide treatment decisions. CD4 cell counts are fundamentally important, however, and techniques to reduce their cost will hopefully increase their availability.[87]

There are no widely accepted standards for laboratory monitoring of ARV therapy. Most would repeat the viral load within several weeks of treatment initiation to both assess and support prescription adherence. At the same visit, side-effects can be discussed as they contribute to longer-term non-adherence and may be reduced by regimen alteration or the prescription of other drugs.

The goal of initial ARV therapy, reducing plasma viral load below assay detection limits, is commonly achieved within 12 weeks, but may require 24 weeks of treatment, especially if the pre-treatment baseline viral load was extremely high.[88] Non-adherence should be suspected if the plasma viral load fails to fall quickly, or if it plateaus above detection levels. Prolonged viremia in the face of ARV exposure will result in drug resistance selection, limiting treatment benefits.

Laboratory testing shortly after ARV initiation is also useful to detect drug toxicity. Early adverse effects of ARV drugs include hepatotoxicity, dyslipidemias, hyperbilirubinemia and anemia. There are no specific guidelines for toxicity monitoring which should be driven by the specific agents used and host susceptibility, and, of course, any interval clinical signs or symptoms.

The frequency of clinical and laboratory monitoring varies after plasma HIV titers fall below detection limits. Many practitioners ask patients to be seen every three to four months if all is going well. With very stable patients, this interval can gradually be extended, but usually to no longer than every 6 months. Each visit should address potential drug toxicity and problems specific to HIV disease. Medication adherence should be assessed and reinforced at each visit as should safe HIV transmission risk behavior.

Experimental Strategies in Initial ARV Therapy

Patients on successful ARV regimens with high CD4 cell counts have often temporarily discontinued therapy. The CD4 cell count usually falls very slowly in such cases, especially if the prior CD4 nadir was not very depressed.[89] Those observations have lead to prospective clinical trials in which ARV treatment is stopped until the CD4 count falls to a pre-specified level. In the Italian BASTA trial, treatment was stopped at a CD4 cell count above 800/mm^3 and was reinstated when the CD4 count fell below 400/mm^3,[90] while the SMART study (recently halted due to inferior outcome with treatment interruption) aimed to keep the CD4 count between 250 mm^3 and 350/mm^3. Current trials are exploring this concept more fully. If positive, such studies might lead to early ARV use while the CD4 cell count is still in a higher range. This strategy might avoid any irreversible immune damage associated with a CD4 cell count fall to low levels. If the off-treatment intervals were substantially longer than the on-treatment periods, the overall cost of treatment might also be reduced. Such a strategy would require care in drug discontinuation to prevent resistance selection. If CD4 testing was available, this strategy could find application in some resource constrained settings.

Induction-maintenance

Interest continues in the concept of beginning ARV therapy with more complex and potentially toxic regimens, followed by a shift to a simpler combination.[91,92] This might be especially attractive in those at higher treatment failure risk such as with a very low baseline CD4 cell count or high levels of viremia. It might also allow the shorter-term use of drugs, such as stavudine that cause severe toxicity with prolonged use, and it is possible that less potent combinations such as those with only three nucleosides may maintain adequate viremia suppression once 'full' suppression is achieved by a more aggressive combination. This remains unproven and an appropriate subject for clinical trials.

Viral Failure

Current ARV regimens are sufficiently potent to suppress viremia in almost all patients.[1] If this does not happen, several causes should be examined. First, the patient may have been infected at baseline with HIV already harboring drug resistance. This can be due to non-disclosed prior treatment or to having acquired ARV-resistant HIV. Resistance as a cause of treatment failure can be reduced with baseline resistance testing, if available.

Another consideration is poor drug exposure due to malabsorption or drug interaction. The former is rare and drug interactions can be avoided by a careful baseline drug history, again including non-prescription products. Of non-ARV drugs, interactions threatening ARV response are most common with gastric acid blockers, especially the potent proton pump inhibitors[85] and with antituberculosis therapy, where rifomycin interactions with protease inhibitors are common.[93]

The most common cause of initial ARV failure is poor medication adherence.[36,94] Non-adherence can be intermittent or nearly continuous. It can involve the entire regimen or only selected agents. Non-adherence can be seen with the first doses prescribed or can occur at any later point, even after prolonged periods of excellent compliance. It may reflect a lack of appropriate baseline counseling, the onset of drug side-effects, or interval substance or alcohol misuse. It, finally, may represent 'treatment fatigue.'

ARV drug resistance often accompanies virologic failure and every case of insufficient suppression or rebound viremia should prompt genotype testing if possible. Virologic failure of the first or even second regimen should prompt an immediate reattempt to again suppress viremia below detection limits. As dictated by circumstances, this may involve adherence support or a change of one or more drugs to reduce side-effects or to correct for resistance mutations. Resuppression in early failure is typically straightforward if non-adherence is the cause and can be corrected.

Virologic failure in the face of multiple resistance mutations is much more difficult to reverse. Non-nucleoside reverse transcriptase resistance mutations affect the entire drug class. Certain mutations in the nucleoside and protease classes also cause extensive cross-resistance. Each case of such 'late failure' is so unique in terms of prior drugs used, toxicity experienced and drug resistance patterns seen that broad generalizations are inescapable (and thus of limited practical value) in suggesting management strategies. One key issue is whether full viremia suppression is still a reasonable goal in the specific patient's care. If so, a new drug regimen designed to resupress viremia should be initiated. If not, continued therapy is usually preferred to full discontinuation. Brief discontinuation to allow wild type HIV outgrowth followed by reinitiation – often termed strategic or structured treatment interruption – is of unproven value.[95,96] Certain resistance mutations – especially those in the nucleoside reverse transcriptor class may decrease HIV fitness, as estimated by *in vitro* replication capacity.[97] Regimen selection aimed at limiting HIV fitness is increasingly popular – and understandable, given the limited options – but of unproven value.[98,99] (See Ch. 15 for a fuller discussion of this biology.)

Specific Management Approaches in Virologic Failure

Non-adherence to Prescribed Regimen

A crucial question is whether the patient simply stopped all medications or stopped only selected drugs. Also key, is whether non-adherence was intermittent or continuous. Was non-adherence triggered by side-effects or inconvenience of the prescribed regimen? Finally and critically, did non-adherence result in resistance selection? In all these cases, the need for rigorous adherence should be stressed along with practical advice on how this can be achieved. Absent toxicity or resistance, the ARV regimen originally prescribed can be continued if adherence can be re-established, and if significant resistance mutations have not yet been selected.

Toxicity to Selected Drugs

ARV side-effects range from minor inconveniences to life-threatening in severity (see Ch. 17 for an expanded discussion of ARV toxicity). Some are transient, others continue over time. Some can be ameliorated with other medications while others are not treatable. Serious side-effects may require permanent avoidance of the offending drug. Hypersensitivity reactions to abacavir or idiosyncratic nevirapine hepatotoxicity are examples of this extreme. On the other hand, some side-effects are temporary and the drug can be continued. Examples here are early CNS side-effects with efavirenz or most rashes with efavirenz or nevirapine. Yet another general toxicity type is that which can be controlled with additional medications if the offending ARV cannot be easily substituted. Zidovudine associated

anemia can be reversed at least partially by recombinant erythropoietin and hyperlipidemias can be controlled, although often only partially, with diet, exercise or statins. In these cases, the ARV causing the side-effect can either be continued, along with the additional medication, or can be replaced with one not having this toxicity. Finally, some ARV side-effects are chronic and essentially irreversible. Stavudine-associated peripheral lipoatrophy and diarrhea second to nelfinavir continue as long as these agents are prescribed. In these situations, the drug causing the side-effect can either be continued or not, depending on severity and patient tolerance. With lipoatrophy, little reversal is seen even with prolonged discontinuation, while nelfinavir-associated diarrhea promptly resolves when the drug is stopped.

An important aspect of ARV toxicity is the effect of 'minor' but chronic treatment side-effects. Over time, these can lead to non-adherence. Patients should be asked specifically about the impact of chronic low-level gastrointestinal or CNS toxicity. If present, changing to other drugs should be considered.

Topics in 'Late' Salvage ARV Therapy

Adding a New Drug to a 'Failing' Regimen

The approval of a new drug adds hope for viremia control in those with ongoing viremia and multiple drug resistance. Adding a single new drug, whether of a new and non-cross resistant class as with enfuvirtide, or with less cross resistance like tipranavir is, itself, of limited value. Unless a new drug can be used with at least one, or preferably two, other active agents, its introduction is rapidly followed by drug resistance selection. Guidelines, therefore increasingly suggest the earlier use of such new agents to improve the hope of re-suppression of viremia with more durable clinical benefits.[2]

'Partial Treatment'

If viremia suppression below detection limits is an unrealistic goal, ongoing ARV use may yet be of clinical utility. The resistance mutations of certain drugs seem to impair HIV 'fitness' and thus *in vivo* virulence, and some drugs may have partial residual antiviral activity even with what appears to be high phenotypic resistance. Discontinuing all ARV therapy in advanced stage HIV disease is often followed by rapid CD4 cell count declines. In contrast,

145

relative CD4 cell count stability, has been seen when some drugs are continued.[100] Typically, this continued therapy includes, at a minimum, two NRTIs and often a PI. In these cases, drugs to be continued should be well tolerated and ones which maintain an impaired HIV replication capacity. It should be stressed, however, that this area is the subject of ongoing research and is of unproven efficacy.

ARV Treatment Approaches in Resource-constrained Settings

There is no difference in the goal of ARV therapy in resource-limited settings, but the access to drugs and monitoring tests may necessitate very different choices. Otherwise, preferred agents may not be available and the low cost of certain generic fixed-dose combinations may require their use even if they contain more toxic ARV drugs. In many countries, important drugs like protease inhibitors are too expensive for common use while stavudine is used because of its low cost even though its associated lipoatrophy is well known. Drugs like ritonavir that require refrigerated storage may be impractical where electrical power and appliances are limited. Common co-infections, especially tuberculosis, also pose a problem in ARV therapy. Drugs needed for tuberculosis therapy, rifampicins particularly, interact with protease inhibitors.

Laboratory tests may also be unavailable in many settings. ARV therapy can be effectively initiated on the basis of clinical condition but is substantially aided by CD4 test results. HIV viral load testing is much less important in initiating ARV therapy, but is of clear utility in managing subsequent treatment failure.

WHO Guidelines suggest ARV initiation when the CD4 falls below $200/mm^3$ or in symptomatic persons.[80] Clinical or CD4 improvements are then followed as evidence of treatment benefit and ARV therapy is continued until either shows progressive disease. The choice of ARV regimens in many countries is severely limited, often consisting primarily of generic fixed-dose combinations. Secondary regimens are even more constrained. Initial regimens often are non-nucleoside based and protease inhibitors may not be available for salvage. CD4 testing is more widely available than HIV viral load testing and resistance tests are generally unavailable. Each element of this discussion, however, is changing rapidly as more international funding for HIV care is reaching many countries most affected by the HIV epidemic.

References

1. Bartlett JA, DeMasi R, Quinn J, et al. Overview of the effectiveness of triple combination therapy in antiretroviral-naive HIV-1 infected adults. AIDS 2001; 15:1369–1377.
2. Yeni PG, Hammer SM, Hirsch MS, et al. Treatment for adult HIV infection: 2004 recommendations of the International AIDS Society – USA Panel. JAMA 2004; 292:251–265.
3. Wood E, Hogg RS, Harrigan PR, et al. When to initiate antiretroviral therapy in HIV-1 infected adults: a review for clinicians and patients. Lancet Infect Dis 2005; 5:407–414.
4. Panel on Clinical Practices for Treatment of HIV Infection. Guidelines for the use of antiretroviral agents in HIV-1-infected adults and adolescents. April 2005; 7:1.
5. Wong JK, Hezareh M, Gunthard HF, et al. Recovery of replication-competent HIV despite prolonged suppression of plasma viremia. Science 1997; 278:1291–1295.
6. Finzi D, Blankson J, Siliciano JD, et al. Latent infection of CD4+ T cells provides a mechanism for lifelong persistence of HIV-1, even in patients on effective combination therapy. Nat Med 1999; 5:512–517.
7. Raffanti SP, Fusco JS, Sherrill BH, et al. Effect of persistent moderate viremia on disease progression during HIV therapy. J Acquir Immune Defic Syndr 2004; 37:1147–1154.
8. Hejdeman B, Lenkei R, Leandersson AC, et al. Clinical and immunological benefits from highly active antiretroviral therapy in spite of limited viral load reduction in HIV type 1 infection. AIDS Res Hum Retroviruses 2001; 17:277–286.
9. Pantaleo G, Graziosi C, Fauci AS. New concepts in the immunopathogenesis of human immunodeficiency virus infection. N Engl J Med 1993; 328:327–335.
10. Soriano V, Castilla J, Gomez-Cano M, et al. The decline in CD4+ T lymphocytes as a function of the duration of HIV infection, age at seroconversion, and viral load. J Infect May 1998; 36:307–311.
11. Deeks SG, Kitchen CM, Liu L, et al. Immune activation set point during early HIV infection predicts subsequent CD4+ T-cell changes independent of viral load. Blood 2004; 104:942–947.
12. Rosenberg E, Cotton D. Primary HIV infection and the acute retroviral syndrome. AIDS Clin Care 1997; 9:19, 23–25.
13. Schacker T, Hughes J, Shea T, et al. Biological and virological characteristics of primary HIV infection. Ann Intern Med 1998; 128:613–620.
14. Bacchetti P, Moss AR. Incubation period of AIDS in San Francisco. Nature 1989; 338:251–253.
15. Buchbinder S, Vittinghoff E. HIV-infected long-term nonprogressors: epidemiology, mechanisms of delayed progression, and clinical and research implications. Microbes Infect 1999; 1:1113–1120.
16. Petrucci A, Dorrucci M, Alliegro MB, et al. How many HIV-infected individuals may be defined as long-term nonprogressors? A report from the Italian Seroconversion Study. Italian Seroconversion Study Group (ISS). J Acquir Immune Defic Syndr Hum Retrovirol Mar 1997; 14:243–248.
17. Wang HG, Williams RE, Lin PF. A novel class of HIV-1 inhibitors that targets the viral envelope and inhibits CD4 receptor binding. Curr Pharm 2004; 10:1785–1793.
18. Berger EA, Murphy PM, Farber JM. Chemokine receptors as HIV-1 coreceptors: roles in viral entry, tropism, and disease. Annu Rev Immunol 1999; 17:657–700.
19. Carrington M, Dean M, Martin MP, O'Brien SJ. Genetics of HIV-1 infection: chemokine receptor CCR5 polymorphism and its consequences. Hum Mol Genet 1999; 8:1939–1945.
20. Wu L, Gerard NP, Wyatt R, et al. CD4-induced interaction of primary HIV-1 gp120 glycoproteins with the chemokine receptor CCR-5. Nature 1996; 384:179–183.
21. Chen CH, Matthews TJ, McDanal CB, et al. A molecular clasp in the human immunodeficiency virus (HIV) type 1 TM protein determines the anti-HIV activity of gp41 derivatives: implication for viral fusion. J Virol Jun 1995; 69:3771–3777.

22. Kilby J, Hopkins S. Venetta T, et al. Potent suppression of HIV-1 replication in humans by T-20, a peptide inhibitor of gp41-mediated virus entry. Nat Med 1998; 4:1302–1307.

23. Gomez C, Hope TJ. The ins and outs of HIV replication. Cell Microbiol 2005; 7:621–626.

24. Gotte M. Inhibition of HIV-1 reverse transcription: basic principles of drug action and resistance. Expert Rev Anti Infect Ther 2004; 2 707–716.

25. Sharma PL, Nurpeisov V, Hernandez-Santiago B, et al. Nucleoside inhibitors of human immunodeficiency virus type 1 reverse transcriptase. Curr Top Med Chem 2004; 4:895–919.

26. Balzarini J. Current status of the non-nucleoside reverse transcriptase inhibitors of human immunodeficiency virus type 1. Curr Top Med Chem 2004; 4:921–944.

27. Sluis-Cremer N, Temiz NA, Bahar I. Conformational changes in HIV-1 reverse transcriptase induced by nonnucleoside reverse transcriptase inhibitor binding. Curr HIV Res 2004; 2:323–332.

28. Tronchet JM, Seman M. Nonnucleoside inhibitors of HIV-1 reverse transcriptase: from the biology of reverse transcription to molecular design. Curr Top Med Chem 2003; 3:1496–1511.

29. Pommier Y, Johnson AA, Marchand C. Integrase inhibitors to treat HIV/AIDS. Nat Rev Drug Discov 2005; 4:236–248.

30. Walmsley S, Bernstein B, King M, et al. Lopinavir-ritonavir versus nelfinavir for the initial treatment of HIV infection. N Engl J Med 2002; 346:2039–2046.

31. Scott JD. Simplifying the treatment of HIV infection with ritonavir-boosted protease inhibitors in antiretroviral-experienced patients. Am J Health Syst Pharm 2005; 62:809–815.

32. Li F, Goila-Gaur R, Salzwedel K, et al. PA-457: a potent HIV inhibitor that disrupts core condensation by targeting a late step in Gag processing. Proc Natl Acad Sci U S A 2003; 100:13555–13560.

33. Stopak K, Greene WC. Protecting APOBEC3G: a potential new target for HIV drug discovery. Curr Opin Investig Drugs 2005; 6:141–147.

34. Gulick RM, Ribaudo HJ, Shikuma CM, et al. Triple-nucleoside regimens versus efavirenz-containing regimens for the initial treatment of HIV-1 infection. N Engl J Med 2004; 350:1850–1861.

35. Hirsch MS, Brun-Vezinet F, Clotet B, et al. Antiretroviral drug resistance testing in adults infected with human immunodeficiency virus type 1: 2003 recommendations of an International AIDS Society-USA Panel. Clin Infect Dis 2003; 37:113–128.

36. Bartlett JA. Addressing the challenges of adherence. J Acquir Immune Defic Syndr 2002; 29:S2–S10.

37. Pujari SN, Patel AK, Naik E, et al. Effectiveness of generic fixed-dose combinations of highly active antiretroviral therapy for treatment of HIV infection in India. J Acquir Immune Defic Syndr 2004; 37:1566–1569.

38. Moore RD, Forney D. Anemia in HIV-infected patients receiving highly active antiretroviral therapy. J Acquir Immune Defic Syndr 2002; 29:54–57.

39. Semba RD, Shah N, Klein RS, et al. Prevalence and cumulative incidence of and risk factors for anemia in a multicenter cohort study of human immunodeficiency virus-infected and -uninfected women. Clin Infect Dis 2002; 34:260–266.

40. Liu X, Schinazi RF. Hepatitis B virus resistance to lamivudine and its clinical implications. Antivir Chem Chemother 2002; 13:143–155.

41. Fischer KP, Gutfreund KS, Tyrrell DL. Lamivudine resistance in hepatitis B: mechanisms and clinical implications. Drug Resist Updat 2001; 4:118–128.

42. Peyriere H, Reynes J, Rouanet I, et al. Renal tubular dysfunction associated with tenofovir therapy: report of 7 cases. J Acquir Immune Defic Syndr 2004; 35:269–273.

43. Ray AS, Olson L, Fridland A. Role of purine nucleoside phosphorylase in interactions between 2',3'-dideoxyinosine

and allopurinol, ganciclovir, or tenofovir. Antimicrob Agents Chemother 2004; 48:1089–1095.

44. Lacombe K, Pacanowski J, Meynard JL, et al. Risk factors for CD4 lymphopenia in patients treated with a tenofovir/didanosine high dose-containing highly active antiretroviral therapy regimen. AIDS 2005; 19:1107–1108.

45. Taburet AM, Piketty C, Chazallon C, et al. Interactions between atazanavir-ritonavir and tenofovir in heavily pretreated human immunodeficiency virus-infected patients. Antimicrob Agents Chemother 2004; 48:2091–2096.

46. Khanlou H, Yeh V, Guyer B, et al. Early virologic failure in a pilot study evaluating the efficacy of therapy containing once-daily abacavir, lamivudine, and tenofovir DF in treatment-naive HIV-infected patients. AIDS Patient Care STDS 2005; 19:135–140.

47. Perez-Elias MJ, Moreno S, Gutierrez C, et al. High virological failure rate in HIV patients after switching to a regimen with two nucleoside reverse transcriptase inhibitors plus tenofovir. AIDS 2005; 19:695–698.

48. Moyle GJ, DeJesus E, Cahn P, et al. Abacavir once or twice daily combined with once-daily lamivudine and efavirenz for the treatment of antiretroviral-naive HIV-infected adults: results of the Ziagen Once Daily in Antiretroviral Combination Study. J Acquir Immune Defic Syndr 2005; 38:417–425.

49. Clay PG. The abacavir hypersensitivity reaction: a review. Clin Ther 2002; 24:1502–1514.

50. Hewitt RG. Abacavir hypersensitivity reaction. Clin Infect Dis 2002; 34:1137–1142.

51. Anon. d4T plus ddI: warning for pregnant women. AIDS Treat News 2001; 358:8.

52. Barrios A, Rendon A, Negredo E, et al. Paradoxical CD4+ T-cell decline in HIV-infected patients with complete virus suppression taking tenofovir and didanosine. AIDS 2005; 19:569–575.

53. Tung MY, Mandalia S, Bower M, et al. The durability of virological success of tenofovir and didanosine dosed at either 400 or 250 mg once daily. HIV Med 2005; 6:151–154.

54. Podzamczer D, Ferrer E, Gatell JM, et al. Early virological failure with a combination of tenofovir, didanosine and efavirenz. Antivir Ther 2005; 10:171–177.

55. Maitland D, Moyle G, Hand J, et al. Early virologic failure in HIV-1 infected subjects on didanosine/tenofovir/efavirenz: 12-week results from a randomized trial. AIDS 2005; 19:1183–1188.

56. Joly V, Flandre P, Meiffredy V, et al. Increased risk of lipoatrophy under stavudine in HIV-1-infected patients: results of a substudy from a comparative trial. AIDS 2002; 16:2447–2454.

57. Simpson DM, Tagliati M. Nucleoside analogue-associated peripheral neuropathy in human immunodeficiency virus infection. J Acquir Immune Defic Syndr 1995; 9:153–161.

58. Fortin C, Joly V. Efavirenz for HIV-1 infection in adults: an overview. Expert Rev Anti Infect Ther 2004; 2:671–684.

59. Bangsberg D, Weiser S, Guzman D, et al. 95% adherence is not necessary for viral suppression in less than 400 copies/mL in the majority of individuals on NNRTI regimens. 12th Conference on Retroviruses and Opportunistic Infections, Boston, MA: 22–25 February 2005.

60. Mofenson LM. Efavirenz reclassified as FDA pregnancy category D. AIDS Clin Care 2005; 17:17.

61. Montaner JS, Cahn P, Zala C, et al. Randomized, controlled study of the effects of a short course of prednisone on the incidence of rash associated with nevirapine in patients infected with HIV-1. J Acquir Immune Defic Syndr 2003; 33:41–46.

62. Metry DW, Lahart CJ, Farmer KL, et al. Stevens-Johnson syndrome caused by the antiretroviral drug nevirapine. J Am Acad Derm 2001; 44:S354–S357.

63. Martinez E, Blanco JL, Arnaiz JA, et al. Hepatotoxicity in HIV-1-infected patients receiving nevirapine-containing antiretroviral therapy. AIDS 2001; 15:1261–1268.

64. Kaplan SS, Hicks CB. Safety and antiviral activity of lopinavir/ritonavir-based therapy in human

immunodeficiency virus type 1 (HIV-1) infection. J Antimicrob Chemother Jun 2005; 56:273–276.

65. Valerio L, Fontas E, Pradier C, et al. Lopinavir/ritonavir combination and total/HDL cholesterol ratio. J Infect 2005; 50:229–235.

66. Havlir DV. O'Marro SD. Atazanavir: new option for treatment of HIV infection. Clin Infect Dis 2004; 38:1599–1604.

67. Johnson M, Grinsztejn B, Rodriguez C, et al. Atazanavir plus ritonavir or saquinavir, and lopinavir/ritonavir in patients experiencing multiple virological failures. AIDS 2005; 19:685–694.

68. Murphy RL, Sanne I, Cahn P, et al. Dose-ranging, randomized, clinical trial of atazanavir with lamivudine and stavudine in antiretroviral-naive subjects: 48-week results. AIDS 2003; 17:2603–2614.

69. Olyaei AJ. deMattos AM, Bennett WM. Renal toxicity of protease inhibitors. Curr Opin Nephrol Hypertens 2000; 9:473–476.

70. Garcia-Silva J, Almagro M, Pena-Penabad C, et al. Indinavir-induced retinoid-like effects: incidence, clinical features and management. Drug Saf 2002; 25:993–1003.

71. Autar RS, Ananworanich J, Apateerapong W, et al. Pharmacokinetic study of saquinavir hard gel caps/ ritonavir in HIV-1-infected patients: 1600/100 mg once-daily compared with 2000/100 mg once-daily and 1000/ 100 mg twice-daily. J Antimicrob Chemother Oct 2004; 54:785–790.

72. Chapman TM, Plosker GL. Perry CM. Fosamprenavir: a review of its use in the management of antiretroviral therapy-naive patients with HIV infection. Drugs 2004; 64:2101–2124.

73. Arvieux C, Tribut O. Amprenavir or fosamprenavir plus ritonavir in HIV infection: pharmacology, efficacy and tolerability profile. Drugs 2005; 65:633–659.

74. Timmermans S, Tempelman C, Godfried MH, et al. Nelfinavir and nevirapine side-effects during pregnancy. AIDS 2005; 19:795–799.

75. Lalezari JP, Henry K, O'Hearn M, et al. Enfuvirtide, an HIV-1 fusion inhibitor, for drug-resistant HIV infection in North and South America. N Engl J Med 2003; 348:2175–2185.

76. Lazzarin A, Clotet B, Cooper D, et al. Efficacy of enfuvirtide in patients infected with drug-resistant HIV-1 in Europe and Australia. N Engl J Med 2003; 348:2186–2195.

77. Mallal S, Nolan D, Witt C, et al. Association between presence of HLA-B*5701, HLA-DR7 and HLA-DQ3 and hypersensitivity to HIV-1 reverse-transcriptase inhibitor abacavir. Lancet 2002; 359:727–732.

78. Strain MC, Little SJ, Daar ES, et al. Effect of treatment, during primary infection, on establishment and clearance of cellular reservoirs of HIV-1. J Infect Dis 2005; 191:1410–1418.

79. Kaufmann DE, Lichterfeld M, Altfeld M, et al. Limited durability of viral control following treated acute HIV infection. PLoS Med 2004; 1:e36.

80. Hammer SM, Turmen T, Vareldzis B, et al. Antiretroviral guidelines for resource-limited settings: the WHO's public health approach. Nat Med 2002; 8:649–650.

81. Pakker NG, Kroon ED, Roos MT, et al. Immune restoration does not invariably occur following long-term HIV-1 suppression during antiretroviral therapy. INCAS Study Group AIDS 1999; 13:203–212.

82. Garcia F, Lazzari E De, Plana M, et al. Long-term CD4+ T-cell response to highly active antiretroviral therapy according to baseline CD4+ T-cell count. J Acquir Immune Defic Syndr 2004; 36:702–713.

83. Holmberg SD, Palella FJ Jr., Lichtenstein KA, et al. The case for earlier treatment of HIV infection. Clin Infect Dis 2004; 39:1699–1704.

84. Strategies for Management of Antiretroviral Therapy (SMART) Study Group. CD4+ count-guided interruption of antiretroviral treatment. N Engl J Med 2006; 355:2283–2296.

85. McNicholl IR. Drug interactions among the antiretrovirals. Curr Infect Dis Rep 2004; 6:159–162.

86. Gupta SK, Eustace JA, Wunston JA, et al. Guidelines for the management of chronic kidney disease in HIV-infected patients: recommendations of the HIV Medicine Association of the Infectious Diseases Society of America. Clin Infect Dis 2005; 40:1559–1585.

87. Stevens G, Rekhviashvili N, Scott LE, et al. Evaluation of two commercially available, inexpensive alternative assays used for assessing viral load in a cohort of human immunodeficiency virus type 1 subtype C-infected patients from South Africa. J Clin Microbiol Feb 2005; 43:857–861.

88. Lepri AC, Miller V, Phillips AN, et al. The virological response to highly active antiretroviral therapy over the first 24 weeks of therapy according to the pre-therapy viral load and the weeks 4–8 viral load. AIDS 2001; 15:47–54.

89. Mussini C, Bedini A, Borghi V, et al. CD4 cell-monitored treatment interruption in patients with a CD4 cell count > 500 × 106 cells/l. AIDS 2005; 19:287–294.

90. Maggiolo F, Ripamonti D, Gregis G, et al. Effect of prolonged discontinuation of successful antiretroviral therapy on CD4 T cells: a controlled, prospective trial. AIDS 2004; 18:439–446.

91. Markowitz M, Hill-Zabala C, Lang J, et al. Induction with abacavir/lamivudine/zidovudine plus efavirenz for 48 weeks followed by 48-week maintenance with abacavir/ lamivudine/zidovudine alone in antiretroviral-naive HIV-1-infected patients. J Acquir Immune Defic Syndr 2005; 39:257–264.

92. Kelly M. Induction-maintenance antiretroviral strategies to reduce long-term toxicity. J HIV Ther 2003; 8:11–14.

93. CDC. Updated guidelines for the use of rifabutin or rifampin for the treatment and prevention of tuberculosis among HIV-infected patients taking protease inhibitors or nonnucleoside reverse transcriptase inhibitors. Centers for Disease Control and Prevention. MMWR 2000; 49:185–189.

94. Nieuwkerk PT, Oort FJ. Self-reported adherence to antiretroviral therapy for HIV-1 infection and virologic treatment response: a meta-analysis. J Acquir Immune Defic Syndr 2005; 38:445–448.

95. Lawrence J, Mayers DL, Hullsiek KH, et al. Structured treatment interruption in patients with multidrug-resistant human immunodeficiency virus. N Engl J Med 2003; 349:837–846.

96. Katlama C, Dominguez S, Gourlain K, et al. Benefit of treatment interruption in HIV-infected patients with multiple therapeutic failures: a randomized controlled trial (ANRS 097). AIDS 2004; 18:217–226.

97. Wainberg MA. The impact of the M184V substitution on drug resistance and viral fitness. Expert Rev Anti Infect Ther 2004; 2:147–151.

98. Barbour JD, Grant RM. The clinical implications of reduced viral fitness. Curr Infect Dis Rep 2004; 6:151–158.

99. Bates M, Wrin T, Huang W, et al. Practical applications of viral fitness in clinical practice. Curr Opin Infect Dis 2003; 16:11–18.

100. Ledergerber B, Lundgren JD, Walker AS, et al. Predictors of trend in CD4-positive T-cell count and mortality among HIV-1-infected individuals with virological failure to all three antiretroviral-drug classes. Lancet 2004; 364:51–62.

CHAPTER 14

Development and Transmission of HIV Drug Resistance

Mark A. Wainberg
Marco Petrella

Introduction

HIV-1 drug resistance has emerged as a major factor that limits the effectiveness of antiviral drugs in treatment regimens. Many studies have shown that the development and transmission of drug-resistant HIV-1 is largely a consequence of incompletely suppressive antiretroviral regimens; HIV-1 drug resistance can significantly diminish the effectiveness and duration of benefit associated with combination therapy for the treatment of HIV/AIDS.[1-6] Resistance-conferring mutations in both the HIV-1 reverse transcriptase (RT) and protease (PR) genes may precede the initiation of therapy due to both spontaneous mutagenesis and the spread of resistant viruses by sexual and other means. However, it is also generally believed that multiple drug mutations to any single or combination of antiretroviral agents (ARVs) are required in order to produce clinical resistance to most ARVs and that these are in fact selected following residual viral replication in the presence of incompletely suppressive drug regimens.[7-9]

In the case of the protease inhibitors (PIs),[10-12] and most nucleoside analog reverse transcriptase inhibitors (NRTIs), the development of progressive high-level phenotypic drug resistance follows the accumulation of primary resistance-conferring mutations in each of the HIV-1 PR and RT genes.[13-15] Non-nucleoside reverse transcriptase inhibitors (NNRTIs) have low genetic barriers for the development of drug resistance and, frequently, a single

primary drug resistance mutation to any one NNRTI may be sufficient to confer high-level phenotypic drug resistance to this entire class of ARVs.[16,17]

Furthermore, differences have also been reported in regard to the development and evolution of antiretroviral drug resistance between subtype B HIV-1 and several group M non-B subtypes. Non-B subtypes, e.g, subtype C HIV-1 variants, are known to possess naturally occurring polymorphisms at several RT and PR codons that are implicated in drug resistance.[18,19] In some studies, the presence of these polymorphisms did not significantly reduce susceptibility to ARVs in phenotypic resistance assays or limit the effectiveness of an initial antiretroviral therapy regimen for a period of up to 18 months.[18,20] However, it has also been suggested that polymorphisms at resistance positions may sometimes facilitate selection of novel pathways leading to drug resistance, especially with incompletely suppressive antiretroviral regimens.[18] This, in turn, may have important clinical implications with respect to choice of effective antiretroviral therapy. This warrants increased genotypic surveillance on a worldwide basis, as the prevalence of non-B HIV-1 infection is increasing rapidly.

As illustrated in Figures 14.1–14.3, it has been possible to select numerous drug resistance mutations for all licensed ARVs and multiple investigational agents such as the HIV-1 integrase and other inhibitors that are currently undergoing clinical testing.[5,6,21] In view of the hypervariability of HIV-1 and limitation of existing antiretroviral combinations

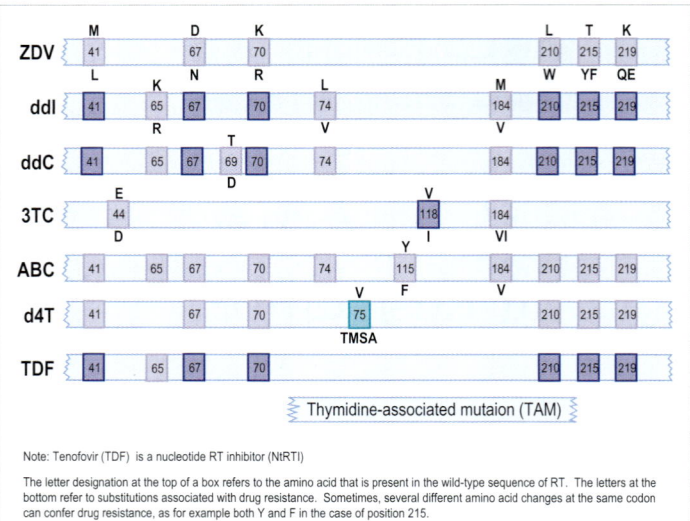

Figure 14.1 Chart of common mutations associated with HIV drug resistance.

Note: Tenofovir (TDF) is a nucleotide RT inhibitor (NtRTI)

The letter designation at the top of a box refers to the amino acid that is present in the wild-type sequence of RT. The letters at the bottom refer to substitutions associated with drug resistance. Sometimes, several different amino acid changes at the same codon can confer drug resistance, as for example both Y and F in the case of position 215.

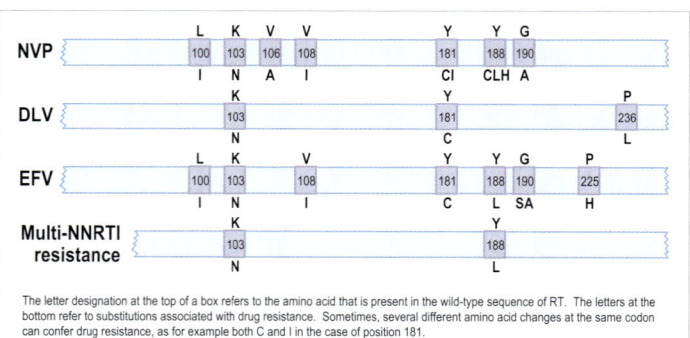

Figure 14.2 Chart of common NNRTI mutations associated with HIV drug resistance.

The letter designation at the top of a box refers to the amino acid that is present in the wild-type sequence of RT. The letters at the bottom refer to substitutions associated with drug resistance. Sometimes, several different amino acid changes at the same codon can confer drug resistance, as for example both C and I in the case of position 181.

to completely suppress viral replication, it is essential that new anti-HIV drug discovery initiatives focus on the identification of new therapeutic targets and the development of antiretroviral agents with more robust genetic barriers and a broader spectrum of activity against drug-resistant HIV-1 variants.

Generation of HIV-1 Drug Resistance

Resistance mutations to ARVs may arise spontaneously as a result of the error-prone replication of HIV-1 and, in addition, are selected both *in vitro* and *in vivo* by pharmacological pressure.[22-24] The high rate of spontaneous mutation in HIV-1 has been largely attributed to the absence of a 3'->5'exonuclease proof-reading mechanism. Sequence analyses of

HIV-1 DNA have detected several types of mutations including base substitutions, additions and deletions.[22] The frequency of spontaneous mutation for HIV-1 varies considerably as a result of differences among viral strains studied *in vitro*.[25] Overall mutation rates for wild-type laboratory strains of HIV-1 have been reported to range from 97×10^{-4} to 200×10^{-4} per nucleotide for the HXB2 clonal variant of HIV-1 to as high as 800×10^{-4} per nucleotide for the HIV-1 NY5 strain.[22,25]

In addition to the low fidelity of DNA synthesis by HIV-1 RT, other interdependent factors that affect rates of HIV mutagenesis include RT processivity, viral replication capacity, viral pool size, and availability of target cells for infection.[26-29] It follows that an alteration in any or combination of these factors might influence the development of HIV drug resistance. There is also data showing that thymidine analog mutations (TAMs) in RT can significantly

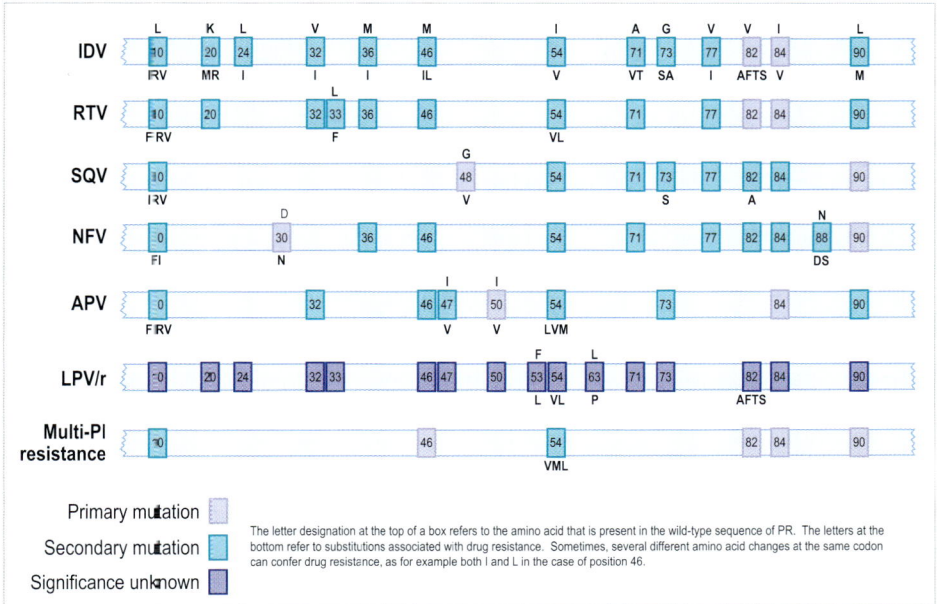

Figure 14.3 Chart of common PR mutations associated with HIV drug resistance.

increase the likelihood of further mutant HIV-1 distributions and evolution of drug resistance; furthermore, this can happen in the presence or absence of concomitant nucleoside RT inhibitors (NRTIs).[30,31]

Inhibitors of Reverse Transcriptase

The reverse transcriptase (RT) enzyme is encoded by the HIV *pol* gene and is responsible for the transcription of double-stranded proviral DNA from viral genomic RNA. Two categories of drugs have been developed to block RT; these are nucleoside analog RT inhibitors (NRTIs) that act to arrest DNA chain elongation by acting as competitive inhibitors of RT and non-nucleoside RT inhibitors (NNRTIs) that act as non-competitive antagonists of enzyme activity by binding to the catalytic site of RT. NRTIs are administered to patients as precursor compounds that are phosphorylated to their active triphosphate form by cellular enzymes. These compounds lack a 3' hydroxyl group (OH) necessary for elongation of viral DNA. These analogs can compete effectively with normal deoxynucleotide triphosphate (dNTP) substrates for binding to RT and incorporation into viral DNA.[32,33]

NNRTI antiviral activity is incompletely understood but is known to involve the binding of these non-competitive inhibitors to a hydrophobic pocket close to the catalytic site of RT.[34,35] NNRTI inhibition reduces the catalytic rate of polymerization without affecting nucleotide binding or nucleotide-induced conformational change.[36] NNRTIs are particularly active at template positions at which the RT enzyme naturally pauses. NNRTIs do not seem to influence the competition between dideoxynucleoside triphosphates (ddNTPs) and the naturally occurring dNTPs for insertion into the growing proviral DNA chain.[37]

Both types of RT inhibitors have been shown to successfully diminish plasma viral burden in HIV-1 infected subjects. However, monotherapy with all drugs has led to drug resistance. Patients who receive combinations of three or more drugs are less likely to develop resistance, since these 'cocktails' can suppress viral replication with much greater efficiency than single drugs or two drugs in combination. Although mutagenesis is less likely to happen in this circumstance, it can still occur, and the emergence of drug-resistant breakthrough viruses has been demonstrated in patients receiving highly active antiretroviral therapy (HAART).[38,39] Furthermore, the persistence of reservoirs of latently infected cells represents another major impediment to currently applied anti-HIV chemotherapy.[40] Replication of HIV might resume once therapy is stopped or interrupted and, therefore, eradication of a latent reservoir of 10^5 cells might take as long as 60 years, a goal that is not practical with currently available drugs and technology.[40,41]

Resistance to 3TC ((-)-2′, 3′-dideoxy-3′-thiacytidine, lamivudine) develops quickly whereas resistance to other NRTIs commonly appears only after about six months of therapy. Phenotypic resistance is detected by comparing the IC_{50} (or drug concentration capable of blocking viral replication by 50%) of pretreatment viral isolates with those obtained after therapy. Thus, higher IC_{50} values obtained after several months of treatment reflect a loss in viral susceptibility to antiretroviral agents (ARVs). Selective polymerase chain reaction (PCR) analysis of the RT genome confirms that the number of mutations associated with drug resistance increases concomitantly with increases in IC_{50} values.

Mutations associated with drug resistance have been reported in response to the use of any single NRTI or NNRTI.[42] However, not all drugs elicit the same mutagenic response; sensitivity and resistance patterns must be considered on an individual drug basis. For example, patients on 3TC monotherapy may develop high-level, i.e. 1000-fold resistance within weeks, whereas 6 months or more are often required in order for sensitivity to ZDV to drop by 50–100-fold. In contrast, HIV may appear to remain reasonably sensitive, even after prolonged monotherapy, to four of the other commonly used nucleoside analogs: ddI (didanosine), ddC (zalcitabine), d4T (stavudine) and ABC (abacavir). In the case of ZDV, increases in IC_{50} below 3-fold are regarded as nonsignificant, while 10–50-fold increases usually represent partial resistance, and increases above 50-fold denote high-level resistance.

Patient resistance to nucleoside analogs can often develop independently of the dose of drug that is administered. Tissue culture data have shown that HIV-1 resistance can be easily demonstrated against each of NRTIs, NNRTIs and PIs, by gradually increasing the concentration of compound in the tissue culture medium.[43,44] Cell lines are especially useful in this regard, since HIV replication occurs very efficiently in such hosts. Tissue culture selection provides an effective pre-clinical means of studying HIV mutagenesis, especially since the same resistance-conferring mutations that arise in cell culture also appear clinically. Owing to the high turnover and mutation rate of HIV-1, the retroviral quasi-species will also include defective virions and singly mutated drug-resistant variants that are present prior to commencement of therapy. Multiple mutated variants appear later, because it requires time to accumulate multiple mutations within a single viral genome, and they are not commonly found in the retroviral pool of untreated patients. An exception to this involves cases of new infection with drug-resistant viruses transmitted from extensively treated individuals. Patients with advanced infection have a higher viral load and a broader range of quasi-species than newly-infected individuals. Such patients are often immunosuppressed and may also have diminished ability to immunologically control viral replication, possibly leading to more rapid development of drug resistance.

Site-directed mutagenesis has shown that a variety of RT mutations encode HIV resistance to both NRTIs and NNRTIs. Crystallographic and biochemical data have demonstrated that mutations conferring resistance to NNRTIs are found in the peptide residues that make contact with these compounds within their binding pocket.[34,35]

Resistance-encoding mutations to NRTIs are found in different regions of the RT enzyme, probably due to the complexity of nucleoside incorporation, which involves several distinct steps. These mutations can decrease RT susceptibility to nucleoside analogs. A summary of primary RT mutations has been published elsewhere.[42]

It has also been shown that a family of insertion and deletion mutations between codons 67 and 70 can cause resistance to a variety of NRTIs including ZDV, 3TC, ddI, ddC, and d4T. Usually, these insertion mutations confer multidrug resistance when present in a ZDV-resistant background. Another less frequently observed resistance mutation, K65R, has been shown to be associated with prior treatment with ABC-containing regimens and results in reduced antiviral susceptibility to both ABC and the acyclic RT nucleotide analog tenofovir (TDF). Hence, resistance to these antiretroviral agents can develop via genetic pathways involving either the TAMs or K65R as hallmark drug resistance mutations.[45] In recent years, the proportion of genotyped clinical samples containing K65R has increased from <1% to almost 4%, reflecting the increased use of TDF in treatment regimens.

Diminished sensitivity to NNRTIs appears quickly both in culture selection protocols and in patients.[34,37] NNRTIs share a common binding site, and mutations that encode NNRTI resistance are located within the binding pocket that makes drug contact.[34,35,37-44,46-49] This explains the finding that extensive cross-resistance is observed among all currently approved NNRTIs.[49,50] A substitution at codon 181 (tyrosine to cysteine) (Y181C) is a common mutation that encodes cross-resistance among many

NNRTIs.[46,51,52] Replacement of Y181 by a serine or histidine also conferred HIV resistance to NNRTIs.[53] A mutation at amino acid 236 (proline to leucine) (P236L), conferring resistance to a particular class of NNRTIs that include delavirdine, can also diminish resistance to nevirapine and other NNRTIs, particularly if a Y181C mutation is also present in the same virus.[54] Other important substitutions are Y188C and Y188H that can also confer NNRTI resistance.

Another drug resistance mutation, namely K103N (lysine to asparagine), is commonly observed and is responsible for reduced susceptibility to all approved NNRTIs.[46,51,52] Substitution of K103N results in alteration of interactions between NNRTIs and RT. The K103N mutation shows synergy with Y181C in regard to resistance to NNRTIs, unlike antagonistic interactions involving Y181C and P236L.[55]

Resistance to NNRTIs is also observed in cell-free enzyme assays.[51,53,56-58] Both Y181I and Y188L mediate decreased sensitivity to NNRTIs without affecting either substrate recognition or catalytic efficiency, supporting the idea that resistance to NNRTIs is attributable to diminished ability of these drugs to be bound by RT.

Protease Inhibitors

Drug-resistant viruses have been observed in the case of all protease inhibitors (PIs) developed to date.[11,12,59] In addition, some strains of HIV have displayed cross-resistance to a variety of PIs after either clinical use or in vitro drug exposure.[11,12,59] In general, the patterns of mutations observed with PIs are more complex than those observed with RT antagonists. First, a greater number of mutations within the protease (PR) gene are involved. This involves greater variability, as well, in temporal patterns of appearance of different mutations and the manner in which different combinations of mutations can give rise to phenotypic resistance. These data suggest that the PR enzyme can adapt more easily than RT to pressures exerted by anti-viral drugs. At least 40 mutations in PR have been identified as responsible for resistance to PIs.[11,12,59]

Certain mutations within the PR gene are more important than others and can confer resistance, virtually on their own, to at least certain PIs.[11,12,59] One mutation, in particular, D30N, is probably unique to nelfinavir (NFV), a potent HIV protease inhibitor. However, a variety of other mutations may confer cross-resistance among multiple drugs within the PI family. In addition, wide arrays of secondary mutations have been observed, that, when combined with primary mutations, can cause increased levels of resistance to occur. On the other hand, the presence of certain secondary mutations on their own may not lead to drug resistance, and, in this context, some of these amino acid changes should be considered to represent naturally-occurring polymorphisms. In addition, it should be noted that resistance to PIs can also result from mutations within the substrates of the PR enzyme, i.e. the Gag and Gag-Pol precursor proteins of HIV. A variety of studies have now shown that mutations at cleavage sites within these substrates can be responsible for drug resistance, both in tissue culture as well as in treated patients. However, the full clinical significance of cleavage site mutations in regard to PR resistance is not yet understood.

Antiretroviral Drug Resistance in Non-B Subtypes of HIV-1 Group M

Genotypic divergence of *Pol* gene sequences between different HIV-1 subtypes is only beginning to be investigated, although the RT and PR enzymes are the main targets of antiretroviral therapy.[60-64] Group O and HIV-2 viruses carry natural polymorphisms Y181C and Y181I that confer intrinsic resistance to NNRTIs.[65-67] Subtype F isolates, showing 11% nucleotide sequence variation from subtype B and group M viruses, have also been reported to have reduced sensitivity to some NNRTIs while retaining susceptibility to others such as nevirapine and delavirdine, NRTIs and PIs.[68,69] In contrast, the drug sensitivity of subtype C isolates from treatment-naive patients in Zimbabwe was reported to be similar to that of subtype B isolates.[69,70] Recent studies conducted with Ethiopian subtype C clinical isolates showed natural resistance to NNRTIs in one case and resistance to ZDV in another, due to natural polymorphisms at positions G190A and K70R, respectively.[71] Another study reported no differences in drug susceptibility among subtypes A, B, C, and E; subtype D viruses showed reduced susceptibility due to rapid growth kinetics.[72] High prevalence (i.e. 94%) of a valine polymorphism (GTG) at position 106 in RT from subtype C HIV-1 clinical isolates has also been reported.[73] In tissue culture experiments, selection of subtype C with efavirenz (EFV) was associated with development of high-level (i.e. 100–1000-fold) phenotypic resistance to all NNRTIs. This was a consequence of a V106M mutation that arose in place of the V106A substitution that is more commonly seen with subtype B viruses.[73] This V106M mutation conferred broad cross-resistance to all currently approved NNRTIs and was selected on the basis of differential codon usage at position 106 in RT, due to redundancy in the genetic code.

Genotypic diversity and drug resistance may be particularly relevant in establishing treatment strategies against African and Asian strains. First, since many antiviral drugs have been designed based on sequences of subtype B RT and PR enzymes, and drug resistance profiles, if not responses, may be different for non-B viral strains. Second, drug resistance may develop more rapidly in resource-poor countries if only sub-optimal therapeutic regimens are available. Global phenotypic and genotypic screening of non-B subtypes is warranted so as not to jeopardize the outcome of recently introduced antiretroviral treatments.[74]

Transmission of HIV Drug-resistance

As stated, highly active antiretroviral therapy (HAART), including drugs that inhibit the RT and PR enzymes of HIV-1, has resulted in declining morbidity and mortality.[75] The failure to completely suppress viral replication allows for the development of genotypic changes in HIV-1 that confer resistance to each of the three major classes of antiretroviral drugs.[76–78] Cumulative data indicate that single drug-resistant variants can be transmitted to approximately 10–15% of newly-infected persons in western countries in which ARVs have been available for many years, with transmission of dual and triple-class multidrug resistance (MDR) observed in 3–5% of cases.[79–82]

There is concern that the transmission of MDR viruses in primary HIV-1 infection (PHI) may limit future therapeutic options. Treatment failure has been observed in several individuals harboring MDR infections.[82-84] Some reports have shown an impaired fitness of transmitted MDR variants compared with wild-type (WT) infections acquired in PHI,[85] and the mutations that were transmitted in such patients persisted in the absence of treatment.[85] This persistence differs from the rapid outgrowth of WT viruses in established infections upon treatment interruption, due to the selective growth advantage and fitness of WT variants.[85–87] Taken together, these findings suggest that archival WT viruses may not exist in MDR infections transmitted during PHI.

Several reports have also documented cases of inter-subtype superinfection (A/E and B) in recently infected intravenous drug users (IDU).[88,89] Other studies have failed to confirm superinfection follow-ing IDU exposure, suggesting that superinfection is a relatively rare event.[90,91] Several subsequent reports demonstrated superinfection in subtype B infections. In one case, a WT superinfection arose following a primary MDR infection.[92,93]

It is important to assess the virological consequences of transmission of drug resistant variants in primary infection, as well as the time to disappearance of resistant virus in those patients not initially treated.

Genotypic analysis indicates that a single dominant HIV-1 species can persist for more than 2 years in circulating plasma and peripheral blood mononuclear cells (PBMC), regardless of route of transmission. Resistant and MDR infections can persist for 2–7 years following PHI.

Superinfection with a second MDR strain in a patient originally infected with a MDR strain from an identified source partner has also been described.[94] In spite of a rapid decline in plasma viremia suggestive of an effective immune response, this patient was susceptible to a second infection which occurred concomitant with a dramatic rise in viral load. Five other subtype B superinfections have been described, as well as three intersubtype A/E and B superinfections.[88,89,92,93,95,96] Six of the seven superinfections described have occurred in the first year following initial infection.

Many have attributed superinfection to co-infection during primary infection. Two longitudinal studies involving IDU populations ($n = 37$ in both studies) indicated that superinfection is a rare phenomenon that was not observed during 1–12 years of follow-up spanning 215 and 1072 total years of exposure.[92,93] However, it is not known whether any patients were recruited within the first year of HIV-1 exposure in these studies. In the case of the MDR infections cited above, identification of the source partner of infection argues against co-infection.[94]

Findings of HIV-1 superinfection are a matter of concern insofar as such results challenge the assumption that immune responses can protect against re-infection. Of course, the impaired viral fitness of the initial MDR infection described above may be a factor in permitting superinfection. The initial MDR strain showed a 13-fold impaired replicative capacity from a WT variant strain from the isolated source partner following a treatment interruption. Fitness considerations may also have been important in a WT superinfection of an initial MDR infection and cases of subtype B superinfection following A/E infections that elicited low-level viremia.[88,89]

In newly infected individuals, multi-mutated viruses conferring MDR may represent a new determinant of virological outcome. Persistence of MDR in the absence of treatment raises serious issues regarding HIV-1 management. For recently infected MDR patients, drug resistance analysis and viral fitness may provide useful information in regard to ultimate therapeutic strategies.

It is interesting to note that the presence of the M184V mutation in reverse transcriptase, associated with high-level resistance to 3TC, seems to have been associated with the persistence of low viral load. In two PHI cases, rebounds to a high level of plasma viremia occurred only at times when the M184V mutation in RT could no longer be detected. A third PHI patient maintained low plasma viremia over 5 years, and his virus also contained the M184V mutation throughout this time. In an additional individual, high viral loads were present at times after primary infection in spite of the M184V mutation, but virus could only be isolated from this individual in coculture experiments after loss of the M184V mutation.[94] These data are consistent with previous findings on loss of fitness conferred by the M184V mutation in reverse transcriptase, alongside multiple other pleiotropic effects, including diminished processivity, diminished rates of nucleotide excision, and diminished rates of initiation of reverse transcription.[97-99]

Other studies suggest that despite reduced ARV susceptibility, MDR infections may be of some immunological and virological benefit due to the impaired replicative capacity of MDR variants.[100-103] Moreover, in all cases, RT assays and competitive fitness assays showed MDR viruses to have compromised replicative capacity. The absence of genotypic changes in these viruses over time further supports the concept of expansion of predominant MDR quasi-species during primary infection. Recombination events can also occur in this period. It is also important to point out that the replication fitness of a given virus vs its transmission fitness may represent two very different concepts.

Antiretroviral therapy (ART), by reducing HIV-1 replication, has been shown not only to impact significantly on morbidity and mortality but also to reduce the spread of HIV-1.[104,105] Treatment effectiveness is hampered by the development of drug resistant (DR) strains, leading inexorably to virological failure.[76] The transmissibility of DR strains is not fully understood and may differ from that of wild-type (WT) strains for at least two reasons: first, the relative fitness of DR strains compared with WT in the absence of therapy and second, the degree to which partially active therapies can reduce viral load in persons harboring resistant viruses.[80,106] As a con-

sequence of widespread use of ART in North America, the transmission of DR strains in recently infected (RI) individuals has increased from 3.8% in 1996 to 14% in 2000. Such an increase of primary DR is of public health concern since a clear association between DR and early treatment failure has been reported.[82] However, several groups in Europe and Australia have reported a recent stable or decreasing trend in DR transmission for reverse transcriptase (RT) and/or protease inhibitors (PI),[107,108] and have attributed this decline to the widespread use of suppressive triple ARV regimens since 1996. This presupposes that transmission of drug resistant variants may have earlier been more common due to the widespread use of suboptimal biotherapy or even monotherapy regimens prior to 1996 and the likelihood that these suboptimal regimens may have selected for drug resistance mutations with very high frequency.[108]

Conclusion

The accumulation of specific resistance-conferring mutations is associated with the development of phenotypic resistance to anti-HIV drugs which can significantly diminish the effectiveness and longevity of antiretroviral therapy. Cross-resistance among drugs of the same class also occurs frequently and is most problematic with NNRTIs due to their lower genetic barrier for rapid selection of drug resistance compared with other classes of ARVs. There is now also data indicating that cross-resistance among the NRTIs may in fact be more widespread than was initially thought.[109] Furthermore, the emergence of new drug resistance mutations is helping to establish new mutant distributions with additional pathways for developing cross-resistance to ARVs.[110] These new patterns of cross-resistance together with increasing transmission of multi-drug resistant HIV-1 variants are problematic and seriously limit the number of effective treatment options that are now available for long-term management of HIV-infection.

Additional strategies, in addition to new drug discovery programs, are urgently required to help curb the development of drug-resistant HIV-1. One possible approach that merits further consideration is based on the maintenance of specific fitness-attenuating drug mutations in therapeutic regimens for HIV-1 infection.[110,111] The M184V substitution in RT has been extensively studied in this regard because of its ability to impair viral replication capacity, while limiting the development of subsequent drug resistance mutations in HIV-1 RT, e.g. TAMs and the Q151M multi-drug complex resistance mutation associated with use of AZT and d4T.[112,113] Of course, restricted evolution of drug resistance in these circumstances may also result from other alterations of RT function by M184V.[97] One recent study has shown that viruses containing the M184V mutation may be transmitted less frequently than viruses containing other mutations associated with drug resistance,[99] perhaps because M184V compromises viral replicative capacity. Further work on these and other topics is needed to improve our understanding of HIV drug resistance in the context of clinical relevance, successful antiviral chemotherapy, and likelihood of transmission of resistant strains.[114]

References

1. Quiros-Roldan E, Signorini S, Castelli F, et al. Analysis of HIV-1 mutation patterns in patients failing antiretroviral therapy. J Clin Lab Anal 2001; 15:43–46.
2. Rousseau M, Vergne L, Montes B, et al. Patterns of resistance to antiretroviral drugs in extensively treated HIV-1-infected patients with failure of highly active antiretroviral therapy. J Acquir Immune Defic Syndr 2001; 26:36–43.
3. Winters M, Baxter J, Mayers D, et al. Frequency of antiretroviral drug resistance mutations in HIV-1 strains from patients failing triple drug regimens. The Terry Beirn Community Programs for Clinical Research on AIDS. Antivir Ther 2000; 1:57–63.
4. Lorenzi P, Opravil M, Hirschel B, et al. Impact of drug resistance mutations on virologic response to salvage therapy. Swiss HIV Cohort Study AIDS 1999; 13:17–21.
5. D'Aquila R, Schapiro J, Brun-Vézinet F, et al. Drug resistance mutations in HIV-1. Top HIV Med 2002; 10:21–25.
6. Yeni P, Hammer S, Carpenter C, et al. Antiretroviral treatment for adult HIV infection in 2002: updated recommendations of the International AIDS Society-USA Panel. JAMA 2002; 288:222–235.
7. de Jong M, Schuurman R, Lange J, et al. Replication of a pre-existing resistant HIV-1 subpopulation in vivo after introduction of a strong selective drug pressure. Antivir Ther 1996; 1:33–41.
8. Mayers D. Prevalence and incidence of resistance to zidovudine and other antiretroviral drugs. Am J Med 1997; 102:70–75.
9. Balotta C, Berlusconi A, Pan A, et al. Prevalence of transmitted nucleoside analogue-resistant HIV-1 strains and pre-existing mutations in pol reverse transcriptase and protease region: outcome after treatment in recently infected individuals. Antivir Ther 2000; 5:7–14.
10. Molla A, Korneyeva M, Gao Q, et al. Ordered accumulation of mutations in HIV protease confers resistance to ritonavir. Nat Med 1996; 2:760–766.
11. Condra J. Virologic and clinical implications of resistance to HIV-1 protease inhibitors. Drug Resist Updat 1998; 1:292–299.
12. Deeks S. Failure of HIV-1 protease inhibitors to fully suppress viral replication. Implications for salvage therapy. Adv Exptl Med Biol 1999; 458:175–182.
13. Frost S, Nijhuis M, Schuurman R, et al. Evolution of lamivudine resistance in human immunodeficiency virus type 1-infected individuals: the relative roles of drift and selection. J Virol 2000; 74:6262–6268.
14. Gotte M, Wainberg MA. Biochemical mechanisms involved in overcoming HIV resistance to nucleoside inhibitors of reverse transcriptase. Drug Resist Updat 2000; 3:30–38.
15. Loveday C. International perspectives on antiretroviral resistance. Nucleoside reverse transcriptase inhibitor resistance. J Acquir Immune Defic Syndr 2001; 26:10–24.
16. Deeks S International perspectives on antiretroviral resistance. Nonnucleoside reverse transcriptase inhibitor resistance. J Acquir Immune Defic Syndr 2001; 26:25–33.
17. Bacheler L, Jeffrey S, Hanna G, et al. Genotypic correlates of phenotypic resistance to efavirenz in virus isolates from patients failing nonnucleoside reverse transcriptase inhibitor therapy. J Virol 2001; 75:4999–5008.
18. Holguin A, Soriano V. Resistance to antiretroviral agents in individuals with HIV-1 non-B subtypes. HIV Clin Trials 2002; 3:403–411.
19. Kantor R, Zijenah L, Shafer R, et al. HIV-1 subtype C reverse transcriptase and protease genotypes in Zimbabwean patients failing antiretroviral therapy. AIDS Res Hum Retroviruses 2002; 18:1407–1413.
20. Alexander C, Montessori V, Wynhoven B, et al. Prevalence and response to antiretroviral therapy of non-B subtypes of HIV in antiretroviral-naive individuals in British Columbia. Antivir Ther 2002; 7:31–35.
21. Wei X, Decker J, Liu H, et al. Emergence of resistant human immunodeficiency virus type 1 in patients receiving fusion inhibitor (T-20) monotherapy. Antimicrob Agents Chemother 2002; 46:1896–1905.
22. Roberts J, Bebenek K, Kunkel T. The accuracy of reverse transcriptase from HIV-1. Science 1988; 242:1171–1173.
23. Preston B, Dougherty J. Mechanisms of retroviral mutation. Trends Microbiol 1996; 4:16–21.
24. Menendez-Arias L. Molecular basis of fidelity of DNA synthesis and nucleotide specificity of retroviral reverse transcriptases. Prog Nucl Acid Res Mol Biol 2002; 71:91–147.
25. Rezende L, Drosopoulos W, Prasad V. The influence of 3TC resistance mutation M184I on the fidelity and error specificity of human immunodeficiency virus type 1 reverse transcriptase. Nucl Acids Res 1998; 26:3066–3072.
26. Coffin J. HIV population dynamics in vivo: implication for genetic variation, pathogenesis, and therapy. Science 1995; 267:483–489.
27. Drosopoulos W, Rezende L, Wainberg M, et al. Virtues of being faithful: can we limit the genetic variation in human immunodeficiency virus? J Mol Med 1998; 76:604–612.
28. Colgrove R, Japour A. A combinatorial ledge: reverse transcriptase fidelity, total body viral burden, and the implications of multiple-drug HIV therapy for the evolution of antiviral resistance. Antiviral Res 1999; 41:45–56.
29. Overbaugh J, Bangham C. Selection forces and constraints on retroviral sequence variation. Science 2001; 292:1106–1109.
30. Mansky L. HIV mutagenesis and the evolution of antiretroviral drug resistance. Drug Resist Updat 2002; 5:219–223.
31. Mansky L, Le Rouzic E, Benichou S, et al. Influence of reverse transcriptase variants, drugs, and Vpr on human immunodeficiency virus type 1 mutant frequencies. J Virol 2003; 77:2071–2080.
32. Furman P, Fyfe J. St. Clair M, et al. Phosphorylation of 3′-azido-3′ deoxythymidine and selective interactions of the 5′-triphosphate with human immunodeficiency virus reverse transcriptase. Proc Natl Acad Sci USA 1986; 83:8333–8337.
33. Hart G, Orr D, Penn C, et al. Effects of (-) 2′-deoxy-3′-thiacytidine (3TC) 5′-triphosphate on human immunodeficiency virus reverse transcriptase and mammalian DNA polymerases alpha, beta and gamma. Antimicrob Agents Chemother 1992; 37:918–920.
34. Ding J, Das K, Moereels H, et al. Structure of HIV-1 RT/TIBO R 86183 complex reveals similarity in the binding of diverse non-nucleoside inhibitors. Nat Struct Biol 1995; 2:407–415.

35. Wu J, Warren T, Adams J, et al. A novel dipyridodiazepinone inhibitor of HIV-1 reverse transcriptase acts through a nonsubstrate binding site. Biochemistry 1991; 30:2022–2026.

36. Spence R, Kati W, Anderson K, et al. Mechanism of inhibition of HIV-1 reverse transcriptase by non-nucleoside inhibitors. Science 1995; 267:988–992.

37. Gu Z, Quan Y, Li Z, et al. Effects of non-nucleosides inhibitors of human immunodeficiency virus type 1 in cell-free recombinant reverse transcriptase assay. J Biol Chem 1995; 270:31046–31051.

38. Gunthard H, Wong J, Ignacio C, et al. Human immunodeficiency virus replication and genotypic resistance in blood and lymph nodes after a year of potent antiretroviral therapy. J Virol 1998; 72:2422–2428.

39. Palmer S, Shafer R, Merigan T. Highly drug-resistant HIV-1 clinical isolates are cross-resistant to many antiretroviral compounds in current clinical development. AIDS 1999; 13:661–667.

40. Finzi D, Blankson J, Siliciano J, et al. Latent infection of CD4+ T cells provides a mechanism for lifelong persistence of HIV-1, even in patients on effective combination therapy. Nat Med 1997; 5:512–517.

41. Wong J, Hezareh M, Gunthard H, et al. Recovery of replication-competent HIV despite prolonged suppression of plasma viremia. Science 1997; 278:1291–1295.

42. Schinazi R, Larder B, Mellors J. Mutations in retroviral genes associated in drug resistance. Intl Antiviral News 1997; 5:129–142.

43. National Institute for Allergy and Infectious Disease (NIAIDS). ACTG virology manual for HIV laboratories. Bethesda, MD: NIAIDS.

44. Japour A, Mayers D, Johnson V, et al. A standardized peripheral mononuclear assay for determination of drug susceptibilities of clinical human immunodeficiency virus type 1 isolates. Antimicrob Agents Chemother 1993; 37:1095–1101.

45. Winston A, Mandalia S, Pillay D, et al. The prevalence and determinants of the K65R mutation in HIV-1 reverse transcriptase in tenofovir-naive patients. AIDS 2002; 16:2087–2089.

46. Richman D, Shih C, Lowy I, et al. Human immunodeficiency virus type 1 mutants resistant to non-nucleoside inhibitors of reverse transcriptase arise in cell culture. Proc Natl Acad Sci USA 1991; 88:11241–11245.

47. Vandamme A, Debyser Z, Pauwels R, et al. Characterization of HIV-1 strains isolated from patients treated with TIBO R82913. AIDS Res Hum Retroviruses 1994; 10:39–46.

48. Chong K, Pagano P, Hinshaw R. Bisheteroarylpiperazine reverse transcriptase inhibitor in combination with 3′-azido-3′-deoxythymidine or 2′,3′-dideoxycytidine synergistically inhibits human immunodeficiency virus type 1 replication in vitro. Antimicrob Agents Chemother 1994; 38:288–293.

49. Esnouf R, Ren J, Ross C, et al. Mechanism of inhibition of HIV-1 reverse transcriptase by non-nucleoside inhibitors. Nat Struct Bio 1995; 2:303–308.

50. Fletcher R, Arion D, Borkow G, et al. Synergistic inhibition of HIV-1 reverse transcriptase DNA polymerase activity and virus replication in vitro by combinations of carboxanilide non-nucleoside compounds. Biochemistry 1995; 34:10106–10112.

51. Byrnes V, Sardana V, Schleif W, et al. Comprehensive mutant enzyme and viral variant assessment of human immunodeficiency virus type 1 reverse transcriptase resistance to non-nucleoside inhibitors. Antimicrob Agents Chemother 1993; 37:1576–1579.

52. Balzarini J, Karlsson A, Perez-Perez M, et al. Treatment of human immunodeficiency virus type 1 (HIV-1)-infected cells with combinations of HIV-1-specific inhibitors results in different resistance pattern than does treatment with single-drug therapy. J Virol 1993c; 67:5353–5359.

53. Sardana V, Emini E, Gotlib L, et al. Functional analysis of HIV-1 reverse transcriptase amino acids involved in resistance to multiple non-nucleoside inhibitors. J Biol Chem 1992; 267:17526–17530.

54. Dueweke T, Pushkarskaya T, Poppe S, et al. A mutation in reverse transcriptase of bis(heteroaryl) piperazine-resistant human immunodeficiency virus type 1 that confers increased sensitivity to other nonnucleoside inhibitors. Proc Natl Acad Sci USA 1993; 90:4713–4717.

55. Nunberg J, Schleif W, Boots E, et al. Viral resistance to human immunodeficiency virus type 1-specific pyridinone reverse transcriptase inhibitors. J Virol 1991; 65:4887–4892.

56. Jonckheere H, Taymans J, Balzarini J, et al. Resistance of HIV-1 reverse transcriptase against [2′, 5′, bis-O-(tert-butyldimethylsily-3′-spiro5″-(4″amino-1″,2″-oxathiole-2″,2″-dioxide)] (TSAO) derivatives is determined by the mutation Glu138-Lys on the p51 subunit. J Biol Chem 1994; 269:25255–25258.

57. Loya S, Bakhanashvili M, Tal R, et al. Enzymatic properties of two mutants of reverse transcriptase of human immunodeficiency virus type 1 (tyrosine 181-isoleucine and tyrosine 188-leucine), resistant to nonnucleoside inhibitors. AIDS Res Hum Retroviruses 1994; 10:939–946.

58. Boyer P, Currens M, McMahon J, et al. Analysis of non-nucleoside drug-resistance variants of human immunodeficiency virus type 1 reverse transcriptase. J Virol 1993; 67:2412–2420.

59. Murphy R. New antiretroviral drugs, Part I: PIs. AIDS Clin Care 1999; 11:35–37.

60. Haesevel M de, Decourt J, Deeleys R, et al. Genomic cloning and complete sequence of a highly divergent African Human Immunodeficiency Virus isolate. J Virol 1994; 68:1586–1596.

61. Cornelissen M, Burg R Van Den, Zorgdrager F, et al. Pol Gene diversity of five Human Immunodeficiency Virus type 1 subtypes: evidence for naturally occurring mutations that contribute to drug resistance, limited recombination patterns, and common ancestry for subtypes B and D. J Virol 1997; 71:6348–6358.

62. Gao Q, Gu Z, Salomon H, et al. Generation of multiple drug resistance by sequential in vitro passage of the Human Immunodeficiency Virus type 1. Arch Virol 1994; 36:111–122.

63. Shaafer R, Winters M, Palmer S, et al. Multiple concurrent reverse transcriptase and protease mutations and multi-drug resistance of HIV-1 isolates from heavily treated patients. Ann Intern Med 1998; 128:906–911.

64. Becker-Pergola G, Kataaha P, Johnston-Dow L, et al. Analysis of HIV type 1 Protease and reverse transcriptase in anti-retroviral drug-naïve Ugandan adults. AIDS Res Hum Retroviruses 2000; 8:807–813.

65. Descamps D, Collin G, Loussert-Ajaka I, et al. HIV-1 group O sensitivity to antiviral drugs. AIDS 1995; 9:977–978.

66. Descamps D, Collin G, Letourneur F, et al. Susceptibility of human immunodeficiency virus type 1 group O isolates to antiretroviral agents: in vitro phenotypic and genotypic analysis. J Virol 1997; 71:8893–8898.

67. Tantillo C, Ding A, Jacobs-Molina R, et al. Locations of anti-AIDS drug binding sites and resistance mutations in three-dimensional structure of HIV-1 reverse transcriptase. Implications for mechanisms of drug inhibition and resistance. J Mol Biol 1994; 243:369–387.

68. Apetrei C, Descamps D, Collin G, et al. Human Immunodeficiency Virus type 1 subtype F reverse transcriptase sequence and drug susceptibility. J Virol 1998; 72:3534–3538.

69. Shafer R, Eisen J, Merigan TC, et al. Sequence and drug susceptibility of subtype C reverse transcriptase from Human Immunodeficiency Virus type 1 seroconverters in Zimbabwe. J Virol 1997; 71:5441–5448.

70. Birk B, Sonnerborg A. Variations in HIV-1 pol gene associated with reduced sensitivity to anti-retroviral drugs in treatment-naïve patients. AIDS 1998; 12:2369–2375.

71. Loemba H, Brenner B, Parniak M, et al. Genetic divergence of human immunodeficiency virus type 1 Ethiopian clade C reverse transcriptase (RT) and rapid development of

resistance against nonnucleoside inhibitors of RT. Antimicrob Agents Chemother 2002; 46:2087–2094.

72. Palmer S, Alaeus A, Albert J, et al. Drug susceptibility of subtypes A, B, C, D and E Human Immunodeficiency Virus type 1 primary isolates. AIDS Res Hum Retroviruses 1998; 14:157–162.

73. Brenner B, Turner D, Oliveira M, et al. A V106M mutation in HIV-1 clade C viruses exposed to efavirenz confers cross-resistance to non-nucleoside reverse transcriptase inhibitors. AIDS 2003; 17:1–5.

74. Petrella M, Brenner B, Loemba H, et al. HIV drug resistance and implications for the introduction of antiretroviral therapy in resource-poor countries. Drug Resist Updat 2001; 4:339–346.

75. Palella FJ, Delaney KM, Moorman AC, et al. Declining morbidity and mortality among patients with advanced human immunodeficiency virus infection. N Engl J Med 1998; 338:853–860.

76. Wainberg MA, Friedland G. Public health implications of antiretroviral therapy and HIV drug resistance. JAMA 1998; 279:1977–1983, 279:2000–2002, 280:1745–1746.

77. Hirsch MS, Brun-Vézinet F, Clotet B, et al. Antiretroviral drug resistance testing in adults with human immunodeficiency virus type 1: 2003 recommendations of an International AIDS Society – USA panel. Clin Infect Dis 2003; 37:113–128.

78. D'Aquila RT, Schapiro JM, Brun-Vezinet F, et al. Drug resistance mutations in HIV-1. Top HIV Med 2003; 11:92–96.

79. Salomon H, Wainberg MA, Brenner BG, et al. Prevalence of HIV-1 viruses resistant to antiretroviral drugs in 81 individuals newly infected by sexual contact or intravenous drug use. AIDS 2000; 14:17–23.

80. Yerly S, Kaiser L, Race E, et al. Transmission of antiretroviral-drug-resistant HIV-1 variants. Lancet 1999; 354:729–733.

81. Boden D, Hurley A, Zhang L, et al. HIV-1 drug resistance in newly infected individuals. JAMA 1999; 282:1135–1141.

82. Little SJ, Holte S, Routy JP, et al. Antiretroviral-drug resistance among patients recently infected with HIV. N Engl J Med 2002; 347:385–394.

83. Hecht GM, Grant RM, Petropoulos CJ, et al. Sexual transmission of an HIV-1 variant resistant to multiple reverse-transcriptase and protease inhibitors. N Engl J Med 1998; 339:307–311.

84. Gandhi RT, Wurcel A, Rosenberg ES, et al. Progressive reversion of human immunodeficiency virus type 1 resistance mutations in vivo after transmission of a multiply drug-resistant virus. Clin Infect Dis 2003; 37:1693–1698.

85. Brenner BG, Routy JP, Petrella M, et al. Persistence and fitness of multidrug-resistant of human immunodeficiency virus type 1 acquired in primary HIV infection. J Virol 2002; 76:1753–1761.

86. Verhofstede C, Wanzeele FV, Van Der Gucht B, et al. Interruption of reverse transcriptase inhibitors or a switch from reverse transcriptase to protease inhibitors resulted in a fast reappearance of virus strains with a reverse transcriptase inhibitor-sensitive genotype. AIDS 1999; 13:2541–2546.

87. Devereux HL, Youle M, Johnson MA, Loveday C. Rapid decline in detectability of HIV-1 drug resistance mutations after stopping therapy. AIDS 1999; 13:123–127.

88. Jost S, Bernard MC, Kaiser L, et al. A patient with HIV-1 superinfection. N Engl J Med 2002; 347:731–736.

89. Ramos A, Hu DJ, Nguyen L, et al. Intersubtype human immunodeficiency virus type 1 superinfection following seroconversion to primary infection in two injecting intravenous drug users. J Virol 2002; 76:7444–7452.

90. Gonzales MJ, Delwart E, Rhee SY, et al. Lack of detectable human immunodeficiency virus type 1 superinfection during 1072 person-years of observation. J Infect Dis 2003; 188:397–405.

91. Tsui R, Herring BL, Barbour JD, et al. Human immunodeficiency virus type 1 superinfection was not detected following 215 years of injection drug user exposure. J Virol 2004; 78:94–103.

92. Altfeld M, Allen TM, Yu XG, et al. HIV-1 superinfection despite broad CD8+ T-cell responses containing replication of the primary infection. Nature 2002; 420:434–439.

93. Koelsch KK, Smith DM, Little SJ, et al. Clade B HIV-1 superinfection with wild-type virus after primary infection with drug-resistant clade B virus. AIDS 2003; 17:11–16.

94. Brenner B, Routy JP, Quan Y, et al.; Co-Investigators of the Quebec Primary Infection Study. Persistence of multidrug resistant HIV-1 in primary infection leading to superinfection. AIDS 2004; 18:1653–1660. [Erratum in AIDS 2004; 18:2107.]

95. Allen T, Altfeld M. HIV-1 superinfection. J Allergy Clin Immunol 2003; 112:829–835.

96. Smith D, Wong J, Hightower, et al. Incidence of HIV superinfection following primary infection. 11th Conference on Retroviruses and Opportunistic Infections; 8–11 February 2004.

97. Petrella M, Wainberg MA. Might the M184V mutation in HIV-1 RT confer clinical benefit? AIDS Rev 2002; 4:224–2332.

98. Turner D, Brenner B, Routy JP, et al. Diminished representation of HIV-1 variants containing select drug resistance-conferring mutations in primary HIV-1 infection. JAIDS 2004; 37:1627–1631.

99. Wainberg MA, Hsu M, Gu Z, et al. Effectiveness of 3TC in HIV clinical trials may be due in part to the M184V substitution in 3TC-resistant HIV-1 reverse transcriptase. AIDS 1996; 10(Suppl 5):S3–S10.

100. Baxter JD, Mayers DL, Wentworth DN, et al. A randomized study of antiretroviral management based on plasma genotypic antiretroviral resistance testing in patients failing therapy. CPCRA 046 Study Team for the Terry Beirn Community Programs for Clinical Research on AIDS. AIDS 2000; 14:83–93.

101. Colgrove RC, Pitt J, Chung PH, et al. Selective vertical transmission of HIV-1 antiretroviral resistance mutations. AIDS 1998; 12:2281–2288.

102. Dickover RE, Garratty EM, Plaeger S, et al. Perinatal transmission of major, minor, and multiple maternal human immunodeficiency virus type 1 variants in utero and intrapartum. J Virol 2001; 75:2194–2203.

103. Verhofstede C, Wanzeele FV, Van Der Gucht B, et al. Interruption of reverse transcriptase inhibitors or a switch from reverse transcriptase to protease inhibitors resulted in a fast reappearance of virus strains with a reverse transcriptase inhibitor-sensitive genotype. AIDS 1999; 13:2541–2546

104. Quinn TC, Wawer MJ, Sewankambo N, et al. Viral load and heterosexual transmission of human immunodeficiency virus type 1. Rakai Project Study Group. N Engl J Med 2000; 342:921–929.

105. Yerly S, Vora S, Rizzardi P, et al. Swiss HIV cohort study. Acute HIV infection: impact on the spread of HIV and transmission of drug resistance. AIDS 2001; 15:2287–2292.

106. Phillips A. Will the drugs still work? Transmission of resistant HIV. Nat Med 2001; 7:993–994.

107. Chaix ML, Descamps D, Harzic M, et al. Stable prevalence of genotypic drug resistance mutations but increase in non-B virus among patients with primary HIV-1 infection in France. AIDS 2003; 17:2635–2643.

108. Ammaranond P, Cunningham P, Oelrichs R, et al. No increase in protease resistance and a decrease in reverse transcriptase resistance mutations in primary HIV-1 infection: 1992-2001. AIDS 2003; 17:264–267.

109. Kuritzkes D. Drug resistance. Navigating resistance pathways. AIDS Read 2002; 12:395–400, 407.

110. Nijhuis M, Deeks S, Boucher C. Implications of antiretroviral resistance on viral fitness. Curr Opin Infect Dis 2001; 14:23–28.

111. Brenner B, Turner D, Wainberg M. HIV-1 drug resistance: can we overcome? Expert Opin Biol Ther 2002; 2:751–761.

112. Ait-Khaled M, Rakik A, Griffin P, et al. Mutations in HIV-1 reverse transcriptase during therapy with abacavir,

lamivudine and zidovudine in HIV-1-infected adults with no prior antiretroviral therapy. Antivir Ther 2002; 7:43–51.

113. Ait-Khaled M, Stone C, Amphlett G, et al. M184V is associated with a low incidence of thymidine analogue mutations and low phenotypic resistance to zidovudine and stavudine. AIDS 2002; 16:1686–1689.

114. Daar ES, Richman DD. Confronting the emergence of drug resistant HIV type 1: Impact of antiretroviral therapy on individual and population resistance. AID Res Hum Retroviruses 2005; 21:343–357.

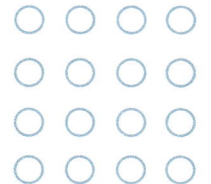

CHAPTER 15

Clinical Implications of HIV Fitness and Virulence

Jason D. Barbour
Steven G. Deeks

Introduction

The capacity of HIV to replicate and cause progressive immunodeficiency depends on a complex and continuously evolving relationship between the virus and its host. Strong selective pressures, including neutralizing antibodies, cytotoxic T cells and antiretroviral therapy, act to prevent viral replication. Through rapid genotypic evolution, HIV evolves to evade these selection pressures, eventually leading to a virus which is most fit to replicate in a given individual. At the same time, there is a strong selective pressure operating at the population level leading to the maintenance of virus that retains the ability to be transmitted between individuals. Of note, there is no strong selective pressure *in vivo* leading to a virus population that rapidly kills its host. Indeed, there likely exists selection at both the virus and host levels, which leads over time to a more benign relationship in which both can co-exist.[1,2] This complex relationship between viral replication ('fitness') and disease progression ('virulence' or 'pathogenicity') is the focus of this chapter.

There is no consistent definition for viral fitness, replicative capacity or virulence.[3] In this review, fitness refers to the capacity of one virus to replicate in a defined environment as compared with a second virus. Hence, fitness *per se* is not a fixed attribute for any given viral species. For example, the drug-resistant variant is more fit than the drug-susceptible wild-type variant in antiretroviral-treated individuals while the wild-type variant is often more fit than

the resistant variant in the absence of antiretroviral treatment. Replicative capacity generally refers to the inherent capacity of a virus to replicate in vitro in the absence of any selection pressures. High throughput commercially available assays are now available which provide an estimate of the degree to which patient-derived reverse transcriptase and protease can support viral replication. Virulence (or pathogenicity) is a distinct process from viral fitness and replicative capacity. Whereas fitness and replicative capacity focus on replication, virulence focuses on the inherent capacity of a virus to cause disease. In HIV infected individuals, virulence is often measured, based on the relative capacity of a virus to deplete CD4+ T-cell counts. As will be discussed here, studies of variation in HIV have revealed that distinct portions of the HIV-1 genome, and stages of its life cycle, may differentially affect viral fitness, replicative capacity, and virulence.

Genetic Diversity of HIV-1

HIV-1 is well suited to rapid adaptation to any obstacle to viral replication. Several factors account for this rapid viral diversification, including a low fidelity (high error rate) of reverse transcriptase, rapid recombination of portions of genetically distinct HIV-1 genomes (which leads to rapid viral evolution), high plasticity of several HIV enzymes, and perhaps the cytidine deaminase APOBEC3G which modifies genetic sequences.

High Error Rate of Reverse Transcriptase

HIV-1 ensures sequence diversity in each generation via reverse transcriptase – which is error prone[4] – making about 1 error per 10 kilobases of nucleotide,[5] the approximate length of the HIV-1 genome. As a billion or more viral particles are generated each day in an infected host, every point variant possible is likely generated in each viral life cycle.

Recombination

HIV-1 genomes are known to frequently recombine.[6] The HIV-1 reverse transcriptase may pause and disengage from the RNA template when generating the viral DNA, which will be integrated into the host genome. Once disengaged, the reverse transcriptase may re-engage the same RNA template, or a distinct template from a genetically distinct HIV-1 genome. The resulting hybrid genome is a recombinant and may possess unique phenotypic characteristics. For example, a virus with a highly efficient reverse transcriptase might recombine with a viral genome coding for an envelope of high affinity for CCR5, leading to high level replication *in vivo*. Circulating recombinant forms of HIV-1 likely arose via such a mechanism.

Partial Inhibition of APOBEC3G by HIV-1 Vif Protein

APOBEC proteins are cytidine deaminases which induces nucleotide changes in the nucleotide sequence of viruses.[7] There are at least 11 APOBEC proteins in humans, with APOBEC 3G and APOBEC 3F believed to be most active against HIV-1. Left unchecked, APOBEC causes hypermutation within the HIV genome thereby rendering all progeny replication incompetent. HIV-1 partially inhibits APOBEC through its Vif protein, which appears to bind to and degrade the enzyme.[8] Although Vif effectively suppresses APOBEC activity, there remains evidence of persistent activity since signature G to A nucleotide changes are readily observed across the genome of virus over time.[7] Theoretically, by only partially evading A3G activity, the rate at which mutations appear within the viral genome is enhanced. Sequence diversity ensures novel variants are produced in each generation – some of which may have a fitness advantage to host obstacles to replication, such as mutation of CTL epitopes, or change in sites within targets of antiretroviral therapy.

Determinants of Virulence: Role of Immune Activation

Simian immunodeficiency virus (SIV) replicates to high levels in its natural hosts (e.g. sooty mangabeys and African Green Monkeys) but does not cause progressive immunodeficiency and increased mortality, and therefore might be considered to be highly fit but non-pathogenic.[9,10] When this same virus is used to experimentally infect non-natural hosts (e.g. macaques), high level replication and rapid disease progression occur. That infection by highly related viral strains between closely related primate species should differ fundamentally in their capacity to damage the infected host suggests that virus/host interactions vary between species, and that this interaction largely defines the relative virulence of SIV (and by extension HIV).

HIV and SIV evolve to adapt to changing host barriers to its replication, and in addition maintain and expand its fitness in the human host by altering the host environment, a process known as 'niche construction.'[11] HIV-1 niche construction theoretically includes the induction of high level T-cell activation (which provides more targets for viral replication), down modulation of MHC expression, alteration of T-cell maturation phenotypes, and depleting and re-organizing lymphoid organs. These changes to the host immune system contribute directly to progressive immunodeficiency independent of any direct cytopathic effect which HIV/SIV has on CD4[+] T cells. For example, T-cell activation, which is the most proximal known measure of disease progression risk and death in humans,[12] may be an essential component of HIV-1 niche construction, inducing the proliferation of target cells, and in turn fueling viral diversification leading to escape from adaptive immune responses, and opportunities for transmission to a new host.

The degree to which SIV and/or HIV causes immune activation may be the critical determinant of virulence *in vivo*.[13,14] SIV infections in its natural hosts are characterized by high level viral replication, but not high level T-cell activation, or other markers of immune dysregulation seen in HIV infection of humans. Sooty mangabeys and its species specific SIV may have co-evolved over tens of thousands of years to allow limited or selected niche construction by SIV, as evidenced by the lack of high level T-cell activation. No such balance appears to exist in HIV-1 infection of humans which expanded into humans less than 100 years ago.[15]

High-throughput Measurements of Replicative Capacity

The strengths and limitations of assays that measure viral fitness and/or replicative capacity are reviewed elsewhere.[16,17] Most of these assays are labor-intensive and are best applied to small well-characterized cohorts. Such assays are not likely to be developed for clinical management. However, with minor modifications, commercially available phenotypic drug susceptibility assays can measure the relative capacity of HIV to replicate in the absence of drug.[18-20] The PhenoSense *Pol* replication capacity assay utilizes viral test vectors that involve extraction of HIV-1 RNA from the plasma of infected persons, followed by RT-PCR amplification of a gene segment containing the terminal 18 codons of *Gag*, all of the *Pro*, and a portion of the reverse transcriptase reading frame.[18] Viral protease-reverse transcriptase *Pol* replication capacity values are expressed as a percentage of the amount of replication of the NL4-3 reference vectors analyzed in parallel in every run. Values <100% have lowered *Pol* replication capacity compared with NL4-3, as well as the average wild-type virus drawn from a patient in chronic infection. Although these assays are standardized and amenable to high-throughput studies, there are significant limitations. In particular, these assays only measure a limited part of the viral genome and do not directly compete the test virus against the control virus.

Antiretroviral Drug Pressure and Changes in Fitness and Virulence

There is growing recognition that antiretroviral therapy selects for mutations that impair the inherent ability of HIV to replicate. This appears to be particularly true for the protease inhibitor class, where drug resistance-related mutations are known to negatively affect the enzymatic activity of protease.[21-25] The negative impact of these changes on replicative capacity offset by compensatory mutations with protease and the substrates for this enzyme (e.g. Gag).[21,26-30] Resistance mutations associated with nucleoside analog exposure also appear to reduce viral fitness (M184V, K65R and T215Y mutations have been most consistently associated with reduced replicative capacity).[31-37] Resistance mutations associated with non-nucleoside reverse transcriptase inhibitors do not appear to dramatically impact viral fitness, perhaps because these mutations do not occur near the active site of the enzyme.[38-40] The relationship between drug exposure and changes in viral replicative capacity and/or fitness has been extensively reviewed elsewhere and will not be discussed further here.[16,17,31,41-44]

The clinical significance of reduced replicative capacity has been extensively studied in antiretroviral-treated patients experiencing an incomplete virologic response to therapy. Such individuals often maintain HIV RNA levels which are below pre-treatment baseline levels despite the emergence of drug-resistant variants. This is typically associated with durable immunologic and perhaps clinical benefit.[45-51] The rate at which CD4+ T-cell counts decline is slower in patients with protease inhibitor-resistant virus compared to those with wild-type HIV (Fig. 15.1)[52]; this difference persists even after controlling for the level of HIV RNA.[47,52] These findings suggested that the relationship between HIV-1 replication and its virulence for CD4+ T cells had been altered in the context of virologic failure, perhaps as a consequence of a reduced ability of the resistant virus to cause thymic dysfunction,[50,53] T-cell activation[54] or T-cell death.[55-59] When patients with drug-resistant virus interrupt therapy, HIV RNA levels often increase rapidly. This increase is temporally associated with release from the latent reservoir of wild-type HIV, which clearly outcompetes the drug-resistant variant in absence of antiretroviral drug pressure.[19,60-63] This increase is also associated with rapid CD4+ T-cell loss; although to what degree this loss can be fully explained by change in HIV RNA levels vs a change in 'virulence' remains unknown.

Replicative Capacity and Virulence in Antiretroviral-treated Patients

The degree of increase in protease inhibitor resistance experienced during early virologic failure of a protease inhibitor-based regimen has been directly correlated with change in viral *Pol* replication capacity.[26] In addition, a direct relationship was observed between the change in *Pol* replication capacity due to drug resistance mutations and the degree of virologic suppression that was achieved. Despite ongoing evolution towards higher protease inhibitor resistance the virus did not develop compensatory mutations to recover *Pol* replication capacity or replicate at high levels in the blood (Fig. 15.2). The patients that sustained partial virologic suppression maintained elevated CD4+ T-cell counts over the period of observation. These results strongly suggested that the basis for the CD4+ T-cell benefit was related to

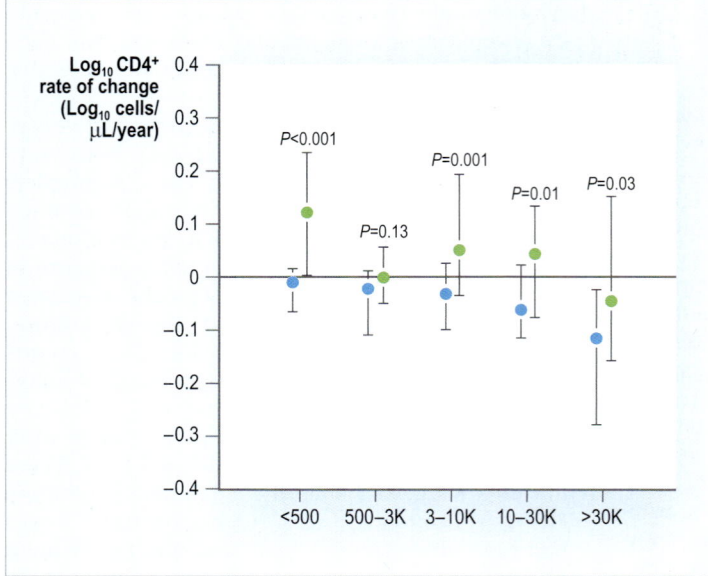

Figure 15.1 Change in specific virulence of HIV-1 among patients in long-term virologic failure of a PI-based regimen. Circles represent average annual $\log_{10}$ CD4+ T-cell loss rates (y-axis) among patients in long-term virologic failure by plasma HIV-1 RNA levels (x-axis). Squares represent average CD4+ loss rates among untreated HIV-1-infected adults.[52]

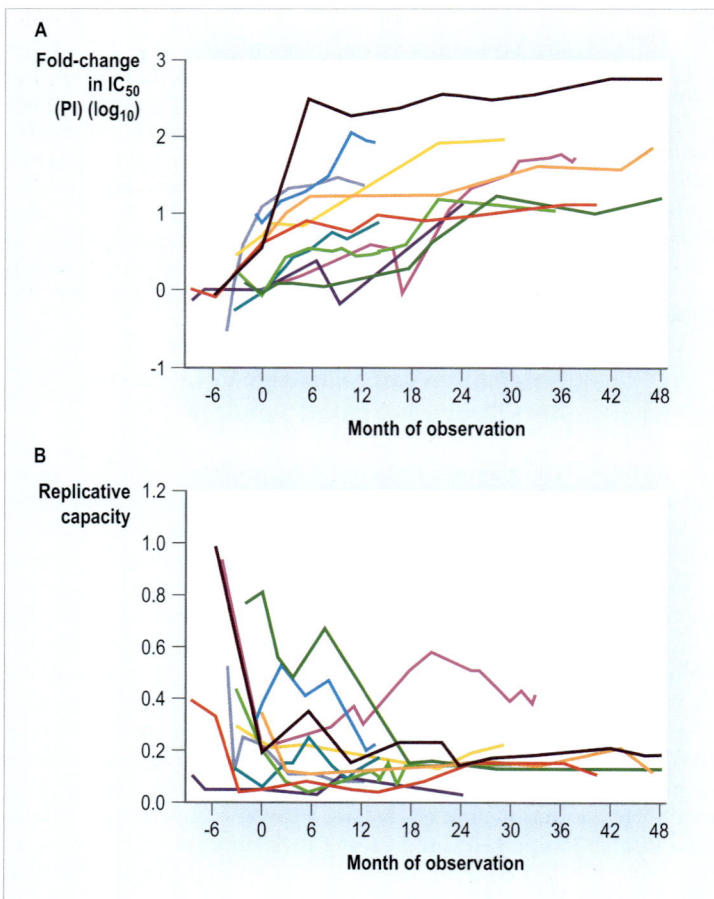

Figure 15.2 *Pol* replication capacity values decline as phenotypic resistance to the prescribed protease inhibitor rises. (A) Despite continuing evolution towards higher PI resistance, *Pol* replicative capacity scores remained durably lowered over the period of observation, indicating (B) no compensatory mutations had occurred within the *Pol* construct that might raise replication capacity.[26]

the change in *Pol* replication capacity, due to development of drug resistance mutations. This result has been observed by other groups.[64,65]

Viral Fitness and Replication Capacity in Antiretroviral-untreated Individuals

Disease progression rates vary widely among untreated HIV-1 infected individuals and at least part of this variation has been linked to HLA Class I allelic variations.[66] However, there is accumulating evidence of the contribution of viral phenotype to variation in disease progression (as defined by either viral load or CD4+ T-cell loss). In a study of 20 HIV infected patients with wild-type HIV interrupting an effective regimen, viral replicative capacity – as defined by an assay which measured *in vitro* replication kinetics – was associated with the off-therapy viral load set-point.[67] In a study using dual competition fitness assays, HIV variants from patients with delayed disease progression were less fit than those found in patients who progressed to AIDS rapidly.[68] Virus isolates from rapid progressors out-competed those from slow progressors; this effect appeared to be predicted by the level of viral replication *in vitro* and *in vivo*. These observations are generally consistent with previous studies suggesting a link between low replicative capacity and long-term non-progression.[68–71]

Because most fitness assays are labor intensive, most studies to date have been limited by a small sample size. In a study of 191 recently infected individuals, replicative capacity – as defined by a single cycle recombinant virus assay – varied widely (Fig. 15.3).[72] Patients bearing HIV-1 variants in the lowest quartile of observed *Pol* replicative capacity values (<43% of wild-type average HIV-1) had significantly elevated CD4+ T-cell counts (Fig. 15.3). Notably, the low *Pol* replicative capacity viruses fell into the same range of values as those observed in patients in long-term virologic failure of a protease inhibitor-based regimen with durably elevated CD4+ T-cell counts. Thus, it appears there is natural variation in the virulence of distinct strains among treatment-naive individuals; for reasons which remain to be defined, this variation in virulence appears to be linked to genetic variation within the *Pol* gene.[73]

Comparable observations were made linking replication capacity and outcome in chronically infected hemophiliacs. Among HIV-infected hemophiliacs with wild-type HIV or NRTI-resistant HIV, a replication capacity <69% (the lower quartile) was associated with reduced rates of progression to AIDS/death.[74] Collectively, these observations suggest that replication capacity provides prognostic information regarding disease progression in untreated individuals, and that this effect persists even after controlling for viral load and other important co-variables.

Impact of Co-receptor Tropism on Fitness and Virulence

The most variable region of the HIV-1 genome is the viral envelop (Env). This protein mediates the entry

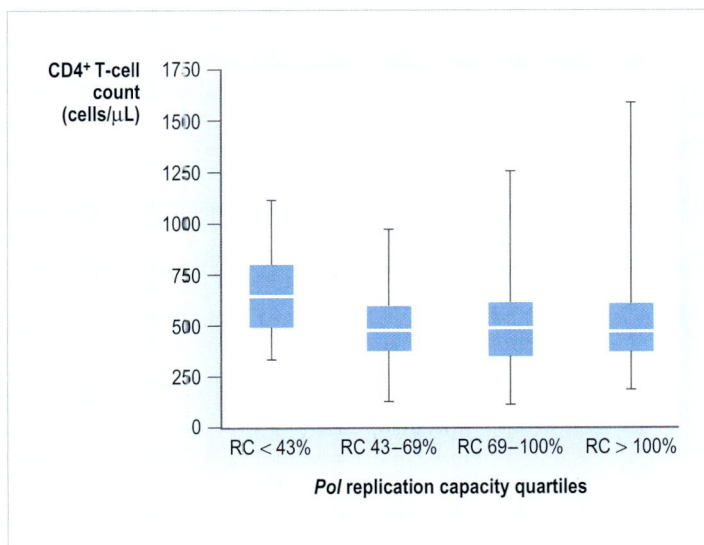

Figure 15.3 Patients bearing a virus of *Pol* replicative capacity lower than 43% of wild-type control had significantly higher CD4+ T-cell counts at study entry, compared with those bearing viruses in any category >43% of wild-type control.[72]

of HIV-1 into target cells via engagement with the CD4 receptor and either the CCR5 or CXCR4 co-receptor. The viral envelop differs to a remarkable degree across patient viral isolates and even within a single patient. The expressed protein varies in amino acid composition, and significant length polymorphisms exist throughout Env. Changes in Env are associated with changes in viral fitness,[75] as well as changes in the route of HIV transmission, co-receptor utilization, and perhaps virulence.[76,77]

Work performed in the early 1990s demonstrated that some patient-derived viruses induce the formation of multi-nucleated cell aggregates or syncytia *in vitro*, and that the presence of such viruses was associated with a more rapid disease progression.[78,79] Subsequently, it was shown that viruses which utilize the co-receptor CXCR4 ('X4 variants') often induce this phenotype while viruses that utilize the co-receptor CCR5 ('R5 variants') generally do not.[80] The CXCR4 (X4) utilizing variants are associated with high HIV-1 RNA (hence considered fit) and may be associated with more rapid CD4+ depletion than R5 viruses, after controlling for HIV RNA levels (and hence may be considered more virulent).[81]

The complex and often conflicting relationship between viral fitness and virulence may be best illustrated by co-receptor tropism. Although both viruses can replicate at high titer *in vivo*, R5 virtues tend to dominate, particularly in early HIV infection. This dominance of R5 occurs even though some *in vitro* data suggest that X4 variants may have greater infectivity. When R5 and X4 were competed *in vitro*, it was observed that X4 caused a rapid depletion of its target cells, leading to diminishing amount of virus production over time. Hence, the X4 variant may destroy, rather than preserve, its own niche for replication.[82] This tendency of X4 utilizing variants to destroy its own niche may explain why X4 variants appear only temporally in some patients, and may not appear in others.[83] This tendency may also explain why X4 emergence was only transient in monkeys even in the presence of drugs designed to inhibit replication of R5 virus.[84]

HIV-1 Entry Inhibitors: Impact on Fitness and Virulence

An additional source of genetic and phenotypic selection for viruses is the use of antiretroviral compounds. Compounds which seek to interrupt viral entry into the cell – either by engaging the virus, the target co-receptor, or an intermediate configuration of the virus and molecule (fusion) – present replica-

tion barriers to the virus. Drug selected mutations that allow HIV to replicate in presence of entry inhibitors often have significant impact on replicative capacity and may even affect clinical virulence.[85-87]

The fusion inhibitor, T-20 (enfuvirtide) blocks entry of HIV-1 into target cells by impeding a conformational change in the gp41 protein of HIV-1. Enfuvirtide is associated with significant virologic suppression, and is now being widely used in clinics in North America and Europe as a component of combination antiretroviral therapy.[88] Resistance to enfuvirtide has now been observed among treated patients,[89] and may confer lowered fitness.[90,91] However, it is not yet clear if the *in vitro* findings will be associated with alterations upon *in vivo* fitness and virulence. Our clinical experience with these compounds is limited, and information on changes in virulence among resistant variants is not definitive. More experience with these compounds will be necessary to gauge effects on viral diversity, fitness and virulence.

Virulence Modulation as an Evolutionary Strategy

Has HIV-1 evolved towards a lower virulence in humans over the course of what we believe is an approximately 75-year-old zoonosis? There is evidence that humans who carry rare allele forms of HLA Class I A and B loci have an advantage in controlling HIV-1 infection.[92] This effect is presumably due to the progressive HIV-1 genetic escape from the more common HLA restricted alleles. The existence of non-pathogenic SIV infections in primate species, such as the sooty mangabey, suggests that adaptation occurred in these species – either by the virus, the host or both.

Viruses take different strategies to persist in human populations that include modulation of virulence. Herpes simplex virus 2 (HSV-2) is hyperendemic in the Americas, Europe, Africa and parts of Asia (at least 25% of the US adult population is sero-positive for HSV-2).[93] Yet only 1 in 50 HSV-2 infected persons suffer from recurrent genital ulcer disease. Hence, HSV-2 is fit for humans, as it replicates in humans and is readily transmitted but appears to be infrequently virulent in immunocompetent hosts. HSV-2 represents a sexually transmitted infection that is fit, highly transmissible but not clinically virulent for most individuals. HIV-1 is highly virulent for humans, but is likely a relatively new infection in humans, the best estimates dating its zoonotic transfer from *pan troglodytes* (chimpanzee) to humans around 1930 in West Africa.[15] HSV-2, by contrast, is likely a long-standing hyper-endemic infections of humans, and may have had significant period of time to modulate its virulence to extend the life of the host, and preserve opportunities for transmission.

Primate lentiviral infections vary in virulence across host species.[9] Among humans there is substantial variation in virulence of different circulating strains of HIV-1.[68,72,94] This variation may be the result of the collective force of selection pressures from the immune system responses of outbred human populations, and – more recently – antiretroviral compounds. HIV-1 of lowered virulence may be less likely to induce symptomatology of acute infection, such as acute retroviral syndrome, leading patients to be unaware they are ill. Once infected, regardless of knowledge of status the strains of lowered virulence are associated with slower CD4+ T-cell loss, thus prolonging the window of clinical latency, and providing more opportunities for transmission of HIV-1. The impact of altered virulence on a population level may be difficult to predict.

Conclusion

Fitness studies – both recombinant and whole genome – allow an opportunity to dissect the segments of the viral life cycle which contribute most directly to virulence, allowing us greater insight into the still unresolved question of how HIV induces progressive rapid CD4+ T-cell loss, immunodeficiency, morbidity and death in the vast majority of those infected with HIV-1. Careful pathogenesis-oriented assessments regarding the impact of fitness/replicative capacity on disease outcomes independent of HIV RNA levels may allow for the development of assays with more precision in prediction of specific measures of clinical virulence. Once developed, these measures might assist in predicting subsequent rate of CD4+ T-cell loss, the occurrence of unrecoverable immune system impairments, time to AIDS, virologic and immunologic responses to treatment, and even specific medical sequelae such as dementia.

References

1. Brander C, Walker BD. Gradual adaptation of HIV to human host populations: good or bad news? Nat Med 2003; 9:1359–1362.

2. Deeks SG, Walker BD. The immune response to AIDS virus infection: good, bad, or both? J Clin Invest 2004; 113:808–810.

3. Deeks SG. Treatment of antiretroviral-drug-resistant HIV-1 infection. Lancet 2003; 362:2002–2011.

4. Preston BD, Poiesz BJ, Loeb LA. Fidelity of HIV-1 reverse transcriptase. Science 1988; 242:1168–1171.

5. Mansky LM, Temin HM. Lower in vivo mutation rate of human immunodeficiency virus type 1 than that predicted from the fidelity of purified reverse transcriptase. J Virol 1995; 69:5087–5094.

6. Shriner D, Rodrigo AG, Nickle DC, et al. Pervasive genomic recombination of HIV-1 in vivo. Genetics 2004; 167:1573–1583.

7. Yu Q, Konig R, Pillai S, et al. Single-strand specificity of APOBEC3G accounts for minus-strand deamination of the HIV genome. Nat Struct Mol Biol 2004; 11:435–442.

8. Stopak K, Noronha C de, Yonemoto W, et al. HIV-1 Vif blocks the antiviral activity of APOBEC3G by impairing both its translation and intracellular stability. Mol Cell 2003; 12:591–601.

9. Kaur A, Grant RM, Means RE, et al. Diverse host responses and outcomes following simian immunodeficiency virus SIVmac239 infection in sooty mangabeys and rhesus macaques. J Virol 1998; 72:9597–9611.

10. Silvestri G, Sodora DL, Koup RA, et al. Nonpathogenic SIV infection of sooty mangabeys is characterized by limited bystander immunopathology despite chronic high-level viremia. Immunity 2003; 18:441–452.

11. Laland KN, Odling-Smee FJ, Feldman MW. Evolutionary consequences of niche construction and their implications for ecology. Proc Natl Acad Sci U S A 1999; 96:10242–10247.

12. Giorgi JV, Hultin LE, McKeating JA, et al. Shorter survival in advanced human immunodeficiency virus type 1 infection is more closely associated with T lymphocyte activation than with plasma virus burden or virus chemokine coreceptor usage. J Infect Dis 1999; 179: 859–870.

13. Silvestri G, Feinberg MB. Turnover of lymphocytes and conceptual paradigms in HIV infection. J Clin Invest 2003; 112:821–824.

14. Grossman Z, Meier-Schellersheim M, Sousa AE, et al. CD4+ T-cell depletion in HIV infection: are we closer to understanding the cause? Nat Med 2002; 8:319–323.

15. Korber B, Muldoon M, Theiler J, et al. Timing the ancestor of the HIV-1 pandemic strains. Science 2000; 288:1789–1796.

16. Quinones-Mateu ME, Arts EJ. Fitness of drug resistant HIV-1: methodology and clinical implications. Drug Resist Updat 2002; 5:224–233.

17. Nijhuis M, Deeks S, Boucher C. Implications of antiretroviral resistance on viral fitness. Curr Opin Infect Dis 2001; 14:23–28.

18. Petropoulos CJ, Parkin NT, Limoli KL, et al. A novel phenotypic drug susceptibility assay for human immunodeficiency virus type 1. Antimicrob Agents Chemother 2000; 44:920–928.

19. Deeks SG, Wrin T, Liegler T, et al. Virologic and immunologic consequences of discontinuing combination antiretroviral-drug therapy in HIV-infected patients with detectable viremia. N Engl J Med 2001; 344:472–480.

20. Bonhoeffer S, Chappey C, Parkin NT, et al. Evidence for positive epistasis in HIV-1. Science 2004; 306:1547–1550.

21. Mammano F, Petit C, Clavel F. Resistance-associated loss of viral fitness in human immunodeficiency virus type 1: phenotypic analysis of protease and gag coevolution in protease inhibitor-treated patients. J Virol 1998; 72:7632–7637.

22. Martinez-Picado J, Savara AV, Sutton L, et al. Replicative fitness of protease inhibitor-resistant mutants of human immunodeficiency virus type 1. J Virol 1999; 73:3744–3752.

23. Nijhuis M, Schuurman R, de Jong D, et al. Increased fitness of drug resistant HIV-1 protease as a result of acquisition of compensatory mutations during suboptimal therapy. AIDS 1999; 13:2349–2359.

24. Bleiber G, Munoz M, Ciuffi A, et al. Individual contributions of mutant protease and reverse transcriptase to viral infectivity, replication, and protein maturation of antiretroviral drug-resistant human immunodeficiency virus type 1. J Virol 2001; 75:3291–3300.

25. Resch W, Ziermann R, Parkin N, et al. Nelfinavir-resistant, amprenavir-hypersusceptible strains of human immunodeficiency virus type 1 carrying an N88S mutation in protease have reduced infectivity, reduced replication capacity, and reduced fitness and process the Gag polyprotein precursor aberrantly. J Virol 2002; 76:8659–8666.

26. Barbour JD, Wrin T, Grant RM, et al. Evolution of phenotypic drug susceptibility and viral replication capacity during long-term virologic failure of protease inhibitor therapy in human immunodeficiency virus-infected adults. J Virol 2002; 76:11104–11112.

27. Myint L, Matsuda M, Matsuda Z, et al. Gag non-cleavage site mutations contribute to full recovery of viral fitness in protease inhibitor-resistant human immunodeficiency virus type 1. Antimicrob Agents Chemother 2004; 48:444–452.

28. Resino S, Bellon JM, Gurbindo MD, et al. CD38 expression in CD8+ T cells predicts virological failure in HIV type 1-infected children receiving antiretroviral therapy. Clin Infect Dis 2004; 38:412–417.

29. Zennou V, Mammano F, Paulous S, et al. Loss of viral fitness associated with multiple Gag and Gag-Pol processing defects in human immunodeficiency virus type 1 variants selected for resistance to protease inhibitors in vivo. J Virol 1998; 72:3300–3306.

30. Watkins T, Resch W, Irlbeck D, et al. Selection of high-level resistance to human immunodeficiency virus type 1 protease inhibitors. Antimicrob Agents Chemother 2003; 47:759–769.

31. Clavel F, Hance AJ. HIV drug resistance. N Engl J Med 2004; 350:1023–1035.

32. Goudsmit J, de Ronde A, Ho DD, et al. Human immunodeficiency virus fitness in vivo: calculations based on a single zidovudine resistance mutation at codon 215 of reverse transcriptase. J Virol 1996; 70:5662–5664.

33. Harrigan PR, Bloor S, Larder BA. Relative replicative fitness of zidovudine-resistant human immunodeficiency virus type 1 isolates in vitro. J Virol 1998; 72:3773–3778.

34. Wainberg MA, Drosopoulos WC, Salomon H, et al. Enhanced fidelity of 3TC-selected mutant HIV-1 reverse transcriptase. Science 1996; 271:1282–1285.

35. White KL, Margot NA, Wrin T, et al. Molecular mechanisms of resistance to human immunodeficiency virus type 1 with reverse transcriptase mutations K65R and K65R+M184V and their effects on enzyme function and viral replication capacity. Antimicrob Agents Chemother 2002; 46: 3437–3446.

36. Back NK, Nijhuis M, Keulen W, et al. Reduced replication of 3TC-resistant HIV-1 variants in primary cells due to a processivity defect of the reverse transcriptase enzyme. Embo J 1996; 15:4040–4049.

37. Weber J, Chakraborty B, Weberova J, et al. Diminished replicative fitness of primary human immunodeficiency virus type 1 isolates harboring the K65R mutation. J Clin Microbiol 2005; 43:1395–1400.

38. Smerdon SJ, Jager J, Wang J, et al. Structure of the binding site for nonnucleoside inhibitors of the reverse transcriptase of human immunodeficiency virus type 1. Proc Natl Acad Sci USA 1994; 91:3911–3915.

39. Dykes C, Fox K, Lloyd A, et al. Impact of clinical reverse transcriptase sequences on the replication capacity of HIV-1 drug-resistant mutants. Virology 2001; 285:193–203.

40. Joly V, Descamps D, Peytavin G, et al. Evolution of human immunodeficiency virus type 1 (HIV-1) resistance mutations in nonnucleoside reverse transcriptase inhibitors (NNRTIs) in HIV-1-infected patients switched to antiretroviral therapy without NNRTIs. Antimicrob Agents Chemother 2004; 48:172–175.

41. Barbour JD, Grant RM. The clinical implications of reduced viral fitness. Curr Infect Dis Rep 2004; 6:151–158.

42. Quinones-Mateu ME, Arts EJ. HIV-1 fitness: implications for drug resistance, disease progression, and global epidemic evolution. In: Kuiken C, Foley B, Hahn B, et al., eds. HIV sequence compendium 2001. Los Alamos, NM: Theoretical Biology and Biophysics Group, Los Alamos National Laboratory; 2001:134–170.

43. Bates M, Wrin T, Huang W, et al. Practical applications of viral fitness in clinical practice. Curr Opin Infect Dis 2003; 16:11–18.

44. Erickson JW, Gulnik SV, Markowitz M. Protease inhibitors: resistance, cross-resistance, fitness and the choice of initial and salvage therapies. AIDS 1999; 13:189–204.

45. Kaufmann D, Pantaleo G, Sudre P, Telenti A. CD4-cell count in HIV-1-infected individuals remaining viraemic with highly active antiretroviral therapy (HAART). Swiss HIV Cohort Study Lancet 1998; 351:723–724.

46. Le Moing V, Thiebaut R, Chene G, et al. Predictors of long-term increase in CD4(+) cell counts in human immunodeficiency virus-infected patients receiving a protease inhibitor- containing antiretroviral regimen. J Infect Dis 2002; 185:471–480.

47. Ledergerber B, Lundgren JD, Walker AS, et al. Predictors of trend in CD4-positive T-cell count and mortality among HIV-1-infected individuals with virological failure to all three antiretroviral-drug classes. Lancet 2004; 364:51–62.

48. Deeks SG, Barbour JD, Grant RM, Martin JN. Duration and predictors of CD4 T-cell gains in patients who continue combination therapy despite detectable plasma viremia. AIDS 2002; 16:201–207.

49. Grabar S, Le Moing V, Goujard C, et al. Clinical outcome of patients with HIV-1 infection according to immunologic and virologic response after 6 months of highly active antiretroviral therapy. Ann Intern Med 2000; 133: 401–410.

50. Lecossier D, Bouchonnet F, Schneider P, et al. Discordant increases in CD4+ T cells in human immunodeficiency virus- infected patients experiencing virologic treatment failure: role of changes in thymic output and T cell death. J Infect Dis 2001; 183:1009–1016.

51. Piketty C, Weiss L, Thomas F, et al. Long-term clinical outcome of human immunodeficiency virus-infected patients with discordant immunologic and virologic responses to a protease inhibitor-containing regimen. J Infect Dis 2001; 183:1328–1335.

52. Deeks SG, Barbour JD, Martin JN, et al. Sustained CD4+ T cell response after virologic failure of protease inhibitor-based regimens in patients with human immunodeficiency virus infection. J Infect Dis 2000; 181:946–953.

53. Stoddart CA, Liegler TJ, Mammano F, et al. Impaired replication of protease inhibitor-resistant HIV-1 in human thymus. Nat Med 2001; 7:712–718.

54. Deeks SG, Hoh R, Grant RM, et al. CD4+ T cell kinetics and activation in human immunodeficiency virus-infected patients who remain viremic despite long-term treatment with protease inhibitor-based therapy. J Infect Dis 2002; 185:315–323.

55. Chavan S, Kodoth S, Pahwa R, et al. The HIV protease inhibitor Indinavir inhibits cell-cycle progression in vitro in lymphocytes of HIV-infected and uninfected individuals. Blood 2001; 98:383–389.

56. Estaquier J, Lelievre JD, Petit F, et al. Effects of antiretroviral drugs on human immunodeficiency virus type 1-induced CD4(+) T-cell death. J Virol 2002; 76:5966–5973.

57. Phenix BN, Angel JB, Mandy F, et al. Decreased HIV-associated T cell apoptosis by HIV protease inhibitors. AIDS Res Hum Retroviruses 2000; 16:559–567.

58. Sloand EM, Maciejewski J, Kumar P, et al. Protease inhibitors stimulate hematopoiesis and decrease apoptosis and ICE expression in CD34(+) cells. Blood 2000; 96:2735–2739.

59. Weichold FF, Bryant JL, Pati S, et al. HIV-1 protease inhibitor ritonavir modulates susceptibility to apoptosis of uninfected T cells. J Hum Virol 1999; 2:261–269.

60. Miller V, Sabin C, Hertogs K, et al. Virological and immunological effects of treatment interruptions in HIV-1 infected patients with treatment failure. AIDS 2000; 14:2857–2867.

61. Lawrence J, Mayers DL, Hullsiek KH, et al. Structured treatment interruption in patients with multidrug-resistant human immunodeficiency virus. N Engl J Med 2003; 349:837–846.

62. Izopet J, Massip P, Souyris C, et al. Shift in HIV resistance genotype after treatment interruption and short-term antiviral effect following a new salvage regimen. AIDS 2000; 14:2247–2255.

63. Devereux HL, Emery VC, Johnson MA, et al. Replicative fitness in vivo of HIV-1 variants with multiple drug resistance-associated mutations. J Med Virol 2001; 65:218–224.

64. Sarmati L, Nicastri E, Montano M, et al. Decrease of replicative capacity of HIV isolates after genotypic guided change of therapy. J Med Virol 2004; 72:511–516.

65. Sufka SA, Ferrari G, Gryszowka VE, et al. Prolonged CD4+ cell/virus load discordance during treatment with protease inhibitor-based highly active antiretroviral therapy: immune response and viral control. J Infect Dis 2003; 187:1027–1037.

66. O'Brien SJ, Gao X, Carrington M. HLA and AIDS: a cautionary tale. Trends Mol Med 2001; 7:379–381.

67. Trkola A, Kuster H, Leemann C, et al. Human immunodeficiency virus type 1 fitness is a determining factor in viral rebound and set point in chronic infection. J Virol 2003; 77:13146–13155.

68. Quinones-Mateu ME, Ball SC, Marozsan AJ, et al. A dual infection/competition assay shows a correlation between ex vivo human immunodeficiency virus type 1 fitness and disease progression. J Virol 2000; 74:9222–9233.

69. Kwa D, Vingerhoed J, Boeser B, et al. Increased in vitro cytopathicity of CC chemokine receptor 5-restricted human immunodeficiency virus type 1 primary isolates correlates with a progressive clinical course of infection. J Infect Dis 2003; 187:1397–1403.

70. Campbell TB, Schneider K, Wrin T, et al. Relationship between in vitro human immunodeficiency virus type 1 replication rate and virus load in plasma. J Virol 2003; 77:12105–12112.

71. Blaak H, Brouwer M, Ran LJ, et al. In vitro replication kinetics of human immunodeficiency virus type 1 (HIV-1) variants in relation to virus load in long-term survivors of HIV-1 infection. J Infect Dis 1998; 177:600–610.

72. Barbour J, Segal MR, Wrin T, et al. Higher CD4+ T-cell counts associated with low viral pro/pol replication capacity among treatment naive adults in early HIV-1 infection. 11th Conference on Retroviruses and Opportunistic Infections, San Francisco, CA: 2004.

73. Segal MR, Barbour JD, Grant RM. Relating HIV-1 sequence variation to replication capacity via trees and forests. Statistical applications in genetics and molecular biology. San Francisco, CA: Center for Bioinformatics and Molecular Biostatistics; 2004.

74. Daar E, Kesler K, Lail A, et al. HIV Co-receptor tropism (CRT) and replication capacity (RC) predict HIV progression. 43rd ICAAC, Chicago, IL: 2003.

75. Rangel HR, Weber J, Chakraborty B, et al. Role of the human immunodeficiency virus type 1 envelope gene in viral fitness. J Virol 2003; 77:9069–9073.

76. Moore JP, Kitchen SG, Pugach P, Zack JA. The CCR5 and CXCR4 coreceptors–central to understanding the transmission and pathogenesis of human immunodeficiency virus type 1 infection. AIDS Res Hum Retroviruses 2004; 20:111–126.

77. Etemad-Moghadam B, Rhone D, Steenbeke T, et al. Membrane-fusing capacity of the human immunodeficiency virus envelope proteins determines the efficiency of CD+ T-cell depletion in macaques infected by a simian-human immunodeficiency virus. J Virol 2001; 75:5646–5655.

78. Koot M, Keet IP, Vos AH, et al. Prognostic value of HIV-1 syncytium-inducing phenotype for rate of CD4+ cell depletion and progression to AIDS. Ann Intern Med 1993; 118:681–688.

79. Richman DD, Bozzette SA. The impact of the syncytium-inducing phenotype of human immunodeficiency virus on disease progression. J Infect Dis 1994; 169:968–974.

80. Alkhatib G, Combadiere C, Broder CC, et al. CC CKR5: a RANTES, MIP-1alpha, MIP-1beta receptor as a fusion cofactor for macrophage-tropic HIV-1. Science 1996; 272:1955–1958.

81. Connor RI, Sheridan KE, Ceradini D, et al. Change in coreceptor use coreceptor use correlates with disease progression in HIV-1–infected individuals. J Exp Med 1997; 185:621–628.

82. Schweighardt B, Roy AM, Meiklejohn DA, et al. R5 human immunodeficiency virus type 1 (HIV-1) replicates more efficiently in primary CD4+ T-cell cultures than X4 HIV-1. J Virol 2004; 78:9164–9173.

83. Shankarappa R, Margolick JB, Gange SJ, et al. Consistent viral evolutionary changes associated with the progression of human immunodeficiency virus type 1 infection. J Virol 1999; 73:10489–10502.

84. Wolinsky SM, Veazey RS, Kunstman KJ, et al. Effect of a CCR5 inhibitor on viral loads in macaques dual-infected with R5 and X4 primate immunodeficiency viruses. Virology 2004; 328:19–29.

85. Moore JP, Doms RW. The entry of entry inhibitors: a fusion of science and medicine. Proc Natl Acad Sci USA 2003; 100:10598–10602.

86. Kilby JM, Eron JJ. Novel therapies based on mechanisms of HIV-1 cell entry. N Engl J Med 2003; 348:2228–2238.

87. Reeves JD, Gallo SA, Ahmad N, et al. Sensitivity of HIV-1 to entry inhibitors correlates with envelope/coreceptor affinity, receptor density, and fusion kinetics. Proc Natl Acad Sci USA 2002; 99:16249–54.

88. Lalezari JP, Henry K, O'Hearn M, et al. Enfuvirtide, an HIV-1 fusion inhibitor, for drug-resistant HIV infection in North and South America. N Engl J Med 2003; 348:2175–2185.

89. Wei X, Decker JM, Liu H, et al. Emergence of resistant human immunodeficiency virus type 1 in patients receiving fusion inhibitor (T-20) monotherapy. Antimicrob Agents Chemother 2002; 46:1896–1905.

90. Lu J, Sista P, Giguel F, et al. Relative replicative fitness of human immunodeficiency virus type 1 mutants resistant to enfuvirtide (T-20). J Virol 2004; 78:4628–4637.

91. Reeves JD, Lee FH, Miamidian JL, et al. Enfuvirtide resistance mutations: impact on human immunodeficiency virus envelope function, entry inhibitor sensitivity, and virus neutralization. J Virol 2005; 79:4991–4999.

92. Trachtenberg E, Korber B, Sollars C, et al. Advantage of rare HLA supertype in HIV disease progression. Nat Med 2003; 9:928–935.

93. Smith JS, Robinson NJ. Age-specific prevalence of infection with herpes simplex virus types 2 and 1: a global review. J Infect Dis 2002; 186 (Suppl):3–28.

94. Barbour JD, Hecht FM, Wrin T, et al. Higher CD4+ T-cell counts associated with low viral pol replication capacity among treatment-naive adults in early HIV-1 infection. J Infect Dis 2004; 190:251–256.

CHAPTER 16

Pharmacology of Antiretroviral Drugs

Concepta Merry
Charles W. Flexner

Introduction

There may be no discipline in modern medicine in which clinical pharmacology is more relevant than in the care of the HIV-infected patient. Many patients currently take at least three antiretroviral (ARV) drugs, medications for the prophylaxis and treatment of opportunistic infections, and often a variety of medications for supportive care of pain, depression, and other concomitant illnesses. Selecting appropriate medications and constructing an effective ARV regimen can be difficult in this era of polypharmacy. In addition to contending with drug resistance, the clinician is faced with food effects, proper spacing of medications, drug-drug interactions, overlapping toxicities, and patient adherence with the regimen.

It is essential to ensure optimal dosing for patients, as high drug concentrations may be associated with more frequent adverse effects and low drug concentrations may be associated with the development of treatment failure.[1,2] Sub-therapeutic drug concentrations can promote the emergence of resistant forms HIV, and thus result in treatment failure.[3] Development of resistance compromises the response of the patient to future therapeutic interventions and may result in the transmission of resistant virus, which is more expensive and difficult to treat.

The main role of clinical pharmacology is to describe, quantify and predict drug concentrations and response in order to design safe and effective regimens. The application of clinical pharmacology to HIV treatment is intended to optimize outcomes for individual patients and to prevent the emergence of drug-resistant virus.

Antiretroviral Drugs

There are currently four classes of drugs available for the treatment of HIV infection: the nucleoside and nucleotide reverse transcriptase inhibitors, the non-nucleoside reverse transcriptase inhibitors, the protease inhibitors and the fusion inhibitors.

1. Nucleoside (NRTI) and nucleotide (NtRTI) reverse transcriptase inhibitors
2. Non-nucleoside reverse transcriptase inhibitors (NNRTI)
3. Protease inhibitors (PI)
4. Fusion inhibitors (FI)

While there are 22 different licensed antiretroviral preparations (Table 16.1), in practice the patient can only benefit from a smaller number of drugs used in combination. For example:

- Zalcitabine (ddC) is rarely prescribed because of toxicity and inconvenience[4]
- Fosamprenavir is a prodrug of amprenavir[4]
- Ritonavir is a potent protease inhibitor with intrinsic antiretroviral activity. It is poorly tolerated and is now prescribed mainly to boost the concentrations of other protease inhibitors

- Resistance to any single ARV may confer cross-resistance to other drugs in the same class, e.g. patients who develop resistance to nevirapine are also resistant to efavirenz.[5]

Principles of Clinical Pharmacology Relevant to the Optimal Prescribing of ARVs

In the following section, the principles of clinical pharmacology relevant to the optimal prescribing of ARV therapy in every day clinical practice are described. The practical application of pharmacological principles is summarized as Treatment Guidelines in the text below.

Pharmacokinetic definitions

Figure 16.1 summarizes the key pharmacokinetic parameters which characterize orally administered drugs. There are limited data on the correlation between different pharmacokinetic parameters and clinical outcome for HIV-infected patients.

- Trough concentration: the concentration of drug in the blood immediately before the next dose is administered, although this does not necessarily represent the lowest concentration during a dosing interval.
- Minimum concentration (C_{min}): the lowest concentration of drug in the blood following the administered dose. The lowest drug concentration frequently occurs immediately before the next dose is administered; for these drugs, the minimum concentration and the trough concentration are identical. However, some drugs such as nelfinavir (NFV) have delayed absorption and the drug concentration falls even lower following the administered dose until the next dose is absorbed. Low minimum drug concentrations may be associated with increased risk of virologic failure for some ARVs.[1] Low minimum drug concentrations may also occur due to drug-drug interactions or non-adherence.
- Peak concentration (C_{max}): the maximum concentration of drug measured in the blood following the administered dose. High peak concentrations correlate with drug toxicity for indinavir and possibly ritonavir.[6]

Table 16.1 Licensed antiretroviral drugs

NRTI and NtRTI[a]	NNRTI[a]	PI[a]	FI[a]
AZT	EFV	SQV	T-20
d4T	NVP	RTV	
3TC	DLV	IDV	
ddC		APV	
ddl		Fos-APV	
FTC		ATV	
ABC		NFV	
TDF		TPV	
		LPV/rtv	
		DRV	

[a]NRTI, nucleoside reverse transcriptase inhibitor; NtRTI, nucleotide reverse transcriptase inhibitor; NNRTI, non-nucleoside reverse transcriptase inhibitor; PI, protease inhibitor; FI, fusion inhibitor; AZT, zidovudine; EFV, efavirenz; SQV, saquinavir; T-20, enfuvirtide; d4T, stavudine; NVP, nevirapine; RTV, ritonavir; 3TC, lamivudine; DLV, delavirdine; IDV, indinavir; ddC, dideoxycytidine; APV, amprenavir; ddl, didanosine; Fos-APV, fosamprenavir; FTC, emtricitabine; ATV, atazanavir; ABC, abacavir; NFV, nelfinavir; TDF, tenofovir; TPV, tipranavir; LPV/rtv, lopinavir/ritonavir coformulation; DRV, darunavir.

Figure 16.1 A summary of the key pharmacokinetic parameters which characterize orally administered drugs.

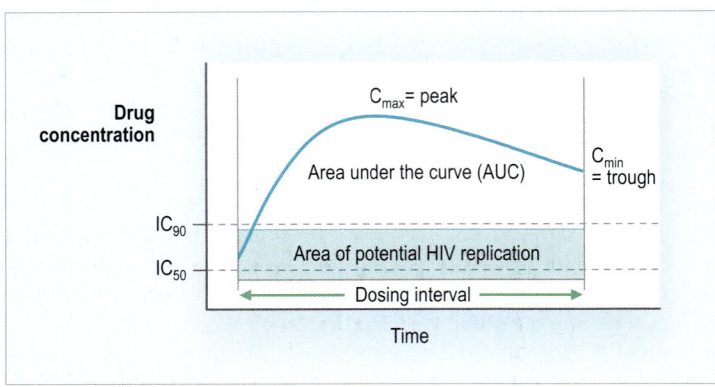

- Half-life ($T_{1/2}$): the length of time it takes for the concentration of drug in the plasma to fall by 50%. This is important clinically, as different constituents of a triple drug regimen may have different half-lives. Therefore, if the clinician stops all drugs at the same time, the drug with the shortest half-life is eliminated first, followed by the drug with the second shortest half-life, followed by the drug with the longest half-life. This exposes the patient's virus sequentially to triple therapy, dual therapy, and ultimately monotherapy. Drugs such as efavirenz and nevirapine have long half-lives and may pose a significant risk for the development of resistance under these circumstances. Therefore it is prudent to stop the individual components of a triple regimen at different times depending on the respective half-lives of the constituent drugs: e.g. a patient receiving a combination of d4T plus 3TC plus nevirapine should stop the nevirapine on day 1 and continue the d4T plus 3TC for at least 2 weeks to provide effective triple therapy as the nevirapine is eliminated from the body. The optimal interval between stopping NNRTIs and the other antiretroviral drugs in the regimen is not known. This is further complicated by the fact that certain ethnic groups, such as African-Americans, have an increased prevalence of genetic polymorphisms that result in a slower rate of clearance of NNRTIs such as efavirenz.[7] This raises logistical issues in Africa, where many patients receive a generically manufactured fixed dose combination of d4T plus 3TC plus nevirapine (Triommune®). For such patients, it may be preferable to stop the Triommune and continue the patient for 1 week on either a fixed dose dual combination of d4T plus 3TC or individually manufactured d4T plus 3TC. However, this approach is often unpopular with patients, as prescribing the individual component drugs increases the drug acquisition costs.

Guideline 1: Avoid Accidental Exposure to Functional Monotherapy when Stopping ARVs

- Area under the curve (AUC): measure of the total net exposure of a patient to a drug over the dosing interval, usually based on plasma concentrations
- Steady-state: point at which the input mass of drug is equivalent to the mass eliminated

from the body by clearance during any unit of time. For a drug administered every half-life, this takes approximately five half-lives to achieve.

Intracellular Phosphorylation

The NRTI's are prodrugs which are converted by host cellular enzymes in the cytoplasm to an active triphosphate. Occasionally, there may be competition for intracellular phosphorylation pathways by similar NRTI's; this can result in clinically relevant drug interactions. For example, zidovudine (azidothymidine; AZT) has been shown to impair the intracellular phosphorylation of stavudine (d4T) in vitro; when these two drugs were combined in clinical trials, this combination was associated with unfavorable outcomes as compared to using either drug without the other, or with other regimens containing two NRTIs.[8]

Guideline 2: Avoid Prescribing d4T with AZT

Tenofovir is also a prodrug which is converted intracellularly to the active diphosphate. Since tenofovir starts with a single phosphate group, the diphosphate of this drug is analogous to an NRTI triphosphate. Purine nucleoside phosphorylase (PNP) is an enzyme responsible in part for the catabolic metabolism of ddI. The activity of PNP is inhibited by tenofovir and tenofovir monophosphate, resulting in increased plasma concentrations of ddI.[9] Use of a reduced dose of enteric coated ddI (250 mg/day), with or without food, produces plasma ddI concentrations similar to that achieved with standard ddI dosing of 400 mg/day in the absence of tenofovir.[10] Since ddI is the only ARV known to be cleared by the PNP pathway, it is unlikely that other drug interactions will occur through this mechanism.

Guideline 3: Reduce Dose of ddI to 250 mg Daily if Co-prescribed with Tenofovir, or Avoid this Combination Altogether

Emtricitabine (FTC) is an analog of 3TC, and therefore these drugs should not be co-prescribed.[4]

Guideline 4: Avoid Prescribing 3TC with FTC

The combination of d4T with ddI is also no longer recommended as it is associated with unacceptably high levels of clinical toxicity, especially peripheral neuropathy and pancreatitis.[4]

Guideline 5: Avoid Prescribing d4T with ddI

Drug Transport Proteins

In addition to metabolism, which refers to chemical biotransformation usually mediated by enzymes in the liver, many drugs are subject to cellular influx or efflux mediated by drug transport proteins. The best known of these, P-glycoprotein (P-gp), is the product of the *mdr1* (multidrug resistance) gene first described as producing broad cross-resistance to certain kinds of cancer chemotherapy. P-gp is expressed in epithelial cells lining the intestinal mucosa, contributing to efflux of drugs back into the intestinal lumen.[11] P-gp therefore contributes to the low bioavailability of certain drugs, for example some HIV protease inhibitors. P-gp is also present in cells making up the blood-brain barrier, and can limit central nervous system penetration of drugs via efflux back into the systemic circulation. Several HIV protease inhibitors are substrates for and inhibitors of P-gp. Protease inhibitor concentrations in the CNS could be increased by inhibiting P-gp mediated efflux.[12] However, high-level expression of P-gp also inhibits HIV replication in vitro. Cells expressing P-gp produce up to 70-fold less HIV than control cells, which is thought to reflect inhibition of HIV entry and/or membrane fusion.[13] Although increased expression of P-gp may lead to decreased intracellular ARV concentrations, P-gp expression may make these same cell less susceptible to HIV infection by interfering with virus entry into the cells, thus counterbalancing low drug concentrations.

Cytochrome P450 Enzymes

Cytochrome P-450 (CYP) enzymes are ubiquitous in higher vertebrates and are the major protective mechanism for chemical detoxification of xenobiotics, including drugs. This system consists of more than 12 families of enzymes common to all mammals.[14] In humans, the CYP1, CYP2, and CYP3 families are primarily responsible for drug metabolism, with the CYP3A subfamily accounting for metabolism of the largest number of drugs, including most HIV protease inhibitors and NNRTIs. CYP450-mediated drug metabolism largely takes place in the liver, although CYP enzymes are also present in other sites, including the intestinal wall. Intestinal drug metabolism contributes to the first-pass metabolism of many orally administered drugs, including saquinavir. Drugs may interact with CYP450 enzymes in one of three ways: (1) as a substrate, (2) as an inducer, and/or (3) as an inhibitor. Inhibitors of CYP3A4 can reduce drug metabolism in the intestinal tract and slow hepatic clearance, thus increasing systemic concentrations. Inducers of CYP metabolism accelerate clearance and decrease absorption and/or systemic concentrations.

Enzyme Inhibition and Boosted Protease Inhibitor Therapy

Inhibitors of CYP-mediated biotransformation can be used to decrease the rate of hepatic clearance and increase concentrations of drugs subject to metabolism by the same pathway. HIV protease inhibitors can be CYP inducers, inhibitors and substrates. As a consequence, these drugs can increase the concentrations of co-administered metabolized drugs, and are subject to having their own concentrations increased by other CYP inhibitors. Most of the currently approved HIV protease inhibitors are metabolized primarily by CYP3A4. The number and magnitude of potential drug interactions associated with these agents varies widely as a function of the relative potency of enzyme inhibiton and induction.

Saquinavir was the first protease inhibitor licensed for use in HIV-infection in the U.S. The original formulation of this drug, a hard gel capsule, had low oral bioavailability. Ritonavir, the second HIV protease inhibitor licensed for use in the U.S., was poorly tolerated at the initially recommended dose of 600 mg twice daily, producing frequent nausea and vomiting. Ritonavir is a very potent inhibitor of CYP3A4, and as a result combined administration of saquinavir and ritonavir produced a mean 20-fold increase in steady-state saquinavir concentrations. Ritonavir affects saquinavir concentrations in two ways: first, by improving oral bioavailability through inhibition of intestinal CYP3A4 and possibly P-gp, and second, by inhibiting hepatic CYP 3A4 and thus decreasing systemic clearance.[15]

Fortunately, ritonavir is much better tolerated at lower doses, which retain most of the CYP 3A4 inhibition of higher dose ritonavir. Today, ritonavir is used mainly as a pharmacokinetic booster of other HIV protease inhibitors, and not for its own intrinsic antiretroviral properties.

Guideline 6: Low Doses of Ritonavir are Used as a Pharmacokinetic Booster to Raise the Concentrations of Other HIV Protease Inhibitors, and Not for the Intrinsic Antiviral Properties of the Drug Itself

Combining a low doses of ritonavir with most available HIV protease inhibitors improves the concentrations of the active PI, and may also allow a reduced dosing and dosing frequency of the co-administered drug.

Kaletra® is a fixed-dose combination of the protease inhibitor lopinavir with a low dose of ritonavir 400/100 mg twice daily, abbreviated LPV/r. [It is customary to use a lower case 'r' when abbreviating The low doses of ritonavir used as a PK enhancer, e.g. ritonavir boosted saquinavir would be written SQV/r 1000/200 mg twice daily.] For dosing recommendations for ritonavir-boosted PI regimens, please consult the web sites recommended at the end of this chapter.

The current formulation of ritonavir is heat labile and thus requires refrigeration. This makes the use of this drug in resource limited settings difficult, especially for migrant groups and in countries with an unpredictable power supply. There have been reports of suboptimal ritonavir concentrations as a result of improperly refrigerated medication.[16,17] A new heat stable formulation of ritonavir is in development, but has not yet been approved.

Guideline 7: The Current Formulation of Ritonavir is Heat Labile and Requires Refrigeration

Amprenavir, nelfinavir, and indinavir are less potent inhibitors of CYP3A4 than ritonavir. All of these drugs increase the mean rifabutin AUC approximately 2-fold, but can be coadministered if the rifabutin dose is decreased by 50%.[4,18] On the other hand, ritonavir increases the rifabutin AUC 4-fold; coadminstration of these drugs has been associated with clinically significant adverse effects including an increased incidence of uveitis.[19] In contrast, the clarithromycin AUC is increased by 77% with ritonavir and 53% with indinavir. Because clarithropmycin has a broada therapeutic index, no dosage adjustment is recommended for patients with normal renal function.[4,18] Azithromycin is primarily excreted by the biliary route and does not interact with inhibitors of CYP3A.[20] HIV patients who are taking protease inhibitors but require MAC prophylaxis may take azithromycin or clarithromycin instead of rifabutin.[4,18] Patients who have failed multiple prior ARV regimens may be treated with a combination of two different protease inhibitors plus ritonavir in order to take advantage of the lack of cross-resistance between certain PI's, and the chance to treat with two active agents instead of one. So-called double-boosted or dual-boosted PI regimens utilize ritonavir to increase the concentrations of two ARV drugs at the same time The pharmacokinetics of such regimens may be complex and difficult to predict, since there is the potential for both PI's to interact with ritonavir and with each other. For current recommendations on dosing of double-boosted protease inhibitor regimens, please see the websites recommended at the end of this chapter.[4,21,22]

Metabolic Enzyme Induction

Enzyme induction refers to an increase in the rate of hepatic metabolism, mediated by increased transcription of mRNA encoding the genes for drug metabolizing enzymes. This leads to a decrease in the concentrations of drugs metabolized by the same enzyme. Rifampin and rifabutin are classic examples of enzyme inducers. Both drugs can cause decreases in plasma concentrations of many concomitant medications including protease inhibitors. The Centers for Disease Control and Prevention (CDC) have issued guidelines for concomitant use of rifampin or rifabutin with HIV protease inhibitors in patients requiring treatment for tuberculosis.[18] Rifampin should be avoided with all single HIV protease inhibitors and is contraindicated in patients receiving twice daily saquinavir plus ritonavir due to high rates of hepatotoxicity.[23]

Guideline 8: Rifampin is Contraindicated in Patients Receiving Twice-daily Ritonavir-boosted Saquinavir Therapy

Rifabutin can be given with indinavir or nelfinavir, but only if the rifabutin dose is reduced and the PI dose is modestly increased.[18]

Nevirapine is a mild to moderate hepatic enzyme Inducer. This NNRTI decreases the AUC of saquinavir and indinavir by 27% and 28%, respectively, but has a minimal effect on ritonavir and nelfinavir.[24,25] Efavirenz is both a P450 inducer and inhibitor. This NNRTI decreases concentrations of amprenavir, saquinavir, and indinavir, and can only be combined with these drugs by increasing their dose, or by adding ritonavir as a PK enhancer.[26]

In addition to being inhibitors of CYP3A4, ritonavir and nelfinavir are moderate hepatic enzyme inducers. They can increase so-called Phase 2 enzymes such as hepatic glucuronosyl transferase, as well as CYP activity. Both PI's decrease the AUC of the oral contraceptive ethinyl estradiol by about 40%. Patients taking ritonavir or nelfinavir must use alternative forms of birth control.[27] It is important to keep in mind that the doses of many concomitant medications will need to be adjusted when starting an enzyme inhibitor and/or inducer like ritonavir or nelfinavir. However, if the enzyme inhibitor or inducer is discontinued, drug doses will need to return to baseline levels.

Some drugs that are inhibitors or substrates for CYP3A4 also inhibit drug transporters like P-glycoprotein. Because the tissue distribution and substrate specificity of CYP3A4 and P-glycoprotein overlap substantially, the relative contribution of each to pharmacokinetic drug-drug interactions is often difficult to quantify.[14] The precise effect of these two pathways on ARV pharmacokinetics remains to be determined in most cases.

Drug–Food Interactions

A number of environmental influences, besides concomitant medications, can influence pharmacokinetics. An especially important influence is food. Food can either increase or decrease the bioavailability of several drugs commonly used in HIV-infected patients. Furthermore. drug-food interactions may require a modification of the scheduling of administration of drugs during the day, and this can have a major effect on the quality of life of patients. Didanosine tablets and sachets are formulated with a buffer that requires administration on an empty stomach because a low gastric pH leads to degradation of the drug.[28] Although not buffered, didanosine enteric coated capsules must also be given on an empty stomach because administration with food decreases bioavailability. Fortunately, the bioavailability of most other NRTI's is not significantly altered by food.[29]

Specific food restrictions of ARV's are summarized in Table 16.2. This information must be incorporated into the counseling required for patients starting or modifying many ARV regimens. This can be particularly difficult for patients in the resource-limited setting, who may only have one meal per day, or for patients who observe religious periods of fasting. Such local factors must be considered by programs which aim to expand access to ARV therapy in resource limited settings such as Sub-Saharan Africa.

Guideline 9: Consider Drugs that do not have Food Restrictions for Patient Populations in Resource-limited Settings

Traditional Medicines

Herbal remedies and nutritional supplements are widely used in HIV-infected patients, although the

Table 16.2 Recommendations for food restrictions for approved antiretrovirals

Take with food	Take on empty stomach	Avoid taking with high fat meals
TDF	IDV[a]	EFV
SQV	ddI	APV
RTV		
NFV		
LPV/rtv		
ATV		

[a]IDV can also be taken with a light, low-fat snack.

potential pharmacokinetic effects of these compounds are often ignored. Some herbal therapies contain ingredients capable of CYP inhibition or induction and have been implicated in drug interactions. For example, St John's wort contains a potent inducer of CYP 3A4, and decreases the AUC of indinavir by over 50%.[30] There is also evidence that St John's wort decreases nevirapine concentrations by a similar magnitude.[31] The mechanism of this interaction appears to involve both induction of CYP3A4 and P-glycoprotein.[32] Patients taking HIV protease inhibitors and non-nucleoside reverse transcriptase inhibitors should be instructed to avoid St John's wort or any dietary supplement containing this herb.

Some nutritional supplements may also contain ingredients capable of affecting the concentrations of co-admninistered ARV's. Raw garlic inhibits the activity of CYP3A4 in vitro and in animals.[33] One study conducted in healthy volunteers found that garlic capsules taken b.i.d. for 3 weeks led to a mean decrease in the saquinavir AUC of approximately 50%, probably as a consequence of reduced bioavailability.[34] Other herbs with reported in vitro effects on CYP450- mediated metabolism include silymarin (milk thistle), ginseng, and skullcap, although clinical pharmacokinetic interaction data with these agents are contradictory or lacking.[35] Traditional and herbal medicines need to be added to the list of agents capable of causing significant drug interactions. Clinicians need to record information about use of these agents when taking medical histories, and consider them when adverse events or treatment failure appear with no other identifiable cause.

This is particularly important in the resource limited setting, where the majority of patients consult traditional healers in preference to medical doctors. It is important to include traditional healers in efforts

Table 16.3 Antiretroviral drugs whose clearance is altered in patients with renal or hepatic insufficiency

Renal insufficiency	Hepatic insufficiency
ddI	ABC
FTC	APV
3TC	ATV
NVP	Fos-APV
D4T	IND
TDF	NVP
ddI	RTV

to expand access to ARV in the resource limited setting, as they are key opinion leaders in the communities and have a significant impact on the health belief model for patients. Furthermore, the metabolism of many components of the traditional herbal medicines may be inhibited by drugs such as ritonavir. It is possible therefore, that western medicines may be responsible for reduced clearance and heretofore unseen side effects of traditional medicines.

Renal and Hepatic Impairment

Since the majority of drugs are eliminated by renal or hepatic clearance, diseases altering the function of these organs can effect the concentrations of drugs. Table 16 3 lists ARVs for which the prescribing information recommends dose modification in the setting of renal or hepatic impairment. It is important to continuously monitor patients and adjust the drug doses accordingly to any identified changes in renal and hepatic function.

In particular, patients with HIV-related renal dysfunction may have marked improvements in renal function once started on effective ARV therapy. For further guidelines on dosing, please consult websites at the end of this chapter.[4,21,22]

Low Weight Individuals

There are limited data on the optimal dosing of antiretrovirals in low weight adults. This is particularly important in malnourished patients with advanced HIV disease in Africa, who may have a low body mass index, and also in many Asian patients who naturally tend to have lower body weights. It is currently recommended that the doses of d4T and ddI be reduced in patients who weigh <60 kg.[29,36] It is

unclear if the dose of ddI should be reduced to 200 mg/day in patients weighing <60 kg who are also receiving tenofovir, and it may be prudent to avoid this combination in such patients. It is important to continuously monitor weight, as patients who have been very ill may gain significant weight once they respond to ARV therapy.

Guideline 10: Continuously Monitor the Need for Dose Modification in Patients with Hepatic or Renal Impairment or Low Body Weight

Pediatrics

Growth and development may result in rapid changes in the activity of some drug metabolizing enzymes. In addition, changes in body surface area and liver blood flow can alter the elimination of metabolized drugs. Other developmental changes that can effect drug concentrations include changes in gastric function, intestinal motility, percentage body fat, concentrations of plasma proteins and renal function.

Guideline 11: Doses of Drugs Need to be Frequently Monitored in Children or Adolescents

Unfortunately, there are limited data on the dosing of some ARVs in children. Generation of such data is essential to ensure the safe and effective rollout of ARVs in children in the resource limited setting. Unlike the developed world, children represent a significant proportion of HIV-infected individuals in the developing world. More rational pediatric dosing recommendations are not sufficient. There is an urgent need to develop pediatric formulations of more ARVs. For example, it is a common practice in Africa for mothers to crush a fixed dose combination of Triommune® with a coconut or stone and to guess as to the correct proportion of the pill to give the child.

Pregnancy

ARVs are administered during pregnancy both to treat the mother and to reduce the risk of mother-to-child transmission of HIV disease. Avoiding teratogenic drugs like efavirenz during pregnancy is an obvious concern. In addition, the concentrations of some medications may be altered during pregnancy. Available data suggest that the concentrations of saquinavir, nelfinavir and indinavir, measured at various time points during pregnancy, are on average lower than those in the non-pregnant woman.[37,38] The mechanism for the difference in pharmacokinetic profiles during pregnancy is multifactorial. Possible contributors include induction of hepatic drug metabolizing enzymes, changes in gastrointestinal transit times, increases in body water and fat, and changes in expression of drug transporters such as P-gp.[38]

Guideline 12: Efavirenz is Associated with a Possible Risk of Teratogenicity and is Not Recommended for Women of Child Bearing Years who Wish to get Pregnant. This Drug Should be Avoided During Pregnancy[39]

A single dose of nevirapine given to the mother and newborn has been shown to reduce transmission of HIV infection from 45% to 16%.[40] Such an approach is inexpensive and practical in the resource limited setting, where the majority of women deliver out of hospital. However, a single dose of nevirapine has a longer half-life (>2 days) than steady-state nevirapine, as it has not had ample time to induce its own metabolism. Lingering drug concentrations may thus select for resistant virus. One recent study suggested that exposure to single-dose nevirapine at delivery may increase the risk of failing subsequent nevirapine treatment because of drug resistance.[41]

Guideline 13: It is Recommended that Patients who Receive Single Dose Nevirapine to Prevent Mother-to-Child Transmission should also Receive a Short Course of Two Other Drugs such as AZT Plus 3TC, to Prevent Prolonged Exposure to Nevirapine Monotherapy[41]

The optimal duration of the additional drugs has not been determined, but a recent study suggests a minimum of 2 weeks to prevent the emergence of resistance.[42]

In nevirapine-naive pregnant women with CD4 cell counts of >250 cells/mm³, it is not recommended to initiate a nevirapine containing regimen, as this has been associated with significant and sometimes fatal hepatotoxicity.[4]

Guideline 14: Nevirapine is Not Recommended for Nevirapine-naive Pregnant Women[4] with a CD4 Cell Count of >250 cells/mm³

Ethnic variations in pharmacokinetics

The influence of genetic factors on drug metabolism and drug concentrations is an important area of clinical research, particularly as ARVs are being initiated in different geographic regions. The field of pharmacogenetics identifies specific genetic traits that might explain interindividual differences in drug concentrations. Emerging data suggest differences in drug concentrations of ARVs in certain ethnic groups.[7] For example, Africans and other ethnic groups may have reduced clearance of nevirapine and prolonged exposure after a single dose given to prevent mother-to-child transmission of HIV.[42]

Conclusion

Clinical pharmacology is an integral part of the management of patients with HIV infection. The availability of ARVs in the resource limited setting raises new logistical and prescribing issues which need to be addressed in order to ensure optimal outcomes for patients in diverse regions.

References

1. Burger D, Hugen P, Reiss P, et al. ATHENA Cohort Study Group. Therapeutic drug monitoring of nelfinavir and indinavir in treatment-naive HIV-1-infected individuals. AIDS 2003; 17:1157–1165.
2. Li RC, Zhu M, Schentag JJ. Achieving an optimal outcome in the treatment of infections. The role of clinical pharmacokinetics and pharmacodynamics of antimicrobials. Clin Pharm 1999; 37:1–16.
3. Molla A, Korneyeva M, Gao Q, et al. Ordered accumulation of mutations in HIV protease confers resistance to ritonavir. Nat Med 1996; 2:760–766.
4. NIH. Online. Available: www.aidsinfo.nih.gov/guidelines.
5. Antinori A, Zaccarelli M, Cingolani A, et al. Crossresistance among nonnucleoside reverse transcriptase inhibitors limits recycling efavirenz after nevirapine failure. AIDS Res Hum Retroviruses 2002; 18:835–838.
6. Gatti G, Di Biagio A, Casazza R, et al. The relationship between ritonavir plasma levels and side-effects: implications for therapeutic drug monitoring. AIDS 1999; 13:2083–2089.
7. Ribaudo H, Clifford D, Gulick R. Relationship between efavirenz pharmacokinetics, side effects, drug discontinuation, virological response and race. Results from ACTG A5095 A5097. 11th Conference on Retroviruses and Opportunistic Infections, San Francisco, CA: 8–11 February 2004.
8. Hoggard PG, Kewn S, Barry MG, et al. Effects of drugs on 2′,3′-dideoxy-2′,3′-didehydrothymidine phosphorylation in vitro. Antimicrob Agents Chemother 1997; 41:1231–1236.
9. Ray A, Oslon L, Fridland A. Mechanism of the drug interactions between 2′,3′-dideoxyinosine and allopurinol, ganciclovir or tenofovir. 5th International Workshop on Clinical Pharmacology of HIV Therapy, Italy: 2004.
10. Kearney BP, Isaacson E, Sayre J, et al. Didanosine and tenofovir DF drug-drug interaction: assessment of didanosine dose reduction. 10th Conference on Retroviruses and Opportunistic Infections, Boston, MA: 10–14 February 2003; Abstract 533.

11. Fojo AT, Ueda K, Slamon DJ, et al. Expression of multidrug resistance gene in human tumors and tissues. Proc Natl Acad Sci USA 1987; 84:265–269.

12. Khaliq Y, Gallicano K, Venance S, et al. Effect of ketoconazole on ritonavir and saquinavir concentrations in plasma and cerebrospinal fl uid from patients infected with human immunodefi ciency virus. Clin Pharmacol Ther 2000; 68:637–646.

13. Flexner C, Speck RR. Role of multidrug transporters in HIV pathogenesis. 8th Conference on Retroviruses and Opportunistic Infections, Chicago, IL: February 2001.

14. Benet LZ, Kroetz DL, Sheiner LB. Pharmacokinetics: dynamics of drug absorption, distribution, and elimination. In: Hardman JG, Limbird LE, eds. The pharmacological basis of therapeutics. 9th edn. New York: McGraw-Hill; 1996.

15. Drewe J, Gutmann H, Fricker G, et al. HIV protease inhibitor ritonavir: a more potent inhibitor of P-glycoprotein than the cyclosporine analog SDZ PSC 833. Biochem Pharmacol 1999; 57:1147–1152.

16. Penzak SR, Acosta EP, Turner M, et al. Antiretroviral drug content in products from developing countries. Clin Infect Dis 2004; 38:1317–1319.

17. Coakley P, Merry C, Kityo C, et al. The pharmacokinetics of saquinavir plus ritonavir in Ugandan patients receiving ritonavir boosted saquinavir hard gel and soft gel. 7th International Congress on Drug Treatment in HIV Infection, Glasgow: 2004.

18. Centers for Disease Control and Prevention. Clinical update: impact on HIV protease inhibitors on the treatment of HIV-infected tuberculosis patients with rifampin. MMWR 2000; 49:185–189.

19. Cato A, Cavanaugh JH, Shi H, et al. Assessment of multiple doses of ritonavir on the pharmacokinetics of rifabutin. XIth International Conference on AIDS, Vancouver, BC: 7–12 July 1996; Abstract MoB174.

20. Honig PK, Wortham DC, Zamani K, et al. Comparison of the effects of the macrolide antibiotics erythromycin, clarithromycin, and azithromycin on terfenadine steadystate pharmacokinetics and electrocardiographic parameters. Drug Invest 1994; 7:148.

21. Online. Available: www.hivpharmacology.com

22. Online. Available: www.hiv-druginteractions.org

23. Grange S, Schutz M, Schmitt C, et al. Unexpected hepatotoxicity observed in a healthy volunteer study on the effects of multiple doses of ritonavir-boosted saquinavir and vice Ch016-X2882.indd 178 11/17/2006 3:19:09 PM versa. 6th International Workshop on Clinical Pharmacology of HIV therapy, Québec: 28–30 April 2005.

24. Murphy R, Gagnier P, Lamson M, et al. Effect of nevirapine on pharmacokinetics of indinavir and ritonavir in HIV-1 patients. 4th Conference on Retroviruses and Opportunistic Infections, Washington, DC: 22–26 January 1997; Westover Management Group.

25. Sahai J, Cameron W, Salgo M, et al. Drug interaction between saquinavir and nevirapine. 4th Conference on Retroviruses and Opportunistic Infections, Washington, DC: 22–26 January 1997; Westover Management Group.

26. Barry M, Mulcahy F, Merry C. Pharmacokinetics and potential interactions amongst antiretroviral agents used to treat patients with HIV infection. Clin Pharm 1999; 36:289–304.

27. Ouellet D, Hsu A, Qian J, et al. Effect of ritonavir on the pharmacokinetics of ethinyl estradiol in healthy female volunteers. XIth International Conference on AIDS, Vancouver, BC: 7–12 July 1996.

28. Knupp CA, Milbrath R, Barbhaiya RH. Effect of time of food administration on the bioavailability of didanosine from a chewable tablet formulation. J Clin Pharmacol 1993; 33:568.

29. Videx EC. (Didanosine) product monograph. Princeton, NJ: Bristol Myers-Squibb; 2001. 30. Piscitelli SC, Burstein AH, Chaitt D, et al. St. John's wort and indinavir concentrations. Lancet 2000; 355:547–548.

31. Maat MMR de, Hoetelmans RMW, Mathot RAA, et al. Drug Interaction between St. John's wort and nevirapine. AIDS 2001; 15:420–421.

32. Roby CA, Anderson GD, Kantor E, et al. St. John's Wort: effect on CYP3A4 activity. Clin Pharmacol Ther 2000; 67:451–457.

33. Laroche M, Choudhri S, Gallicano K, Foster B. Severe gastrointestinal toxicity with concomitant ingestion of ritonavir and garlic. Can J Infect Dis 1998; 9 (Suppl A):471.

34. Piscitelli SC, Burstein AH, Welden N, et al. The effect of garlic supplements on the pharmacokinetics of saquinavir. Clin Infect Dis 2002; 34:234–238.

35. Lee LS, Andrade ASA, Flexner C. Natural health product-antiretroviral drug interactions: pharmacokinetic and pharmacodynamic effects. Clin Infect Dis 2006; 43:1052–1059.

36. Zerit→(Stavudine) product monograph. Princeton, NJ: Bristol Myers-Squibb; 2002.

37. van Heeswijk RP, Khaliq Y, Gallicano KD, et al. The pharmacokinetics of nelfi navir and M8 during pregnancy and post partum. Clin Pharmacol Ther 2004; 76:588–597.

38. Kosel BW, Beckerman KP, Hayashi S, et al. Pharmacokinetics of nelfi navir and indinavir in HIV-1-infected pregnant women. AIDS 2003; 17:1195–1199.

39. Fundaro C, Genovese O, Rendeli C, et al. Myelomeningocele in a child with intrauterine exposure to efavirenz. AIDS 2002; 16:299–300. [Erratum in: AIDS 2002; 16:1443.]

40. Lallemant M, Jourdain G, Le Coeur S, et al. Perinatal HIV prevention trial (Thailand) investigators. Single-dose perinatal nevirapine plus standard zidovudine to prevent mother-to-child transmission of HIV-1 in Thailand. N Engl J Med 2004; 351:217–228.

41. Lockman S, Shapiro RL, Smeaton LM, Wester C, Thior I, Stevens L, Chand F, Makhema J, Moffat C, Asmelash A, Ndase P, Arimi P, van Widenfelt E, Mazhani L, Novitsky V, Lagakos S, Essex M. Response to antiretroviral therapy after a single, peripartum dose of nevirapine. N Engl J Med. 2007; 356:135-47.

42. Cressey TR, Jourdain G, Lallemant MJ, et al. Persistence of nevirapine exposure during the postpartum period after intrapartum single-dose nevirapine in addition to zidovudine prophylaxis for the prevention of mother-to-child transmission of HIV-1. J Acquir Immune Defic Syndr 2005; 38:283–288.

CHAPTER 17

Complications Resulting from Antiretroviral Therapy for HIV Infection

David Nolan
Simon Mallal
Peter Reiss

Introduction

The treatment of HIV infection has passed through a number of distinct phases over the almost 25-year history of the HIV/AIDS pandemic, accompanied by significant shifts in both patients' and clinicians' perceptions of antiretroviral drug toxicity. Prior to the introduction of 'highly active antiretroviral therapy' (HAART) regimens around 1996 – and even in the early years of the HAART era – any concerns regarding long-term drug toxicities were dramatically outweighed by the obvious short-term benefits and improved survival associated with these combination drug regimens. However, a number of recent developments have provided a more central role for antiretroviral drug toxicity in shaping HIV management. These include a recognition that adverse events associated with antiretroviral treatment are an important source of morbidity and even mortality, threatening to outweigh AIDS-related events in frequency and overall detrimental effects on quality of life even in advanced HIV disease[1]; and evidence that numerous HAART regimens provide equivalent effectiveness in the treatment of HIV infection, so that choice of therapy is often directed by the differential risk of drug toxicity associated with individual HIV drugs. The improved long-term prognosis of HIV disease has also focused attention on the potential for drug therapy to increase the risk of prevalent diseases (most notably cardiovascular disease) among those who have survived with HIV infection for many years. Finally, it is now apparent that certain long-term HIV drug toxicities provide an ongoing burden of disease that once established are difficult to reverse. In this context, there is an ongoing need not only to prevent these complications wherever possible, but also to develop effective treatment strategies for those affected by these complications of therapy for HIV.

Antiretroviral drug toxicities cover a broad spectrum, due in part to the large number of drugs used routinely for HIV treatment. These drug side-effects will be considered in turn, with an emphasis on clinical management based on an understanding of individual drug toxicity profiles. The influence of host and disease-related factors in determining the risk of these adverse effects will also be considered.

'Lipodystrophy Syndrome': Body Composition and Metabolic Complications

The 'lipodystrophy syndrome' represents a cluster of antiretroviral therapy complications first recognized among HAART recipients in 1998. The clinical syndrome incorporates lipoatrophy (pathological loss of subcutaneous fat), as well as metabolic complications including dyslipidemia and insulin resistance that may be accompanied by abdominal or localized fat accumulation (Fig. 17.1A–D). While defining lipodystrophy has been a perennial topic for debate

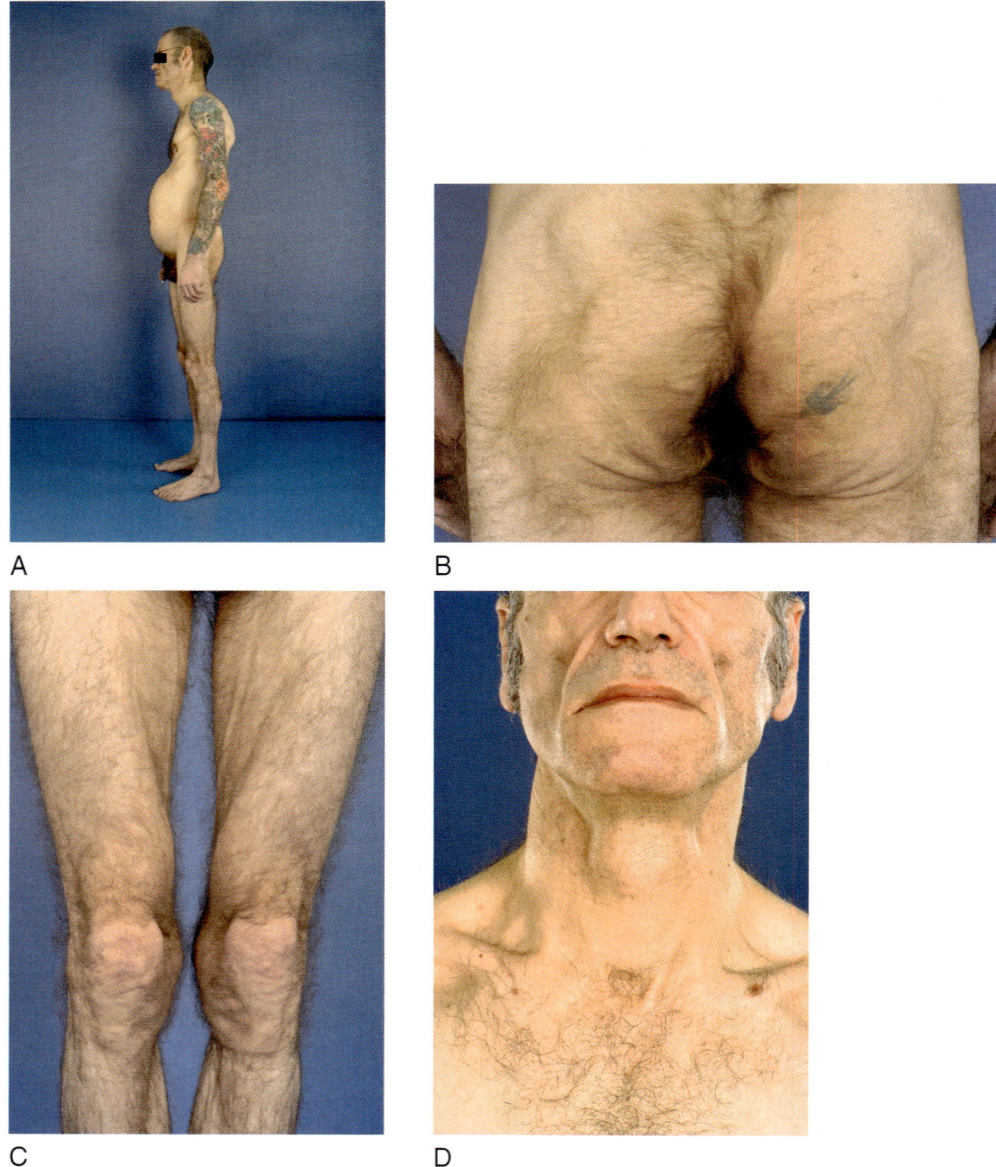

A B

C D

Figure 17.1 (A) Abnormal fat distribution with joint peripheral lipoatrophy and abdominal fat accumulation. (B) Subcutaneous fat atrophy of buttocks in the same patient. (C) Subcutaneous fat atrophy of the legs in the same patient. (D) Facial subcutaneous fat atrophy in the same patient.

among researchers in this field, examining the component features of the syndrome separately appears to represent the most pragmatic approach to clinical management. This is most apparent in the case of lipoatrophy, as this complication appears to be quite distinct from other lipodystrophy manifestations in terms of its risk factor profile.

Lipoatrophy: Dominant Contribution of NRTI Therapy

Lipoatrophy is extremely uncommon in the general community, and is therefore strongly and specifically linked to antiretroviral therapy.[2] The unusual nature of these body changes also makes lipoatrophy highly stigmatizing because of its rarity and its visual associations with illness.

Thymidine analog NRTI therapy alone is sufficient to cause lipoatrophy and is an independent risk factor for its occurrence in HAART-treated individuals. Clinical trials data have demonstrated that risk of clinically apparent lipoatrophy is approximately 40–50% among those treated with stavudine over 30 months, compared with 10–20% in zidovudine-treated individuals. Longitudinal studies have also demonstrated that body fat tends to remain stable or even increase in the first 6–12 months of therapy, and then to decline over the subsequent 12–24 months among patients receiving zidovudine or stavudine-based treatment. These studies also reveal that some degree of fat loss is common in patients receiving these drugs, so that lipoatrophy can be viewed as a pathological process of variable severity, rather than a phenomenon that can be readily defined as 'present' or 'absent.' In this context, the ability to recognize milder forms of lipoatrophy, and to assess the rate of fat loss in the critical period from 6–24 months after commencing treatment with stavudine or zidovudine, may allow for therapeutic intervention before fat loss becomes severe.

Alternative NRTI and nucleotide analog drugs such as abacavir, tenofovir and emtricitabine have not been associated with lipoatrophy in clinical studies. The specific associations between lipoatrophy and stavudine or zidovudine NRTI therapy have also been underlined by the demonstration that substituting abacavir or tenofovir in patients with clinically apparent lipoatrophy has been associated with statistically significant improvements in fat wasting.[3,4] Replacement of stavudine or zidovudine-containing therapy by complete NRTI and nucleotide-sparing, protease inhibitor-containing therapy including lopinavir/r plus an NNRTI (either efavirenz or nevirapine) has recently been demonstrated to likewise result in modest improvement in limb fat wasting. These particular regimens may however be associated with increases in plasma triglyceride and cholesterol and their virologic potency remains to be determined. However, increases in limb fat resulting from these switch strategies are often limited and not apparent to either clinicians or patients, so it would seem prudent to focus on prevention of lipoatrophy as fat restoration appears to be a slow and possibly incomplete process. In contrast, over 30 trials investigating HIV protease inhibitor discontinuation as a therapeutic strategy[5] have failed to demonstrate beneficial effects on reversing lipoatrophy, although metabolic abnormalities such as dyslipidemia and insulin resistance and occasionally intraabdominal visceral fat accumulation may improve.

The differential effects of NRTI therapy on lipoatrophy risk are associated with their different propensity to cause mitochondrial DNA depletion and mitochondrial toxicity specifically in adipocytes (fat-storing cells).[6] Accordingly, histopathology of subcutaneous adipose tissue from patients with lipoatrophy has revealed pronounced mitochondrial abnormalities, and increased adipocyte apoptosis that improves after discontinuing stavudine therapy in favor of abacavir,[7] but not after switching HIV protease inhibitor therapy.[8] Peripheral blood mitochondrial DNA content unfortunately does not appear to provide a clinically useful surrogate marker for mitochondrial toxicity in adipose tissue, so that assessing and monitoring disease progression continues to rely on DEXA scans or clinical assessment of body composition.

Choice of NRTI therapy is therefore the primary management decision that affects risk of lipoatrophy, irrespective of which additional drugs are also used in creating a HAART regimen (e.g. NNRTI or HIV protease inhibitor therapy). However, host factors are also important in determining the severity of lipoatrophy among patients receiving stavudine or zidovudine, with decreased risk of lipoatrophy among those aged <35–40 years, and among white vs non-white racial groups. With regard to the influence of HIV disease itself, low pre-treatment CD4+ T-cell count ($<100 \times 10^6$/L) is associated with increased risk of lipoatrophy while on treatment, irrespective of the virological or immunological response to therapy. This argues against recommending delayed introduction of HIV treatment due to concerns regarding drug toxicities.

Beyond the Prevention of Lipoatrophy: Therapeutic Options?

For those individuals affected by lipoatrophy, reversal of fat loss remains a slow process with gradual improvement measured over years. Removing stavudine and/or zidovudine treatment where possible represents a therapeutic strategy that can at least halt disease progression, but definitive treatments beyond that are limited at present. In the case of facial lipoatrophy, the dermal filler poly-L-lactic acid ('Newfill') has now been approved by the US Food and Drug Administration (FDA) for this indication, and has proved safe and effective over one year follow-up. The use of high-fat or high-energy diets to promote fat gain in patients with lipoatrophy cannot be supported, even after the causative NRTI drug has been removed. In this circumstance, the end-organ damage to subcutaneous adipose tissue depots means that this fat tissue is unable to effectively take-up dietary fat, thereby increasing the risk of unwanted side-effects such as visceral/abdominal fat accumulation and hypertriglyceridemia.

Dyslipidemia, Insulin Resistance and Cardiovascular Risk. Dynamic Effects of Environment, HIV Infection and Specific Antiretroviral Drugs

There is an increasing appreciation of the complexity that underlies associations between antiretroviral therapy and metabolic complications such as dyslipidemia and insulin resistance, although considering specific 'treatment phases' can help to clarify these issues. A central issue here is that many of the metabolic endpoints that are considered are common in the general population and are therefore subject to many genetic (non-modifiable) and environmental (potentially modifiable) effects that are not specific to HIV infection nor its treatment. This is not to downplay the important role that HIV drugs have in the pathogenesis of metabolic complications, but to place these effects in a broader clinically relevant context.

The 'Pre-treatment' Phase: Background Risk and the Influence of HIV Infection

The 'Metabolic Syndrome' incorporates lipid parameters (high triglyceride and low HDL-cholesterol values), abdominal obesity, and evidence of impaired glucose tolerance into a clinical entity that is present in more than 30% of adults (both male and female) in population studies.[9] This metabolic phenotype has a striking resemblance to the metabolic complications that have been incorporated into the 'lipodystrophy syndrome.' Both are characterized by the presence of high levels of triglyceride-enriched lipoproteins, which manifests as an atherogenic lipid profile including high triglyceride, high apolipoprotein CIII, B and E and elevated 'non-HDL' cholesterol levels.[10,11] Importantly, this syndrome is associated with a significantly increased risk of cardiovascular disease, even after adjustment for known cardiovascular risk factors including LDL-cholesterol levels.[9] As may be expected, a diet high in saturated fat and calories and low in dietary fiber along with a sedentary lifestyle are significant risk factors for its development.

With regard to the influence of HIV infection on metabolism, studies going back more than a decade have demonstrated that advancing HIV disease and immune deficiency is accompanied by changes in lipoprotein metabolism characterized by decreased levels of total, LDL-cholesterol (LDL-c) and HDL-cholesterol (HDL-c) as well as decreased apolipoprotein B.[12] These metabolic parameters fall in parallel with CD4+ T-cell counts, while progression to AIDS is associated with elevated triglyceride levels and an increase in more atherogenic small dense low density lipoprotein particles.[13] Early stage untreated HIV infection therefore represents a relatively low cholesterol state, while more advanced disease and the presence of AIDS may be associated with a more pro-atherogenic lipid profile.

The 'Treatment' Phase: Metabolic Complications of Specific Antiretroviral Drugs

The use of any effective treatment regimen may counteract these changes in plasma lipoproteins associated with HIV infection *per se* and to some extent restore plasma lipoprotein levels to those present prior to acquisition of infection.

There is now however definitive evidence that treatment with selected HIV protease inhibitors can rapidly induce significant metabolic abnormalities, including but not limited to changes in plasma lipids and lipoproteins, in both HIV-infected and HIV-negative subjects, although it must also be acknowledged that metabolic effects of these drugs can no longer be considered 'class effects.' For example, indinavir has been shown to induce significant insulin resistance following short-term drug exposure in healthy control subjects,[14] while lopinavir therapy under similar conditions is associated with elevated triglyceride levels but no significant impact on insulin sensitivity.[15] Newer HIV protease inhibitors, such as atazanavir do not appear to have any unfavorable effects on lipid or glucose metabolism,[16] paving the way for *intra-class* PI switching strategies in response to treatment-induced dyslipidemia.

Turning to NNRTI drugs, there is now little doubt that nevirapine, and to a lesser extent, efavirenz stand out as having specific and potentially anti-atherogenic effects on HDL-cholesterol levels. For example, in the large 2NN trial nevirapine therapy was associated with a 42.5% increase of HDL-cholesterol while efavirenz had a more modest effect on HDL-cholesterol (33.7%).[17] These differences remained, or even increased, after adjusting for changes in HIV-1 RNA and CD4+ cell levels, indicating an independent effect of the drugs on lipids that could not be explained by suppression of HIV-1 infection. Accordingly, the use of nevirapine in 'PI switching' studies has been associated with favorable effects on dyslipidemia and insulin resistance.[5] Hence, in patients with established cardiovascular risk factors, and particularly those with existing cardiovascular disease, NNRTI-containing regimens appear to be a rational treatment choice.

Monitoring and Managing Metabolic Complications

Large-scale cardiovascular disease studies have consistently shown that combination antiretroviral therapy for HIV is associated with an increased risk of cardiovascular disease endpoints,[18,19] with the presence of traditional cardiovascular risk factors also being important additional independent predictors of cardiovascular events within HIV-infected patient populations. It therefore seems prudent to assess and manage global cardiovascular risk in all HIV-infected patients, with particular attention to baseline (pre-treatment) values and metabolic responses to HIV treatment. Given that HDL-c levels as well as total and LDL-cholesterol levels are modulated by progressive HIV infection, and the importance of the 'non-HDL' cholesterol fraction in determining cardiovascular risk in the context of the metabolic syndrome, it may be useful to monitor the non-HDL cholesterol fraction (total cholesterol minus HDL-c) in these individuals in order to capture the total burden of atherogenic triglyceride-rich lipoproteins.

What lipid-lowering therapy can be offered to patients experiencing metabolic complications, particularly when alternative HAART regimens are not available due to problems of resistance or intolerance? Early studies suggest that pravastatin treatment resulted in an approximately 20% reduction in total and non-HDL cholesterol levels, which may be indirectly compared with the effects of switching from PI therapy to nevirapine over 24 weeks in a European study, where non-HDL cholesterol levels fell by 15%. However, the difficulties in achieving standard goals of lipid-lowering therapy according to National Cholesterol Education Program (NCEP) guidelines have also been noted in the ACTG 5087 study, which compared pravastatin with fenofibrate as single agents, and also combined these drugs when NCEP target levels were not reached. Combined treatment was required for approximately 75% of the subjects in each treatment arm, and resulted in composite goal values (LDL, HDL and TG levels) in only ≈ 5% of recipients, although goal HDL-c and triglyceride values were achieved in ≈ 60% and ≈ 50% of cases. Non-HDL cholesterol decreased by ≈ 18% in the combined therapy group. Guidelines have been established for the assessment and treatment of lipid abnormalities in HIV-infected subjects,[20] which recommend the use of standard treatment approaches based on global cardiovascular risk assessment. Among those with existing cardiovascular disease or markedly increased risk (>20% 10-year predicted risk), statin drugs are recommended for their prognostic and survival benefit, irrespective of the baseline lipid values.[21]

Other NRTI-associated Complications

Lactic Acidosis and Hyperlactatemia

Lactic acidosis is probably the most recognizable feature of mitochondrial dysfunction in clinical disease, in which loss of mitochondrial oxidative function leads to increased reliance on 'anaerobic' metabolism and the inevitable accumulation of lactate (and thus, of acid). In the setting of NRTI therapy, there is now an appreciation of a spectrum of clinical disease associated with elevated systemic lactate levels.[22] At one end of this spectrum is a relatively common syndrome of mild, asymptomatic, nonprogressive hyperlactatemia (generally <2.5 mmol/L), which appears to represent a 'compensated' homeostatic system in which elevated lactate production is balanced by effective mechanisms of lactate clearance. While the degree of hyperlactatemia appears to be greater in the presence of stavudine or didanosine therapy compared with zidovudine or abacavir, this syndrome appears to be benign irrespective of the choice of NRTI therapy.

In contrast, lactic acidosis and hepatic steatosis represents a relatively uncommon (1–2/1000 person-years) but life-threatening clinical syndrome in which lactate homeostasis is completely 'decompensated,' allowing the rapid, progressive accumulation of lactate and development of acidosis in affected patients. A critical aspect of lactic acidosis is its unpredictability, as it typically occurs in patients who have been on stable NRTI regimens for months or even years, and is not heralded by increased lactate levels before the development of the fulminant syndrome. Host risk factors for NRTI-associated lactic acidosis include concurrent liver disease, female gender, and obesity, and while the majority of reported cases in recent years have involved stavudine-based HAART, cases involving zidovudine therapy also occur. The cornerstone of management of this condition is early recognition of the clinical manifestations: abdominal symptoms including nausea, vomiting, anorexia, abdominal pain and distension, fatigue, with biochemical evidence of hepatocellular liver dysfunction and lactate level generally >5 mmol/L. These clinical and laboratory abnormalities should lead to prompt cessation of NRTI therapy. A more recently identified clinical syndrome accompanying lactic acidosis is progressive, severe neuromuscular weakness mimicking the Guillain–Barré syndrome. Overall, the mortality associated with NRTI-associated lactic acidosis remains unacceptably high, at around 50%.

An 'intermediate' syndrome has also been described, characterized by symptomatic hyperlactatemia or hepatic steatosis without systemic acidosis, which is almost uniformly associated with stavudine therapy (incidence ≈ 13/1000 person-years). In this setting, lactate levels and symptoms can be controlled following modification of NRTI therapy to zidovudine or abacavir.

Pancreatitis

There is a differential diagnosis for pancreatitis occurring in an HIV-infected individual that includes severe HIV protease inhibitor-induced hypertriglyceridemia, and the effects of other drugs such as pentamidine. A diagnosis of pancreatitis includes clinical symptoms of abdominal pain combined with elevated serum amylase levels, thus excluding cases of isolated hyperamylasemia which have been associated with moderate to severe immune deficiency where the relationship between this biochemical abnormality and pancreatitis is uncertain.

The most comprehensive data concerning risk factors for NRTI-associated pancreatitis comes from the Johns Hopkins AIDS Service cohort ($n = 2613$ cases),[23] with supporting data from the ACTG 5025 study. In these analyses, didanosine and stavudine were associated with roughly equivalent risk of pancreatitis, with estimated incidence rates of 0.8 and 1.1 cases per 100 person-years, respectively. Combining these drugs increased risk approximately 2-fold, while concurrent didanosine and hydroxyurea use increased relative risk approximately 8-fold, including several fatal cases. More recently, cases of pancreatitis have been reported with concurrent use of didanosine and tenofovir – including with reduced doses of didanosine (250 mg/day) – presumably due to the ability of tenofovir to 'boost' didanosine effects *in vivo*.[24]

Neuropathy

Neuropathic changes frequently do not come to the attention of clinicians as the symptoms are of gradual onset, and clinical signs of nerve damage are not generally sought in clinical practice. Hence, the prevalence – and potential long-term impact – of neuropathy is likely to be underestimated. In this instance, there is a definite contribution of HIV disease *per se* to the pathogenesis of a form of distal sensory neuropathy that is clinically and electrophysiologically indistinguishable from so-called 'toxic neuropathy from antiretroviral drugs.'[25] It is therefore difficult to dissect out the relative contribution of disease-associated and drug-associated factors in the syndrome, as these effects are likely to be synergistic. The clinical syndrome common to both HIV-associated and toxic sensory polyneuropathy is dominated by peripheral pain and dysesthesia, with rare motor involvement.

The greatest risk of treatment-induced neuropathy has been associated with zalcitabine NRTI therapy, which induced neuropathy in approximately one-third of patients receiving low-dose therapy (2.25 mg/day), and almost universally at higher doses in clinical trials. Stavudine and didanosine have also been associated with increased risk of neuropathy in the large Johns Hopkins AIDS Service cohort study. Compared with a crude incidence rate of 6.8 cases per 100 person-years for didanosine, stavudine use was associated with a relative risk of 1.4, while concurrent use of these drugs further increased risk (3.5-fold relative risk compared with didanosine alone). Concurrent hydroxyurea therapy had an additional effect (7.8-fold relative risk compared with didanosine alone).

Reversal of established neuropathy appears to be a slow process that is dependent on cessation of the offending NRTI drug. The identification of L-carnitine deficiency, and the use of L-acetyl-carnitine therapy, may also have beneficial effects on nerve regeneration, while lamotrigine therapy has also been associated with improved pain symptoms in the context of NRTI-associated toxic polyneuropathy. As with any clinical neuropathy, a search for contributing factors such as diabetes, excessive alcohol consumption, and vitamin deficiencies (e.g. thiamine, B_{12}, and folate) should be undertaken; ideally, prior to initiating NRTI therapy.

Hematological Complications of NRTI Therapy

These complications have assumed less importance in clinical management in the HAART era, reflecting the fact that HIV disease severity – and particularly the presence of one or more AIDS-defining illnesses – contributes significantly to the risk of anemia and other hematological events (e.g. thrombocytopenia, neutropenia) in untreated individuals. Nevertheless, zidovudine therapy has been associated with increased risk of anemia in HAART recipients compared with other NRTI drugs (relative risk ≈ 1.15), suggesting that this drug should be used with caution when hemoglobin levels are low prior to treatment. This may be particularly relevant when initiating antiretroviral therapy in resource poor countries where patients may be more prone to have reduced hemoglobin levels as a result of concomitant parasitic infection (malaria, hookworm), malnutrition or genetically determined hemoglobinopathies.

Recent studies have also suggested that combined full-dose didanosine and tenofovir treatment may contribute to a targeted toxicity against lymphocytes, resulting in reduced CD4+ T-cell counts, despite the presence of undetectable viral loads,[26] affecting >50% of patients receiving this drug combination in one clinical trial. Hence, drug toxicity should be considered as a potential explanation when there is significant discordance between virological suppression and CD4+ T-cell responses on HAART while employing this particular combination of antiretrovirals.

Tenofovir Renal Safety

The renal safety of tenofovir has been a topic of interest for some time now, following a number of reports (involving >30 cases) of significant renal toxicity with renal tubular damage and/or acute renal failure. In the large Gilead 903 study in which patients were selected for normal renal function at baseline, no evidence of significant renal toxicity could be identified over a 3-year treatment period using serum creatinine measures.[27] However, a recent study has observed reductions in glomerular filtration rate (≈ 10%) along with ≈ 20% increase in rate of proteinuria >130 mg/day.[28] Hence, simple measurements of serum creatinine may not be sufficient to capture the true effects of this drug on renal function. Further clinical data are awaited, but

in the meantime, it would be prudent to carefully consider more stringent assessments of glomerular filtration rate (as well as markers of renal tubular toxicity such as hypophosphatemia). Here, calculated methods such as the Cockcroft–Gault equation that adjust for body weight and gender may be useful for monitoring purposes. In addition, it would seem prudent to only use tenofovir with caution in patients with already compromised renal function. When doing so, proper dose adjustment needs to be employed.

Abacavir Hypersensitivity Reactions

Abacavir hypersensitivity reactions are the most frequent adverse events associated with use of this drug, consistently affecting ≈ 8% of abacavir-exposed individuals in clinical trials. The syndrome is characterized by the onset within the first 6 weeks of abacavir treatment of constitutional symptoms (fever, malaise, lethargy), with frequent involvement of the skin (rash) and/or gastrointestinal tract (nausea, vomiting, abdominal pain, diarrhea); although the wide array of clinical symptoms that may signify abacavir hypersensitivity can lead to uncertainty in the diagnostic classification. A history of definite abacavir hypersensitivity precludes any further use of abacavir because rechallenge can evoke more rapid onset and severe reactions. In this respect, a definitive diagnosis of abacavir hypersensitivity may be facilitated by the use of epicutaneous patch testing (Fig. 17.2).[29]

Genetic risk factors have proven highly predictive of abacavir hypersensitivity, so that carriage of the *HLA-B*5701* genetic marker is associated with >70% risk of developing abacavir hypersensitivity reactions, while the risk of abacavir hypersensitivity reactions among those who are negative for this HLA marker is less than 1%. Prospective genetic testing for *HLA-B*5701* would therefore stratify patients into high-risk and low-risk groups, allowing for a more rational and cost-effective approach to abacavir prescribing.[30]

Other HIV Protease Inhibitor-associated Complications

These adverse effects tend to be strongly associated with individual drugs within the HIV protease inhibitor (PI) class, rather than representing drug 'class effects.'

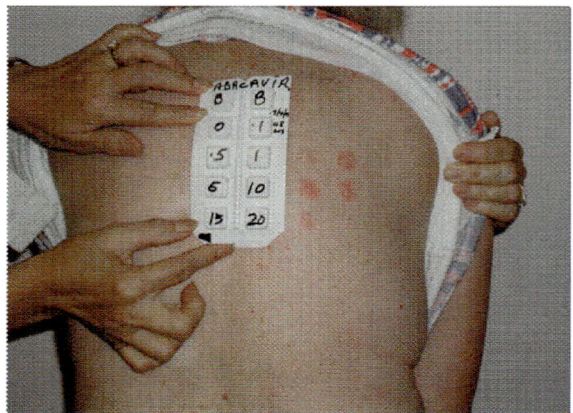

Figure 17.2 Abacavir hypersensitivity demonstrated by erythematous and vesicular skin changes in response to a range of abacavir concentrations (as shown) in a petrolatum vehicle.

Abnormal Liver Function/Liver Enzyme Abnormalities

Atazanavir and indinavir have been shown to cause reversible unconjugated hyperbilirubinemia (via UDP-glucuronosyltransferase inhibition), particularly in those who are genetically prone to Gilbert's syndrome. The prevalence of this asymptomatic abnormality correlates well with the ability of these drugs to inhibit the relevant enzyme (clinical jaundice ≈ 10% with atazanavir, <1% with indinavir), and does not represent hepatic cell damage.

Full-dose (but not low-dose) ritonavir has been associated with increased risk of hepatoxicity as defined by transaminase elevation (i.e. >5-fold elevation of ALT and/or AST levels), with a relative risk of approximately four compared with other PI drugs. However, the presence of chronic viral hepatitis (i.e. hepatitis B or C) and/or alcohol abuse remain the most important risk factors for such hepatoxicity on HAART, which may reflect altered hepatic drug metabolism as well as the restoration of pathogenic inflammatory responses to hepatitis viruses following successful HIV therapy.[31]

Gastrointestinal Intolerance

Persistent diarrhea is a relatively frequent complication of nelfinavir therapy, affecting 20–50% of recipients. Of the other PI drugs, lopinavir and fosamprenavir have also been associated with diarrhea, particularly in the early weeks of treatment (incidence ≈ 10%). Diarrhea seems to be much less

of a problem with the use of (ritonavir-boosted) atazanavir.

Nephrolithiasis

Indinavir is associated with risk of renal calculus formation, affecting >10% of recipients. Indinavir-induced renal calculi (which are radiolucent) generally respond to hydration, diuresis and urinary acidification. Indinavir is also associated with 'retinoid' side-effects, including dry lips and skin (≈ 30%), and hair and nail changes including paronychia (≈ 5%).

Toxicity Profiles of NNRTI Drugs: Efavirenz and Nevirapine

The NNRTI drugs efavirenz and nevirapine have proven to be highly effective HIV drugs that carry minimal risk of lipodystrophic side-effects. Moreover, there is evidence that PI-to-NNRTI switching strategies have proved to be more tolerable overall (particularly in relation to gastrointestinal side-effects) as well as improving patients' metabolic status. Such broad statements need to be interpreted with caution, however, given an awareness of the individual toxicity profiles of drugs within both the NNRTI and PI drug classes.

Efavirenz Therapy and Central Nervous System Side-effects

The efficacy of efavirenz-containing regimens, and the much lower likelihood of severe hepatic and skin toxicities that may be associated with nevirapine treatment, has led to the adoption of efavirenz as recommended first line therapy for HIV in various treatment guidelines. The most frequent adverse effects associated with this drug relate to cognitive and neuropsychiatric function, affecting ≈ 15% of efavirenz recipients within 1 month of initiating treatment. While these side-effects generally resolve in the early stages of treatment, cohort studies have identified ongoing symptoms including dizziness, sadness, irritability, nervousness and mood changes, impaired concentration and abnormal dreams.[32] Suicidal ideation has also been reported in a minority of patients, indicating that neuropsychiatric manifestations may be severe in some cases. While this list would appear to constitute a significant burden of toxicity, it was interesting to note that patients on efavirenz or nevirapine regimens consistently report equivalent improvements in quality of life.

Nevirapine Toxicity Profile

Although quality of life and overall toxicity burden appear to be equivalent for efavirenz and nevirapine treatment, the toxicity profile of nevirapine is demonstrably different to efavirenz, as observed in the 2NN trial in which treatment-associated rash (Figs 17.3, 17.4) and hepatotoxicity emerged as a relatively rare but potentially life-threatening toxicity.[33] On the other hand, central nervous system disturbances are infrequent with nevirapine use, and beneficial effects on lipid profiles appear to be more marked, both when using nevirapine as part of first-line therapy or after switching from PI therapy.

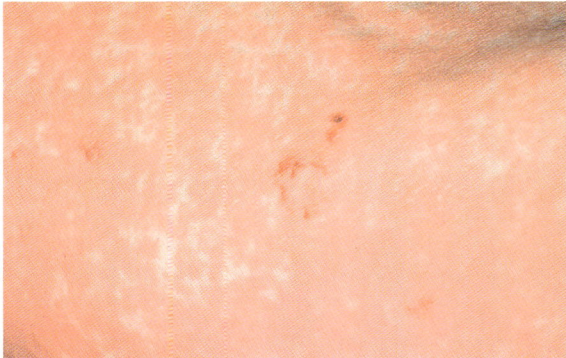

Figure 17.3 Maculopapular rash in a patient with light skin receiving nevirapine.

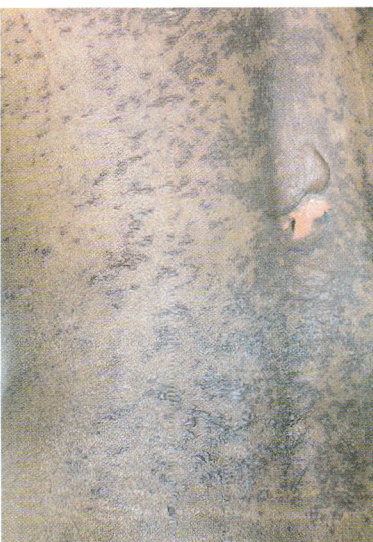

Figure 17.4 Maculopapular rash in a patient with dark skin receiving nevirapine.

Safety data compiled by Boehringer–Ingelheim relating to nevirapine therapy have clearly demonstrated that severe (grade 3–4) hepatotoxicity and rash occur during the early phase of treatment (within 12 weeks of treatment initiation) in ≈ 5% of nevirapine recipients, and that low CD4$^+$ T-cell counts are relatively protective against the development of these severe toxicity syndromes. This is now reflected in a new FDA and European Medicines Agency (EMEA) label for nevirapine that recommends against the initiation of nevirapine in adult females with CD4$^+$ cell counts >250 cells/mm^3 or in adult males with CD4$^+$ cell counts >400 cells/mm^3 unless the benefit outweighs the risk. In this context, a recent study has identified that a combination of host genetic susceptibility (carriage of *HLA-DRB1*0101*) and sufficiently high CD4$^+$ T cells (>25%) identified a proportion of the treated population at high risk of nevirapine hypersensitivity,[34] suggesting that in future it may be possible to predict a patient's ability to tolerate nevirapine therapy with a greater certainty than is currently available.

Conclusions

- The toxicity profiles of antiretroviral drugs can to some extent, be grouped according to the nucleoside reverse transcriptase inhibitor (NRTI), protease inhibitor (PI) and non-nucleoside reverse transcriptase inhibitor (NNRTI) drug classes, but important distinctions have also emerged between drugs within each of these classes. Hence, the notion of 'class effects' (e.g. PI drugs and metabolic complications) can no longer be applied usefully when considering the toxicity profiles of antiretroviral drug regimens.

- Lipoatrophy, which is the major clinical component of the 'lipodystrophy syndrome', is strongly associated with the use of thymidine analog NRTI drugs stavudine and (to a lesser extent) zidovudine. Use of alternative drug regimens, along with the judicious use of stavudine/zidovudine in those with favorable host factors (e.g. CD4 >100, age <35 years, non-white racial origin, males) and appropriate monitoring for early manifestations of fat loss, are strategies to be exploited in order to render lipoatrophy a largely preventable side effect of HIV treatment. It is important that these insights are also taken into account when prioritizing first-line treatment regimens for use in resource-poor settings.

- The toxicity profiles of newer NRTI drugs such as tenofovir and abacavir need to be carefully considered and further researched, so that reduced risk of lipoatrophy is not traded off against increased risk of other toxicities. In the case of tenofovir, renal safety remains an issue that has not been satisfactorily resolved to date. Abacavir hypersensitivity syndrome is better understood, representing a drug hypersensitivity syndrome with a strong genetic basis (*HLA-B*5701*).

- The contribution of PI drug therapy to metabolic complications appears to be highly specific to individual drugs, with evidence that newer agents such as atazanavir are not associated with direct effects on metabolism.

- The Metabolic Syndrome has been recognized in recent years as a distinct clinical entity that is associated with an increased risk of cardiovascular disease and mortality. This syndrome is highly prevalent in the adult population (>30%), and increases in prevalence and severity with age, and therefore represents a common underlying disorder in HIV-infected patients that may be unmasked/accelerated by therapy with selected PI drugs. This syndrome also shares many characteristics with the metabolic phenotype observed in the 'lipodystrophy syndrome,' so much can be learned from this disease model regarding the assessment and management of lipid abnormalities and overall cardiovascular risk.

- The NNRTI drugs efavirenz and nevirapine are characterized by a low risk of lipodystrophic side-effects, potentially beneficial effects on lipid metabolism (nevirapine > efavirenz) and good overall tolerability. While the prevalence of adverse events is similar with these two drugs, their toxicity profiles are quite different, however, with a predominance of neuropsychological side-effects with efavirenz compared with problems of rash and hepatitis associated with nevirapine.

- Drug toxicity represents not only a short-term issue affecting choice of HIV therapy, but is also associated with a burden of disease that can require long-term assessment and management. For example, an increased understanding of the pathogenesis of lipoatrophy has revealed that clinical loss of fat reflects widespread loss of adipocytes (fat cells) within the adipose tissue, which suggests that reversal of the disease process is likely to be slow and/or incomplete

even after the offending drugs are removed. Similarly, increasing predisposition towards the Metabolic Syndrome through the use of PI drugs may be associated with long-term cardiovascular disease risk. In this context, there is an ongoing need for treatment as well as prevention options to be explored.

References

1. Reisler RB, Han C, Burman WJ, et al. Grade 4 events are as important as AIDS events in the era of HAART. J Acquir Immune Defic Syndr 2003; 34:379–386.
2. Palella FJ Jr., Cole SR, Chmiel JS, et al. Anthropometrics and examiner-reported body habitus abnormalities in the multicenter AIDS cohort study. Clin Infect Dis 2004; 38:903–907.
3. Carr A. Workman C, Smith DE, et al. Abacavir substitution for nucleoside analogs in patients with HIV lipoatrophy: a randomized trial. JAMA 2002; 288:207–215.
4. Moyle G, Sabin CA, Cartledge J, et al. A randomized comparative trial of tenofovir DF or abacavir as replacement for a thymidine analogue in persons with lipoatrophy. AIDS 2006; 20:2043–2050.
5. Dreschler H. Powderly WG. Switching effective antiretroviral therapy: a review. Clin Infect Dis 2002; 35:1219–1230.
6. Nolan D, Hammond E, James I, et al. Contribution of nucleoside-analogue reverse transcriptase inhibitor therapy to lipoatrophy from the population to the cellular level. Antivir Ther 2003; 8:617–626.
7. McComsey GA, Paulsen DM, Lonergan JT, et al. Improvements in lipoatrophy, mitochondrial DNA levels and fat apoptosis after replacing stavudine with abacavir or zidovudine. AIDS 2005; 19:15–23.
8. Domingo P, Matias-Guiu X, Pujol RM, et al. Switching to nevirapine decreases insulin levels but does not improve subcutaneous adipocyte apoptosis in patients with highly active antiretroviral therapy-associated lipodystrophy. J Infect Dis 2001; 184:1197–1201.
9. Ford ES. The metabolic syndrome and mortality from cardiovascular disease and all-causes: findings from the National Health and Nutrition Examination Survey II Mortality Study. Atherosclerosis 2004; 173:309–314.
10. Petit JM, Duong M, Florentin E, et al. Increased VLDL-apoB and IDL-apoB production rates in nonlipodystrophic HIV-infected patients on a protease inhibitor-containing regimen: a stable isotope kinetic study. J Lipid Res 2003; 44:1692–1697.
11. Sekhar RV, Jahoor F, White AC, et al. Metabolic basis of HIV-lipodystrophy syndrome. Am J Physiol Endocrinol Metab 2002; 283:332–337.
12. Grunfeld C, Pang M, Doerrler W, et al. Lipids, lipoproteins, triglyceride clearance, and cytokines in human immunodeficiency virus infection and the acquired immunodeficiency syndrome. J Clin Endocrinol Metab 1992; 74:1045–1052.
13. Grunfeld C, Kotler DP, Hamadeh R, et al. Hypertriglyceridemia in the acquired immunodeficiency syndrome. Am J Med 1989; 86:27–31.
14. Noor MA, Lo JC, Mulligan K, et al. Metabolic effects of indinavir in healthy HIV-seronegative men. AIDS 2001; 15:11–18.
15. Lee GA, Seneviratne T, Noor MA, et al. The metabolic effects of lopinavir/ritonavir in HIV-negative men. AIDS 2004; 18:641–649.
16. Noor MA, Parker RA, O'Mara E, et al. The effects of HIV protease inhibitors atazanavir and lopinavir/ritonavir on insulin sensitivity in HIV-seronegative healthy adults. AIDS 2004; 18:2137–2144.

17. Van Leth F, Phanuphak P, Stroes E, et al. Nevirapine and Efavirenz elicit different changes in lipid profiles in antiretroviral-therapy-naive patients infected with HIV-1. PLoS Med 2004; 1:e19.

18. D'Arminio Monforte A, Sabin CA, Phillips AN, et al. Cardio- and cerebrovascular events in HIV-infected persons. AIDS 2004; 18:1811–1817.

19. Friis-Moller N. Sabin CA, Weber R, et al. Combination antiretroviral therapy and the risk of myocardial infarction. N Engl J Med 2003; 349:1993–2003.

20. Dube MP, Stein JH, Aberg JA, et al. Guidelines for the evaluation and management of dyslipidemia in human immunodeficiency virus (HIV)-infected adults receiving antiretroviral therapy: recommendations of the HIV Medical Association of the Infectious Disease Society of America and the Adult AIDS Clinical Trials Group. Clin Infect Dis 2003; 37:613–627.

21. Heart Protection Study Collaborative Group. MRC/BHF Heart Protection Study of cholesterol lowering with simvastatin in 20,536 high-risk individuals: a randomised placebo-controlled trial. Lancet 2002; 360:7–22.

22. John M, Mallal S. Hyperlactatemia syndromes in people with HIV infection. Curr Opin Infect Dis 2002; 15:23–29.

23. Moore RD, Keruly JC, Chaisson RE. Incidence of pancreatitis in HIV-infected patients receiving nucleoside reverse transcriptase inhibitor drugs. AIDS 2001; 15:617–620.

24. Kirian MA, Higginson RT, Fulco PP. Acute onset of pancreatitis with concomitant use of tenofovir and didanosine. Ann Pharmacother 2004; 38:1660–1663.

25. Keswani SC, Pardo CA, Cherry CL, et al. HIV-associated sensory neuropathies. AIDS 2002; 16:2105–2117.

26. Negredo E, Molto J, Burger D, et al. Unexpected CD4 cell count decline in patients receiving didanosine and tenofovir-based regimens despite undetectable viral load. AIDS 2004; 18:459–463.

27. Gallant JE, Staszewski S, Pozniak AL, et al. Efficacy and safety of tenofovir DF vs stavudine in combination therapy in antiretroviral-naive patients: a 3-year randomized trial. JAMA 2004; 292:191–201.

28. Mauss S, Berger F, Schmutz G. Antiretroviral therapy with tenofovir is associated with mild renal dysfunction. AIDS 2005; 19:93–95.

29. Phillips EJ, Sullivan JR, Knowles SR, et al. Utility of patch testing in patients with hypersensitivity syndromes associated with abacavir. AIDS 2002; 16:2223–2225.

30. Hughes DA, Vilar FJ, Ward CC, et al. Cost-effectiveness analysis of HLA B*5701 genotyping in preventing abacavir hypersensitivity. Pharmacogenetics 2004; 14:335–342.

31. Sulkowski MS. Drug-induced liver injury associated with antiretroviral therapy that includes HIV-1 protease inhibitors. Clin Infect Dis 2004; 38 (Suppl):90–97.

32. Lochet P, Peyriere H, Lotthe A, et al. Long-term assessment of neuropsychiatric adverse reactions associated with efavirenz. HIV Med 2003; 4:62–66.

33. Van Leth F, Phanuphak P, Ruxrungtham K, et al. Comparison of first-line antiretroviral therapy with regimens including nevirapine, efavirenz, or both drugs, plus stavudine and lamivudine: a randomised open-label trial, the 2NN Study. Lancet 2004; 363:1253–1263.

34. Martin AM, Nolan D, James I, et al. Predisposition to nevirapine hypersensitivity associated with HLA-DRB1*0101 and abrogated by low CD4 T-cell counts. AIDS 2005; 19:97–99.

CHAPTER 18

HIV Immune Reconstitution Inflammatory Syndrome

Paul R. Bohjanen

David R. Boulware

Introduction

As increasing numbers of HIV-infected people worldwide begin antiretroviral therapy (ART), more experience is being developed with the normal course of immune reconstitution and the pathologic. In a subset of those initiating ART, a harmonious gradual reconstitution of the immune system does not occur, but instead, an abrupt transition to a pathologic inflammatory state occurs that is associated with clinical deterioration. In this abnormal inflammatory state, patients clinically worsen despite an otherwise excellent classic response to ART as evidenced by decreased HIV viral load and increased CD4 T-cell counts. This clinical worsening in these patients is due to the development of a paradoxical inflammatory response by the immune system to a variety of infectious or non-infectious antigens. This paradoxical inflammatory response has been termed HIV immune reconstitution inflammatory syndrome (IRIS). Alternative names have been used to describe this clinical entity including immune reconstitution Syndrome and immune reconstitution disease. Differing nomenclature, differing clinical scenarios, and perhaps differing pathogenic mechanisms make it difficult to define IRIS as a single clinical entity, and IRIS probably represents a variety of inflammatory syndromes that occur following the initiation of ART.

There are two common pathologic scenarios of IRIS presentation (Box 18.1), which we describe here

as immune reconstitution syndrome (also known as paradoxical IRIS) and immune reconstitution disease (also known as unmasking IRIS). As the immune system reconstitutes, inflammation develops in response to either infectious or non-infectious antigens. The result is either a new diagnosis of an opportunistic infection (OI) or apparent clinical relapse of a previously treated infection. Immune reconstitution disease occurs following the initiation of ART due to worsening of an active or latent OI and infectious pathogens are present. An example of immune reconstitution disease or unmasking is the activation of latent tuberculosis following the initiation of ART. Immune reconstitution syndrome is the paradoxical clinical recrudescence of a successfully treated infection. In this scenario, a symptomatic relapse occurs despite microbiologic treatment success and sterile cultures. Within the published literature, case reports of IRIS events have been associated with a wide variety of opportunistic infections, malignancies, and autoimmune disorders.

Among previously treated infections, differentiating IRIS from disease relapse is often impossible based on the clinical presentation. Patients with IRIS may have identical symptoms to their prior initial presentation of an infection or they may exhibit clinical worsening despite adequate antimicrobial therapy. Importantly, among patients with IRIS recrudescence, microbiologic culture data is often negative, and the pathologic process is inflammatory and not microbiologic in etiology. Distinguishing IRIS from treatment failure, antimicrobial resistance,

---

Box 18.1

Immune reconstitution inflammatory syndrome pathologic scenarios

- Immune reconstitution disease (unmasking IRIS)
  - Occult, subclinical opportunistic infection
  - Unmasked by ART
  - Infectious pathogens present
- Immune reconstitution syndrome (paradoxical IRIS)
  - Clinical recrudescence of a successfully treated infection
  - Symptomatic relapse despite microbiologic treatment success.
  - Antigen driven immune activation
  - Sterile cultures

Box 18.2

Proposed criteria for diagnosis of immune reconstitution inflammatory syndrome

Evidence of response to ART with either:

- CD4[+] T-cell count increase
- Virologic response with >1 $\log_{10}$ copies/mL decrease in HIV RNA.

Infectious or Inflammatory condition temporally related to the initiation of ART
Symptoms can not be explained by either:

- A newly acquired infection
- Expected clinical course of a previously recognized and successfully treated infectious agent
- Side-effects of ART

---

or non-compliance is critical. Although criteria for the diagnosis of IRIS have been proposed, no unified clinical case definition of IRIS has been formalized.[1] General criteria for the diagnosis of IRIS are presented in Box 18.2.

HIV Pathogenesis and the Beneficial Effects of ART

For the majority of HIV-infected patients initiating ART, immune reconstitution is of great benefit. A hallmark of HIV pathogenesis is the gradual destruction of the immune system over a period of many years leading to increased susceptibility to opportunistic infections and the development of AIDS. In untreated HIV-infected patients, ongoing viral replication leads to the destruction of millions of CD4[+] T cells each day.[2] In the early stages of HIV infection, HIV-specific immune responses help to limit viral replication, and the destruction of CD4[+] T cells is balanced by the generation of new CD4[+] T cells.[2,3] The ongoing viral replication over a period of years, however, leads to chronic immune cell activation and inflammation, resulting in scarring and destruction of the normal lymph node architecture.[4,5] The number of circulating CD4[+] T cells gradually decreases as the regenerative capacity of the immune system can no longer keep up with the ongoing loss of lymphatic tissue and the destruction of CD4[+] T cells. Over a period of many years, this destruction of the immune system results in increased susceptibility to OIs and the development of AIDS.

The major goal of ART therapy for HIV infection is to suppress viral replication to prevent further

deterioration and to allow regeneration of the immune system. Even patients with advanced AIDS often exhibit improved functioning of their immune system after the initiation of ART, a phenomenon referred to as immune reconstitution. As virologic control over HIV is established following initiation of ART, immune reconstitution occurs in two phases. First, there is redistribution, proliferation, and a reduction in apoptosis of existing T cells from lymphatic tissues into blood resulting in an initial increase in CD4 T-cell counts during the first 3 weeks. These redistributed cells are predominantly pre-existing memory CD4[+] cells (CD45RA[-]RO[+]).[6] This is followed by a less-pronounced but steady increase in naive CD4[+] cells (CD45RA[+]) of thymic origin.[6] Decreases in the expression of cell surface markers of activation (HLA-DR, CD38) on CD4 and CD8 T cells correlate with viral suppression,[7,8] suggesting that the chronic immune activation that occurs during HIV infection is reversed by ART. Lymphocyte proliferative responses to *Candida* normalize within 3 months, and T-cell specific responses to HIV and protein antigens, such as tetanus toxoid, improve during the first year of therapy.[6] This improved immunity makes HIV-infected patients less susceptible to opportunistic infections, and several studies have shown that primary or secondary prophylaxis against various opportunistic infections can be safely discontinued in patients who have sustained increases in CD4 counts and/or sustained viral suppression following the initiation of ART.[9–12]

IRIS Pathogenesis

Although most patients show clinical improvement following initiation of ART, the subset of patients who develop IRIS experience clinical worsening, as a pathologic consequence of their improvement in immune function. In immune reconstitution disease, the clinical deterioration after starting ART is due to an improving immune system interacting with organisms that were already present in the body prior to the initiation of ART. In this clinical scenario, patients with advanced HIV are unable to mount an effective immune response against pathogens that are present, but ART leads to an improvement in their immune function, and therefore pathogens that were previously not recognized by the immune system are unmasked and evoke an inflammatory response. The transition from subclinical, occult infection to symptomatic inflammation in patients with immune reconstitution disease depends on improved immune function, but the inflammatory response may actually be exaggerated compared with the response that occurs in patients with normal immune systems. The homeostatic mechanisms that normally limit immune activation may have been damaged as a result of HIV-induced immune destruction leading to exaggerated inflammation.

In contrast to immune reconstitution disease, in which an active infection is unmasked, immune reconstitution syndrome is the recrudescence of an infection that had been successfully treated. Immune reconstitution syndrome is caused by activation of the immune system against persisting antigens present as debris or dead organisms following the initiation of ART. As in immune reconstitution disease, the inflammatory response that occurs in these patients may be exaggerated compared with the response in patients with normal immune function. We do not currently know if all IRIS disease recrudescence occurs via the same pathogenic mechanism, or if distinctly different mechanisms exist. In acute onset IRIS occurring within days to weeks after ART initiation, is there a different pathogenesis vs IRIS occurring months to years later? Is the difference in timing solely explainable by a variable time period needed for the restoration of T-cell specific cellular immunity targeted toward a particular immunologic antigen? How much does the role of innate immunity contribute? Clearly, activation of the immune system occurs in all forms of IRIS, but it is unknown whether the responses that occur in different clinical scenarios are due to appropriate antigen-specific responses, exaggerated antigen-specific responses, or non-specific inflammatory responses that are triggered as a result of immune dysregulation. Because patients with advanced HIV often exhibit non-specific immune activation as they progress to AIDS,[13] it is possible that this non-specific inflammation becomes exaggerated in a subset of patients as they respond to ART. Although existing data is limited, histopathology from a few published case reports of IRIS showed that mononuclear inflammatory cells with or without a granulomatous pattern of inflammation were observed in inflamed tissues from patients with IRIS.[14,15] Also, TNF-α expression and genetic polymorphisms appear to be involved in developing IRIS.[1,16] Most reported cases of Immune Reconstitution Disease associated with mycobacteria develop within the first 3 months of HAART when CD45Ro memory lymphocyte redistribution occurs.[17] Recirculation of the previously sequestered CD45Ro cell population may provide the opportunity for relevant pathogen-specific cells to gain access to sites of infection and engage in the host inflammatory response to foreign antigens. Mycobacterial antigens that trigger TB-associated IRIS may be in the form of viable organisms, dead organisms, or residual antigen. After TB treatment, antigens persist long after microbiologic sterility. For example, mycobacterial DNA and cell wall components persist in host tissues for weeks after initiation of anti-mycobacterial therapy.[18,19]

Timing

The timing of the occurrence of IRIS after ART initiation is quite variable. The range reported in the literature is from 2 days to 5 years (Table 18.1). In the largest case series of 57 patients with cryptococcal, tuberculosis (TB), or *Mycobacterial avium* complex (MAC) induced IRIS in Houston, TX, the median time of onset was 46 days.[20] Based in part on this, the consensus of expert opinion is that the majority of IRIS is likely to occur within the first 2 months after ART.[20] While certainly the majority (>50%) probably occurs during the first 2 months, this certainly does not exclude later presentation, whereby at least 30% may present beyond the first 2 months.[20] Among published cases-series of IRIS, the average time to onset of IRIS is 56 days from ART initiation. Even if one excludes the French cryptococcal IRIS experience in which the onset of IRIS occurred much later than most other studies, the average time to onset of IRIS is 44 days; however, the range remains expansive.[21] Of course, the first several weeks of treatment for an OI is also when disease relapse is most likely

Table 18.1 Alternate timing of onset of IRIS from ART initiation

Condition	Location	IRIS cases (n)	Prevalence rate (%)	Onset (days)[b]	Range (days)	Follow-up (years)[a]	Reference
Cryptococcus	Houston, TX	18	31	30	3–330	1.5	26
Cryptococcus	France	12	10	240	60–1110	2	21
TB	Chennai, India	11	8	42	10–89	0.5	31
TB	France	16	43	12	2–114	3[b]	22
Cryptococcus, TB, or MAC	Houston, TX	57	32%	46	3–658	2.2	20
MAC	Vancouver	51	13	21	7–700	2.4[b]	58
Kaposi sarcoma	Seattle, WA	19[c]	N/A	35[a]	21–∞	N/A	70
Any	Holland	17	2	72	2–319	<1	85
Any	London	44	22	84	21–168	0.5	51
All[d]		227	13	56	2–1110	1.75	

MAC, *Mycobacterium avium* complex. [a]mean, [b]median, [c]including 10 patients from the literature, [d]weighted totals presented. Houston cryptococcal data is not double counted.

due to therapy failure, *de novo* drug resistance, or poor compliance. In cases of therapeutic failure, a microbiologic culture should still reveal continued presence of an organism, whereas in cases of IRIS, follow-up cultures should be sterile.

Risk Factors for IRIS

The factors associated with an increased risk of developing IRIS include both the timing and response to HIV ART as well as burden of disease. Non-modifiable IRIS risk factors include being ART naive with a >2 log drop in HIV-1 RNA viral load at 90 days of ART and a >50 cells/µL CD4 count increase at 90 days.[20] These factors are unfortunately not very useful for practicing clinicians, as the majority of IRIS occurs within 60 days of ART. The vast majority, but not all, of patients who develop IRIS tend to have a baseline pre-ART CD4 count <100 cells/µL; however, having a CD4 count <100 cells/µL is not an independent risk factor. Neither baseline CD4 absolute count or HIV-1 RNA viral load are consistently predictive for the development of IRIS after treatment of a known OI.[20-22] Gender may be a risk factor with men perhaps having a 2–3-fold higher risk.[20,21,23]

Unmasking a subclinical infection is more likely at CD4 counts <200 cells/µL as is the risk of all OIs in general; however once the CD4 count <200 cells/µL, the absolute level has not been predictive.[20-23] Certain genetic cytokine polymorphisms may be protective or contribute toward IRIS.[24]

One of the findings with the highest positive predictive value, based on the available data, is an increase in the CD4 percentage of ≥12% in the first 30 days of ART.[22] This occurred in nearly half of patients with HIV-associated IRIS due to TB in France, but in none of patients without IRIS.[22] Similarly, a rapid increase in the CD4 : CD8 ratio of >0.33 within 30 days in patients with TB co-infection appeared to be always pathogenic.[22,25]

Timing of Initiating ART

An important but poorly understood modifiable risk factor for IRIS is the timing of ART initiation in patients with IRIS-associated OIs. Patients started on ART within 2 months of an OI appear to have anywhere from 0 to up to a 6-fold increase in the risk of developing IRIS.[20,21,23] This finding is based on retrospective data, and there are no prospective, randomized studies that identify the optimal timing of ART initiation following an OI. Some experts recommend deferring ART by at least 8 weeks for patients with a significant OI, such as TB or cryptococcal meningitis; however, consensus is not universal.[21,26] Among patients who initiated ART within 30 days of an OI, 66% did well without developing IRIS.[20] When ART was initiated within 60 days of a diagnosis of cryptococcal meningitis, 80% did well clinically.[21] The biologic rationale for delaying therapy would be to provide prolonged therapy against a known opportunistic infection and standard prophylaxis prior to starting ART. This therapy would decrease microbial antigen burden, and theoretically, less antigen would be present to stimulate the recovering immune system. While certainly the relative risk of IRIS is increased with earlier initiation of therapy, individual patient circumstances should still guide the rationale of care. In each patient, the risk of developing IRIS should be weighed against the patient's need for ART. If ART is to be started within 2 months of an OI, a discussion of IRIS risk with the patient and close monitoring would be warranted.

Greater burden of disease may also be a risk factor. Patients with disseminated cryptococcal fungemia appear to have a 6-fold higher risk of subsequently developing IRIS.[21] Some 70% of patients with cryptococcal IRIS did not have a sterile follow-up culture at 2 weeks, 2-times greater than those not developing IRIS.[21] Similarly, those patients with a cryptococcal antigen titer >1:1024 had an increased risk of IRIS.[21] Patients with disseminated TB infection involving both pulmonary and extrapulmonary sites,[27] were 3.5-fold more likely to develop IRIS compared with pulmonary TB alone.[28]

The clearance of antigen following treatment of an infection is a much slower phenomena than microbiologic sterility. For example, in HIV-infected patients with pneumococcal bacteremia, 40% still had detectable pneumococcal c-polysaccharide antigen in their urine at 1 month.[29] Those with higher initial levels of antigen were more likely to have persistence (60% vs 20%). Similarly, mycobacterial DNA persists beyond culture viability by 1–2 months on average and up to 9 months.[19,30] This type of

antigen persistence may explain some cases of later-onset IRIS.

Common Clinical Immune Reconstitution Inflammatory Syndromes

The clinical presentation of an IRIS patient is sometimes quite similar to that of the fundamental opportunistic infection. Increasingly, this blurs the distinction between the relative contributions of a pathogenic infection vs the immune response in contributing to the patient's symptoms. Two of the best-described IRIS-associated infections include tuberculosis and cryptococcal meningitis. Other common IRIS conditions are presented (Table 18.2).

Tuberculosis IRIS

Occasionally, patients with HIV-related TB experience a temporary exacerbation of symptoms, signs or radiographic manifestations of TB after initiating ART and anti-TB treatment. Signs and symptoms are variable in intensity but may include high fever, lymphadenopathy, TB abscesses, expanding central nervous system lesions, and worsening of CXR findings. TB IRIS can be severe with rapid progression, development of respiratory failure, and death occurring within as little time as 10 days.

Anecdotally and in published case series, tuberculosis (TB) is the most common condition to result in IRIS. This is undoubtedly influenced by one-third

Table 18.2 Frequent immune reconstitution inflammatory syndromes

Condition	Clinical features	Laboratory features
CMV	Blurred vision	Vitritis, uveitis
Cryptococcus	Meningitis, mediastinitis	Sterile culture, decreased CRAG, elevated CSF pressure in 50%
Herpes viruses	Classic dermatologic lesions of HSV or VZV of various intensity	PCR positive
Hepatitis B or C	Acute hepatitis Rapid development of cirrhosis Difficult to distinguish from hepatotoxicity	HBV/HCV viral load variable. Increased LFTs
M. avium complex	Lymphadenitis, draining sinuses Pulmonary-thoracic disease Abdominal lymphadenopathy	Granulomatous reaction, paucity of organisms, rare hypercalcemia. Fever 66%. Prior diagnosis 25%
M. tuberculosis	Lymphadenitis, pneumonitis	Paucity of AFB, PCR positive

of the world's population having latent TB infection (LTBI).[31] The retrospective, prevalence rate varies between 8% and 36% for the development of TB IRIS among patients started on ART with previously known active TB disease.[20,28,32] In these patients, excluding resistant TB and therapy failure or non-compliance is crucial. Acid fast bacillus (AFB) cultures should ideally have sterilized, although depending on the acuity of onset of IRIS, this may or may not have occurred. The World Health Organization (WHO) treatment guidelines prioritize TB treatment over HIV therapy to prevent further TB transmission.[33] When clinically possible, the WHO recommends deferring ART therapy until TB treatment is either complete or through the initial 2-month phase of intensive TB therapy.[33] This strategy is meant to minimize side-effects and drug interactions, improve patient compliance, and simplify management of side-effects such as hepatotoxicity.

The incidence of unmasked TB disease among those started on ART without prior active TB is unknown but probably varies with the prevalence of latent TB in the population. Defining the incidence of TB IRIS in patients without active TB is further complicated by the high rates of anergy to tuberculosis skin tests in late stage HIV infection. Extra-pulmonary manifestations of TB are frequently seen in TB-associated IRIS.[17,34,35] Common manifestations and scenarios include: fever (88%), development of new lymphadenopathy (69%), splenic abscess (19%), new arthritis or Pott's disease (19%), worsening of pulmonary symptoms such as cough, or progression of radiologic infiltrates (13%).[22] Notably, the diagnosis of TB IRIS needs to be made in conjunction with the presence of microbiologic susceptible organisms and known adherence to anti-TB medications. Invoking a diagnosis of IRIS, based on treatment failure only is unwise. Depending on the severity of symptoms, patients have done well with observation, non-steroidal anti-inflammatory drugs (NSAIDs), or corticosteroids in retrospective studies and case reports.[17,22,36]

Paradoxical IRIS reactions are thought to be due to restoration of cell-mediated immune responses to mycobacterial antigens. This can be associated with conversion from pretreatment tuberculin skin test (TST) anergy to a positive response following anti-TB treatment.[37] Paradoxical clinically worsening after starting anti-TB therapy can occur even without administration of ART.[38] In HIV-seronegative South Africans with pulmonary TB, additional weight loss and functional deterioration often occurred during the first weeks of anti-TB treatment.[39] In a case series

among HIV-seropositive patients, 7% of those treated for TB clinically worsened without receiving ART.[28]

In persons with TB IRIS-associated clinical deterioration, TNF-α expression temporally increased.[39] The increase in TNF-α was unique as a marker of deterioration since other markers of immune activation including interleukin-2 receptor, interferon-gamma, interleukin-6, and TNF-α receptor all decreased.[39] The increase in TNF-α expression may result from macrophage activation in response to release of mycobacterial cell wall antigens during treatment.[39,40] TNF-α may play a pathogenic role to drive the inflammation that leads to clinical deterioration. Similarly, following anti-TB therapy of HIV-infected patients in Ghana, macrophage activation, as assessed by CD14 expression, increased during the first month of treatment while other markers of inflammation such as C-reactive protein (CRP) and the T-cell activation marker CD25 decreased progressively after the initiation of anti-TB therapy.[40] Immunologic assays, such as the QuantiFeron© test, which quantifies interferon-gamma production in response to M. tuberculosis antigen stimulation, may help elucidate the contribution of T-cell specific immunity to the development of IRIS.

Studies in the pre-HIV era indicated a benefit of corticosteroids in the setting of severe TB infection, such as meningitis, pleural, and pericardial TB.[41] Considering that more than 2 billion people in the world are latently infected with TB, and at least 12 million are co-infected with HIV and TB, the published case-series literature consists of <500 patients with HIV and TB co-infection.[20,22,31,42] Large prospective clinical studies are still needed to define the true incidence, clinical severity, and best treatment approaches for TB-associated IRIS.

Cryptococcal Meningitis IRIS

There have been two retrospective studies of cryptococcal meningitis IRIS conducted among patients in France and Houston, Texas.[21,26] Among 179 patients receiving ART described cumulatively, the incidence of IRIS is reported between 10% and 30%. In cryptococcal IRIS, patients' clinical presentation is identical to what is expected in treatment failure and relapse. In IRIS, a culture-negative meningitis occurs, thought to be triggered by the presence of residual antigen in the CSF. WBC and protein counts in the cerebral spinal fluid (CSF) are also elevated in IRIS but are indistinguishable from what occurs in standard cryptococcal meningitis. The spectrum of cryptococcal disease in IRIS can also be atypical. Lymphadenopathy and mediastinitis have been reported.[43] Cryptococcomas in the brain parenchyma have also been reported.[15,44] In these cases, a paucity of organisms is usually recovered but copious granulomatous inflammation exists.

Of persons with IRIS, 80% will have a CSF WBC cell count <100 cells/μL.[26] The CSF glucose level is usually in the low normal range. In persons with cryptococcal meningitis, increased intracranial pressure (ICP) of >20 cm H_2O is very common. An elevated ICP occurs in 50% of individuals and pressures >35 cm H_2O occur in 25% of individuals.[45] In cases of IRIS, the ICP is equally or even more elevated than with culture positive cryptococcal meningitis. More than 75% of patients with IRIS will have a CSF opening pressure >30 cm H_2O, and the average is 45 cm H_2O.[26]

Obtaining a culture is critical to differentiate treatment failure or relapse from IRIS. In the developing world, where amphotericin B alone (without flucytosine) is often used as treatment, the failure rate is relatively high, at up to 35%. In cases of IRIS, the CSF cryptococcal antigen (CRAG) titer usually decreases dramatically following initiation of anticryptococcal therapy.[21,26] The average level of the CSF CRAG titer in patients with culture positive cryptococcal meningitis is 1:2048. Whereas in culture negative IRIS patients, the CRAG titer averages 1:128 in the CSF.[26,46] In patients with IRIS, 75% will have a CSF CRAG titer ≤1:256, where as in culture positive meningitis 75% of CRAG titers are ≥1:256.[26]

Hepatitis

Hepatitis B virus (HBV) and hepatitis C virus (HCV) co-infection with HIV are common conditions worldwide, especially in Asia or among illicit drug use (IDU) populations. Differentiating between what is hepatotoxicity due to ART vs an IRIS event is difficult. At present, there are no reliable markers to distinguish the two, and hepatitis-associated IRIS is probably under-recognized. The pathogenesis of hepatitis-associated IRIS appears to be immune mediated. As immune reconstitution occurs, the immune system may target hepatitis viruses causing an increase destruction of infected hepatocytes. The spectrum of hepatitis may range from mild asymptomatic disease to fulminant hepatic necrosis and death. Stopping ART is warranted in severe cases. For Hepatitis B, initiation of anti-hepatitis B therapy prior to the initiation of ART may theoretically reduce the risk of IRIS; however even with this strategy, hepatitis IRIS can still occur.[47] The change in

HBV viral load in IRIS is variable: the viral load may be decreased due to improved immunologic control or increased due to fulminant hepatic necrosis.[47,48]

HLA class-II antigen presentation to $CD4^+$ T cells is the basis for host viral defense. In the setting of IRIS, decreasing antigen presentation theoretically would be ideal. Chloroquine has been shown to decrease cell surface HBV antigen presentation *in vitro*.[49] Case reports document severe flares of chronic hepatitis B infection with hepatic insufficiency after discontinuation of chloroquine given for malaria prophylaxis or rheumatoid arthritis therapy.[50] Adjunct chloroquine therapy could potentially be used in patients co-infected with HBV or HCV in the first few weeks after the initiation of ART to prevent IRIS, although this approach has not yet been studied.

Dermatologic IRIS

A wide variety of dermatologic manifestations of IRIS may occur during immune recovery. In a recent case series, dermatologic IRIS conditions were 4-fold more frequently diagnosed than all other IRIS conditions.[51] Some more common dermatologic IRIS conditions include herpes simplex virus (HSV), genital warts, molluscum contagiosum, varicella zoster, and eosinophilic folliculitis.[51,52] Eosinophilic folliculitis anecdotally is a very common skin complaint that occurs after ART. Among dermatology clinic patients on ART, 82% were diagnosed with eosinophilic folliculitis.[52] Of the IRIS dermatologic events, half were new presentations of previously unrecognized infections or conditions.[51] Therapy is targeted at the underlying pathology. For eosinophilic dermatitis, itraconazole has been used for its anti-eosinophilic effect, and topical permethrin has also been used.[53]

Other Common Clinical Scenarios

There is a wide variety of case reports documenting IRIS events in numerous OIs, but few case series. Whether this is because of more sporadic occurrence of the OIs themselves, or whether the incidence of IRIS with other OIs is lower or less severe, is unknown.

Pneumocystis *jiroveci* Pneumonia (PCP)

PCP was perhaps the prototypical condition in which the role of inflammation in the disease process was first elucidated.[54,55] Corticosteroid administration is now part of the standard therapy for persons with Pa_{O2} <70 mmHg.[56] Once ART is started, however, paradoxical reactions characteristic of IRIS can occur with or after a treated PCP infection. Wislezi and colleagues' experience with PCP revealed that those developing paradoxical reactions typically had severe PCP infections with newly identified late-stage HIV infection.[57] After starting ART, some patients subsequently developed PCP IRIS between 7 and 17 days after PCP diagnosis. Patients with PCP IRIS initially responded well to PCP therapy but subsequently, after starting ART, worsened developing high-grade fever and acute respiratory failure. In this case series, patients began ART early after the diagnosis of PCP (1 to 16 days). In such cases, lung pathologic findings and analysis of bronchoalveolar lavage fluid show a severe inflammatory reaction associated with the persistence of only rare *P. jiroveci* cysts. All the patients improved after discontinuation of HAART or steroid re-introduction, or both.

Mycobacterium avium complex

In one case series, 30% of patients with *M. avium* complex (MAC) subsequently developed IRIS upon ART initiation with a cumulative incidence rate of 15 episodes per 100 patient years.[20] MAC accounted for 20% of all IRIS events; however this condition may be overrepresented due to the time period of the study, 1997–2000.[20] The incidence of MAC in North America and Europe has decreased considerably in the ART era; however for persons presenting with CD4 counts <50 cells/μL MAC is still a risk. In a Canadian case series from 1993 through 2004, the cumulative incidence of IRIS among those starting ART with CD4 counts <100 cells/μL or <50 cells/μL was 3.5% and 3.6%, respectively.[58] In the Canadian series, 75% were new diagnoses and 40% were receiving prior MAC prophylaxis. The most common IRIS feature is localized lymphadenitis, usually cervical, abdominal, or mediastinal.[20,36,58] Lymphadenitis occurs in >75% of IRIS events.[20,58] Disseminated disease with positive mycobacterial blood cultures is rare in the setting of IRIS (<10%), except for abdominal disease (25%).[58] Other atypical presentations may include: prolonged fever of unknown origin (FUO), hepatosplenomegaly, abscess, or hypercalcemia. Fever is more common in abdominal or pulmonary disease.[58] In one case series, 2/10 patients with MAC IRIS-associated lymphadenitis also had pronounced hypercalcemia.[20] The hypercalcemia may be caused by unregulated 1,25-hydroxyvitamin D production as part of a granulomatous immune response.

Once again, the most serious differential diagnosis is treatment failure due to the development of drug resistance.[59] To differentiate IRIS from resistance, obtaining tissue for AFB staining, culture, and resistance testing is essential. PCR probes are also commonly used in clinical practice for diagnostic purposes; however, PCR might not distinguish IRIS from persistent infection. Among HIV-seronegative persons treated for TB, 25% have PCR-positive sputum after two and four months of antimycobacterial therapy.[18]

Cytomegalovirus (CMV)

Prior to ART, CMV retinitis occurred principally among HIV-infected patients with <50 CD4+ T cells/μL. With successful ART, anti-CMV therapy typically can be withdrawn safely once CD4 cells rise above 100–150 cells/μL.[11] As the immune system reconstitutes, restored CMV-specific IgG antibody and CD8+ responses are usually protective. Among persons with CMV, the CMV viral load declines in blood when starting ART with the median time to CMV suppression being 3 months (range 1–10 months).[60] However, immune recovery can uncommonly lead to a CMV IRIS. Manifestations of CMV IRIS include uveitis, retinitis, vitritis, cystic macular edema, or papillitis.[61] The most common condition, vitritis, presents with acute onset of visual blurring.[62] The median onset may be quite delayed at near 18 months with a wide range.[61,63] Differentiation of an immune reconstitution retinitis from CMV cytopathic retinitis by ophthalmologic appearance is impossible. CMV IRIS typically resolves with watchful waiting in contrast to viral retinitis. Expert opinion advises screening for subclinical eye disease prior to ART initiation. Whether this approach is truly beneficial is unknown.

Progressive Multifocal Leukoencephalopathy (PML)

ART-induced immune restoration is beneficial for patients with AIDS-related progressive multifocal leukoencephalopathy (PML) and is the primary treatment available. Restoration of JC virus-specific CD4+ T-cell responses are associated with clearance of JC virus from the cerebrospinal fluid.[64] However, in some instances, immune reconstitution may cause paradoxical clinical deterioration and an IRIS event.[65,66] In one case series, 19% of PML cases developed IRIS 21–55 days after ART was initiated.[67] Case reports suggest the CNS lesions in PML IRIS have an acute perivenous leukoencephalitis that are devoid of JC virus by PCR.[65] These IRIS lesions can exist simultaneously with classic PML lesions that have active inflammatory changes with abundant JC virus and perivascular infiltration by CD8+ lymphocytes.[65] While classical PML lesions are non-contrast enhancing on MRI, IRIS lesions are inflammatory and can demonstrate enhancement.[67] Prognosis is poor since ART is the treatment of choice for PML, and stopping of ART would lead to progression of the PML. Corticosteroids do not appear to be of benefit.[65,66]

Autoimmune Diseases

Autoimmune diseases presenting or exacerbating temporally after ART initiation are an uncommon, but recognized phenomena.[1,68] Through 2005, 32 cases have been individually described with sarcoidosis and autoimmune thyroid disease being most common.[69] Among a prospective cohort of 395 HIV-infected patients followed longitudinally at the Cleveland Clinic from 1989 to 2000, a dramatic decline has occurred in autoimmune problems such as reactive arthritis, psoriatic arthritis, and connective tissue disease with ART.[69] Thus while autoimmune IRIS can occur, the immune dysregulation that occurs in advanced HIV is a larger relative risk. ART provides an approximately two-thirds relative risk reduction in the incidence of new autoimmune disease during the first 3–5 years of ART.[69]

Malignancy

Kaposi sarcoma (KS) is an AIDS-defining condition that typically improves with immune reconstitution; however, clinical flares and worsening can occur shortly after starting ART.[70] The timing of onset appears to be similar, within the first 2–3 months of ART. In patients with IRIS, cutaneous KS lesions may initially expand or become painful; visceral KS-associated IRIS may be fatal. Most hematological malignancies such as lymphoma have improved outcome with successful immune reconstitution, but an IRIS syndrome may mimic relapse of a malignancy.[71]

IRIS in resource-limited regions

In the past few years, ART therapy has become much more widely available in many resource-limited regions of the world, including sub-Saharan Africa

and parts of Asia. As a result, IRIS is emerging as an important complication of HIV therapy in resource-limited regions. Because of the limited availability of antiretroviral medications, often only patients with the most advanced disease are treated, and these patients are at risk for developing IRIS. Patients in resource-poor regions are at particularly high risk because of the high prevalence of infections that are associated with IRIS, including tuberculosis, cryptococcal meningitis, and hepatitis B. As antiretroviral medications continue to be introduced into resource poor regions, we should expect that the incidence of IRIS will increase. It is important to perform clinical research in these regions to determine the magnitude of the IRIS problem and to identify the best evidence-based management strategies.

Treatment of Immune Reconstitution Inflammatory Syndrome

No randomized controlled trials have evaluated treatment of IRIS. Anecdotal experiences have used different therapeutic strategies depending on the severity of disease (Table 18.3). For mild cases, observation alone with close clinical and appropriate laboratory monitoring may suffice. For moderate cases of inflammation, non-steroidal anti-inflammatory drugs (NSAIDs) have been effective at successfully ameliorating symptoms.[15,20,21] For severe cases, several strategies have been employed. Corticosteroids, such as dexamethasone, have been utilized.[15,20] For IRIS induced lymphadenopathy, such as is common with TB IRIS, debulking the antigenic burden via lymph node drainage may be a viable diagnostic and therapeutic approach.[20,36] In episodes of culture negative cryptococcal meningitis IRIS, a combination of mechanical drainage via repeat

Table 18.3 Treatment strategies for IRIS

Clinical severity	Treatment options
Mild	Observation
Moderate	NSAIDs
Severe	Corticosteroids Temporary cessation of ART Surgical debulking
Potential alternative strategies	Chloroquine Thalidomide Leflunomide

No treatment has been prospectively studied in immune reconstitution inflammatory syndrome patients.

lumbar punctures for alleviation of elevated intra-cranial pressure and corticosteroids have been used.[26]

Reports in the literature show that corticosteroids have been used to treat IRIS, but there have been no randomized controlled trials. As well, there have been some difficulties in interpreting the reported studies. For example, in one series, 5/8 persons with MAC-associated IRIS experienced relapse when ste-roids were tapered or stopped.[51] Although the WHO has recommended prednisone (1–2 mg/kg for 1–2 weeks, then gradually decreasing doses) for TB IRIS when severe paradoxical reactions occur, they also indicate there is no evidence for this.[31]

The concept of prophylaxis to prevent IRIS is purely speculative at present. However, if the inci-dence of IRIS for common opportunistic infections, such as TB, is prospectively found to be in the range of 10–30%, prophylaxis during the first 3–6 months of ART is an obvious next step. A prophylactic agent would need to have the necessary properties of being an anti-inflammatory with excellent tolerability and without any drug–drug interactions so as not to interfere with ART compliance or effectiveness.

Alternative Therapies and Future Possibilities

Alternative therapeutic approaches include the use of thalidomide, chloroquine, or leflunomide for treating IRIS. Experience with these agents as treat-ment for IRIS is negligible, and further investigation is warranted; however, each agent has properties making them an attractive potential alternative to the side-effects of corticosteroids.

Thalidomide

Thalidomide (α-N-phthal-imidoglutarimide) attenu-ates TNF-α induced NF-kappa-β activation.[72] Previ-ously, thalidomide has been used for the treatment of HIV-associated aphthous ulcers and wasting syn-drome.[73,74] In persons with CD4 counts of 200 500 cells/μL, thalidomide doses of 150 mg daily were well tolerated.[75] In combination with dexametha-sone, thalidomide decreases expression of TNF-α, TGF-β, IL-1β.[76] Pentoxifylline also has anti-TNF activ-ity and could be a potential therapy for IRIS through similar mechanisms.[77]

Chloroquine

Chloroquine's mechanism of action is as a weak base that accumulates in intracellular vesicles, raising their pH and affecting the activity of enzymes involved in the endosomal processing pathway for post-translational protein modification. The result of this is multi-factorial. First, post-translation protein misfolding occurs resulting in decreased infectious virus production. This has been shown with HIV and HBV in *in vitro* and *in vivo* models.[78,79] Second, cytokines, which are also proteins, that mediate inflammation such as TNF-α, interleukin-1 (IL-1), IL-6, and IL-12 are also reduced.[80,81] Third, for fungal organisms, such as histoplasmosis and cryptococ-cus, the elevated intracellular pH is hostile and *in vitro* appears to interfere with normal pathogenesis of the organisms and results in increased immune system killing. Furthermore, chloroquine is concen-trated intracellularly and in lymphatic tissues.

Leflunomide

Leflunomide is a novel immunosuppressant used for rheumatoid arthritis that blocks nuclear factor kappa B (NF-KB) induced cellular activation. NF-KB is a transcription factor activated in response to inflammatory stimuli and its induced expression is a rate limiting step for cellular activation and nuclear transcription.[82] Leflunomide decreases HIV replication by 75% *in vitro* and decreases the expres-sion of the cytokines TNF-α and IL-1 as well as the expression of the cell surface molecules CD4 and CCR5.[83] An ongoing NIH trial is evaluating lefluno-mide's anti-HIV efficacy.[84] This agent may have the advantage of inhibiting HIV as well as preventing IRIS.

Immunomodulatory aspects of each of these med-ications make them potential agents for use in either preventing or treating IRIS. In particular, chloro-quine's 60-year safety record, pharmacokinetics, affordability, and worldwide availability make chlo-roquine a particularly viable candidate for future investigation in the treatment and prophylaxis of IRIS. Thalidomide's history as a well known terato-gen will likely limit investigation into its use and limit its applications in women.

Limitations of Current Knowledge

There are several significant limitations that temper one's ability to interpret the present published litera-ture from the first decade of experience with ART. The largest limitation is that all of the data to date regarding IRIS are retrospective. There are ongoing prospective studies; however at present, many inher-ent biases exist for interpretation of existing data. First, there is an information bias in extracting patient data retrospectively. Second, there is a selection bias for inclusion in the case series. For example, most studies excluded patients lost to follow-up. In the largest series, 17% were lost to follow-up.[20] Third, the decision to initiate ART during the time period of these studies (1996 to ≈ 2000–2002) is an unknown confounder. Present US guidelines do not recommend ART typically among those with CD4 >350 cells/μL; however in the time period for these studies' data collection, more patients were given therapy. Among the French cryptococcal experience, 50% were excluded either due to unknown HIV status or not receiving ART.[21] Fourth, almost all of the published experience exists in developed countries where <10% of the world's burden of HIV infection exists. How applicable this IRIS experience is to resource-limited countries is unknown.

Conclusion

IRIS is a newly recognized complication of HIV ART. Two common clinical scenarios occur. First, ART may unmask pre-existing subclinical disease. This is best termed 'immune reconstitution disease'. Second, a successfully treated opportunistic infection may have a paradoxical clinical recrudescence in the presence of sterile microbiologic cultures, a phenomenon known as 'immune reconstitution syndrome'. In this scenario, the inflammation following immune recovery targets non-infectious residual antigens that persist following a prior treated infection. The onset of IRIS is variable. Most, but not all cases occur within the first 12 weeks of initiating ART. The true incidence of IRIS is unknown, but IRIS appears to be an emerging issue in HIV therapy, especially in resource-limited regions. Optimal timing for the initiation of ART after the diagnosis of an opportunistic infection is unknown. Limited retrospective data suggests early initiation of ART within 2 months of an opportunistic infection may increase the risk of IRIS up to 6-fold; however, this degree of risk has not been found in all studies. The best approaches to treatment of IRIS are also unknown, but anti-inflammatory agents or corticosteroids are the anecdotal cornerstones of therapy.

References

1. French MA, Price P, Stone SF. Immune restoration disease after antiretroviral therapy. AIDS 2004; 18:1615–1627.
2. Perelson AS, Neuman AU, Markowitz M, et al. HIV-1 dynamics in vivo: virion clearance rate, infected cell life-span, and viral generation time. Science 1996; 271:1582–1586.
3. Ogg GS, Jin X, Bonhoeffer S, et al. Quantitation of HIV-1-specific cytotoxic T lymphocytes and plasma load of viral RNA. Science 1998; 279:2103–2106.
4. Schacker TW, Nguyen PL, Martinez E, et al. Persistent abnormalities in lymphoid tissues of human immunodeficiency virus-infected patients successfully treated with highly active antiretroviral therapy. J Infect Dis 2002; 186:1092–1097.
5. Schacker TW, Reilly C, Beilman GJ, et al. Amount of lymphatic tissue fibrosis in HIV infection predicts magnitude of HAART-associated change in peripheral CD4 cell count. AIDS 2005; 19:2169–2171.
6. Connick E, Lederman MM, Kotzin BL, et al. Immune reconstitution in the first year of potent antiretroviral therapy and its relationship to virologic response. J Infect Dis 2000; 181:358–363.
7. Landay AL, Bettendorf D, Chan E, et al. Evidence of immune reconstitution in antiretroviral drug experienced patients with advanced HIV disease. AIDS Res Hum Retroviruses 2002; 18:95–102.
8. Al-Harthi L, Voris J, Patterson BK, et al. Evaluation of the impact of highly active antiretroviral therapy on immune recovery in antiretroviral naive patients. HIV Med 2004; 5:55–65.
9. El-Sadr WM, Burman WJ, Grant LB, et al. Discontinuation of prophylaxis for Mycobacterium avium complex disease in HIV-infected patients who have a response to antiretroviral therapy. Terry Beirn Community Programs for Clinical Research on AIDS. N Engl J Med 2000; 342:1085–1092.
10. Furrer H, Egger M, Opravil M, et al. Discontinuation of primary prophylaxis against Pneumocystis carinii pneumonia in HIV-1-infected adults treated with combination antiretroviral therapy. Swiss HIV Cohort Study N Engl J Med 1999; 340:1301–1306.
11. Tural C, Romeu J, Sirera G, et al. Long-lasting remission of cytomegalovirus retinitis without maintenance therapy in human immunodeficiency virus-infected patients. J Infect Dis 1998; 177:1080–1083.
12. Vibhagool A, Sungkanuparph S, Mootsikapun P, et al. Discontinuation of secondary prophylaxis for cryptococcal meningitis in human immunodeficiency virus-infected patients treated with highly active antiretroviral therapy: a prospective, multicenter, randomized study. Clin Infect Dis 2003; 36:1329–1331.
13. Sousa AE, Carneiro J, Meier-Schellersheim M, et al. CD4 T cell depletion is linked directly to immune activation in the pathogenesis of HIV-1 and HIV-2 but only indirectly to the viral load. J Immunol 2002; 169:3400–3406.
14. Hoffman C, Horst H-A, Albrecht H, et al. Progressive multifocal leukoencephalopathy with unusual inflammatory response during antiretroviral therapy. J Neurol Neurosurg Psychiatry 2003; 74:1142–1144.
15. York J, Bodi I, Reeves I, et al. Raised intracranial pressure complicating cryptococcal meningitis: immune reconstitution inflammatory syndrome or recurrent cryptococcal disease. J Inf 2005; 51:165–171.
16. Stone SF, Price P, French MA. Immune restoration disease: a consequence of dysregulated immune responses after HAART. Curr HIV Res 2004; 2:235–242.
17. Shelburne SA. III, Hamill RJ, Rodriguez-Barradas MC et al., Immune reconstitution inflammatory syndrome: emergence of a unique syndrome during highly active antiretroviral therapy. Medicine (Baltimore) 2002; 81:213–227.
18. Velayati AA, Bakayev VV, Bahrmand AR. Use of PCR and culture for detection of Mycobacterium tuberculosis in specimens from patients with normal and slow responses to chemotherapy. Scand J Infect Dis 2002; 34:163–166.
19. Kennedy N, Gillespie SH, Saruni AO, et al. Polymerase chain reaction for assessing treatment response in patients with pulmonary tuberculosis. J Infect Dis 1994; 170:713–716.
20. Shelburne SA, Visnegarwala F, Darcourt J, et al. Incidence and risk factors for immune reconstitution inflammatory

syndrome during highly active antiretroviral therapy. AIDS 2005; 19:399–406.

21. Lortholary O, Fontanet A, Memain N, et al. Incidence and risk factors of immune reconstitution inflammatory syndrome complicating HIV-associated cryptococcosis in France. AIDS 2005; 19:1043–1049.

22. Breton G, Duval X, Estellat C, et al. Determinants of immune reconstitution inflammatory syndrome in HIV type 1-infected patients with tuberculosis after initiation of antiretroviral therapy. Clin Inf Dis 2004; 39:1709–1712.

23. Olalla J, Pulido F, Rubio R, et al. Paradoxical responses in a cohort of HIV-1-infected patients with mycobacterial disease. Int J Tuberc Lung Dis 2002; 6:71–75.

24. Price P, Morahan G, Huang D, et al. Polymorphisms in cytokine genes define subpopulations of HIV-1 patients who experienced immune restoration diseases. AIDS 2002; 16:2043–2047.

25. Barry SM, Lipman MC, Deery AR, et al. Immune reconstitution pneumonitis following Pneumocystis carinii pneumonia in HIV-infected subjects. HIV Med 2002; 3:207–211.

26. Shelburne SA, Darcourt J, White CA, et al. The Role of Immune Reconstitution Inflammatory Syndrome in AIDS-related Cryptococcus neoformans disease in the era of highly active antiretroviral therapy. Clin Inf Dis 2005; 40:1049–1053.

27. McCormack JG. Miliary tuberculosis with paradoxical expansion of intracranial tuberculomas complicating HIV infection in a patient receiving highly active antiretroviral therapy. Clin Infec Dis 1998; 26:1008–1009.

28. Wendel KA, Alwood KS, Gachuhi R, et al. Paradoxical worsening of tuberculosis in HIV-infected persons. Chest 2001; 120:193–197.

29. Boulware DR, Merrifield C, Daley CL, et al. Rapid diagnosis of Streptococcus pneumoniae infection among HIV-infected adults by urine antigen detection and CRP. Unpublished data.

30. Moore DF, Curry JI, Knott CA, et al. Amplification of rRNA for assessment of treatment response of pulmonary tuberculosis patients during antimicrobial therapy. J Clin Microbiol 1996; 34:1745–1749.

31. WHO. Global Plan to Stop TB. Geneva: World Health Organization; 2001.

32. Narita M, Ashkin D, Hollender ES, et al. Paradoxical worsening of tuberculosis following antiretroviral therapy in patients with AIDS. Am J Respir Crit Care Med 1998; 158:157–161.

33. WHO. Treatment of tuberculosis: guidelines for national programmes (WHO/CDS/TB/2003.313). Geneva: World Health Organization; 2003.

34. Race EM, Adelson-Mitty J, Kriegel GR, et al. Focal mycobacterial lymphadenitis following initiation of protease-inhibitor therapy in patients with advanced HIV-1 disease. Lancet 1998; 351:252–255.

35. Hirsch HH, Kaufmann G, Sendi P, et al. Immune reconstitution in HIV-infected patients. Clin Infect Dis 2004; 38:1159–1166.

36. Lawn SD, Bekker LG, Miller RF. Immune reconstitution disease associated with mycobacterial infections in HIV-infected individuals receiving antiretrovirals. Lancet Infect Dis 2005; 5:361–373.

37. Markman M, Eagleton LE. Paradoxical clinical improvement and radiographic deterioration in anergic patients treated for far advanced tuberculosis. N Engl J Med 1981; 305:167.

38. Chien JW, Johnson JL. Paradoxical reactions in HIV and pulmonary TB. Chest 1998; 114:933–936.

39. Bekker LG, Maartens G, Steyn L, et al. Selective increase in plasma tumor necrosis factor-alpha and concomitant clinical deterioration after initiating therapy in patients with severe tuberculosis. J Infect Dis 1998; 178:580–584.

40. Lawn SD, Labeta MO, Arias M, et al. Elevated serum concentrations of soluble CD14 in HIV- and HIV+ patients with tuberculosis in Africa: prolonged elevation during anti-tuberculosis treatment. Clin Exp Immunol 2000; 120:483–487.

41. Alzeer AH, Fitzgerald JM. Corticosteroids and tuberculosis: risks and use as adjunct therapy. Tubercle Lung Dis 1993; 74:6–11.

42. Kumarasamy N, Chaguturu S, Mayer KH, et al. Incidence of immune reconstitution syndrome in HIV/tuberculosis co-infected patients after initiation of generic antiretroviral therapy in India. J AIDS 2004; 37:1574–1577.

43. Trevenzoli M, Cattelan AM, Rea F, et al. Mediastinitis due to cryptococcal infection: a new clinical entity in the HAART era. J Infect 2002; 45:173–179.

44. Cattelan AM, Trevenzoli M, Sasset L, et al. Multiple cerebral cryptococcomas associated with immune reconstitution in HIV-1 infection. AIDS 2004; 18:349–351.

45. Graybill JR, Sobel J, Saag M, et al. Cerebrospinal fluid hypertension patients with AIDS and cryptococcal meningitis. 37th Interscience Conference on Antimicrobial Agents and Chemotherapy, Toronto, ON, Canada: 1997; Washington, DC: American Society for Microbiology; 1997.

46. Sobel JD. Practice guidelines for the treatment of fungal infections. Clin Infect Dis 2000; 30:652.

47. Drake A, Mijch A, Sasadeusz J. Immune reconstitution hepatitis in HIV and hepatitis B coinfection, despite lamivudine therapy as part of HAART. Clin Infect Dis 2004; 39:129–132.

48. Perrillo R. Acute flares in chronic Hepatitis B: the natural and unnatural history of an immunologically mediated liver disease. Gastroenterology 2001; 120:1009–1022.

49. Penna A, Fowler P, Bertoletti A, et al. Hepatitis B virus (HBV)-specific cytotoxic T-cell (CTL) response in humans: characterization of HLA class II-restricted CTLs that recognize endogenously synthesized HBV envelope antigens. J Virol 1992; 66:1193–1198.

50. Helbling B, Reichen J. Reactivation of hepatitis B following withdrawal of chloroquine. Schweiz Med Wochenschr 1994; 124:759–762.

51. Ratnam I, Chiu C, Kandala NB, et al. Incidence and risk factors for immune reconstitution inflammatory syndrome in an ethnically diverse HIV type 1-infected cohort. Clin Infect Dis 2006; 42:418–427.

52. Rajendran PM, Dolev JC, Heaphy MR Jr, et al. Eosinophilic folliculitis: before and after the introduction of antiretroviral therapy. Arch Derm 2005; 141:1227–1231.

53. Maurer TA. Dermatologic manifestations of HIV infection. Top HIV Med 2005; 13:149–154.

54. Gagnon S, Boota AM, Fischl MA, et al. Corticosteroids as adjunctive therapy for severe Pneumocystis carinii pneumonia in the acquired immunodeficiency syndrome. A double-blind, placebo-controlled trial. N Engl J Med 1990; 323:1444–1450.

55. Dean GL, Williams DI, Churchill DR, et al. Transient clinical deterioration in HIV patients with Pneumocystis carinii Pneumonia after starting highly active antiretroviral therapy: Another case of immune restoration inflammatory syndrome. Am J Respir Crit Care Med 2002; 165:1670–1670.

56. Wachter RM, Luce JM. Respiratory failure from severe Pneumocystis carinii pneumonia: entering the third era. Chest 1994; 106:1313–1315.

57. Wislez M, Bergot E, Antoine M, et al. Acute respiratory failure following HAART introduction in patients treated for Pneumocystis carinii pneumonia. Am J Respir Crit Care Med 2001; 164:847–851.

58. Phillips P, Bonner S, Gataric N, et al. Nontuberculous Mycobacterial immune reconstitution syndrome in HIV-infected patients: spectrum of disease and long term follow-up. Clin Inf Dis 2005; 41:1483–1497.

59. Heifets L. Susceptibility testing of mycobacterium avium complex isolates. Antimicrob Agents Chemother 1996; 40:1759–1767.

60. Deayton J, Mocroft A, Wilson P, et al. Loss of cytomegalovirus (CMV) viraemia following highly active antiretroviral therapy in the absence of specific anti-CMV therapy. AIDS 1999; 13:1203–1206.

61. Cassoux N, Lumbroso L, Bodaghi B, et al. Cystoid macular oedema and cytomegalovirus retinitis in patients with HIV disease treated with highly active antiretroviral therapy. Br J Ophthalmol 1999; 83:47–49.

62. Deayton JR, Wilson P, Sabin CA, et al. Changes in the natural history of cytomegalovirus retinitis following the introduction of highly active antiretroviral therapy. AIDS 2000; 14:1163–1170.

63. Lin DY, Warren JF, Lazzeroni LC, et al. Cytomegalovirus retinitis after initiation of highly active antiretroviral therapy in HIV infected patients: natural history and clinical predictors. Retina 2002; 22:268–277.

64. Gasnault J, Kahraman M, de Goer Herve MG, et al. Critical role of JC virus-specific CD4 T-cell responses in preventing progressive multifocal leukoencephalopathy. AIDS 2003; 17:1443–1449.

65. Vendrely A, Bienvenu B, Gasnault J, et al. Fulminant inflammatory leukoencephalopathy associated with HAART-induced immune restoration in AIDS-related progressive multifocal leukoencephalopathy. Acta Neuropathol 2005; 109:449–455.

66. Silva MT, Pacheco MC Jr, Vaz B. Inflammatory progressive multifocal leukoencephalopathy after antiretroviral treatment. AIDS 2006; 20:469–471.

67. Cinque P, Bossolasco S, Brambilla AM, et al. The effect of highly active antiretroviral therapy-induced immune reconstitution on development and outcome of progressive multifocal leukoencephalopathy: study of 43 cases with review of the literature. J Neurovirol 2003; 9:73–80.

68. Viani RM. Sarcoidosis and interstitial nephritis in a child with acquired immunodeficiency syndrome: implications of immune reconstitution syndrome with an indinavir-based regimen. Pediatr Infect Dis J 2002; 21:435–438.

69. Calabrese LH, Kirchner E, Shrestha R. Rheumatic complications of human immunodeficiency virus infection in the era of highly active antiretroviral therapy: emergence of a new syndrome of immune reconstitution and changing patterns of disease. Semin Arthritis Rheum 2005; 35:166–174.

70. Leidner RS, Aboulafia DM. Recrudescent Kaposi's sarcoma after initiation of HAART: a manifestation of immune reconstitution syndrome. AIDS Patient Care Stds 2005; 19:635–644.

71. Robertson P, Scadden DT. Immune reconstitution in HIV infection and its relationship to cancer. Hematol Oncol Clin North Am 2003; 17:703–716.

72. Yagyu T, Kobayashi H, Matsuzaki H, et al. Thalidomide inhibits tumor necrosis factor-alpha-induced interleukin-8 expression in endometriotic stromal cells, possibly through suppression of nuclear factor-kappa? activation. J Clin Endocrinol Metab 2005; 90:3017–3021.

73. Jacobson JM, Greenspan JS, Spritzler J, et al. Thalidomide for the treatment of oral aphthous ulcers in patients with human immunodeficiency virus infection. N Engl J Med 1997; 336:1487–1493.

74. Reyes-Teran G, Sierra-Madero JG, del Martinez Cerro V, et al. Effects of thalidomide on HIV-associated wasting syndrome: a randomized, double-blind, placebo-controlled clinical trial. AIDS 1996; 10:1501–1507.

75. Wohl DA, Aweeka FT, Schmitz J, et al. Safety, tolerability, and pharmacokinetic effects of thalidomide in patients infected with human immunodeficiency virus: AIDS Clinical Trials Group 267. J Infect Dis 2002; 185: 1359–1363.

76. Hatjiharissi E, Terpos E, Papaioannou M, et al. The combination of intermediate doses of thalidomide and dexamethasone reduces bone marrow micro-vessel density but not serum levels of angiogenic cytokines in patients with refractory/relapsed multiple myeloma. Hematol Oncol 2004; 22:159–168.

77. Lima V, Brito GA, Cunha FQ, et al. Effects of the tumour necrosis factor-alpha inhibitors pentoxifylline and thalidomide in short-term experimental oral mucositis in hamsters. Eur J Oral Sci 2005; 113:210–217.

78. Tsai WP, Nara PL, Kung HF, et al. Inhibition of human immunodeficiency virus infectivity by chloroquine. AIDS Res Hum Retrovir 1990; 6:481–489.

79. Savarino A, Gennero L, Sperber K, et al. The anti-HIV-1 activity of chloroquine. J Clin Virol 2001; 20:131–135.

80. Rayne F, Vendeville A, Bonhoure A, et al. The ability of chloroquine to prevent tat-induced cytokine secretion by monocytes is implicated in its in vivo anti-HIV-1 activity. J Virol 2004; 78:12054–12057.

81. Hong Z, Jiang Z, Liangxi W, et al. Chloroquine protects mice from challenge with CpG ODN and LPS by decreasing proinflammatory cytokine release. Int Immunopharmacol 2004; 4:223–234.

82. Manna SK, Aggarwal BB. Immunosuppressive leflunomide metabolite (A77 1726_ blocks TN-dependent nuclear factor-KB activation and gene expression. J Immunol 1999; 162:2095–2102.

83. Schlapfer E, Fischer M, Ott P, et al. Anti-HIV-1 activity of leflunomide: a comparison with mycophenolic acid and hydroxyurea. AIDS 2003; 17:1613–1620.

84. National Institute of Allergy and Infectious Diseases. Effect of leflunomide on T cell proliferation in HIV-infected patients. Online. Available: ClinicalTrials.gov identifier, NCT00101374.

85. de Boer MGJ, Kroon FP, Kauffman RH, Vriesendorp R. Immune restoration in HIV-infected individuals receiving highly active antiretroviral therapy: clinical and immunological characteristics. Netherlands J Med 2003; 61:408–412.

CHAPTER 19

Adherence to HIV Antiretroviral Therapy in Resource-limited Settings

Jayne Byakika-Tusiime
Catherine Orrell
David Bangsberg

Introduction

The Joint United Nations Programme on HIV/AIDS (UNAIDS) estimates that 39.4 million people are living with the human immunodeficiency virus (HIV). Some 90% of these are from developing countries. Sub-Saharan Africa is the worst affected region with 25.4 million people infected.[1] Nearly 6 million people worldwide are in need of treatment but <10% of these were receiving treatment as of June 2004.[2] Lack of access to HIV treatment is a global health emergency that is being handled by several global organizations and funding bodies. Increases in international financial support and a decrease in the cost of treatment and monitoring tests have improved access to therapy.

While expanding access to HIV/AIDS treatment to resource-limited settings is recognized as a global health priority, there is concern that widespread antiretroviral use could lead to widespread drug resistance.[3–5] Data from the developed world indicates that up to 10% of incident infections and 50% of prevalent infections carry resistant virus,[6,7] which compromises treatment response.[8] Limiting drug resistance is especially important in resource-limited settings where there are limited options for second-line regimens.

Suboptimal adherence leading to incomplete viral suppression is the primary predictor of drug resistance.[9–11] Some have suggested that extreme poverty in resource-limited settings will lead to suboptimal adherence and the global transmission of drug resistant virus.[12] This chapter reviews the levels and barriers of adherence to antiretroviral therapy as they pertain to resource-limited settings.

Levels of Adherence in Resource-rich Settings

Most of our understanding of adherence to HIV antiretroviral therapy comes from studies in resource-rich settings. While adherence to early single protease inhibitor regimens available in 1996 required >95% adherence for reliable viral suppression,[13] most populations studied fall short of this goal. Suboptimal adherence rates have been reported in: a large multicenter clinical trial (85% adherence by self-report);[14] patients from a veterans and university hospital (75% by electronic medication monitoring);[13] among the marginally housed (73% by pill count, 67% by electronic medication monitoring);[15] among those with serious mental illness (66% by electronic medication monitoring);[16] among predominately minority women (64% by electronic medication monitoring);[17] and among inner-city residents with a history of injection drug use (80% by pill count, 53% by electronic medication monitoring).[18,19] While many of the studies in the USA are in populations with significant barriers to adherence, studies in broader populations in Canada and Europe report similar rates of adherence,[20,21] with one exception.[22]

In all, average adherence to antiretroviral therapy, using the best measures is approximately 70%[23] and declines over time[15,24] in resource-rich countries.

Predictors of Adherence in Resource-rich Settings

A number of factors have been associated with non-adherence to ART in resource-rich settings. Predictors of adherence may be related to the patient, regimen, disease, and health care setting/provider characteristics.[25,26]

Patient-related psychosocial determinants are better predictors of adherence than demographic determinants. These include psychiatric morbidity (particularly depression), active drug or alcohol use, stressful life events, lack of social support, and poor health literacy.[27-29] Studies report conflicting evidence about the association between sociodemographic factors and adherence behavior. When an association is found, the direction is towards lower levels of adherence with younger age, non-white race/ethnicity, and lower income, which may be due to uncontrolled confounding by other factors. Gender, educational level, insurance status, and HIV risk factors generally are not associated with adherence behavior.[24,27,29,30]

Factors related to the treatment regimen include the number of pills prescribed, the complexity of the regimen (dosing frequency and food restrictions), the specific type of antiretroviral drugs, and the short and long-term medication side-effects. Greater regimen complexity (dosing frequency and food instructions), pill burden and side-effects are associated with non-adherence.[31,32] Once-daily regimens may improve adherence behavior, but this has not yet been adequately examined. Other studies report that the 'fit' of the regimen into an individual's daily routine is another important determinant of adherence.[33,34]

Disease-related predictors include: stage and duration of HIV infection. A few studies describe a relationship between HIV-related symptoms and non-adherence.[35-37] Other studies describe an association between a lower CD4 count and non-adherence, although this finding is seen less consistently across studies.[27,28,35,38] Two studies describe increased adherence in those with a history of opportunistic infections.[39,40] The authors postulate that experience with illness increases the motivation to adhere.

Provider-related determinants include a trusting provider-patient relationship[41,42] and provider experience.[43] Ease of access to medication refills, presence of a social worker, and availability of afternoon clinics have been associated with good adherence.[44] Aspects of the clinical setting that may influence adherence include access to ongoing primary care, involvement in a dedicated adherence program, availability of transportation and child care, pleasantness of the clinical environment, convenience in scheduling appointments, perceived confidentiality, and satisfaction with past experiences in the health care system. Dissatisfaction with prior experience in the health care system has been associated with non-adherence.[34] While several provider and health system factors are associated with good adherence, individual providers have rarely preformed better than random at predicting individual adherence behavior.[27,45-47]

Levels of Adherence in Resource-limited Settings

Several groups voiced concerns about the ability of patients in resource-limited settings to maintain the high level of adherence required to obtain adequate viral suppression and hence prevent the emergence of resistant strains of the virus.[4,5,48] Some have suggested that extreme poverty will be associated with poor adherence.[49] Others have argued that comprehensive adherence programs should be in place prior to expanding antiretroviral access in developing countries.[50,51]

Contrary to early concerns, adherence in developing countries has been found to be generally better than adherence in developed countries. Most studies done in resource-limited settings have found adherence levels of greater than 90% with the majority of them from sub-Saharan Africa.[52-67] Orrell found that 48-week clinic-based pill count adherence was 93.5% in 289 individuals attending a public hospital HIV clinic and receiving free ART through Phase III studies.[53] In a cohort of Senegalese adults, mean adherence was 91% by clinic-based pill count and self-report.[57] In a 12-week study of 34 ART-naive, HIV-positive Ugandans purchasing therapy, mean adherence as measured by electronic medication monitoring caps, home-based unannounced pill count, and patient report ranged from 91–94%.[52] Similarly, Byakika and co-workers found 97.3–99.8% unannounced pill count adherence in individuals receiving free therapy in the Mother to Child Transmission Program in Kampala, Uganda.[65] A multi-center trial of 60 ARV naive patients in Cameroon to determine the effectiveness and safety of a generic fixed dose combination of nevirapine, stavudine and lamivudine documented a mean self reported adherence of 99%[60] and confirmed by antiretroviral drug level concentrations.

The remaining studies done in sub-Saharan Africa rely on patient-reported measures of adherence. These studies generally find levels of patient-reported adherence comparable to resource-rich settings. Laurent et al, in a cohort of Senegalese HIV-infected adults followed for a median of 30 months, reported good adherence (80–90%) linked with comparably good biologic and clinical outcomes.[57] In a prospective one-arm trial to determine the effectiveness of once-a-day HAART in 40 treatment-naive Senegalese adults, 95% of the patients reported taking all their tablets in the previous 3 days.[64] In a prospective observational study in Senegal among 58 treatment naive patients, 87.9% of the participants reported >80% adherence, however, only those who had the capacity to adhere to ART and contribute to the subsidized treatment, according to a social survey, were included in the study. In spite of the generally good adherence, the general trend was declining adherence with time.[68] In a study of 7812 HIV-infected South Africans enrolled in a private sector HIV/AIDS disease management program, adherence to ART was >70% for 3908 patients.[69] In a study of 66 patients at an adult clinic in Soweto, South Africa, 88% of the patients reported >95% adherence.[54] A cross-sectional study of 304 self-paying patients in Kampala, Uganda, found >95% adherence in 68% of the patients measured by self-report.[56] Results of the assessment of the first national program to provide ART in Uganda showed that patients took their drugs 'about as prescribed' in 88% instances.[63] In a randomized controlled trial in Mombasa, Kenya to determine the efficacy and acceptability of an alarm device for improving medication compliance among women in resource-limited countries, 66% of women reported >95% compliance.[70] One of the few studies to find levels of adherence comparable with resource-rich settings was a cross-sectional study of 109 self-paying patients on ART in Botswana, where only 54% of the patients reported >95% adherence.[58] Similarly, Akam reported 68% of doses taken in Cameroon.

Studies in resource-limited settings outside Africa also find levels of adherence generally equivalent to or better than resource-rich settings. In a 50-month study of 182 HIV-infected Brazilians receiving free ART, Brigido and co-workers found that only 41% of the patients had optimal adherence by self-report over 30 days.[62] However, Remien and his co-workers, found that 82% of 200 individuals on free ART in public health care systems in Rio de Janeiro[71] reported >90% adherence.[72] In a retrospective study of 161 Chinese HIV-infected patients who had been on ART for at least 1 year, over 95% of the patients reported taking more than 95% of their medications.[67] In a cross-sectional study of 310 HIV positive patients on ART in India, mean 4-day adherence for those paying for therapy was 96.4%, while that of patients receiving free therapy was 80.5%.[66]

In addition to chronic treatment for symptomatic disease, short-course antiretroviral therapy to prevent maternal-to-child transmission is an important part of antiretroviral therapy delivery in resource-limited countries. In a randomized clinical trial in Kenya to study compliance with antiretroviral regimens to prevent perinatal HIV-1 transmission, 86% of the participants reported taking at least 80% of the antepartum doses of the Thai-CDC regimen although only 44% reported taking at least 80% of the expected intrapartum doses. A total of 91% of the women reported taking the maternal dose before delivery and 97% reported giving the infant dose.[73]

Barriers to Adherence in Resource-limited Settings

Many of the barriers associated with non-adherence in resource-rich settings also apply to resource-limited settings. These include frequency of dosing,[53] younger age,[53,66] being single,[56] depression,[66] male gender,[54] forgetfulness,[58,62,67] being too busy or away from home,[58,67] regimen complexity,[54] psychosocial factors,[67] intolerance, alcohol consumption and lack of belief in efficacy of ART.[62] Nonetheless, there are many additional barriers that are unique to resource-limited settings such as the cost of medication, long distance to the treatment centers, stigma, medication stock outs, and speaking a different language from the health care providers.

The cost of antiretroviral medications is the most frequently cited barrier to adherence in resource-limited settings.[54–56,58] Even with the recent great cost reductions in drug prices many patients cannot sustain self-pay therapy. Until recently, there were very few HIV/AIDS treatment centers in resource-limited settings. Patients travel long distances to the few available centers and incur substantial cost during transport to clinic or pharmacy. Individuals on fully subsidized therapy face financial barriers in transport to clinic or pharmacy required to maintain therapy. Weiser and co-workers in Botswana and Brigido and co-workers in Brazil found that distance to clinic was associated with non-adherence.[58,62] In Botswana, non-adherence due to difficulties in transport and difficulty paying for medication lead to large gaps in treatment rather than day-to-day missed doses.[58] If cost was removed as a barrier adherence, the proportion of adherent individuals in Bostwana increased from 54% to 74%. Byakika-Tusiime and co-workers found that inability to purchase therapy was the most significant predictor of incomplete adherence.[56] Those earning <US$50/month on self-pay therapy were almost three times more likely, than greater income levels, to achieve <95% adherence. In the Soweto study, self-paying patients were on dual therapy because they could not afford the recommended triple therapy.[54] In the Senegalese cohort, adherence rose from 83% to 93% when the cost of the drugs was reduced.[55] Van Oosterhout and co-workers found drug shortage in the hospital and financial constraints as the main barriers to adherence in Malawi.[74] Akam reported that 53% of individuals on self-pay therapy in Thailand discontinue treatment due to financial constraints.[75] With the exception of one study,[66] financial barriers to securing therapy is one of the most consistent barriers to reliable antiretroviral use in resource-limited settings. These studies raise the question as to whether failure to access therapy due to logistical or financial constraints should be considered non-adherence? Adherence, commonly defined as 'taking medication as prescribed,' presumes access to therapy. As such, failure to access therapy should be distinguished from failure to adhere in future studies.

Stigma remains an important problem in many resource-limited settings. Stigma has been associated with non-adherence in Soweto[54] and Botswana.[58] In the Soweto study, the odds of obtaining >95% adherence decreased considerably with an increased fear of stigmatization (rejection or violence or both) by the patient's sexual partner. A total of 15% of patients in the Botswana study claimed that stigma interfered with their ability to take medication. Stigma usually posed a barrier for patients who thought they could not take their treatments at home or at work due to fear of detection and for patients who felt uncomfortable going to the clinic for tests and medication refills as a result of confidentiality concerns.

Language and literacy can be important barriers to adherence in resource-limited settings. Many HIV-infected individuals in resource-limited settings are illiterate or have very low education. While patients attending regional health centers may speak local languages, English is the medium of communication in many health facilities. Patients may misunderstand the instructions given about their medications leading to missing their doses. Orrell and co-workers found that speaking a different language from the healthy facility staff was a predictor of incomplete adherence.[53]

Differing Levels of Adherence in Resource-rich and Resource-limited Settings

Why are levels of adherence in resource-limited settings higher than in resource-rich settings? While this is largely unknown, it is clear that severe poverty does not preclude excellent adherence and there are several potential explanations for why levels of adherence may be exceptional in many resource-limited settings. People receiving therapy in resource-limited settings generally start therapy at later stages of disease and may have more dramatic improvements in health and functional status with initiation of therapy. These improvements likely reinforce early adherence to therapy. HIV+ parents who have lost spouses and other relatives due to HIV may be caring for large numbers of dependent children, which has been described as a central motivation for adherence.[76] Because patients on self-pay therapy often secure funds from extended family networks, there is, by necessity, strong social support to adhere to therapy.[76] Finally, active drug use is an important barrier to adherence in resource-rich settings. While opiate use is present in many resource-limited settings, active stimulant use, which has a particularly deleterious impact on adherence, is uncommon.[41,77]

Are the current levels of adherence reported in resource-limited settings sustainable? Gill and co-workers have argued that early reports of high adherence may be misleading.[78] Early reports may indeed overestimate adherence due to the intense selection bias of individuals with early access to HIV therapy. As treatment expands, population estimates of adherence may fall. Most studies have looked at patients who recently initiated HIV therapy. Adherence is often highest early in treatment due to amelioration of HIV-related symptoms and improvement in health status. As treatment continues, improvements in health plateaus and chronic complications of therapy such as neuropathy or lipodystrophy become more frequent and more severe.[79] Adherence in resource-rich settings tends to decline over time,[80] and some reports suggest similar declines of adherence with long-term treatment in resource-limited settings. Because of the possible selection bias and short-term follow-up, early reports may describe a 'honeymoon effect,' which will wane as treatment access expands and patients continue treatment for decades.[57,68] While levels of adherence in resource-limited settings may fall from these early estimates, they have a long way to fall before they reach the levels found in resource-rich settings.

Conclusion

Levels of adherence to ART in resource-limited settings are comparable with or even better than levels in resource-rich settings. Early reports of adherence may decline as treatment expands and patient's clinical response plateaus in the setting of long-term side-effects. Few studies have addressed barriers to antiretroviral therapy, but cost of therapy and transport is a major barrier to reliable access to therapy. Mechanisms to sustain current levels of adherence and monitor for future declines in adherence will be important in preserving optimal treatment responses and limited the development of drug resistance.

References

1. UNAIDS. AIDS epidemic update: 2004. Geneva: Joint United Nations Programme on HIV/AIDS (UNAIDS) and World Health Organization (WHO); 2004.
2. WHO. The World Health Report 2004: Changing history. Geneva: World Health Organization; 2004.
3. Stevens WKS, Corrah T. Antiretroviral therapy in Africa. Br Med J 2004; 328:280–282.
4. Harries ADND, Hargreaves NJ, Kaluwa O, et al. Preventing antiretroviral anarchy in Africa. Lancet 2001; 358:410–414.
5. Popp D, Fisher JD. First, do no harm: a call for emphasizing adherence and HIV prevention interventions in active antiretroviral therapy programs in the developing world. AIDS 2002; 16:676–678.
6. Little SJ, Holte S, Routy JP, et al. Antiretroviral-drug resistance among patients recently infected with HIV. N Engl J Med 2002; 347:385–394.
7. Wensing AM, Boucher CA. Worldwide transmission of drug-resistant HIV. AIDS Rev 2003; 5:140–155.
8. Little SJ, Routy P, Daar ES, et al. Antiretroviral drug susceptibility and response to initial therapy among recently HIV-infected subjects in North America. 8th Conference on Retroviruses and Opportunistic Infections, Chicago: 2001.
9. Bangsberg DR, Moss AR, Deeks SG. Paradoxes of adherence and drug resistance to HIV antiretroviral therapy. J Antimicrob Chemother 2004; 53:696–699.
10. King MS, Brun SC, Kempf DJ. Relationship between adherence and the development of resistance in antiretroviral-naive HIV-1-infected patients receiving lopinavir/ritonavir or nelfinavir. J Infect Dis 2005; 191:2046–2052.
11. Harrigan PR, Hogg RS, Dong WW, et al. Predictors of HIV drug-resistance mutations in a large antiretroviral-naive

cohort initiating triple antiretroviral therapy. J Infect Dis 2005; 191:339–347.
12. Popp D, Fisher JD. First, do no harm: a call for emphasizing adherence and HIV prevention interventions in active antiretroviral therapy programme in the developing world. AIDS 2002; 16:676–678.
13. Paterson DL, Swindells S, Mohr J, et al. Adherence to protease inhibitor therapy and outcomes in patients with HIV infection. Ann Intern Med 2000; 133:21–30.
14. Mannheimer S, Friedland G, Matts J, et al. The consistency of adherence to antiretroviral therapy predicts biologic outcomes for human immunodeficiency virus-infected persons in clinical trials. Clin Infect Dis 2002; 34:1115–1121.
15. Bangsberg DR, Hecht FM, Charlebois ED, et al. Adherence to protease inhibitors, HIV-1 viral load, and development of drug resistance in an indigent population. AIDS 2000; 14:357–366.
16. Wagner GJ, Kanouse DE, Koegel P, et al. Adherence to HIV antiretrovirals among persons with serious mental illness. AIDS Patient Care STDS 2003; 17:179–186.
17. Howard AA, Arnsten JH, Lo Y, et al. A prospective study of adherence and viral load in a large multi-center cohort of HIV-infected women. AIDS 2002; 16:2175–2182.
18. McNabb J, Ross JW, Abriola K, et al. Adherence to highly active antiretroviral therapy predicts virologic outcome at an inner-city human immunodeficiency virus clinic. Clin Infect Dis 2001; 33:700–705.
19. Arnsten JH, Demas PA, Farzadegan H, et al. Antiretroviral therapy adherence and viral suppression in HIV-infected drug users: comparison of self-report and electronic monitoring. Clin Infect Dis 2001; 33:1417–1423.
20. Hogg RS, Heath K, Bangsberg D, et al. Intermittent use of triple-combination therapy is predictive of mortality at baseline and after 1 year of follow-up. AIDS 2002; 16:1051–1058.
21. Knobel H, Alonso J, Casado JL, et al. Validation of a simplified medication adherence questionnaire in a large cohort of HIV-infected patients: the GEEMA Study. AIDS 2002; 16:605–613.
22. Walsh JC, Mandalia S, Gazzard BG. Responses to a 1 month self-report on adherence to antiretroviral therapy are consistent with electronic data and virological treatment outcome. AIDS 2002; 16:269–277.
23. Bangsberg DR, Deeks SG. Is average adherence to HIV antiretroviral therapy enough? J Gen Intern Med 2002; 17:812–813.
24. Mannheimer S, Friedland G, Matts J, et al. The consistency of adherence to antiretroviral therapy predicts biologic outcomes for human immunodeficiency virus-infected persons in clinical trials. Clin Infect Dis 2002; 34:1115–1121.
25. Reiter GS, Stewart KE, Wojtusik L, et al. Elements of success in HIV clinical care: multiple interventions that promote adherence. Top HIV Med 2000; 8:5.
26. Ickovics JR, Meade CS. Adherence to antiretroviral therapy among patients with HIV: a critical link between behavioral and biomedical sciences. J Acquir Immune Defic Syndr 2002; 31(Suppl):98–102.
27. Paterson DL, Swindells S, Mohr J, et al. Adherence to protease inhibitor therapy and outcomes in patients with HIV infection. Ann Intern Med 2000; 133:21–30.
28. Stone VE. Strategies for optimizing adherence to highly active antiretroviral therapy: lessons from research and clinical practice. Clin Infect Dis 2001; 33:865–872.
29. Turner BJ, Laine C, Cosler L, et al. Relationship of gender, depression, and health care delivery with antiretroviral adherence in HIV-infected drug users. J Gen Intern Med 2003; 18:248–257.
30. Fogarty L, Roter D, Larson S, et al. Patient adherence to HIV medication regimens: a review of published and abstract reports. Patient Educ Couns 2002; 46:93–108.
31. Maggiolo F, Ripamonti D, Arici C, et al. Simpler regimens may enhance adherence to antiretrovirals in HIV-infected patients. HIV Clin Trials 2002; 3:371–378.

32. Stone VE, Jordan J, Tolson J, et al. Perspectives on adherence and simplicity for HIV-infected patients on antiretroviral therapy: self-report of the relative importance of multiple attributes of highly active antiretroviral therapy (HAART) regimens in predicting adherence. J Acquir Immune Defic Syndr 2004; 36:808–816.

33. Gifford AL, Bormann JE, Shively MJ, et al. Predictors of self-reported adherence and plasma HIV concentrations in patients on multidrug antiretroviral regimens. J Acquir Immune Defic Syndr 2000; 23:386–395.

34. Chesney MA. Factors affecting adherence to antiretroviral therapy. Clin Infect Dis 2000; 30 (Suppl 2):S171–S176.

35. Gifford AL, Bormann JE, Shively MJ, et al. Predictors of self-reported adherence and plasma HIV concentrations in patients on multidrug antiretroviral regimens. J Acquir Immune Defic Syndr 2000; 23:386–395.

36. Wagner GJ. Predictors of antiretroviral adherence as measured by self-report, electronic monitoring, and medication diaries. AIDS Patient Care STDS 2002; 16:599–608.

37. Holzemer WL, Corless IB, Nokes KM, et al. Predictors of self-reported adherence in persons living with HIV disease. AIDS Patient Care STDS 1999; 13:185–197.

38. Gordillo V, Amo J del, Soriano V, et al. Sociodemographic and psychological variables influencing adherence to antiretroviral therapy. AIDS 1999; 13:1763–1769.

39. Gao X, Nau DP, Rosenbluth SA, et al. The relationship of disease severity, health beliefs and medication adherence among HIV patients. AIDS Care 2000; 12:387–398.

40. Singh N, Squier C, Sivek C, et al. Determinants of compliance with antiretroviral therapy in patients with human immunodeficiency virus: prospective assessment with implications for enhancing compliance. AIDS Care 1996; 8:261–269.

41. Ingersoll K. The impact of psychiatric symptoms, drug use, and medication regimen on non-adherence to HIV treatment. AIDS Care 2004; 16:199–211.

42. Russell J, Krantz S, Neville S. The patient-provider relationship and adherence to highly active antiretroviral therapy. J Assoc Nurses AIDS Care 2004; 15:40–47.

43. Delgado J, Heath KV, Yip B, et al. Highly active antiretroviral therapy: physician experience and enhanced adherence to prescription refill. Antivir Ther 2003; 8:471–478.

44. Gross R, Zhang Y, Grossberg R. Medication refill logistics and refill adherence in HIV. Pharmacoepidemiol Drug Saf 2005; 14:789–793.

45. Gross R, Bilker WB, Friedman HM, et al. Provider inaccuracy in assessing adherence and outcomes with newly initiated antiretroviral therapy. AIDS 2002; 16:1835–1837.

46. Bangsberg D, Hecht F, Clague H, et al. Provider assessment of adherence to HIV antiretroviral therapy. J Acquir Immune Defic Syndr 2001; 26:435–442.

47. Murri R, Ammassari A, Trotta MP, et al. Patient-reported and physician-estimated adherence to HAART: social and clinic center-related factors are associated with discordance. J Gen Intern Med 2004; 19:1104–1110.

48. Stevens W, Kaye S, Corrah T. Antiretroviral therapy in Africa. Br Med J 2004; 328:280–282.

49. Donnelly J. Prevention urged in AIDS fight; Natsio says funds should spend less on HIV treatment. Boston: Boston Globe; 2001.

50. Popp D, Fisher JD. First, do no harm: a call for emphasizing adherence and HIV prevention interventions in active antiretroviral therapy programs in the developing world. AIDS 2002; 16:676–678.

51. Stevens W, Kaye S, Corrah T. Antiretroviral therapy in Africa. Br Med J 2004; 328:280–282.

52. Oyugi JH, Byakika-Tusiime J, Charlebois ED, et al. Multiple validated measures of adherence indicate high levels of adherence to generic HIV antiretroviral therapy in a resource-limited setting. J Acquir Immune Defic Syndr 2004; 36:1100–1102.

53. Orrell C, Bangsberg DR, Badri M, et al. Adherence is not a barrier to successful antiretroviral therapy in South Africa. AIDS 2003; 17:1369–1375.

54. Nachega JB, Stein DM, Lehman DA, et al. Adherence to antiretroviral therapy in HIV-infected adults in Soweto, South Africa. AIDS Res Hum Retroviruses 2004; 20:1053–1056.

55. Laniece I, Ciss M, Desclaux A, et al. Adherence to HAART and its principal determinants in a cohort of Senegalese adults. AIDS 2003; 17 (Suppl):103–108.

56. Byakika-Tusiime J, Oyugi JH, Tumwikirize WA, et al. Adherence to HIV antiretroviral therapy in HIV+ Ugandan patients purchasing therapy. Int J STD AIDS 2005; 16:38–41.

57. Laurent C, Ngom Gueye NF, Ndour CT, et al. Long-term benefits of highly active antiretroviral therapy in Senegalese HIV-1-infected adults. J Acquir Immune Defic Syndr 2005; 38:14–17.

58. Weiser SWW, Bangsberg D, Thior I, et al. Barriers to antiretroviral adherence for patients living with HIV infection and AIDS in Botswana. J Acquir Immune Defic Syndr 2003; 34:281–288.

59. Laurent C, Meilo H, Guiard-Schmid JB, et al. Antiretroviral therapy in public and private routine health care clinics in Cameroon: lessons from the Doula antiretroviral (DARVIR) initiative. Clin Infect Dis 2005; 41:108–111.

60. Laurent C, Kouanfack C, Koulla-Shiro S, et al. Effectiveness and safety of a generic fixed-dose combination of nevirapine, stavudine, and lamivudine in HIV-1-infected adults in Cameroon: open-label multicentre trial. Lancet 2004; 364:29–34.

61. Remien RH, Hirky AE, Johnson MO, et al. Adherence to medication treatment: a qualitative study of facilitators and barriers among a diverse sample of HIV+ men and women in four US cities. AIDS Behav 2003; 7:61–72.

62. Brigido LF, Rodrigues R, Casseb J, et al. Impact of adherence to antiretroviral therapy in HIV-1-infected patients at a university public service in Brazil. AIDS Patient Care STDS 2001; 15:587–593.

63. Weidle PJ, Malamba S, Mwebaze R, et al. Assessment of a pilot antiretroviral drug therapy programme in Uganda: patients' response, survival, and drug resistance. Lancet 2002; 360:34–40.

64. Landman R, Schiemann R, Thiam S, et al. Once-a-day highly active antiretroviral therapy in treatment-naive HIV-1-infected adults in Senegal. AIDS 2003; 17:1017–1022.

65. Byakika J, Oyugi JH, Musoke P, et al. Adherence approaches 100% with excellent viral load suppression when all HIV-infected Ugandan household members receive antiretroviral treatment. 12th Conference on Retroviruses and Opportunistic Infections, Boston, MA: 2005.

66. Pujari SSA, Sengar R, Garg R, et al. Adherence to antiretroviral therapy (ART) and its principal determinants in HIV-infected adults in India. 12th Conference on Retroviruses and Opportunistic Infections Boston, MA: February 2005.

67. Fong OW, Ho CF, Fung LY, et al. Determinants of adherence to highly active antiretroviral therapy (HAART) in Chinese HIV/AIDS patients. HIV Med 2003; 4:133–138.

68. Laurent C, Diakhate N, Gueye NF, et al. The Senegalese government's highly active antiretroviral therapy initiative: an 18-month follow-up study. AIDS 2002; 16:1363–1370.

69. Nachega JHM, Lo M, Omer S, et al. Adherence to antiretroviral therapy assessed by pharmacy claims and survival in HIV-infected South Africans. 12th Conference on Retroviruses and Opportunistic Infections, Boston, MA: 2005.

70. Frick PA, Lavreys L, Mandaliya K, et al. Impact of an alarm device on medication compliance in women in Mombasa, Kenya. Int J STD AIDS 2001; 12:329–333.

71. Barroso PF, Schechter M, Gupta P, et al. Adherence to antiretroviral therapy and persistence of HIV RNA in semen. J Acquir Immune Defic Syndr 2003; 32:435–440.

72. Remien RH, Bastos FI, Berkman A, et al. Universal access to antiretroviral therapy may be the best approach to 'Do no harm' in developing countries: the Brazilian experience. AIDS 2003; 17:786–787.

73. Kiarie JN, Kreiss JK. Richardson BA, et al. Compliance with antiretroviral regimens to prevent perinatal HIV-1 transmission in Kenya. AIDS 2003; 17:65–71.

74. Oosterhout JJ van, Bodasing N, Kumwenda JJ, et al. Evaluation of antiretroviral therapy results in a resource-poor setting in Blantyre, Malawi. Trop Med Int Health 2005; 10:464–470.

75. Akam A. Ant -retroviral adherence in a resource poor setting. XV International AIDS Conference, Bangkok: 30 March –2 April 2004.

76. Crane J, Kawuma A. Oyugi J, et al. The Price of adherence: Qualitative findings from patients purchasing fixed-dose combination generic HIV antiretroviral therapy in Kampala, Uganda. AIDS Behav 2006; 10:437–442.

77. Moss AR, Hahn JA, Perry S, et al. Adherence to highly active antiretroviral therapy in the homeless population in San Francisco: a prospective study. Clin Infect Dis 2004; 39:1190–1198.

78. Gill CJ, Hamer DH, Simon JL, et al. No room for complacency about adherence to antiretroviral therapy in sub-Saharan Africa. AIDS 2005; 19:1243–1249.

79. Ammassari A, Antinori A, Cozzi-Lepri A, et al. Relationship between HAART adherence and adipose tissue alterations. J Acquir Immune Defic Syndr 2002; 31 (Suppl):140–144.

80. Howard AA, Arnsten JH, Lo Y, et al. A prospective study of adherence and viral load in a large multi-center cohort of HIV-infected women. AIDS 2002; 16:2175–2182.

SECTION THREE: DISEASES ASSOCIATED WITH HIV INFECTION

CHAPTER 20

Oral Complications of HIV Infection

John S. Greenspan
Deborah Greenspan

Introduction

Oral lesions have been recognized as prominent features of the acquired immunodeficiency syndrome (AIDS) and human immunodeficiency virus (HIV) infection since the beginning of the epidemic, and continue to be important.[1,2] Some of these changes are reflections of reduced immune function manifested as oral opportunistic conditions, which are often the earliest clinical features of HIV infection. Some, in the presence of known HIV infection, are highly predictive of the ultimate development of the full syndrome, whereas others represent the oral features of AIDS itself. The particular susceptibility of the mouth to HIV disease is a reflection of a wider phenomenon. Oral opportunistic infections occur in a variety of conditions in which the teeming and varied micro-flora of the mouth take advantage of local and systemic immunologic and metabolic imbalances. They include oral infections in patients with primary immunodeficiency, leukemia, and diabetes, and those resulting from radiation therapy, cancer chemotherapy, and bone marrow suppression. Oral lesions seen in association with HIV infection are classified in Table 20.1, and our general approach to the diagnosis and management of oral HIV disease is summarized in Table 20.2. Standardized definitions and diagnostic criteria for these lesions have been established.[3,4]

In the prospective cohorts of HIV-infected homosexual and bisexual men in San Francisco, hairy leukoplakia was the most common oral lesion (20.4%), and pseudomembranous candidiasis the next most common (5.8%).[5] The relationships between prevalence of oral lesions and CD4 cell count or HIV viral load shows fairly close correlations.[6-10] These lesions occur at an early stage after seroconversion and are predictors of progression.[11] Oral lesions are also common in HIV-infected women[9,10,12,13] and children.[14,15] While their overall frequency has fallen with the introduction of antiretroviral therapy, including HAART (high activity antiretroviral therapy), changes in their nature and relative frequency have been seen, with major decreases in Kaposi's sarcoma, lymphoma, oral candidiasis and hairy leukoplakia; no changes in aphthous ulcers and often increases in oral papillomavirus warts.[16-19] However, oral lesions are more common in people who smoke cigarettes.[20]

Candidiasis

The pseudomembranous form of oral candidiasis (thrush) was described in the first group of AIDS patients and is a harbinger of the full-blown syndrome in HIV-positive individuals.[21,22] We have shown that both oral candidiasis and hairy leukoplakia predict the development of AIDS in HIV-infected patients independently of CD4 counts.[23] However, it is not well recognized that oral candidiasis can take several forms, some of them with subtle clinical appearances.[24] The most common form, pseudomembranous candidiasis, appears as removable white plaques on any oral mucosal surface (Fig. 20.1). These plaques may be as small as 1–2 mm or may be

Table 20.1 Oral lesions in HIV infection

Fungal	Bacterial	Viral	Neoplastic	Autoimmune/idiopathic
Candidiasis: 　pseudomembranous, 　erythematous, 　angular cheilitis Histoplasmosis Cryptococcosis Penicillinosis	Periodontal disease Necrotizing stomatitis Tuberculosis MAC Bacillary angiomatosis Other	Herpes simplex Chicken pox Herpes zoster Cytomegalovirus 　lesions Hairy leukoplakia HPV lesions	Kaposi's sarcoma Non-Hodgkin's 　lymphoma Hodgkin's 　lymphoma Lip cancer	Salivary gland disease Aphthous ulcers ITP Other

extensive and widespread. They can be wiped off, leaving an erythematous or even bleeding mucosal surface.

The erythematous form (Fig. 20.2) is seen as smooth red patches on the hard or soft palate, buccal mucosa, or dorsal surface of the tongue. These lesions may seem insignificant and may be missed unless a thorough oral mucosal examination is performed in good light.

Angular cheilitis (Fig. 20.3), due to *Candida* infection, presents as erythema, cracks and fissures at the corner of the mouth. We have found that erythematous candidiasis is as serious a prognostic indicator of the development of AIDS as pseudomembranous candidiasis.[24]

Denture stomatitis is frequently a form of erythematous candidiasis that occurs in association with the fitting surface of dentures. Clinically it appears as a smooth red area, often demarcating the outline of the denture on the palate. *Candida* also colonizes/inhabits the fitting surface of a plastic denture, and if the fitting surface of the denture is pressed into a *Candida* culture plate, prolific growth of colonies of the fungus will subsequently be seen.

Diagnosis of oral candidiasis involves potassium hydroxide preparation of a smear from the lesion (Fig. 20.4). Culture provides information about the species involved. However, because a positive candidal culture can be obtained from over 50% of the normal population, culture is usually not useful for diagnosis. It may be helpful in cases of oral candidiasis unresponsive to antifungal therapy to determine *Candida spp* and/or possible azole resistant candidiasis.

Treatment

Oral candidiasis in patients with HIV infection can be treated with oral or systemic therapy and sometimes a combination of both.

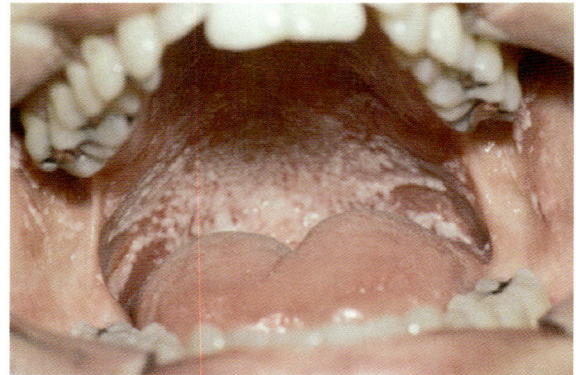

Figure 20.1 Pseudomembranous candidiasis.

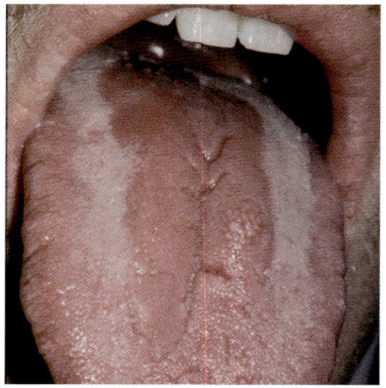

Figure 20.2 Erythematous candidiasis.

Oral topical agents include troches, tablets, creams and suspensions. For an oral topical agent to be effective, adequate contact time is crucial. Suspensions are therefore probably not the best first choice. It is also important that sucrose is not used as a flavoring agent for several reasons, most particularly because of the risk of development of caries and

Table 20.2 Diagnosis and management of oral HIV disease

Condition	Diagnosis	Management
Fungal		
Candidiasis	Clinical appearance KOH preparation Culture	Antifungals Treatment for 2 weeks with systemic or topical agents Topical creams for angular cheilitis
Histoplasmosis	Biopsy	Systemic therapy
Geotrichosis	KOH preparation Culture	Polyene antifungals
Cryptococcosis	Culture Biopsy	Systemic therapy
Aspergillosis	Culture Biopsy	Systemic therapy
Bacterial		
Linear gingival erythema	Clinical appearance	Plaque removal, chlorhexidine
Necrotizing ulcerative periodontitis	Clinical appearance	Plaque removal, debridement, povidone-iodine, metronidazole, chlorhexidine
Necrotizing stomatitis	Clinical appearance Culture and biopsy (to exclude other causes)	Débridement, povidone-iodine, metronidazole, chlorhexidine
Mycobacterium avium complex	Culture Biopsy	Systemic therapy
Klebsiella stomatitis	Culture	Systemic therapy (based on antibiotic sensitivity testing)
Viral		
Herpes simplex	Clinical appearance Immunofluorescence on smears	Most cases are self-limiting Oral acyclovir or valacyclovir
Herpes zoster	Clinical appearance	Oral or intravenous acyclovir
Cytomegalovirus ulcers	Biopsy, immunohistochemistry for CMV	Ganciclovir
Hairy leukoplakia	Clinical appearance Biopsy; in situ hybridization for Epstein–Barr virus	Not routinely treated Oral acyclovir or valacyclovir for severe cases
Warts	Clinical appearance Biopsy	Excision
Neoplastic		
Kaposi's sarcoma	Clinical appearance	Palliative surgical or laser excision for some bulky or unsightly lesions; intralesional chemotherapy or sclerosing agents; radiation therapy; chemotherapy
Non-Hodgkin's lymphoma	Biopsy	Chemotherapy
Squamous cell carcinoma	Biopsy	Excision or radiation therapy or both
Other		
Recurrent aphthous ulcers	History Clinical appearance Biopsy (to exclude other causes)	Topical steroids, such as fluocinonide mixed 50/50 with orobase, applied to lesions 4 times a day Thalidomide for most severe cases
Immune thrombocytopenic purpura	Clinical appearance Hematological work-up	
Salivary gland disease	History, clinical appearance, salivary flow measurements Biopsy (to exclude other causes) needle or labial salivary gland biopsy)	Salivary stimulants or change in systemic medication or both Consider use of Salagen or Evoxac Topical fluorides, toothpastes and rinses

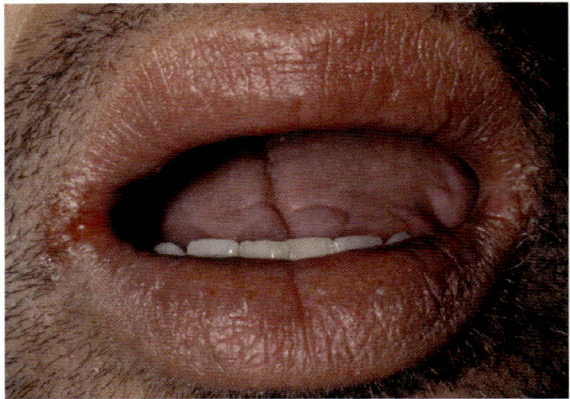

Figure 20.3 Angular cheilitis.

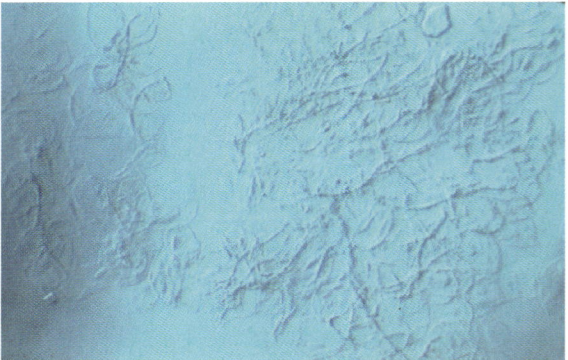

Figure 20.4 Potassium hydroxide preparation. Fungal hyphae and blastospores.

the possibility of increased dental plaque production. For intraoral candida lesions, effective agents include[25] topical antifungal agents, including nystatin vaginal tablets (Mycostatin), 100 000 units t.i.d., dissolved slowly in the mouth; nystatin oral pastilles (Mycostatin), 200 000 units, one pastille five times daily; or clotrimazole oral tablets (Mycelex), 10 mg, one tablet five times daily. Amphotericin oral lozenge (10 mg); one to be dissolved slowly in the mouth three times per day, is an effective topical antifungal that is available in some countries, such as the UK and parts of Europe, but not in the USA. The effectiveness of topical medications depends on adherence to recommended dosing regimens. Topical tablets, troches and pastilles need adequate saliva to be effective. For those people with dry mouth, sipping a little water before use and occasionally during use of the medication can be helpful. When S topical medications containing sucrose or dextrose,

which have the potential to cause caries, are used, daily topical fluoride rinses should be used by those taking these medications frequently.

For those individuals who find it difficult to use these medications 4–5 times a day, systemic therapy can be considered. The azoles are frequently used for systemic therapy. There are many drug interactions, so care must be taken before these drugs are prescribed.

Fluconazole (Diflucan) is a systemic antifungal agent. The recommended dose is a 100 mg tablet, once daily for 14 days. Oral fluconazole is an effective antifungal agent that does not depend on gastric pH for absorption. Side-effects include nausea and skin rash. Two 100 mg tablets are used on the first day, followed by one 100 mg tablet daily until the lesions disappear. Fluconazole is also available as an oral suspension, 10 mg/mL, and 10 mL used as a swish and swallow once per day.[26] Itraconazole is a systemic, triazole antifungal agent and is available as a capsule and suspension. Itraconazole oral solution has been evaluated in clinical trials as being an effective agent in the treatment of oral candidiasis, and salivary levels of itraconazole persist up to 8 h after dosing. Oral itraconazole suspension, 20 mL, taken once or twice a day for 2 weeks is useful in cases that do not respond to fluconazole or clotrimazole. Antifungal therapy should be maintained for 2 weeks, and some patients may need maintenance therapy because of frequent relapse.

In the years before HAART was widely used, many cases of oral candidiasis resistant to fluconazole were reported. Such complications are rare in patients on HAART. Factors associated with the development of resistance include CD4 count <100, previous use of fluconazole and the emergence of new resistant strains of *C. albicans* or the emergence of strains such as *C. glabrata*, *C. tropicalis* and *C. krusei* which are inherently less sensitive to fluconazole.[27] However, in most cases, fluconazole is an extremely well tolerated and an effective anti-fungal agent.

For patients who develop oral candidiasis that appears unresponsive to therapy, treatment choices include higher doses of fluconazole, itraconazole 200–400 mg/day, itraconazole suspension 20 mL once or twice daily, or amphotericin oral lozenges if available, and if none of these are successful, intravenous amphotericin B may be needed. Voriconazole is a newer antifungal agent and may be useful in patients with resistant disease, rather than as first line therapy, as it is associated with more side-effects than fluconazole.

Angular cheilitis usually responds to topical antifungal creams, such as nystatin-triamcinolone

(Mycolog), clotrimazole (Mycelex), or ketoconazole (Nizoral). Patients with both intraoral candidiasis and angular cheilitis benefit from treatment with topical creams for the corners of the mouth as well as treatment for their intraoral lesions. Patients with denture stomatitis should be asked to remove their dentures before using intraoral topical medications and the dentures should be left out at night and left in a solution of three or four drops of bleach in a denture bowl. The dentures should be thoroughly rinsed and cleaned before placing them in the mouth.

Occasionally, other and unusual oral fungal lesions are seen. They include histoplasmosis,[28] geotrichosis,[29] aspergillosis,[30] and cryptococcosis.[31]

Gingivitis and Periodontitis

Unusual forms of gingivitis and periodontal disease[32] are seen in association with HIV infection, notably in groups where antiretroviral therapy is not available such as in many geographic areas with high HIV prevalences. The gingivae may show a fiery red marginal line, known as linear gingival erythema, even in mouths showing absence of significant accumulations of plaque.[33] In early reports in the US and Europe, the periodontal disease, necrotizing ulcerative periodontitis, occurred in approximately 30–50% of AIDS clinic patients[34] but was rarely seen in asymptomatic HIV-positive individuals.[35] It resembles, in some respects, acute necrotizing ulcerative gingivitis (ANUG) superimposed on rapidly progressive periodontitis (Fig. 20.5) and is frequently

seen in African AIDS patients. Thus, there may be halitosis and a history of rapid onset. There is necrosis of the tips of interdental papillae, with the formation of cratered ulcers. However, in contrast to patients with ANUG, these patients complain of spontaneous bleeding and severe, deep-seated pain that is not readily relieved by analgesics. There may be rapid progressive loss of gingival and periodontal soft tissues and extraordinarily rapid destruction of supporting bone. Teeth may, therefore, loosen and even exfoliate. The periodontal disease often demonstrates alarming severity and a rapid rate of progression not seen by the majority of practicing dentists and periodontists prior to the AIDS epidemic. Exposure and even sequestration of bone may occur, producing necrotizing stomatitis lesions[36] similar to the noma seen in severely malnourished people in the Second World War, and more recently in developing countries in association with malnutrition and chronic infection, such as malaria. The pathologic and microbiologic features of these remarkable periodontal lesions are well documented.[37] Standard therapy for gingivitis and periodontitis is ineffectual. Instead, the therapeutic regimen that is effective[38] involves thorough debridement and curettage, followed by application of a combination of topical antiseptics, notably povidone-iodine (Betadine) irrigation followed with chlorhexidine (Peridex or PerioGard) mouthwashes, sometimes supplemented with a 4- to 5-day course of antibiotics, such as metronidazole (Flagyl) 250 mg q.i.d., Augmentin 250 mg (1 tab t.i.d.), or clindamycin 300 mg t.i.d. Treatment will fail if thorough local removal of bacteria and diseased hard and soft tissue is not achieved during the initial treatment phase and maintained long term. Our impression has been that the diagnosis and management of the periodontal complications of HIV/AIDS are challenging and are less likely to be successful unless carried out by, or under the supervision of, experienced dental health professionals.

Other Bacterial Lesions

A few cases have occurred of oral mucosal lesions associated with unusual bacteria, including *Klebsiella pneumoniae* and *Enterobacter cloacae*.[39] These have been diagnosed using aerobic and anaerobic cultures and have responded to antibiotic therapy based on *in vitro* sensitivity assays. Oral ulcers caused by *Mycobacterium avium* have also been described,[40] as have the lesions of bacillary angiomatosis.[41]

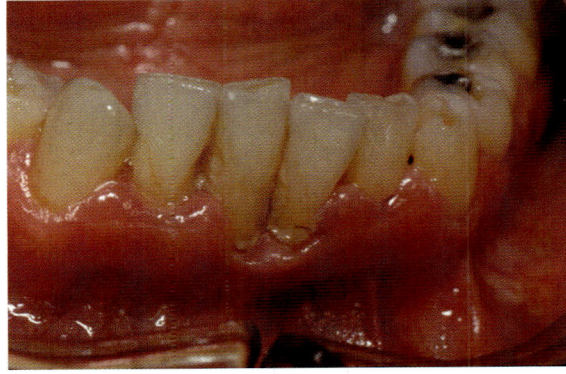

Figure 20.5 Necrotizing ulcerative periodontitis in HIV infection.

Herpes Simplex

Oral lesions due to herpes simplex virus (HSV; see Ch. 39) were a common feature of HIV infection and are still occasionally seen. Diagnosis is usually made from the clinical appearance. The condition usually occurs as recurrent intraoral lesions with crops of small, painful vesicles that ulcerate. These lesions commonly appear on the hard palate or gingiva. Intraoral recurrent herpes simplex rarely occurs on keratinized mucosa. Smears from the lesions may reveal giant cells, and HSV can be identified using monoclonal antibodies and immunofluorescence. The lesions usually heal within 5–7 days, although they may recur in patients with lesions that have been present for 1–2 days treatment with acyclovir or valacyclovir. For those with frequent recurrence, it may be considered appropriate to treat them with oral acyclovir as soon as symptoms are reported. Usually, one 200 mg capsule of acyclovir taken five times a day is effective. Acyclovir-resistant herpes of the lips and perioral structures have been described.[42] For herpes labialis, treatment with penciclovir topical cream applied to the lesions every 2 h for 4 days or the OTC preparation Abreva may be effective. For multiple lip lesions, systemic therapy may result in quicker resolution of the lesions.

Herpes Zoster

Both chickenpox and herpes zoster (shingles; see Ch. 39) have occurred in association with HIV infection.[43] In orofacial zoster, the vesicles and ulcers follow the distribution of one or more branches of the trigeminal nerve on one side. Facial nerve involvement with facial palsy (Ramsay Hunt syndrome) also may occur. Prodromal symptoms may include pain referred to one or more teeth, which often prove to be vital and noncarious. The ulcers usually heal in 2–3 weeks, but pain may persist. Oral acyclovir in doses up to 4 g/day for 7–10 days or valacyclovir 1 g t.i.d. for 7 days may be used in severe cases, but occasionally patients must be hospitalized to receive intravenous acyclovir therapy.

Cytomegalovirus Ulcers

Oral ulcers caused by cytomegalovirus (CMV; see Ch. 39) occasionally occur.[44] These ulcers can occur on any oral mucosal surface, and diagnosis is made by biopsy and immunohistochemistry. Oral ulcers due to CMV are usually seen in the presence of dis-seminated disease, but cases have occurred in which the oral ulcer was the first presentation. Whether to treat with ganciclovir or foscarnet depends on the severity of the viral infection, and a full work-up is indicated. Ulcers simultaneously infected by both HSV and CMV also occur.[44]

Hairy Leukoplakia

First seen on the tongue in homosexual men,[45,46] hairy leukoplakia has since been described in several oral mucosal locations, including the buccal mucosa, soft palate, and floor of mouth, and in all risk groups for AIDS. Hairy leukoplakia produces white thickening of the oral mucosa, often with vertical folds or corrugations (Fig. 20.6). The lesions range in size from a few millimeters to involvement of the entire dorsal surface of the tongue. The differential diagnosis includes pseudomembranous candidiasis, idiopathic leukoplakia, smoker's leukoplakia, epithelial dysplasia or oral cancer, white sponge nevus, and the plaque form of lichen planus. Biopsy reveals epithelial hyperplasia with a thickened parakeratin layer, showing surface irregularities, projections resembling 'hairs,' vacuolated prickle cells, and very little inflammation.[47] Epstein–Barr virus (EBV) can be identified in vacuolated and other prickle cells and in the cells of the superficial layers of the epithelium using cytochemistry, electron microscopy, Southern blotting, and *in situ* hybridization.[47,48] For cases in which biopsy is not considered appropriate (e.g. hemophiliacs, children, large-scale epidemiologic studies), we and others have used cytospin and filter *in situ* hybridization techniques.[49] Langerhans' cells are sparse or absent from the lesion.[50] Hairy leukoplakia is not premalignant.[51] Indeed, the keratin

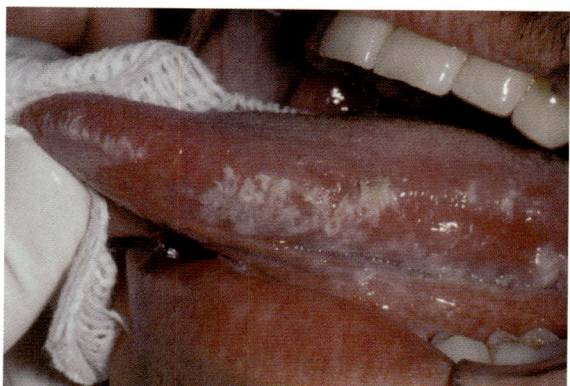

Figure 20.6 Hairy leukoplakia.

profile of the lesion suggests reduced, rather than increased, cell turnover.[52]

Almost all patients with hairy leukoplakia are HIV-positive and in the absence of modern antiretroviral therapy, many subsequently develop AIDS (median time 24 months) and die (median time 44 months).[23,53,54] Rare cases have been described in HIV-negative individuals, usually in association with immunosuppression associated with organ transplantation.[55] Hairy leukoplakia has not been seen other than on mucosal surfaces other than that of the mouth.[56]

Hairy leukoplakia apparently is an EBV-induced benign epithelial thickening. High doses of oral acyclovir appear to reduce the lesion clinically,[25,57] however, these effects are soon reversed after cessation of acyclovir therapy. Hairy leukoplakia occasionally may regress spontaneously.[58]

It is not clear whether hairy leukoplakia is caused by direct infection or reinfection of maturing epithelial cells by EBV from the saliva, by EBV-infected B cells infiltrating the epithelium, or by latent infection of the basal cell layer.[59] EBV variants, unusual EBV types, and even multiple strains of EBV have been found in the lesion.[60] HL is a fertile model for studies of EBV gene expression.[61,62]

Warts

Oral lesions caused by human papillomavirus (HPV)[63] can occur as single or multiple papilliferous warts with multiple white and spike-like projections, as pink cauliflower-like masses (Fig. 20.7), as single projections, or as flat lesions resembling focal epithelial hyperplasia. In patients with HIV infection, we have seen numerous examples of each type. Southern blot hybridization has rarely revealed (as might

be expected) HPV types 6, 11, 16, and 18, which usually are associated with anogenital warts, but HPV type 7, which usually is found in butcher's warts of the skin, or HPV types 13 and 32, previously associated with focal epithelial hyperplasia.[64] Novel HPV types are also found.[65]

Sexual transmission thus seems non-involved in these warts. Instead, they may be attributable to activation of latent HPV infection or perhaps autoinfection from skin and face lesions. Histologically dysplastic warts due to novel HPV types have also been described[66] but are not associated with malignant transformation. Informed histopathological diagnosis is important because these benign lesions have sometimes been mistakenly diagnosed as premalignant dysplasia or even well differentiated carcinoma.

If large, extensive, or otherwise troublesome, as is the case in significant numbers of patients who are on antiretroviral therapy and present to specialized clinics with oral warts, these lesions can be removed using surgical or laser excision. In many cases, we have seen recurrence after therapy and even extensive spread throughout the mouth. Furthermore, our impression is that not only the frequency and severity, but also the response to therapy of oral warts are worse in patients receiving HAART. Topical agents such as podofilox (Condylox) and imiquimod (Aldara) have been tried, but there have been no published placebo controlled studies showing efficacy with oral warts.

Neoplastic Disease

Kaposi's Sarcoma

Kaposi's sarcoma (KS; see Ch. 40) in patients with AIDS produces oral lesions in many cases.[67,68] The lesions occur as red or purple macules, papules, or nodules (Fig. 20.8). Occasionally, the lesions are the same color as the adjoining normal mucosa. Although frequently they are asymptomatic, pain may occur because of traumatic ulceration with inflammation and infection. Bulky lesions may be visible or may interfere with speech and mastication. Diagnosis involves biopsy.

Lesions at the gingival margin frequently become inflamed and painful because of plaque accumulation. Excision, by surgical means or by laser, is readily performed and can be repeated if the lesion again produces problems. Local radiation therapy has been used to reduce the size of such lesions. Oral

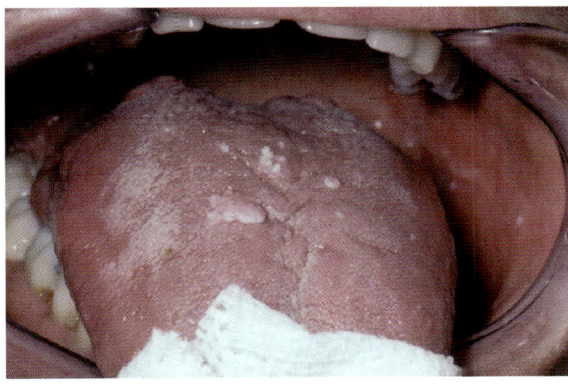

Figure 20.7 Papillomavirus warts.

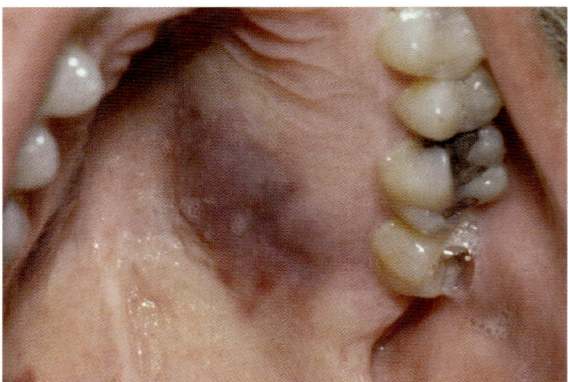

Figure 20.8 Kaposi's sarcoma.

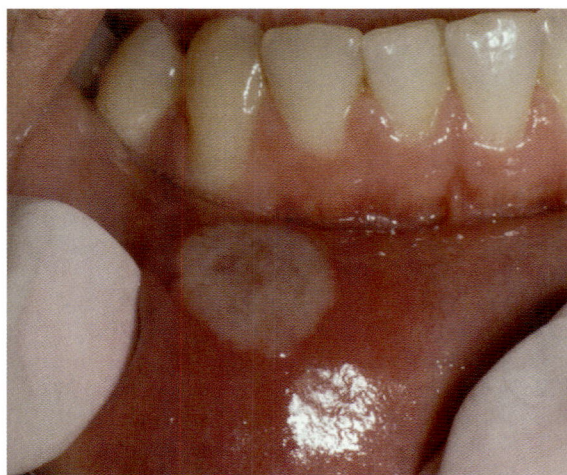

Figure 20.9 Recurrent aphthous ulcer.

lesions usually regress when patients receive chemotherapy for aggressive KS, and individual lesions may respond to local injection of vinblastine[69] or sclerosing agents.[70]

Lymphoma

Although not seen as frequently as with oral KS, oral lesions are a feature in patients with HIV-associated lymphoma (see Ch. 40).[71] A biopsy may prove that poorly defined alveolar swellings, discrete oral masses or non-healing ulcers in individuals who are HIV-positive are non-Hodgkin's lymphoma. No treatment is provided for the oral lesions separate from the systemic chemotherapy regimen that usually is used in such cases.

Carcinoma

On the issue of possible relationships between oral cancer and HIV infection, some studies indicate an increased risk of lip cancer, while one suggests an increase in several epithelial malignancies including tongue cancer. Frisch[72] examined cancer registry data from 11 US areas and found an association between HIV infection and lip cancer (relative risk 3.1 (1.9–4.8). Grulich and co-workers[73] in Australia, found increases in lip cancer of 2.6 times the standard incidence rate. Demopoulos and co-workers[74] used cancer registry files at Bellevue Hospital in New York City and compared cancers in HIV positive and negative individuals. HIV positives with cancer were on average over a decade younger than HIV negatives (47.6 years versus 60.3 years; $P = 0.04$). The cancers in HIV-infected people included lung, skin, penis, larynx, tongue, colon and rectum. These findings indicate that we cannot exclude the possibility that these epithelial malignancies may be seen as HIV infected people survive much longer under the influence of current and emerging antiretroviral therapy.

Other Lesions

Recurrent aphthous ulcers (RAU) are a common finding in the normal population. There is an impression,[75] not substantiated by prospective studies of incidence, that RAU are more common among HIV-positive individuals. These lesions occur as recurrent crops of small (1–2 mm) to large (1 cm) ulcers (Fig. 20.9) on the non-keratinized oral and oropharyngeal mucosa. They can interfere significantly with speech and swallowing and may present considerable problems in diagnosis. Location of RAU on the non-keratinized mucosa help in the differential diagnosis between RAU and HSV, as HSV lesions usually occur on keratinized mucosa. History may also be helpful, as typically those with RAU have experienced episodes of lesions occurring on areas such as the buccal mucosa, lateral margin of the tongue or floor of mouth, over many years often starting in childhood. When they are large and persistent, biopsy may be indicated to exclude lymphoma. The histopathologic features of RAU are those of non-specific inflammation. Treatment with topical steroids is often effective in reducing pain and accelerating healing. Valuable agents include fluocinonide (Lidex), 0.05% ointment, mixed with equal parts of Orabase applied to the lesion up to six times daily, or clobetasol (Temovate), 0.05% mixed with equal parts of Orabase applied three times daily. These are particularly effective treatments for early lesions. Dexamethasone (Decadron) elixir, 0.5 mg/mL used as a rinse and expectorated, is also helpful, particularly when the location of the lesion makes it difficult for the patient to apply fluocinonide. Thalidomide, in defined protocols, has been found to be useful in very severe cases of steroid-resistant ulcers,[76] but lower continuing doses do not prevent recurrences.[77]

Immune thrombocytopenic purpura may produce oral mucosal ecchymoses or small blood-filled lesions. Spontaneous gingival bleeding may occur. Diagnosis by hematological evaluation is usually straightforward, but, as with any systemic condition presenting as oral lesions, full work-up is indicated.

Salivary gland enlargement, predominantly involving the parotids is seen in pediatric AIDS patients[14] (Fig. 20.8) and among adults (Fig. 20.10) who are HIV-positive. This is one feature of the diffuse infiltrative lymphocytosis syndrome (DILS).[50,78,79] HIV-infected children with parotid enlargement progress less rapidly than those without that condition.[80] No specific cause for HIV-associated salivary gland disease has been determined, although viral causes are suspected. The salivary gland enlargement of DILS in adults may be accompanied by elevated CD-8 counts and labial salivary gland biopsy shows a CD-8 lymphocytic infiltrate, reminiscent of the focal lymphocytic sialadenitis of Sjögren's syndrome, where however the infiltrate is predominantly of CD4 cells. Diagnosis to exclude lymphoma, leukemia, and other causes of salivary gland enlargement may involve labial salivary gland

biopsy and major salivary gland needle biopsy. Some of these cases show xerostomia. Furthermore, the latter condition may be seen in association with HIV infection in the absence of salivary gland enlargement. The patient may complain of oral dryness, and there may be signs of xerostomia, such as lack of pooled saliva, failure to elicit salivary expression from Stensen's or Wharton's ducts, and obvious mucosal dryness. Tests of salivary function, notably stimulated parotid flow-rate determination, show reduced salivary flow. Some of these cases are attributable to side-effects of the many medications that reduce salivation. Stimulation of salivary flow by use of sugar-free candy or sugar-free chewing gum or the use of Salagen or Evoxac may alleviate some of the discomfort. Topical fluorides and other preventive dentistry approaches are used to reduce the frequency of caries.

Conclusion

The oral manifestations of HIV infection occur as a variety of opportunistic infections, neoplasms, and other lesions. Some of them are common, perhaps the most common, features of HIV disease and are highly predictive of the development of AIDS. Their pattern, nature and relative frequency appear to change in those on retroviral therapy. Clinicians caring for HIV-infected persons should become familiar with the diagnosis and management of this group of conditions.

The oral lesions of HIV infection present challenges of diagnosis and therapy. They also offer unrivaled opportunities to investigate the epidemiology, cause, pathogenesis, and treatment of mucosal diseases. As the epidemic progresses, it can be expected that further lesions will be observed and that additional rational and effective therapeutic approaches will be developed.

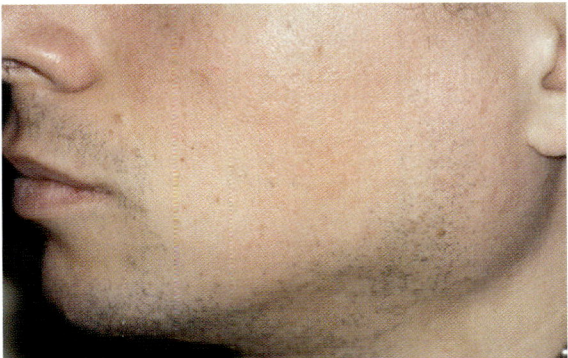

Figure 20.10 Parotid enlargement as part of diffuse infiltrative lymphocytosis syndrome (DILS).

References

1. Gottlieb MS, Schroff R, Schantez HM. Pneumocystis carinii pneumonia and mucosal candidiasis in previously healthy homosexual men: evidence of a new acquired cellular immunodeficiency. N Engl J Med 1981; 305:1425–1431.
2. Leigh JE, Shetty K, Fidel PL Jr. Oral opportunistic infections in HIV-positive individuals: review and role of mucosal immunity. AIDS Patient Care STDS 2004; 18:443–456.
3. EC-Clearinghouse on Oral Problems Related to HIV Infection and WHO Collaborating Centre on Oral Manifestations of the Human Immunodeficiency Virus. Classification and diagnostic criteria for oral lesions in HIV infection. J Oral Pathol Med 1993; 22:289–291.
4. Greenspan JS, Barr CE, Sciubba JJ, et al; The USA Oral AIDS Collaborative Group. Oral manifestations of HIV infection:

definitions, diagnostic criteria and principles of therapy. Oral Surg Oral Med Oral Pathol 1992; 73:142–144.

5. Feigal DW, Katz MH, Greenspan D, et al. The prevalence of oral lesions in HIV-infected homosexual and bisexual men: three San Francisco epidemiological cohorts. AIDS 1991; 5:519–525.

6. Patton LL. Sensitivity, specificity, and positive predictive value of oral opportunistic infections in adults with HIV/AIDS as markers of immune suppression and viral burden. Oral Surg Oral Med Oral Pathol Oral Radiol Endod 2000; 90:182–188.

7. Chattopadhyay A, Caplan DJ, Slade GD, et al. Incidence of oral candidiasis and oral hairy leukoplakia in HIV-infected adults in North Carolina. Oral Surg Oral Med Oral Pathol Oral Radiol Endod 2005; 99:39–47.

8. Chattopadhyay A, Caplan DJ, Slade GD, et al. Risk indicators for oral candidiasis and oral hairy leukoplakia in HIV-infected adults. Commun Dent Oral Epidemiol 2005; 33:35–44.

9. Greenspan D, Komaroff E, Redford M, et al. Oral mucosal lesions and HIV viral load in the Women's Interagency HIV Study (WIHS). J Acquir Immune Defic Syndr 2000; 25:44–50.

10. Greenspan D, Gange S, Phelan JA, et al. Reduced incidence of oral lesions in HIV-1 infected women: changes with highly active antiretroviral therapy. J Dent Res 2004; 83:145–150.

11. Hilton JF, Donegan E, Katz MH, et al. Development of oral lesions in human immunodeficiency virus-infected transfusion recipients and hemophiliacs. Am J Epidemiol 1997; 145:164–174.

12. Shiboski CH, Hilton JF, Neuhaus JM, et al. Human immunodeficiency virus-related oral manifestations and gender. A longitudinal analysis. The University of California, San Francisco Oral AIDS Center Epidemiology Collaborative Group. Arch Intern Med 1996; 156:2249–2254.

13. Tappuni AR. Fleming GJ The effect of antiretroviral therapy on the prevalence of oral manifestations in HIV-infected patients: a UK study. Oral Surg Oral Med Oral Pathol Oral Radiol Endod 2001; 92:623–628.

14. Flanagan MA, Barasch A, Koenigsberg SR, et al. Prevalence of oral soft tissue lesions in HIV-infected minority children treated with highly active antiretroviral therapies. Pediatr Dent 2001; 22:287–291.

15. Exposito-Delgado AJ, Vallejo-Bolanos E, Martos-Cobo EG. Oral manifestations of HIV infection in infants: a review article. Med Oral Patol Oral Cir Bucal 2004; 9:410–420.

16. Patton LL, McKaig R, Strauss R, et al. Changing prevalence of oral manifestations of human immuno-deficiency virus in the era of protease inhibitor therapy. Oral Surg Oral Med Oral Pathol Oral Radiol Endod 2000; 89:299–304.

17. Schmidt-Westhausen AM, Priepke F, et al. Decline in the rate of oral opportunistic infections following introduction of highly active antiretroviral therapy. J Oral Pathol Med 2000; 29:336–341.

18. Ramirez-Amador V, Esquivel-Pedraza L, Sierra-Madero J, et al. The changing clinical spectrum of human immunodeficiency virus (HIV)-related oral lesions in 1,000 consecutive patients. A 12-year study in a referral center in Mexico. Medicine 2003; 82:39–50.

19. Greenspan D, Canchola AJ, MacPhail LA, et al. Effect of highly active antiretroviral therapy on frequency of oral warts. Lancet 1991; 357:1411–1412.

20. Palacio H, Hilton JF, Canchola AJ, et al. Effect of cigarette smoking on HIV-related oral lesions. J Acquir Immune Defic Syndr Hum Retrovirol 1997; 14:338–342.

21. Klein RS, Harris CA, Small CR, et al. Oral candidiasis in high-risk patients as the initial manifestation of the acquired immunodeficiency syndrome. N Engl J Med 1984; 311:354–358.

22. Murray HW, Hillman AD, Rubin BY, et al. Patients at risk for AIDS-related opportunistic infections. N Engl J Med 1985; 313:1504–1510.

23. Katz MH, Greenspan D, Westenhouse J, et al. Progression to AIDS in HIV-infected homosexual and bisexual men with hairy leukoplakia and oral candidiasis. AIDS 1992; 6:95–100.

24. Dodd CL, Greenspan D, Katz MH, et al. Oral candidiasis in HIV infection: pseudomembranous and erythematous candidiasis show similar rates of progression to AIDS. AIDS 1991; 5:1339–1343.

25. Greenspan D, Shirlaw PJ. Management of the oral mucosal lesions seen in association with HIV infection. Oral Dis 1997; 3(Suppl):229–234.

26. Pons V, Greenspan D, Debruin M. Therapy for oropharyngeal candidiasis in HIV-infected patients: a randomized, prospective multicenter study of oral fluconazole versus clotrimazole troches. Multicenter Study Group. J Acquir Immune Defic Syndr 1993; 6:1311–1316.

27. Heald AE, Cox GM, Schell WA, et al. Oropharyngeal yeast flora and fluconazole resistance in HIV-infected patients receiving long-term continuous versus intermittent fluconazole therapy. AIDS 1996; 10:263–268.

28. Heinic G, Greenspan D, MacPhail LA, et al. Oral Histoplasma capsulatum in association with HIV infection: a case report. J Oral Pathol Med 1992; 21:85–89.

29. Heinic GS, Greenspan D, MacPhail LA, et al. Oral Geotrichum candidum infection in association with HIV infection. Oral Surg Oral Med Oral Pathol 1992; 73:726–728.

30. Shannon MT, Sclaroff A, Colm SJ. Invasive aspergillosis of the maxilla in an immunocompromised patient. Oral Surg Oral Med Oral Pathol 1990; 70:425–427.

31. Glick M, Cohen SG, Cheney RT, et al. Oral manifestations of disseminated Cryptococcus neoformans in a patient with acquired immunodeficiency syndrome. Oral Surg Oral Med Oral Pathol 1987; 64:454–459.

32. Robinson PG. The significance and management of periodontal lesions in HIV infection. Oral Dis 2002; 8(Suppl):91–97.

33. Lamster I, Grbic J, Fine J, et al. A critical review of periodontal disease as a manifestation of HIV infection. Proceedings of the Second International Workshop on Oral Manifestations of HIV Infection, Chicago. Chicago: Quintessence Publishing Co.; 1994.

34. Masouredis CM, Katz MH, Greenspan D, et al. Prevalence of HIV-associated periodontitis and gingivitis in HIV-infected patients attending an AIDS clinic. J Acquir Immune Defic Syndr 1992; 5:479–483.

35. Winkler JR, Herrera C, Westenhouse J, et al. Periodontal disease in HIV-infected and uninfected homosexual and bisexual men [letter]. AIDS 1992; 6:1041–1043.

36. Williams CA, Winkler JR, Grassi M, Murray PA. HIV-associated periodontitis complicated by necrotizing stomatitis. Oral Surg Oral Med Oral Pathol 1990; 69:351–355.

37. Zambon JJ, Reynolds H, Smutko J, et al. Are unique bacterial pathogens involved in HIV-associated periodontal diseases? Proceedings of the Second International Workshop on Oral Manifestations of HIV Infection, Chicago. Chicago: Quintessence Publishing Co.; 1994.

38. Palmer GD. Periodontal therapy for patients with HIV infection. Proceedings of the Second International Workshop on Oral Manifestations of HIV Infection, Chicago. Chicago: Quintessence Publishing Co.; 1994.

39. Schmidt-Westhausen A, Fehrenbach FJ, Reichart PA. Oral Enterobacteriaceae in patients with HIV infection. J Oral Pathol 1990; 19:229–231.

40. Volpe F, Schimmer A, Barr C. Oral manifestations of disseminated Mycobacterium avium-intracellulare in a patient with AIDS. Oral Surg 1985; 60:567–570.

41. Speight PM. Epithelioid angiomatosis affecting the oral cavity as a first sign of HIV infection. Br Dent J 1991; 171:367–370.

42. Erlich KS, Mills J, Chatis P, et al. Acyclovir-resistant herpes simplex virus infections in patients with the acquired immunodeficiency syndrome. N Engl J Med 1989; 320:293–296.

43. Schiodt M, Rindum J, Bygbert I. Chickenpox with oral manifestations in an AIDS patient. Dan Dent J 1987; 91:316–319.

44. Heinic GS, Northfelt DW, Greenspan JS, et al. Concurrent oral cytomegalovirus and herpes simplex virus infection in association with HIV infection: a case report. Oral Surg Oral Med Oral Pathol 1993; 75:488–494.

45. Greenspan D, Greenspan JS, Conant M, et al. Oral "hairy" leucoplakia in male homosexuals: evidence of association with both papillomavirus and a herpes-group virus. Lancet 1984; 2:831–834.

46. Greenspan JS, Greenspan D, Palefsky JM. Oral hairy leukoplakia after a decade. Epstein-Barr Virus Report 1995; 2:123–128.

47. Greenspan JS, Greenspan D, Lennette ET, et al. Replication of Epstein–Barr virus within the epithelial cells of hairy leukoplakia, an AIDS-associated lesion. N Engl J Med 1985; 313:1564–1571.

48. DeSouza YG, Greenspan D, Felton JR, et al. Localization of Epstein–Barr virus DNA in the epithelial cells of oral hairy leukoplakia using in-situ hybridization on tissue sections [Letter]. N Engl J Med 1989; 320:1559–1560.

49. DeSouza YG, Freese UK, Greenspan D, et al. Diagnosis of Epstein–Barr virus infection in hairy leukoplakia by using nucleic acid hybridization and noninvasive techniques. J Clin Microbiol 1990; 28:2775–2778.

50. Schiodt M, Dodd CL, Greenspan D, et al. Natural history of HIV-associated salivary gland disease. Oral Surg Oral Med Oral Pathol 1992; 74:326–331.

51. Daniels TE, Greenspan D, Greenspan JS, et al. Absence of Langerhans cells in oral hairy leukoplakia, an AIDS-associated lesion. J Invest Dermatol 1987; 89:178–182.

52. Williams DM, Leigh IM, Greenspan D, et al. Altered patterns of keratin expression in oral hairy leukoplakia: prognostic implications. J Oral Pathol Med 1991; 20:167–171.

53. Greenspan D, Greenspan JS, Hearst NG, et al. Oral hairy leukoplakia; human immunodeficiency virus status and risk for development of AIDS. J Infect Dis 1987; 155:475–478.

54. Greenspan D, Greenspan JS, Overby G, et al. Risk factors for rapid progression from hairy leukoplakia to AIDS: a nested case control study. J Acquir Immune Defic Syndr 1991; 4:652–658.

55. Itin P, Rufli I, Fudlinser R, et al. Oral hairy leukoplakia in a HIV-negative renal transplant patient: a marker for immunosuppression. Dermatologica 1988; 17:126–128.

56. Hollander H, Greenspan D, Stringari S, et al. Hairy leukoplakia and the acquired immunodeficiency syndrome. Ann Intern Med 1986: 104:892.

57. Resnick L, Herbst JHS, Ablashi DV, et al. Regression of oral hairy leukoplakia after orally administered acyclovir therapy. JAMA 1988; 259:384–388.

58. Katz MH, Greenspan D, Heinic GS, et al. Resolution of hairy leukoplakia: an observational trial of zidovudine versus no treatment [Letter]. J Infect Dis 1991; 164:1240–1241.

59. Becker J, Leser U, Marschall M, et al. Expression of proteins encoded by Epstein–Barr virus trans-activator genes depends on the differentiation of epithelial cells in oral hairy leukoplakia. Proc Natl Acad Sci USA 1991; 88:8332–8336.

60. Walling DM, Edmiston SN, Sixbey JW, et al. Coinfection with multiple strains of the Epstein-Barr virus in human immunodeficiency virus-associated hairy leukoplakia. Proc Natl Acad Sci USA 1992; 89:6560–6564.

61. Palefsky JM, Penaranda ME, Pierik LT, et al. Epstein–Barr virus BMRF-2 and BDLF-3 expression in hairy leukoplakia. Oral Dis 1997; 3(Suppl):171–176.

62. Penaranda ME, Lagenaur LA, Pierik LT, et al. Expression of Epstein–Barr virus BMRF-2 and BDLF-3 genes in hairy leukoplakia. J Gen Virol 1997; 78:3361–3370.

63. Hagensee ME, Cameron JE, Leigh JE, et al. Human papillomavirus infection and disease in HIV-infected individuals. Am J Med Sci 2004; 328:57–63.

64. Greenspan D, Villiers EM de, Greenspan JS, et al. Unusual HPV types in the oral warts in association with HIV infection. J Oral Pathol 1988; 17:482–487.

65. Volter C, He Y, Delius H, et al. Novel HPV types in oral papillomatous lesions from patients with HIV infection. Int J Cancer 1996; 66:453–456.

66. Regezi JA, Greenspan D, Greenspan JS, et al. HPV-associated epithelial atypia in oral warts in HIV+ patients. J Cutan Pathol 1994; 21:217–223.

67. Regezi JA, MacPhail LA, Daniels TE. Oral Kaposi's sarcoma: a 10-year retrospective histopathologic study. J Oral Pathol Med 1993; 22:292–297.

68. Ficarra G, Berson AM, Silverman S, et al. Kaposi's sarcoma of the oral cavity: a study of 134 patients with a review of the pathogenesis, epidemiology, clinical aspects, and treatment. Oral Surg Oral Med Oral Pathol 1988; 66:543–550.

69. Epstein JB, Scully C. Intralesional vinblastine for oral Kaposi's sarcoma in HIV infection. Lancet 1989; 2:1100–1101.

70. Lucatoto FM, Sapp JP. Treatment of oral Kaposi's sarcoma with a sclerosing agent in AIDS patients. Oral Surg Oral Med Oral Pathol 1993; 75:192–198.

71. Ziegler JL, Beckstead JA. Volberding PA, et al. Non-Hodgkins lymphoma in 90 homosexual men: relation to generalized lymphadenopathy and the acquired immunodeficiency syndrome. N Engl J Med 1984; 311:565–570.

72. Frisch M, Biggar RJ, Engels EA, et al; AIDS-Cancer Match Registry Study Group. Association of cancer with AIDS-related immunosuppression in adults. JAMA 2001; 285:1736–1745.

73. Grulich AE, Li Y, McDonald A, et al. Rates of non-AIDS-defining cancers in people with HIV infection before and after AIDS diagnosis. AIDS 2002; 16:1155–1161.

74. Demopoulos BP, Vamvakas E, Ehrlich JE, et al. Non-acquired immunodeficiency syndrome-defining malignancies in patients infected with human immunodeficiency virus. Arch Pathol Lab Med 2003; 127:589–592.

75. MacPhail LA, Greenspan JS. Oral ulceration in HIV infection: investigation and pathogenesis. Oral Dis 1997; 3(Suppl):190–193.

76. Jacobson JM, Greenspan JS, Spritzler J, et al. Thalidomide for the treatment of oral aphthous ulcers in patients with human immunodeficiency virus infection. National Institute of Allergy and Infectious Diseases AIDS Clinical Trials Group. N Engl J Med 1997; 336:1487–1493.

77. Jacobson JM, Greenspan JS, Spritzler J, et al. Thalidomide in low intermittent doses does not prevent recurrence of human immunodeficiency virus-associated aphthous ulcers. J Infect Dis 2001; 183:343–346.

78. Itescu S, Dalton J, Zhang HZ, et al. Tissue infiltration in a CD8 lymphocytosis syndrome associated with human immunodeficiency virus-1 infection has the phenotypic appearance of an antigenically driven response. J Clin Invest 1993; 91:2216–2225.

79. Itescu S, Brancato LJ, Winchester R. A sicca syndrome in HIV infection: association with HLA-DR5 and CD8 lymphocytosis [Letter]. Lancet 1989; 2:466–468.

80. Leggott PJ. Oral manifestations of HIV infection in children. Oral Surg Oral Med Oral Pathol 1992; 73:187–192.

CHAPTER 21

Ocular Manifestations

James P. Dunn

Introduction

The ocular manifestations of HIV/AIDS can be categorized into five areas: non-infectious retinal microvasculopathy, ocular infections, neuroophthalmologic disorders, ocular neoplasms, and ocular side-effects of systemic medications. Ocular complications, most commonly, cytomegalovirus (CMV) retinitis, are a significant cause of diminished quality of life in patients with HIV/AIDS.[1-3] In the pre-HAART era, up to 49.1 events of vision loss to 20/200 or worse, occurred per 100 eye-years, and the rate of legal blindness, with visual acuity loss in the better-seeing eye to 20/200 or worse, ranged up to 14.8 per 100 patient-years (PY). Most cases of severe visual loss were associated with retinitis involving the macula or optic nerve. Others were due to retinal detachment, which occur in about one-third of eyes with CMV retinitis per year.[1] A more recent study conducted after the introduction of HAART found that in patients affected with CMV retinitis, about one-third of eyes had suffered visual impairment (visual acuity of 20/50 or worse) at the time of diagnosis, and almost one-fifth had a visual acuity of 20/200 or worse.[3] Recognition of the ocular manifestations of HIV/AIDS is critical, as they may be the first sign of advanced immunosuppression, may provide clinical confirmation of systemic disease suspected elsewhere, and early diagnosis may minimize the ocular morbidity by allowing prompt therapy. Reducing the incidence of ocular opportunistic infections with HAART is also important, given that CMV retinitis is the most expensive AIDS-related condition.[4] The average cost of treating a single episode of CMV retinitis in the pre-HAART era was nearly US$20 000. In a recent study that adjusted for HAART usage and concomitant AIDS-defining illnesses, it was determined that oral anti-CMV therapy saved US$7185 per treatment period over i.v. therapy, while intraocular anti-CMV therapy saved US$6866 over i.v. therapy per treatment period.[5]

Non-infectious Retinal Microvasculopathy

The most common ocular manifestation of HIV/AIDS is a non-infectious retinal microvasculopathy, sometimes called 'AIDS retinopathy' or 'background HIV retinopathy'. The prevalence is correlated with the degree of immunosuppression.[6] Patients with CD4 cell counts >200 cells/mL are rarely affected, but well over half of patients with CD4 cell counts <50 cells/mL have clinically evident retinopathy, and virtually all patients with advanced AIDS are found to have at least some microvascular abnormalities when fluorescein angiography is performed. Cotton-wool spots (infarcts of the superficial nerve fiber layer, Figure 21.1) are the most common feature, but flame-shaped and dot-blot hemorrhages, Roth spots, and capillary non-perfusion can also be seen. Affected patients rarely have impaired visual acuity, and there is no pain, redness, or photophobia. Occasionally, cotton-wool spots near the macular can cause small scotomata. On the other hand, psychophysical testing in patients with AIDS may demonstrate impaired color vision and contrast sensitivity, suggesting a cumulative effect of nerve fiber layer infarcts.

Cotton-wool spots are evanescent; as the superficial retinal edema clears, the feathery white lesions disappear, leaving subtle depressions in the retina

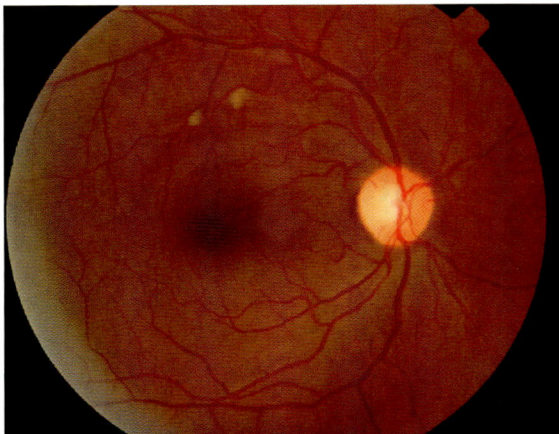

Figure 21.1 Non-infectious retinal microvasculopathy (background HIV retinopathy), right eye. Note the cotton-wool spots superior to the fovea.

Box 21.1

Ocular Infections

I. Corneal and conjunctival infections
   a. Molluscum contagiosum virus
   b. Herpes zoster ophthalmicus
   c. Herpes simplex virus
   d. Microsporidiosis
   e. Fungal keratitis
   f. Bacterial keratitis.
II. Retinal and choroidal infections
   a. Cytomegalovirus retinitis
   b. Progressive outer retinal necrosis
   c. Acute retinal necrosis
   d. Toxoplasmosis retinitis.
III. Central nervous system infections
   a. Cryptococcosis
   b. Toxoplasmosis
   c. Progressive multifocal leukoencephalopathy
   e. Varicella zoster.
IV. Other infections
   a. Syphilis
   b. Tuberculosis.

that can sometimes be detected with careful contact lens biomicroscopy. New lesions may develop in patients who remain immunosuppressed, but patients who respond to HAART usually regain a normal-appearing fundus. Non-infectious retinal microvasculopathy in HIV-infected patients is more extensive than that found in patients who are iatrogenically immunosuppressed.[7]

The significance of detecting non-infectious retinal microvasculopathy is that it serves as a clinical marker of advanced immunosuppression. Affected patients are at greater risk for ocular opportunistic infections such as CMV retinitis, and some investigators recommend routine dilated ophthalmoscopic examinations at 3–6-month intervals to detect early evidence of infection. Non-infectious microvasculopathy must be distinguished from other causes of cotton-wool spots and retinal hemorrhages, such as diabetes, hypertension, and pancreatitis, as well as from infectious retinitis such as CMV retinitis or metastatic *Candida* endophthalmitis. The characteristic feathery border of the cotton-wool spots, lack of uveitis, and the absence of progression of lesions over several weeks in non-infectious microvasculopathy is usually sufficient to distinguish these entities clinically.

The cause of the microvasculopathy is not known, although it is generally agreed that infection with HIV (which has been identified in most ocular tissues in infected patients) in and of itself does not account for the changes. Vascular sludging due to hypergammaglobulinemia, immunoglobulin deposition with immune complex formation, and local release of

cytotoxic substances, have all been suggested as causative factors.

In contrast, retinal macrovasculopathy (retinal vein or retinal artery occlusions) occurs in only about 1% of patients with HIV/AIDS.[8] As with non-infectious microvasculopathy, the cause is not known. Visual loss, however, may be severe. There is no specific therapy; control of vasculopathic risk factors such as hypertension, diabetes, or dyslipidemia is indicated.

Ocular Infections

Infections in patients with HIV/AIDS (Box 21.1) can be categorized by their location (lid, conjunctival, or corneal versus retinal or choroidal) and by their frequency. The prevalence of some ocular infections is markedly increased in HIV-infected individuals (e.g. CMV retinitis), while others do not appear to be more common (e.g. herpes simplex keratitis). Two important principles to bear in mind are: (1) ocular infections in this population may be polymicrobial, particularly in the retina or choroid, and (2) the clinical findings may be very different from that seen in immunocompetent individuals. An 11-year retrospective study[9] examined the incidence of CMV retinitis, herpes zoster ophthalmicus, *Pneumocystis* choroidopathy, herpes simplex keratitis, *Toxoplasma* retinitis, fungal retinitis, ocular syphilis, and ocular lymphoma in all patients at San Francisco General Hospital. Only CMV retinitis, herpes zoster ophthalmicus, and, to a lesser extent, *Toxoplasma* retinitis showed both an elevated risk ratio and rate difference among patients who were HIV-positive compared with patients who were HIV-negative. Molluscum contagiosum and herpes zoster are also more common in HIV-infected patients. However, the conjunctival flora in patients with AIDS does not appear to be different from that in HIV-negative individuals.[10]

Molluscum Contagiosum

Molluscum contagiosum virus (MCV) is a poxvirus that produces characteristic waxy, umbilicated, keratinized lesions on the skin and, rarely, the conjunctiva or mucous membranes. The lesions spread by direct contact. In immunocompetent individuals, children are most commonly affected; the facial and periocular MCV lesions tend to be single or limited to a small number, but can cause a severe follicular conjunctivitis. In contrast, HIV-infected patients often have multiple lesions, often confluent, but rarely develop conjunctivitis. In large lesions, the differential diagnosis includes disseminated cryptococcosis or histoplasmosis and bacillary angiomatosis. Treatment is usually based on cosmetic indications, as the lesions may be quite disfiguring. Treatment options include surgical excision, cryoablation, or chemocautery, but the most effective therapy is HAART; immune recovery may result in dramatic disappearance of the lesions.

Herpes Simplex

Herpes simplex virus (HSV) can cause cutaneous, conjunctival, or corneal lesions. Eyelid lesions usually manifest as vesicular eruptions that cross dermatomal distributions; there may be ulceration of the eyelid margin. Keratitis takes the form of epithelial keratitis (dendritic lesions or geographic ulcerations) or stromal ulceration. Ocular involvement is usually unilateral. Treatment with topical trifluridine (Viroptic) for 10–14 days is usually effective; many clinicians recommend oral acyclovir (Zovirax) or valacyclovir (Valtrex) for secondary prophylaxis to reduce the risk of recurrence.

Varicella Zoster

Varicella zoster infection can cause conjunctivitis, keratitis, iritis, scleritis, and retinitis (see below).

Herpes zoster ophthalmicus (HZO) may be multidermatomal, but V_1 is the most commonly affected dermatome. Corneal involvement, uveitis, and postherpetic neuralgia are more common in HZO in HIV-infected patients compared with HIV-negative patients. Treatment includes intravenous acyclovir or valacyclovir. Zoster ophthalmicus may represent an early and ominous sign of HIV infection, and HIV testing should be considered in any young adult presenting with HZO.

Several factors may increase the risk of ocular surface disease in patients with AIDS, including dry eye, trauma, exposure keratopathy (including drug-induced stupor), use of topical corticosteroids to treat uveitis, and the use of crack cocaine, the smoke from which may have both a neurotrophic and toxic effect on corneal epithelium. There are a number of ocular surface infections (too numerous to mention here) that have been reported only anecdotally in patients with AIDS. For reasons that are unclear, certain infections such as corneal microsporidiosis appear to be less common now than 10 or 15 years ago. Any patient with keratitis or conjunctivitis that appears atypical, rapidly progressive, or unresponsive to empiric therapy should undergo cultures and stains.

Infections of the retina and choroid are a significant cause of morbidity in patients with HIV/AIDS. In the pre-HAART era, CMV retinitis occurred in about 30% of patients with AIDS and constituted about 80–90% of all CMV infections. Currently, however, the risk is about 5% or less. CMV retinitis remains by far the most common of these infections, because HAART is associated with a marked reduction in all ocular opportunistic infections. Patients at greatest risk are those with a CD4 count <25 cells/mL.[6]

Symptoms of CMV retinitis include floaters, photopsias, and visual field deficits without pain, redness, or photophobia. Up to half of affected patients are asymptomatic. Retinitis is unilateral at the time of diagnosis in about two-thirds of patients; half of these patients will develop contralateral retinitis within 6 months if not treated.[1]

CMV retinitis is usually diagnosed clinically. The characteristic appearance is a dry, granular-appearing border around lesions that may show a mixture of hemorrhage and necrosis (fulminant/edematous retinitis, Figure 21.2) or necrosis without hemorrhage (indolent/granular retinitis, Figure 21.3). About 20% of patients have a striking perivascular sheathing that may be evident in the retina well away from areas of retinitis. Lesions may be single or multiple. There is usually a mild anterior chamber

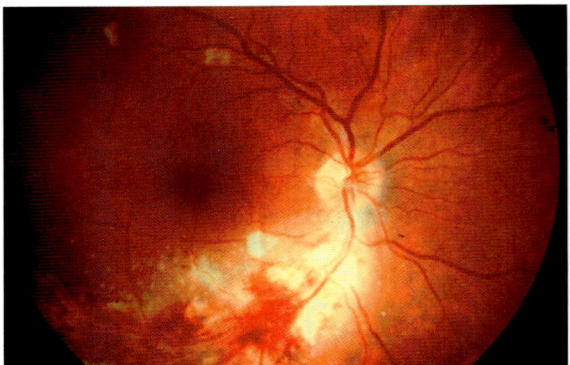

Figure 21.2 Fulminant/hemorrhagic CMV retinitis along the inferotemporal arcade, right eye. Note the cotton-wool spots along the superotemporal arcade (concurrent non-infectious microvasculopathy).

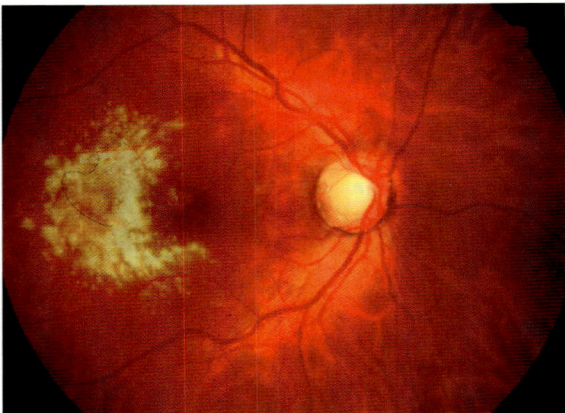

Figure 21.3 Indolent/granular CMV retinitis in the temporal macula, right eye. Note the absence of hemorrhage but the presence of the characteristic granular-appearing border of the lesion.

uveitis and vitreitis. The retinitis is slowly progressive; untreated lesions progresses on average about 25 μm/day. Therefore, the risk to vision is much greater from lesions near the fovea or optic nerve.

Affected retina is non-functional and does not regenerate. Vision loss from CMV retinitis may result from macular necrosis, optic nerve involvement (CMV papillitis or optic neuritis), retinal detachment, or retinal edema at the leading edge of active lesions. Retinal detachments occurred in up to 50% of patients within a year of diagnosis in the pre-HAART era; in patients treated with HAART, the overall risk of detachment is lower, but remains similar in patients with a CD4+ count below 50 cells/mL.[11,12]

Untreated CMV retinitis is relentlessly progressive and results in complete loss of vision with total retinal necrosis and optic nerve atrophy. There are a number of drugs used to treat CMV retinitis: ganciclovir, valganciclovir, cidofovir, foscarnet, and fomivirsen. Formulations of these drugs and their side-effects are given in Table 21.1. Randomized clinical trials in the pre-HAART era indicated comparable efficacy of intravenous ganciclovir and foscarnet[13]; both treatments were initially effective, but relapse was almost inevitable (50% within 3 months), and lifelong therapy was needed. The median survival after the diagnosis of CMV retinitis was 8–12 months. A major drawback to the use of intravenous ganciclovir and foscarnet is the need for daily therapy; patients treated with these drugs require placement of a permanent indwelling catheter.

Relapse (progression) of CMV retinitis is noted clinically as whitening of a previously inactive-appearing border and migration of the border edge.

It is usually caused by inadequate intraocular drug penetration into the eye. This problem may be overcome by placement of an intraocular ganciclovir implant, which in randomized controlled trials has been proven more effective than intravenous ganciclovir.[14] The implant delivers intraocular drug concentrations roughly 4-fold higher than can be achieved with intravenous ganciclovir. However, the implant must be given with systemic anti-CMV therapy to reduce the risk of contralateral and visceral CMV disease.[14] Complications of ganciclovir implantation have included endophthalmitis, retinal detachment, vitreous hemorrhage, cataract, and hypotony.[15] There is no significant difference in the risk of retinal detachment in eyes treated with a ganciclovir implant compared with eyes treated with systemic anti-CMV therapy.[11] Transient decreases in visual acuity may occur postoperatively, as a result of postoperative cycloplegia, vitreous hemorrhage, or temporary astigmatism. Rare complications include scleritis and implant extrusion.

Valganciclovir, a pro-drug of oral ganciclovir, is the systemic drug usually given because of its once-daily maintenance regimen and its comparable efficacy to intravenous ganciclovir.[16] CMV retinitis is associated with an increased risk for mortality even after adjusting for demographic, immunologic, HIV virologic, and treatment factors,[17] so that oral anti-CMV therapy is usually indicated in patients with unilateral CMV retinitis.

Fomivirsen (Vitravene), an oligonucleotide antisense compound, was approved by the FDA in 1998 for intravitreal injection every other week for induc-

Table 21.1 Drugs used to treat CMV retinitis

Drug	Form	Mechanism of action	Side-effects	Comments
Ganciclovir (Cytovene)	Intravenous	Anti-CMV DNA polymerase	Bone marrow suppression, nausea	Comparable efficacyto i.v. foscarnet
Ganciclovir (Cytovene)	Oral	Anti-CMV DNA polymerase	Bone marrow suppression, nausea, diarrhea	Limited bioavailability; rarely used
Ganciclovir (Vitrasert)	Intraocular implant	Anti-CMV DNA polymerase	Hemorrhage, endophthalmitis, hypotony, cataract	More effective than i.v. ganciclovir
Valganciclovir (Valcyte)	Oral	Anti-CMV DNA polymerase	Bone marrow suppression, nausea, diarrhea	Has replaced p.o. ganciclovir and has largely replaced i.v. ganciclovir
Cidofovir (Vistide)	Intravenous (i.v.)	Anti-CMV DNA polymerase	Renal insufficiency, uveitis, hypotony	Must be given concurrently with probenecid
Foscarnet (Foscavir)	Intravenous (i.v.)	Anti-CMV DNA polymerase	Renal insufficiency, electrolyte abnormalities, penile ulcers	Requires indwelling catheter; comparable efficacy to i.v. ganciclovir
Fomivirsen (Vitravene)	Intravitreous injection	Antisense oligonucleotide	Uveitis, glaucoma, pigmentary retinopathy	Taken off the market in 2003 due to poor sales

tion, then once monthly for maintenance therapy. The drug showed promise in treating ganciclovir-resistant CMV retinitis. Ocular toxicity, especially retinal pigment epitheliopathy, uveitis, and glaucoma were reported.[18] The drug was withdrawn from the market by the manufacturer in 2003 because of weak sales.

Viral drug resistance occurs in 20–30% of patients treated with systemic anti-CMV therapy after 6–12 months of therapy. Patients with ganciclovir-resistant strains of CMV in the blood or urine (defined phenotypically as an IC50 >6.0 µmol/L and genotypically as the occurrence of a cytomegalovirus UL97 gene mutation known to confer ganciclovir resistance) tend to have a poorer visual prognosis and have an increased risk of retinitis progression.[19] Low-level resistance is caused by mutations in the CMV UL97 gene, which codes for a protein kinase necessary for the uptake of ganciclovir into infected cells. High-level resistance is caused by mutations in the UL54 gene, which codes for CMV DNA polymerase. Mutations found in the blood generally correlate with those obtained from vitreous specimens. Viral drug resistance testing in patients with CMV retinitis has not achieved the same clinical usage found in HIV testing.

The use of HAART increases the efficacy of specific anti-CMV therapy, so the ganciclovir implant may no longer be as critical in maintaining good visual outcomes.[20] In a recent large, multi-center study,[21] the overall rate of retinitis progression was 0.10/person-years (PY); among those with CD4 cell counts <50 cells/mL, it was 0.58/PY, compared with 0.02/PY among those with CD4 cell counts of ≥200/mL (P <0.0001). Significant risk factors for retinitis progression included a low CD4 cell count, positive CMV load, longer time from AIDS diagnosis, and low Karnofsky score. These findings compare favorably with the rate of retinitis progression of approximately 3.0/PY reported in the pre-HAART era. However, the study also confirmed that retinitis progression can occur even among patients with high CD4 cell counts and presumed immune recovery, so that continued ophthalmologic follow-up of patients with immune recovery is recommended to detect early retinitis progression. Data from the same cohort indicated that the risk of retinal detachment and of second-eye involvement was substantially lower in patients with CMV retinitis treated with HAART than in historical control patients from the pre-HAART era, but the benefit was mostly limited to those patients with a CD4 count >50 cells/mL.[12] A randomized clinical trial comparing intravenous cidofovir to the ganciclovir implant plus oral ganciclovir in patients with CMV retinitis, most of whom were taking HAART, found no significant differences in visual outcomes,[22] although the side-effect profiles vary between the two treatment regimens, as expected (Table 21.1). Eventually, sustained immune recovery from HAART alone is sufficient in many patients to suppress CMV retinitis, even after discontinuation of anti-CMV therapy.

In a large study of patients initially presenting with unilateral CMV retinitis (91% of whom were subsequently treated with anti-CMV therapy), involvement of the second eye occurred in 26.1%/PY (19.6% within the first 6 months), less than half the rate previously reported in untreated groups.[23] Initial CD4 cell counts >12 cells/mL and use of HAART were associated with 64% and 46% reduction in incidence. The benefit from HAART was limited to those patients who developed immune recovery of a degree expected to restore innate control of CMV (a rise in the CD4 cell count by >50 cells/mL to a level >100 cells/mL). The risk of contralateral retinitis was highest when CD4 cell counts were very low and in the months immediately after the diagnosis of CMV retinitis.

The differential diagnosis of CMV retinitis includes necrotizing herpetic retinitis (progressive outer retinal necrosis and acute retinal necrosis), syphilitic retinitis, toxoplasmosis retinitis, metastatic *Candida* retinitis, background HIV retinopathy, and non-Hodgkin's lymphoma.[24] In most cases, the diagnosis is made clinically, but occasionally PCR testing from vitreous or aqueous specimens may be necessary.

Retinal Detachment

Retinal detachment is common in eyes with CMV retinitis[1,11-13] and even more common in eyes with necrotizing herpetic retinopathy (see below). Surgical repair usually necessitates vitrectomy with silicone oil tamponade, with a high risk of subsequent development of cataract.[25] Visually significant posterior capsular opacification tends to occur rapidly following cataract surgery.

Immune Recovery Uveitis

Immune recovery uveitis (IRU), a syndrome of iritis, vitreitis, and macular edema, occurs in some patients with CMV retinitis who have developed a substantial degree of immune recovery (generally regarded as an increase in the CD4 cell count by >50 cells/mL or a sustained increase in the CD4 cell count to >100 cells/mL). The condition occurs only in eyes with CMV retinitis. Immune recovery uveitis is now a leading cause of visual impairment in patients with AIDS.[2] Initial treatment of CMV retinitis with the ganciclovir implant may reduce the risk of IRU com-

pared with patients treated with intravenous cidofovir. Treatment of IRU consists of periocular and/or oral corticosteroids for macular edema and vitrectomy for structural complications such as epiretinal membrane formation.[26] Mild macular edema may resolve spontaneously, but more severe disease may be recalcitrant to treatment. There are conflicting data as to whether resuming anti-CMV therapy is beneficial[27]; however, one small study that performed PCR of blood, aqueous, and vitreous specimens in patients with IRU did not find detectable CMV, suggesting that there is not ongoing viral replication in the vitreous body and aqueous humor of these patients.[28]

All currently approved drugs for the treatment of CMV retinitis are virostatic only. In the pre-HAART era, discontinuation of therapy due to drug toxicity invariably resulted in the progression of the retinitis. However, in patients with sustained immune recovery due to HAART (generally defined as a sustained increase in the CD4 cell count to >100 cells/mL or an increase of >50 cells/mL from baseline), anti-CMV therapy can usually be safely discontinued if the retinitis has been inactive for more than 3 months.[29] Some authors believe that a longer course of anti-CMV therapy prior to discontinuation because of immune recovery may decrease the risk of immune recovery uveitis.[30]

Progressive Outer Retinal Necrosis

Progressive outer retinal necrosis (PORN) is a variant of necrotizing herpetic retinopathy that occurs in patients with advanced immunosuppression and is nearly always caused by varicella zoster virus.[31] Affected patients may complain of eye pain with movement as a result of optic nerve involvement even before the retinal lesions are visible. Retinal findings include multifocal necrotic lesions that rapidly coalesce and spread much faster than CMV retinitis. There is minimal or no vitreous inflammation; the retinal vasculature appears normal but a 'cracked mud' perivascular pattern, caused by early removal of necrotic debris or edema by retinal tissue, is characteristic. The majority of patients become legally blind within 1 month due to retinal detachment, optic neuropathy, or widespread retinal necrosis. Retinal and vitreous hemorrhage is common and may also compromise vision. Treatment usually consists of combination antiviral therapy, such as valacyclovir plus foscarnet, but long-term retention of vision is unlikely if the patient does not respond to HAART.

Acute Retinal Necrosis

Acute retinal necrosis (ARN) is another variant of necrotizing herpetic retinopathy characterized by marked anterior and intermediate uveitis, retinal arteritis, papillitis of the optic disc, and retinal and choroidal occlusive vasculitis.[32] Affected patients usually have a CD4 cell count >60 cells/mL and a history of dermatomal zoster or herpes simplex virus dermatitis. There is a high risk of retinal detachment and blindness, although aggressive therapy with intravenous acyclovir or foscarnet and early laser retinopexy to prevent extension of peripheral detachments may result in good vision.

Ocular Toxoplasmosis

The incidence of ocular toxoplasmosis has declined markedly due to the widespread use of HAART as well as trimethoprim-sulfamethoxazole for primary prophylaxis against central nervous system toxoplasmosis. Ocular findings in patients with AIDS may differ considerably from that in immunocompetent patients. Multifocal or bilateral involvement, absence of pre-existing chorioretinal scars, and evidence of systemic toxoplasmosis infection are all much more common in patients with AIDS.[33] Toxoplasmosis retinitis may mimic CMV retinitis, but can usually be distinguished by the presence of a smooth, non-granular border, relative absence of retinal hemorrhage, and prominent vitreous and anterior chamber inflammation. Treatment is similar to that used in immunocompetent individuals, but long-term secondary prophylaxis may be necessary.

Syphilis

Syphilis and tuberculosis are usually considered in the differential diagnosis of intraocular infection. Syphilis can cause uveitis, optic neuropathy, and necrotizing retinitis. Serologic testing with RPR and FTA-ABS should be performed in any HIV-infected patient with uveitis, and CSF VDRL should be performed if there are associated neuroophthalmic signs or symptoms. Treatment with high-dose intravenous penicillin for 10–14 days (12–24 million units/day) is recommended for HIV-positive patients with ocular syphilis. *Ocular tuberculosis* is rare in the USA, despite the resurgence of TB in the HIV-infected population. Ocular involvement may include panuveitis and choroidopathy. Multi-drug therapy is usually effective.

Neuroophthalmic Manifestations

Neuroophthalmic Complications

Neuroophthalmic complications are relatively uncommon manifestations of HIV/AIDS, occurring in <10% of patients. Patients treated with HAART have a lower incidence of opportunistic intracranial infections.[34] A variety of clinical findings, including visual impairment, cranial nerve palsies, papillary abnormalities, optic neuropathies (papilledema, optic neuritis, optic atrophy), and visual field defects may occur.[35] Cryptococcal meningitis and intracranial toxoplasmosis are the most common underlying causes. Serologic testing, laboratory testing (including lumbar puncture), and imaging studies are often necessary to confirm the diagnosis and allow appropriate therapy. Occasionally, biopsy of brain tissue may be necessary (e.g. to distinguish between intracranial toxoplasmosis and non-Hodgkin's lymphoma). Suspicion of an infectious etiology (e.g. intracranial zoster) by PCR testing of cerebrospinal fluid can be very helpful.

Progressive Multifocal Leukoencephalopathy

Progressive multifocal leukoencephalopathy (PML) is caused by the JC virus. Ocular manifestations include homonymous visual field defects, occipital blindness, and nuclear and supranuclear palsies. Symptoms may improve in patients who begin HAART and develop immune recovery. The differential diagnosis includes lymphoma and intracranial zoster.

Neoplasms

Ophthalmic neoplasms in HIV-infected patients are much less common than similar tumors occurring elsewhere.[36] Kaposi sarcoma and squamous cell carcinoma affect the eyelid or conjunctiva, whereas non-Hodgkin's lymphoma can involve the retina, choroid, or orbit.

Kaposi Sarcoma

Kaposi sarcoma (KS) is a tumor of endothelial origin. Human herpes virus 8 has been identified as the causative agent. Although KS was once found in up to 30% of patients with AIDS, ocular involvement was less common than oral, pulmonary, cutaneous, or gastrointestinal disease. Today, ocular KS is rare. Lesions are seen most often in the inferior conjunctival cul-de-sac, where they can mimic non-clearing subconjunctival hemorrhage, or on the eyelid, where they manifest as raised, purplish, nodules. As with many virally-mediated diseases in patients with AIDS, HAART is the most effective definitive therapy.[36] Palliative therapy for eyelid or conjunctival disease is usually undertaken for cosmetic reasons or because of secondary eyelid abnormalities (e.g. entropion); options include radiation, surgical excision, systemic or intralesional chemotherapy, or cryoablation. Systemic ganciclovir, used to treat CMV retinitis, reduces the risk of KS.

Ocular Squamous Cell Carcinoma

Ocular squamous cell carcinoma (SCC) usually involves the limbal area and presents as a gelatinous or scaly lesion with variable leukoplakia. It may be associated with human papillomavirus infection. The incidence appears to be greater in sub-Saharan Africa than in the USA. HIV-infected patients with conjunctival SCC are at increased risk of life-threatening metastatic disease. Treatment consists of wide excision with freeze–thaw cryotherapy to the adjacent margins, often with application of a topical antimetabolite such as mitomycin-C.

B-cell Non-Hodgkin's Lymphoma

B-cell non-Hodgkin's lymphoma (NHL) is associated with Epstein–Barr infection. The incidence of primary central nervous system lymphoma has decreased in the era of HAART. Ocular NHL is rare, but can occur in the retina, choroid, or orbit. Retinal involvement is associated with central nervous system NHL, while choroidal involvement is associated with systemic NHL. Within the eye, NHL may cause a necrotizing retinitis that is in the differential diagnosis for CMV, toxoplasmosis, or syphilitic retinitis. The prognosis is poor, despite new combination regimens of intrathecal and intraocular chemotherapy.

Ocular Side-effects of Systemic Medications

Rifabutin (*Mycobutin*)

Rifabutin (*Mycobutin*) is used in the treatment of and prophylaxis against mycobacterial infections. Acute uveitis with or without hypopyon formation can occur as a result of this drug, particularly when given at daily doses exceeding 600 mg and when ethambutol and clarithromycin are given concurrently.[37] Patients may present with acute pain, redness, and photophobia mimicking HLA-B27-associated uveitis or even endophthalmitis. Discontinuation of the drug and aggressive topical and/or periocular corticosteroid therapy is effective. Some patients have been able to resume rifabutin therapy successfully after resolution of the uveitis. Asymptomatic peripheral corneal endothelial deposits have also been associated with rifabutin therapy. The pathophysiologic mechanism of the uveitis and endothelial deposits is unknown.

Cidofovir (Vistide)

Cidofovir (*Vistide*), used in the treatment of CMV retinitis, can cause an acute or indolent anterior and intermediate uveitis, usually after the patient has received 3–5 doses.[38] Posterior synechiae formation occurs in over half of affected patients, and hypotony is common. It is essential to recognize the uveitis as early as possible, because continued cidofovir treatment can result in worsening of the uveitis and irreversible vision loss. Patients taking other nephrotoxic medications are at greatest risk. Discontinuation of cidofovir and treatment with topical corticosteroids is usually effective. Cidofovir should be resumed only with great caution in any affected patient.

Several drugs can cause optic neuropathy, of which ethambutol (*Myambutol*) is the best known. Findings include decreased color vision and central or centrocecal scotomata, usually 3–6 months after initiating therapy. Patients taking more than 15 mg/kg per day and those with renal insufficiency are at greatest risk. There is no specific treatment; discontinuation of the drug usually results in slow but variable visual recovery. Sildenafil (*Viagra*) has recently been associated with anterior ischemic optic neuropathy (AION), and other drugs used to treat erectile dysfunction probably carry a similar risk. However, patients taking these drugs generally have other risk factors for AION, such as diabetes, hypertension, and dyslipidemia, and a causative effect of sildenafil has not been proven; whether HIV-infected patients taking the drug are at increased risk is not known.

Interferon-α

Interferon-α can cause an ischemic retinopathy manifesting as cotton-wool spots, retinal hemorrhages, arteriolar occlusion, and capillary non-perfusion. Vision usually remains good, and the retinopathy typically resolves after discontinuation of the drug. Didanosine, an antiretroviral nucleotide analogue, may cause a peripheral pigmentary retinopathy. Children appear to be more susceptible than adults. The macula is usually spared, so that central visual acuity remains intact.

Conclusion

Ocular manifestations of AIDS are common and potentially blinding. The widespread use of HAART has resulted in a marked reduction in the incidence of ocular infections and improved the outcome of treatment in many of these disorders. Discontinuation of specific anti-infective therapy may be possible in patients with CMV retinitis and toxoplasmosis, but immune recovery may precipitate intraocular inflammation and vision-threatening macular edema in patients with CMV retinitis. Clinical recognition of ocular infections or neoplastic disorders may provide important information in the diagnosis and treatment of systemic diseases.

References

1. Holbrook JT, Jabs DA, Weinberg DV, et al. Visual loss in patients with cytomegalovirus retinitis and acquired immunodeficiency syndrome before widespread availability of highly active antiretroviral therapy. Arch Ophthalmol 2003; 121:99–107.
2. Jabs DA. AIDS and ophthalmology in 2004. Arch Ophthalmol 2004; 122:1040–1042.
3. Kempen JH, Martin BK, Wu AW, et al. The effect of cytomegalovirus retinitis on the quality of life of patients with AIDS in the era of highly active antiretroviral therapy. Ophthalmology 2003; 110:987–995.
4. Moore RD, Chaisson RE. Cost-utility analysis of prophylactic treatment with oral ganciclovir for cytomegalovirus retinitis. J Acquir Immune Defic Syndr Hum Retrovirol 1997; 16:15–21.
5. Mahadevia PJ, Gebo KA, Pettit K, et al. The epidemiology, treatment patterns, and costs of cytomegalovirus retinitis in the post-HAART era among a national managed-care population. J Acquir Immune Defic Syndr 2004; 36:972–977.
6. Jabs DA. Ocular manifestations of HIV infection. Trans Am Ophthalmol Soc 1995; 93:623–683.
7. Glasgow BJ, Weisberger AK. A quantitative and cartographic study of retinal microvasculopathy in acquired immunodeficiency syndrome. Am J Ophthalmol 1994; 118:46–56
8. Dunn JP, Yamashita A, Kempen JH, et al. Retinal vascular occlusion in patients infected with human immunodeficiency virus. Retina 2005; 25:759–766.
9. Hodge WG, Seiff SR, Margolis TP. Ocular opportunistic infection incidences among patients who are HIV positive compared to patients who are HIV negative. Ophthalmology 1998; 105:895–900.
10. Gritz DC, Scott TJ, Sedo SF, et al. Ocular flora of patients with AIDS compared with those of HIV-negative patients. Cornea 1997; 16:400–405.
11. Kempen JH, Jabs DA, Dunn JP, et al. Retinal detachment risk in cytomegalovirus retinitis related to the acquired immunodeficiency syndrome. Arch Ophthalmol 2001; 119:33–40.
12. Jabs DA, Van Natta ML, Thorne JE, et al. Course of cytomegalovirus retinitis in the era of highly active antiretroviral therapy: 2. Second eye involvement and retinal detachment. Ophthalmology 2004; 111:2232–2239.
13. Studies of the Ocular Complications of AIDS Research Group. Foscarnet-Ganciclovir Cytomegalovirus Retinitis Trial. 4. Visual outcomes. Studies of Ocular Complications of AIDS Research Group in collaboration with the AIDS Clinical Trials Group. Ophthalmology 1994; 101:1250–1261.
14. Martin DF, Kuppermann BD, Wolitz RA, et al. Oral ganciclovir for patients with cytomegalovirus retinitis treated with a ganciclovir implant. Roche Ganciclovir Study Group N Engl J Med 1999; 340:1063–1070.
15. Dunn JP, Van Natta M, Foster G, et al. Complications of ganciclovir implant surgery in patients with cytomegalovirus retinitis: the Ganciclovir Cidofovir Cytomegalovirus Retinitis Trial. Retina 2004; 24:41–50.
16. Cvetkovic RS. Wellington K. Valganciclovir: a review of its use in the management of CMV infection and disease in immunocompromised patients. Drugs 2005; 65:859–878.
17. Jabs DA, Holbrook JT, Van Natta ML, et al. Risk factors for mortality in patients with AIDS in the era of highly active antiretroviral therapy. Ophthalmology 2005; 112:771–779.
18. Vitravene Study Group. Safety of intravitreous fomivirsen for treatment of cytomegalovirus retinitis in patients with AIDS. Am J Ophthalmol 2002; 133:484–498.
19. Jabs DA, Martin BK, Forman MS, et al. Cytomegalovirus resistance to ganciclovir and clinical outcomes of patients with cytomegalovirus retinitis. Am J Ophthalmol 2003; 135:26–34.
20. Kempen JH, Jabs DA, Wilson LA, et al. Risk of vision loss in patients with cytomegalovirus retinitis and the acquired immunodeficiency syndrome. Arch Ophthalmol 2003; 121:466–476.
21. Jabs DA, Van Natta ML, Thorne JE, et al. Course of cytomegalovirus retinitis in the era of highly active antiretroviral therapy: 1. Retinitis progression. Ophthalmology 2004; 111:2224–2231.
22. Studies of Ocular Complications of AIDS Research Group. The AIDS Clinical Trials Group. The ganciclovir implant plus oral ganciclovir versus parenteral cidofovir for the treatment of cytomegalovirus retinitis in patients with acquired immunodeficiency syndrome: The Ganciclovir Cidofovir Cytomegalovirus Retinitis Trial. Am J Ophthalmol 2001; 131:457–467.
23. Kempen JH, Jabs DA, Wilson LA, et al. Incidence of cytomegalovirus (CMV) retinitis in second eyes of patients with the acquired immune deficiency syndrome and unilateral CMV retinitis. Am J Ophthalmol 2005; 139:1028–1034.
24. Davis JL. Differential diagnosis of CMV retinitis. Ocul Immunol Inflamm 1999; 7:159–166.
25. Tanna AP, Kempen JH, Dunn JP, et al. Incidence and management of cataract after retinal detachment repair with silicone oil in immune compromised patients with cytomegalovirus retinitis. Am J Ophthalmol 2003; 136:1009–1015.
26. El-Bradey MH, Cheng L, Song MK, et al. Long-term results of treatment of macular complications in eyes with immune recovery uveitis using a graded treatment approach. Retina 2004; 24:376–382.
27. Kosobucki BR, Goldberg DE, Bessho K, et al. Valganciclovir therapy for immune recovery uveitis complicated by macular edema. Am J Ophthalmol 2004; 137:636–638.
28. Siqueira RC, Cunha A, Orefice F, et al. PCR with the aqueous humor, blood leukocytes and vitreous of patients affected by cytomegalovirus retinitis and immune recovery uveitis. Ophthalmologica 2004; 218:43–48.
29. Whitcup SM, Fortin E, Lindblad AS, et al. Discontinuation of anticytomegalovirus therapy in patients with HIV

infection and cytomegalovirus retinitis. JAMA 1999;
282:1633–1637.

30. Jabs DA, Bolton SG, Dunn JP, et al. Discontinuing
anticytomegalovirus therapy in patients with immune
reconstitution after combination antiretroviral therapy. Am
J Ophthalmol 1998; 126:817–822.

31. Engstrom RE, Holland GN, Margolis TP, et al. The
progressive outer retinal necrosis syndrome. A variant of
necrotizing herpetic retinopathy in patients with AIDS.
Ophthalmology 1994; 101:1488–1502.

32. Duker JS. BLumenkranz MS. Diagnosis and management
of the acute retinal necrosis (ARN) syndrome. Surv
Ophthalmol 1991; 35:327–343.

33. Holland GN, Engstrom RJ, Glasgow BJ, et al. Ocular
toxoplasmosis in patients with the acquired
immunodeficiency syndrome. Am J Ophthalmol 1988;
106:653–657.

34. Sacktor N. The epidemiology of human immunodeficiency
virus-associated neurological disease in the era of highly

active antiretroviral therapy. J Neurovirol 2002;
8(Suppl):115–121.

35. Vrabec TR. Posterior segment manifestations of HIV/AIDS.
Surv Ophthalmol 2004; 49:131–157.

36. Goedert JJ. The epidemiology of acquired
immunodeficiency syndrome malignancies. Semin Oncol
2000; 27:390–401.

37. Shafran SD, Singer J, Zarowny DP, et al. Determinants of
rifabutin-associated uveitis in patients treated with
rifabutin, clarithromycin, and ethambutol for
Mycobacterium avium complex bacteremia: a multivariate
analysis. Canadian HIV Trials Network Protocol 010 Study
Group. J Infect Dis 1998; 177:252–255.

38. Akler ME, Johnson DW, Burman WJ, et al. Anterior uveitis
and hypotony after intravenous cidofovir for the treatment
of cytomegalovirus retinitis. Ophthalmology 1998;
105:651–657.

CHAPTER 22

Global HIV and Dermatology

Toby Maurer

Staphylococcal Aureus Skin Infections

Staphylococcus aureus (*S. aureus*) is the most common cutaneous bacterial infection in a person with HIV disease.[1] Community acquired infections of subcutaneous and deep tissues are common throughout the world.[2] In the Caribbean Islands and Africa, bacterial infection in HIV has been documented to represent up to 40% of all skin diseases as either primary infection or secondary superinfection of eczema or scabies.[3] However, the frequency of bacterial disease of the skin is decreasing with changing economic standing and wider access to antimicrobials.[4] In Nigeria, Gondor, Kenya, and Ethiopia, eczematous diseases have replaced bacterial infections as the leading cause of cutaneous disease.[5]

High rates of *S. aureus* carriage of HIV-infected patients when compared with control populations has been noted and presumably serves as a risk factor for soft tissue and recurrent infections.[6] *S. aureus* in the skin can manifest in many ways including bullous impetigo, ecthyma, folliculitis, abscesses, and furuncles. Occasionally, large areas of follicles are involved forming a violaceous plaque. The plaque may or may not be studded with pustules. Rarely, abscess of the muscle (pyomyositis) may occur as well as deep tissue involvement in the form of necrotizing fasciitis.

With the widespread use of trimethoprim-sulfamethoxazole for the prophylaxis of Pneumocystis carinii pneumonia, there as been a marked increase of resistant *S. aureus*. Methicillin resistant *Staphylococcus aureus* (MRSA) is becoming an increasing problem in the HIV-infected patient. Risk factors for the development of MRSA in HIV includes CD4 counts $<100/mm^3$, previous hospitalizations, high risk sexual practices, drug-using behaviors and environmental exposures.[7]

Treatment

Knowing the organism and its sensitivities is imperative where at all possible. Increasing resistance to β-lactam drugs and fluoroquinolones has been reported. Erythromycin, clindamycin, sulfamethoxazole, gentamicin, and intravenous vancomycin are still used. Tetracycline drugs are being used with more frequency.[8] Linezolid is an expensive alternative and should be reserved for cases in which there is documented resistance to the above mentioned antibiotics.[9] Incision and drainage of abscesses is critical. Hibiclens and Betadine washes may have a role but can often dry out the skin, leading to eczematous eruptions that are prone to secondary bacterial infections. Mupirocin ointment reduces carriage rates in HIV and prevents relapses but there is concern of emerging mupirocin resistance.[10] Rifampin can be used in combination with other antibiotics to reduce carriage rates of *S. aureus* and act synergistically with other antibiotics but cannot be used with many of the antiretroviral medications, particularly the protease inhibitors, because of drug–drug interactions.[11] In Mali, an algorithm for treatment of skin diseases was developed. Patients were first evaluated for signs of pyoderma by looking for presence of yellow crusts, pus, sores or blisters. Depending on the degree of pyoderma, patients were treated with topical antiseptics or oral antibiotics and returned for a follow-up visit. Abscesses were incised and drained and not treated with antibiotics. The use of this algorithm correctly identified pyodermas and secondarily infected eczemas 96–98% of the time, and decreased the use of steroids and antifungals.[12]

Bacillary Angiomatosis

Bacillary angiomatosis (BA), a treatable opportunistic infection, can present as vascular, easily friable lesions or subcutaneous lesions in patients with advanced HIV disease. The agents causing this infection have been classified as Bartonella and at least 15 species have been identified worldwide and are associated with different vectors.[13,14] Cutaneous manifestations of BA in the HIV-infected population are primarily caused by two species, *B. henselae* and *B. quintana*.[15,16] Epidemiologically, *B. henselae* has been associated with cat and flea exposure. *B. quintana* has been associated with low income, homelessness, and exposure to lice.[17] BA has been reported in South America, Europe, India, and Africa.[13,18–21] Seroprevalence studies have been done to show that the organism is present in Japan in HIV-infected subjects.[22] In countries where Kaposi's sarcoma (KS) is prevalent, BA may be under recognized as it can mimic the vascular lesions typically associated with KS. Lesions of BA have also been confused with pyogenic granuloma and lymphoma.[23]

Bacillary angiomatosis initially was considered a disorder of the skin, but systemic involvement is common. Visceral disease may present as osseous lesions, hepatic and splenic tumors, lymph node disease, pulmonary lesions, brain lesions, bone marrow, and widespread fatal systemic involvement. Bacillary angiomatosis can present as bacteremia and endocarditis in HIV-infected patients.[16] Lesions should be biopsied and examined with hematoxylin and eosin staining and Warthin–Starry silver staining which reveals the organisms. Culture, indirect fluorescent antibody testing and polymerase chain reaction can be performed on lesions and serum. Immunohistochemical staining for anti-HHV8 can be used to differentiate KS from BA.[24]

Treatment with erythromycin or doxycycline for at least 3 months is recommended even though cutaneous lesions resolve in 3–4 weeks. Relapses can occur if treatment is not continued appropriately. Severely ill patients should be treated with i.v. doxycycline with either gentamicin or rifampin for at least 4 months.

Pigmentation

HIV infection is associated with pigment disorders, both hyperpigmentation and hypopigmentation. Hyperpigmentation has been reported in HIV-infected persons with background pigment. Advanced HIV infection and immunosuppression has also been associated with more diffuse hyperpigmentation. In a Chinese HIV-infected population in Malaysia, hyperpigmentation was the most common skin disorder representing 36% of the whole group studied.[25] Pigmentation is most commonly seen in the sun-exposed areas but becomes more diffuse over the body. Photodistributed hyperpigmentation has been noted with CD4 counts <100 and may be the presenting sign of HIV infection.[26] Hyperpigmentation has also been linked with eczematous features, both in the acute and chronic form.[27]

Several reasons for hyperpigmentation have been postulated.[28] Medications used for the treatment and prophylaxis of AIDS-related conditions can cause photosensitivity.[29] These drugs include trimethoprim-sulfamethoxazole, azithromycin, dapsone, ketoconazole and anti-tuberculosis drugs. Antiretroviral medications like indinavir, saquinavir, and efavirenz have been associated with photosensitivity.[30] Zidovudine (AZT) may result in the hyperpigmentation of the nails, oral mucosa, and skin and appears to be related to increased melanogenesis and not to drug deposition or photosensitivity.[31] Concomitant diseases in HIV-infected individuals, such as *Porphyria cutanea tardae*, which causes photosensitivity and *Mycobacteria avium intracellulare* are affecting the adrenal glands and causing adrenal suppression, can eventuate in hyperpigmentaiton.[32] Sunscreen (SPF15 or higher) and avoidance of sun exposure can improve the hyperpigmentation.

Pigmented oral lesions are not uncommon, particularly in India and Africa.[14] Similar oral lesions are noted in Caucasians with HIV infection who have not been on any medications.

Hypopigmentation in HIV infection in the form of vitiligo has been reported. Vitiligo has been considered to be an autoimmune disorder like alopecia areata possibly reflecting concomitant B-cell dysfunction in HIV infection. Vitiligo has also been reported in persons with increasing CD4 cell counts on antiretroviral therapy.[33]

Syphilis

Worldwide, there has been a dramatic increase in the reported number of cases of syphilis in recent years.[34-38] The majority of cases in large urban settings have been in men, particularly men having sex with men.[39,40] In Europe and the USA, the overall proportion of syphilis patients co-infected with HIV is 50%.[41] Over 70% of these co-infected patients were already aware of their HIV infection at the time that they were diagnosed with syphilis.[37,42-45] Methamphetamine use has been implicated in the rising incidence of syphilis in the USA and Europe, particularly with cases of reinfection of syphilis.[46,47] Among women with syphilis and HIV, sex work, limited or no use of condoms, and alcohol and drug use were found to be risk factors.[34,37] Screening of syphilis, even in asymptomatic HIV-infected patients, is recommended.[48,49]

Primary and secondary cutaneous presentations of syphilis are similar in HIV and non-HIV-infected individuals.[50] Lesions include chancres, sometimes with rapid evolution to secondary stages, papulosquamous lesions on the trunk and palmar/plantar regions, patchy alopecia and osteochondritis of the sternal region.[51-53] Uveitis with or without rash is another common manifestation.[54] Oral lesions are also common.[14] Tertiary cutaneous lesions are characterized by verrucous or hyperkeratotic nodules. Lues maligna has been reported in HIV infection.[55] Skin biopsies or dark field microscopy of cutaneous lesions demonstrates spirochetes and establishes the diagnosis.[49] Negative serologic tests may not be adequate to rule out secondary syphilis as HIV infection my delay development of serologic evidence of *T. pallidum*. However, for the majority of patients, serologic testing is adequate.[56]

Central nervous system involvement may manifest early in HIV and relapse in CNS may be more common even after standard treatment. Clinicians should carefully follow HIV-infected patients who have been treated with standard therapies for early syphilis. If CNS signs or symptoms develop, clinicians should perform appropriate evaluation for early CNS relapse, including lumbar puncture and VDRL of the cerebrospinal fluid.[57]

The CDC recommends treating primary and secondary syphilis with 2.4 million units of benzathine penicillin given intramuscularly at a single session. Some specialists recommend benzathine penicillin 2.4 million units weekly for 2 or 3 weeks. In late latent disease, three doses of benzathine penicillin are recommended 1 week apart. For penicillin-allergic patients, doxycycline and tetracycline are recommended. Erythromycin is not recommended. Treatment failures have been noted with Azithromycin.[58] Since the relapse rate of neurosyphilis is approximately 17% in patients treated with standard

regimens, HIV-infected patients should be evaluated clinically and serologically for treatment failure at 3, 6, 9, 12, and 24 months after therapy. Although of unproven benefit, some specialists recommend a CSF examination 6 months after therapy.[56]

HIV-infected patients who meet the criteria for treatment failure should be managed in the same manner as HIV-negative patients (i.e. a CSF examination and re-treatment). CSF examination and re-treatment also should be strongly considered for patients whose nontreponemal test titers do not decrease fourfold within 6–12 months of therapy. Most specialists would re-treat patients with benzathine penicillin G administered as three doses of 2.4 million units i.m. each at weekly intervals, if CSF examinations are normal.[56]

Patients with neurosyphilis should be treated with crystalline penicillin G, 2.4 million units intravenously every 4 h for at least 10 days.[56]

Itching

Itching is a common complaint among HIV-infected patients. Pruritus without a rash is less common than originally thought and can be associated with concomitant systemic diseases like hepatitis C, chronic renal failure, lymphomas, and methamphetamine use. When a pruritic dermatitis is noted, a careful history and physical examination usually reveals a primary dermatologic condition for which standard treatment for the underlying condition can proceed. Included in this heterogenous group of diseases are xerosis, eczema, seborrheic dermatitis, psoriasis, *S. aureus* folliculitis, eosinophilic folliculitis, prurigo nodularis, pruritic papular eruption (PPE) of HIV, arthropod assaults and scabies and drug rashes. Biopsy and cultures of lesions can be helpful in distinguishing these conditions.[27]

As early as 1983, there have been reports from sub-Saharan Africa, Haiti, Brazil and Thailand, of intensely pruritic papules and nodules that begin on the extensor surfaces of the extremities and subsequently involve the trunk and face.[59-62] These lesions have not been reported in Europe or America. These lesions are often the presenting sign of HIV and appear before other opportunistic infections. This eruption has been correlated with CD4 counts that were generally low. Biopsy findings have included a mild to moderate dermal perivascular and periadnexal infiltrate. Early lesions biopsied in Uganda have revealed histology consistent with arthropod bites.[63] It has been hypothesized that this condition represents an altered and hyperactive immune response to arthropod bites.[64,65] Cytokine profiles of individuals with PPE, show lower levels of interleukin 2 and γ-interferon arguing for a dysregulated immune system.[66] Potent topical steroids and ultraviolet light have been of some benefit.[67] Anecdotally, with immune reconstitution from antiretroviral therapy (ART), this eruption resolves.[63,68]

Eosinophilic folliculitis (EF) has been reported in Southeast Asia, India, Europe and North America.[14,27,69,70] This disease presents with urticarial papules and nodules on the scalp, neck, face, upper chest and back of HIV-infected persons who have usually had a nadir CD4 count under 100 and with a current CD4 count <200. This condition can also be seen in individuals who are starting an antiretroviral regimen and are experiencing immune reconstitution. The pathogenesis of EF remains elusive.[71] Histologically, there is a predominant perifollicular infiltrate of eosinophils.[68,72] Treatment options include waiting out the immune reconstitution period (the first 12 weeks of ART therapy), potent topical steroids and antihistamines, itraconazole, UVB therapy, and isotretinoin.[73]

Prurigo nodularis has been reported globally and is characterized by pruritic dome-shaped nodules initially presenting on the photoexposed areas of the extremities and eventually involving the trunk.[27] These nodules are bilateral and symmetric and appear in persons with background pigment, usually with CD4 counts <100. The incessant rubbing and scratching of these lesions can lead to lichenification of the skin as well as pigment change, both hyper and hypopigmentation. A search for an underlying, treatable condition like scabies or eczema is warranted.[12,74] Immune reconstitution with ART has been helpful. Potent topical steroids and antihistamines are of benefit. Ultraviolet light and thalidomide have been somewhat helpful when other therapies have failed.[75]

Scabies is noted globally and usually present with pruritic papules with accentuation in the intertriginous areas, genitalia and fingerwebs.[12,74] With advancing immunosuppression, the infestation may become more widespread and refractory to treatment.[76] Crusted scabies may also occur with advanced HIV and presents with thick crusts that are nonpruritic and are teeming with mites.[77] Of particular challenge, are outbreaks of scabies in institutional settings like orphanages, hospitals and hospice settings.[3] Topical treatment of scabies is with benzyl benzoate 10%, sulfirim 2% (in Europe) permethrin 5% cream (available in the USA and UK). Gammabenzene hexachloride (lindane) is contraindicated in HIV as it has been associated with the development

of peripheral neuropathies. Oral ivermectin can also be used for treatment of scabies in an institution or for crusted scabies. Treatment of contacts and proper cleaning of garments and linens is essential in treatment, particularly in institutional settings.[78,79]

Cutaneous Tuberculosis

Cutaneous and intraoral tuberculosis in HIV-infected patients has been described most frequently in India, Brazil, Thailand and Africa.[14,80-84] The majority of cases have been associated with pulmonary disease. In several cases, unsuspected pulmonary disease was discovered on chest X-ray and sputum samples after the diagnosis of cutaneous disease was made. This was particularly true for tuberculosis in the oral cavity.[83] Lesions can present as single or multiple lesions and as infiltrated plaques, nodules or papillomas. Scrofuloderma is also a presentation.[85] Cutaneous TB can mimic fungal or bacterial infections, KS, neoplastic processes and herpetic infections and should be considered in the differential diagnosis of these diseases. Biopsy and tissue culture confirm the diagnosis.[80,86] An id reaction in the form of papulonecrotic id, has been described in a patient with immune reconstitution.[87,88]

Mycobacterium avium complex (MAC) infrequently presents with skin manifestations although it as been reported to form single or multiple nodules and cervical lymphadenitis in persons whose CD4 counts are <200.[89] A search for systemic disease should be undertaken with blood cultures and bone marrow aspirates for culture. MAC is seen more frequently in the developed world and has been infrequently reported in Trinidad and Kenya.[90]

Leishmania

Leishmania, cutaneous, mucocutaneous, and visceral have been reported in HIV co-infected persons.[91-93] This is a protozoan disease transmitted by the sandfly and occurs in HIV-infected patients who live in or have traveled to endemic areas for leishmania. In Spain, around the Mediterranean basin, there is a high prevalence of visceral leishmaniasis (kala-azar) among HIV-infected patients.[94,95] Immunosuppression can lead to progression from otherwise asymptomatic disease to the classic forms of the disease. While most patients with leishmania and HIV have CD4 counts <200, many of these patients represent relapses of leishmania with a waning immune system. These patients had been treated previously with standard therapies for leishmania. Patients can present with a few spontaneously healing lesions, diffuse non-healing lesions, mucocutaneous lesions or localized or diffuse hyperpigmentation. Diagnosis is made by biopsy of tissue looking for amastigotes in lesions.[93] Bone marrow can be biopsied in cases of suspected visceral involvement.[91] However, it should be noted that in persons with visceral leishmaniasis, any skin lesion (not only those of leishmania) can harbor amastigotes and is due to general involvement of the macrophages systemically.[96] Culture of tissue is standard so that the species of leishmania can be identified and correct therapy can proceed particularly for Leishmania braziliensis and panamensis so that the risk of mucocutaneous disease can be reduced.[92] Local therapy can be used for localized lesions and includes cryotherapy and paromycin ointment. Proven therapies include antimonials, pentamidine, amphoteric B, interferon with antimony and miltefosine.[97] All HIV-infected patients should be carefully monitored after treatment to insure that treatment was successful and that relapses do not occur.

Leprosy

Studies have indicated that HIV infection does not affect the clinical presentation of leprosy.[98] Continued immunosuppression with HIV infection may cause a relapse of leprosy in persons already treated and leprosy itself may accelerate the progression of HIV.[99] Several reports document inflammatory and vasculoulcerative reactions of leprosy within 2–6 months after starting ART.[100-102] This is thought to be part of the immune-reconstitution syndrome and has been documented particularly in patients whose CD4 counts were <100 when initiating ART. Occasionally, anti-inflammatory medications have been used in addition to leprosy and HIV medications with varying success. It has also been noted that while leprosy may worsen during the first few weeks of ART when there is immune reconstitution, lesions improve with appropriate multi-drug therapy for leprosy.

Nocardia

Nocardiosis is a localized infection or disseminated infection caused by an aerobic actinomyces that is geographically distributed worldwide. It has been reported in HIV-infected patients the USA, Africa, and Thailand.[103-104] There are fewer reports of nocardia and HIV infection from Europe although there have been recent reports from Spain and France. Nocardia predominantly affects the pulmonary system. Skin is the second most common site of infection and presents as cutaneous or subcutaneous abscesses.[105] Intravenous drug use has been identified as a risk factor in HIV-infected patients. Most HIV-infected patients with nocardia have CD4 cell counts <200 with the majority having a known diagnosis of AIDS at the time of infection.[106] Diagnosis can be made by using a modified acid fast stain on tissue or by culturing tissue, fluid or blood.[106] The treatment of choice is trimethoprim-sulfamethoxazole. Sensitivities to cultured material can be done. In a recent study from Thailand, patients who were resistant to Sulfa-TMP succumbed to death.[103] Imipenem, amikacin, minocycline, amoxicillin-clavulanic acid, and third generation cephalosporins have been proposed with unclear outcomes. Where possible, debridement of skin lesions is indicated as adjunctive therapy to antibiotics. Previous studies have reported that most patients respond to therapy in an average of 4 months. Cessation of therapy can be followed by recurrence and progression of disease in spite of reinitiation of therapy. Some authors have suggested that lifelong therapy should be instituted in the treatment of nocardia in HIV co-infected patients, particularly those who have evidence of advanced HIV disease. It is unclear what role ART has in this group of patients.

Penicillium

Penicilliosis marneffei is a common fungal infection presenting in HIV co-infected persons in Southeast Asia, particularly Thailand and the Southern part of China.[25,107,108] Presenting symptoms include molluscum-like skin lesions, acneiform and folliculocentric lesions with fever, anemia, and weight loss. Diagnosis can be established by analysis of blood and bone marrow aspirates with Wright stain. Touch smears of tissue as well as biopsies of lymph node and skin can be used to establish a diagnosis. Tissue culture is definitive and reveals a dimorphic fungus. CD4 counts are usually <100 in patients presenting with this diagnosis. Mortality is very high for untreated patients. Treatment consists of amphotericin B or itraconazole.[107]

Primary HIV

Acute retroviral syndrome (ARS) or primary HIV infection may be the presenting sign in 40–90% of patients. It is often asymptomatic and non-specific. ARS consists of a mononucleosis-like illness with fever, lymphadenopathy, pharyngitis, and neurologic symptoms. The skin rash includes a maculopapular exanthema, oral and genital ulcers, and infiltrated plaques on the chest and back.[109,110] There should be a high index of suspicion for HIV infection in patients presenting with these symptoms.[111] Patients with primary HIV infection may be highly infectious because of the presence of high viral burden in blood and genital secretions.[112] Diagnosis can be made by finding positive plasma HIV RNA and negative HIV antibody.[113] Treatment with ART early in this phase of may decrease the severity of the disease, alter the initial viral set point and reduce the rate of viral replication. However, therapy may cause drug toxicities and potential resistance if therapy fails.[110]

Drug Eruptions

In spite of drug–drug interactions with antiretroviral drugs, there are very few cutaneous drug reactions to protease inhibitors or nucleoside reverse transcriptase inhibitors (NRTIs), with the exception of abacavir.[114] About 5% of patients will develop a hypersensitivity reaction to abacavir within the first 8 weeks of treatment.[115] This has been characterized as a morbilliform dermatitis, lymphadenopathy with or without fever, gastrointestinal symptoms, respiratory symptoms, myalgia, or malaise. A recent study found that history of allergy to nevirapine and being naive to ART increased the risk of developing abacavir hypersensitivity.[115] Cutaneous side-effects to protease inhibitors are few and occur within the first 4 months of treatment, with the majority of reactions occurring within the first 4 weeks.[116] Hypersensitivity reactions have been reported frequently with the non-nucleoside reverse transcriptase inhibitors (NNRTIs) nevirapine and efavirenz, usually presenting as a maculopapular rash with or without fever developing 1–3 weeks after initiation of the drug. Drug photosensitivity has been reported with efavirenz. Amprenavir has a similar cutaneous hypersensitivity profile to that of the NNRTIs.[117] Nevirapine rash and systemic symptoms may be related to HLA type and depletion of CD4 cells. Rash alone was not found to be related to HLA type.[118] Antihistamine or prednisone pretreatments do not appear to decrease the development of NNRTI drug eruptions.[119,120] Nevirapine has been associated with Steven's–Johnson syndrome and toxic epidermal necrolysis and thus it has been recommended that this drug

and others in its class be discontinued upon first signs of rash.[121]

Sulfonamide rashes and drug hypersensitivity are common among HIV-infected patients presenting with a wide variety of cutaneous reactions.[122] Clindamycin has also been implicated as a common antibiotic causing cutaneous reactions.[123] The mechanism of hypersensitivity reactions and antibiotics in HIV has been explored and includes the inability of HIV-infected cells to deal with reactive metabolites of these drugs. Desensitization protocols for sulfonamides may allow for continued use of the drug.

Psoriasis

Psoriasis in HIV has been reported since the early days of the epidemic.[27,61] It presents in HIV as in non-HIV-infected persons with large marginated silvery-scaled plaques. Often, there is nail pitting. Arthritis may be a component of psoriasis, particularly in HIV disease presenting as a Reiter's-like syndrome.[124] These patients have a high prevalence of HLA B27 or B7 CREG antigens. Psoriasis may appear early in HIV infection and can be exacerbated by declining CD4 cell count and increasing viral load. It has been noted that there is a higher frequency of inverse psoriasis in HIV with lesions presenting in the flexural areas. Oral and genital areas can be involved. In KwaZulu-Natal, South Africa, psoriasis affected young black patients and was the most frequent reason for admission to dermatology wards.[125] Pruritus can be a frequent problem with psoriasis and can lead to secondary S. aureus infections. With the advent of ART, it appears that psoriasis in HIV co-infection is easier to treat with topical agents and standard therapies.[126] Topical treatment includes topical steroids and Vitamin D analogs (calcipotriene). In persons who have not yet started ART or are intolerant to ART, acitretin has been efficacious at low doses.[127] Transaminases and triglycerides should be monitored in these patients particularly if they are on ARTs. Acitretin has been reported to aid in the arthritic component of Reiter's-like arthritis.[124] Ultraviolet light can be used in HIV co-infected psoriasis with no evidence of adverse affect in CD4 counts. Methotrexate had been contraindicated early in the epidemic because there was a higher rate of mortality associated with this drug in HIV-infected patients but the evidence points to a cohort effect of patients being treated at that time.[128] The role and side-effects of biologics has yet to be elucidated in the treatment of psoriasis in HIV.[129]

Seborrheic dermatitis

Seborrheic dermatitis is an inflammatory eruption usually affecting the scalp and central areas of the face, particularly around the eyebrows and nasolabial folds. Early in the AIDS epidemic, the prevalence of this disease ranged from 40–80%, whereas in the non-immunosuppressed population, the prevalence approximated 5%.[27,84] A larger number of patients with advanced disease present with seborrheic dermatitis as compared with those with early stage disease however, seborrheic dermatitis can be seen throughout the spectrum of disease. Seborrheic dermatitis has been noted worldwide.[130-132] One study noted that persons on ART had less seborrheic dermatitis than those who were not on ART and that as CD4 counts increased on ART, seborrheic dermatitis was reduced by half compared with those not treated by ART.[133,134] With HIV infection, occasionally seborrheic dermatitis will occur on the center of the chest, axilla, and groin. The scale is usually fine, loose or waxy, on red or pink, poorly defined patches. Pruritus is generally mild. In individuals with a background pigment in their skin, seborrheic dermatitis can appear as hypopigmented areas. When seborrheic dermatitis presents in the groin or axilla, it can be intensely red and can present like inverse psoriasis. This morphology has been termed sebopsoriasis. The etiology of seborrheic dermatitis remains unclear but it appears that the Malassezia species (*Pityrosporum ovale*) may play a role.[135]

Treatment consists of mild topical steroids (e.g. 1% hydrocortisone ointment) and topical imidazoles cream (clotrimazole or ketoconazole), applied together twice daily, which reduces both the inflammatory response and the amount of *Pityrosporum ovale*. For the scalp, tar, zinc, ketoconazole, or selenium sulfide shampoos can be used. Because seborrheic dermatitis is a chronic condition, maintenance therapy is required, which usually consists of therapy with these agents twice weekly.[136]

Candida

Oral candidiasis has been associated with HIV early in the epidemic. It can present in the oropharynx and esophagus as erythematous or white plaques, with or without erosions.[137] *Candida* can cause an angular cheilitis in HIV-infected individuals and has been noted to be exacerbated by immune reconstitution.[88] *Candida* in the ano-genital area can be a presenting sign of HIV. While it has been documented that patients with CD4 counts <300 and high viral load have a higher incidence of developing *Candida*, *Candida* has been seen throughout the spectrum of HIV disease. It has been noted that with the administration of ART, *Candida* can be decreased by half.[133] In several studies however, oral candidiasis indicated a poor prognosis in spite of the use of ART. However, it may be that candidiasis in those individuals, is an indicator of failure to ART treatment. While *Candida albicans* is the most common organism causing oral candidiasis, there has been an emergence of non-albicans species.[138] In addition, there is more evidence for fluconazole resistant *Candida*. Initial treatment of *Candida* should include clotrimazole troches on an episodic basis. For more severe *Candida* or *Candida* not responding to episodic treatment with troches, itraconazole and amphotericin can be used. The use of caspofungin against *Candida* strains is being explored. Fluconazole prophylaxis should be avoided because of emerging resistance.[139]

Intertriginous Infections

Either *Candida* or tinea can cause intertriginous infections. *Candida* usually presents with bright red, slightly eroded plaques, often with satellite pustules. In males, the scrotum is often involved. Tinea is usually pruritic. The scrotum is spared. Tinea may extend to large parts of the body. Tinea and *Candida* should be diagnosed by examination of the scales with potassium hydroxide. Topical treatment is usually adequate with twice daily applications of an imidazole cream. Candidal lesions may be moist, so drying soaks with Burow's solution 1:20 may be helpful. Treatment with topical antifungals should be continued for 3–4 weeks and may be required for intermittent relapses. Occasionally, a secondary bacterial infection may be responsible for non-healing erosions in the groin area. Refractory intertriginous eruptions may be caused by seborrheic dermatitis or psoriasis.

Candidal Infection of the Nails

Candida or tinea may affect the nails. *Candida* often presents with erythema around the nailbed (paronychia). The cuticle may be lost and the nail plate may become ridged. The paronychia of *Candida* should be differentiated from the paronychia seen with indinavir (a sterile paronychia). With *Candida*, there is usually a concomitant pseudomonal infection presenting with a greenish hue to the nail. Topical imidazole or thymol 2–4% twice daily can be used. The pseudomonal infection can be treated with gentamicin or tobramycin solution. In refractory cases, oral antifungals and oral antipseudomonal drugs can be used for 1 month.

Tinea Infection of the Nails, Feet, and Hands

Tinea infection of the nails is very common in HIV and has been reported to be prevalent in around 20%–35% of HIV-infected patients. ART may not change the prevalence of onychomycosis.[140] Tinea of the nail does not present with a paronychia but rather involves the nail plate. Nails become opaque and thickened and often split. Tinea of the soles of the feet or toe webs is also common. Occasionally, the palms are involved with scaly plaques. Tinea can spread to the hairy areas, especially on the face and lower legs presenting like plaques of folliculitis. Direct examination of skin scrapings and culture for identification of species is helpful.

Tinea of the palms and soles and localized areas of the body can be treated with topical imidazoles or terbinafine. For tinea involving hair follicles, oral antifungals are required for approximately 1 month. For nails, oral antifungals are required but should be used when there is nail discomfort. Relapse rates for tinea of the nails is high and transaminase elevation and drug–drug interactions should be taken into consideration with use of these agents. Oral terbinafine can be used continuously for 3 months at a dose of 250 mg q.d. Itraconazole can be pulsed at 400 mg q.d. × 7 days per month for 3 months. Griseofulvin, a 12–18-month course can also be used with a lower success rate and a higher recurrence rate but may be the least hepatotoxic of the oral agents. The efficacy rates and relapse rates of onychomycosis in the HIV-infected population bear further study.

Superficial Onychomycosis

In many countries throughout the world, superficial mycoses account for up to 50% of dermatologic disease in HIV-infected patients. *Tinea corporis* is characterized by well-demarcated plaques of scale with central clearing. For extensive areas of involvement, it has been argued that oral antifungals are more effective than topicals and can be used for shorter periods of time.[141]

Deep (Systemic) Fungal Infections

Systemic infections reported in HIV include cryptococcus, histoplasmosis, sporotrichosis, aspergillosis, coccidiomycosis, actinomycosis, phaeohyphomycosis, and chromoblastomycosis.

Cryptococcosis

Approximately 6% of patients with HIV disease and cryptococcus present with skin lesions. By definition, these patients have systemic disease marked by positive serum cryptococcal antigen tests. A systemic work-up should be done to include involvement of central nervous system disease. Patients presenting with cryptococcus have CD4 counts under 200. Skin lesions can occur anywhere on the body and present as pearly 2–5 mm translucent papules that resemble molluscum. However, unlike molluscum, they present over a short period of time.[142] Another presentation includes larger gelatinous plaques usually with umbilicated areas. Diagnosis is established by skin biopsy and culture. Treatment is with systemic antifungals that include amphotericin B, flucytosine, fluconazole, itraconazole. Maintenance therapy should be continued for life. The role of successful ART therapy is unknown with regard to maintenance therapy.

Histoplasmosis

The incidence of disseminated histoplasmosis is between 5% and 20% in patients with AIDS living in endemic areas.[143] Histoplasma-endemic areas include Texas, the Ohio and Mississippi River Valleys in the USA, Mexico, Panama and South America.[144-146] The organism involved is *Histoplasmosis capsulatum*. Skin involvement occurs in 10–17% of patients with advanced HIV disease (CD4 <100). The cutaneous lesions are not specific and present as erythematous macule, papules, maculopapular lesions, pustules, acneiform lesions, ulcerations, and plaques.[147] The diagnosis should be suspected in persons living in or from endemic areas who present with fever, respiratory symptoms, weight loss, and diarrhea. Sepsis, disseminated intravascular coagulopathy, and renal failure can be seen. Histologic analysis of the skin may demonstrate granulomas. Organisms are seen with methamine silver stain. Bone marrow is positive in 75% of cases and blood culture is positive in 50–70% of cases. In those who survive, relapse is common and therefore requires lifelong maintenance treatment. *Histoplasma duboisii* has been identified in the African continent, both West and Central African countries and presents most commonly with mucocutaneous lesions from 38% to 82% of cases. Cutaneous lesions tend to be papules with ulceration and crusting. It has been postulated that histoplasmosis is probably an underdiagnosed systemic disease in Africa. Histoplasmosis has also been described in Europe, particularly in persons who come from areas where histoplasmosis is known to exist.

Sporotrichosis

Sporotrichosis in HIV can disseminate either from local lesions or from asymptomatic pulmonary infections that spread hematogenously to the skin and joints. Sporotrichosis has been reported worldwide. It can present with widespread cutaneous ulcers and subcutaneous nodules. Disseminated sporotrichosis occurs in patients with CD4 counts <200 and in alcoholics. Skin biopsies and cultures establish the diagnosis. Amphotericin B and itraconazole are used for treatment. Potassium iodide solution (SSKI) should not be used in patients with HIV and sporotrichosis. Like the other systemic fungal diseases, lifelong therapy is needed to prevent relapses.[148]

Aspergillus

Cutaneous aspergillus can occur as a primary or secondary infection. The latter is from hematogenous spread of underlying structures. Primary cutaneous aspergillus is associated with local skin injury (from tape and intravenous catheter sites) and neutropenia.[149] Lesions can appear as erythematous indurations with overlying pustules or ulcers. Treatment includes local debridement and amphotericin B or itraconazole.[150]

Cancrum Oris

Noma or cancrum oris is an infectious disease that starts as necrotizing ulcerative gingivitis, progresses with tumefaction and destroys adjacent structures around and deep to the area.[151] It occurs in countries where there is extreme poverty, malnutrition and HIV. It tends to occur in children and young adults (2–16).[152] It has been reported in South America and Africa in the HIV-infected population.[153] Local

debridement and antibiotics are established treatments.

Recurrent Aphthous Stomatitis

Aphthoses in HIV-infected patients can be larger and more difficult to treat. They can occur intraorally or in the anogenital region. They can be extremely painful and the diagnosis should be established by biopsy to rule out other infectious causes or neoplasms. The worst of these has been seen in patients who present with profound neutropenia as well as HIV disease with CD4 counts <200. Local injection with steroids, application of high potency steroids and thalidomide can be useful in the treatment of these ulcers.[154]

Eczematous Dermatitis

Eczematous dermatitis, both in the form of atopic dermatitis and xerosis can present in both children and adults infected with HIV. In one series, 50% of infants with advanced HIV disease had atopic dermatitis.[155] Adults with a previous history of atopic disease may also note recurrence of atopy in advanced disease. They may develop atopic dermatitis when previously they had only respiratory symptoms.[27] In countries where there is a large HIV-infected population, the incidence of eczema is increasing.[4,74] Dry skin and eczema has been reported in up to 56% of AIDS patients. The TH1/TH2 imbalance in patients with HIV has been proposed as the explanation of this prevalent disease in HIV. Evidence from an American cohort of women with HIV suggests that if the CD4 count was <200 before ART was initiated, atopic dermatitis continues in spite of ART.[140] Clinically, atopic dermatitis is characterized by scaly plaques, particularly in flexural areas. The distribution of atopic dermatitis may differ with ethnicity. In Black Africans, atopic dermatitis involves the extensor surfaces, affecting the elbow and wrist joints. The face is predominantly involved. Treatment for xerosis and atopic dermatitis is the same as in the non-HIV-infected population and consists of emollients, topical steroid, sedating antihistamines and avoidance of soap and water.

Human Papillomavirus

Cutaneous warts are seen more frequently in HIV-infected men and women. They have been noted to be more extensive and more difficult to treat than warts in the non-immunocompromised patients. Unusual wart types and reports of epidermodysplasia verruciformis have been reported in HIV-infected individuals.[156,157] The warts themselves rarely cause symptoms unless they are on the soles of the feet and around the fingernails, where there have been reports of excruciating pain. With the introduction of ART, intraoral warts were noted to increase in incidence. ART has not reduced the number or severity of warts and remains of concern to patients.[158]

Treatment of warts in HIV patients is the same as in the non-HIV-infected patient and has an approximately 50% success rate. Relapse of warts is especially common. Destructive modes of therapy include liquid nitrogen every 3 weeks, salicylic acid, laser, and excision. Immunomodulating therapy in the form of imiquimod has had less than promising results on cutaneous warts. Topical cidofovir has been used but is very expensive to formulate.[159]

Malignancies of the Skin

The non-AIDS defining cancers in HIV include basal cell cancers, squamous cell cancers and melanomas. Several studies have documented that the incidence of these cancers in HIV exceeds the incidence of these cancers in the general population.[2,160–162] Risk factors for development of these cancers include Caucasian/non-Hispanic race, increasing age, longer duration of HIV infection independent of age and history of opportunistic infections. Low CD4 counts or low CD4 nadirs do not seem to be significant for tumor initiation as these tumors have been noted to develop throughout the range of CD4 counts. However, there is some recent evidence that those patients who did not receive ART were at risk of developing cancer compared to those who did receive ART.[163] The role of ART however is unclear with regard to the incidence of cancer. Some studies have shown that the incidence of cancer remains the same in the pre-ART and post-ART era. The diagnosis of basal cell cancer and squamous cell cancer is the same in the HIV-infected patient as in the non-HIV-infected patient.[164] For basal cell cancers on the face, surgical excision is recommended. Curettage and dessication for tumors on the body is recommended. Squamous cell carcinomas should be excised regardless of location. These tumors usually present on sun-exposed skin as non-healing tumors.

The diagnostic criteria for melanoma also apply in HIV as in non-HIV infection.[165] It has been suggested that there be a high index of suspicion for melanoma in an otherwise banal appearing but rapidly growing melanocytic nevus in an HIV-infected individual.[164] Basal cell and squamous cell cancers should be treated in the same manner as non-melanoma skin cancers in the general population. Radiation treatment should be avoided in the treatment of squamous cell cancers in HIV. Close follow-up for metastatic squamous cell cancer is recommended. Tumor surveillance may be altered in the HIV-infected patient. Similarly, in HIV-infected patients with melanoma, tumors may be more aggressive independent of CD4 count. ART may maintain the immune and tumor surveillance systems and therefore ART therapy is suggested in persons with HIV regardless of CD4 count. Again, close follow-up for recurrent or metastatic tumors is recommended in persons with melanoma and HIV, as there is a higher incidence of metastases and recurrence. Sentinel node biopsies should be considered at shallower thicknesses of the original melanoma than what is usually recommended in the non-HIV-infected patient.

References

1. Castano-Molina C, Cockerell CJ. Diagnosis and treatment of infectious diseases in HIV-infected hosts. Dermatol Clin 1997; 15:267–283.
2. Barro-Traore F, Traore A, Konate I, et al. [Epidemiological features of tumors of the skin and mucosal membranes in the department of dermatology at the Yalgado Ouedraogo National Hospital, Ouagadougou, Burkina Faso.] Sante 2003; 13:101–104.
3. Geoghagen M, Pierre R, Evans-Gilbert T, et al. Tuberculosis, chickenpox and scabies outbreaks in an orphanage for children with HIV/AIDS in Jamaica. West Indian Med J 2004; 53:346–351.
4. Hartshorne ST. Dermatological disorders in Johannesburg, South Africa. Clin Exp Dermatol 2003; 28:661–665.
5. Nnoruka EN. Skin diseases in South-east Nigeria: a current perspective. Int J Dermatol 2005; 44:29–33.
6. Shapiro M, Smith KJ, James WD, et al. Cutaneous microenvironment of human immunodeficiency virus (HIV)-seropositive and HIV-seronegative individuals, with special reference to Staphylococcus aureus colonization. J Clin Microbiol 2000; 38:3174–3178.
7. Lee NE, Taylor MM, Bancroft E, et al. Risk factors for community-associated methicillin-resistant Staphylococcus aureus skin infections among HIV-positive men who have sex with men. Clin Infect Dis 2005; 40:1529–1534.
8. Ruhe JJ, Monson T, Bradsher RW, et al. Use of long-acting tetracyclines for methicillin-resistant Staphylococcus aureus infections: case series and review of the literature. Clin Infect Dis 2005; 40:1429–1434.
9. Ellis MW, Lewis JS 2nd. Treatment approaches for community-acquired methicillin-resistant Staphylococcus aureus infections. Curr Opin Infect Dis 2005; 18:496–501.
10. Kluytmans JA, Wertheim HF. Nasal carriage of Staphylococcus aureus and prevention of nosocomial infections. Infection 2005; 33:3–8.
11. Niemi M, Backman JT, Fromm MF, et al. Pharmacokinetic interactions with rifampicin: clinical relevance. Clin Pharmacokinet 2003; 4:819–850.

12. Mahe A, Faye O, N'Diaye HT, et al. Definition of an algorithm for the management of common skin diseases at primary health care level in sub-Saharan Africa. Trans R Soc Trop Med Hyg 2005; 99:39–47.

13. Frean J, Arndt S, Spencer D. High rate of Bartonella henselae infection in HIV-positive outpatients in Johannesburg, South Africa. Trans R Soc Trop Med Hyg 2002; 96:549–550.

14. Lanjewar DN, Bhosale A, Iyer A. Spectrum of dermatopathologic lesions associated with HIV/AIDS in India. Indian J Pathol Microbiol 2002; 45:293–298.

15. Koehler JE. Bartonella-associated infections in HIV-infected patients. AIDS Clin Care 1995; 7:97–102.

16. Koehler JE, Sanchez MA, Tye S, et al. Prevalence of Bartonella infection among human immunodeficiency virus-infected patients with fever. Clin Infect Dis 2003; 37:559–566.

17. Plettenberg A, Lorenzen T, Burtsche BT, et al. Bacillary angiomatosis in HIV-infected patients–an epidemiological and clinical study. Dermatology 2000; 201:326–331.

18. Lanjewar DN, Bhosale A, Iyer A. Spectrum of dermatopathologic lesions associated with HIV/AIDS in India. Indian M Pathol Microbiol 2002; 45:293–298.

19. Minga KA, Goeri I, Boka MB, et al. Bacillary angiomatosis in an adult infected with HIV-1 at an early stage of immunodepression Abidjan, Cote d'Ivoire. Bull Soc Pathol Exot 2002; 95:34–36.

20. Ciervo A, Petrucca A, Ciarrocchi S, et al. Molecular characterization of first human Bartonella strain isolated in Italy. J Clin Microbiol 2001; 39:4554–4557.

21. Gazineo JL, Trope BM, Maceira JP, et al. Bacillary angiomatosis: description of 13 cases reported in five reference centers for AIDS treatment in Rio de Janeiro, Brazil. Rev Inst Med Trop Sao Paulo 2001; 43:1–6.

22. Tsukahara M, Tsuneoka H, Goto M, et al. Seroprevalence of Bartonella henselae among HIV-1 infected patients in Japan. Kansenshogaku Zasshi 1999; 73:1241–1242.

23. Rosales CM, McLaughlin MD, Sata T, et al. AIDS presenting with cutaneous Kaposi's sarcoma and bacillary angiomatosis in the bone marrow mimicking Kaposi's sarcoma. AIDS Patient Care STDS 2002; 16:573–577.

24. Cheuk W, Wong KO, Wong CS, et al. Immunostaining for human herpesvirus 8 latent nuclear antigen-1 helps distinguish Kaposi sarcoma from its mimickers. Am J Clin Pathol 2004; 121:335–342.

25. Jing W, Ismail R. Mucocutaneous manifestations of HIV infection a retrospective analysis of 145 cases in a Chinese population in Malaysia. Int J Dermatol 1999; 38:457–463.

26. Wong SN, Khoo LS. Chronic actinic dermatitis as the presenting feature of HIV infection in three Chinese males. Clin Exp Dermatol 2003; 28:265–268.

27. Gelfand JM, Rudikoff D. Evaluation and treatment of itching in HIV-infected patients. Mt Sinai J Med 2001; 68:298–308.

28. Bilu D, Mamelak AJ, Nguyen RH, et al. Clinical and epidemiologic characterization of photosensitivity in HIV-positive individuals. Photodermatol Photoimmunol Photomed 2004; 20:175–183.

29. Joyner S, Lee D, Hay P, et al. Hydroxyurea-induced nail pigmentation in HIV patients. HIV Med 1999; 1:40–42.

30. Terheggen F, Frissen J, Weigel H, et al. Nail, hair and skin hyperpigmentation associated with indinavir therapy. Aids 2004; 18:1612.

31. Rahav G, Maayan S. Nail pigmentation associated with zidovudine: a review and report of a case. Scand J Infect Dis 1992; 24:557–561.

32. Grover C, Kubba S, Bansal S, et al. Pigmentation: a potential cutaneous marker for AIDS. J Dermatol 2004; 31:756–760.

33. Antony FC, Marsden RA. Vitiligo in association with human immunodeficiency virus infection. J Eur Acad Dermatol Venereol 2003; 17:456–458.

34. Gutierrez-Gallardo MC, Valle GF do, Sa FC, et al. Clinical characteristics and evolution of syphilis in 24 HIV+

individuals in Rio de Janeiro, Brazil. Rev Inst Med Trop Sao Paulo 2005; 47:153–157.

35. Gare J, Lupiwa T, Suarkia DL, et al. High prevalence of sexually transmitted infections among female sex workers in the eastern highlands province of Papua New Guinea: correlates and recommendations. Sex Transm Dis 2005; 32:466–473.

36. Hesketh T, Tang F, Wang ZB, et al. HIV and syphilis in young Chinese adults: implications for spread. Int J STD AIDS 2005; 16:262–266.

37. Amo J del, Gonzalez C, Losana J, et al. Influence of age and geographical origin in the prevalence of high risk human papillomavirus in migrant female sex workers in Spain. Sex Transm Infect 2005; 81:79–84.

38. Nnoruka EN, Ezeoke AC. Evaluation of syphilis in patients with HIV infection in Nigeria. Trop Med Int Health 2005; 10:58–64.

39. Ryder N, Bourne C, Rohrsheim R. Clinical audit: adherence to sexually transmitted infection screening guidelines for men who have sex with men. Int J STD AIDS 2005; 16:446–449.

40. Dougan S, Elford J, Rice B, et al. Epidemiology of HIV among black and minority ethnic men who have sex with men in England and Wales. Sex Transm Infect 2005; 81:345–350.

41. Lautenschlager S. Sexually transmitted infections in Switzerland: return of the classics. Dermatology 2005; 210:134–142.

42. Bij AK van der, Stolte IG, Coutinho RA, et al. Increase of sexually transmitted infections. not HIV, among young homosexual men in Amsterdam: are STIs still reliable markers for HIV transmission? Sex Transm Infect 2005; 81:34–37.

43. Sasse A, Defraye A, Ducoffre G. Recent syphilis trends in Belgium and enhancement of STI surveillance systems. Euro Surveill 2004; 9:6–8.

44. Cowan S. Syphilis in Denmark-Outbreak among MSM in Copenhagen, 2003–2004. Euro Surveill 2004; 9:25–27.

45. Marcus U, Bremer V, Hamouda O. Syphilis surveillance and trends of the syphilis epidemic in Germany since the mid-90s. Euro Surveill 2004; 9:11–14.

46. Wong W, Chaw JK, Kent CK, et al. Risk factors for early syphilis among gay and bisexual men seen in an STD clinic: San Francisco, 2002–2003. Sex Transm Dis 2005; 32:458–463.

47. Fenton KA, Imrie J. Increasing rates of sexually transmitted diseases in homosexual men in Western Europe and the United States: why? Infect Dis Clin North Am 2005; 19:311–331.

48. Cohen CE, Winston A, Asboe D, et al. Increasing detection of asymptomatic syphilis in HIV patients. Sex Transm Infect 2005; 81:217–219.

49. Gilleece Y, Sullivan A. Management of sexually transmitted infections in HIV positive individuals. Curr Opin Infect Dis 2005; 18:43–47.

50. Sanchez MR. Infectious syphilis. Semin Dermatol 1994; 13:234–242.

51. Ortega KL, Rezende NP, Watanuki F, et al. Secondary syphilis in an HIV positive patient. Med Oral 2004; 9:33–38.

52. Baniandres Rodriguez O, Nieto Perea O, Moya Alonso L, et al. [Nodular secondary syphilis in a HIV patient mimicking cutaneous lymphoma]. Med Interna 2004; 21:241–243.

53. Dave S, Gopinath DV, Thappa DM. Nodular secondary syphilis. Dermatol Online J 2003; 9:9.

54. Doris JP, Saha K, Jones NP, et al. Ocular syphilis: the new epidemic. Eye 2006; 20:703–705.

55. Passoni LF, Menezes JA de, Ribeiro SR, et al. Lues maligna in an HIV-infected patient. Rev Soc Bras Med Trop 2005; 38:181–184.

56. Centers for Disease Control and Prevention. Sexually transmitted diseases treatment guidelines 2002. MMWR 2002; 51:1–98.

57. Chan DJ. Syphilis and HIV co-infection: when is lumbar puncture indicated? Curr HIV Res 2005; 3:95–98.

58. Centers for Disease Control and Prevention (CDC). Azithromycin treatment failures in syphilis infections – San Francisco, California, 2002–2003. MMWR 2004; 53:197–198.

59. Colebunders R, Mann JM, Francis H, et al. Generalized papular pruritic eruption in African patients with human immunodeficiency virus infection. AIDS 1987; 1:117–121.

60. Bason MM, Berger TG, Nesbitt LT Jr. Pruritic papular eruption of HIV-disease. Int J Dermatol 1993; 32:784–789.

61. Sivayathorn A, Srihra B, Leesanguankul W. Prevalence of skin disease in patients infected with human immunodeficiency virus in Bangkok, Thailand. Ann Acad Med Singapore 1995; 24:528–533.

62. Ishii N, Nishiyama T, Sugita Y, et al. Pruritic papular eruption of the acquired immunodeficiency syndrome. Acta Dermatol Venereol 1994; 74:219–220.

63. Resneck JS Jr, van Beek M, Furmanski L, et al. Etiology of pruritic papular eruption with HIV infection in Uganda. JAMA 2004; 292:2614–2621.

64. Penneys NS, Nayar JK, Bernstein H, et al. Chronic pruritic eruption in patients with acquired immunodeficiency syndrome associated with increased antibody titers to mosquito salivary gland antigens. J Am Acad Dermatol 1989; 21:421–425.

65. Rosatelli JB, Roselino AM. Hyper-IgE, eosinophilia, and immediate cutaneous hypersensitivity to insect antigens in the pruritic papular eruption of human immunodeficiency virus. Arch Dermatol 2001; 137:672–673.

66. Aires JM, Rosatelli JB, de Castro Figueiredo JF, et al. Cytokines in the pruritic papular eruption of HIV. Int J Dermatol 2000; 39:903–906.

67. Pardo RJ, Bogaert MA, Penneys NS, et al. UVB phototherapy of the pruritic papular eruption of the acquired immunodeficiency syndrome. J Am Acad Dermatol 1992; 26:423–428.

68. McCalmont TH, Altemus D, Maurer T, et al. Eosinophilic folliculitis. The histologic spectrum. Am J Dermatopathol 1995; 17:439–446.

69. Ho MH, Chong LY, Ho TT. HIV-associated eosinophilic folliculitis in a Chinese woman: a case report and a survey in Hong Kong. Int J STD AIDS 1998; 9:489–493.

70. Hayes BB, Hille RC, Goldberg LJ. Eosinophilic folliculitis in 2 HIV-positive women. Arch Dermatol 2004; 140:463–465.

71. Teofoli P, Barbieri C, Pallotta S, et al. Pruritic eosinophilic papular eruption revealing HIV infection. Eur J Dermatol 2002; 12:600–602.

72. Holmes RB, Martins C, Horn T. The histopathology of folliculitis in HIV-infected patients. J Cutan Pathol 2002; 29:93–95.

73. Ellis E, Scheinfeld N. Eosinophilic pustular folliculitis: a comprehensive review of treatment options. Am J Clin Dermatol 2004; 5:189–197.

74. Nnoruka EN. Current epidemiology of atopic dermatitis in south-eastern Nigeria. Int J Dermatol 2004; 43:739–744.

75. Maurer T, Poncelet A, Berger T. Thalidomide treatment for prurigo nodularis in human immunodeficiency virus-infected subjects: efficacy and risk of neuropathy. Arch Dermatol 2004; 140:845–849.

76. Thappa DM, Karthikeyan K. Exaggerated scabies: a marker of HIV infection. Indian Pediatr 2002; 39:875–876.

77. Brites C, Weyll M, Pedroso C, et al. Severe and Norwegian scabies are strongly associated with retroviral (HIV-1/HTLV-1) infection in Bahia, Brazil. AIDS 2002; 16:1292–1293.

78. Buffet M, Dupin N. Current treatments for scabies. Fundam Clin Pharmacol 2003; 17:217–225.

79. Osborne GE, Taylor C, Fuller LC. The management of HIV-related skin disease. Part I: infections. Int J STD AIDS 2003; 14:78–88.

80. Pandhi D, Reddy BS, Chowdhary S, et al. Cutaneous tuberculosis in Indian children: the importance of screening for involvement of internal organs. J Eur Acad Dermatol Venereol 2004; 18:546–551.

81. Kenyon TA, Creek T, Laserson K, et al. Risk factors for transmission of Mycobacterium tuberculosis from HIV-infected tuberculosis patients, Botswana. Int J Tuberc Lung Dis 2002; 6:843–850.

82. Chiewchanvit S, Mahanupab P, Walker PF. Cutaneous tuberculosis in three HIV-infected patients. J Med Assoc Thai 2000; 83:1550–1554.

83. Miziara ID. Tuberculosis affecting the oral cavity in Brazilian HIV-infected patients. Oral Surg Oral Med Oral Pathol Oral Radiol Endod 2005; 100:179–182.

84. Hira SK, Wadhawan D, Kamanga J, et al. Cutaneous manifestations of human immunodeficiency virus in Lusaka, Zambia. J Am Acad Dermatol 1988; 19:451–457.

85. High WA, Evans CC, Hoang MP. Cutaneous miliary tuberculosis in two patients with HIV infection. J Am Acad Dermatol 2004; 50:S110–S113.

86. Chapman AL, Munkanta M, Wilkinson KA, et al. Rapid detection of active and latent tuberculosis infection in HIV-positive individuals by enumeration of Mycobacterium tuberculosis-specific T cells. AIDS 2002; 16:2285–2293.

87. Alsina M, Campo P, Toll A, et al. Papulonecrotic tuberculide in a human immunodeficiency virus type 1-seropositive patient. Br J Dermatol 2000; 143:232–233.

88. Jevtovic DJ, Salemovic D, Ranin J, et al. The prevalence and risk of immune restoration disease in HIV-infected patients treated with highly active antiretroviral therapy. HIV Med 2005; 6:140–143.

89. Boyd AS, Robbins J. Cutaneous Mycobacterium avium intracellulare infection in an HIV+ patient mimicking histoid leprosy. Am J Dermatol 2005; 27:39–41.

90. Mahaisavariya P, Chaiprasert A, Khemngern S, et al. Nontuberculous mycobacterial skin infections: clinical and bacteriological studies. J Med Assoc Thai 2003; 86:52–60.

91. Bosch RJ, Rodrigo AB, Sanchez P, et al. Presence of Leishmania organisms in specific and non-specific skin lesions in HIV-infected individuals with visceral leishmaniasis. Int J Dermatol 2002; 41:670–675.

92. Choi CM. Lerner EA. Leishmaniasis: recognition and management with a focus on the immunocompromised patient. Am J Clin Dermatol 2002; 3:91–105.

93. Bittencourt A, Silva N, Straatmann A, et al. Post-kala-azar dermal leishmaniasis associated with AIDS. Braz J Infect Dis 2002; 6:313–316.

94. Agostoni C, Dorigoni N, Malfitano A, et al. Mediterranean leishmaniasis in HIV-infected patients: epidemiological, clinical, and diagnostic features of 22 cases. Infection 1998; 26:93–99.

95. Barrio J, Lecona M, Cosin J, et al. Leishmania infection occurring in herpes zoster lesions in an HIV-positive patient. Br J Dermatol 1996; 134:164–166.

96. Gallego MA, Aguilar A, Plaza S, et al. Kaposi's sarcoma with an intense parasitization by Leishmania. Cutis 1996; 57:103–105.

97. Schraner C, Hasse B, Hasse U, et al. Successful treatment with miltefosine of disseminated cutaneous leishmaniasis in a severely immunocompromised patient infected with HIV-1. Clin Infect Dis 2005; 40:e120–e124.

98. Pereira GA, Stefani MM, Araujo Filho JA, et al. Human immunodeficiency virus type 1 (HIV-1) and Mycobacterium leprae co-infection: HIV-1 subtypes and clinical, immunologic, and histopathologic profiles in a Brazilian cohort. Am J Trop Med Hyg 2004; 71:679–684.

99. Rath N, Kar HK. Leprosy in HIV infection: a study of three cases. Indian J Lepr 2003; 75:355–359.

100. Pignataro P, Rocha Ada S, Nery JA, et al. Leprosy and AIDS: two cases of increasing inflammatory reactions at the start of highly active antiretroviral therapy. Eur J Clin Microbiol Infect Dis 2004; 23:408–411.

101. Couppie P, Abel S, Voinchet H, et al. Immune reconstitution inflammatory syndrome associated with HIV and leprosy. Arch Dermatol 2004; 140:997–1000.

102. Visco-Comandini U, Longo B, Cuzzi T, et al. Tuberculoid leprosy in a patient with AIDS: a manifestation of immune restoration syndrome. Scand J Infect Dis 2004; 36:881–883.

103. Mootsikapun P, Intarapoka B, Liawnoraset W. Nocardiosis in Srinagarind Hospital, Thailand: review of 70 cases from 01996–02001. Int J Infect Dis 2005; 9:154–158.

104. Jones N, Khoosal M, Louw M, et al. Nocardial infection as a complication of HIV in South Africa. J Infect 2000; 41:232–239.

105. Uttamchandani RB, Daikos GL, Reyes RR, et al. Nocardiosis in 30 patients with advanced human immunodeficiency virus infection: clinical features and outcome. Clin Infect Dis 1994; 18:348–353.

106. Javaly K, Horowitz HW, Wormser GP. Nocardiosis in patients with human immunodeficiency virus infection. Report of 2 cases and review of the literature. Medicine (Baltimore) 1992; 71:128–138.

107. Supparatpinyo K, Khamwan C, Baosoung V, et al. Disseminated Penicillium marneffei infection in southeast Asia. Lancet 1994; 344:110–113.

108. Duong TA. Infection due to Penicillium marneffei, an emerging pathogen: review of 155 reported cases. Clin Infect Dis 1996; 23:125–130.

109. Porras-Luque JI, Valks R, Casal EC, et al. Generalized exanthem with palmoplantar involvement and genital ulcerations. Acute primary HIV infection. Arch Dermatol 1998; 134:1279–1282.

110. Sun HY, Chen MJ, Hung CC, et al. Clinical presentations and virologic characteristics of primary human immunodeficiency virus type-1 infection in a university hospital in Taiwan. J Microbiol Immunol Infect 2004; 37:271–275.

111. Kobayashi S, Segawa S, Kawashima M, et al. A case of symptomatic primary HIV infection. J Dermatol 2005; 32:137–142.

112. Daar ES, Moudgil T, Meyer RD, et al. Transient high levels of viremia in patients with primary human immunodeficiency virus type 1 infection. N Engl J Med 1991; 324:961–964.

113. Taiwo BO, Hicks CB. Primary human immunodeficiency virus. South Med J 2002; 95:1312–1317.

114. Duval X, Journot V, Leport C, et al. Incidence of and risk factors for adverse drug reactions in a prospective cohort of HIV-infected adults initiating protease inhibitor-containing therapy. Clin Infect Dis 2004; 39:248–255.

115. Chirouze C, Hustache-Mathieu L, Rougeot C, et al. [Risk factors for Abacavir-induced hypersensibility syndrome in the real world.] Pathol Biol (Paris) 2004; 52:529–533.

116. Rotunda A, Hirsch RJ, Scheinfeld N, et al. Severe cutaneous reactions associated with the use of human immunodeficiency virus medications. Acta Dermatol Venereol 2003; 83:1–9.

117. Phillips EJ, Kuriakose B, Knowles SR. Efavirenz-induced skin eruption and successful desensitization. Ann Pharmacother 2002; 36:430–432.

118. Martin AM, Nolan D, James I, et al. Predisposition to nevirapine hypersensitivity associated with HLA-DRB1 and abrogated by low CD4 T-cell counts. AIDS 2005; 19:97–99.

119. Wit FW, Wood R, Horban A, et al. Prednisolone does not prevent hypersensitivity reactions in antiretroviral drug regimens containing abacavir with or without nevirapine. AIDS 2001; 15:2423–2429.

120. Launay O, Roudiere L, Boukli N, et al. Assessment of cetirizine, an antihistamine, to prevent cutaneous reactions to nevirapine therapy: results of the Viramune Zyrtec double-blind, placebo-controlled trial. Clin Infect Dis 2004; 38:66–72.

121. Fagot JP, Mockenhaupt M, Bouwes-Bavinck JN, et al. EuroSCAR Study Group. Nevirapine and the risk of Steven's-Johnson syndrome or toxic epidermal necrolysis. AIDS 2001; 15:1843–1848.

122. Slatore CG, Tilles SA. Sulfonamide hypersensitivity. Immunol Allergy Clin North Am 2004; 24:477–490.

123. Wijsman JA, Dekaban GA, Rieder MJ. Differential toxicity of reactive metabolites of clindamycin and sulfonamides in HIV-infected cells: influence of HIV infection on clindamycin toxicity in vitro. J Clin Pharmacol 2005; 45:346–351.

124. Utikal J, et al. Reiter's syndrome-like pattern in AIDS-associated psoriasiform dermatitis. J Eur Acad Dermatol Venereol 2003; 17:114–116.

125. Mosam A, et al. The impact of human immunodeficiency virus/acquired immunodeficiency syndrome (HIV/AIDS) on skin disease in KwaZulu-Natal, South Africa. Int J Dermatol 2004; 43:782–783.

126. Fischer T, Schworer H, Vente C, et al. Clinical improvement of HIV-associated psoriasis parallels a reduction of HIV viral load induced by effective antiretroviral therapy. AIDS 1999; 13:628–629.

127. Blanche P. Acitretin and AIDS-related Reiter's disease. Clin Exp Rheumatol 1999; 17:105–106.

128. Maurer TA, Zackheim HS, Tuffanelli L, et al. The use of methotrexate for treatment of psoriasis in patients with HIV infection. J Am Acad Dermatol 1994; 31:372–375.

129. Aboulafia DM, Bundow D, Wilske K, et al. Etanercept for the treatment of human immunodeficiency virus-associated psoriatic arthritis. Mayo Clin Proc 2000; 75:1093–1098.

130. Tzung TY, Yang CY, Chao SC, et al. Cutaneous manifestations of human immunodeficiency virus infection in Taiwan. Kaohsiung J Med Sci 2004; 20:216–224.

131. Pitche P, Tchangai-Walla K, Napo-Koura G, et al. [Prevalence of skin manifestations in AIDS patients in the Lome-Tokoin University Hospital (Togo)]. Sante 1995; 5:349–352.

132. Wiwanitkit V. Prevalence of dermatological disorders in Thai HIV-infected patients correlated with different CD4 lymphocyte count statuses: a note on 120 cases. Int J Dermatol 2004; 43:265–268.

133. Dunic I, Vesic S, Jevtovic DJ. Oral candidiasis and seborrheic dermatitis in HIV-infected patients on highly active antiretroviral therapy. HIV Med 2004; 5:50–54.

134. Muhammad B, Eligius L, Mugusi F, et al. The prevalence and pattern of skin diseases in relation to CD4 counts among HIV-infected police officers in Dar es Salaam. Trop Doct 2003; 33:44–48.

135. Pechere M, Krischer J, Remondat C, et al. Malassezia spp carriage in patients with seborrheic dermatitis. J Dermatol 1999; 26:558–561.

136. Gupta AK, Bluhm R. Seborrheic dermatitis. J Eur Acad Dermatol Venereol 2004; 18:13–26.

137. Melo NR, Taguchi H, Jorge J, et al. Oral Candida flora from Brazilian human immunodeficiency virus-infected patients in the highly active antiretroviral therapy era. Mem Inst Oswaldo Cruz 2004; 99:425–431.

138. Lattif AA, Banerjee U, Prasad R, et al. Susceptibility pattern and molecular type of species-specific Candida in oropharyngeal lesions of Indian human immunodeficiency virus-positive patients. J Clin Microbiol 2004; 42:1260–1262.

139. Goldman GH, da Silva Ferreira ME, dos Reis Marques E, et al. Evaluation of fluconazole resistance mechanisms in candida albicans clinical isolates from HIV-infected patients in Brazil. Diagn Microbiol Infect Dis 2004; 50:25–32.

140. Maurer T, Rodrigues LK, Ameli N, et al. The effect of highly active antiretroviral therapy on dermatologic disease in a longitudinal study of HIV type 1-infected women. Clin Infect Dis 2004; 38:579–584.

141. Millikan LE. Role of oral antifungal agents for the treatment of superficial fungal infections in immunocompromised patients. Cutis 2001; 68:6–14.

142. Manfredi R, Mazzoni A, Nanetti A, et al. Morphologic features and clinical significance of skin involvement in patients with AIDS-related cryptococcosis. Acta Dermatol Venereol 1996; 76:72–74.

143. Ramdial P, Mosam A, Dlova NC, et al. Disseminated cutaneous histoplasmosis in patients infected with human immunodeficiency virus. J Cutan Pathol 2002; 29:215–225.

144. Calza L, Manfredi R, Donzelli C, et al. Disseminated histoplasmosis with atypical cutaneous lesions in an Italian HIV-infected patient: another autochthonous case. HIV Med 2003; 4:145–148.

145. Lo Cascio G, Ligozzi M, Maccacaro L, et al. Diagnostic aspects of cutaneous lesions due to Histoplasma capsulatum in African AIDS patients in nonendemic areas. Eur J Clin Microbiol Infect Dis 2003; 22:637–638.

146. Gutierrez ME, Canton A, Sosa N, et al. Disseminated histoplasmosis in patients with AIDS in Panama: a review of 104 cases. Clin Infect Dis 2005; 40:1199–1202.

147. Couppie P, Roussel M, Thual N, et al. [Disseminated histoplasmosis: an atypical ulcerous form in an HIV-infected patient.] Ann Dermatol Venereol 2005; 132:133–135.

148. Rocha MM, Dassin T, Lira R, et al. Sporotrichosis in patient with AIDS: report of a case and review. Rev Iberoam Micol 2001; 18:133–136.

149. Shetty D, Giri N, Gonzalez CE, et al. Invasive aspergillosis in human immunodeficiency virus-infected children. Pediatr Infect Dis J 1997; 16:216–221.

150. Stanford D, Boyle M, Gillespie R. Human immunodeficiency virus-related primary cutaneous aspergillosis. Australas J Dermatol 2000; 41:112–116.

151. Ibeziako SN, Nwolisa CE, Nwaiwu O. Cancrum oris and acute necrotising gingivitis complicating HIV infection in children. Ann Trop Paediatr 2003; 23:225–226.

152. Faye O, Keita M, N'diaye HT, et al. [Noma in HIV-infected adults]. Ann Dermatol Venereol 2003; 130:199–201.

153. Chidzonga MM. HIV/AIDS orofacial lesions in 156 Zimbabwean patients at referral oral and maxillofacial surgical clinics. Oral Dis 2003; 9:317–322.

154. Gileva OS, Sazhina MV, Gileva ES, et al. Spectrum of oral manifestations of HIV/AIDS in the Perm region (Russia) and identification of self-induced ulceronecrotic lingual lesions. Med Oral 2004; 9:212–215.

155. Rudikoff D. The relationship between HIV infection and atopic dermatitis. Curr Allergy Asthma Rep 2002; 2:275–281.

156. Palefsky JM. Cutaneous and genital HPV-associated lesions in HIV-infected patients. Clin Dermatol 1997; 15:439–447.

157. Degener AM, Laino L, Pierangeli A, et al. Human papillomavirus-32-positive extragenital Bowenoid papulosis (BP) in a HIV patient with typical genital BP localization. Sex Transm Dis 2004; 31:619–622.

158. Rodrigues LK, Maurert BT. Cutaneous warts in HIV-positive patients undergoing highly active antiretroviral therapy. Arch Dermatol 2001; 137:1103–1104.

159. Toutous-Trellu L, Hirschel B, Piguet V, et al. [Treatment of cutaneous human papilloma virus, poxvirus and herpes simplex virus infections with topical cidofovir in HIV positive patients]. Ann Dermatol Venereol 2004; 131:445–449.

160. Cooley TP. Non-AIDS-defining cancer in HIV-infected people. Hematol Oncol Clin North Am 2003; 17:889–899.

161. Allardice GM, Hole DJ, Brewster DH, et al. Incidence of malignant neoplasms among HIV-infected persons in Scotland. Br J Cancer 2003; 89:505–507.

162. Rabkin CS, Biggar RJ, Horm JW. Increasing incidence of cancers associated with the human immunodeficiency virus epidemic. Int J Cancer 1991; 47:692–696.

163. Clifford GM, Polesel J, Rickenbach M, et al. Cancer risk in the Swiss HIV Cohort Study: associations with immunodeficiency, smoking, and highly active antiretroviral therapy. J Natl Cancer Inst 2005; 97: 425–432.

164. Wilkins K, Dolev JC, Turner R, et al. Approach to the treatment of cutaneous malignancy in HIV-infected patients. Dermatol Ther 2005; 18:77–86.

165. Calista D. Five cases of melanoma in HIV positive patients. Eur J Dermatol 2001; 11:446–449.

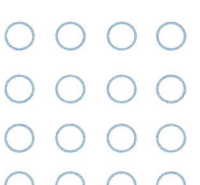

CHAPTER 23

Gastrointestinal Disorders in HIV

Michael H. Serlin
Douglas Dieterich

Introduction

Gastrointestinal disease in human immunodeficiency virus (HIV) spans the entire GI tract from the mouth to the rectum. The spectrum of gastrointestinal symptoms in HIV ranges from odynophagia and dysphagia, to nausea and vomiting, to abdominal pain and finally diarrhea and tenesmus. As with normal hosts, gastrointestinal disorders are very common in HIV patients, whether it be from opportunistic infections secondary to the patient's immunosuppressed status, medication induced, or through other etiologies. Almost all HIV and AIDS patients have some gastrointestinal complaints throughout the course of their illness. With the dramatic changes in HIV care because of highly active antiretroviral therapy (ART) in the mid-1990s, the incidence of opportunistic infections are decreasing, and as a result, the clinical picture of gastrointestinal illnesses in HIV is changing. The evaluation of the HIV patient with gastrointestinal complaints requires a thorough history and physical exam, in addition to selected studies, in order to diagnose the correct disease and treat accordingly.

Esophageal Disorders

Patients with HIV and AIDS typically can have upper gastrointestinal symptoms, which can range from dysphagia, or difficulty swallowing, to odynophagia, or the feeling of pain upon swallowing. At least one-third of patients with HIV before the ART era had esophageal complaints,[1] and the incidence increased with the progression of the disease. Most of the symptoms in these patients are secondary to opportunistic infections caused by the patient's immunosuppressed state, and related to the degree of immunosuppression. The most common etiologies of esophageal pathology and esophagitis in AIDS patients (Table 23.1) are *Candida* species, herpes simplex virus (HSV), and cytomegalovirus (CMV).[2] In addition, there is also an entity of idiopathic esophageal ulcers (IEU) that is also seen in HIV patients, which may be immunologically mediated,[3] or caused by HIV itself.[4] Other etiologies of esophageal complaints include malignancy (especially lymphoma and Kaposi's sarcoma) and other noninfectious causes. However, with the introduction of protease inhibitors (PIs) in 1996 and ART, and the decreased incidence of AIDS, more esophageal complaints in HIV these days are related to common etiologies like gastroesophageal reflux disease (GERD) than opportunistic infections.[5]

In addition to the most common symptoms of dysphagia and odynophagia, other symptoms can also suggest esophageal disease in HIV patients, like chest pain, nausea, vomiting, anorexia and weight loss. The symptoms can be acute or have a more chronic, progressive course. In addition, dysphagia is often associated with candidal esophagitis, whereas odynophagia is generally symptomatic of esophageal ulcerative disease. Patients can have both dysphagia and odynophagia, and because they also may have more than one illness concurrently, it is

Table 23.1 Esophageal diseases in HIV patients

Etiology	Symptoms	Diagnosis	Endoscopic appearance	Treatment
Candida	Dysphagia Odynophagia	Response to empiric fluconazole. Endoscopy	Creamy whitish-yellow adherent plaques 'shaggy appearance'	Fluconazole 200 mg p.o., then 100 mg p.o. q.d. Clotrimazole troches. Amphotericin B i.v. 0.3– 0.5 mg/kg per day. Caspofungin i.v. 70 mg × 1; 50 mg/day.
CMV	Odynophagia Dysphagia	Endoscopy with biopsy (inclusions on pathology)	Single or multiple ulcers; giant ulcers; diffuse esophagitis	Ganciclovir i.v. 5– 10 mg/kg per day. Foscarnet i.v. 90 mg/kg b.i.d. Valganciclovir p.o. 900 mg/day. Cidofovir 5 mg/kg weekly.
HSV	Odynophagia Dysphagia Chest pain Nausea/vomiting	Endoscopy with biopsy (from ulcer edge)	Well-circumscribed 'volcano' ulcer; 1–3 mm vesicles	Acyclovir p.o./i.v. 15– 30 mg/kg per day. Valacyclovir p.o. 1 g b.i.d. Famciclovir 500 mg b.i.d. Foscarnet i.v. 40 mg/kg b.i.d.
Idiopathic esophageal ulcers (IEU)	Odynophagia	Endoscopy with biopsy. Diagnosis of exclusion	Variable	Prednisone p.o. 40 mg/day. Thalidomide p.o. 200 mg/day.
GERD	Dyspepsia Belching Nocturnal cough	Endoscopy. Therapeutic and behavioral management	Esophagitis. Hiatal hernia	Oral H_2 blockers. Oral proton pump inhibitors. Behavioral modifications.
Malignancy (Kaposi's sarcoma and lymphoma most common)	Dysphagia Weight loss Hematemesis	Endoscopy with biopsy. Radiology (CT scan)	Variable. Neoplastic mass	Antiretroviral therapy. Surgery. Chemotherapy. Radiation.
Pill-esophagitis	Dyspepsia odynophagia	History Endoscopy	Variable ulcerations	Behavior or pharmaceutical modification.

CMV, cytomegalovirus; HSV, herpes simplex virus; GERD, gastroesophageal reflux disease; H_2, histamine-2. Adapted with permission from Sande MA, Volberding PA, eds. Medical Management of AIDS, 6th edn. Philadelphia: WB Saunders.

imperative to pursue a thorough investigation as to the etiology of esophageal complaints in HIV patients.

The evaluation of HIV patients with esophageal symptoms does not definitively need to include endoscopy with biopsy, but this is the gold standard, as it allows the physician to visualize the esophageal lumen, and to biopsy affected sites (Fig. 23.1). The history and physical exam is obviously important, as it may lead to a discovery of GERD, or pill-induced esophagitis. In addition, patients with disseminated CMV (e.g. CMV retinitis) with esophageal symptoms (especially odynophagia) may respond to CMV anti-viral therapy in the absence of diagnostic endoscopy and biopsy. The most common sign on physical exam

that relates to esophageal complaints is oral thrush, which can be suggestive of esophageal candidiasis in patients with esophageal complaints. In these patients, especially those with only dysphagia (or dysphagia and odynophagia, but not those with solely odynophagia) it may be beneficial to document the response from an empiric trial of oral fluconazole, as opposed to endoscopy.[6] If there is a symptomatic response to the fluconazole, then it can be presumed the patient had candidal esophagitis and proceed accordingly.

In addition to history and physical exam, there are other ways to evaluate esophageal complaints. Barium esophagography is relatively insensitive and non-specific and should not be used for diagnostic

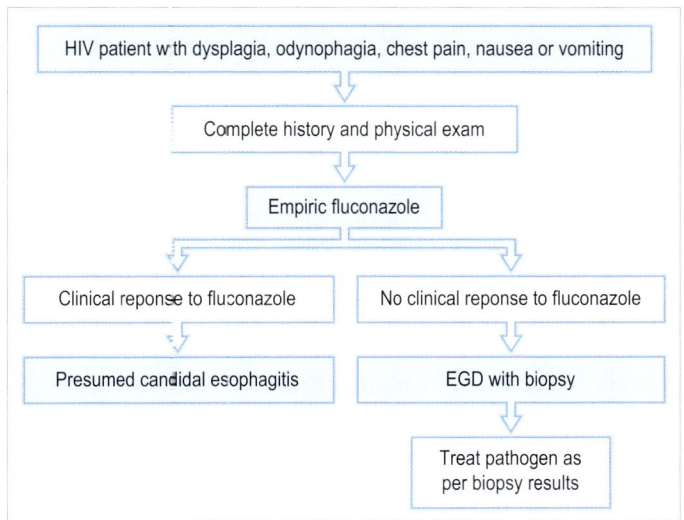

Figure 23.1 Algorithm in the approach to the HIV patient with esophageal complaints.

purposes, but the most characteristic finding in candidal esophagitis is diffuse mucosal irregularity resulting in a 'shaggy' appearance mimicking diffuse ulceration.[7] CMV and IEU may appear as well circumscribed ulcers that may be shallow or deep, and are indistinguishable on barium swallow.[8] Of course, radiography can determine a neoplastic origin to dysphagia in patients with malignancies. Another form of evaluation is brush cytology, where a cytology brush is passed through a nasogastric tube and obtains tissue for viral cultures and immunohistochemistry. Unfortunately, this leads to large sampling error, because it is done blindly without visualization of the lumen, and misses diagnoses (as patients may have two infectious processes, and IEU cannot be diagnosed). Viral culture and cytologic brushings add little in the evaluation of AIDS patients with esophagitis over endoscopy with biopsy.[9] Endoscopy with biopsy generally yields a viral or fungal diagnosis based on culture and hematoxylin and eosin staining (which will exclude a viral etiology); only after several biopsy samples do not show any etiology of the ulcerations can a tentative, exclusionary diagnosis of IEU be made.

Candidal esophagitis is the most common cause of esophagitis in HIV patients, especially in patients with complaints of dysphagia, or odynophagia and dysphagia.[10] The fungal isolate is generally *Candida albicans*, though other species of *Candida* can also affect the esophagus. It should be suspected in patients with a CD4+ lymphocyte count of <100 cells/mm³ (though can occur at any CD4+ count), and esophageal symptoms with or without

thrush, which can be absent in 30% of patients.[11] In patients with HIV and new onset symptoms, an empiric trial of standard dosed fluconazole is an effective strategy, as 82% of patients in a prospective study responded. If there is no response, endoscopy can be pursued.[6] In patients that fail empiric antifungal therapy, the most common etiology (in 77% of the patients) is ulcerative esophagitis as opposed to persistent candidiasis.[12] Fluconazole is the drug of choice for candidiasis, with a loading dose of 200 mg orally followed by 100 mg daily from 10–14 days. Clotrimazole troches are also successful, as topical treatment of esophageal candidiasis,[13] but nystatin is not.[14] Itraconazole and ketoconazole are efficacious systemic therapies, but not as effective as fluconazole.[15,16] Amphotericin B is also a helpful therapy, but is generally used only in azole-resistant patients because of the toxicity of the medication. Low-dose amphotericin (0.3–0.5 mg/kg per day for 7–14 days) is usually adequate. Caspofungin can also be used in candidal esophagitis, and is felt to be as efficacious as fluconazole and well tolerated.[17] However, it is only available in intravenous form and is more expensive, but may be the drug of choice for azole-resistant mucosal candidiasis because of the relative lack of toxicity compared with amphotericin B. Primary prophylaxis of candidal disease is not recommended because of the non-life-threatening nature of the disease, the effectiveness of acute therapy, and the risk of antifungal resistance.

While *Candida* is the most common esophageal pathogen, it can also occur in addition to ulcerative esophagitis in HIV patients. CMV esophagitis is the most common etiology of odynophagia in HIV patients and therefore esophageal ulcerations, up to 45% of patients in one prospective study.[18] Fever and substernal chest pain can be reported in addition to odynophagia, and thrush can be concomitant, but dysphagia is very uncommon. The diagnosis of CMV is best made by endoscopy and biopsy, with the pathology showing viral cytopathic effect in the gastrointestinal mucosa via intranuclear inclusions. Immunohistochemistry is also helpful for confirmation, as viral cultures are less sensitive and specific.[19]

CMV is the most common viral pathogen in the esophagus in HIV patients, and esophagitis is the most common extraocular manifestation of CMV.[20] It can appear as a diffuse esophagitis, single or multiple ulcers, or giant ulcers involving the whole esophagus, and generally occurs when the CD4+ lymphocyte count is <50. It may be discovered only after treatment for *Candida*, as they may exist concurrently in 20% of patients.[21] The incidence of CMV esophagitis has declined dramatically in the ART era. Treatment for CMV esophagitis involves a wide array of antiviral medications, namely ganciclovir, valganciclovir, foscarnet, and cidofovir. Ganciclovir was the first agent used to combat CMV and has the most data behind it; the response rate is about 70–80%. It is given intravenously in a 2–4 week induction period, 5–10 mg/kg per day, but has dose limiting side-effects, mainly bone marrow suppression (and resultant neutropenia and thrombocytopenia). Oral ganciclovir can also be used as maintenance therapy, but the data is limited. Intravenous foscarnet (90 mg/kg b.i.d., 2–3 weeks) is seen as equally effective to intravenous ganciclovir in the treatment of CMV esophagitis, but comes with a nephrotoxic side-effect profile; however, randomized studies have shown equal efficacy and safety.[22] Foscarnet is generally used in cases of clinical failure after ganciclovir induction.[23] Oral valganciclovir (900 mg/day) has not been tested in CMV esophagitis, but does have 60% of the bioavailability of intravenous ganciclovir. Cidofovir also can treat CMV, but is not typically used because of nephrotoxicity.

HSV esophagitis is a relatively uncommon cause of esophageal ulceration in HIV patients compared with CMV and IEU. The endoscopic appearance is described as being well circumscribed and having a 'volcano' like appearance, distinguishing them from the ulcers seen in CMV infection, which tend to be linear or longitudinal and are deeper.[24] Treatment is with oral acyclovir (15–30 mg/kg per day), though if patients have difficulty with swallowing, intravenous acyclovir can be used. Valacyclovir and famci-

clovir can also be used because of their efficacy and convenient dosing schedules. Foscarnet intravenously (40 mg/kg b.i.d.) is used in cases of acyclovir resistance.[25] Secondary prophylaxis with valacyclovir (500–1000 mg/day) is recommended in patients with frequent relapses.

Idiopathic esophageal ulcers (IEU) are a diagnosis of exclusion if none of the pathologic, fungal, or viral studies return a diagnosis. The treatment of idiopathic esophageal ulcers is done with oral corticosteroids, generally starting at 40 mg of oral prednisone daily.[26] If the patient cannot take medications orally, then the corticosteroids can be given intravenously. In addition, thalidomide can also be used for IEU if corticosteroids are not efficacious.[27]

In addition to the infections and ulcerations discussed above, there are other esophageal issues in HIV, namely motility and neuropathic issues. There is a form of HIV neuropathy that could lead to gastrointestinal complaints, like gastroparesis. These would be treated symptomatically, with prokinetic agents like metoclopramide. Additionally, in patients with both symptomatic esophageal complaints, as well as those that are asymptomatic, there are findings of esophageal motility abnormalities. This is probably because of the neurotropic nature of HIV leading to autonomic dysfunction in the gastrointestinal neurologic plexus.[2]

Gastric Disorders

The problems associated with the stomach in HIV patients are similar to the stomach problems of non-HIV infected individuals. Opportunistic infections that affect HIV patients typically do not affect the stomach. Symptoms and presentation are often related to abdominal pain, nausea or vomiting. The most common manifestations of gastric illness in HIV patients is like the general population, namely GERD, peptic ulcer disease (PUD) and gastritis. Care needs to be used when prescribing Histamine-2 (H_2) blockers or proton-pump inhibitors (PPIs), however, as these medications can interact with ART, especially PPIs. Work-up is the same as with the general population, and endoscopy with biopsy is the gold standard for diagnosis. *Helicobacter pylori*, a common cause of peptic ulcer disease in non-HIV positive patients, seems to have a decreased incidence in HIV patients compared with the general population; CMV may actually be the leading cause of PUD in HIV patients.[28] As far as actual HIV-related gastric pathology, gastric lymphoma, Kaposi's sarcoma, and some of the opportunistic organisms (e.g. CMV, tuberculosis, toxoplasmosis, and cryptococcosis) can be seen. In addition, dyspepsia, nausea and vomiting can all be related to the side-effects of various anti-retroviral medications.

Diarrhea

One of the most common complaints of HIV patients is diarrhea. The reasons for diarrhea are multifold, but most commonly relate to opportunistic infection and antiretroviral medications. A more in depth coverage of diarrheal illness in HIV patients is discussed later in Ch. 65: *Etiology and Management of Diarrhea in HIV-infected Patients and Impact on Antiretroviral Therapy*, but an overview will follow here. As with esophageal disease, the incidence of opportunistic infections has decreased in the ART era, though the incidence of chronic diarrhea has remained steady even in the ART era.[29] The evaluation of diarrhea includes a thorough history and physical, as much can be determined from just eliciting the patient's history of symptoms. If the diarrhea occurs with upper abdominal cramps, or bloating, this suggests an upper intestinal source, or enteritis. Bloody diarrhea, tenesmus, and lower abdominal cramping imply colonic involvement. In addition, patients with a history of receptive anal intercourse have a higher involvement of colitis and sexually transmitted pathogens (e.g. gonorrhea, HSV, etc.) in the anorectal area. Homosexual or bisexual men have a 3-fold higher incidence of diarrhea than patients in other risk groups. Obviously, travel and diet history can also be important in the histories of HIV patients with diarrhea. As with other aspects of HIV, opportunistic infections tend to be more common in the setting of lower CD4− lymphocyte counts (and therefore greater immunosuppression).

The diagnostic studies involved in the work-up of diarrhea in the HIV patient are similar to those in the general population. In addition to history and physical exam (exam specifically adds little to diagnosis, other than evidence of malnutrition), the first route of investigation is often the stool examination. The tests to order include bacterial culture, *clostridium difficile* toxin assay, as well as looking for ova and parasites, especially *Isospora*, *Cryptosporidium*, and *Microsporidia*. These generally need to be specified as potential pathogens when the sample is sent to microbiology when looking at ova and parasites. In addition, a gram stain or methylene blue stain for fecal leukocytes can also be helpful, as evidence of fecal leukocytes may point towards a picture of colitis. Another form of non-invasive testing is blood

cultures and serologies, which can be helpful for the diagnosis of systemic opportunistic infections like *Mycobacterium avium intracellulare* (MAI) or viral etiologies like CMV. Especially in the patients who have diarrhea and fever, MAI may be a possibility. However, with all of these etiologies, a diagnosis may be treated, and symptoms may still persist as secondary infections may also be present. For colitis, a barium enema or abdominal radiography may detail the presence of a toxic megacolon, a complication of *Clostridium difficile* colitis.

In addition to the non-invasive studies listed above, in the absence of a diagnosis, the workup for diarrhea should include some invasive studies as well. The first step is generally a flexible sigmoidoscopy, which can give visualization of the colon (to diagnose or rule out pseudomembranous colitis, among other etiologies) and provide tissue for biopsy. Abnormal tissue should be biopsied, but if the mucosa is normal then random tissue can be sent. The flexible sigmoidoscopy is better than the alternatives as it does not require sedation. If small intestinal etiology is suspected, an EGD (going past the second portion of the duodenum) can help determine the cause of the diarrhea through biopsies of the small bowel, sent not only for pathology, but also electron microscopy and culture analysis. If the flexible sigmoidoscopy is non-diagnostic, and there is still no diagnosis from other studies, a colonoscopy can be performed so more biopsies can be done to rule out opportunistic infections, especially in the ileum. This is rarely done, however, and in general, the absence of definitive diagnosis leads to treatment and evaluation (as will be discussed later).

Infections of the Small Intestine (Enteritis)

The symptoms associated with enteritis are typically associated with diarrhea and prolonged malabsorption leading to malnutrition. This is generally because of opportunistic infections, and, similar to other pathologies in HIV patients, the incidence of enteritis has decreased in the highly active antiretroviral therapy (ART) era. The main symptoms of enteritis are copious voluminous diarrhea (>2 L/day) with dehydration and malabsorption, as opposed to colitis, which is a bloody, painful diarrhea. The work-up of enteritis is detailed above, but specifically should include stool studies, and, if non-diagnostic, esophagogastroduodenoscopy (EGD) with biopsy. The etiologies of enteritis in HIV patients are multifold, and include bacterial, viral, fungal, and parasitic pathogens. These can be diagnosed by the stool studies detailed earlier.

Parasites may be the most common etiology for enteritis, especially in those patients not on ART and greatly immunosuppressed. Parasites are typically diagnosed through stool analysis for ova and parasites, including direct fluorescent antibody (DFA), enzyme-linked immunosorbent assay (ELISA) or polymerase chain reaction (PCR). Light microscopy can be used, though PCR can be diagnostic at much lower levels of parasitic infection. *Cryptosporidium parvum* is the most commonly identifiable pathogen in AIDS related persistent diarrhea, especially in patients with CD4+ lymphocyte counts <200. It is typically treated with paromomycin 1500–3000 mg every 6–8 h orally, or Azithromycin 900–1200 mg four times a day, though albendazole 400 mg twice a day has also shown to be effective. Nitazoxanide (1 g twice daily for at least 2 weeks) can also be used in the treatment of cryptosporidiosis, but a cure is generally not possible if the CD4+ lymphocyte count is <50. However, a study with children showed no benefit to nitazoxanide at all in HIV+ children (just HIV seronegative ones).[30] Hyperimmune bovine colostrums can also be used, but typically not to cure the parasitic infection.[31]

Microsporidiosis is the next most commonly identifiable refractory diarrhea in HIV patients. This can be treated with albendazole as well (400–1600 mg every 12 h orally) but most cases are poorly responsive to treatment and require indefinite therapy. *Isospora belli* is rare in the USA, but is more common in developing countries. Trimethoprim-sulfamethoxazole, one double strength tablet every 6 h for 10 days is the treatment of choice, but pyrimethamine 50–75 mg four times daily (with folinic acid 5 mg orally four times daily) is acceptable for patients with allergies to sulfa medications.[32] Lastly, *Giardia lamblia* and amoebic dysentery can also occur in HIV patients, at the same incidence as the general population, and can be treated with metronidazole 750 mg thrice daily for 5–10 days, or tinidazole 2 g orally once for giardiasis, 3 days for amebic dysentery.[30] For strongyloidosis, thiabendazole 25 mg/kg twice daily orally is the drug of choice. Albendazole seems to be active against all of the parasitic organisms associated with diarrhea in HIV patients, and could be the first line of therapy when parasitic infection is suspected, pending microbiological study.

With all of the aforementioned parasites, treatment cannot only be targeted at the pathogen, but also at the diarrheal symptoms, with the use of somatostatin analogs like octreotide to try to reduce the amount of diarrhea. In addition, since the parasites are both more common and more chronic at lower CD4+ lymphocyte counts, ART, which reduces the degree of immunosuppression, can also be curative. Opioids such as tincture of opium or codeine can provide symptomatic relief in cases of severe diarrhea through its constipating actions, as well as pain relief.[33] Bulking agents, lactose-free diets, and antidiarrheal medications like diphenoxylate with atropine or loperamide are also beneficial in treating diarrheal symptoms.

Viral infection in HIV patients can cause diarrhea, typically through colitis, but also rarely through an enteritis. CMV, in addition to causing esophagitis, can also affect the GI tract through diarrheal illness, and runs the spectrum from asymptomatic carriage to severe diarrheal illness including appendicitis, bleeding and perforation. It typically occurs in the setting of severe immunosuppression with a CD4+ lymphocyte count <100. The diagnosis of CMV enterocolitis is best made through demonstrating a viral cytopathic effect in tissue specimens, but viral stool cultures can also signify disease (though are less sensitive). The treatment for CMV enterocolitis is mainly ganciclovir and foscarnet, as described earlier in the esophagitis section. Valganciclovir may not achieve adequate bioavailability because of the enterocolitis.

Other viruses can affect the HIV patient gastrointestinal tract, including rotavirus, adenovirus, Norwalk virus, or unusually, picornaviruses, and coronaviruses. These tend to be less common than the other pathologies previously described, and are difficult to diagnose as well. Adenovirus can cause a hemorrhagic colitis; acute diarrhea is seen in patients with only adenovirus in stools, but patients with adenovirus on biopsy specimen generally have a chronic diarrhea.[34] HSV can cause diarrhea via systemic infection in end-stage HIV patients, or can cause a colitis and proctitis through HIV mucosal lesions. HSV can be treated with acyclovir, valacyclovir, famciclovir, or, if acyclovir resistant, foscarnet (as previously described in the esophagitis section).

In addition, HIV itself may be a cause of HIV enteropathy and a diarrheal pathogen, and may be identified in gut tissue in up to 40% of patients, but this is controversial. Idiopathic AIDS enteropathy, on the other hand, is the term used for a chronic diarrhea in an AIDS patient that is without identifiable pathogen or diagnosis (despite intensive investigation). Mucosal hyperproliferation is noted on biopsy. For these etiologies, in addition to ART to increase CD4+ lymphocyte count and reduce immunosuppression, should be treated symptomatically with bulking agents, antidiarrheals, and opioids. The combination of antidiarrheal therapy with ART has been shown to be more beneficial than antidiarrheal therapy alone in HIV patients with chronic diarrhea.[35]

Other agents that can cause enteritis include *Mycobacterium avium intracellulare* (MAI) and *Pneumocystis jiroveci* (PCP). Small intestinal disease is the most common site of gastrointestinal luminal involvement by MAI.[36] It is often seen with diffuse small bowel infiltration (mimicking Whipple's Disease) and causes severe malabsorption in patients with CD4+ lymphocyte counts of <50. If a malabsorptive diarrhea occurs with fever and night sweats, in addition to weight loss, MAI must be considered, and blood cultures or a bone marrow biopsy may be diagnostic for disseminated MAI infection. Diagnosing MAI enteritis is more difficult, however, as a positive stool is not diagnostic for gastrointestinal disease (though can suggest subsequent disseminated disease).[37] An endoscopic biopsy and acid-fast staining can show acid-fast bacilli and give an ideal diagnosis. Treatment is with a multitude of options, using combinations of clarithromycin 500 mg twice daily, ethambutol 800–1200 mg orally daily, azithromycin 600 mg daily, rifampin 600 mg daily, rifabutin 300 mg daily, amikacin 15 mg/kg three times weekly, and ciprofloxacin 750 mg twice daily. These can reduce, but not eradicate, MAI. Luminal tuberculosis can also occur as an example of extrapulmonary involvement, but is rare; in contrast to MAI, it can generally be treated to cure with antituberculous therapy. *Pneumocystis jiroveci* (PCP) can also be seen as the cause of diarrhea in HIV patients, but is very uncommon, especially in the setting of PCP prophylaxis for AIDS patients; treatment is with antipneumocystis therapy,[38] generally with trimethoprim-sulfamethoxazole.

Colitis

Bacterial infections in HIV patients typically cause a picture of colitis instead of enteritis, with bloody diarrhea and tenesmus. The most common bacterial pathogens seen in HIV patients include salmonellae, Shigella, *E. coli*, *Campylobacter jejuni*, and *Clostridium difficile*. Salmonellosis is 100 times more common in HIV patients than in immunocompetent hosts,[39] and recurrent salmonella bacteremia establishes the diagnosis of AIDS in an HIV patient. The diagnosis is straightforward, as salmonella can normally be cultured in stool specimens in addition to blood culture results. Salmonella gastroenteritis can present with either watery diarrhea or dysentery (mucopurulent diarrhea) with or without fever, abdominal pain, or nausea and vomiting. Though the diarrhea may be self-limited, the treatment is generally ciprofloxacin 500 mg orally twice a day, for 2–4 weeks, for eradication.

Shigella has a similar presentation to salmonellosis, with a similar wide spectrum of presentation of illness. It does come with a high rate of severe complications, including anemia, hypoglycemia, sepsis, hemolytic uremic syndrome, disseminated intravascular coagulopathy and renal failure, with which mortality obviously increases. It also can be treated with ciprofloxacin 500–750 mg twice a day orally for 5–7 days, and is diagnosed by stool culture as well.

Campylobacter jejuni generally presents as a watery diarrhea, and its incidence is probably decreased due to widespread PCP prophylaxis with trimethoprim-sulfamethoxazole. It is typically harder to culture from stool, and may be diagnosed by endoscopic biopsy. Antimicrobial therapy is not essential, though erythromycin 250–500 mg orally four times daily, or ciprofloxacin 500 mg orally twice a day for 5–7 days may reduce the duration of the illness. *E. Coli* may be seen (in any of several strains), and, like the other enteric bacterial diarrheal illnesses, can be treated with a fluoroquinolone like ciprofloxacin. As illustrated, in cases of suspected bacterial diarrhea, ciprofloxacin would cover most enteric pathogens and would be the empiric drug of choice.

Clostridium difficile is seen in HIV patients not only in the presence of antibiotic therapy, but also in the absence of recent antibiotic therapy. The most common antibiotics that cause *C. difficile* are clindamycin, ampicillin, cephalosporins and aminoglycosides. The clinical presentations and response to therapy are not different in HIV patients than in patients without HIV. Diagnosis is made by detecting *C. difficile* toxin in stool assay, and treatment is with metronidazole 250–500 mg orally every 6–8 h for 10–14 days, or tinidazole, in addition to stopping the offending initial antibiotic therapy. In resistant cases, oral vancomycin 250 mg every 6 h can be used, as can rifaximin 200 mg three times daily, though it is not as effective as vancomycin. In cases of suspected *C. difficile* without diagnosis via stool toxin assay, a flexible sigmoidoscopy can look for pseudomembranous colitis, which can be diagnostic for *C. difficile*.

Fungal etiologies of diarrhea in HIV patients are relatively rare, but can occur in patients with immunocompromised states and low CD4+ lymphocyte counts. Gastrointestinal histoplasmosis appears to be the most commonly described fungal etiology of diarrhea in HIV patients, and typically occurs in the setting of a systemic infection. Diagnosis is made by fungal culture and smear of tissue or blood,[40] and treatment is with amphotericin B 0.5–1 mg/kg per day intravenously initially, with maintenance therapy with itraconazole 200 mg orally daily. Coccidiomycosis and cryptococcosis are also rare, and occur in the presence of systemic infections as well. In addition, as candidal infections are the most common opportunistic infections of HIV patients, a dehydrating diarrhea can also occur as a manifestation of the infection.

Obviously, not all causes of diarrhea in HIV patients are secondary to opportunistic infections. Several noninfectious etiologies of diarrhea in HIV patients can occur as well, including the most common, drug-induced diarrhea. The most common drugs that cause diarrhea in HIV patients are nucleoside reverse transcriptase inhibitors (NRTIs) and protease inhibitors (PIs). With protease inhibitors, diarrhea is the most common side-effect reported with nelfinavir and saquinavir, most commonly occurs at the initiation of treatment, and is a cause of cessation of therapy and lack of adherence to treatment.[41] Newer agents like lopinavir-ritonavir seem to cause less diarrhea than older PIs like nelfinavir.[42] Treatment is generally guided towards treatment of symptoms, namely with bulking agents or antidiarrheals like loperamide.

Other causes of diarrhea in HIV patients include inflammatory bowel disease, including Crohn's disease and ulcerative colitis, neither of which have increased incidence in HIV patients. Treatment is tailored according to the disease process itself, though an active disease process may decrease CD4+ lymphocyte count; this may be reversed by colectomy.[43] In addition, AIDS related illnesses that are noninfectious but can also cause diarrhea and gastrointestinal issues include lymphoma and Kaposi's sarcoma, both of which are diagnosed by biopsy. Infiltration of the mucosal tract by the neoplasm can lead to diarrhea and weight loss.

Anorectal Disease

Anorectal disease is a big component of HIV gastrointestinal care, especially among homosexual males. Interestingly, the incidence of anorectal pathology in HIV patients has not been affected by ART.[44] Many anorectal pathologies are seen in HIV patients, including anal fistulas and fissures, perirectal abscesses, ulcerations and proctitis (Box 23.1). In addition, anal neoplasms as a result of human papillomavirus (HPV) and other etiologies can also occur.

Anorectal carcinoma has an increased incidence in both HIV patients and among homosexual males, and is the fourth most common malignancy seen in HIV;[45] HIV+ homosexual men have twice the incidence than HIV negative homosexual men. Anal squamous cell carcinoma is frequently associated with squamous intraepithelial neoplasia and HPV, much like cervical carcinoma, and can be detected by anorectal cytology, similar to Papanicolaou smears.[46] The gold standard for diagnosis of anorectal neoplastic disease is still anoscopy with biopsy, though anorectal cytology can be useful as a screening test.

In addition to anal carcinoma, other anorectal symptoms are common in the HIV population, especially among homosexual males. Anal condyloma is the most common HIV related anal pathology, and is associated with HPV infection; treatment options include a variety of surgical options, including cryotherapy. The four most common infectious causes of proctitis in men who have sex with men are gonorrhea, herpes simplex, chlamydia and syphilis.[47] Gonorrhea and chlamydia are typically treated together with ceftriaxone 125 mg i.m. once and azithromycin 1 g orally once; fluoroquinolones, oral cephalospo-

---

Box 23.1

Differential diagnosis in anorectal disease in HIV patients

Bacterial

- *Neisseria gonorrhea*
- *Chlamydia trachomatis* (including Lymphogranuloma venereum)
- *Treponema pallidum* (syphilis)
- *Shigella*
- *Salmonella*
- *E. coli*

Viral

- Herpes Simplex (HSV)
- Human Papillomavirus (HPV)
- Cytomegalovirus (CMV)

Other

- Anorectal carcinoma
- Crohn's disease
- Ulcerative colitis
- Radiation proctitis
- Anal fissures
- Anal fistulas
- Perirectal abscess.

rins and doxycycline (100 mg orally twice a day for 7 days) can also be used. Primary syphilis is treated with benzathine penicillin G 2.4 million units i.m. once (or doxycycline 100 mg twice daily for 2 weeks if penicillin allergic). HSV infections, as described earlier with esophagitis and colitis, can also cause perianal and rectal ulcerations, with associated symptoms of tenesmus, pain, and bleeding. Treatment is with antiherpetic medications like acyclovir, valacyclovir, or famciclovir, as explained earlier, with foscarnet in acyclovir-resistant cases. Other etiologies of proctitis include lymphogranuloma venereum, as well as other causes of colitis detailed above; clinical overlap can also happen in HIV patients. In addition to a thorough physical examination, all patients with anorectal symptoms should have anoscopy and sigmoidoscopy with mucosal biopsy to look for fissures, perirectal abscesses, and fistulas in addition to searching for opportunistic infections, with microbiological studies sent for viral, fungal and bacterial cultures.

References

1. Connolly GM, Hawkins D, Harcourt-Webster JN, et al. Oesophageal symptoms, their causes, treatment and prognosis in patients with AIDS. Gut 1989; 30:1033–1039.
2. Zalar AE, Olmos MA, Piskorz EL, et al. Esophageal motility disorders in HIV patients. Dig Dis Sci 2003; 48:962–967.
3. Bach MC, Valenti AJ, Howell DA. Odynophagia from aphthous ulcers of the pharynx and esophagus in AIDS. Ann Intern Med 1988; 109:338–339.
4. Kotler DP, Reka S, Orenstein JM, et al. Chronic idiopathic esophageal ulceration in AIDS: characterization and treatment with corticosteroids. J Clin Gastroenterol 1992; 15:284–290.
5. Monkemuller KE, Call SA, Lazenby AJ, et al. Declining prevalence of opportunistic gastrointestinal disease in the era of combination antiretroviral therapy. Am J Gastroenterol 2000; 95:457–462.
6. Wilcox CM, Alexander LN, Clark WS, et al. Fluconazole compared with endoscopy for human immunodeficiency virus- infected patients with esophageal symptoms. Gastroenterology 1996; 110:1803–1809.
7. Dolin R, Masur H, Saag MS. AIDS therapy. 2nd edn. Edinburgh: Churchill Livingstone; 2002.
8. Wilcox CM, Straub RF, Schwartz DA. Prospective endoscopic characterization of cytomegalovirus esophagitis in patients with AIDS. Gastrointest Endosc 1994; 40:481.
9. Wilcox CM, Rodgers W, Lazenby A. Prospective comparison of brush cytology, viral culture, and histology for the diagnosis of ulcerative esophagitis in AIDS. Clin Gastroenterol Hepatol 2004; 2:564–567.
10. Bini EJ, Micale PL, Weinshel EH. Natural history of HIV-associated esophageal disease in the era of protease inhibitor therapy. Dig Dis Sci 2000; 45:1301–1307.
11. Wilcox CM, Straub RF, Clark WS. Prospective evaluation of oropharyngeal findings in human immunodeficiency virus-infected patients with esophageal ulcer. Am J Gastroenterol 1995; 90:1938.
12. Wilcox CM, Straub RF, Alexander LN, et al. Etiology of esophageal disease in human immunodeficiency virus-infected patients who fail antifungal therapy. Am J Med 1996; 101:599–604.
13. Koletar SL, Russell JA, Fass RJ, et al. Comparison of oral fluconazole and clotrimazole troches as treatment of oral candidiasis in patients infected with human immunodeficiency virus. Antimicrob Agents Chemother 1990; 34:2267.
14. Pons V, Greenspan D, Lozada-Nur F. Oropharyngeal candidiasis in patients with AIDS: randomized comparison of fluconazole versus nystatin oral suspensions. Clin Infect Dis 1997; 24:1204–1207.
15. Barbaro G, Barbarini G. Calderon, et al. Fluconazole versus itraconazole for Candida esophagitis in AIDS. Gastroenterology 1996; 111:1169–1177.
16. Laine L, Dretler RH, Conteas CN, et al. Fluconazole compared with ketoconazole for the treatment of candida esophagitis in AIDS: a randomized trial. Ann Intern Med 1992; 117:655.
17. Villanueva A, Gotuzzo E, Arathoon EG, et al. A randomized double-blind study of caspofungin versus fluconazole for the treatment of esophageal candidiasis. Am J Med 2002; 113:294–299.
18. Wilcox CM, Schwartz DA, Clark WS. Esophageal ulceration in human immunodeficiency virus infection: causes, response to therapy, and long-term outcome. Ann Intern Med 1995; 123:143–149.
19. Goodgame RW, Genta RM, Estrada R, et al. Frequency of positive tests for cytomegalovirus in AIDS patients: endoscopic lesions compared with normal mucosa. Am J Gastroenterol 1993; 88:338.
20. Cheung TW, Teich SA. Cytomegalovirus infection in patients with HIV infection. Mt Sinai J Med 1999; 66:113–124.
21. Laine L, Bonacini M. Sattler F, et al. Cytomegalovirus and Candida esophagitis in patients with AIDS. J Acquir Immune Defic Syndr 1992; 5:605–609.
22. Parente F, Bianchi Porro G. Treatment of cytomegalovirus esophagitis in patients with acquired immune deficiency syndrome: a randomized controlled study of foscarnet versus ganciclovir. Ital Cytomegalovirus Study Group Am J Gastroenterol 1998; 93:317–322.
23. Dieterich DT, Poles MA, Dicker M, et al. Foscarnet treatment of cytomegalovirus gastrointestinal infections in acquired immunodeficiency syndrome patients who have failed ganciclovir induction. Am J Gastroenterol 1993; 88:542–548.
24. McBane RD, Gross JB Jr. Herpes esophagitis: clinical syndrome, endoscopic appearance, and diagnosis in 23 patients. Gastrointest Endosc 1991; 37:600–603.
25. Verdonck LF, Cornelissen JJ, Smit J, et al. Successful foscarnet therapy for acyclovir-resistant mucocutaneous infection with herpes simplex virus in a recipient of allogeneic BMT. Bone Marrow Transplant 1993; 11:177–179.
26. Wilcox CM, Schwartz DA. A pilot study of oral corticosteroid therapy for idiopathic esophageal ulcerations associated with human immunodeficiency virus infection. Am J Med 1992; 93:131–134.
27. Jacobson JM, Spritzler J, Fox L, et al. Thalidomide for the treatment of esophageal aphthous ulcers in patients with human immunodeficiency virus infection. National Institute of Allergy and Infectious Disease AIDS Clinical Trials Group. J Infect Dis 1999; 180:61–67.
28. Chiu HM, Wu MS, Hung CC. Low prevalence of Helicobacter pylori but high prevalence of cytomegalovirus-associated peptic ulcer disease in AIDS patients: Comparative study of symptomatic subjects evaluated by endoscopy and CD4 counts. J Gastroenterol Hepatol 2004; 19:423–428.
29. Call SA, Heudebert G, Saag M, et al. The changing etiology of chronic diarrhea in HIV-infected patients with CD4 cell counts less than 200 cells/mm^3. Am J Gastroenterol 2000; 95:3142–3146.
30. Amadi B, Mwiya M, Musuku J, et al. Effect of nitazoxanide on morbidity and mortality in Zambian children with cryptosporidiosis: a randomised controlled trial. Lancet 2002; 360:1375–1380.

31. Miao YM, Gazzard BG. Management of protozoal diarrhoea in HIV disease. HIV Med 2000; 1:194–199.

32. Mitra AK, Hernandez CD, Hernandez CA, et al. Management of diarrhea in HIV-infected patients. Int J STD AIDS 2001; 12:630–639.

33. Meyer M. Palliative care and AIDS: 2 – Gastrointestinal symptoms. Int J STD AIDS 1999; 10:495–507.

34. Thomas PD, Pollok RCG, Gazzard BG. Enteric viral infections as a cause of diarrhoea in the acquired immunodeficiency syndrome. HIV Med 1999; 1:19–24.

35. Bini EJ, Cohen J. Impact of protease inhibitors on the outcome of human immunodeficiency virus-infected patients with chronic diarrhea. Am J Gastroenterol 1999; 94:3553–3559.

36. Gray JR, Rabeneck L. Atypical mycobacterial infection of the gastrointestinal tract in AIDS patients. Am J Gastroenterol 1989; 84:1521.

37. Chin DP, Hopewell PC, Yajko DM, et al. Mycobacterium avium complex in the respiratory or gastrointestinal tract and the risk of M. avium complex bacteremia in patients with human immunodeficiency virus infection. J Infect Dis 1994; 169:289.

38. Bellomo AR, Perlman DC, Kaminsky DL, et al. Pneumocystis colitis in a patient with the acquired immunodeficiency syndrome. Am J Gastroenterol 1992; 87:759–761.

39. Hsu RB, Tsay YG, Chen RJ, et al. Risk factors for primary bacteremia and endovascular infection in patients without acquired immunodeficiency syndrome who have nontyphoid salmonellosis. Clin Infect Dis 2003; 36:829–834.

40. Wheat LJ, Connoly-Stringfield PA, Baker RL, et al. Disseminated histoplasmosis in the acquired immune deficiency syndrome: Clinical findings, diagnosis, and treatment, and review of the literature. Medicine 1990; 69:361.

41. Sherman DS, Fish DN. Management of protease inhibitor-associated diarrhea. Clin Infect Dis 2000; 30:908–914.

42. Guest JL, Ruffin C, Tschampa JM, et al. Differences in rates of diarrhea in patients with human immunodeficiency virus receiving lopinavir-ritonavir or nelfinavir. Pharmacotherapy 2004; 24:727–735.

43. Sharpstone DR, Duggal A, Gazzard BG. Inflammatory bowel disease in individuals seropositive for the human immunodeficiency virus. Eur J Gastroenterol Hepatol 1996; 8:575–578.

44. Gonzalez-Ruiz C, Heartfield W, Briggs B, et al. Anorectal pathology in HIV/AIDS-infected patients has not been impacted by highly active antiretroviral therapy. Dis Colon Rectum 2004; 47:1483–1486.

45. Rabkin CS, Yellin F. Cancer incidence in a population with a high prevalence of infection with human immunodeficiency virus type 1. J Natl Cancer Inst 1994; 86:1711–1716.

46. Friedlander MA, Stier E, Lin O. Anorectal cytology as a screening tool for anal squamous lesions: cytologic, anoscopic, and histologic correlation. Cancer 2004; 102:19–26.

47. Klausner JD, Kohn R, Kent C. Etiology of clinical proctitis among men who have sex with other men. Clin Infect Dis 2004; 38:300–302.

CHAPTER 24

Primary Neurological Manifestation of HIV/AIDS

David B. Clifford

Mesfin Teshome Mitike

Introduction

As the AIDS pandemic unfolds, the number of people living with human immunodeficiency virus (HIV) infection continues to soar. Two-thirds of infected persons are in Africa, where the epidemic exploded during the 1990s, and one-fifth are in Asia, where the epidemic has been growing rapidly in recent years. As of the end of 2003, between 34.6 million and 42.3 million people throughout the world were living with HIV infection, and more than 20 million had died of acquired immunodeficiency syndrome (Joint United Nations Program on HIV/AIDS, Geneva, July 2004). In that year alone, about 4.8 million people became infected with HIV, and an estimated 2.9 million died of AIDS. The global statistics makes it clear that the burden remains greatest in Africa, although it is home to only 11% of the world population. Sadly, direct evidence about specific manifestations of the epidemic are largely unknown where it is most prevalent. This is especially true of neurological complications of HIV/AIDS representing an important spectrum of primary complications of HIV in developed nations. Our descriptions in this chapter are thus based on observations made before and after availability of antiretroviral therapy (ART) in the western world. Observations from the developing world are only beginning to emerge to determine whether behavior of the disease in the developing world will replicate the experience from the West. While no firm evidence contradicts this expectation, the importance of viral and host genetics in determining disease manifestations is undeniable, as is knowledge that these factors are different in various portions of the world. It is also certain that co-infections influence the course of HIV disease, and these are well known to differ in the developing world, again providing factors that may well alter the natural history of HIV neurological disease.

NeuroAIDS issues may be conveniently considered as primary complications, including conditions that are in some way directly the consequence of the HIV infection, or secondary complications (Box 24.1). The primary complications include HIV-associated dementia (HAD), also known as AIDS dementia complex (ADC), HIV-associated cognitive motor disorders, HIV-associated myelopathy and HIV-associated peripheral neuropathy. Secondary complications result as a consequence of the immunodeficient state of the host (Box 24.1). Neurological infections that fall into this category include cryptococcal meningitis, toxoplasma encephalitis, cytomegalovirus encephalitis and radiculomyelitis, progressive multifocal leukoencephalopathy, and varicella zoster complications. This chapter will focus on the primary neuroAIDS complications, while many of the secondary complications are described elsewhere in the text.

The frequency of neurological complications has changed as the epidemic has evolved, being profoundly impacted by therapeutic practices and perhaps by varying underlying risks in various affected populations. Both the primary HIV-

Primary HIV-associated neurological complications:

- HIV-associated dementia (HAD)
- HIV-associated cognitive motor disorder
- HIV-associated myelopathy
- HIV-associated peripheral neuropathy.

Notable secondary neurological complications:

- Cryptococcal meningitis
- Toxoplasma encephalitis
- Cytomegalovirus encephalitis and radiculomyelitis
- Progressive multifocal leukoencephalopathy
- Varicella zoster (shingles)
- Neurosyphilis
- M. tuberculosis meningitis.

associated complications and the secondary complications occur more frequently in advanced stages of HIV, when the immune system is most impaired. HAD, HIV-associated myelopathy, and peripheral neuropathy are all seen most commonly after the CD4+ lymphocyte count drops below 200 cells/μL. Often primary neurological manifestations are not noticed when early development of opportunistic illnesses supervene, masking the anticipated course of disease progression. As more subjects in developing countries are managed to prevent and treat secondary complications, we anticipate a rapid emergence of clinical recognition of primary HIV-associated neurological complications. Furthermore, with more successful HIV therapy, most patients retain a higher level of immunity, live longer, and the prevalence of HAD actually increases again in populations of long-term survivors.

Diagnostic rules in the setting of HIV deserve some special cautions. While in most of medicine, a single disease should be sought to understand most patient's complaints, in AIDS, neurological complications often are superimposed on an ongoing process with a different etiology. Drug toxicity may add other facets to neurological conditions. Clinical features often reflect the sum of deficits from multiple pathophysiologic perturbations. In addition, AIDS patients are susceptible to the same neurological diseases as patients who do not have HIV infection and thus the clinician must not always leap to unusual diagnoses in the setting of HIV disease, considering as well conditions common in the immunocompetent population.

Pathophysiology, Pathogenesis, and Genetics

Primary HIV-associated complications result from infection in the nervous system, and respond to anti-retroviral therapy. The mechanism by which HIV infection leads to HAD is likely multifactorial and is a subject of intense research. HIV enters the brain and CSF almost immediately after systemic infection. HIV is thought to enter the brain via HIV-infected monocytes, which then differentiate into macrophages. The virus can be recovered from the nervous system throughout the illness. However, productive HIV infection is almost exclusively localized in monocytes and macrophages and probably occurs most commonly late in the disease. Neurons are rarely if ever infected, and astroglial cells, while they may be infected, do not seem to support replication, and the consequences of their infection remain uncertain. It seems likely that much of the pathological consequence of the HIV infection in the brain is secondary to the infection rather than being directly correlated to the extent of viral load in the CNS. Thus, pathological studies suggest that cytokine production is more closely linked with the degree of HAD than the viral load.[1] However, replicative HIV infection in the CNS, reflected by increasing HIV RNA viral loads in the CSF, has been loosely associated with primary HAD.[2] The pathologic impact of the infection is seen early in the deep gray matter of the brain, in white matter, and eventually is reflected in the cortex resulting in loss of neurons and simplified dendritic structures.[3]

While most people are susceptible to HIV, infections require both CD4 receptors and chemokine receptors. Viral isolates may evolve in a host from CCR5 receptor dependent (R5) to a virus with different cellular tropism using the CXCR4 (X4) co-receptors. Considerable evidence suggests that the primary brain isolates are of the R5 class consistent with the fact that these are the predominant receptors on monocytes and macrophages, the primary cells with replicative infection in the brain. It is interesting that some people are protected from HIV infection by a genetic mutation in the CCR5 chemokine receptor that prevents it from participating as a co-receptor for cellular infection. Understanding the factors selecting the subset of HIV-infected persons who develop neurological disease is a fundamental problem of great significance. There are likely to be both host and viral factors that predispose to development of the primary HIV complications. Understanding these should provide greater understanding of the diseases as well as opportunities to protect people from their consequences.

HIV-associated Dementia (HAD)

Clinical Features

HAD is part of a spectrum of motor, cognitive and behavioral problems that develop in advancing HIV infection (Box 24.2). Early signs and symptoms are subtle and may be overlooked. Historically, patients often present with insidious onset of reduced work productivity, poor concentration, mental slowing, and forgetfulness. The cognitive decline is often characterized by slowed thought and speech, which the patient as well as examiners may recognize. Habits of reading and recreation are impacted early, and productivity drops. Apathy and withdrawal from hobbies and social activities are common and must be differentiated from depression. Motor slowing is also typical, and has provided convenient means of documenting advancing neurological involvement. Imbalance, clumsiness and weakness

are common motor complaints. Behavioral changes are less common, but may be dramatic manifestations of the neurological involvement. Flattened affect is typical, and develops even without overt affective disorder. Other manifestations include sleep disturbance, psychosis and seizures. Occasional frank psychotic episodes develop.

As the disease advances, global dementia with memory loss and language impairment develops, culminating in a virtual vegetative state. Neuropsychological evaluation reveals features suggestive of a subcortical dementia, such as is seen in Parkinson's disease. Early in the course of CNS disease, patients develop psychomotor slowing, memory loss, and word-finding difficulties. As the stage of the disease advances, severe psychomotor retardation and language impairment become obvious, leading to akinetic mutism. Clinicians sometimes comment on parallels with Parkinson's disease, and indeed the earliest regions of the brain affected in HIV include the basal ganglia.[4] Recent studies reveal loss of dopamine transporters in basal ganglia correlate with progressive cognitive disability. The greater dopamine transporter decrease in the putamen than in the caudate parallels that are observed in Parkinson's disease.[5]

Neurological examination at early stages of the disease may be normal or reveal subtle changes best documented by formalized neuropsychological testing and referred to as minor cognitive motor disorder (MCMD). Sometimes patients fluctuate between normal performance and MCMD. However, some subjects progress to more advanced disease including more obvious clinical phenotype with frontal release signs, tremor, motor weakness, hyperreflexia, clonus, spasticity and poor coordination. These signs reflect more severe encephalitis as well as a concomitant presence of vacuolar myelopathy and/or neuropathy. As terminal stage is approaching worsening psychomotor retardation and dementia with apraxia, paraplegia leaves the patient bed ridden. Death ensures in a few months time.

Diagnosis

There is no simple test to diagnose HAD. Diagnosis of primary HIV disease is achieved by ruling out alternative causes and recognizing patterns of illness associated with primary disease. These conditions are generally encountered when the HIV disease is advanced, as defined by low CD4 lymphocyte counts (most often below 350 cells/μL) and systemic evidence of immunodeficiency in other areas coin-

---

Box 24.2

Salient clinical features of HIV-associated dementia

Cognitive changes:

- Reduced concentration, inability to focus thoughts or finish tasks
- Decreased reading, less interest in TV
- Decreased memory, making lists, needing reminders
- Speech changes, slowing, sometimes word finding difficulty

Motor changes:

- Slow initiation of movement
- Imbalance, clumsiness
- Weakness
- Sometime myoclonus
- Changes in bladder function, urgency, incontinence

Behavioral changes:

- Personality changes, flat affect
- Depressed appearance
- Sleep disturbance, generally hypersomnia
- Rarely psychotic thought.

ciding with most opportunistic infection. While cognitive impairment in recent years is seen with higher mean CD4 count than a decade ago,[6] it remains problematic to ascribe neurologic problems to these disorders if the viral disease is extremely well controlled and the immune system is relatively intact. Investigations encompass staging of the disease and define current disease control by current and nadir CD4 count and viral load measurement including CSF viral loads. MR and CT imaging studies are most important for ruling out alternative diagnoses, but may support a diagnosis of HAD when typical atrophy or white matter disease is demonstrated (Fig. 24.1). MR spectroscopy has been extensively used in the research setting seeking non-invasive means of monitoring CNS disease. Markers of gliosis or inflammation appear to occur early with late loss of neuronal markers. Some reports correlate these measures with treatment as well as disease progression, but to date MRS has been of little practical use in tracking the CNS disease in the clinic. Functional MRI is not yet widely available, but early studies suggest that before performance deteriorates, recruitment patterns change suggesting that the tasks are more difficult and require recruitment of more brain activity in affected individuals. Position emission tomography (PET) may show abnormalities in subcortical metabolism early with advancing hypometabolism globally in later stages. It is expensive and limited to selected laboratory centers.

CSF is rarely completely normal but the mild lymphocytic cellular response and mild elevation of protein that is most often encountered is not at all diagnostic. Elevated immunoglobulins, not rarely with oligoclonal banding, may be detected. Careful analysis of CSF helps to exclude other etiologic causes of altered neurologic status. In untreated patients, more elevated HIV viral loads in CSF are typical but not diagnostic of primary HIV neurological disease, but the association of cognitive impairment with viral load appears even less reliable in the era of HAART.

For clinical and research purposes, the Memorial Sloan Kettering (MSK) staging system developed by Dr Richard Price and colleagues has been widely employed to stage primary neuroAIDS (Table 24.1). The staging system summarizes a continuum of neurological dysfunction ranging from no impairment (ADC stage 0) and sub-clinical disease (ADC stage 0.5) to profound global dysfunction, leaving the patient essentially vegetative (ADC stage 4). Severity is based on the degree to which neurologic impairment interferes with the patient's ability to work or conduct activities of daily living. There is a critical need for better validated measures of early neuroAIDS disease, particularly means of determining which subjects may suffer progressive deterioration and thus be better candidates for interventions and trials.

Treatment

There is no specific therapy available for cognitive decline in AIDS. Optimal therapy of HIV is a uniform goal once the diagnosis is established, although it is still not clear when ARVs are best introduced during the course of the disease. The central importance of antiretroviral therapy with relation to CNS manifestations is undeniable. Prior to introduction of antiretrovirals, the prevalence of HAD was typically at least 60–70% in advanced disease.[7] Introduction of zidovudine was associated with clearcut improvement in cognitive performance,[8] and in a small placebo controlled trial of high doses of zidovudine in subjects with active dementia.[9] In early years of HIV therapy, incidence of HAD dropped to ≈7% per year with roughly 20% prevalence in the population.[10] HAD has become rare in patients responding well to ARV with controlled viral loads, with estimated incidence now much less than 5%. Thus, amelioration of marked cognitive impairment can be added to the other major benefits of effective antiretroviral therapy. However, even the lower incidence of dementia, when coupled with much longer survival, has resulted in stable or even increasing numbers of cognitively impaired

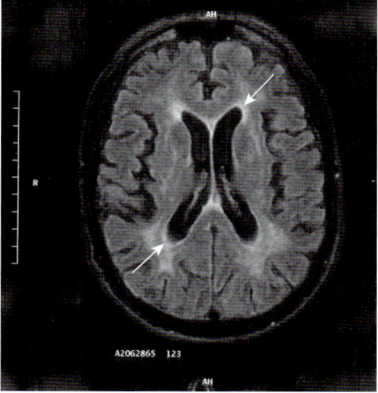

Figure 24.1 MR scan of a patient with HIV-associated dementia. Note the marked, widespread cortical atrophy, ventricular enlargement and diffuse changes in the subcoritcal white matter (arrows)

Table 24.1 Memorial Sloan Kettering scale: clinical staging of the AIDS dementia complex (ADC)

Stage (ADC)	Characteristics
Stage 0 (normal)	Normal mental and motor function.
Stage 0.5 (equivocal/ subclinical)	Either minimal or equivocal symptoms of cognitive or motor dysfunction characteristic of ADC, or mild signs (snout response, slowed extremity movements), but without impairment of work or capacity to perform activities of daily living (ADL). Gait and strength are normal.
Stage 1 (mild)	Unequivocal evidence (symptoms, signs, neuropsychological test performance) of functional intellectual or motor impairment characteristic ADC, but able to perform all but the more demanding aspects of work or ADL. Can walk without assistance.
Stage 2 (moderate)	Cannot work or maintain the more demanding aspects of daily life, but able to perform basic activities of self-care. Ambulatory, but may require a single prop.
Stage 3 (severe)	Major intellectual incapacity (cannot follow news or personal events, cannot sustain complex conversation, considerable slowing of all output) or motor disability (cannot walk unassisted, requiring walker or personal support, usually with slowing and clumsiness of arms as well).
Stage 4 (end stage)	Nearly vegetative. Intellectual and social comprehension and output are at a rudimentary level. Nearly or absolutely mute. Paraparetic or paraplegic with double (urinary and bowel) incontinence.

As used in AIDS Clinical Trials Group protocols.

patients in some clinics, and less improvement in prevalence of neurologic impairment than is desirable.[11] Early studies in Uganda support the prevalence of neurologic impairment in less developed settings and reinforce the importance of introducing ARV as soon as possible.[12]

Antiretroviral drugs vary in their penetrance of the CNS compartment with several, particular protease inhibitors probably having limited access to the brain. It remains uncertain how important it is that therapy be tailored for CNS penetration, but emerging evidence suggests that this characteristic of therapy may be important to consider.[13,14] Neuroprotective strategies distinct from ARV are under investigation, but none have been demonstrated to be effective beyond HIV therapy.[15]

At present, many experts delay ARV until the CD4 count falls below 350 cells/μL or until viral load is quite high, predicting rapid disease progression. However, there is general support for aggressive and consistent use of combined antiretroviral treatment once symptomatic disease, including neurological disease, is identified. The current challenge for therapeutic development resides in balancing the degree and durability of viral response with the cost and complications of the therapy, including side-effects and secondary toxicities. Eventually, efficient strategies for the best use of these drugs must consider the short-term viral response, and also the ability to continue to construct treatment for decades into the future. Treatment of HIV within the CNS in theory

may be even more difficult than systemic infection, since the virus is harbored in longer lived cells and may be exposed to lower and less effective levels of ARV. The quantity of information on CNS efficacy of HIV therapy is suboptimal. CNS penetration of antiretroviral is in part governed by protein binding. For instance, only small fractions of serum levels of protease inhibitors (PI) compounds are achieved in the CSF and presumably also the brain. Other drugs are actively transported out of the central compartment.[16] Despite these theoretical concerns, decline in the incidence of neurological complication has closely followed improvement in systemic HIV therapy. Thus, the clinician's first task is to construct the most effective and best tolerated HIV therapy overall. The importance of constructing a relatively more brain penetrating regimen remains to be proved. However, it is rational to use the best penetrating brain regimen if primary neuroAIDS complications are suspected. Based primarily on CSF penetration (which is not necessarily the same as brain penetration) optimal nucleoside reverse transcriptase inhibitors (NRTI) include zidovudine, stavudine and abacavir. Nevirapine appears to cross the blood–brain barrier well[17] and is theoretically a favorable drug from none nucleoside reverse transcriptase inhibitors (NNRTI) class, but there is documentation of therapeutic efficacy with efavirenz.[18] From the PI class of ARV, indinavir is the least protein bound and has best evidence of efficacy in the CNS.[19]

Measuring the efficacy for primary neuroAIDS therapy remains more challenging than systemic therapy. In cases of clear-cut neurological impairment, a rather dramatic clinical improvement may at times be noted, and the benefits of therapy are easily appreciated. However, with more subtle disabilities, it is much harder to document a response to therapy. For clinical trial development of treatment, repeated well validated neuropsychometric measures to reflect the clinical response to therapy are generally employed. Viral load in CNS, which generally is lower than systemic values, has poor correlation with severity of neurological disease and often provides little guidance for therapy.

Driven by the concern that viral infection is not eliminated from brain by antiviral therapy, considerable effort has been placed in pathophysiologically oriented protective strategies to block presumed neurotoxic damage.[15] To date, small controlled studies have evaluated the toxicity, safety and tolerability of different presumed protective drugs and failed to demonstrate marked neuroprotective properties. Only selegiline has appeared to be both safe and to demonstrate some neurocognitive benefit in an auditory learning task.[20] Selegiline is undergoing further evaluation, while such agents as minocycline appear poised for additional neuroprotective analysis.[21] At present no adjuvant therapy can be recommended outside of the clinical trial setting.

HIV Neuropathy

Clinical Features

Peripheral nerve damage is one of the most common neurological complications of HIV infection and its treatment. HIV-associated sensory neuropathy (HIV-SN) is a major source of morbidity among AIDS patients. Of these, the distal sensory neuropathies, which occur in the advanced stage of HIV disease, are the most common, affecting approximately 30% of AIDS patients. It is important, however, to recognize that other forms of peripheral nerve diseases occur in HIV infections related to other infectious agents and immune mediated damages, which potentially are also treatable. We emphasize the most common forms of HIV-SN, distal sensory polyneuropathy (DSP) and antiretroviral toxic neuropathy (ATN). These two forms are phenotypically identical. They present as a length-dependent neuropathy with distal to proximal development of symptoms. A mixture of negative symptoms of

numbness and sensory loss along with the positive dysesthetic and painful sensations is typical of the severe spectrum of this disorder. The symptoms are typically described as painful numbness, aching, or burning. Symptoms are generally worse at night and can be aggravated by innocuous stimuli, such as bed sheets or wearing shoes. Abnormalities on neurological examination are generally limited to sensory nerve fibers and include reduced or absent ankle reflexes and increased vibratory and pin sensation thresholds.

Diagnosis

As with HAD, it is necessary to come to the diagnosis of HIV-associated neuropathy only by finding typical presentation and ruling out alternative diagnoses. No secure test assures the diagnosis of HIV-associated PN. The typical pattern of distal sensory loss with almost completely sensory involvement of PN is typical, and asymmetric neuropathies, or those with substantial motor involvement suggest an alternative diagnosis. Physiologic testing may be of limited value in HIV-SN. Affected patients can often test normally on routine nerve conduction study. This reflects the prominent small caliber sensory nerve involvement in HIV-SN while nerve conduction tests preferentially evaluate larger nerve fibers. Skin biopsy and visualization of epidermal nerve fibers is a useful diagnostic tool in research settings and theoretically could allow monitoring treatment aimed at nerve regeneration.[22] Reduction in fiber density, increased frequency of fiber varicosities and fiber fragmentation are prominent features of skin biopsy from patients with HIV-SN. While this clearly is associated with HIV itself in advanced disease, the clinical syndrome is often caused by dideoxynucleoside drugs used to treat HIV including didanosine (DDI), stavudine (D4T), and zalcitabine (DDC). While both DSN and ATN can co-exist in a single patient, temporal profile of symptoms in relation to introduction and termination of neurotoxic medications can help in distinguishing the active pathophysiologic process.

Often the typical picture of disease becomes evident when other predisposing conditions for neuropathy are present in the history of the patient. The risk of developing the neuropathy may be further enhanced by concurrent impact of diabetes or nutritional deficient states, especially vitamin B_{12} and thiamine deficiency. DSP is associated with advanced HIV disease, with lower CD4 count and higher viral load being risk factors. An association between viral set point and the subsequent development of HIV-SN has been suggested. Advancing age is also a risk factor, and increasingly note in the developed world in relation to neuropathy. While the incidence of most neurological complications of HIV has fallen dramatically over the past decade, HIV-SN has become more prevalent, coinciding among other reasons with the widespread use of dideoxynucleoside drugs. ATN has subsequently emerged as a common cause of HIV-SN. ATN symptoms typically begin from a few weeks to 6 months after introduction of toxic medications, depending on the NRTI and dose used as well as underlying risks for neuropathy. Symptoms may continue to worsen after discontinuation of the offending agent, followed by at least partial improvement in most but not all patients over a period of weeks to months.

The main pathologic features that characterize DSP and ATN include 'dying back' axonal degeneration of long axons in distal regions, loss of unmyelinated fibers, and variable degree of macrophage infiltration in peripheral nerve and dorsal root ganglia. Marked activation of macrophages as well as the effect of proinflammatory cytokines appears to be the main immunopathogenic factor in DSP.[23] Interference with DNA synthesis and mitochondria abnormalities produced by nucleoside antiretroviral drugs has been postulated as pathologic factors involved in ATN.

Treatment

Treatment for HIV-SN includes optimizing the environment for the nerves by assuring optimal nutritional status and minimal toxic insults. Practically, it is common to be left with only symptomatic therapy options. In case of ATN, the suspected agent should be discontinued if possible, or the dose reduced if that can be done without jeopardizing viral control. Sadly, because development of resistant virus is a life-threatening risk of suboptimal dosing of ARV, this strategy is often impossible. Several drugs, normally effective in symptomatic therapy for neuropathic pain, are apparently ineffective in HIV-SN. Currently, the only therapies shown to be effective in randomized, placebo controlled clinical trials to have efficacy against pain are lamotrigine[24] and recombinant human nerve growth factor.[25] The effects were modest and inconsistent for both and the latter is not commercially available, so there remains a serious need for more effective therapy for this disorder. Clinicians have generally found that gabapentin in higher doses of 1800–

3600 mg/day have provided the best advantage for chronic pain control, but it is often necessary to employ long-acting narcotic drugs to provide reasonable quality of life in the face of troubling pain.

One additional neuromuscular syndrome may prove of importance in developing countries due to widespread use of stavudine. A recently described syndrome termed the neuromuscular weakness syndrome is a life-threatening neuromuscular sequelae typically occurring several weeks subsequent to lactic acidosis associated with d-drug toxicity.[26] Over several weeks, even after the lactic acidosis is cleared, the patients develop severe weakness and subacute painful neuropathic symptoms. Reflexes are markedly depressed, and muscle biopsies suggest mitochondrial myopathy as well as neuropathic changes. Eye movements may be restricted. Supportive therapy, and avoidance of mitochondrial toxins allow recovery of many of these patients, but notable mortality has been associated with this condition.

HIV-1 Associated Vacuolar Myelopathy

Clinical Features

Vacuolar myelopathy is the most common chronic myelopathy associated with HIV infection. It occurs during the late stage of HIV infection, when CD4 counts are very low. It is often seen in conjunction with AIDS dementia complex, peripheral neuropathies, opportunistic CNS, and peripheral nervous system infections. In the early years of HIV when therapy was quite limited, myelopathy was clinically noted in up to 20% of adult HIV patients, while pathologic study of the spinal cord indicated involvement in over half of AIDS autopsies. Pathophysiologic data is limited but it has been suggested that infiltration and/or involvement of the cord with HIV-infected cells secreting neurotoxic factors, neurotoxic HIV proteins, or less likely direct viral involvement and impaired ability to utilize vitamin B_{12} could underlie this devastating disorder. The vacuolar degeneration of heavily myelinated tracts including the corticospinal tract results in progressive spastic diplegia (paraplegia), often with substantial bladder involvement and sensory ataxia. Sensory involvement is less typical and difficult to separate from associated peripheral neuropathy. However, both dorsal column and spinothalamic sensory deficits are often appreciated in these patients. Neurologic bladder complaints are typical.

Diagnosis

Laboratory studies focus on exclusion of treatable causes like vitamin B_{12} deficiency and compressive myelopathy. It is critical in this case not to ascribe serious myelopathy to HIV without imaging the cord for treatable compressive lesions. Negative imaging studies with MRI and normal level for vitamin level are cornerstone for inclusion and consideration of the disease.

Treatment

Treatment for myelopathy is probably best addressed by optimized ARV. The high prevalence of this disorder in untreated HIV disease is substantially different from the experience in the era of highly active therapy where myelopathy is very rarely encountered in successfully treated subjects. A recent effort to collect cases of active myelopathy in the USA led by the Neurologic AIDS Research Consortium did not find enough cases in major medical centers to undertake treatment trials. It is also found that when the treatment is started in patients beginning to demonstrate myelopathy, that it is arrested and partially reversed in many cases. In addition to ARV treatment, care in nutrition is very important, an aspect of therapy that it can be anticipated will be of particular importance in the developing world where diets may be marginal.

Conclusion

Primary neurological complications at every level of the nervous system have been a significant part of the impact of HIV infection in developed countries. While these manifestations may be veiled by the acute illnesses complicating untreated disease, they are almost surely present in the much larger group of people suffering HIV in developing countries, and are likely to be noted more prominently as therapy is introduced. Because the actual manifestations of these disease are likely to be dependent both on viral and host genetics, both of which may have significant differences in various parts of the world, it will be critical to monitor the presentation and course of these complications in the different settings where this disease is prevalent.

References

1. Wesselingh SL, Power C, Glass JD, et al. Intracerebral cytokine messenger RNA expression in acquired immunodeficiency syndrome dementia. Ann Neurol 1993; 33:576–582.
2. Ellis RJ, Hsia K, Spector SA, et al. Cerebrospinal fluid human immunodeficiency virus Type 1 RNA levels are elevated in neurocognitively impaired individuals with acquired immunodeficiency syndrome. Ann Neurol 1997; 42:679–688.
3. Sá MJ, Madeira MD, Ruela C, et al. AIDS does not alter the total number of neurons in the hippocampal formation but induces cell atrophy: a stereological study. Acta Neuropathol 2000; 99:643–653.
4. Rottenberg DA, Moeller JR, Strother SC, et al. The metabolic pathology of the AIDS dementia complex. Ann Neurol 1987; 22:700–706.
5. Wang GJ, Chang L, Volkow ND, et al. Decreased brain dopaminergic transports in HIV-associated dementia patients. Brain 2004; 127:2452–2458.
6. Dore GJ, Correll PK, Li Y, et al. Changes to AIDS dementia complex in the era of highly active antiretroviral therapy. AIDS 1999; 13:1249–1253.
7. Navia BA, Jordan BD, Price RW. The AIDS dementia complex: I. Clinical features. Ann Neurol 1986; 19:517–524.
8. Schmitt FA, Bigley JW, McKinnis R, et al. Neuropsychological outcome of zidovudine (AZT) treatment of patients with AIDS and AIDS-related complex. N Engl J Med 1988; 319:1573–1578.
9. Sidtis JJ, Gatsonis C, Price RW, et al. Zidovudine treatment of the AIDS dementia complex: Results of a placebo-controlled trial. Ann Neurol 1993; 33:343–349.
10. McArthur JC, Hoover DR, Bacellar H, et al. Dementia in AIDS patients: Incidence and risk factors. Neurology 1993; 43:2245–2252.
11. Sacktor N, McDermott MP, Marder K, et al. HIV-associated cognitive impairment before and after the advent of combination therapy. J Neurovirol 2002; 8:136–142.
12. Sacktor NC, Wong M, Nakasujja N, et al. The International HIV Dementia Scale: a new rapid screening test for HIV dementia. AIDS 2005; 19:1367–1374.
13. Letendre SL, McCutchan JA, Childers ME, et al. Enhancing antiretroviral therapy for human immunodeficiency virus cognitive disorders. Ann Neurol 2004; 56:416–423.
14. Cysique LA, Maruff P, Brew BJ. Antiretroviral therapy in HIV infection: are neurologically active drugs important? Arch Neurol 2004; 61:1699–1704.
15. Clifford DB. Human immunodeficiency virus-associated dementia. Arch Neurol 2000; 57:321–324.
16. Choo EF, Leake B, Wandel C, et al. Pharmacological inhibition of P-glycoprotein transport enhances the distribution of HIV-1 protease inhibitors into brain and testes. Drug Metab Disposition 2000; 28:655–660.
17. Glynn SL, Yazdanian M. In vitro blood-brain barrier permeability of nevirapine compared to other HIV antiretroviral agents. J Pharm Sci 1998; 87:306–310.
18. Tashima K, Caliendo AM, Ahmad M, et al. Cerebrospinal fluid human immunodeficiency virus type 1 (HIV-1) suppression and efavirenz drug concentrations in HIV-1-infected patients receiving combination therapy. J Infect Dis 1999; 180:862–864.
19. Martin C, Sönnerborg A, Svensson JO, et al. Indinavir-based treatment of HIV-1 infected patients: efficacy in the central nervous system. AIDS 1999; 13:1227–1232.
20. The Dana Consortium on the Therapy of HIV Dementia and Related Cognitive Disorders. A randomized, double-blind, placebo-controlled trial of deprenyl and thioctic acid in human immunodeficiency virus-associated cognitive impairment. Neurology 1998; 50:645–651.
21. Zink MC, Uhrlaub J, DeWitt J, et al. Neuroprotective and anti-human immunodeficiency virus activity of minocycline. JAMA 2005; 293:2003–2011.

22. Polydefkis M, Yiannoutsos CT, Cohen BA, et al. Reduced intraepidermal nerve fiber density in HIV-associated sensory neuropathy. Neurology 2002; 58:115–119.

23. Keswani SC, Pardo CA, Cherry CL, et al. HIV-associated sensory neuropathies. AIDS 2002; 16:2105–2117.

24. Simpson DM, McArthur JC, Olney R, et al. Lamotrigine for HIV-associated painful sensory neuropathies. Neurology 2003; 60:1508–1514.

25. McArthur JC, Yiannoutsos C, Simpson DM, et al. A phase II trial of nerve growth factor for sensory neuropathy associated with HIV infection. Neurology 2000; 54:1080–1088.

26. Simpson D, Estanislao L, Evans S, et al. HIV-associated neuromuscular weakness syndrome. AIDS 2004; 18:1403–1412.

CHAPTER 25

Psychiatric Barriers and the International AIDS Epidemic

Alex Thompson
Jessica Long
Andrew Angelino
Glenn Treisman

Introduction

The classic triad of infectious disease involves looking at the factors of host, agent, and environment when trying to analyze the causes and successful interventions regarding an epidemic. Previous world pandemics have had different vectors of spread and different host vulnerabilities than the HIV/AIDS epidemic. The primary vector of spread for HIV is behavioral, and is specifically related to behaviors involving intimate contact and blood or secretion contact. When the epidemic was first detected, the vulnerable host groups were identified as Homosexuals, Heroin addicts, Haitians, and Hemophiliacs (the 4-H group), which allowed certain behaviors to be considered as vectors for the agent. In the early years of the epidemic, doctors began to recognize that mental health and psychiatric disorders played a role in the spread of this virus in the USA and in developed countries. Massive educational efforts in the developed countries slowed the epidemic to some extent, but it continued to spread among those who were unable to modify their behavior. Subsequent work has suggested that psychiatric disorders play an important role in both the spread of the virus through the risk behaviors that they provoke, and that these disorders impact treatment response as well, by affecting compliance with treatment, willingness to accept treatment, and the resources to obtain treatment (Fig. 25.1).

Economically disadvantaged people have limited access to psychiatric treatment. Chronic mental illness tends to run in families and to deplete economic resources, resulting in economic 'downward drift' of those most likely to get serious mental disorders. This results in decreased mental healthcare available to those with more severe mental illness. This has been recognized both in developed countries and the rest of the world.[1,2] This complicates the treatment of HIV, as those in countries most severely affected by HIV have the most limited resources for mental health treatment and the most limited resources for HIV treatment. For instance, by the end of 2003, only 7% of those in need of antiretroviral treatment in developing countries had such access.[3] Similarly, according to the WHO World Mental Health Consortium, 35.5–50.3% of serious cases of mental illness in developed countries and 76.3–85.4% of cases in less developed countries received no treatment in the 12 months prior to its survey.[4] An estimated 450 million people worldwide suffer from psychiatric and neurological disorders.[5] In 2001, the World Health Organization focused its annual report on mental health. The WHO estimates that neuropsychiatric disorders contribute 31% of all years of life lived with disability worldwide and by region: 18% in Africa; 43% in the Americas; 27% in the

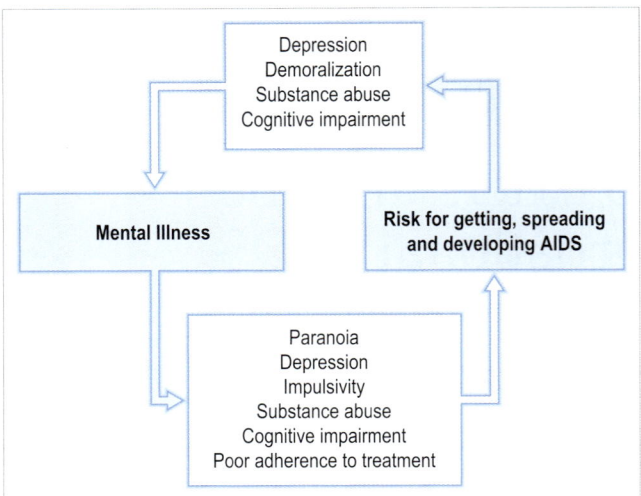

Figure 25.1 Psychiatric disorders play an important role in both the spread of the virus through behavior and the impact on treatment response.

Eastern Mediterranean; 43% in Europe; 27% in Southeast Asia; and 31% in the Western Pacific. Major depression is the leading cause of disability worldwide and ranks fourth (just behind HIV/AIDS) in the global burden of disease, and it is expected to rise to the number two spot by 2020. In fact, among global estimates of years of life lived with disability for all ages, unipolar depression ranks first, and five other psychiatric morbidities rank in the top 20 causes (HIV/AIDS is ranked number 18). For both sexes, ages 15–44, unipolar depression, alcohol use disorders, and schizophrenia constitute the three leading causes and bipolar disorder is the fifth leading cause (HIV/AIDS is the seventh). At any one time, the WHO estimates a point prevalence of 10% of neuropsychiatric conditions among adults worldwide. Treatment of mental disorders is associated with considerable stigma across most cultures and economic circumstances, and in the USA, psychiatric treatment tied to HIV treatment has been far more successful than when the services were provided independently. The intersections of HIV and mental illness deserve examination in discussions regarding prevention, treatment, and prognosis of persons with HIV. Mental illnesses are unique in their effects upon not only the disease course of HIV, but also the perpetuation of the epidemic and failure of treatment. Additionally, HIV itself is unique in its manifestations and increased risk of mental illness.

The disparity of mental health resources in countries with HIV cannot be overstated. According to the Global Summary of the HIV and AIDS Epidemic, December 2004, Africa has 25.4 million adults and children living with HIV (64.5% of the world's total).[6]

The estimated 3.1 million newly-infected adults and children in Africa represented 63.3% of the World's total, while the 2.3 million AIDS deaths in adults and children represented about three-quarters of the world's total. There is much disparity among the countries in Africa regarding prevalence. For instance, in southern Africa, all seven countries have prevalence rates above 17%. In western Africa, no country has a prevalence higher than 10%, with most falling between 1% and 5%. The prevalence in central and east Africa appears to fall somewhere between these two areas at 4–13%.[3]

Mental health country profiles were done in Kenya, Uganda, and Zambia. In Kenya, with a population of 30 million, there are 50 psychiatrists (only 15 of which work in the public sector). Prior research had estimated a psychiatric morbidity of about 45% in a primary care clinic in Nairobi. Another study at an STD clinic in Nairobi found a psychiatric morbidity of 75% in those with HIV compared with 36% in those who were HIV negative.[7] As of 2002, Uganda had a population of 24.7 million people for whom there were 12 psychiatrists and little access to special mental healthcare in the country.[8] In Zambia, with a population of about 10 million, there are about 260 total mental health workers in the country.[9] In Tanzania, just 10 psychiatrists served its population of 30 million in 2001. For comparison's sake, in the UK, according to World Bank statistics in 2002, there were 8082 psychiatrists for its population of 60 million.[10]

Asia, with 60% of the world's population, is experiencing rapid spread of HIV. Outside of South Africa, India has the highest number of its population living with HIV. Three-quarters of its over 1 billion inhabitants live in rural areas, most of which are not well served by formal or specialized health-care services. A meta-analysis of epidemiological studies regarding mental illness in India found a prevalence of 58.2/1000. For a country considered developing based on economic parameters, India has a large number of healthcare providers. However, most of these providers are found in urban areas, while most of the population is placed rurally, and statistically there are just four psychiatrists per million people.[11] Similarly, Thailand, a country with a population of over 61 million, has approximately 351 psychiatrists with over half of them located in Bangkok, averaging about six psychiatrists per 1 million people.[12] In Malaysia, with a population of 24 million, there are 145 psychiatrists that help run 30 mental health wards of 20–100 beds each.[13] A survey done in 2000 found Nepal, a country of 24 million people, to have a total of 27 psychiatrists, no child or geriatric psychiatrists, four neurologists, five psychiatric nurses, and five clinical psychologists.[14] In Pakistan, for its population of over 140 million people, there are 342 psychiatrists as of the year 2000, when there were but 65 in 1980.[15]

For all countries, the importance of unique cultural values and beliefs also play a role in mental health research and treatment. Mental illness is something that carries a high stigma and is often felt to be due to punishment from ancestors or possession from spirits. For example, in Uganda, those who are mentally ill are not eligible for employment or voting. There is frequent use of traditional healers and the importance of traditional healers in ongoing policy development and community mental health treatment is high. Almost all persons with mental illness in Uganda and 70–80% of those with a mental illness in Zambia will consult a traditional healer as first line of care.[7,8]

The purpose of addressing the issues raised in the country mental health profiles is to provide a parallel view of the deficits of mental health coverage in the areas devastated by HIV. As we will now address, there is significant psychiatric comorbidity in HIV/AIDS. The presence of a major mental illness both increases the likelihood of behaviors that put one at risk for HIV infection and limits the effectiveness of focused treatment on HIV and AIDS.

Psychiatric disorders differ in etiology, pathology, and treatment. Although in the USA there has been a great focus on 'disease' psychiatry and the use of disease-based criteria for conditions (such as those used in the DSM-IV), many psychiatric conditions are not diseases and do not fit well into this model,

but still have a huge impact on HIV infection. We will discuss psychiatric diseases, which are presumed to involve lesion-type pathology in the brain first, and then discuss problems of addictive behavior and problems of temperament and endowment. We would like to acknowledge that problems originating in a person's experience have a profound influence on their ability to accept treatment as well. For instance, those persons who have experienced misuse at the hands of trusted paternal figures will have trust issues when accessing medical care, and those with disordering sexual experiences at vulnerable developmental stages have a risk for developing high risk sexual behaviors including promiscuity and prostitution. Although there is a literature involving HIV and these kinds of problems, it is mostly beyond the scope of this discussion.

Chronic Mental Illness and HIV Infection

A subset of patients with chronic mental illnesses such as recurrent severe major depression, schizophrenia, and bipolar affective disorder have been studied together as a high risk population, and this group has been shown to have increased HIV-risk behaviors in every population that has been studied, although these have mostly been in developed countries. The prevalence rate of HIV among the chronically mentally ill in the USA has been estimated to be between 4% and 20%.[16–20] A study examining 234 patients attending community mental health clinics in Melbourne, Australia, found that patients with mental illness were more likely to participate in unprotected casual sex and injection drug use when compared with the general population.[21] There are many other studies supporting the notion that those with chronic mental illness have a higher rate of behaviors that put them at risk for HIV.[22–26]

To worsen matters, mental illness impairs a patient's ability to adhere to complicated medication regimens necessary to suppress viral replication and HIV disease. Successful treatment requires consistently taking at least 90% of prescribed antiretroviral medications.[27,28] It is known that not just dose adherence, but schedule adherence is necessary for the complete suppression of the virus. Studies have shown a wide variety of adherence rates ranging from 32% to over 80%, depending on the group studied and the length of time over which adherence is being monitored. A study of 115 patients in a Los Angeles HIV clinic found 3-day, 1-week, and 1-month adherence success rates (taking 95% of doses) of 58.3, 34.8, and 26.1%, respectively. Three-day adherence was strongly related to mental health, social support, patient physician relationship, and side-effects.[29] Another study that did not exclude the mentally ill estimated sustained viral suppression in only 25–40% of patients.[30]

Mood Disorders in HIV/AIDS

Affective disorders (mood disorders), particularly major depression, are the most common comorbid psychiatric conditions in patients suffering from HIV disease. The prevalence of major depression in those with HIV in the USA has been estimated at 15–40%.[31-34] The prevalence exceeds 50% in persons with HIV seeking psychiatric treatment.[31] When addressing the diagnosis of depression, one must consider other options such as demoralization, dementia, and delirium, all common comorbidities in those with HIV and AIDS. While checklists can be useful for screening, a detailed history that addresses areas such as mood, self attitude, vital sense, hedonic capacity, and neurovegetative symptoms will make the diagnosis clear.[35] The importance of diagnosing and treating depression rests in the ability to improve quality of life, decrease high-risk behaviors, and improve medication compliance.

It has been difficult to show that bipolar disorder has a statistically significant prevalence in patients with HIV, but it is clear that advanced HIV can trigger a mania-like state which has been described as AIDS mania. In one study of a large clinical cohort, 8% of patients with AIDS had mania which is 10 times the expected 6-month prevalence in the general population.[36] AIDS mania appears to be a unique type of mania associated with the late stage of HIV infection with an appearance similar to a delirium. The predominant mood appears to be irritability and an involved work-up for delirium (Box 25.1) needs to be completed prior to making this diagnosis.[35]

This issue is complicated in the global community by different standards and beliefs regarding mental illness. A researcher with a depression inventory will have little luck in diagnosing or understanding mental illness in culturally unique communities. An excellent example of this was described in a study from Uganda that looked at local perceptions of the impact HIV had on mental health. Key informants described two local syndromes, *Yo'kwekyawa* (translated as 'hating oneself') and *Okwekubaziga* (translated as 'pitying oneself'), as resulting from HIV infection. Both of these encompass many aspects of what we understand as major depression and give

Box 25.1	
'I WATCH DEATH' mnemonic for delirium	
Infectious	Sepsis, encephalitis, meningitis, syphilis, urinary tract infection, pneumonia
Withdrawal	Alcohol, barbiturates, sedatives-hypnotics
Acute metabolic	Acidosis, electrolyte disturbance, hepatic or renal failure
Trauma	Head trauma, burns
CNS disease	Hemorrhage, CVA, vasculitis, seizures, tumor
Hypoxia	Acute hypoxia, chronic lung disease, hypotension
Deficiencies	B_{12}, hypovitaminosis, niacin, thiamin
Environmental	Hypothermia, hyperthermia, endocrinopathies
Acute Vascular	Hypertensive emergency, subarachnoid hemorrhage, sagittal vein thrombosis
Toxins/drugs	Medications, street drugs, alcohol, pesticides, industrial poisons
Heavy metals	Lead, mercury

Source: Cohen BJ. Theory and practice of psychiatry. Oxford: Oxford University Press; 2003:110.

strength to the notion that those affected with HIV anywhere in the world are likely to have similar mental health manifestations (like depression), though they may not describe it in a manner familiar to the western world.[37]

AIDS Delirium and Dementia

AIDS dementia is described elsewhere in this volume, but can present as a depressive-like illness because of the profound apathy that often accompanies it. AIDS dementia is also often associated with AIDS mania. Delirium can mimic any psychiatric disorder, and has a poor prognosis if not detected. Delirium and dementia are frequently present in the late stage of HIV disease. Delirium is a state of global cerebral dysfunction, and is characterized by an 'altered level of consciousness' and a 'waxing and waning course.' Often presenting a diagnostically frustrating picture, a delirious patient may seem normal when the attending doctor comes around and then at night, may become agitated and difficult to care for. AIDS delirium presents itself with waxing and waning levels of consciousness, inattentiveness, trouble concentrating, memory, behavioral, and perceptual abnormalities. Delirium in AIDS can reflect metabolic disturbances, electrolyte imbalance, encephalitis, sepsis, or a side-effect of medications.[38] Additionally, immunocompromised patients are at risk for infections, which may present with neuropsychiatric symptoms and are associated with the chronic condition of AIDS dementia. Progressive multifocal leukoencephalopathy (PML), cytomegalovirus encephalitis, cryptococcal meningitis, toxoplasmosis, and varicella-zoster virus encephalitis are just some of the many central nervous system infections HIV patients may acquire that present with neuropsychiatric symptoms including diminished cognitive functioning, depressed mood, and Parkinsonian and fine-motor movement disturbances.[39] Delirium is a serious medical illness and requires diagnosis if it is to be treated with the appropriate aggressiveness. This is important, as delirium has been found to be related to decreased survival when it presents in a patient with AIDS.[40]

AIDS dementia is a subcortical dementia similar to the dementias that present in patients with Parkinson's and Huntington's diseases. Patients present with profound psychomotor slowing, accompanied by impairments in mood, memory, and movement (the subcortical triad). It is the subtle change in these areas (psychomotor slowing, fine motor task skills, and memory) that make up what is called the minor cognitive motor disorder (MCMD), a syndrome felt to be a very early stage of AIDS-associated dementia. AIDS dementia is usually associated with profound apathy, but may be complicated by a spectrum of symptoms including irritability, hyperactivity, agitation, insomnia, euphoria, and psychosis (this may accompany AIDS mania).[35] Some investigators have suggested that up to two-thirds of AIDS patients have an HIV-associated dementia.[41] Unlike the other subcortical dementias, there is effective treatment for HIV-associated dementia with aggressive HAART (highly active antiretroviral therapy).

HIV and Substance Abuse

Addictive behaviors are a problem throughout the world. The susceptibility to addiction is clearly complex, involving cultural, social, psychological, genetic, and psychiatric factors. For some time, addictions in the Western hemisphere have been regarded as diseases, a useful concept in some ways, namely in de-stigmatizing patients who suffer from these chronic problems. While there is some evidence of brain pathology that may perpetuate certain

substance use disorders, there is also a paradigm for describing behaviors that become self-perpetuating as a result of recruitment of the brain's normal reward systems (see McHugh[42] for more discussion). Intravenous drug use holds a premier place in the discussion of substance abuse, as it is a direct route of infection and spread of HIV. It is a major player in the ongoing AIDS epidemic in Asia, Eastern Europe, Latin America, and developed countries. From India to China, HIV prevalence in communities of IDUs have increased from 0 to 50% in as quickly as 6 months time; and the map of HIV spread throughout Southeast Asia by virus strain, not coincidentally, follows heroin trafficking patterns in the area.[43]

Other substance use disorders play an important role in the transmission of HIV through the promotion of high-risk behaviors. Clearly, regardless of the country, behavior is the most common vector of HIV transmission, and has a substantial impact on the perpetuation of the epidemic. A behavior is a goal directed coordinated series of actions; something one does. Behaviors occur in response to the environment, and are followed by an environmental response, but may also be followed by an internally mediated reward signal within the brain, which is then likely to increase the behavior. It is conditioning by this reward that 'drives' behaviors such as the insertion of a needle into your arm, 'chasing the dragon,' visiting a brothel, or having high-risk sex. There is some response within the brain that was positive and responds with the message, 'hey...do that again...that felt good.'

Behaviors involve the brain's internal reward circuitry. The behavior releases reward neurotransmitters in the brain leading to a sense of pleasure. With the waning of the pleasure comes an urge, or craving, to accomplish the behavior that originated in the good feelings. Such a positive feedback loop can be very helpful when increasing the frequency of behaviors needed for survival such as sleeping, eating, and sex. However, such a loop, if not tightly regulated, can lead to an excessive focus on a particular behavior. If you eat enough or sleep enough, you lose interest in that activity temporarily. The loop is 'off.' Drugs and alcohol can activate this loop and can drive it out of control. Genetics, environment, and circumstances all play a role in both the likelihood of using the drugs and the degree of reward they provoke. Other psychiatric illnesses also play a role in determining the likelihood of using drugs and the vulnerability of the reinforcement loop to get out of control. Understanding these things can help reduce the stigma associated with addiction and motivate the change necessary to stop the devastating behaviors (see Treisman and Angelino for further discussion).

Personality, Temperament, and HIV

Since the time of ancient medicine, those interested in healing and illness have recognized differences in personality types and the likely behaviors associated with those types. The four humors of Greek medicine: melancholic, choleric, sanguine, and phlegmatic, retain utility as personality descriptors today. We have added a variety of ways to view these same features, from describing their theoretical origins in experiences from a Freudian point of view (oral, anal), to describing them in terms of their impact on others (antisocial, avoidant), to describing their behavioral characteristics (risk-taking, pleasure-seeking). In each set of descriptors, one can see that careful, anxious and risk-avoidant people are at lower risk for HIV, while those who are risk-taking, emotion-driven, and unconcerned with their own well-being are at higher risk. One can also see that those who are unconcerned about their responsibilities to others might knowingly continue to spread HIV with little regard for the impact they have on others. A limited amount of research has been done in this area regarding HIV, mostly in Western cultures and developed cultures, but is never-the-less of crucial importance to stopping the HIV epidemic. People with certain personality types are 'vulnerable' to situations that might expose them to HIV, and need adequate coaching in advance to help them avoid the trap their vulnerabilities might set for them.

Lastly, psychiatric disorders often compound each other in comorbid situations. Major depression increases the likelihood of alcohol abuse, and alcohol abuse worsens major depression. People who are risk-taking or severely anxious are also more likely to overuse alcohol, and their depression makes their anxiety or risk-taking worse. Each of these features seems to compound risk for HIV and related conditions, such as Hepatitis C, STDs, and a host of other behaviorally transmitted infections.

Conclusion

The need for the recognition and treatment of mental illness in the global fight against HIV/AIDS is paramount: mental and behavior disorders are not only more likely to be seen in those infected with HIV but are important risk factors for HIV acquisition and transmission. Furthermore, these disorders deplete their victims economically and interfere with treatment by impairing adherence. The complex interplay of HIV/AIDS and mental illness can be daunting. However, it offers a unique and necessary opportunity for both prevention and improved therapy. There is evidence that local treatment programs for mental illness can be efficient and cost effective in developing countries.[44] By addressing the psychiatric morbidities surrounding HIV, we may not only reduce the global burden of disease but may prevent further spread of AIDS. We have low rates of diagnosis and treatment of the mentally ill with HIV and low rates of HAART compliance necessary to suppress the HIV and prevent the development of resistant virus. Such facts make the situation in developing countries seem that much more desperate. In locales with limited medical, financial, and human resources, it seems unlikely we will make inroads into recognizing and managing the mentally ill suffering from HIV disease and AIDS when most have no access to the treatment for the underlying disease. What that leaves us with is hope and the clear view of our responsibilities as physicians and human beings.

References

1. David Satcher. Mental health: a report of the surgeon general. 92nd Annual NAACP Convention, New Orleans, LA: 1999.
2. WHO. WHO resource book on mental health, human rights and legislation. Geneva: World Health Organization; 2005.
3. UNAIDS. Report on the global AIDS epidemic: Executive summary. Baltimore, MD: UNAIDS; 2004. Online. Available: www.unaids.org
4. The WHO World Mental Health Survey Consortium. Prevalence, severity, and unmet need for treatment of mental disorders in the World Health Organization world mental health surveys. JAMA 2004; 291:2581–2590.
5. WHO. World Health Report 2001: Mental health: new understanding, new hope. Geneva: World Health Organization; 2001.
6. UNAIDS. Global summary of the HIV and AIDS epidemic. Geneva, Switzerland: UNAIDS; 2004. Online. Available: www.unaids.org
7. Kiima DM, Njenga FG, Okonji MM, et al. Kenya mental health country profile. Int Rev Psychiatry 2004; 16:48–53.
8. Ndyanabangi S, Basangwa D, Lutakome J, et al. Uganda country mental health profile. Int Rev Psychiatry 2004; 16:54–62.
9. Mayeya J, Chazulwa R, Mayeya PN, et al. Zambia mental health country profile. Int Rev Psychiatry 2004; 16:63–72.
10. Njenga F. Focus on Psychiatry in East Africa. Br J Psychiatry 2002; 181:354–359.
11. Khandelwal SK, Jhingan HP, Ramesh S, et al. India mental health country profile. Int Rev Psychiatry 2004; 16:126–141.
12. Siriwanarangsun P, Liknapichitkul D, Khandelwal SK. Thailand mental health country profile. Int Rev Psychiatry 2004; 16:150–158.
13. Parameshvara Deva M. Malaysia mental health country profile. Int Rev Psychiatry 2004; 16:167–176.
14. Regmi SK, Pokharel A, Ojha SP, et al. Nepal mental health country profile. Int Rev Psychiatry 2004; 16:142–149.
15. Karim S. Pakistan mental health country profile. Int Rev Psychiatry 2004; 16:83–92.

16. Cournos F, Empfield M, Horwath E, et al. HIV seroprevalence among patients admitted to two psychiatric hospitals. Am J Psychiatry 1991; 48:1225–1230.

17. Empfield M, Cournos F, Meyer I, et al. HIV seroprevalence among homeless patients admitted to a psychiatric inpatient unit. Am J Psychiatry 1993; 150:47–52.

18. Meyer I, McKinnon K, Cournos F, et al. HIV seroprevalence among long-stay patients in a state psychiatric hospital. Hosp Community Psychiatry 1993; 44:282–284.

19. Susser E, Valencia E, Conover S. Prevalence of HIV infection among psychiatric patients in a New York City men's shelter. Am J Public Health 1993; 83:568–570.

20. Rosenberg SD, Goodman LA, Osher FC, et al. Prevalence of HIV, hepatits B, and hepatitis C in people with severe mental illness. Am J Gastroenterol 2001; 91:31–37.

21. Davidson S, Judd F, Jolley D, et al. Risk factors for HIV/AIDS and hepatitis C among the chronic mentally ill. Aust N Z J Psychiatry 2001; 35:203–209.

22. Kelly JA, Murphy DA, Bahn GR, et al. AIDS/HIV risk behaviour among the chronic mentally ill. Am J Psychiatry 1992; 149:886–889.

23. Cournos F, Guido JR, Coomaraswamy S, et al. Sexual activity and risk of HIV infection among patients with schizophrenia. Am J Psychiatry 1994; 151:228–232.

24. Coverdale JH, Turbott SH, Roberts H. Family planning needs and STD risk behaviours of female psychiatric out-patients. Br J Psychiatry 1997; 171:69–72.

25. Volavka J, Convit A, O'Donnell J, et al. Assessment of risk behaviors for HIV infection among psychiatric inpatients. Hosp Community Psychiatry 1992; 43:482–485.

26. Otto-Salaj LL, Stevenson LY. Influence of psychiatric diagnoses and symptoms on HIV risk behavior in adults with serious mental illness. AIDS Read 2001; 206:197–204, 206–208.

27. Moreno A, Perez-Elias MJ, Casado JL, et al. Effectiveness and pitfalls of initial highly active antiretroviral therapy in HIV-infected patients in routine clinical practice. Antiviral Ther 2000; 5:243–248.

28. Paterson DL, Swindells S, Mohr J, et al. Adherence to protease inhibitor therapy and outcomes in patients with HIV infection. Ann Intern Med 2000; 133:21–30.

29. Murphy DA, Marelich WD, Hoffman D, et al. Predictors of antiretroviral adherence. AIDS CARE 2004; 16:471–484.

30. Lucas GM, Chaisson RE, Moore RD. Highly active antiretroviral therapy in a large urban clinic: risk factors for virologic failure and adverse drug reactions. Ann Intern Med 1999; 131:81–87.

31. Work Group on HIV/AIDS. Practice guidelines for the treatment of patients with HIV/AIDS. Am J Psychiatry 2000; 157:11.

32. Atkinson JH Jr, Grant I, Kennedy CJ, et al. Prevalence of psychiatric disorders among men infected with human immunodeficiency virus: a controlled study. Arch Gen Psychiatry 1988; 45:859–864.

33. Perkins DO, Stern RA, Golden RN, et al. Mood disorders in HIV infection: prevalence and risk factors in a non epicenter of the AIDS epidemic. Am J Psychiatry 1994; 151:233–236.

34. Treisman GJ, Fishman M, Schwartz J, et al. Mood disorders in HIV infection. Depress Anxiety 1998; 7:178–187.

35. Treisman GJ, Angelino AF. The psychiatry of AIDS. Baltimore, Maryland: Johns Hopkins University Press; 2004.

36. Lyketsos CG, Hanson AL, Fishman M, et al. Manic syndrome early and late in the course of HIV. Am J Psychiatry 1993; 150:326–327.

37. Wilk CM, Bolton P. Local perceptions of the mental health effects of the Uganda acquired immunodeficiency syndrome epidemic. J Nerv Ment Dis 2002; 190: 394–397.

38. Uldall KK, Berghuis JP. Delirium in AIDS patients: recognition and medication factors. AIDS Patient Care STDS 1997; 11:435–441.

39. Redington JJ, Tyler KL. Viral infections of the nervous system, 2002: update on diagnosis and treatment. Arch Neurol 2002; 59:712–718.

40. Uldall KK, Ryan R, Berghuis JP, et al. Association between delirium and death in AIDS patients. AIDS Patient Care STDS 2000; 14:95–100.

41. Navia BA, Jordan BD, Price RW. The AIDS dementia complex: I. clinical features. Ann Neurol 1986; 19:517–524.

42. McHugh PR, Slavney PR. The perspectives of psychiatry, second edition. Baltimore, MD: Johns Hopkins University Press; 1998.

43. Cohen J. Asia and Africa: on different trajectories? Science 2004; 304:1932–1938.

44. Patel V, Saraceno B, Kleinman A. Beyond evidence: the moral case for international mental health. Am J Psychiatry 2006; 163:1312–1315.

CHAPTER 26

Cardiovascular Complications of HIV Infection

James H. Stein

Introduction

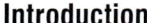

Since the first description of acquired immune deficiency syndrome (AIDS) in 1981, human immunodeficiency virus (HIV) infection and AIDS have reached worldwide epidemic proportions.[1] In the year 2000, over 36 million adults and children were estimated to be living with HIV infection or AIDS, and over 5 million individuals are expected to be newly infected with HIV.[2] Over 16 million individuals have died of AIDS, and each day more than 16 000 people are newly infected.[3] Sub-Saharan Africa has been most tragically affected by this epidemic and over 23 million individuals currently are living with HIV and AIDS.[2]

In the USA, there are an estimated 900 000 individuals living with HIV infection and approximately 40 000 new infections occurring each year.[4] With the advent of highly active antiretroviral therapy (HAART), there has been a dramatic decline in death from AIDS and a slowing of the progression from HIV to AIDS, so more people are living with AIDS in the USA than ever before.[4] Nevertheless, the use of HAART also has been associated with cardiac toxicity. This chapter will review cardiovascular complications in patients with HIV infection, specifically focusing on complications related to HIV infection, AIDS, and their treatment. The common cardiovascular complications observed in HIV-infected patients are outlined in Box 26.1.

Although there have been multiple reports of rare cardiovascular complications and isolated case reports, this chapter will focus on common manifestations.

Cardiomyopathy and Congestive Heart Failure

Dilated cardiomyopathy, myocarditis, and their complication of congestive heart failure are among the most common complications of HIV infection. Before the advent of HAART, the incidence of dilated cardiomyopathy among patients with HIV infection was 15.9/1000 cases.[5] The prevalence of cardiomyopathy among patients with HIV infection has been reported to be as high as 15%.[6] In a 4-year prospective echocardiographic study survey of 296 patients with HIV infection, dilated cardiomyopathy was associated with a CD4 cell count of <100 mm³ and reduced survival time. In that study, the median survival was 101 days (95% confidence intervals [CI], 42–146) for patients with dilated cardiomyopathy compared with 472 days (95% CI, 383–560) for HIV-positive patients without left ventricular systolic dysfunction.[6] Dilated cardiomyopathy tends to occur late in the course of HIV infection. At autopsy, myocarditis has been described in up to 30% of patients.[7] It is likely that myocarditis and dilated cardiomyopathy represent a continuum of disease progression.

The development of dilated cardiomyopathy is a powerful adverse prognostic indicator. In multivariate analysis, the hazard ratio for death in patients

---

Box 26.1

Common cardiovascular complications observed in patients with HIV infection

- Cardiomyopathy and congestive heart failure
- Pericardial disease
- Pulmonary hypertension
- Endocarditis
- Neoplasms
- Coronary artery disease

Box 26.2

Common causes of HIV-associated dilated cardiomyopathy[5]

- Myocarditis: HIV, Coxsackie virus Group B, Epstein–Barr virus, cytomegalovirus, echovirus, *Toxoplasma gondii*
- Autoimmunity
- Metabolic: Selenium, vitamin B_{12}, carnitine deficiency
- Endocrine: Thyroid hormone, growth hormone, adrenal insufficiency, hyperinsulinemia

---

with HIV-associated cardiomyopathy compared with idiopathic dilated cardiomyopathy, approaches 6.0.[8] Similarly, among children with vertically transmitted HIV infection in the Pediatric Pulmonary and Cardiovascular Complications of HIV Study, predictors of adverse outcomes included impaired left ventricular function, increased left ventricular thickness, heart rate, and blood pressure.[9]

The pathogenesis of dilated cardiomyopathy is an area of intense study (Box 26.2). HIV may damage cardiac myocytes by a direct cytolytic effect or through an 'innocent bystander' reaction.[10] Infection of myocardial cells by HIV-1 has been demonstrated in a patchy distribution.[11] The mechanism by which HIV infection enters cardiac myocytes is not clear; however, it has been hypothesized that 'reservoir' cells such as dendritic cells may mediate the interaction between HIV-1 and myocytes and may activate cytokines that contribute to tissue damage.[8] Indeed, reservoir cells also are present in the cerebral cortex and may lead to chronic cytokine release and tissue destruction, accounting for the increased rate of death due to congestive heart failure in patients with HIV-associated encephalopathy.[12,13] Although HIV has been detected in cardiac tissue, it remains unclear if HIV or a secondary viral infection such as cytomegalovirus, Group B Coxsackie virus, Epstein–Barr virus, or adenovirus mediate the high incidence of myocarditis among HIV-infected patients.

It appears that immunologic mechanisms contribute to HIV-associated dilated cardiomyopathy. Uncontrolled hypergammaglobulinemia from T-helper cell dysfunction and increased concentrations of circulating immune complex have been associated with cardiac inflammation.[7] HIV protein transcription also may alter the surface of cardiac myocytes with induction of cell-surface immunogenetic proteins that may lead to cardiac autoantibodies that could trigger cardiac destruction. Cardiac specific

autoantibodies have been demonstrated in up to 30% of patients with HIV-associated cardiomyopathy.[14,15]

Nutritional abnormalities also may play a role in some patients, especially late in HIV infection. Deficiencies of selenium, vitamin B_{12}, and carnitine have been reported and associated with left ventricular dysfunction.[5,16] Other metabolic and endocrine abnormalities that have been associated with cardiac dysfunction include hypothyroidism, growth hormone deficiency, hypoadrenalism, and hyperinsulinism.[7,17]

Several drugs used by patients with HIV infection have been associated with dilated cardiomyopathy. The nucleoside reverse transcriptase inhibitor zidovudine has been associated with dilated cardiomyopathy both in children and adults.[18,19] Cardiac mitochondrial destruction and inhibition of mitochondrial DNA replication also has been described in transgenic mice.[20] This association was not observed, however, in the Pediatric Pulmonary and Cardiovascular Complications of HIV study, in which infants with vertically transmitted HIV infection who were followed from birth to age 5 years with serial echocardiograms did not demonstrate an association between left ventricular dysfunction and exposure to zidovudine. It appears that neither didanosine nor zalcitabine prevent or cause dilated cardiomyopathy.[5]

Drugs that are used to treat complications of HIV infection also have been associated with dilated cardiomyopathy. These medications include the antifungal agent amphotericin B, which in addition to being associated with cardiomyopathy may cause hypertension and bradycardia. Doxorubicin, which is used to treat Kaposi's sarcoma, is a well-known cause of cardiomyopathy. Foscarnet treatment of cytomegalovirus infection may cause cardiomyopathy as well. Erythropoietin-α commonly causes hypertension. Interferon-α, an immunomodulator that is used as an antineoplastic and antiviral agent, can also cause cardiomyopathy; however, arrhythmia and myocardial ischemia are more common.[7] Finally, as survival with HIV infection increases and risk factors for atherosclerosis develop due to aging and the use of HAART, myocardial infarction and coronary atherosclerosis are increasingly common phenomena that may contribute to left ventricular systolic dysfunction, as discussed below. Although left ventricular dysfunction is a harbinger of a poor outcome related to AIDS patients, patients may die of progressive left ventricular dysfunction or arrhythmias. Several medications used by HIV-infected patients predispose to arrhythmias, including those mentioned above (amphotericin B, interferon-α) and other agents such as ganciclovir, which can cause ventricular tachycardia. Agents that prolong the QT interval and therefore predispose to torsades de pointes include pentamidine, pyrimethamine, and trimethaprim-sulfamethoxazole.[7]

Pericardial Disease

Pericardial effusion is one of the most common clinically relevant cardiac complications in patients with HIV infection. Pericardial effusion can have a wide range of manifestations including the asymptomatic effusion incidentally detected by echocardiography or routine chest imaging, cardiac tamponade, acute or chronic pericarditis, and uncommonly, constrictive pericardial disease. A review of 15 autopsy and echocardiographic studies that included 1139 HIV-infected patients revealed that approximately 21% had a pericardial effusion, most of which were without an identifiable cause and were asymptomatic.[21] In another study, a 9% annual incidence of cardiac tamponade in AIDS patients with pericardial effusion was reported.[22] In a prospective study of 231 male subjects, serial echocardiograms performed every 3–6 months revealed an approximately 11% annual incidence of pericardial effusion.[22] Pericardial effusions resolved spontaneously in approximately 42% of patients.[22] Although most of the effusions were small and asymptomatic, the survival of AIDS patients with pericardial effusion was shorter (36% at 6 months) than individuals without effusions (93% at 6 months, relative risk 2.2, 95% CI, 1.2–4, $P = 0.01$).[22]

Most pericardial effusions in patients with HIV infection are idiopathic. Culture of pericardial fluid usually is unrevealing; however, opportunistic infections and neoplasms can be diagnosed (Box 26.3).

Box 26.3

Common causes of HIV-associated pericardial effusion

- Idiopathic: Capillary leak
- Malignant: Kaposi's sarcoma, lymphoma
- Infectious: Bacterial – *Staphylococcus*, *Streptococcus*, *Proteus*, *Nocardia*, *Pseudomonas*, *Klebsiella*, *Enterococcus*, *Listeria*, *Mycobacteria*
- Viral: HIV, herpes simplex virus, cytomegalovirus
- Fungal/Protozoan: *Cryptococcus*, *Histoplasma*, *Toxoplasma*
- Hypothyroidism

Increased production of cytokines such as interleukin-2 and a tumor necrosis factor in patients with end-stage HIV infection has been associated with capillary leak syndrome, which also can be seen in patients with AIDS-wasting and malnutrition. Indeed, asymptomatic pericardial effusion may be due to advanced immune dysfunction despite a relatively preserved CD4 count.[22] Pericardial effusions due to Kaposi's sarcoma and malignant lymphomas may occur; however, infectious causes are more common. In published cases of cardiac tamponade in patients with HIV infection, over one-quarter were due to mycobacterium tuberculosis, 17 were purulent and related to the bacteria in Box 26.3, and 8% were due to mycobacterium intracellulare. Lymphoma and Kaposi's sarcoma were associated with approximately 5% of the effusions. Cytomegalovirus was associated with approximately 3% of the cases.[21,22]

Pulmonary Hypertension

The incidence of HIV-associated pulmonary hypertension is approximately 1 in 200 compared with 1 in 200 000 in the general population.[23] Patients with HIV-associated pulmonary hypertension appear to progress more rapidly and to have a worse 1-year survival than individuals without HIV infection who develop primary pulmonary hypertension.[23,24] HIV infection is regarded as a risk factor for the development of pulmonary hypertension. Pulmonary hypertension in patients with HIV does not appear to be associated with the CD4 cell count or a history of pulmonary infection. Plexogenic lesions have been found in the majority of patients with HIV-associated pulmonary hypertension, which may represent an arteriopathy directly related to

HIV infection or a 'bystander' effect. Alveolar macrophages frequently are affected with HIV and release tissue necrosis factor-alpha, super-oxide anions and proteolytic enzymes which are directly toxic, chemotactic factors that further induce inflammatory cell infiltration. They also enhance leukocyte adherence to the endothelium and promote endothelial proliferation.[5,7] An HIV-envelope glycoprotein, Gp-120, stimulates production of endothelin-1, an important vasoconstrictor, and TNF-α.[23] In addition to primary pulmonary hypertension, secondary causes due to talc exposure in injection drug users, chronic liver disease, interstitial lung disease, and coagulopathies also may contribute to HIV-associated pulmonary hypertension. Right ventricular hypertrophy and failure are uncommon, but are known sequelae of pulmonary hypertension.

Endocarditis

In patients with HIV infection, the most common endocardial lesion is non-bacterial thrombotic endocarditis ('marantic' endocarditis).[7,25] Non-bacterial thrombotic endocarditis is characterized by the presence of fibrin-rich collections of platelets and erythrocytes that adhere to valves, forming a fibrin mesh with relatively little inflammatory reaction. It has been identified in 3–5% of patients with HIV infection and is most common in patients with HIV wasting or end-stage AIDS.[7,25] Systemic embolism is common, but most episodes are clinically silent. The diagnosis of non-bacterial thrombotic endocarditis is usually made post mortem.

Infective endocarditis occurs at a similar rate among patients with HIV infection, as in other groups of individuals at increased risk such as intravenous drug users.[5] Estimates of the prevalence of endocarditis range from 6.3% to 34% of HIV-infected patients who use intravenous drugs.[5] Intravenous drug users frequently have right-sided valvular infections due to *Staphylococcus aureus*, *Streptococcus pneumonia*, and *Streptococcus viridans*.[5,26] Other causes include *Hemophilus influenza*, *Candida albicans*, *Aspergillus fumigatus*, and *Cryptococcus neoformans*.[5] Although presentations of infectious endocarditis usually are similar, survival with endocarditis is worse in individuals with HIV infection.

Neoplasms

The most common cardiac neoplasms in HIV-infected patients are non-Hodgkin's lymphoma and Kaposi's sarcoma. Although malignant lymphomas of the heart are rare, in the pre-HAART era lymphomas were identified in 5–10% of patients with HIV infection, which is a 60–100 times higher prevalence than expected in the general population.[7,27] HIV-associated lymphomas are typically derived from B-lymphocytes and are of high grade. Metastatic lymphomas of the heart are more common than primary cardiac lymphomas, which tend to be rare. Most patients have disseminated disease at the time of their initial presentation, although some patients may have primary lymphomas involving only the pericardium.[27] In general, AIDS-associated lymphomas are found in patients with low CD4 cell counts; however, non-Hodgkin's lymphoma may occur in patients with less advanced immune suppression. The prognosis of patients with HIV-associated cardiac non-Hodgkin's lymphoma is poor, although remission has been observed in patients treated with combination chemotherapy.

Autopsy studies estimated the prevalence of Kaposi's sarcoma involving the heart at rates of 12–28%.[5] Most of the autopsies were performed in individuals who are homosexual or bisexual and demonstrated that cardiac involvement usually was due to disseminated Kaposi's sarcoma with metastases involving the pericardium.[28,29] Metastases to sub-epicardial adipose tissue adjacent to major coronary arteries has been described.[28,29] Most findings related to Kaposi's sarcomas are at autopsy; however, bloody pericardial effusions may be discovered by imaging or pericardiocentesis in patients with advanced disease.

Coronary Artery Disease

With the advent of HAART, survival with HIV infection has improved dramatically and there is increasing epidemiological overlap between patients with HIV infection and those at risk for coronary artery disease. Overlapping risk factors include increasing age, a high prevalence of tobacco use, and a disproportionate increase in the number of individuals of African or Hispanic descent.[30] Risk factors for coronary artery disease, including hypertension, hyperlipidemia, hyperglycemia, and central obesity develop in the majority of patients receiving HAART.[30]

It is important to recognize that before HAART, coronary artery disease had been identified in young adults postmortem and was felt to be associated with HIV-1 infection, cytomegalovirus, or other inflammatory disorders such as hypersensitivity vasculitis,

Kawasaki disease, Takayasu's arteritis, and polyarteritis nodosa.[5,31,32] Before HAART, the prevalence of hypertension in patients with HIV infection was estimated to be as high as 25%.[33] An increased prevalence of hypertension also has been described in the HAART era and is associated with lipodystrophy and HAART-related metabolic syndrome.[34]

In the absence of HAART, a dyslipidemia characterized by hypocholesterolemia with low levels of low-density lipoprotein cholesterol, low levels of high-density lipoprotein cholesterol, and hypertriglyceridemia was identified.[35,36] The hypertriglyceridemia in patients with AIDS is associated with increased concentrations of very low-density lipoproteins, likely due to delayed clearance resulting in the presence of small, dense LDL particles.[35-37] Hypertriglyceridemia is prominent as AIDS progresses and is a marker of increasing viral load.[35] With the advent of HAART and specifically in the presence of HIV protease inhibitors, hyperlipidemia has become more common and more severe.[38-41] In the Swiss HIV cohort, hypercholesterolemia and hypertriglyceridemia were 1.7- to 2.3-fold more likely in individuals on HAART that contained a protease inhibitor.[42] Severe hypercholesterolemia (>240 mg/dL) and hypertriglyceridemia (>500 mg/dL) were identified, respectively in >60% and >70% of subjects receiving HIV protease inhibitors, with incident rate ratios of 2.8 and 6.1 attributed to use of these medications.[41] The dyslipidemia associated with HIV protease inhibitors is characterized by an increase in very low-density lipoproteins and intermediate-density lipoproteins as well as the presence of small LDL particles.[43,44] Several mechanisms by which HAART could lead to dyslipidemia have been proposed (Box 26.4).[45]

Several studies have shown increased prevalence of subclinical atherosclerosis in patients receiving HAART.[30] With one exception, several studies also have demonstrated endothelial dysfunction in individuals receiving HAART.[30,44] Although it remains controversial as to whether or not HAART, or a component of HAART (such as protease inhibitors) directly causes cardiovascular disease, it is clear that their associated risk factors are major contributors.[30,46] To date, two prospective studies[47,48] have associated use of HAART with cardiovascular events and four of five retrospective studies have had similar findings, albeit with study-specific limitations.[30,49-53]

The Infectious Disease Society of America and the Adult AIDS Clinical Trials Group have provided guidelines for the evaluation and management of dyslipidemia in HIV-infected adults receiving anti-

---

Box 26.4

Possible mechanisms for protease inhibitor-associated dyslipidemia[45]

Impaired lipoprotein clearance
- Inhibition of LDL receptor-related protein with down-regulation of the LDL receptor
- Abnormal regulation of apo C-III[a]
  - Inhibition of lipoprotein lipase
  - Impaired lipoprotein-cell surface interactions
  - Impaired cellular retinoic acid binding protein-1

Increased hepatic cholesterol and triglyceride synthesis
- Increased hepatocyte accumulation of sterol regulatory element binding protein-1c[a]
  - Decreased proteasome activity
  - Improved nutritional status
  - Impaired cellular retinoic acid binding protein-1
- Increased hepatic substrate delivery[a]

[a]May be exacerbated by insulin resistance.
LDL, low-density lipoprotein.

---

retroviral therapy.[54] These guidelines draw heavily upon the National Cholesterol Education Program Adult Treatment Panel III guidelines.[54] A subsequent implications paper should be considered in conjunction with them.[55] These topics have been reviewed extensively elsewhere[30] and a summary of these guidelines is provided in Figure 26.1.

Conclusion

HIV infection and AIDS have reached global epidemic proportions. Although HAART is very effective at improving survival with HIV infection, it is not widely available in some parts of the world that have been greatly affected by AIDS. In patients who are unable to receive HAART, end-stage complications of AIDS that affect the heart, including dilated cardiomyopathy, myocarditis, pericardial effusion, pulmonary hypertension, endocarditis, and involvement of the heart with neoplasms are not uncommon. In parts of the world where HAART is used frequently, complications relating to aging and use of HAART such as coronary artery disease and its risk factors such as diabetes mellitus, hyperlipidemia, hypertension, and obesity are prevalent, leading to overlapping epidemiology and disease manifestations.

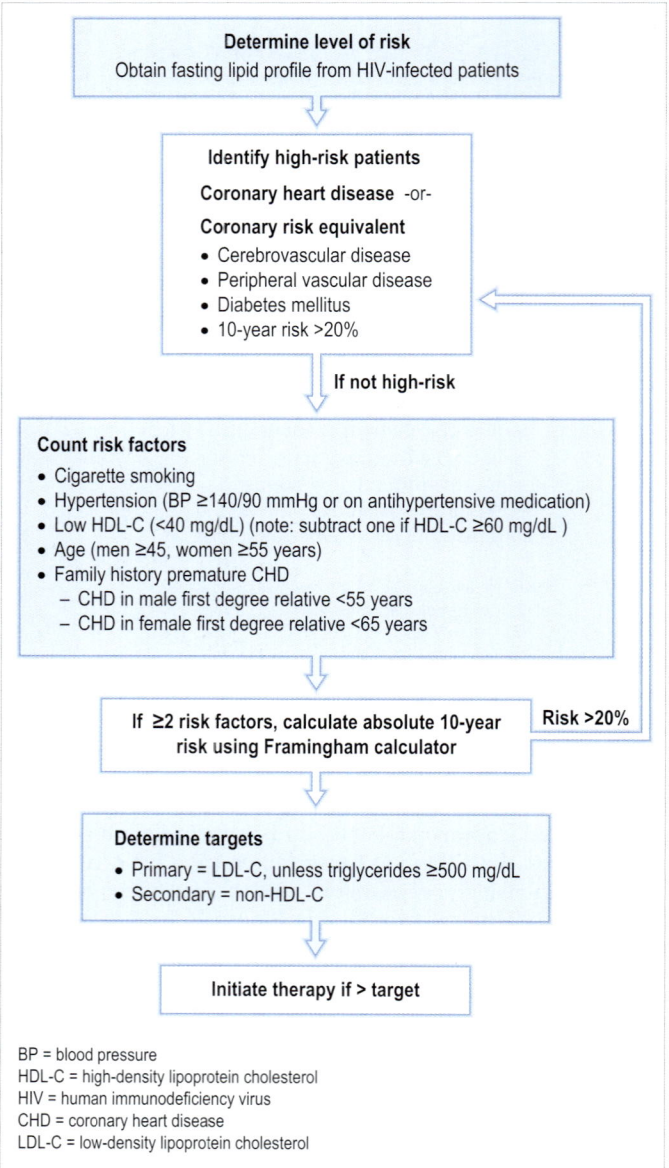

Figure 26.1 Summary of the Infectious Disease Society of America/Adult AIDS Clinical Trials Group Guidelines for evaluation and management of dyslipidemia.[30,54]

References

1. Sepkowitz KA. AIDS – the first 20 years. N Engl J Med 2001; 344:1764–1772.
2. CDC. HIV/AIDS Surveillance Report. Centers for Disease Control and Prevention, 2000; 12:No 1.
3. National Center for HIV, STD and TB Prevention. The global AIDS program: philosophy. Updated 21 September 2004. Online. Available: www.cdc.gov/nchstp/od/gap/philosophy.htm (accessed 16 November 2004).
4. CDC. HIV/AIDS update: A glance at the HIV epidemic. Online. Available: www.cdc.gov/nchstp/od/new/At-a-Glance.pdf (accessed 16 November 2004).
5. Barbaro G. Cardiovascular manifestations of HIV infection. Circulation 2002; 106:1420–1425.
6. Currie PF, Jacob AJ, Foreman AR, et al. Heart muscle disease related to HIV infection: prognostic implications. Br Med J 1994; 309:1605–1607.
7. Rerkpattanapipat P, Wongpraparut N, Jacobs LE, et al. Cardiac manifestations of acquired immunodeficiency syndrome. Arch Intern Med 2000; 160:602–608.
8. Barbaro G, Di Lorenzo G, Soldini M, et al. Intensity of myocardial expression of inducible nitric oxide synthase influences the clinical course of human immunodeficiency virus-associated cardiomyopathy. Gruppo Italiano per lo Studio Cardiologico dei pazienti affetti da AIDS (GISCA). Circulation 1999; 100:933–939.

9. Lipshultz SE, Easley KA, Orav EJ, et al. Left ventricular structure and function in children infected with human immunodeficiency virus: the prospective P2C2 HIV Multicenter Study. Pediatric Pulmonary and Cardiac Complications of Vertically Transmitted HIV Infection (P2C2 HIV) Study Group. Circulation 1998; 97:1246–1256.

10. Barbaro G, Di Lorenzo G, Grisorio B, et al. Incidence of dilated cardiomyopathy and detection of HIV in myocardial cells of HIV-positive patients. Gruppo Italiano per lo Studio Cardiologico dei pazienti affetti da AIDS. N Engl J Med 1998; 339:1093–1099.

11. Barbaro G, Di Lorenzo G, Grisorio B, et al. Cardiac involvement in the acquired immunodeficiency syndrome: a multicenter clinical-pathological study. Gruppo Italiano per lo Studio Cardiologico dei pazienti affetti da AIDS Investigators. AIDS Res Hum Retroviruses 1998; 14:1071–1077.

12. Cooper ER, Hanson C, Diaz C, et al. Encephalopathy and progression of human immunodeficiency virus disease in a cohort of children with perinatally acquired human immunodeficiency virus infection. Woman and Infants Transmission Study Group. J Pediatr 1998; 132:808–812.

13. Barbaro G, Di Lorenzo G, Soldini M, et al. Clinical course of cardiomyopathy in HIV-infected patients with or without encephalopathy related to the myocardial expression of tumour necrosis factor-alpha and nitric oxide synthase. AIDS 2000; 14:827–838.

14. Yunis NA, Stone VE. Cardiac manifestations of HIV/AIDS: a review of disease spectrum and clinical management. J Acquir Immune Defic Syndr Hum Retrovirol 1998; 18:145–154.

15. Currie PF, Goldman JH, Caforio AL, et al. Cardiac autoimmunity in HIV related heart muscle disease. Heart 1998; 79:599–604.

16. Jacob AJ, Sutherland GR, Bird AG, et al. Myocardial dysfunction in patients infected with HIV: prevalence and risk factors. Er Heart J 1992; 68:549–553.

17. Barbaro G. Pathogenesis of HIV-associated heart disease. AIDS 2003; 17(Suppl):12–20.

18. Herskowitz A, Willoughby SB, Baughman KL, et al. Cardiomyopathy associated with antiretroviral therapy in patients with HIV infection: a report of six cases. Ann Intern Med 1992; 116:311–313.

19. Domanski MJ, Sloas MM, Follmann DA, et al. Effect of zidovudine and didanosine treatment on heart function in children infected with human immunodeficiency virus. J Pediatr 1995. 127:137–146.

20. Lewis W, Grupp IL, Grupp G, et al. Cardiac dysfunction occurs in the HIV-1 transgenic mouse treated with zidovudine. Lab Invest 2000; 80:187–197.

21. Estok L, Wallach F. Cardiac tamponade in a patient with AIDS: a review of pericardial disease in patients with HIV infection. Mt Sinai J Med 1998; 65:33–39.

22. Heidenreich PA, Eisenberg MJ, Kee LL, et al. Pericardial effusion in AIDS. Incidence and survival. Circulation 1995; 92:3229–3234.

23. Mesa RA, Edell ES, Dunn WF, et al. Human immunodeficiency virus infection and pulmonary hypertension: two new cases and a review of 86 reported cases. Mayo Clin Proc 1998; 73:37–45.

24. Petitpretz P, Brenot F, Azarian R, et al. Pulmonary hypertension in patients with human immunodeficiency virus infection. Comparison with primary pulmonary hypertension. Circulation 1994; 89:2722–2727.

25. Kaul S, Fishbein MC, Siegel RJ. Cardiac manifestations of acquired immune deficiency syndrome: a 1991 update. Am Heart J 1991; 122:535–544.

26. Nahass RG, Weinstein MP, Bartels J, et al. Infective endocarditis in intravenous drug users: a comparison of human immunodeficiency virus type 1-negative and -positive patients. J Infect Dis 1990; 162:967–970.

27. Aboulafia DM, Bush R, Picozzi VJ. Cardiac tamponade due to primary pericardial lymphoma in a patient with AIDS. Chest 1994; 106:1295–1299.

28. Lewis W. AIDS: cardiac findings from 115 autopsies. Prog Cardiovasc Dis 1989; 32:207–215.

29. Silver MA, Macher AM, Reichert CM, et al. Cardiac involvement by Kaposi's sarcoma in acquired immune deficiency syndrome (AIDS). Am J Cardiol 1984; 53: 983–985.

30. Stein JH. Managing cardiovascular risk in patients with HIV infection. J Acquir Immun Defic Syndr 2005; 38:115–123.

31. Tabib A, Greenland T, Mercier I, et al. Coronary lesions in young HIV-positive subjects at necropsy. Lancet 1992; 340:730.

32. Constans J, Marchand JM, Conri C, et al. Asymptomatic atherosclerosis in HIV-positive patients: A case-control ultrasound study. Ann Med 1995; 27:683–685.

33. Aoun S, Ramos E. Hypertension in the HIV-infected patient. Curr Hypertens Rep 2000; 2:478–481.

34. Sattler FR, Qian D, Louie S, et al. Elevated blood pressure in subjects with lipodystrophy. AIDS 2001; 15:2001–2010.

35. Grunfeld C, Pang M, Doerrler W, et al. Lipids, lipoproteins, triglyceride clearance, and cytokines in human immunodeficiency virus infection and the acquired immunodeficiency syndrome. J Clin Endocrinol Metab 1992; 74:1045–1052.

36. Feingold KR, Krauss RM, Pang M, et al. The hypertriglyceridemia of acquired immunodeficiency syndrome is associated with an increased prevalence of low density lipoprotein subclass pattern B. J Clin Endocrinol Metab 1993; 76:1423–1427.

37. Hellerstein MK, Grunfeld C, Wu K, et al. Increased de novo hepatic lipogenesis in human immunodeficiency virus infection. J Clin Endocrinol Metab 1993; 76: 559–565.

38. Carr A, Samaras K, Burton S, et al. A syndrome of peripheral lipodystrophy, hyperlipidaemia and insulin resistance in patients receiving HIV protease inhibitors. AIDS 1998; 12:51–58.

39. Dube MP, Sattler FR. Metabolic complications of antiretroviral therapies. AIDS Clin Care 1998; 10:41–44.

40. Periard D, Telenti A, Sudre P, et al. Atherogenic dyslipidemia in HIV-infected individuals treated with protease inhibitors. Swiss HIV Cohort Study Circ 1999; 100:700–705.

41. Tsiodras S, Mantzoros C, Hammer S, et al. Effects of protease inhibitors on hyperglycemia, hyperlipidemia, and lipodystrophy: a 5-year cohort study. Arch Intern Med 2000; 160:2050–2056.

42. Fellay J, Boubaker K, Ledergerber B, et al. Prevalence of adverse events associated with potent antiretroviral treatment: Swiss HIV Cohort Study. Lancet 2001; 358:1322–1327.

43. Purnell JQ, Zambon A, Knopp RH, et al. Effect of ritonavir on lipids and post-heparin lipase activities in normal subjects. AIDS 2000; 14:51–57.

44. Stein JH, Klein MA, Bellehumeur JL, et al. Use of human immunodeficiency virus-1 protease inhibitors is associated with atherogenic lipoprotein changes and endothelial dysfunction. Circulation 2001; 104:257–262.

45. Stein JH. Dyslipidemia in the era of HIV protease inhibitors. Prog Cardiovasc Dis 2003; 45:293–304.

46. Depairon M, Chessex S, Sudre P, et al. Premature atherosclerosis in HIV-infected individuals–focus on protease inhibitor therapy. AIDS 2001; 15:329–334.

47. Friis-Moller N, Weber R, Reiss P, et al. Cardiovascular disease risk factors in HIV patients–association with antiretroviral therapy. Results from the DAD study. AIDS 2003; 17:1179–1193.

48. Holmberg SD, Moorman AC, Williamson JM, et al. Protease inhibitors and cardiovascular outcomes in patients with HIV-1. Lancet 2002; 360:1747–1748.

49. Klein D, Hurley LB, Quesenberry JC, et al. Do protease inhibitors increase the risk for coronary heart disease in patients with HIV-1 infection? J Acquir Immune Defic Syndr 2002; 30:471–477.

50. Mary-Krause M, Cotte L, Simon A, et al. Increased risk of myocardial infarction with duration of protease inhibitor therapy in HIV-infected men. AIDS 2003; 17:2479–2486.

51. Currier JS, Taylor A, Boyd F, et al. Coronary heart disease in HIV-infected individuals. J Acquir Immune Defic Syndr 2003; 33:506–512.

52. Bozzette SA, Ake CF, Tam HK, et al. Cardiovascular and cerebrovascular events in patients treated for human immunodeficiency virus infection. N Engl J Med 2003; 348:702–710.

53. Rickerts V, Brodt H, Staszewski S, et al. Incidence of myocardial infarctions in HIV-infected patients between 1983 and 1998: the Frankfurt HIV-cohort study. Eur J Med Res 2000; 5:329–333.

54. Dube MP, Stein JH, Aberg JA, et al. Guidelines for the evaluation and management of dyslipidemia in human immunodeficiency virus (HIV)-infected adults receiving antiretroviral therapy: recommendations of the HIV Medical Association of the Infectious Disease Society of America and the Adult AIDS Clinical Trials Group. Clin Infect Dis 2003; 37:613–627.

55. Grundy SM, Cleeman JI, Merz CN, et al. Implications of recent clinical trials for the National Cholesterol Education Program Adult Treatment Panel III guidelines. Circulation 2004; 110:227–239.

CHAPTER 27

Endocrine Complications of HIV Infection

Melissa E. Weinberg

Joan C. Lo

Carl Grunfeld

Morris Schambelan

Introduction

A wide spectrum of endocrine complications is associated with HIV infection and AIDS. Although these disorders may reflect changes induced by HIV itself, more often they are a consequence of systemic illness, opportunistic infections, neoplasm, body composition changes, and/or HIV-related therapies. The extensive introduction of highly active antiretroviral therapy (HAART) in developed nations has clearly altered the endocrinologic manifestations of HIV. As the incidence of glandular infiltration by opportunistic infections (OIs) and neoplasm declines, increased attention has been directed toward the metabolic complications of therapy. Studies performed in the pre-HAART era remain relevant, however, to the management of patients in many parts of the world where there is limited access to HIV care and to those who become resistant to antiretroviral therapy. A greater understanding of these disorders, especially as the HIV epidemic evolves, is crucial to the ongoing care of HIV-infected patients. This chapter describes the endocrine complications of HIV disease and provides a general approach to management, primarily referencing high-quality review articles, rather than the primary references, due to space limitations.

The Pituitary

Pituitary Pathology

Systematic post mortem examination of the pituitary gland in patients with AIDS, performed before the introduction of HAART, found direct infectious involvement in 12% of adenohypophyses by either cytomegalovirus (CMV) or *Pneumocystis carinii,* rarely involving the neurohypophyses.[1] Since pituitary involvement was always accompanied by generalized and/or cerebral infection, this study may not reflect the situation of patients who do not yet have significant immunosuppression or who are effectively treated with HAART. Additional patients have presented with panhypopituitarism resulting from cerebral toxoplasmosis, and central diabetes insipidus has been reported in an AIDS patient with herpetic meningoencephalitis. Neoplastic infiltration of the pituitary gland is very rare, although one case of pituitary lymphoma in a patient with AIDS has been reported.[2] Hypopituitarism, independent of cause, is treated with physiologic hormone replacement and requires monitoring of hormonal status.

Alterations in Pituitary Function

Studies employing gonadotropin- or thyrotropin-releasing hormones (i.e. GnRH and TRH) have consistently found that the functional reserve of the anterior pituitary is normal. Prolactin levels, in the absence of medication effect, are usually normal and respond to TRH stimulation appropriately.[2] Posterior pituitary function, however, may be abnormal, as an increased incidence of hyponatremia and the syndrome of inappropriate ADH secretion was reported in hospitalized AIDS patients. A primary pituitary disorder cannot be concluded from this study, however, because there were other factors influencing the development of hyponatremia including pulmonary infection (most notably, *Pneumocystis carinii* pneumonia) and treatment with medications (e.g. trimethoprim) that confounded the issue.[3]

Somatotropic Axis

HIV infection *per se* does not appear to affect the somatotropic axis, based on frequent sampling studies among men with asymptomatic HIV infection, clinically stable AIDS, and healthy controls.[4] Growth hormone (GH) and insulin-like growth factor-1 (IGF-1) secretion and action, however, are influenced by nutritional status and body composition; therefore, distinct abnormalities have been observed in patients with AIDS wasting and the HIV-associated lipodystrophy syndrome. AIDS wasting may resemble an acquired GH-resistant state, explaining the decreased levels of IGF-1 and IGF-1 binding protein-3 that have been observed in the setting of increased GH. In contrast, patients with HIV-associated lipodystrophy demonstrate an inverse correlation between GH levels and visceral obesity, consistent with the reduced GH levels found in generalized obesity.[5]

Effects of Antiretroviral Therapy

GH secretion is affected by body composition changes, which may be associated with HAART, but the specific effects of individual agents on the somatotropic axis have not been investigated. Galactorrhea and marked hyperprolactinemia, however, were reported in a series of four patients following initiation of protease inhibitors (PIs) for HAART or post-HIV exposure prophylaxis.[6] Although three of these patients had received medications that may increase serum prolactin levels (metoclopramide or fluoxetine), symptoms resolved only after the protease inhibitors were discontinued. The authors postulated that PIs might either directly cause hyperprolactinemia or, by inhibiting cytochrome P450, enhance the dopamine antagonist effect of other drugs.

The Thyroid

Thyroid Pathology

Clinically significant OIs of the thyroid occur very rarely in patients with AIDS, and the advent of HAART has further reduced the frequency. In a Brazilian autopsy study, two-thirds of thyroids examined demonstrated pathologic changes, even though none of the patients had pre-mortem clinical manifestations of thyroid disease. Indeed, more than one opportunistic agent was found in the majority of specimens.[7] Reported pathogens infecting the thyroid include *Pneumocystis carinii*, cytomegalovirus, *Cryptococcus neoformans*, *Aspergillus fumigatus*, *Rhodococcus equi*, *Haemophilus influenzae*, *Microsporidia*, *Histoplasma capsulatum*, *Paracoccidioides brasiliensis*, *Mycobacterium avium intracellulare* and *Mycobacterium tuberculosis*. *Pneumocystis carinii* thyroiditis is the most common OI of the thyroid, occurring primarily among patients receiving aerosolized pentamidine for *Pneumocystis carinii* pneumonia prophylaxis.[8] Clinical manifestations are variable, and functional testing may reveal transient hyperthyroidism (that may not require treatment) or hypothyroidism.

Neoplastic infiltration of the thyroid is also uncommon in patients with AIDS, though there have been a few cases of Kaposi's sarcoma involving the thyroid gland in patients with pre-existing cutaneous lesions. Primary malignancy, as well as metastatic disease, may also develop in the setting of HIV infection, but only two cases of thyroid lymphoma and one case of thyroid carcinoma have been reported. In addition to invasion of the thyroid gland by infection or neoplasm, other frequent pathologic changes include nonspecific focal chronic inflammation, colloid goiter, and lipomatosis.[7]

Alterations in Thyroid Function

Although asymptomatic HIV patients with stable body weight are usually clinically euthyroid, abnormal thyroid homeostasis is often present in patients with AIDS. In non-thyroidal illness (NTI), inhibition of peripheral T4 to T3 conversion and reduced reverse T3 (rT3) clearance results in low T3 and elevated rT3, usually accompanied by a normal thyroid-stimulating hormone (TSH). The characteristic changes of NTI differ from those observed in AIDS patients who often have higher T3 levels and lower rT3 levels than would generally be expected. The increased thyroid hormone-binding globulin (TBG) levels associated with HIV infection do not explain these findings.[9] The abnormalities of thyroid testing in HIV-infected individuals compared with seronegative patients with NTI are presented in Table 27.1. The maintenance of normal T3 levels among AIDS patients has led to concern that the protective effects that reduction of T3 provides in NTI, such as lowering metabolic rate, ameliorating weight loss, and decreasing protein catabolism, may be compromised. Lower T3 levels are observed, however, during secondary infection and anorexia. Other patients with asymptomatic HIV infection have been reported to demonstrate characteristics of compensated hypothyroidism including mildly elevated 24-h TSH profiles (within the normal range), lower free T4 levels, and a greater TSH response to TRH infusion.[10] These alterations in thyroid hormone physiology may be adaptive to chronic illness, decreased energy intake, or the increased metabolic demands of HIV infection.

Effects of Antiretroviral and other Therapies

Medications such as rifampin, ketoconazole, and ritonavir may alter thyroid function by accelerating the metabolic clearance of thyroid hormone and can precipitate hypothyroidism in patients with marginal thyroid reserve; thus, higher doses of

Table 27.1 Alterations in thyroid function in HIV infection

	Seronegative NTI	HIV-infected, stable	HIV-infected, sick
T3	↓↓	Normal	?↓
RT3	↑	↓	↓ or Normal
TBG	↑	↑	↑↑
T4	Normal or ↓	Normal	Normal
TSH	Normal, may be ↑ curing recovery	Normal	Normal

NTI, non-thyroidal illness. From Sellmeyer and Grunfeld.[2]

thyroxine may be necessary in patients receiving concomitant replacement therapy.[8]

Among patients with hepatitis C infection, treatment with interferon-α (INF-α) has been associated with the development of autoimmune thyroid diseases (AITD) such as Grave's disease (GD) and Hashimoto's thyroiditis, as well as subacute or destructive thyroiditis. Since individuals with either pre-existing or recently detected thyroid autoantibodies (i.e. thyroid peroxidase antibody [TPOAb] and thyroglobulin antibody [TgAb]) are at higher risk for INF-α-induced AITD, practitioners should test TSH, free T4, and thyroid antibodies before initiation of INF-α treatment, followed by measurement of TSH every 8–12 weeks during treatment.[11] IFN-α treatment should be delayed until correction of pre-existing thyroid dysfunction. Even if thyroid dysfunction develops during treatment, IFN-α need not be discontinued unless destructive thyroiditis with severe symptoms refractory to β-blockers or GD requiring high doses of anti-thyroidal medications develops. Although most patients who develop thyroid dysfunction as a result of treatment with INF-a normalize after it is discontinued, a minority of patients continue to require treatment.[11]

Since the introduction of HAART, AITD has been reported as a late complication of immune reconstitution, typically presenting as GD 1–2 years after initiation of therapy.[12] The onset of AITD is temporally consistent with thymic production of naïve CD4+ cells (the 'late' phase of T-cell repopulation), and immune dysregulation in those with genetic predisposition may result in thyroid-specific autoimmunity. AITD manifesting as Hashimoto's thyroiditis could presumably also result from this phenomenon, perhaps explaining the increased prevalence of subclinical hypothyroidism among patients receiving HAART in some series.[13] Patients treated with interleukin-2 (IL-2), a potential new therapy for HIV infection, are also susceptible to both thyroiditis and GD, presumably as a result of a similar immunopathogenesis.[14] Other authors have found that IL-2 stimulates the pituitary-thyroid axis, leading to elevations in free T4 that are in the hyperthyroid range.

Treatment Considerations

The subtle alterations in thyroid function found in HIV-infected individuals must be interpreted in their clinical context. In patients with clinically significant and biochemically confirmed hypothyroidism, low doses of replacement therapy (levothyroxine

25–50 μg daily) should be prescribed initially, with gradual titration and monitoring of TSH levels to avoid exacerbation of cachexia in affected patients. The clinical management for patients with hyperthyroidism and co-existing HIV infection is similar to that for immunocompetent individuals, except that a tender or nodular thyroid gland in a patient with advanced HIV disease should prompt further investigation for an opportunistic infection or malignancy of the thyroid. Diagnostic evaluation includes a fine needle aspiration (FNA) biopsy of the affected gland, and *Pneumocystis carinii* organisms can be demonstrated with Gomori's methenamine silver stain. FNA should also be considered in patients with Kaposi's sarcoma, especially those with disseminated disease, who present with a thyroid nodule in order to identify the rare case of Kaposi's sarcoma of the thyroid.

The Adrenal

Adrenal Pathology

Although pathologic involvement of the adrenal gland was frequently noted during autopsy in the pre-HAART era, clinical adrenal insufficiency was relatively rare. While cytomegalovirus adrenalitis was the most common finding, *Mycobacterium tuberculosis*, *Mycobacterium avium* complex, *Cryptococcus neoformans* and *Toxoplasmosis gondii* were also found to infect the adrenal gland. Other abnormal pathology, including infiltration with Kaposi's sarcoma or lymphoma, hemorrhage, fibrosis, infarction, and focal necrosis were also reported.[8]

Alterations in Adrenal Function

HIV-infected individuals commonly demonstrate characteristic changes in steroid metabolism including an elevation in basal cortisol levels that may be accompanied by decreased responsiveness to ACTH stimulation. Lower levels of ACTH and the adrenal steroid dehydroepiandrosterone (DHEA) are often observed, as well as impaired adrenal reserve of the 17-deoxysteroids (corticosterone, deoxycorticosterone, and 18-OH-deoxycorticosterone).[15] Factors such as cytokines, acting independently of the pituitary gland, may directly enhance cortisol biosynthesis in the absence of an increase in ACTH. In some HIV-infected patients, however, the combination of increased cortisol and ACTH levels suggests hypothalamic activation, although those with late-stage HIV disease often have an attenuated pituitary-adrenal response to corticotropin-releasing hormone (CRH). Compensatory rises in ACTH levels may also develop in those with subclinical adrenal insufficiency due to physiologic hormonal feedback mechanisms. In AIDS patients who present with elevated levels of both cortisol and ACTH but manifest paradoxical Addisonian features, peripheral glucocorticoid resistance may be present.[16]

Dehydroepiandrosterone (DHEA) in HIV Infection

Levels of DHEA, a weak adrenal androgen, decline with advancing age and chronic illness, in contrast to levels of cortisol that remain relatively stable. Interest in DHEA therapy among the HIV community was motivated by studies showing that DHEA inhibits HIV-1 replication and activation *in vitro*. The increased production of cortisol and reduction of DHEA levels may contribute to the unfavorable shift in cytokine production observed during HIV disease progression.[17] Cross-sectional studies that associate low DHEA levels and elevated cortisol to DHEA ratios with advanced HIV infection are insufficient to demonstrate causality. Low serum concentrations of DHEA, however, have been significantly correlated with CD4 cell count, weight loss, and progression to AIDS. Although a small double-blind placebo-controlled clinical trial of oral administration of DHEA (50 mg daily) showed improved quality of life in patients with AIDS without change in CD4 count,[18] DHEA cannot be recommended in the routine treatment of HIV-infected patients until its efficacy has been proven in larger, randomized clinical trials evaluating multiple outcomes.

Effects of Antiretroviral and other Therapies

Although HIV-associated fat redistribution, particularly dorsocervical fat pad enlargement and visceral adiposity, appears phenotypically similar to Cushing's syndrome, overt hypercortisolism has not been found in affected patients.[19] Although the demonstration of both normal diurnal cortisol excretion and normal response to exogenous CRH administration provides additional evidence that the development of lipodystrophy can not be attributed to abnormal cortisol metabolism, others have hypothesized that it may be related to the increased cortisol/DHEA ratio observed in these patients. Iatrogenic Cushing's syndrome, however, can occur in patients treated with ritonavir, when given in conjunction with nasal or inhaled fluticasone (for allergic rhinitis or asthma). Ritonavir administration prolongs the half-life of fluticasone via effects on cytochrome P450, leading to much higher plasma levels of fluticasone than pharmacologically intended and the classic physical manifestations of glucocorticoid excess. Relative adrenal suppression ensues, and associated conditions such as osteoporosis or diabetes may be induced or exacerbated. Practitioners should be aware of this potential interaction in order to avoid delays in diagnosis among patients who have pre-existing body composition changes of ART-associated lipodystrophy that mask the clinical features of Cushing's syndrome.[20]

Multiple medications used to treat HIV disease are known to affect adrenocortical function. Both ketoconazole, by inhibiting cortisol biosynthesis, and rifampin, by increasing the metabolic clearance of cortisol, may lead to adrenal insufficiency in patients with impaired adrenal reserve.[8] Megestrol acetate, a progestational agent used as an appetite stimulant in the treatment of AIDS wasting, has been shown to suppress both the hypothalamic-pituitary-adrenal (HPA) axis and the hypothalamic-pituitary-gonadal (HPG) axis. Due to its intrinsic glucocorticoid-like activity, some patients receiving long-term therapy may develop iatrogenic Cushing's syndrome and/or diabetes mellitus, as well as adrenal failure when treatment is suddenly discontinued. Opiate use, often seen co-existing with HIV infection, can also lead to alterations in the HPA axis with an up to 70% lower cortisol response to ACTH stimulation.[21]

Treatment Considerations

The alterations in steroid metabolism observed in patients with HIV infection may be adaptive to chronic illness and may not require treatment. Estimates of the prevalence of adrenal insufficiency vary considerably, depending on the population studied, whether or not patients manifest clinical signs and symptoms, and the method of diagnostic testing used. Adrenal insufficiency is clearly more common than in the general population, and the diagnosis should be considered in patients who present with malaise, orthostatic hypotension, nausea, abdominal pain, weight loss, hyponatremia, and hypoglycemia. The appropriate method of adrenal function testing, however, is controversial. Although the ACTH stimulation test (administration of 250 µg cosyntropin) is the most widely available, it may not identify all patients with impaired pituitary reserve. In several reported cases, insulin-induced hypoglycemia or the metyrapone test was necessary to confirm the diagnosis of adrenal insufficiency in HIV-infected patients. Others have proposed that stimulatory testing using a lower dose of cosyntropin (1 or 10 µg) will increase the sensitivity to detect HPA axis dysfunction, though the low-dose test may lack specificity in the presence of systemic illness.

Patients with documented adrenal insufficiency should be treated with glucocorticoid replacement therapy and require increased doses during periods of stress. If primary adrenal failure is present with evidence of concomitant mineralocorticoid deficiency (hyperkalemia and metabolic acidosis), the addition of fludrocortisone should be considered. Controversy exists regarding whether patients with elevated basal cortisol levels, but a blunted response to standard single-dose ACTH stimulation, should be treated with glucocorticoid therapy. Some of these patients probably do not require chronic glucocorticoid replacement since they show adequate cortisol response after receiving supraphysiologic ACTH stimulation for three consecutive days.[15] These challenging cases must be evaluated individually, with the goal of minimizing unnecessary glucocorticoid exposure. The administration of short-term, supplementary glucocorticoids to symptomatic patients who demonstrate a sub-normal rise in cortisol levels during periods of stress is reasonable.

The Pancreas

Pancreatic Pathology

Autopsy series show that morphologic abnormalities of the pancreas are common in AIDS patients (up to 90%); however, most of these lesions are asymptomatic.[22] OIs such as mycobacteria, toxoplasmosis, cytomegalovirus, and *Pneumocystis carinii* of the pancreas have been documented, with presentation similar to that of pancreatitis due to other causes.[23] The most common OI reported is pancreatic tuberculosis, presenting with diverse manifestations, such as pancreatic masses mimicking carcinoma, obstructive jaundice, pancreatitis, gastrointestinal bleeding, generalized lymphadenopathy, and may be diagnosed by abdominal computed tomography followed by FNA of the pancreas. HIV-associated neoplasms rarely affect the pancreas, although Kaposi's sarcoma has been reported, successfully treated with intensive antiviral therapy and paclitaxel.[24]

Alterations in Glucose Homeostasis

Prior to the use of HAART, hyperinsulinemic euglycemic clamp studies in stable HIV-infected men show increased rates of insulin clearance and increased insulin sensitivity of peripheral tissues compared with non-infected controls. These findings contrast with those observed in classic sepsis, which is often accompanied by insulin resistance and hyperglycemia. In addition, studies utilizing the insulin tolerance test found no evidence of insulin resistance among ART-naive, HIV-infected individuals. Non-oxidative glucose disposal predominantly accounts for this increased uptake, and it has been hypothesized that the observed rise in hepatic glucose production compensates for the increased disposal, thus maintaining plasma glucose levels within the normal range.[2]

Effects of Antiretroviral and other Therapies

Pentamidine, used in the prevention and treatment of *Pneumocystis carinii*, commonly causes pancreatic β-cell toxicity when administered either intravenously or aerosolized. Acute insulin secretion and hypoglycemia may be followed by β-cell destruction and diabetes mellitus.[8] In addition, acute pancreatitis has been associated with pentamidine, trimethoprim-sulfamethoxazole, the nucleoside analogs ddI and ddC, and ritonavir-induced hypertriglyceridemia. As previously discussed, megestrol acetate has intrinsic glucocorticoid-like activity and has been reported to exacerbate hyperglycemia or cause frank diabetes, although the incidence of this complication is low.

Alterations in glucose metabolism associated with HAART have received increased attention as the individual components of the HIV-associated lipodystrophy syndrome and its associated metabolic abnormalities have been elucidated. This syndrome has been extensively studied and is reviewed elsewhere in this text (Chapter 17). Although early anecdotal reports led to the assumption that PIs were directly responsible for all of these complications, it is now clear that both body composition abnormalities and impaired glucose homeostasis occur in PI-naive patients treated with nucleoside reverse transcriptase inhibitors (NRTIs). Furthermore, when patients with HIV-associated lipodystrophy were compared with seropositive patients without lipodystrophy but with similar duration and modality of ART, studies showed impaired glucose

disposal rates (assessed by hyperinsulinemic euglycemic clamp), non-oxidative glucose metabolism (assessed by indirect calorimetry), and insulin secretion (assessed by frequently sampled intravenous tolerance test).[25]

The prevalence of diabetes among patients taking HAART may be as high as 14%, depending on the population studied and the definition of diabetes used for diagnosis.[26] Impaired glucose tolerance and peripheral insulin resistance are much more common than frank diabetes, affecting up to 60% of those taking PIs. Individual PIs have distinct effects on metabolism and, therefore, must be investigated separately.[27] In studies among healthy volunteers, designed to minimize the confounding factors of HIV infection itself, immune reconstitution, and the changes in body composition resulting from restoration in health, indinavir was shown to induce insulin resistance both acutely and after four weeks of treatment. *In vitro* studies implicate acute blockade of the glucose transporter, GLUT4, in decreasing insulin-mediated glucose uptake. In contrast, treatment with atazanavir has not been found to induce insulin resistance. The results for other members of the medication class, including lopinavir/ritonavir, have been less consistent. Thus, there does not appear to be a 'class effect' of PIs on glucose homeostasis.[27]

The development of hyperglycemia and type 2 diabetes requires not only peripheral insulin resistance, but also impairment in pancreatic β-cell insulin secretion. Treatment with the PIs nelfinavir, indinavir, lopinavir/ritonavir, and saquinavir causes diminished first-phase insulin release, which may lead to postprandial hyperglycemia. *In vitro* studies demonstrate that ritonavir, nelfinavir, and saquinavir impair glucose-mediated insulin secretion by pancreatic β-cells, likely by inducing alterations in the insulin signaling pathway. Results for indinavir have differed, again highlighting the importance of studying PIs individually.[27]

Treatment Considerations

An International AIDS Society – USA panel has published recommendations for managing the metabolic complications of HIV infection including abnormalities in glucose homeostasis.[28] If HAART includes a PI associated with changes in glucose homeostasis, fasting glucose should be monitored before initiation, at the time of a change in therapy, 3 to 6 months after starting or switching therapy, and at least annually during stable therapy. For patients with risk factors for type 2 diabetes or those with severe body composition changes, an OGTT may be considered. If possible, the panel recommends avoiding PIs as initial therapy or switching from PI-based therapy to an acceptable alternative regimen among patients with pre-existing glucose intolerance or those with first-degree relatives with diabetes. Short-term improvements in insulin resistance have been observed in studies that substitute nevirapine, efavirenz, or abacavir for the PI component of HAART regimens.

Treatment of diabetes in HIV-infected patients should emphasize healthy diet, regular exercise, and maintenance of normal body weight. Among the accepted first-line oral medications for diabetes, preference may be given to insulin-sensitizing agents. Both metformin and rosiglitazone lead to improvements in glucose metabolism in HIV-infected patients. Metformin should be avoided in those with a history of renal disease or with lactic acidemia, a recognized adverse effect of NRTIs. In addition, clinicians should be aware of potential interactions between PIs and hypoglycemic agents, such as ritonavir and nelfinavir which induce CYP 2C9 and may reduce concentrations of selected sulfonylureas and rosiglitazone.[28]

Bone

Alterations in Bone Metabolism

Reduced bone mineral density (BMD) may be present in as many as 80% of HIV-infected individuals, though prevalence estimates of osteopenia vary widely and may depend on the presence or absence of ART and lipodystrophy, severity of HIV disease, and pre-existing bone loss risk factors. Some patients with HIV disease and low BMD may have vitamin D insufficiency with secondary hyperparathyroidism and a high bone turnover rate with osteoclast activation.[29] Histomorphometric analyses demonstrate altered bone remodeling in HIV-infected patients.[30] There is evidence from studies of ART-naive, seropositive patients that HIV infection *per se* promotes bone loss. Potential mechanisms for this effect include chronic T-cell activation, which induces pro-inflammatory cytokines that may contribute to osteoclast activation, or direct infection of the bone marrow. Reduced BMD among patients with HIV infection is likely multifactorial, with possible contributions from weight loss, malnutrition, malabsorption (leading to vitamin D deficiency), and hypogonadism, as well as traditional risk factors for

osteoporosis such as gender, low BMI, increased age, increased time from menopause, smoking, and injection drug use.[31] While osteopenia occurs frequently, there are no data showing that reduced BMD increases fracture risk in patients with HIV disease, perhaps because most are young and lack risk factors for falls.[30] Fragility fractures in AIDS patients have been reported, and steps should be taken to anticipate and prevent this complication as the HIV-infected population ages.

Effects of Antiretroviral and other Therapies

Since the introduction of HAART, studies investigating the relationships between accelerated bone loss and specific therapies such as PIs and/or the presence of ART-lipodystrophy have been conflicting.[30] Initial reports of PI-induced osteoporosis have not been well-supported by subsequent longitudinal data that demonstrate relatively stable BMD in patients taking PIs. Other medications used in the treatment of HIV and its complications that may contribute to the development of osteoporosis include corticosteroids, pentamidine, and ketoconazole. Opiates may also contribute to low bone mineral density, as an 11% reduction in lumbar bone mineral density was found in heroin users compared with controls, though this effect may, at least partially, be attributed to associated hypogonadism.[32]

Treatment Considerations

The pharmacologic agents used to treat osteopenia and osteoporosis in HIV-infected patients have primarily been testosterone and bisphosphonates.[31] Although intramuscular injections of testosterone were found to increase lumbar spine BMD in 54 eugonadal men with AIDS wasting compared with those who received placebo,[33] routine use is not yet justified. Several studies show that alendronate (70 mg once-weekly), either alone or in combination with vitamin D and calcium, improves BMD in patients with HIV infection. The studies investigating the effects of switching ART regimen on BMD have been small and of short duration; therefore no clear recommendations can be made. Until further research elucidates the relative contribution of factors associated with HIV-associated bone loss, an International AIDS Society – USA panel does not recommend routine screening for osteoporosis in HIV-infected patients.[28] Those individuals who possess additional risk factors may warrant regional

DXA scanning. If osteoporosis is present or a pathological fracture occurs in the setting of osteopenia, work-up for secondary causes of osteoporosis should be initiated and bisphosphonate therapy considered. In addition, practitioners should encourage patients to address modifiable risk factors (e.g. smoking cessation), to engage in weight-bearing exercise, and to increase intake of calcium and vitamin D.

Osteonecrosis, death of bone resulting from circulatory insufficiency, is recognized as another complication of HIV infection, and may present as either unilateral or bilateral bone or joint pain. Avascular necrosis of the hip was detected by MRI in 4.4% of 339 asymptomatic HIV-infected patients in a cross-sectional study as compared with none of the seronegative controls.[34] The shoulder may also be affected. In some studies, osteonecrosis was associated with prior glucocorticoid use. Unfortunately, surgical intervention remains the only available treatment for symptomatic osteonecrosis.

Reproductive Health in Men

Testicular Pathology

Histopathologic changes in the testes are commonly found in autopsy studies among men with AIDS, usually revealing hypospermatogenesis and atrophy. HIV DNA can be identified by PCR *in situ* hybridization in approximately 30% of residual germ cells. Pathologic damage to the testes during AIDS, such as decreased spermatogenesis and interstitial inflammation, is associated with decreased testosterone and bioavailable testosterone, as well as increased serum gonadotropin levels.[35] Not surprisingly, testicular atrophy is more likely to be found in AIDS patients with lower BMI. In men with AIDS, OIs such as cytomegalovirus, *Toxoplasma gondii*, and *Mycobacterium avium intracellulare* have been found on pathologic examination of testes. AIDS patients are also at greater risk for the development of testicular malignancy, including Kaposi's sarcoma, lymphoma, and germ cell tumors.

Alterations in Sex Hormones

Early in the course of HIV infection, hyperresponsiveness of luteinizing hormone (LH) to infusion of gonadotropin-releasing hormone (GnRH) may explain the normal or, in some cases, elevated total and free testosterone levels.[36] As HIV disease progresses to AIDS, testosterone levels usually decrease. An assessment of free or bioavailable testosterone is necessary in order to diagnose androgen deficiency, since increased sex hormone-binding globulin (SHBG) levels have been observed in this population. Especially in the post-HAART era, direct testicular pathology causing primary hypogonadism is less common than hypogonadotropic (or secondary) hypogonadism in men with HIV. Factors such as chronic illness, altered cytokine profiles, OIs, medications, cachexia and associated malnutrition all may contribute to hypothalamic-pituitary-gonadal (HPG) axis dysfunction. The loss of lean body mass and muscle strength in patients with the AIDS wasting syndrome may be attributable, at least partially, to co-existing hypogonadism. In contrast to the decreased levels of testosterone, serum and urinary levels of estrogens may be elevated in HIV-infected male patients.[37] Although gynecomastia in HIV-infected men may be due to hypoandrogenism and/or elevated estrogen levels, liver disease, and the use of commonly implicated medications, clinicians should bear in mind that gynecomastia is common among healthy men as they age.

Effects of Antiretroviral and other Therapies

A number of medications used in the treatment of HIV and its related disorders affect the reproductive health of men. Systemic glucocorticoid therapy and megestrol acetate, due to its intrinsic glucocorticoid-like activity, can both cause HPG axis suppression. Ketoconazole, particularly at higher doses, and the chronic use of alcohol, opiates, and marijuana impair testosterone production.[21] These drugs, as well as HAART, may lead to gynecomastia in HIV-infected men. Though these body shape changes were initially attributed to PIs, other antiretroviral medications, such as the NNRTI efavirenz, have been associated with gynecomastia among patients taking HAART. Treatment options specifically aimed at reversing gynecomastia induced by HAART have not been systematically evaluated, although a case report describes successful treatment of an HIV-infected man with the selective estrogen receptor modulator tamoxifen.[38]

Sexual dysfunction is a common complaint among men with advanced HIV disease with an estimated prevalence of nearly 60%. Although erectile and ejaculatory dysfunction, as well as loss of libido, are often attributed to low testosterone levels, other factors, including neurologic disease, systemic illness, drug effects, weakness, low energy, and psychosexual issues may also be contributory.[36] Sexual dysfunction has been associated with PI therapy in reports of affected men without any other apparent etiology. In some of these patients in whom endocrinologic investigation was performed, as well as subjects in a different study where HAART was associated with a higher prevalence of low libido, raised serum estradiol levels were observed.[39]

Treatment Considerations

After confirming hypogonadism with repeated morning measurements of testosterone utilizing a reliable laboratory assay and excluding reversible etiologies, symptomatic patients with primary or secondary hypogonadism should be offered therapy with replacement doses of testosterone. Testosterone administration is usually achieved in clinical practice, either by intramuscular injection every 2–3 weeks using testosterone esters (e.g. enanthate and cypionate) or by transdermal delivery through a patch or gel formulation. Although the testosterone patch and gel avoid large fluctuations in circulating testosterone levels resulting from intermittent injections, transdermal routes of administration do not always result in therapeutic testosterone levels at the recommended doses. Clinical assessment of the response and subsequent laboratory monitoring of testosterone concentration should be performed, along with periodic measurements of HDL cholesterol, hematocrit, and prostate-specific antigen. Hypogonadal men with HIV-associated weight loss treated with physiologic testosterone therapy with or without concurrent resistance training show improvement in lean body mass, muscle strength, bone mineral density and quality of life.[40] Given the potential risks, the role of supraphysiologic testosterone therapy or other anabolic steroids in eugonadal men with weight loss cannot be established until long-term safety data are available. Low testosterone levels have also been postulated to partially explain the anemia commonly observed in HIV disease, as supplemental androgens were negatively associated with the presence of anemia.[41] Clinicians should be aware of the drug interaction between sildenafil, used in the treatment of erectile dysfunction, and several PIs (indinavir, ritonavir, saquinavir, and nelfinavir) that can result in elevated levels of sildenafil. In order to avoid the greater risk of sildenafil-related adverse events, low doses should be used cautiously in these patients.

Fertility and Reproductive Issues

Analysis of semen among men with early HIV disease is usually normal and compatible with fertility. In contrast, untreated men with progression to advanced stages of HIV often have both oligospermia and an increased proportion of morphologically abnormal sperm.[36] Antiretroviral therapy with zidovudine does not adversely affect sperm production or quality. Treatment with testosterone or anabolic steroids is associated with azoospermia.

Reproductive Health in Women

Ovarian Function and Alterations in Sex Hormones

In contrast to those describing testicular pathology, there have been no systematic autopsy series reporting pathologic examination of the ovaries. Several case reports in the literature, including presentations of cytomegalovirus oophoritis and ovarian Burkitt's lymphoma, suggest that the ovaries are susceptible to OIs and HIV-associated neoplasms. HIV can directly infect cells and tissues from both the upper and lower female reproductive tract, including the vaginal mucosa, fallopian tubes, uterus, and cervix.[42]

As expected with any chronic illness, women with significant AIDS wasting do report more amenorrhea.[43]

In contrast to initial reports indicating higher rates of menstrual irregularities among HIV-infected women without clinical AIDS, prospective data from two large cohorts failed to confirm this finding. Higher viral loads and lower CD4 cell counts, however, were associated with increased menstrual cycle length and variability.[36] In addition, narcotics, marijuana and chronic alcohol consumption are known to affect menstrual function and ovulation. Similar to findings in men, women with AIDS wasting also demonstrate reduced androgen levels. This hypoandrogenism appears to be a result of shunting of adrenal steroid metabolism away from androgenic pathways toward cortisol production, rather than due to decreased ovarian production of androgens.[44]

Effects of Antiretroviral Therapy

Since the advent of HAART, the specific body composition changes reported as part of the HIV-associated lipodystrophy syndrome, including central fat accumulation (affecting the breasts and abdomen) and peripheral lipoatrophy, usually are not accompanied by abnormalities in endogenous sex hormones. Although a small initial study linking hyperandrogenemia and hyperinsulinemia in HIV-infected women with lipodystrophy suggested that these patients may have characteristic features of the polycystic ovary syndrome, later reports from the same group found reduced free testosterone levels and LH to FSH ratios with normal menstrual function and ovarian morphology by ultrasound.[45] Nonetheless, serum testosterone in the range of an androgen-secreting tumor has been reported in a woman with HIV-associated lipodystrophy syndrome.[46]

Treatment Considerations

Contraception for HIV-infected women should include a combination of barrier method and another form of acceptable contraception. Treatment with oral contraceptives may increase cervical and vaginal shedding of HIV.[36] Nevirapine and ritonavir have been shown to affect the pharmacokinetics of ethinyl estradiol and may lead to reduced contraceptive efficacy when administered in combination with oral contraceptives. Following recent studies showing that women with HIV have lower testosterone levels than healthy non-infected controls, attention has begun to focus on the therapeutic potential of androgen therapy in women, including anabolic steroids. Even though studies show that low-dose twice-weekly transdermal testosterone administration is well-tolerated among HIV-infected women, these preparations are not yet commercially available. While initial reports of women with the AIDS wasting syndrome demonstrated benefits in weight gain, quality of life, and muscle strength with physiologic testosterone replacement, a more recent clinical trial failed to find significant effects on fat-free mass, body weight, or muscle performance.[47] Data regarding the long-term effects of testosterone on multiple other outcomes including cardiovascular disease, body composition, ovarian physiology, sexual function, and quality of life is warranted in order to determine the role of androgen replacement in women.

Fertility and Reproductive Issues

Risk of spontaneous fetal loss may be up to 3-fold higher in HIV-infected women, as a result of

HIV transmission and fetal thymic dysfunction,[48] although these studies were performed in women who did not receive prenatal ART. Lower pregnancy and birth rates, however, may also be partially attributed to prior knowledge of HIV seropositivity, since the rates of therapeutic abortion are also higher. Even though effective ART is available during pregnancy and at delivery for prevention of mother-to-child transmission, there are complex ethical and social issues regarding conception in women with HIV infection. Pregnancy in HIV-infected women does not appear to adversely alter the course of HIV infection or related markers of immune function, based on the results of several large cohort studies performed in developed nations.[36]

Wasting Syndrome

Although the incidence of new AIDS wasting has declined since the introduction of HAART, weight loss and muscle wasting remain significant problems for individuals with HIV infection, particularly in parts of the world without extensive access to HAART. Increased mortality, accelerated disease progression, loss of muscle protein mass, and impairment of strength and functional status have all been associated with wasting.[49] Weight loss that does not meet the CDC case definition of AIDS wasting (>10% of baseline body weight with clinical symptoms) still predicts increased morbidity and mortality in this setting. Wasting is multifactorial and may represent the common endpoint of multiple, related pathophysiologic processes related to the progression of HIV infection including inadequate energy balance, malabsorption, altered cytokine profiles, and metabolic abnormalities such as hypogonadism. AIDS wasting appears to be an episodic process, exacerbated by acute secondary infections that lead to anorexia, extremely diminished caloric intake, and metabolic changes that may synergistically contribute to the loss of lean body mass (LBM).[50] This condition is distinct from the body composition changes known as HIV-associated lipodystrophy, which may be associated with subcutaneous and peripheral fat loss, reviewed elsewhere in this text.

Treatment Considerations

In light of the poor prognosis associated with wasting, clinicians should emphasize the prevention of weight loss by addressing weight and nutritional status as a routine part of both initial and ongoing

HIV care. Patients should be weighed at each visit, as well as encouraged to maintain a nutritional diet with adequate caloric intake and engage in moderate exercise. Those with active weight loss require comprehensive assessment of the potential comorbidities and/or underlying mechanisms described above, including ruling out secondary infection and optimizing antiretroviral therapy. Nutritional counseling should consider psychosocial factors, as access to food, depression, and socioeconomic standing can affect both the quantity and quality of food intake.

Randomized, placebo-controlled trials have investigated a variety of approaches for the treatment of AIDS-associated weight loss such as progressive resistance training (PRT), nutritional supplementation, cytokine suppression, and the administration of appetite stimulants, androgenic steroids, and growth hormone (GH).[49] Dronabinol improves subjective appetite but results in little or no weight gain. Megestrol acetate, a synthetic progestational agent, effectively stimulates appetite and achieves weight gain. Possibly as a result of its potent glucocorticoid-like activity and/or suppression of gonadal steroid production, megestrol acetate predominantly increases fat tissue rather than LBM. Despite the decline in hypogonadism among men with HIV infection since the widespread introduction of HAART, studies continue to show 20% prevalence of hypogonadism among men with AIDS wasting. Physiologic testosterone replacement, which induces gain of LBM, may be considered in these patients. Treatment with anabolic steroids also increases LBM, but it is frequently complicated by the development of abnormal liver enzymes and dyslipidemia. There have been several randomized, placebo-controlled trials investigating GH as a potential therapy for AIDS wasting[51] including a recent study of short-term GH administration at the time of OIs.[50] Adverse effects of GH reported in these trials included arthralgias, myalgias, edema, diarrhea, carpal tunnel compression, and perhaps most importantly, glucose intolerance. Since long-term effects are unknown, clinicians should only consider GH injections for rapid weight loss associated with acute infection or for persistent wasting refractory to other therapies.[49]

References

1. Sano T, Kovacs K, Scheithauer BW, et al. Pituitary pathology in acquired immunodeficiency syndrome. Arch Pathol Lab Med 1989; 113:1066–1070.
2. Sellmeyer DE, Grunfeld C. Endocrine and metabolic disturbances in human immunodeficiency virus infection and the acquired immune deficiency syndrome. Endocr Rev 1996; 17:518–532.
3. Agarwal A, Soni A, Ciechanowsky M, et al. Hyponatremia in patients with the acquired immunodeficiency syndrome. Nephron 1989; 53:317–321.
4. Heijligenberg R, Sauerwein HP, Brabant G, et al. Circadian growth hormone secretion in asymptomatic human immune deficiency virus infection and acquired immunodeficiency syndrome. J Clin Endocrinol Metab 1996; 81:4028–4032.
5. Bhasin S, Singh AB, Javanbakht M. Neuroendocrine abnormalities associated with HIV infection. Neuroendocrinology 2001; 30:749–765.
6. Hutchinson J, Murphy M, Harries R, et al. Galactorrhoea and hyperprolactinaemia associated with protease-inhibitors. Lancet 2000; 356:1003–1004.
7. Lima MK, Freitas LL, Montandon C, et al. The Thyroid in Acquired Immunodeficiency Syndrome. Endocr Pathol 1998; 9:217–223.
8. Hofbauer LC, Heufelder AE. Endocrine implications of human immunodeficiency virus infection. Medicine 1996; 75:262–278.
9. Grunfeld C, Pang M, Doerrler W, et al. Indices of thyroid function and weight loss in human immunodeficiency virus infection and the acquired immunodeficiency syndrome. Metabolism 1993; 42:1270–1276.
10. Hommes MJ, Romijn JA, Endert E, et al. Hypothyroid-like regulation of the pituitary-thyroid axis in stable human immunodeficiency virus infection. Metabolism 1993; 42:556–561.
11. Carella C, Mazziotti G, Amato G, et al. Clinical review 169: Interferon-alpha-related thyroid disease: pathophysiological, epidemiological, and clinical aspects. J. Clin Endocrinol Metab 2004; 89:3656–3661.
12. Jubault V, Penfornis A, Schillo F, et al. Sequential occurrence of thyroid autoantibodies and Graves' disease after immune restoration in severely immunocompromised human immunodeficiency virus-1-infected patients. J Clin Endocrinol Metab 2000; 85:4254–4257.
13. Beltran S, Lescure FX, Desailloud R, et al. Increased prevalence of hypothyroidism among human immunodeficiency virus-infected patients: a need for screening. Clin Infect Dis 2003; 37:579–583.
14. Jimenez C, Moran SA, Sereti I, et al. Graves' disease after interleukin-2 therapy in a patient with human immunodeficiency virus infection. Thyroid 2004; 14:1097–1102.
15. Membreno L, Irony I, Dere W, et al. Adrenocortical function in acquired immunodeficiency syndrome. J Clin Endocrinol Metab 1987; 65:482–487.
16. Mayo J, Collazos J, Martinez E, et al. Adrenal function in the human immunodeficiency virus-infected patient. Arch Intern Med 2002; 162:1095–1098.
17. Clerici M, Galli M, Bosis S, et al. Immunoendocrinologic abnormalities in human immunodeficiency virus infection. Ann NY Acad Sci 2000; 917:956–961.
18. Piketty C, Jayle D, Leplege A, et al. Double-blind placebo-controlled trial of oral dehydroepiandrosterone in patients with advanced HIV disease. Clin Endocrinol (Oxf) 2001; 55:325–330.
19. Lo JC, Mulligan K, Tai VW, et al. 'Buffalo hump' in men with HIV-1 infection. Lancet 1998; 351:867–870.
20. Samaras K, Pett S, Gowers A, et al. Iatrogenic Cushing's syndrome with osteoporosis and secondary adrenal failure in human immunodeficiency virus-infected patients receiving inhaled corticosteroids and ritonavir-boosted protease inhibitors: six cases. J Clin Endocrinol Metab 2005; 90:4394–4398.
21. Cooper OB, Brown TT, Dobs AS. Opiate drug use: a potential contributor to the endocrine and metabolic complications in human immunodeficiency virus disease. Clin Infect Dis 2003; 37:S132–S136.

22. Chehter EZ, Longo MA, Laudanna AA, et al. Involvement of the pancreas in AIDS: a prospective study of 109 post-mortems. AIDS 2000; 14:1879–1886.

23. Keaveny AP, Karasik MS. Hepatobiliary and pancreatic infections in AIDS: Part I. AIDS Patient Care STDS 1998; 12:347–357.

24. Menges M, Pees HW. Kaposi's sarcoma of the pancreas mimicking pancreatic cancer in an HIV-infected patient. Clinical diagnosis by detection of HHV 8 in bile and complete remission following antiviral and cytostatic therapy with paclitaxel. Int J Pancreatol 1999; 26:193–199.

25. Andersen O, Haugaard SB, Andersen UB, et al. Lipodystrophy in human immunodeficiency virus patients impairs insulin action and induces defects in beta-cell function. Metabolism 2003; 52:1343–1353.

26. Brown TT, Cole SR, Li X, et al. Antiretroviral therapy and the prevalence and incidence of diabetes mellitus in the multicenter AIDS cohort study. Arch Intern Med 2005; 165:1179–1184.

27. Lee GA, Rao MN, Grunfeld C. The effects of HIV protease inhibitors on carbohydrate and lipid metabolism. Curr Infect Dis Rep 2004; 6:471–482.

28. Schambelan M, Benson CA, Carr A, et al. Management of metabolic complications associated with antiretroviral therapy for HIV-1 infection: recommendations of an International AIDS Society-USA panel. J Acquir Immune Defic Syndr 2002; 31:257–275.

29. Seminari E, Castagna A, Soldarini A, et al. Osteoprotegerin and bone turnover markers in heavily pretreated HIV-infected patients. HIV Med 2005; 6:145–150.

30. Thomas J, Doherty SM. HIV infection–a risk factor for osteoporosis. J Acquir Immune Defic Syndr 2003; 33:281–291.

31. Qaqish RB. Bone disorders associated with the human immunodeficiency virus: pathogenesis and management. Pharmacotherapy 2004; 24:1331–1346.

32. Pedrazzoni M, Vescovi PP, Maninetti L, et al. Effects of chronic heroin abuse on bone and mineral metabolism. Acta Endocrinol (Copenh) 1993; 129:42–45.

33. Fairfield WP, Finkelstein JS, Klibanski A, et al. Osteopenia in eugonadal men with acquired immune deficiency syndrome wasting syndrome. J Clin Endocrinol Metab 2001; 86:2020–2026.

34. Miller KD, Masur H, Jones EC, et al. High prevalence of osteonecrosis of the femoral head in HIV-infected adults. Ann Intern Med 2002; 137:17–25.

35. Salehian B, Jacobson D, Swerdloff RS, et al. Testicular pathologic changes and the pituitary-testicular axis during human immunodeficiency virus infection. Endocr Pr 1999; 5:1–9.

36. Lo JC, Schambelan M. Reproductive function in human immunodeficiency virus infection. J Clin Endocrinol Metab 2001; 86:2338–2343.

37. Teichmann J, Stephan E, Lange U, et al. Evaluation of serum and urinary estrogen levels in male patients with HIV-infection. Eur J Med Res 1998; 3:533–537.

38. Kegg S, Lau R. Tamoxifen in antiretroviral-associated gynaecomastia. Int J STD AIDS 2002; 13:582–583.

39. Lamba H, Goldmeier D, Mackie NE, et al. Antiretroviral therapy is associated with sexual dysfunction and with increased serum oestradiol levels in men. Int J STD AIDS 2004; 15:234–237.

40. Dobs A. Role of testosterone in maintaining lean body mass and bone density in HIV-infected patients. Int J Impot Res 2003; 15:S21–S25.

41. Behler C, Shade S, Gregory K, et al. Anemia and HIV in the antiretroviral era: potential significance of testosterone. AIDS Res Hum Retroviruses 2005; 21:200–206.

42. Howell AL, Edkins RD, Rier SE, et al. Human immunodeficiency virus type 1 infection of cells and tissues from the upper and lower human female reproductive tract. J Virol 1997; 71:3498–3506.

43. Grinspoon S, Corcoran C, Miller K, et al. Body composition and endocrine function in women with acquired immunodeficiency syndrome wasting. J Clin Endocrinol Metab 1997; 82:1332–1337. Erratum in: J Clin Endocrinol Metab 1997; 82:3360.

44. Grinspoon S, Corcoran C, Stanley T, et al. Mechanisms of androgen deficiency in human immunodeficiency virus-infected women with the wasting syndrome. J Clin Endocrinol Metab 2001; 86:4120–4126.

45. Johnsen S, Dolan SE, Fitch KV, et al. Absence of polycystic ovary syndrome features in human immunodeficiency virus-infected women despite significant hyperinsulinemia and truncal adiposity. J Clin Endocrinol Metab 2005; 90:5596–5604.

46. Dahan MH, Lyle LN, Wolfsen A, et al. Tumor-level serum testosterone associated with human immunodeficiency virus lipodystrophy syndrome. Obstet Gynecol 103.5 Pt 2004; 2:1094–1096.

47. Choi HH, Gray PB, Storer TW, et al. Effects of testosterone replacement in human immunodeficiency virus-infected women with weight loss. J Clin Endocrinol Metab 2005; 90:1531–1541.

48. Shearer WT, Langston C, Lewis DE, et al. Early spontaneous abortions and fetal thymic abnormalities in maternal-to-fetal HIV infection. Acta Paediatr Suppl 1997; 421:60–64.

49. Grinspoon S, Mulligan K; Department of Health and Human Services Working Group on the Prevention and Treatment of Wasting and Weight Loss. Weight loss and wasting in patients infected with human immunodeficiency virus. Clin Infect Dis 2003; 36:S69–S78.

50. Paton NI, Newton PJ, Sharpstone DR, et al. Short-term growth hormone administration at the time of opportunistic infections in HIV-positive patients. AIDS 1999; 13:1195–1202.

51. Mulligan K, Schambelan M. Anabolic treatment with GH, IGF-I, or anabolic steroids in patients with HIV-associated wasting. Int J Cardiol 2002; 85:151–159.

CHAPTER 28

Renal Complications of HIV Infection

Jula K. Inrig
Lynda A. Szczech
Trevor E. Gerntholtz
Paul E. Klotman

Introduction

In the early 1980s, a unique kidney disease was described among HIV-infected patients.[1,2] Patients usually presented with significant proteinuria and rapid progression to end-stage renal disease (ESRD).[2] When initially described, this renal failure was felt due to heroin nephropathy as it clinically appeared similar. As clinicians continued to see renal disease associated with HIV infection, the existence of a distinct disease called HIV-associated nephropathy (HIVAN) was debated. As more patients with HIV infection without a history of heroin use were noted to have renal disease, HIVAN was established as a unique entity.[2] From a once rare complication of HIV infection, HIVAN has emerged as the most common cause of ESRD in HIV-infected patients.[3] In addition, as patients with HIV/AIDS are surviving longer, the prevalence of HIV-infected patients with chronic kidney diseases continues to rise.[4] With up to 42 million people infected with HIV/AIDS worldwide and a prevalence of renal disease in HIV-infected black patients of 3.5–12%, up to 5 million people worldwide may be affected by HIV related kidney disease.[2,5] This chapter will review the epidemiology and clinical course of HIV related renal disease using USA, European, and African studies to compare results based on regions of the world. Such a comparison requires initial insight into methods and infrastructure for delivery of healthcare within regions to provide a framework for the understanding of study comparisons.

Overview of Global Healthcare/Delivery

Healthcare and its delivery vary drastically around the world. In the USA and Europe, healthcare is available to a greater proportion of the population than in many other parts of the world. In Africa, unfortunately, the availability of health services is considerably more limited. The leading cause of death worldwide is infectious disease – 43% in the developing world compared with 1.2% in the developed world (The World Health Report). Many reasons are responsible for this difference including environmental exposures, lack of water treatment, a general lack of public health infrastructure and limited drug availability. Infectious diseases such as tuberculosis and malaria have been longstanding health problems; however, AIDS has recently become a significant epidemic particularly in sub-Saharan Africa and India. Despite the growing AIDS epidemic, limited resources are available for the majority of patients needing therapy. The financial limitations are significant and can be compared based on the annual *per capita* expenditure on health care in different regions. In 2001, annual *per capita* expenditure on healthcare in international dollars was 12 in the Democratic Republic of the Congo, 22 in the Congo, 34 in Afghanistan, 153 in Egypt, and 652 in South Africa; this is in contrast to >2800 in select European countries and >4000 in the USA.[6] Due to limited preventive services in Africa, screening for renal disease is essentially non-existent and because of more pressing and immediate health concerns, screening assumes a lower priority. As a result, patients are often diagnosed late in the course of their disease after presenting to a hospital with another illness or overt nephrotic syndrome. Thus, treatment is limited by late diagnosis, comorbid conditions, and shortage of resources. In contrast, patients in the USA and Europe with known HIV may undergo screening for renal involvement and thus may be offered therapy earlier in the course of their disease.

Epidemiology

One of the first clinical reports of HIVAN occurred in 1984 in the USA.[1] Not surprisingly, the initial description engendered a debate that was focused mainly on whether or not this was a different entity from heroin nephropathy. As both children and patients without a history of heroin use were identified with renal disease and the disease became better defined histologically, the separate term HIVAN emerged to describe the combination of clinical and histological findings. In the early era of HIV, patients with HIVAN were diagnosed late in the course of HIV infection, usually already with AIDS. Predictably, renal survival for those diagnosed with HIVAN was 1–4 months without therapy.[1,2,7,8] With the advent of highly active antiretroviral therapy (HAART) and the decline in mortality from AIDS, kidney diseases have become major contributors to HIV morbidity and mortality and are now the fourth leading cause of death in US AIDS patients.[9]

While no data on global prevalence exists, HIVAN is likely to have the highest prevalence in Africa. According to the 2004 report on the global AIDS epidemic, almost 38 million (range 34.6–42.3 million) people are living with AIDS in the world.[10] Within sub-Saharan Africa alone, nearly 30 million people are currently infected. In the USA, the prevalence of renal disease has been noted to be between 3.5–12% in HIV-infected African Americans.[2,5] If one assumes a similar prevalence among persons of African descent, then up to 3 million patients may have renal disease in sub-Saharan Africa alone. Any estimate of prevalence, however, needs to account for the different mortality rates among HIV-infected patients and its variation by country. Without having an exact estimate, the prevalence of renal disease could be hypothesized to be quite high. One report in 2003 in the Nigerian Journal of Medicine studying the prevalence of renal disease in consecutive patients with AIDS seen in the infection unit suggests that these estimates are conservative. Of 79 patients with AIDS, renal disease was present in 51.8% (41 patients)

as compared with 12.2% (7 patients) of non-HIV-infected controls. Of these 79 patients, 19% ($n = 15$) had azotemia, 25% had proteinuria alone, and 7.6% had both proteinuria and azotemia.[11]

The current leading cause of death from AIDS worldwide is infection; but as HAART becomes more available and survival is prolonged, renal disease will likely become a major secondary cause of mortality and morbidity as it has in the USA. As the mortality rate from AIDS declined in the early 1990s, the number of black patients living with HIV increased significantly. As a result, this 'at risk' group lived longer and HIVAN became one of the most rapidly increasing causes of end-stage renal disease in the USA.[3]

Patterns of Renal Disease in Africa

There is a large variation in the patterns of renal diseases reported in different geographic regions of Africa. Unfortunately, accurate and comprehensive statistics are not available.[12] For example, a single available study of 368 patients with chronic kidney disease (CKD) in Nigeria demonstrate that 62% had an undetermined etiology of renal failure.[13] The prevalence of CKD in sub-Saharan Africa is not known. Data from the South African Dialysis and Transplant registry regarding etiologies of ESRD reflect only patients selected for dialysis. As only patients eligible for transplantation are offered dialysis and few patients with diabetic ESRD are offered dialysis or transplantation due to comorbid conditions, the available data likely does not reflect accurately the spectrum of renal diseases in the population as a whole.

In North Africa, the incidence of renal disease appears to be much higher than in the US, but the prevalence is lower due to higher mortality and fewer available treatment options.[14] The reported annual incidence of ESRD ranges between 34 and 200 patients per million population (pmp) and the respective prevalence ranges from 30–430 patients pmp. Despite the high mortality from ESRD, the prevalence of CKD appears to be increasing. The principle causes of CKD are interstitial nephritis (14–32%), glomerulonephritis (11–24%), diabetes (5–20%), and nephrosclerosis (5–31%). Trends in Egypt suggest an increasing prevalence of interstitial nephropathies and diabetes.[14] FSGS is reported in 23–34% of the glomerulonephritides and is mostly clustered in black patients.[14]

Overall, glomerular disease appears to be more prevalent and more severe in Africa than in Western countries. It has been estimated that between 0.2–2.4% of medical admissions in tropical countries are due to renal disease (0.5% Zimbabwe, 0.2% Kwa Zulu Natal, South Africa; 2.0% in Uganda and 2.4% Nigeria).[15] It has been observed that the majority of these admissions are related to glomerulonephritis which responds poorly to treatment and progresses to ESRD. In addition, glomerulonephritis in South Africa is more frequent in blacks and less frequent in Indians and Caucasians. This is a similar pattern to the distribution of HIVAN. Given the high prevalence of HIV/AIDS in South Africa, it can be postulated that some of these renal disorders may be caused by HIVAN or other HIV-related renal diseases.

Racial Distribution of HIVAN

As demonstrated by US and European epidemiologic and pathologic data, HIVAN has an overwhelmingly higher prevalence in HIV-infected patients of African descent as compared with Caucasians.[5,16-20] With the emergence of HIV throughout the world in the 1980s, a change in the pathologic findings in African patients with nephrotic syndrome was described. A study from Zaire in 1993 reported the pathologic findings of 92 patients with documented nephrotic syndrome systematically biopsied between 1986 and 1989. A total of 41% of these patients were found to have focal and segmental glomerulosclerosis (FSGS) which was a sevenfold increase from previous prevalence rates of FSGS of only 6%. The investigators were uncertain of the cause of the increase in FSGS but proposed that AIDS might be responsible.[21] This study cannot assess the predisposition of blacks to HIVAN but does suggest that HIVAN has become an increasing health problem in this population. Early in the HIV epidemic, epidemiologic data from the United States and Europe noted HIVAN was diagnosed primarily in areas with large populations of HIV-infected black patients.[19] Two series from France and London have reported that 97/102 and 17/17 of patients diagnosed with HIVAN were black, respectively.[22,23]

In contrast to the high rate of HIV-related kidney diseases in predominantly black populated regions, Caucasians are noted to have a much lower prevalence of classic HIVAN. A post mortem analysis of 239 consecutive Swiss patients who died from AIDS between 1981 and 1989 demonstrated renal pathologic findings in 43% of patients, with HIVAN in only 1.7% (4/239) of the patients.[18] Given that 95% of the patients were Caucasians, this study emphasizes the low prevalence of classic HIVAN in Caucasians.

Another study reviewed the pathologic features of 120 consecutively autopsied HIV-infected Caucasian patients in Italy. Of these patients, 68% had pathologic renal changes and none of the renal specimens had classic HIVAN. The most common pathologic abnormality was immune-mediated glomerular diseases (25 patients) and tubulointerstitial lesions (19 patients).[20] A similar study of 26 Caucasian patients in northern Italy with HIV who underwent renal biopsy failed to reveal any lesions of HIVAN. The majority of diagnoses were immune complex-mediated glomerulonephritis.[16] While patients of African descent are at the highest risk for HIVAN, other ethnic groups have renal disease related to other pathologic entities.

Pathologic Findings

HIV-associated nephropathy has pathologic findings similar to idiopathic and heroin-related FSGS, however there are several unique findings that are suggestive of HIV infection.[17] First, in HIVAN there is a tendency for the entire glomerular tuft to sclerose and collapse rather than finding only a segmental glomerular lesion (Fig. 28.1). In the tubules, there is often severe injury with proliferative microcyst formation and tubular degeneration. The tubular disease is characterized by the development of tubular dilation accompanied by flattening and atrophy of the tubular epithelial cells. Electron microscopy can reveal the presence of numerous tubuloreticular structures in the glomerular endothelial cells. The tubuloreticular inclusions are composed of ribonucleoprotein and membrane structures; their synthesis is stimulated by α-interferon. The only other disorder in which these structures are prominently seen is lupus nephritis, which is also associated with chronically high levels of circulating α-interferon. The finding of tubuloreticular inclusion had been noted to be a common pathologic abnormality in the pre-HAART era; however this pathologic abnormality is now found less frequently potentially related to the advent of effective antiviral therapy resulting in reduced levels of plasma interferon.[17,24] In patients with human immunodeficiency virus-1 (HIV-1) infection and kidney disease, several different glomerular syndromes have been described (Box 28.1). The most common pathologic finding is HIVAN. In the USA, the second most common pathologic findings are membranoproliferative GN (often with HCV coinfection) or mesangioproliferative

301

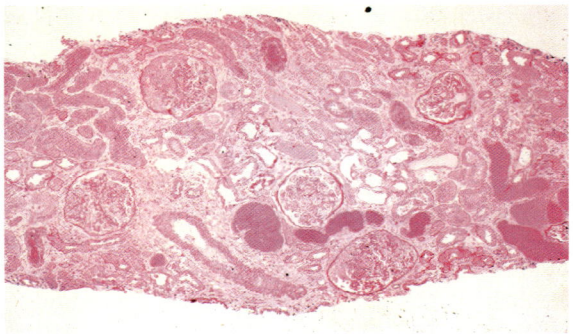

A

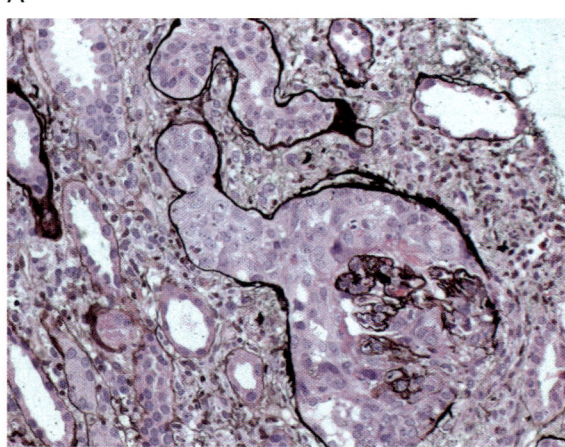

B

Figure 28.1 Kidney biopsy specimens. (A) Low-power view of a biopsy specimen from a patient with HIVAN in the USA. There are 5 glomeruli with collapsing sclerosis and podocyte hyperplasia. The tubules are separated by edema, mild fibrosis and patchy interstitial inflammatory infiltrates. Some tubules show degenerative changes with focal tubular microcysts containing large casts. (B) High-power view of a biopsy specimen from a patient with HIVAN in Brazil. Note the collapsing sclerotic glomerulus, tubular atrophy, and interstitial inflammation. (Courtesy of C.E. Poli de Figueiredo, MD, DPhil, Medical School PUCRS, Porto Alegre, Brazil.)

> **Box 28.1**
>
> **Diagnosis in HIV-infected patients with proteinuria**
>
> - HIV-associated nephropathy[a]
> - Membranoproliferative GN (often with HCV)[a]
> - Mesangioproliferative GN
> - Immune complex GN
> - Membranous nephropathy
> - IgA Nephropathy
> - Post-infectious GN
> - Minimal change disease
> - Diabetic nephropathy
> - Tubulointerstitial nephritis
> - Thrombotic microangiopathy
> - Amyloidosis
>
> [a]Most common pathologic findings.

other GN; 3% had tubulointerstitial nephritis; 3% had acute tubular necrosis and 3% other.[27] However, among hospitalized HIV-infected patients with acute renal failure, the most common diagnosis is acute tubular necrosis.

Clinical Manifestations and Diagnosis

Among patients with HIVAN, severe proteinuria (often in the nephrotic range >3 g/day) with progression to ESRD within 1–4 months of diagnosis was initially described.[1,2,7,8,28] Subsequent data in the setting of monotherapy with zidovudine and HAART suggests a much slower progression.[25,28,29] While early reports suggested that HIVAN was a late manifestation of AIDS, occurring when CD4 counts were well below 200×10^6 cells/L, subsequent data suggests that a lower CD4 count may be associated with a faster progression and greater likelihood of biopsy.[22,25] A case report of HIVAN demonstrates its presence as early as the time of acute HIV seroconversion.[30] Most patients with HIVAN do not have significant peripheral edema and despite the high prevalence of hypertension in blacks, patients with HIVAN are not usually hypertensive. Laboratory data are nonspecific in HIVAN. Serologic studies for glomerular diseases (i.e. ANA, complements, Antistreptolysin O antibodies, ANCA, anti-GBM, cryoglobulins) are usually negative except for in patients with Hepatitis C co-infection. Ultrasonography will typically reveal bilaterally echogenic and enlarged kidneys in contrast to other conditions where the

(GN), followed by immune complex GN, membranous, and IgA nephropathy.[17,25] Less commonly, patients with HIV have been found to have thrombotic microangiopathy, minimal change disease, and amyloidosis.[25,26] This is in comparison to patients seen in Baragwanath, South Africa. Among 64 HIV-infected patients, 39% had classic HIVAN; 14% had immune complex rich 'lupus-like' disease; 38% had other glomerulonephritides (GN) including 13% membranous, 9% post-infectious GN, 6% IgA nephropathy, 5% mesangioproliferative GN, 5%

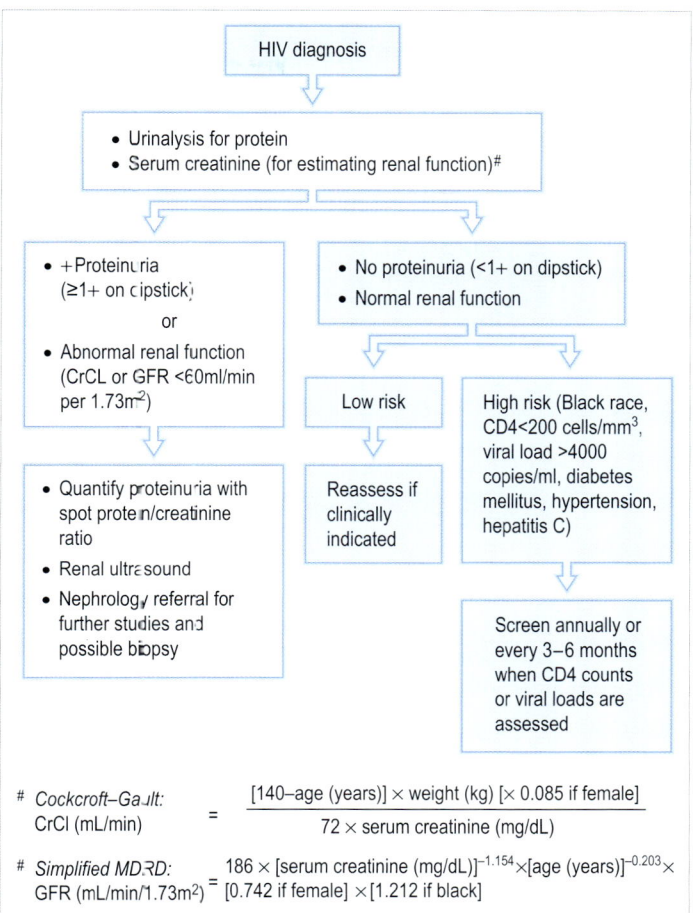

Figure 28.2 Screening algorithm for kidney disease in HIV-infected patients. (Adapted from Gupta SK, Eustace JA, Winston JA, et al. Guidelines for the management of chronic kidney disease in HIV-infected patients: recommendations of the HIV Medicine Association of the Infectious Diseases Society of America. Clin Infect Dis 2005; 40:1559–1585.)

kidneys shrink in size as function deteriorates. Diagnosis of specific histology requires a renal biopsy. Figure 28.3 proposes a screening algorithm for kidney disease in HIV-infected patients.

Pathogenesis

Early in the description of HIVAN, it was uncertain whether HIV-1 caused injury through a direct effect on renal cells or an indirect effect from immune dysregulation. Studies by Bruggeman and co-workers using a murine model of HIVAN, demonstrated that HIV-1 expression in renal epithelial cells is necessary for the development of the HIVAN phenotype.[31] They went on to demonstrate that both tubular and glomerular epithelial cells are infected by HIV-1 in patients with HIVAN.[32] Furthermore, Marras and co-workers demonstrated that the renal tubular epithelial cells support viral replication, subsequent divergence, and act as a separate compartment from blood.[33] Based on a study by Winston and co-workers, renal parenchymal cells can serve as a reservoir for HIV and the presence of the virus can persist in glomerular and tubular epithelial cells despite antiviral therapy.[34]

The mechanisms by which HIV-1 gains entry into epithelial cells remains unclear. The major co-receptors for HIV-1 have not been detected using immunocytochemistry but more sensitive methods including PCR suggest that CD4 and CXCR4 can be detected in cultured renal epithelial cells.[35] The data are less clear for the other co-receptors. Whether the receptors are in sufficiently high density or functional enough to mediate entry into the cell also remains unknown.[35]

The observation that HIV DNA has been found in glomeruli of HIV-infected patients without HIVAN suggests that some additional factor (such as a genetic predisposition) may be required.[36] The pathologic findings of collapsing focal glomerulosclerosis combined with tubular microcystic disease has been thought to be specific to HIVAN. However, a recent report of collapsing GN in seven Caucasian HIV negative patients who were treated with high dose pamidronate suggests that other environmental agents can also induce collapse.[37] Thus, Caucasian patients can develop a collapsing phenotype but the mechanism appears to be different from those observed in response to HIV infection in blacks.

The racial predilection for HIVAN in blacks strongly suggests that genetic factors play an important role in the pathogenesis of HIVAN. In support of this, Gharavi and co-workers assessed the influence of genetic background on the development or progression of HIVAN by crossing the HIVAN transgenic mouse with mice of different genetic backgrounds.[38] These investigators found that the HIVAN phenotype varied from severe renal disease to no renal disease based on the background strain of the mice. In addition, genome-wide analysis of linkage in 185 heterozygous transgenic backcross mice identified a locus on chromosome 3A1-3, HIVAN1, that showed highly significant linkage to renal disease. This locus, HIVAN1, is syntenic to human chromosome 3q25-27, which is an interval showing suggestive evidence of linkage to various nephropathies.[38]

Treatment

Despite the high prevalence of kidney disease in HIV-infected patients, no prospective randomized controlled trials have been performed to assess the effect of various treatments on outcome. However, a number of retrospective analyses have been performed to assess the association between antiretroviral therapy, angiotensin-converting enzyme inhibitors, and steroids and outcomes (Box 28.2).

Antiretroviral Therapy

Initial reports of the efficacy of monotherapy with zidovudine on HIVAN were conflicting. FSGS was noted to develop in many patients despite treatment with zidovudine and thus it was suggested to be of little benefit.[39] Other studies suggested that zidovudine might delay the progression of HIV nephropathy if begun when patients had mild proteinuria and near normal renal function.[28] In a retrospective cohort of 19 patients with a clinical diagnosis of

---

Box 28.2

Management of kidney disease in HIV-infected patients[a]

- Control blood pressure to <130/80, initial agents should be ACE inhibitors for patients with proteinuria
- Prepare for dialysis by placing dialysis access
- Discuss renal transplantation
- If proven HIVAN, treat with HAART
- If patient with HIVAN fails to respond to HAART, consider adding ACE inhibitor (if not already initiated) and/or prednisone

[a]Adapted from Gupta SK, Eustace JA, Winston JA, et al. Guidelines for the management of chronic kidney disease in HIV-infected patients: recommendations of the HIV Medicine Association of the Infectious Diseases Society of America. Clin Infect Dis 2005; 40:1559–1585.

HIVAN, protease inhibitor usage has also been associated with a slower decline in creatinine clearance (−0.08 mL/min per month versus −4.30 mL/min per month for those not administered one of these drugs).[29] In another analysis, among patients with HIVAN, the use of antiretroviral therapy (ART) was associated with a slower progression to end-stage renal disease (HR 0.24, $P = 0.03$).[25] Despite a variety of study designs, it would appear that these reports are generally consistent in that either suppression of viral replication or ART slows the progression of renal disease among patients with HIVAN.

Among HIV-infected patients with renal disease other than HIVAN, a single study suggests that antiretroviral therapy may not be associated with a similar benefit.[25] Additional studies to confirm this are required.

Angiotensin-converting Enzyme Inhibitors

ACE inhibitors have been shown to be efficacious in a variety of renal disorders associated with proteinuria, such as diabetes mellitus. In patients with HIVAN, retrospective analyses suggest that the use of ACE-I is associated with improved renal survival. Kimmel and co-workers reported a delayed progression of renal failure in a retrospective cohort of nine patients with HIVAN compared with a group of controls.[8] Burns and co-workers prospectively evaluated 20 patients with 'early' HIVAN (baseline creatinine <2.0 mg/dL, 177 μmol/L) all of whom were offered fosinopril.[7] In the 12 patients who were compliant with treatment, renal function remained stable at 12 and 24 weeks of follow-up. In the eight untreated patients, serum creatinine increased from 88.4 to 433.2 μmol/L. Long-term effects have also been reported with ACE inhibitors. In a single-center prospective study, 44 patients with biopsy-proven HIVAN and early renal disease (mean serum creatinine <2.0 mg/dL, <177 μmol/L, <50% with proteinuria >3 g/day) were all offered treatment with fosinopril.[40] In the 28 patients who consented to fosinopril, serum creatinine remained stable after a median of 479.5 days of follow-up in all but one patient who progressed to ESRD. All of the 16 patients who refused treatment progressed to ESRD after a median period of 146 days. Initial serum creatinine and proteinuria were similar in both groups but exposure to antiretroviral therapy prior to the study appeared different (57% in the ACE-I group versus 31%, $P = 0.12$) as was CD4 count (172 versus 120 $P = 0.06$).

The potential benefit of ACE-I was also demonstrated by Gertholtz among 64 patients with HIV who underwent renal biopsy in South Africa.[27] In 26 patients with HIVAN, use of an ACE-I was associated with improved renal survival ($P = 0.00026$). All patients progressed to ESRD by 15 weeks of follow-up in the absence of ACE-I compared with 30% with ESRD at 160 weeks of follow-up in the ACE-I treated group. As patients were not randomized to treatment groups, baseline characteristics were different and included a lower creatinine (448 μmol/L versus 1082 μmol/L), higher albumin, and higher cholesterol level in the ACE-I group. ACE-I therapy appeared to have no effect on proteinuria.[27] As only six patients in this cohort were taking antiretrovirals, further research is required to define the benefit of ACE-I among patients using HAART.

Steroids

Initial observations in children with HIVAN suggested corticosteroids to be ineffective. However, later research has found that select patients may respond to therapy.[4,41] In a retrospective cohort, 13 of 21 patients with biopsy proven HIVAN received corticosteroids for one month followed by a steroid taper over several months. Seven patients treated with corticosteroids stayed off dialysis at 6 months of follow-up compared with only one of the non-corticosteroid group ($P = 0.06$).[4] A second group reported a series of 20 patients (17 with biopsy proven HIVAN) who were treated with prednisone 60 mg/day for 2–11 weeks followed by a slow taper.

After a mean follow-up of 44 weeks, eight patients required maintenance dialysis, 11 died from AIDS-related complications, and seven were alive and free from dialysis.[41] Unfortunately, in both groups, infectious related complications were high. Gertholtz retrospectively analyzed patients in South Africa with kidney disease and HIV and found that prednisone had no effect on outcome.[27] Szczech and co-workers retrospectively studied 19 patients with suspected HIVAN or other HIV-related lesions. The five patients who received prednisone experienced an increase in creatinine clearance of 5.57 mL/min per month, whereas the 14 patients who did not receive prednisone experienced a decline in creatinine clearance of 3.32 ml/min per month ($P = 0.003$).[29] Given the small number of observational studies, the short follow-up and the likelihood of relapse and adverse events, definitive conclusions cannot be made regarding the efficacy or safety of steroids for the treatment of HIVAN.

Renal Replacement Therapy

With the rapid progression of renal failure in patients with HIVAN, renal replacement therapy (RRT) becomes the major therapeutic option. Unfortunately, the availability of RRT to patients with ESRD is not uniform globally. The availability of dialysis and transplantation are particularly variable in Africa. According to the Dialysis registry (1994–1998), only 32 patients were on renal replacement therapy in the Congo, seven in Namibia, 350 in Sudan, and >3000 in South Africa. Treatment rates in South Africa are 99 per million population as compared with treatment rates in North Africa which are 30–186.5 per million population (pmp).[12,15] This is in contrast to the 2002 treatment rates in the USA at 1432 per million population[3] and Europe at 438 pmp (Iceland) to 1081 pmp (Spain).[26] Dialysis services are predominantly available only in urban regions in Africa and are thus inaccessible to poorer, rural patients.[12]

In South Africa, there is strict rationing of dialysis due to the lack of resources and funding. The National Health Department has formalized a protocol for the management of ESRD: state facilities will only offer patients long-term dialysis if they are eligible for a kidney transplant. Currently, HIV-infected patients with acute renal failure may be supported by dialysis on a short-term basis but HIV-infected patients are not candidates for renal transplantation and subsequently are not offered long-term dialysis.[12]

Dialysis and transplant programs in the rest of Africa are dependent of the availability of funding and donors. Nigeria, Tanzania, Ethiopia, Cote d'Ivoire, and Cameroon offer very limited dialysis to a small number of patients for short time periods. Peritoneal dialysis is limited due to the high cost of peritoneal fluids and the high rate of peritonitis.[14]

Course and Outcome

In the absence of treatment with antiretroviral therapy, reports from the early 1990s suggest patients' progress to ESRD within 1–4 months of diagnosis.[7,8,28] Subsequent data in the setting of monotherapy with zidovudine and HAART suggests a much slower progression.[25,28,29] Clinical variables associated with increased risk of progressive renal failure include decreased CD4 count[22,25] elevated serum creatinine,[25] increased proteinuria,[22] higher viral HIV-1 viral load[22,25] and the presence of Hepatitis C co-infection.[25]

Patients with a pathologic diagnosis of HIVAN had worse renal survival compared with patients with lesions other than HIVAN. In a cohort of 89 HIV-infected patients with renal disease biopsied between 1995 and 2000, 17 of 47 patients with lesions other than HIVAN required the institution of renal replacement therapy at an average time of 731 days (±642 days) from renal biopsy as compared to 25/42 patients with HIVAN who required initiation of renal replacement therapy at an average time of 254 days (±331 days) from renal biopsy ($P = 0.0003$ comparing time with initiation of renal replacement therapy).[25] The prolonged renal survival of patients with HIVAN as compared to earlier reports is arguably related to a number of factors including the use of ART and HAART.

In a retrospective review of 64 HIV-infected patients in Baragwanath, Africa, who underwent renal biopsy, the investigator could not distinguish a difference in renal or overall survival between patients with HIVAN and those with other pathologic findings. In the 25 South African patients with biopsy proven HIVAN at 28 weeks of follow-up, 9/25 (36%) died, 8/25 (32%) were lost to follow-up and the remaining 8/25 (32%) were free of dialysis. In 27 HIV-infected patients with other pathologic diagnosis at an average of 10–30 weeks of follow-up, 15/27 (55%) died, 3/27 (11%) were lost to follow-up, and the remaining 9/27 (33%) were free of dialysis.[27] Further research to understand the effect of international differences in populations is required to reconcile these conflicting results.

In the USA, ESRD patients with HIVAN have decreased overall survival when compared with other patients with ESRD. In an analysis of 3374 incident patients with ESRD in 1996, patients with a diagnosis of HIVAN ($n = 36$) had a 4.74-fold increased risk of mortality after adjusting for clinical variables other than HIV. The 1-year survival in this cohort of patients with HIVAN was 53%, however more recent data from 1999–2000 report a 1-year survival of up to 74% in dialysis patients with HIVAN which may reflect the benefit of HAART in this patient population.[42] Unfortunately, dialysis is not always available for HIV-infected patients with renal failure; thus, in the absence of other life-threatening illnesses, life expectancy can be drastically shortened.

Conclusion

Kidney disease in HIV-infected patients is common, and HIVAN is the leading cause of CKD, particularly in patients of African descent. Patients with HIVAN are often diagnosed late in the course of their HIV illness and present with proteinuria and renal insufficiency. Without treatment, renal survival is only a few months. However, small clinical trials and epidemiologic data strongly suggest a benefit of HAART therapy in the treatment of HIVAN.[25,28,29] In addition, similar studies have noted ACE-I therapy is associated with improved renal survival.[7,8,27,40] Based on the best available data, if ACE-I and HAART are available, they should be utilized to try to prolong renal survival in these patients. As countries become more developed and HAART becomes more widely available through the World Health Organization AIDS initiative, patients can be anticipated to live longer and an increasing number of HIV-infected patients will have advanced kidney failure. Decisions regarding renal replacement therapy including transplantation are going to become significant issues as cost and resources are limited in a significant number of geographic areas.

References

1. Gardenswartz MH, Lerner CW, Seligson GR, et al. Renal disease in patients with AIDS: a clinicopathologic study. Clin Nephrol 1984; 21:197–204.
2. Rao TK, Filippone EJ, Nicastri AD, et al. Associated focal and segmental glomerulosclerosis in the acquired immunodeficiency syndrome. N Engl J Med 1984; 310:669–673.
3. Renal Data Systems US. USRDS 2003 Annual data report: Atlas of end-stage renal disease in the United States. Bethesda, MD: National Institutes of Health, National

Institute of Diabetes and Digestive and Kidney Diseases; 2003.

4. Eustace JA, Nuermberger E, Choi M, et al. Cohort study of the treatment of severe HIV-associated nephropathy with corticosteroids. Kidney Int 2000; 58:1253–1260.

5. Shahinian V, Rajaraman S, Borucki M, et al. Prevalence of HIV-associated nephropathy in autopsies of HIV-infected patients. Am J Kidney Dis 2000; 35:884–888.

6. WHO. The World Health Report 2004 – Health systems: improving performance, Annex Table 6. Geneva: World Health Organization; 2004.

7. Burns GC, Paul SK, Toth IR, et al. Effect of angiotensin-converting enzyme inhibition in HIV-associated nephropathy J Am Soc Nephrol 1997; 8:1140–1146.

8. Kimmel PL, Mishkin GJ, Umana WO. Captopril and renal survival in patients with human immunodeficiency virus nephropathy Am J Kidney Dis 1996; 28:202–208.

9. Selik RM, Byers RE Jr, Dworkin MS. Trends in diseases reported on U.S. death certificates that mentioned HIV infections, 1987-1999. J Acquir Immune Defic Syndr 2002; 29:378–387.

10. Joint United Nations Programme on HIV/AIDS. Executive Summary: Report on the Global AIDS Epidemic. Geneva: UN; 2004.

11. Agaba EI, Agaba PA, Sirisena ND, et al. Renal disease in the acquired immunodeficiency syndrome in north central Nigeria. Niger J Med 1993; 12:120–125.

12. DoH, South Africa. Nephrology Report 1 and 2: MTS meeting. South Africa: Department of Health; 2003.

13. Mabayoje MO, Bamgboye EL, Odutola TA, et al. Chronic renal failure at the Lagos University Teaching Hospital: A 10 year review. Transplant Proc 1992; 24:1851–1852.

14. Barsoum RS. End-stage renal disease in North Africa. Kidney Int 2003; 3:S111–S114.

15. Naicker S. End-stage renal disease in sub-Saharan and South Africa. Kidney Int 2003; 63:S119–S122.

16. Casanova S, Mazzucco G, Barbiano di Belgiojoso G, et al. Pattern of glomerular involvement in human immunodeficiency virus-infected patients: an Italian study. Am J Kidney Dis 1995; 26:446–453.

17. D'Agati V, Suh JI, Carbone L, et al. Pathology of HIV-associated nephropathy: a detailed morphologic and comparative study. Kidney Int 1989; 35:1358–1370.

18. Hailemariam S, Walder M, Burger HR, et al. Renal Pathology and premortem clinical presentation of Caucasian patients with AIDS: An autopsy study from the era prior to antiretroviral therapy. Swiss Med Wkly 2001; 131:412–417.

19. Monahan M, Tanji N, Klotman PE. HIV-associated nephropathy: An urban epidemic. Semin Nephrol 2001; 21:394–402.

20. Monga G, Mazzucco G, Boldorini R, et al. Renal changes in patients with acquired immunodeficiency syndrome: a post-mortem study on an unselected population in northwestern Italy. Mod Pathol 1997; 10:159–167.

21. Pakasa M, Mangani N, Dikassa L. Focal and segmental glomerulosclerosis in nephrotic syndrome: a new profile of adult nephrotic syndrome in Zaire. Mod Pathol 1993; 62:125–128.

22. Laradi A, Mallet A, Beaufils H, et al. HIV-associated nephropathy: outcome and prognosis factors. Groupe d'Etudes Nephrologiques d'Ile de France. J Am Soc Nephrol 1998; 9:2327–2335.

23. Williams DI, Williams DJ, Williams IG, et al. Presentation, pathology, and outcome of HIV associated renal disease in a specialist centre for HIV/AIDS. Sex Transm Infect 1998; 74:179–184.

24. Stylianou E. Interferons and interferon (IFN-inducible protein 10 during highly active antiretroviral therapy (HAART) – possible immunosuppressive role of IFN-alpha in HIV infection. Clin Exp Immunol 2000; 119:479–485.

25. Szczech LA, Gupta SK, Habash R, et al. The clinical epidemiology and course of the spectrum of renal diseases associated with HIV infection. Kidney Int 2004; 66:1145–1152.

26. ERA-EDTA Registry. 2002 Annual Report. Amsterdam, The Netherlands: Academic Medical Center; 2004: May.

27. Gerntholtz T. The many faces of HIV and kidney disease: clinical and pathological features. Personal communication: Dumisan Mzamane African Institute of Kidney Disease; 2004.

28. Ifudu O, Rao TK, Tan CC, et al. Zidovudine is beneficial in human immunodeficiency virus associated nephropathy. Am J Nephrol 1995; 15:217–221.

29. Szczech LA, Edwards LJ, Sanders LL, et al. Protease inhibitors are associated with a slowed progression of HIV-related diseases. Clin Nephrol 2002; 57:336–341.

30. Levin ML, Palella F, Shah S, et al. HIV-associated nephropathy occurring before HIV antibody seroconversion. Am J Kidney Dis 2001; 37:E39.

31. Bruggeman LA, Dikman S, Meng C, et al. Nephropathy in human immunodeficiency virus-1 transgenic mice is due to renal transgene expression. J Clin Invest 1997; 100:84–92.

32. Bruggeman LA, Ross MD, Tanji N, et al. Renal epithelium is a previously unrecognized site of HIV-1 infection. J Am Soc Nephrol 2001; 11:2079–2087.

33. Marras D, Bruggeman LA, Gao F, et al. Replication and compartmentalization of HIV-1 in kidney epithelium of patients with HIV-associated nephropathy. Nat Med 2002; 8:522–526.

34. Winston JA, Bruggeman LA, Ross MD, et al. Nephropathy and establishment of a renal reservoir of HIV type 1 during primary infection. N Engl J Med 2001; 344:1979–1084.

35. Conaldi PG, et al. HIV-1 kills renal tubular epithelial cells in vitro by triggering an apoptotic pathway involving caspase activation and Fas upregulation. J Clin Invest 1998; 102:2041–2049.

36. Kimmel PL, Ferreira-Centeno A, Farkas-Szallasi T, et al. Viral DNA in microdissected renal biopsy tissue from HIV-infected patients with nephrotic syndrome. Kidney Int 1993; 43:1347–1352.

37. Markowitz GS, Appel GB, Fine PL, et al. Collapsing focal segmental glomerulosclerosis following treatment with high- dose pamidronate. J Am Soc Nephrol 2001; 12:1164–1172.

38. Gharavi AG, Ahmad T, Wong RD, et al. Mapping a locus for susceptibility to HIV-1-associated nephropathy to mouse chromosome 3. Proc Natl Acad Sci USA 2004; 101:2488–2493.

39. Rao TK. Clinical features of human immunodeficiency virus associated nephropathy. Kidney Int 1991; 35:S13–S18.

40. Wei A, Burns GC, Williams BA, et al. Long-term renal survival in HIV-associated nephropathy with angiotensin-converting enzyme inhibition. Kidney Int 2003; 64:1462–1471.

41. Smith MC, Austen JL, Carey JT, et al. Prednisone improves renal function and proteinuria in human immunodeficiency virus-associated nephropathy. Am J Med 1996; 101:41–48.

42. Ahuja TS, Grady J, Khan S. Changing trends in the survival of dialysis patients with human immunodeficiency virus in the United States. J Am Soc Nephrol 2002; 13:1889–1893.

CHAPTER 29

Pneumocystis Pneumonia

J. Lucian Davis
Laurence Huang

Introduction

Prior to the HIV/AIDS epidemic, *Pneumocystis* pneumonia (PCP) was an unusual cause of pneumonia, occurring almost exclusively in immunocompromised persons. In 1981, the description of PCP in previously healthy men who either had sex with other men (MSM) and/or who were injection drug users (IDU) heralded the onset of the HIV/AIDS epidemic that currently affects greater than 40 million people worldwide. Since these initial reports, tremendous advances have occurred in our understanding of HIV infection and PCP. This chapter focuses on the clinical aspects of PCP, our current understanding, and emerging concepts of clinical importance to the global community.

Incidence

Although its incidence has declined dramatically, PCP remains the leading AIDS-defining opportunistic infection in the USA and in the countries that comprise the World Health Organization (WHO) Western European Region.[1] PCP is also a frequent opportunistic infection in HIV-infected patient cohorts, and it is an important cause of HIV-associated mortality.[2] Of concern, PCP is increasingly described in Africa, Asia, and Latin America, regions of the world where >90% of the estimated people living with HIV/AIDS reside and where access to combination antiretroviral therapy and even PCP prophylaxis with trimethoprim-sulfamethoxazole (co-trimoxazole) are limited (Table 29.1). At present, most of the data on PCP in these regions is limited to single institution studies.[3] These studies include different study designs, study populations, diagnostic procedures, and specific criteria for defining PCP (clinical versus microscopic confirmation) that limit firm conclusions. Nevertheless, in contrast to early reports from both clinical and autopsy studies, PCP appears to be a frequent opportunistic infection in HIV-infected people throughout the world, including Africa. Importantly, a substantial proportion of these HIV-infected patients with PCP have been found to have concurrent tuberculosis, a finding that complicates the diagnosis and treatment.[4] As the HIV/AIDS epidemic progresses in these regions, it is increasingly important to develop diagnostic and treatment algorithms that can be used in settings where resources, diagnostic tests, and medications are limited.

Risk Factors for *Pneumocystis* Pneumonia

A CD4-lymphocyte count <200 cells/μL, a history of oropharyngeal candidiasis, and prior PCP are all well-established risk factors for PCP.[5] PCP was perhaps the first disease to document the role of the CD4-lymphocyte count as a tool to assess the risk for the development of an HIV-associated opportunistic infection.[6] Several studies demonstrate that the risk of PCP is increased in persons with a CD4-lymphocyte count <200 cells/μL and that the majority of PCP cases occur in patients whose CD4 count is <200 cells/μL.[6,7] Thus, a CD4 count that is significantly >200 cells/μL argues against the presence of PCP. Unfortunately, CD4-lymphocyte determination is unavailable in many areas of the world and clinicians are left to infer the degree of immunocompromise from indirect measures including absolute lymphocyte count.

Table 29.1 Clinical and autopsy studies of undifferentiated pneumonia in Africa, Asia, and Latin America

Reference	Subjects	Specimen(s)	Stain	Proportion with PCP	Proportion with other lung diseases
Autopsy studies of pneumonia in children in Africa					
Ansari NA et al., Pediatr Infect Dis J 2003	Cross-sectional autopsy study of 35 HIV+ children who died in hospital in Francistown, Botswana, 1997–1998	Lung	MS	31%	CMV 23% TB 11% RSV 11%
Rennert WP et al., Clin Infect Dis 2002	Cross-sectional study of 93 HIV-antibody+ children (CDC AIDS category B & C, advanced) dying of lung disease in Soweto, South Africa, 1998–1999	Core Bx	MS IF Ab	11%	CMV 32% BPNA 14% TB 4.3%
Chintu C et al., Lancet 2002	Cross-sectional autopsy study of 180 HIV+ children dying in hospital in Lusaka, Zambia, 1997–2000	Lung	MS	29%	BPNA 41% CMV 22% TB 18%
Nathoo KJ et al., Trans R Soc Trop Med Hyg 2001	Cross-sectional, autopsy study of 24 HIV-antibody+ children dying of pneumonia in Harare, Zimbabwe, 1995	FNA & Core Bx	Giemsa MS PCR	67%	BPNA 33% CMV 10%
Ikeogu MO et al., Arch Dis Child 1997	Cross-sectional, autopsy study of 122 HIV-antibody+ (43 with clinical AIDS) children dying on arrival to hospital in Bulawayo, Zimbabwe, 1992–1993	Lung	MS	16%	BPNA 86% TB 4%
Lucas SB et al., BMJ 1996	Cross-sectional, autopsy study of 78 HIV+ children dying in hospital in Abidjan, Ivory Coast, 1991–1992	Lung	N/A	14%	BPNA 42% CMV 31% TB 1.3%
Jeena PM et al., Ann Trop Paediatr 1996	Prospective case-control, autopsy of 31 HIV+ infants dying in intensive care units in Durban, South Africa, 1993–1994	ETA Core Bx	MS IF Ab PCR	52%	CMV 29% BPNA 26% TB 3.2%
Clinical studies of pneumonia in children in Africa					
Kouakoussui A et al., Paed Resp Rev 2004	Prospective study of 98 HIV+ children (mean CD4 363) before initiation of antiretroviral therapy in a clinic in Abidjan, Ivory Coast, 2000–2003	N/A	N/A	0.36 per 100 child-months	LRTI 6.07, TB 0.71 per 100
Ruffini DD et al., AIDS 2002	105 HIV+ infants (mean CD4% 20%, 27% on PCP prophylaxis) in hospital with severe pneumonia, 18 undergoing autopsy in Soweto, South Africa, 1999	IS NPA Core Bx	MS IF Ab	49%	CMV 44% Viral 8.3% TB 2.9%
Madhi SA et al., Clin Infect Dis 2002	Cross-sectional study of 231 episodes of pneumonia in 185 HIV+ children (33% on PCP prophylaxis) in hospital in Soweto, South Africa, 2000–2001	IS & NPA	IF Ab	44% of all episodes	Viral 12% BPNA 8.1%
Zar HJ et al., Acta Paediatr 2001	Cross-sectional study of 151 HIV+ children admitted to an intensive care unit with pneumonia in Soweto, South Africa, 1998	NPA IS Lavage	MS IF Ab	9.9%	BPNA 47% CMV 14% TB 7.3%
Madhi SA et al., Clin Infect Dis 2000	Cross-sectional study of 548 HIV-antibody+ infants (25% CDC AIDS class C) in hospital with severe LRTI in Soweto, South Africa, 1997–1998	Clinical	N/A	15%	BPNA 15%

Study	Description	Specimen	Method	PCP	Other findings
Graham SM et al., Lancet 1999	Cross-sectional study of 93 HIV+ children in hospital with severe pneumonia (WHO criteria) in Blantyre, Malawi, 1996	NPA	IF Ab	17%	BPNA 13%
Kamiya Y et al., Arch Dis Child 1997	Cross-sectional study of 19 infants with clinical AIDS and acute LRTI in Lilongwe, Malawi, 1995	NPA	IF Ab	16%	N/A

Autopsy studies of pneumonia in adults in Africa

Study	Description	Specimen	Method	PCP	Other findings
Ansari NA et al., Int J Tuberc Lung Dis 2002	Cross-sectional, autopsy study of 104 HIV+ adults dying in hospital in Francistown, Botswana, 1997–1998	Lung	MS	11%	TB 40%, BPNA 23%, KS 11%
Lucas SB et al., AIDS 1993	Cross-sectional, autopsy study of 247 HIV+ adults dying in hospital in Abidjan, Ivory Coast, 1991–1992	Lung	MS	2.8%	TB 38%, Nocardia 4%
Abouya YL et al., Am Rev Respir Dis 1992	Cross-sectional, autopsy study of 53 HIV+ adults dying on a pulmonary ward in Abidjan, Ivory Coast, 1989	Lung	MS	9.4%	TB 40%, KS 5.7%

Clinical studies of pneumonia in adults in Africa

Study	Description	Specimen	Method	PCP	Other findings
Zouiten F et al., AIDS 2002	Cross-sectional study of 92 HIV+ women seen in a specialty clinic in Tunis, Tunisia, 1986–2001	N/A	N/A	12%	BPNA 25%, TB 6.5%
Corbett EL et al., Clin Infect Dis 2002	Prospective study of 1792 HIV+ adult men in Welkom, South Africa, 599 in hospital, 1998–1999	N/A	MS	1.3%	TB 21%, PNA 17%
Karstaedt AS et al., Trans R Soc Trop Med Hyg 2001	Retrospective case series of 120 adults with AIDS (median CD4 38) in hospital with PCP in Soweto, South Africa, 1996–1998	IS 54% ES 42% BAL 4%	IF Ab	N/A	TB 19%, BPNA 12%
Daley CL et al., Am J Respir Crit Care Med 1996	Cross-sectional study of 127 HIV + adults in hospital with respiratory symptoms in Dar es Salaam, Tanzania, 1991–1993	BAL 25%	N/A	0.8%	TB 75%, BPNA 14%
Sow PS et al., AIDS 1993	Cross-sectional study of 27 HIV+ adults (56%, CD4 <200) in hospital in Dakar, Senegal, 1992	IS	Tol Blue	22%	N/A
Cheval P et al., Med Trop (Mars) 1993	Cross-sectional study of 307 HIV+ patients (78% WHO Stage 3 or 4, advanced AIDS) in hospital in Pointe-Noire, Republic of Congo, 1989–1991	N/A	N/A	4.9%	N/A
Atzori C et al., Trans R Soc Trop Med Hyg 1993	Cross-sectional study of 83 HIV+ adults in hospital for respiratory symptoms in Malenga Makali, Tanzania, 1991	IS	Tol Blue MS	6%	TB 39%
Karstaedt AS, S Afr Med J 1992	Cross-sectional study of 181 HIV + adults (51% with AIDS) in Soweto, South Africa, 1987–1990	N/A	N/A	0.5%	TB 15%
Serwadda D et al., AIDS 1989	Cross-sectional study of 40 HIV+ patients with fever, pulmonary infiltrates in Kampala, Uganda, 1987–1988	BAL	Giemsa MS	0%	BPNA 12%, TB 15%
Carme B et al., Bull Soc Pathol Exot Filiales 1988	Cross-sectional study of 104 HIV+ adults (AIDS WHO Stage 4) on a pulmonary ward in Brazzaville, Republic of Congo, 1986–1987	Clinical[3]	N/A	<8.6%	BPNA 45%, TB 44%

Table 29.1 Clinical and autopsy studies of undifferentiated pneumonia in Africa, Asia, and Latin America—cont'd

Reference	Subjects	Specimen(s)	Stain	Proportion with PCP	Proportion with other lung diseases
Zouiten F et al., AIDS 2002	Cross-sectional study of 92 HIV+ women seen in a specialty clinic in Tunis, Tunisia, 1986–2001	N/A	N/A	12%	BPNA 25% TB 6.5%
Corbett EL et al., Clin Infect Dis 2002	Prospective study of 1792 HIV+ adult men in Welkom, South Africa, 599 in hospital, 1998–1999	N/A	MS	1.3%	TB 21% PNA 17%
Karstaedt AS et al., Trans R Soc Trop Med Hyg 2001	Retrospective case series of 120 adults with AIDS (median CD4 38) in hospital with PCP in Soweto, South Africa, 1996–1998	IS 54% ES 42% BAL 4%	IF Ab	N/A	TB 19% BPNA 12%
Daley CL et al., Am J Respir Crit Care Med 1996	Cross-sectional study of 127 HIV + adults in hospital with respiratory symptoms in Dar es Salaam, Tanzania, 1991–1993	BAL 25%	N/A	0.8%	TB 75% BPNA 14%

Clinical studies of pulmonary disease of undetermined etiology in adults in Africa

Reference	Subjects	Specimen(s)	Stain	Proportion with PCP	Proportion with other lung diseases
Worodria W et al., Int J Tuberc Lung Dis 2003	Cross-sectional study of 83 HIV+ adults with 3-week history of undiagnosed lung disease in hospital in Kampala, Uganda, 1999–2000	BAL	IF Ab	39%	TB 24% BPNA19%
Aderaye G et al., AIDS 2003	Cross-sectional study of 199 HIV+ adults in hospital for undiagnosed lung disease, in Addis Ababa, Ethiopia, 1996	ES	IF Ab PCR	30%	N/A
Lockman S et al., Int J Tuberc Lung Dis 2003	Cross-sectional study of 121 HIV+ adults, most in hospital, with undiagnosed lung disease in Gaborone and Francistown, Botswana, 1997	IS	Tol Blue MS PCR	3.3%	TB 50% BPNA 25%
Chakaya JM et al., East Afr Med J 2003	Cross-sectional study of 51 HIV+ adults in hospital with undiagnosed lung disease in Nairobi, Kenya, 1999–2000	BAL	Tol Blue IF Ab	37%	BPNA 37%
Hargreaves NJ et al., Trans R Soc Trop Med Hyg 2001	Cross-sectional study of 164 HIV+ adults with undiagnosed lung disease in Lilongwe, Malawi, 1997–1999	BAL	IF Ab PCR	9.1%	TB 39%
Mahomed AG et al., East Afr Med J 1999	Cross-sectional study of 67 HIV+ adults with undiagnosed lung disease, IS negative for PCP, in Johannesburg, South Africa, 1985–1992	BAL & TBBx	Tol Blue MS	43%	TB 13%
Dieng Y et al., Dakar Med 1999	Cross-sectional study of 29 HIV+ adults in hospital for undiagnosed lung disease in Dakar, Senegal, 1996–1997	BAL	Tol Blue Giemsa	6.9%	N/A
Malin AS et al., Am J Respir Crit Care Med 1994	Cross-sectional study of 64 HIV+ adults (median CD4 183) in hospital with undiagnosed lung disease in Harare, Zimbabwe, 1992–1993	BAL	Tol Blue Giemsa MS, PCR	33%	TB 39% KS 9.3% CMV 1.6%
Batungwanayo J et al., Am J Respir Crit Care Med 1994	Prospective cohort study of 111 HIV+ adults (42% with AIDS by WHO criteria) with undiagnosed lung disease in Kigali, Rwanda, 1990	BAL & TBBx	Giemsa MS	5%	TB 23% Crypto 11% KS 8.1%

Autopsy studies of pneumonia in adults and children in Asia

Reference	Study	Specimen	Stain	%	Other
Hsiao CH et al., J Microbiol Immunol Infect 1997	Cross-sectional, autopsy study of 16 adults who died in hospital in Taipei, Taiwan, 1986–1996	Lung	N/A	50%	CMV 88% TB 44%
Bhoopat L et al., Asia Pac J Aller Imm 1994	Cross-sectional, autopsy study of 29 children who died with AIDS in Chiang Mai, Thailand, up to 1994	Lung	N/A	66%	CMV 48% TB 3.4%

Clinical studies of pneumonia in adults and children in Asia

Reference	Study	Specimen	Stain	%	Other
Mishra M et al., Indian J Med Microbiol 2006	Cross-sectional study of 1101 HIV+ adults in hospital in Nagpur, India, 1999–2005	IS	Giemsa Tol Blue MS	25%	N/A
Knauer A et al. Wien Klin Wochenschr, 2005	Cross-sectional study of 59 HIV+ adolescents and adults in hospital with interstitial lung disease in Nonthaburi, Thailand, 2002–2003	Clinical	N/A	25%	TB 44% BP 20% Crypto 8.5%
Udwadia ZF et al., JAPI, 2005	Cross-sectional study of 119 HIV+ adults in hospital with lung disease in Mumbai, India, 2000–2003	N/A BAL	N/A	32%	N/A
Sharma SK et al., BMC Infect Dis, 2004	Cross-sectional study of 135 HIV+ adults in hospital for opportunistic disease in New Delhi, India, 2000–2003	Clinical IS	N/A	7.4%	TB 71% (All sites)
Kay Thwe H et al., SE Asian J Trop Med Pub Health 2003	Cross-sectional study of 60 HIV+ adults (mean CD4 132, not on PCP prophylaxis) with ≥2 weeks of dry cough in Waibargi, Myanmar, 2000–2001	IS	Giemsa MS	30%	TB 17%
Usha MM et al., Indian J Pathol Microbiol 2000	Cross-sectional study of 32 HIV+ adults with AIDS and a respiratory complaint in Chennai, India, up to 1997	IS	Tol Blue Giemsa IF Ab	28%	TB 47%
Mathews MS et al., Indian J Chest Dis Allied Sci 2000	Cross-sectional study of 15 adults with AIDS in Vellore, India, 1992–1997	ETA IS	Tol Blue Giemsa IF Ab	33%	N/A
Lumbiganon P et al., J Med Assc Thai 2000	Prospective cohort study of 90 children with AIDS (WHO criteria) in Khon Kaen, Thailand, 1989–1998	N/A	N/A	36 cases	TB 8 cases
Tansuphasawadikul S et al., AIDS 1999	Cross-sectional study of 2261 HIV+ adults (69% AIDS) in hospital in Nonthaburi, Thailand, 1993–1996	Clinical	N/A	4.8%	TB 37% Pen 3.2%

Autopsy studies of pneumonia in adults and children in Latin America

Reference	Study	Specimen	Stain	%	Other
Cury PM et al., Pathol Res Pract 2003	Cross-sectional, autopsy study of 92 adults who died with AIDS in São Paulo, Brazil, 1993–2000	Lung	MS	17%	TB 27% Histo 5.4% Crypto 4.3%
Drut R et al., Pediatr Pathol Lab Med 1997	Retrospective autopsy case series of 74 children registered in a database after dying of AIDS throughout Latin America, 1992–1994	Lung	N/A	20%	BPNA 15% CMV 5.4% Histo 2.7%

Table 29.1 Clinical and autopsy studies of undifferentiated pneumonia in Africa, Asia, and Latin America—cont'd

Reference	Subjects	Specimen(s)	Stain	Proportion with PCP	Proportion with other lung diseases
Mohar A et al., AIDS 1992	Cross-sectional autopsy study of 177 adults who died with AIDS in Mexico City, Mexico, 1984–1989	Lung	MS	24%	TB 25% (all sites)
Michalany J et al., Ann Pathol 1987	Cross-sectional, autopsy study of 15 adults who died with AIDS in São Paulo, Brazil, 1981–1985	Lung	Giemsa MS	13%	CMV 47% TB 20%
Clinical studies of pneumonia in adults in Latin America					
Chernilo S et al., Rev Med Chil 2005	Cross-sectional study of 236 cases of lung disease in 171 HIV+ adults in hospital Santiago, Chile, 1999–2003	BAL	Stain N/A PCR	38%	BP 24% TB 12% KS 3.3%
Villasis-Keever A et al., Arch Med Res 2001	Cross-sectional study of 909 HIV+ adults in an outpatient clinic in Mexico City, Mexico, 1984–1995	N/A	N/A	18%	TB 18% Histo 1.4% (both all sites)
Lambertucci JR et al., Rev Inst Med Trop São Paulo 1999	Cross-sectional study of 55 adults with AIDS in hospital with fever of undetermined etiology in Minas Gerais, Brazil, 1989–1997	Clinical	N/A	15%	TB 33% Histo 3.6% (both all sites)
Fonseca L et al., Int J Epidemiol 1999	Prospective study of 145 asymptomatic HIV+ adults (mean CD4 492) in São Paulo, Brazil, followed for 4 years between 1985 and 1997	N/A	N/A	17%	TB 19%
Santoro-Lopes G et al., J AIDS Hum Retrovirol 1998	Cross-sectional study of 124 HIV+ adults having newly developed AIDS (mean CD4 88) in hospital in Rio de Janeiro, Brazil, 1991–1995	N/A	N/A	14%	N/A
Rodriguez French A et al., Rev Med Panama 1996	Cross-sectional study of 55 adults with AIDS in hospital for respiratory complaints in Panama City, Panama, 1995	ES or IS TTA BAL	Giemsa MS	45%	N/A
Santos B et al., Int J STD AIDS 1994	Cross-sectional study of 224 adults with AIDS in a referral center in Porto Alegre, Brazil, 1986–1991	N/A	N/A	17%	TB 19% (all sites)
Weinberg A et al., Rev Inst Med Trop São Paulo 1993	Cross-sectional study of 35 HIV+ adults with respiratory complaints in São Paulo, Brazil, 1988–1989	ES BAL TBBx	Tol Blue MS	55%	TB 41% CMV 7.4%
Moreira ED Jr et al., Am J Trop Med Hyg 1993	Cross-sectional study of 111 adults with AIDS in an outpatient clinic in Salvador, Brazil, 1989–1991	Clinical TBBx	MS	22%	TB 24% BPNA 22%

Specimen(s): BAL, bronchoalveolar lavage; BW, bronchial wash; Core Bx, core biopsy; ES, expectorated sputum; ETA, endotracheal aspirate; IS, induced sputum; Lavage, blind BW; Lung, fixed lung tissue; NPA, nasopharyngeal aspirate; TBBx, transbronchial biopsy; TTA, transtracheal aspirate.
Stains: MS, methenamine silver; Tol Blue, toluidine blue O; IF Ab, immunofluorescence antibody; PCR, polymerase chain reaction.
Other lung diseases: BPNA, bacterial pneumonia; CMV, cytomegalovirus; Crypto, cryptococcosis; Histo, histoplasmosis; LRTI, lower respiratory tract infection; PCP, *pneumocystis jirovecii* pneumonia; Pen, penicilliosis; RSV, respiratory syncitial virus; TB, tuberculosis; Viral, other viral infection.
All categories: N/A, Not available.

Clinical Presentation

The clinical presentation of PCP in HIV-infected persons differs from the presentation in other immunocompromised persons. In general, HIV-infected patients present with a sub-acute onset and longer symptom duration than other immunocompromised patients.[8] Compared with non-HIV patients, HIV-infected patients with PCP present with a higher arterial oxygen tension and a lower alveolar-arterial oxygen gradient. In addition, bronchoscopy with bronchoalveclar lavage (BAL) examination reveals significantly greater numbers of *Pneumocystis* organisms and fewer neutrophils in HIV-infected patients.[9]

Symptoms and Signs

Classically, patients with PCP present with fever, cough, and dyspnea of 2–4 weeks duration.[10] The cough is usually dry and non-productive, unless a concurrent bacterial infection is present. Fatigue is a frequent complaint whereas chest pain (unless due to an associated pneumothorax), chills, and night sweats are less frequent complaints. Symptoms are often subtle at the onset but are gradually progressive and may be present for weeks and occasionally months before diagnosis.

Physical examination is non-specific for PCP. Vital signs often reveal an oral temperature >38.5°C, tachypnea, and a decreased oxygen saturation. Typically, the pulmonary examination is unremarkable, even in the presence of significant disease and hypoxemia. One maneuver that has been reported to be sensitive for PCP is the elicitation of a cough after deep inspiration. Bilateral fine inspiratory crackles are the most frequent abnormal finding on auscultation.

Laboratory Tests

No current laboratory test is specific for PCP. The serum lactate dehydrogenase (LDH) is usually elevated in patients with PCP.[11] Published studies report the sensitivity of an elevated serum LDH for PCP to range from 82% to 100%. Unfortunately, the serum LDH is a non-specific test and elevations are seen in many pulmonary and non-pulmonary conditions. The arterial blood gas (ABG) is an essential laboratory test in patients with PCP. PCP patients will usually have a decreased arterial oxygen tension, an increased alveolar-arterial oxygen gradient, and a respiratory alkalosis. The ABG should be used to decide whether to admit a patient to the hospital to receive supplemental oxygen, whether to administer adjunctive corticosteroids (PaO_2 <70 mmHg or an alveolar-arterial oxygen gradient >35 mmHg), and to assess response to PCP therapy. More recently, plasma S-adenosylmethionine (SAM) measurement was reported to be a sensitive test for PCP. In one study, plasma SAM concentration was undetectable in 14 of 15 HIV-infected patients with either histologically confirmed or clinically suspected PCP.[12] The median SAM concentration in these patients was significantly lower than that in healthy control subjects or HIV-infected patients without PCP. In addition, serial SAM concentrations appeared to parallel the clinical course of PCP on treatment. Three PCP patients who responded to treatment had a rise in their SAM concentrations to the normal range. Further studies are warranted to confirm these initial results.

Chest Radiograph

The chest radiograph is the cornerstone of the diagnostic evaluation of patients with suspected PCP. Classically, patients with PCP present with bilateral, diffuse, symmetric reticular (interstitial) or granular opacities on their chest radiograph (Fig. 29.1).[13] PCP

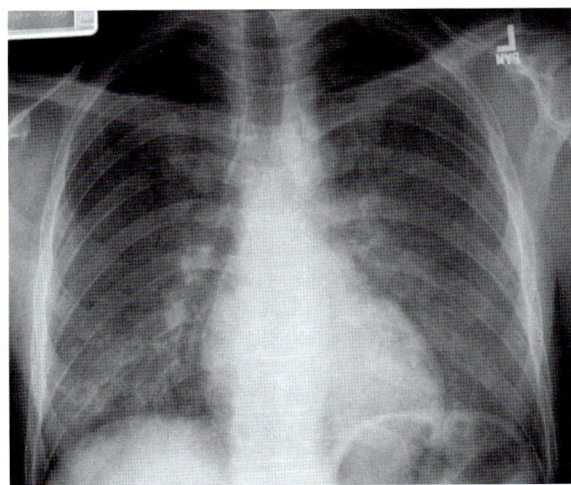

Figure 29.1 Chest radiograph of an HIV-infected person, CD4-lymphocyte count <200 cells/μL demonstrating the characteristic bilateral, diffuse, symmetric reticular-granular opacities of PCP. Bronchoscopy with bronchoalveolar lavage fluid examination revealed *Pneumocystis* organisms.

often begins with central or perihilar opacities and a middle-lower lung zone predominance. As with the classic radiographic presentation, these opacities are bilateral and symmetric and can progress to diffuse involvement if the disease is left undiagnosed and untreated. However, patients with PCP occasionally can present with unilateral, focal, or asymmetric opacities on their chest radiograph and the specific pattern seen is often more important than the exact distribution. Thus, PCP must be considered in any HIV-infected patient who is at risk for PCP, has a compatible clinical presentation, and presents with reticular or granular opacities on chest radiograph, regardless of whether the findings are unilateral or bilateral, focal or diffuse, asymmetric or symmetric. Clearly though, the presence of bilateral, diffuse, and symmetric reticular (interstitial) or granular opacities increases the probability of PCP significantly. In one study, patients who had interstitial infiltrates noted on their radiograph had a 4.4 greater odds of having PCP than those without this pattern and patients who had interstitial infiltrates that involved five or six of the six defined lung zones (upper, middle, and lower lung zones on the right and left lungs) had a 5.3 greater odds of having PCP.[14]

Thin-walled cysts or pneumatoceles are reported in approximately 5–34% of PCP cases. Pneumatoceles may be present at the time of diagnosis, may develop while on therapy, and may persist despite successful therapy. The pneumatoceles may be single or multiple in number and small or large in size. Usually, pneumatoceles are multiple in number and located in the upper lobes. Importantly, the presence of pneumatoceles predisposes patients to the development of pneumothorax, a difficult management problem for clinicians caring for PCP patients. However, pneumothorax may also occur in the absence of radiographically demonstrable pneumatoceles.

Less commonly, patients with PCP may present with a lobar or segmental consolidation, and with cavitary and non-cavitary nodules of varying size. Apical or upper lung zone disease that resembles tuberculosis has been associated with aerosolized pentamidine prophylaxis, although this presentation can also occur in patients receiving other forms of PCP prophylaxis or no preventive therapy. While reported, intrathoracic adenopathy and pleural effusions are rarely due to PCP. The presence of these radiographic findings should prompt a search for an alternate or co-existing process such as bacterial pneumonia, tuberculosis, fungal pneumonia, or pulmonary Kaposi's sarcoma.

Patients with PCP may present with a normal chest radiograph. Published studies report the incidence of this to be in the range of 0–39%. While patients with PCP and a normal chest radiograph have a better prognosis than patients with bilateral diffuse opacities, they often represent a diagnostic challenge and require a timely evaluation before their disease progresses.

There are a few studies on the course of respiratory symptoms and chest radiographic abnormalities in patients successfully treated for PCP.[13,15] Patients with PCP often experience a clinical and radiographic worsening in the first 3–5 days of PCP therapy. In one study of 104 patients with PCP, 46% demonstrated a deterioration in the chest radiograph at 1 week.[13] In this same study, approximately one-third of the patients showed no change in their radiograph over the first 3 weeks. A general rule is that the more severe the PCP, the more prolonged the time to clinical and chest radiographic resolution.

Other Tests

Tests including chest high-resolution computed tomography (presence of ground-glass opacities) (Fig. 29.2), pulmonary function tests (decreased diffusing capacity for carbon monoxide, DLCO), and gallium scanning (increased uptake over the lungs) can all be used in the diagnostic evaluation of patients with suspected PCP.[11] Typically, these studies are performed in patients whose clinical presentation is strongly suggestive of PCP but whose

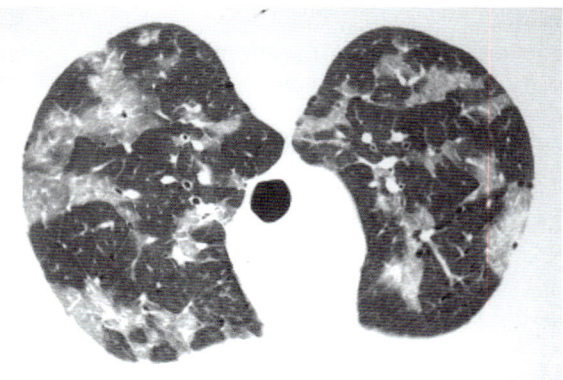

Figure 29.2 Chest high-resolution computed tomographic (HRCT) scan of an HIV-infected person, CD4-lymphocyte count <200 cells/μL, whose chest radiograph was normal. Because of a clinical suspicion for PCP, the patient underwent HRCT, which demonstrated the characteristic patchy ground-glass opacities of PCP. Induced sputum examination revealed *Pneumocystis* organisms.

chest radiograph is normal or minimally abnormal. However, these tests are relatively expensive and typically unavailable in many areas of the world. One simple test for PCP is non-invasive exercise oximetry, since patients with PCP will often have a decline in their oxygen saturation with exertion.

Diagnosis

There is no universally agreed upon approach to the diagnostic evaluation of suspected PCP. Many institutions treat patients with suspected PCP empirically while institutions such as San Francisco General Hospital pursue a definitive microscopic diagnosis (Fig. 29.3).[16] As *Pneumocystis* cannot be routinely cultured, the diagnosis of PCP traditionally relies on microscopic visualization of the characteristic cysts and/or trophic forms on stained respiratory specimens. Typically, these respiratory specimens are obtained from sputum induction or bronchoscopy. However, institutions report different degrees of success with sputum induction and bronchoscopy

with bronchoalveolar lavage (BAL) with and without transbronchial biopsies (TBBx). Recently, advances in polymerase chain reaction (PCR) technology have enabled the use of rapid, non-invasive procedures such as oropharyngeal washing as a method for specimen acquisition. In one study, a non-invasive, 60-s gargle (oropharyngeal wash) specimen paired with a PCR-based quantitative assay had a sensitivity and specificity for PCP of 88% and 85%, respectively.[17] However, in the absence of prospective studies comparing various management and diagnostic strategies, the specific approach to a patient with suspected PCP is often based on the prevalence of PCP, clinician and institutional preferences and experiences, and availability of diagnostic procedures and microbiologic techniques and assays. In areas of the world where tuberculosis is prevalent and where resources are limited, the examination of sputum for acid-fast bacilli may be a prudent diagnostic and public health practice (Fig. 29.4). Studies designed to examine practical, cost-effective diagnostic approaches to the patient with suspected PCP in a resource-limited setting are needed.

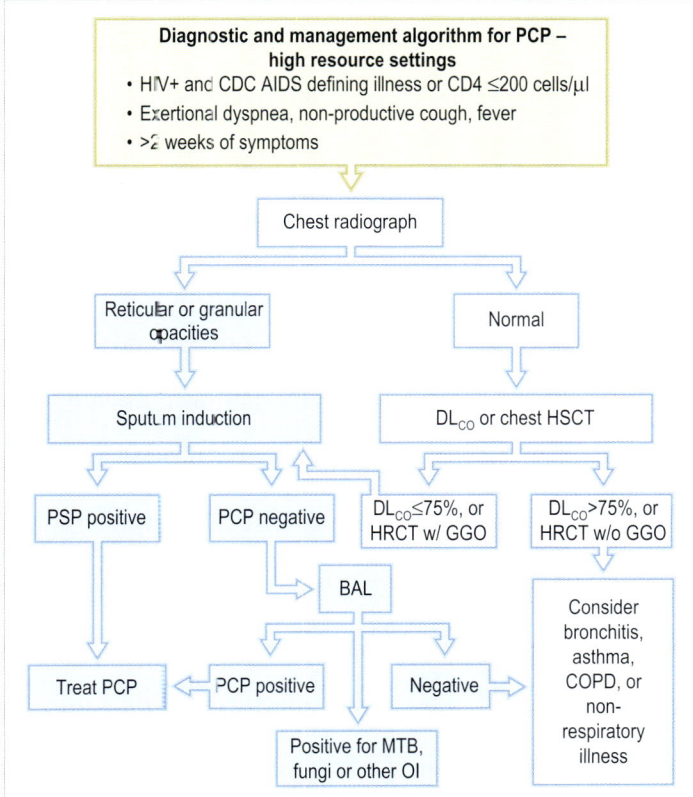

Figure 29.3 Diagnostic algorithm for the evaluation of HIV-infected persons with suspected PCP used at San Francisco General Hospital. CDC, Centers for Disease Control; COPD, chronic obstructive pulmonary disease; DLCO, single-breath diffusing capacity for carbon monoxide; HRCT, high-resolution computed tomography; GGO, ground-glass opacities; BAL, bronchoalveolar lavage; MTB, *Mycobacterium tuberculosis*; OI, opportunistic infection.

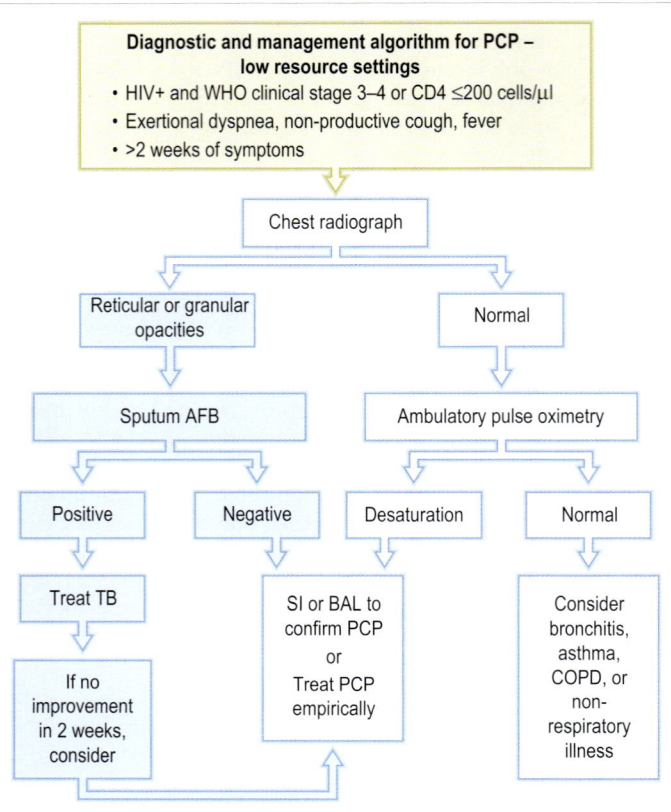

Diagnostic and management algorithm for PCP – low resource settings
- HIV+ and WHO clinical stage 3–4 or CD4 ≤200 cells/μl
- Exertional dyspnea, non-productive cough, fever
- >2 weeks of symptoms

Chest radiograph

Reticular or granular opacities — Normal

Sputum AFB — Ambulatory pulse oximetry

Positive — Negative — Desaturation — Normal

Treat TB

If no improvement in 2 weeks, consider

SI or BAL to confirm PCP or Treat PCP empirically

Consider bronchitis, asthma, COPD, or non-respiratory illness

Figure 29.4 Algorithm for evaluation of HIV-infected persons with suspected PCP in resource-limited settings. AFB, acid-fast bacilli; COPD, chronic obstructive pulmonary disease; SI, sputum induction; BAL, bronchoalveolar lavage; TB, tuberculosis; WHO, World Health Organization.

Treatment

The standard treatment duration for HIV-infected patients with PCP is 21 days.[18] Trimethoprim-sulfamethoxazole is recommended as first-line treatment for PCP (Table 29.2). Trimethoprim and sulfamethoxazole each inhibit an important enzyme in folate metabolism; trimethoprim inhibits dihydrofolate reductase, while sulfamethoxazole inhibits dihydropteroate synthase. Since many microorganisms cannot transport folate into cells as mammalian cells can, most prokaryotes and lower eukaryotes must synthesize folates *de novo*. Thus, the fixed-dose combination of trimethoprim-sulfamethoxazole offers excellent activity against *Pneumocystis* and many other important HIV-associated bacterial and protozoan pathogens. The availability of trimethoprim-sulfamethoxazole in both intravenous and oral formulations, its favorable toxicity profile (compared to intravenous pentamidine), and its low cost are all additional advantages. However, the use of trimethoprim-sulfamethoxazole for PCP prophylaxis has led to concerns over the possible development of

drug resistant *Pneumocystis* as mutations in the dihydropteroate synthase gene are reported in association with prophylaxis use and, in some studies, are associated with increased mortality and increased PCP treatment failure using trimethoprim-sulfamethoxazole.[19–22] Since trimethoprim-sulfamethoxazole is often the only PCP treatment available in many regions of the world, the development of high-level drug resistance may have severe consequences for patients with PCP residing in these resource-limited areas.[23–25]

Intravenous pentamidine isethionate and clindamycin plus primaquine are both effective PCP therapies and should be considered the main alternatives in patients who are allergic to, intolerant of, or failing trimethoprim-sulfamethoxazole.[18] Compared with trimethoprim-sulfamethoxazole, pentamidine has comparable efficacy but is associated with more frequent and severe toxicities that relegate it to second-line status. Clindamycin plus primaquine is reported to be an excellent salvage therapy option for PCP.

Finally, patients with moderate to severe PCP, demonstrated by an oxygen saturation ≤93% or a

Table 29.2 Treatment Options for *Pneumocystis* pneumonia[a]

Treatment regimen	Dose(s), route, frequency	Side-effects
Trimethoprim (TMP)-sulfamethoxazole (SMX) Fixed (1–5 mg) dose	15–20 mg/kg per day (TMP), i.v. or p.o., divided every 6–8 h	GI (nausea, vomiting), rash, fever, cytopenia, elevated liver transaminases, hyperkalemia
Pentamidine isethionate	3–4 mg/kg per day, i.v. (infused slowly over >60 min), once daily	Nephrotoxicity, electrolyte disturbances, pancreatitis, hypo- and hyperglycemia
Clindamycin plus primaquine	300–900 mg, i.v. or p.o., divided every 6–8 h plus 15–30 mg base p.o., once daily	Nausea, vomiting, diarrhea, rash, hemolytic anemia (check G6PD level), methemoglobinemia
Trimetrexate[b] ± Dapsone	45 mg/m² per day, i.v., once daily ±100 mg, p.o., once daily	Cytopenia, rash, fever, elevated liver transaminases, hemolytic anemia (check G6PD level), methemoglobinemia
Trimethoprim plus Dapsone	15 mg/kg per day, p.o., divided every 8 h plus 100 mg, p.o., once daily	Nausea, vomiting, rash, hemolytic anemia (check G6PD level), methemoglobinemia
Atovaquone	750 mg, p.o. (suspension, take with food) twice–thrice daily	Nausea, vomiting, diarrhea, rash

[a]Patients with moderate to severe PCP (PaO₂ <70 mmHg OR an alveolar-arterial oxygen gradient >35 mmHg) should receive adjunctive corticosteroids – either prednisone 40 mg p.o. twice daily ×5 days, then 40 mg p.o. once daily ×5 days, then 20 mg p.o. once daily ×11 days or methylprednisolone equivalent. [b]Trimetrexate must be administered with leucovorin (20 mg/m², p.o., every 6 h). Leucovorin must be continued for 3 days after the last Trimetrexate dose.

PaO_2 <70 mmHg or an alveolar-arterial oxygen gradient >35 mmHg, should receive corticosteroid therapy in addition to specific PCP treatment.[26] Adjunctive corticosteroids, either oral prednisone or intravenous methylprednisolone, should be started at the same time that specific PCP treatment is begun. Several studies document a reduction in respiratory failure and mortality rates in patients randomized to corticosteroids.[26] Thus, the potential survival benefits associated with corticosteroid therapy outweigh the risks of this additional immunosuppressive therapy potentially unmasking an occult opportunistic infection such as tuberculosis.

Prophylaxis

Perhaps the single most effective PCP prevention strategy is the use of combination antiretroviral therapy to increase the CD4-lymphocyte count to above the threshold associated with an increased risk of PCP (200 cells/μL). Multiple studies conclusively demonstrate that the risk of PCP is low in patients whose CD4-lymphocyte count has risen from below to >200 cells/μL as a result of antiretroviral therapy.[5] In these persons, both primary and secondary PCP prophylaxis can be safely discontinued once the CD4-lymphocyte count has remained >200 cells/μL for at least 3 months.[27,28] One exception is that those with a history of PCP that occurred at a CD4-lymphocyte count >200 cells/μL should remain on PCP prophylaxis for life, regardless of the degree of antiretroviral-associated rise in CD4-lymphocyte count.[5]

In regions where antiretroviral therapy is unavailable or in persons who are unable or unwilling to use combination antiretroviral therapy or who are unresponsive to these therapies, PCP prophylaxis is effective at decreasing rates of PCP. Current guidelines recommend that HIV-infected adults and adolescents who have a CD4-lymphocyte count <200 cells/μL or a history of oropharyngeal candidiasis receive primary PCP prophylaxis and those with a history of PCP receive secondary prophylaxis.[5] Adults and adolescents who do not meet these criteria but who have a CD4-lymphocyte percentage of <14% or a prior AIDS-defining illness should be considered for PCP prophylaxis. These recommendations also apply to HIV-infected women who are pregnant. Infants born to HIV-infected mothers should receive prophylaxis at 4–6 weeks of age, until the infant's HIV serostatus can be conclusively deter-

Table 29.3 Prophylaxis options for Pneumocystis pneumonia

Prophylaxis regimen	dose(s), route, frequency	Comment
Trimethoprim (TMP) – sulfamethoxazole (SMX)	1 DS tablet p.o. daily ~ 1 SS tablet p.o. daily > 1 DS tablet p.o. thrice weekly	Regimens listed in recommended order (1st ~ 2nd > 3rd)
Dapsone	100 mg p.o. daily 50 mg p.o. twice daily	May also be combined with pyrimethamine and leucovorin
Atovaquone	1500 mg p.o. daily	
Aerosolized pentamidine	300 mg aerosolized monthly	Via Respirgard II nebulizer

DS, double-strength; SS, single-strength.

mined. Those infants who are subsequently determined to be uninfected with HIV can discontinue prophylaxis. HIV-infected infants and any infant whose HIV serostatus remains unknown should continue to receive prophylaxis for the first year of life. After the first year, the need for subsequent prophylaxis is based on age-specific CD4-lymphocyte count thresholds: for children 1–5 years of age: CD4-lymphocyte count <500 cells/μL or CD4 lymphocyte percentage <15%; children ≥6 years of age: CD4-lymphocyte count <200 cells/μL (as for adults and adolescents) or CD4-lymphocyte percentage <15%. Once started, persons should remain on prophylaxis for life, unless their CD4-lymphocyte counts increase from below to >200 cells/μL for at least 3 months as a result of antiretroviral therapy. As for PCP treatment, trimethoprim-sulfamethoxazole is recommended as first-line prophylaxis against PCP (Table 29.3). Dapsone, atovaquone, and aerosolized pentamidine are all alternatives in patients who are allergic to or intolerant of trimethoprim-sulfamethoxazole.

One final aspect of PCP prevention that warrants additional study is the prevention of exposure to the source of human *Pneumocystis*. Serologic studies suggest that exposure to *Pneumocystis* occurs early in life.[29-31] Unfortunately, the natural reservoir for human *Pneumocystis* remains unknown, although studies in animals and emerging studies in humans indicate that humans are one reservoir.[32] In well-controlled laboratory experiments, animal-to-animal transmission of *Pneumocystis* via aerosol has been conclusively demonstrated to occur under a variety of different conditions.[33-35] Furthermore, immunocompromised laboratory animals may develop PCP after a brief exposure to a same-species animal with PCP. Thus, recommendations for immunocompromised persons to avoid contact with patients with PCP may be reasonable. However, studies in humans also suggest that immuno-

competent as well as immunocompromised persons without clinical PCP may be colonized with human *Pneumocystis* and may serve as an additional source of infection to unsuspecting immunocompromised persons.[36-40] Thus, even if an immunocompromised person avoids contact with a patient with PCP, the person may still be exposed to *Pneumocystis* through someone who is colonized or sub-clinically infected with the organism. Studies to define the epidemiology and transmission of human *Pneumocystis* are needed to identify the potential methods of disease prevention.

Conclusion

The HIV/AIDS epidemic brought prominence and clinical importance to PCP, a previously uncommon pneumonia. In the past 25 years, tremendous advances have occurred in our understanding of HIV infection and PCP. However, gaps in our knowledge remain and continued study of this important disease is still needed.

References

1. Serraino D, Puro V, Boumis E, et al. Epidemiological aspects of major opportunistic infections of the respiratory tract in persons with AIDS: Europe, 1993-2000. Aids 2003; 17:2109–2116.
2. Morris A, Lundgren JD, Masor H, et al. Current epidemiology of *Pneumocystis* pneumonia. Emerg Infect Dis 2004; 10:1713–1720.
3. Worodria W, Okot-Nwang M, Yoo SD, et al. Causes of lower respiratory infection in HIV-infected Ugandan adults who are sputum AFB smear-negative. Int J Tuberc Lung Dis 2003; 7:117–123.
4. Fisk DT, Meshnick S, Kazanjian PH. *Pneumocystis carinii* pneumonia in patients in the developing world who have acquired immunodeficiency syndrome. Clin Infect Dis 2003; 36:70–78.
5. Kaplan JE, Masur H, Holmes KK. Guidelines for preventing opportunistic infections among HIV-infected persons – 2002. Recommendations of the U.S. Public Health Service

and the Infectious Diseases Society of America. MMWR Recomm Rep 2002; 51:1–52.

6. Phair J, Munoz A, Detels R, et al. The risk of *Pneumocystis carinii* pneumonia among men infected with human immunodeficiency virus type 1. Multicenter AIDS Cohort Study Group N Engl J Med 1990; 322:161–165.

7. Stansell JD, Osmond DH, Charlebois E, et al. Predictors of *Pneumocystis carinii* pneumonia in HIV-infected persons. Pulmonary Complications of HIV Infection Study Group. Am J Respir Crit Care Med 1997; 155:60–66.

8. Kovacs JA, Hiemenz JW, Macher AM, et al. Pneumocystis carinii pneumonia: a comparison between patients with the acquired immunodeficiency syndrome and patients with other immunodeficiencies. Ann Intern Med 1984; 100:663–671.

9. Thomas CF, Jr., Limper AH. Pneumocystis pneumonia. N Engl J Med 2004; 350:2487–2498.

10. Kales CP, Murren JR, Torres RA, et al. Early predictors of in-hospital mortality for Pneumocystis carinii pneumonia in the acquired immunodeficiency syndrome. Arch Intern Med 1987; 147:1413–1417.

11. Huang L, Stansell JD. AIDS and the lung. Med Clin North Am 1996; 80 775–801.

12. Skelly M, Hoffman J, Fabbri M, et al. S-adenosylmethionine concentrations in diagnosis of Pneumocystis carinii pneumonia. Lancet 2003; 361:1267–1268.

13. DeLorenzo LJ, Huang CT, Maguire GP, et al. Roentgenographic patterns of *Pneumocystis carinii* pneumonia in 104 patients with AIDS. Chest 1987; 91:323–327.

14. Huang L, Stansell J, Osmond D, et al. Performance of an algorithm to detect Pneumocystis carinii pneumonia in symptomatic HIV-infected persons. Pulmonary Complications of HIV Infection Study Group. Chest 1999; 115:1025–1032.

15. Datta D, Ali SA, Henken EM, et al. *Pneumocystis carinii* Pneumonia: The Time Course of Clinical and Radiographic Improvement. Chest 2003; 124:1820–1823.

16. Huang L, Hecht FM, Stansell JD, et al. Suspected *Pneumocystis carinii* pneumonia with a negative induced sputum examination. Is early bronchoscopy useful? Am J Respir Crit Care Med Jun 1995; 151:1866–1871.

17. Larsen HH, Huang L, Kovacs JA, et al. A prospective, blinded study of quantitative touch-down polymerase chain reaction using oral-wash samples for diagnosis of *Pneumocystis* pneumonia in HIV-infected patients. J Infect Dis 2004; 189:1679–1683.

18. Benson CA, Kaplan JE, Masur H, et al. Treating opportunistic infections among HIV-infected adults and adolescents: recommendations from CDC, the National Institutes of Health, and the HIV Medicine Association/ Infectious Diseases Society of America. MMWR Recomm Rep 2004; 53:1–112.

19. Huang L, Crothers K, Atzori C, et al. Dihydropteroate synthase gene mutations in Pneumocystis and sulfa resistance. Emerg Infect Dis 2004; 10:1721–1728.

20. Beard CB, Roux P, Nevez G, et al. Strain typing methods and molecular epidemiology of *Pneumocystis* pneumonia. Emerg Infect Dis 2004; 10:1729–1735.

21. Stein CR, Poole C, Kazanjian P, et al. Sulfa use, dihydropteroate synthase mutations, and *Pneumocystis jirovecii* pneumonia. Emerg Infect Dis 2004; 10:1760–1765.

22. Crothers K, Beard CB, Turner J, et al. Severity and outcome of HIV-associated *Pneumocystis* pneumonia containing *Pneumocystis jirovecii* dihydropteroate synthase gene mutations. Aids 2005; 19:801–805.

23. Kazanjian PH, Fisk D, Armstrong W, et al. Increase in prevalence of Pneumocystis carinii mutations in patients with AIDS and *P. carinii* pneumonia, in the United States and China. J Infect Dis 2004; 189:1684–1687.

24. Zar HJ, Alvarez-Martinez MJ, Harrison A, et al. Prevalence of dihydropteroate synthase mutants in HIV-infected South African Children with *Pneumocystis jiroveci* Pneumonia. Clin Infect Dis 2004; 39:1047–1051.

25. Iliades P, Meshnick SR, Macreadie IG. Mutations in the *Pneumocystis jirovecii* DHPS gene confer cross-resistance to sulfa drugs. Antimicrob Agents Chemother 2005; 49:741–748.

26. The National Institutes of Health – University of California Expert Panel for Corticosteroids as Adjunctive Therapy for Pneumocystis Pneumonia. Consensus statement on the use of corticosteroids as adjunctive therapy for Pneumocystis pneumonia in the acquired immunodeficiency syndrome. N Engl J Med 1990; 323:1500–1504.

27. Lopez Bernaldo de Quiros JC, Miro JM, Pena JM, et al. A randomized trial of the discontinuation of primary and secondary prophylaxis against Pneumocystis carinii pneumonia after highly active antiretroviral therapy in patients with HIV infection. Grupo de Estudio del SIDA 04/98. N Engl J Med 2001; 344:159–167.

28. Ledergerber B, Mocroft A, Reiss P, et al. Discontinuation of secondary prophylaxis against Pneumocystis carinii pneumonia in patients with HIV infection who have a response to antiretroviral therapy. Eight Eur Study Groups N Engl J Med 2001; 344:168–174.

29. Bishop LR, Kovacs JA. Quantitation of anti-*Pneumocystis jirovecii* antibodies in healthy persons and immunocompromised patients. J Infect Dis 2003; 187:1844–1848.

30. Daly KR, Koch J, Levin L, et al. Enzyme-linked immunosorbent assay and serologic responses to *Pneumocystis jiroveci*. Emerg Infect Dis 2004; 10:848–854.

31. Respaldiza N, Medrano FJ, Medrano AC, et al. High seroprevalence of *Pneumocystis* infection in Spanish children. Clin Microbiol Infect 2004; 10:1029–1031.

32. Kovacs JA, Gill VJ, Meshnick S, et al. New insights into transmission, diagnosis, and drug treatment of *Pneumocystis carinii* pneumonia. JAMA 2001; 286:2450–2460.

33. An CL, Gigliotti F, Harmsen AG. Exposure of immunocompetent adult mice to *Pneumocystis carinii* f. sp. muris by cohousing: growth of *P. carinii* f. sp. muris and host immune response. Infect Immun 2003; 71:2065–2070.

34. Gigliotti F, Harmsen AG, Wright TW. Characterization of transmission of *Pneumocystis carinii* f. sp. muris through immunocompetent BALB/c mice. Infect Immun 2003; 71:3852–3856.

35. Vestereng VH, Bishop LR, Hernandez B, et al. Quantitative real-time polymerase chain-reaction assay allows characterization of Pneumocystis infection in immunocompetent mice. J Infect Dis 2004; 189:1540–1544.

36. Maskell NA, Waine DJ, Lindley A, et al. Asymptomatic carriage of *Pneumocystis jiroveci* in subjects undergoing bronchoscopy: a prospective study. Thorax 2003; 58:594–597.

37. Morris A, Kingsley LA, Groner G, et al. Prevalence and clinical predictors of Pneumocystis colonization among HIV-infected men. AIDS 2004; 18:793–798.

38. Morris A, Sciurba FC, Lebedeva IP, et al. Association of chronic obstructive pulmonary disease severity and Pneumocystis colonization. Am J Respir Crit Care Med 2004; 170:408–413.

39. Totet A, Latouche S, Lacube P, et al. *Pneumocystis jirovecii* dihydropteroate synthase genotypes in immunocompetent infants and immunosuppressed adults, Amiens, France. Emerg Infect Dis 2004; 10:667–673.

40. Medrano FJ, Montes-Cano M, Conde M, et al. *Pneumocystis jirovecii* in general population. Emerg Infect Dis 2005; 11:245–250.

CHAPTER 30

Other HIV-related Pneumonias

John G. Bartlett

Introduction

The lower respiratory tract has been and continues to be a major site of opportunistic infections in patients with HIV infection. The infections that are encountered are quite different in the developed world and in the developing world, based on availability of HAART, *Pneumocystis jiroveci* pneumonia (PCP) prophylaxis and the epidemiology of tuberculosis. There is a substantial spectrum of different pathogens that are involved in pulmonary infections, although the great majority of cases are presumably bacterial or viral and never have a clear etiologic diagnosis. The purpose of this chapter is to review pneumonia with emphasis on appropriate diagnostic studies and treatment. Emphasis will also be placed on the different experiences in distinct geographic areas based on the generalization regarding unique experiences noted above. It should be noted that *Pneumocystis jiroveci* and mycobacteria are discussed elsewhere. The focus of attention here will be on bacterial pathogens and fungi.

Frequency

Bacterial pneumonia was a common cause of HIV-related complications in the pre-HAART era and continued to be a major problem in the developing world. A prospective study of 1100 HIV-infected patients for the 5-year period of 1988 through 1994 in the USA, showed an incidence of approximately 100 cases per 1000 person-years (PY), an incidence about eight times higher than for an age-matched controlled population.[1,2] The major pathogens

encountered in this study of 521 cases of pneumonia (where the likely pathogen was identified) were bacterial infection, 44%; *P. jiroveci*, 42%; tuberculosis, 5%; and other opportunistic infections, 8%. Of the bacterial causes, the most frequent were *S. pneumoniae*, *H. influenzae*, *P. aeruginosa*, and *S. aureus*. Atypical agents were rarely encountered.[3]

Bacterial Pneumonia

There are four bacterial agents that have been associated with HIV infection and immunodeficiency: *S. pneumoniae*, *H. influenzae*, *P. aeruginosa*, and *Nocardia*. This listing does not include mycobacteria, which are discussed elsewhere. Of these, pneumococcal pneumonia is clearly the most frequent and most important (Table 30.1).

Pneumococcal Pneumonia

The frequency of pneumococcal bacteremia is estimated at 150–300 times more common with HIV infection than in persons seronegative for HIV. The increased rate appears to apply to all CD4 cell strata, but is most common in those with low CD4 cell counts.[3] This frequency has changed substantially in developed countries due to the notable impact of HAART and the demonstrated benefit of PCP prophylaxis in reducing these infections.[4,5]

The clinical presentation of pneumococcal pneumonia appears approximately the same for patients with or without HIV infection, except for the high rates of bacteremia. Extrapulmonary involvement (meningitis, septic arthritis, and endocarditis) are

Table 30.1 Correlation of chest X-ray changes and etiology of pneumonia

Change	Common	Uncommon
Consolidation	Pyogenic bacteria, Kaposi's sarcoma, cryptococcosis	*Nocardia, M. tuberculosis, M. kansasii, Legionella, B. bronchiseptica*
Reticulonodular infiltrates	*P. jiroveci, M. tuberculosis,* histoplasmosis, coccidioidomycosis	Kaposi's sarcoma, toxoplasmosis, CMV, leishmania, lymphoid interstitial pneumonitis
Nodule	*M. tuberculosis,* cryptococcosis	Kaposi's sarcoma, *Nocardia*
Cavity	*M. tuberculosis, S. aureus* (IDU), *Nocardia, P. aeruginosa,* cryptococcosis, coccidioidomycosis, histoplasmosis, aspergillosis, anaerobes	*M. kansasii,* MAC, *Legionella, P. carinii,* lymphoma, *Klebsiella, Rhodococcus equi*
Hilar nodes	*M. tuberculosis,* histoplasmosis, coccidioidomycosis, lymphoma, Kaposi's sarcoma	*M. kansasii,* MAC
Pleural effusion	Pyogenic bacteria, Kaposi's sarcoma, *M. tuberculosis* (congestive heart failure, hypoalbuminemia)	Cryptococcosis, MAC, histoplasmosis, coccidioidomycosis, aspergillosis, anaerobes, *Nocardia,* lymphoma, toxoplasmosis, primary effusion lymphoma

infrequent. The classic presentation is sudden onset with chills and fever, usually accompanied by cough, dyspnea, and pleurisy. These symptoms clearly distinguish this pulmonary infection from PCP and TB. The chest X-ray shows the usual focal infiltrate (Table 30.2). Cavity formation, atypical infiltrates, and hilar adenopathy are rare and suggest an alternative diagnosis. Most patients produce sputum, which becomes a diagnostic resource for gram stain, Quellung tests, and culture. As noted, blood cultures are often positive. A new test that appears to be about 80% sensitive and 95% specific in adults with pneumococcal bacteremia is the urinary antigen assay.[6] The treatment of pneumococcal pneumonia is the same for persons with HIV infection as for others. The preferred drugs are summarized in Table 30.2. In Africa, most strains of *S. pneumoniae* appear to respond to betalactams, which are the preferred drugs. In the USA, there is concern about penicillin resistance, but ceftriaxone or cefotaxime are active against about 94% of strains; if there is a reason to suspect resistance or the patient is critically ill, most authorities recommend a fluoroquinolone either alone or in combination with one of the preferred betalactams. One curious observation is that patients who are critically ill with pneumococcal pneumonia with bacteremia involving penicillin-sensitive strains appear to do better when the betalactam is combined with a macrolide compared with the betalactam alone.[7] The reason for this is unclear, but some suspect a role of the antiinflammatory activity of the

macrolide. The duration of therapy is arbitrary; the usual recommended duration is 5–7 days after the patient becomes afebrile. The rate of recurrent pneumococcal pneumonia is high, actually 8–25% within 6 months. These are generally infections involving new strains rather than relapses so longer treatment does not appear to be an advantage.[8,9]

The 23 valent pneumococcal vaccine is commonly recommended for this population, but remains controversial in terms of any demonstrated benefit. In other populations, the only benefit convincingly shown was a 50% reduction in the frequency of pneumococcal bacteremia suggesting that patients with AIDS may continue to be a high priority, at least when the CD4 cell count is sufficiently high for an immunologic response.[10]

Haemophilus influenzae

This organism is second to the pneumococcus as a cause of bacterial pneumonia in patients with HIV infection.[11,12] The frequency of *H. influenzae* bacteremia is magnified by 10–100-fold with HIV. Most cases involve non-typeable strains.[12] This infection is similar to that of pneumococcal pneumonia with an acute onset characterized by fever, cough, sputum production and dyspnea. Chest X-rays usually show a bronchopneumonia. The diagnosis is best established by Gram stain and culture of sputum and culture of blood. About 40% of these strains produce

Table 30.2 Bacterial infections

Agent	Course	Frequency, setting	Typical findings	Diagnosis	Treatment
Gram-negative bacilli	Acute, purulent sputum	Uncommon, except with nosocomial infection or neutropenia. *Pseudomonas aeruginosa* is relatively common in late-stage disease, cavitary disease, or chronic antibiotic exposure (median CD4 50 cells/mm³)	Lobar or bronchopneumonia	Sputum GS and culture (sensitivity is >80%, but specificity is poor)	Need *in vitro* susceptibility tests Long-term ciprofloxacin usually results in relapse and resistance to *P. aeruginosa*
Haemophilus influenzae	Acute, purulent sputum	Incidence is 100-fold higher than in healthy controls; most infections are caused by unencapsulated strains	Bronchopneumonia	Sputum GS and culture (sensitivity of culture is 50%; prior antibiotics usually preclude growth)	Oral: Amox-CA, azithromycin, TMP-SMX, fluoroquinolone, cephalosporin; Intravenous: Cefotaxime, ceftriaxone
Legionella	Acute mucopurulent sputum	Uncommon, HIV-associated risk is debated	Bronchopneumonia; sometimes multiple infiltrates in noncontiguous segments	Sputum culture; urinary antigen (*Legionella pneumophila* serogroup 1)	Fluoroquinolone, macrolide, doxycycline
Nocardia	Chronic or asymptomatic; sputum production	Uncommon; frequency higher with chronic corticosteroid use (median CD4 count 50 cells/mm³)	Nodule or cavity	Sputum or fiber-optic bronchoscopy (FOB); GS, modified acid-fast bacillus (AFB) stain and culture; should alert lab if suspected	Sulfonamide/TMP-SMX
Staphylococcus aureus	Acute, subacute, or chronic; purulent sputum	Uncommon, except with injected drug use and tricuspid valve endocarditis with septic emboli	Bronchopneumonia, cavitary disease, septic emboli with cavities ± effusion	Blood sputum GS and culture (sputum culture is sensitive, but specificity is poor). Blood cultures are nearly always positive with endocarditis.	MSSA: Nafcillin/oxacillin, cefuroxime, TMP-SMX, clindamycin MRSA: TMP-SMX or clindamycin if sensitive; Vancomycin
Streptococcus pneumoniae	Acute, purulent sputum ± pleurisy	Common, all stages HIV infection; incidence is 100-fold higher than in healthy controls; recurrence rate at 6 months is 6–24%; higher with low CD4 counts and with smoking	Lobar or broncho-pneumonia ± pleural effusion	Blood cultures often positive, sputum gram stain (GS), Quellung, culture (sensitivity of culture is 50%; prior antibiotics usually preclude growth)	Oral: Amoxicillin, macrolide, cefdinir, cefprozil, cefpodoxime, fluoroquinolone; Intravenous: Cefotaxime, ceftriaxone, fluoroquinolone

betalactamase so that amoxicillin is often ineffective. The preferred drugs are a third-generation cephalosporin, a betalactam-betalactamase inhibitor, fluoroquinolone, azithromycin or sulfamethoxazole-trimethoprim.[13] The response is generally good and treatment is continued for 5–7 days after the patient becomes afebrile. Trimethoprim-sulfamethoxazole prophylaxis should prevent this infection, but other forms of PCP prophylaxis will not. *H. influenzae* vaccine is not indicated because the rates of this infection are relatively low and the majority involve non-typeable strains.

Staphylococcus aureus

Patients with HIV infection have not been clearly defined as at risk for infections involving *S. aureus*. Those with injection drug use as their risk have increased rates of infections involving *S. aureus* that appear independent of HIV *per se*. Most of these infections are soft tissue infections at injection sites or pyomyositis. Many have tricuspid valve endocarditis involving this organism, which often presents with embolic lesions in the lung. The diagnosis is generally easily established with the characteristic findings on chest X-ray combined with positive blood cultures, echocardiogram, and the clearly associated IDU risk. Patients with HIV infection and this complication generally respond to standard therapy for staphylococcal tricuspid endocarditis, although most urge closer observation and a more prolonged duration of treatment.[14,15] There is a relatively new form of staphylococcal pneumonia that is presently quite rare, but might become far more prevalent and is important to recognize. This is the USA300 strain that was recognized in the late 1990s and is often resistant to all betalactams, but sensitive to most other drugs active versus *S. aureus* including trimethoprim-sulfamethoxazole, clindamycin, doxycycline, and gentamicin. It is most frequently associated with severe soft tissue infections including necrotizing fasciitis and furunculosis. Persons with HIV infection have been defined as at risk for these soft tissue infections, if in the category of MSM or IDU. This organism may also cause pneumonia characterized by a fulminant course, with shock, necrosis of the lung, and empyemas. As noted, the unique strain of *S. aureus* involved in these cases in the USA usually is USA300, although other strains with similar properties are found in other parts of the world. The pathogenic mechanism is not clear, but a characteristic feature of these strains is that they possess the genes for the Panton–Valentine leukocidin as well as the *mec*IV mechanism of methicillin resistance. Optimal treatment of pneumonia is not clear, but many authorities recommend the use of vancomycin or linezolid, often in combination with other drugs such as rifampin or clindamycin.

Pseudomonas aeruginosa

Pneumonia with this organism is infrequent, but it is a serious complication of late stage disease indicating profound immunosuppression.[13,16,17] Most patients have a CD4 cell count <50 cells/mm^3 and some have additional risk factors such as neutropenia or corticosteroid therapy. Many have bacteremia and the mortality rate is relatively high. The organism is usually easy to recover from sputum and refractory to eradication despite aggressive antimicrobial therapy. The usual treatment is a combination of antipseudomonad betalactams combined with tobramycin. The usual temptation is to treat the patient with an oral fluoroquinolone, generally levofloxacin or ciprofloxacin, in an effort to achieve discharge and better life quality, but most will relapse with a fluoroquinolone-resistant strain.

Atypical Agents

Chlamydia pneumoniae and *Mycoplasma pneumoniae* appear to be relatively uncommon in patients with HIV infection.[3,13,18] A major problem is the limited accuracy of the diagnostic test for these two atypical agents. One study reported results with the standard microimmunofluorescence (MIF) serology; nevertheless, *C. pneumonia* accounted for only 13 of 319 (2.5%) of pneumonias in patients with HIV infection.[19] *C. pneumoniae* and *M. pneumoniae* have not been generally associated with infections in compromised hosts and this presumably accounts for the paucity of cases. By contrast, Legionella has a clear association with compromised cell-mediated immunity, so one would expect more cases with HIV infection.[20,21,22] One early report indicated a 50-fold increase in the frequency of Legionnaires' disease with HIV infection, but this has remained an isolated report not substantiated by others. Blatt and co-workers[22] reviewed eight cases of Legionnaires' disease encountered in the HIV Natural History Study of the US Air Force; the median CD4 cell count was 83 cells/mm^3; five cases were nosocomial; six had co-existing pulmonary pathogens; none acquired this infection while receiving prophylaxis with sulfamethoxazole-trimethoprim; and all responded well to standard therapy with a macrolide. The conclusion is that atypical agents play a minimal role in bacterial pneumonia in patients with HIV infection or AIDS.

Diagnostic Approach

Key clues to the probability of a bacterial pneumonia in a patient with HIV infection are the features that characterize bacterial pneumonia in other populations: the rapid pace, the usual clinical features of cough, sputum, and dyspnea, and the X-ray which almost invariably shows a pulmonary infiltrate. Key factors in the assessment are the CD4 cell count (to evaluate susceptibility to opportunistic pathogens), the degree of oxygenation and vital signs (to assess severity of illness), and the characteristic features of the infiltrate. Features on the chest X-ray that suggest specific etiologic causes are summarized in Table 30.1. In many cases, this will be the initial presentation and the CD4 cell count may be pending at the time diagnostic and therapeutic decisions need to be made. In general, the absolute lymphocyte count may be helpful. An absolute lymphocyte count (ALC) of <1200 cells/mm^3 correlates roughly with a CD4 cell count of <200 cells/mm^3. Patients with advanced HIV infection may also demonstrate evidence of chronic disease with anemia, hypoalbuminemia, weight loss, etc. If the diagnosis of HIV is suspected, but never established, the rapid serologic test will notably facilitate making the diagnosis in a timely fashion. This test and the CBC are generally available in virtually all parts of the world. The legal requirements for informed consent will depend on local standards.

In terms of the etiologic diagnosis, standard tests for patients sufficiently sick to require hospitalization are blood cultures and, in many centers, Gram stain and culture of expectorated sputum.[22,23] Although emphasis has been placed on the probability of bacterial pneumonia on patients with rapid and acute illness, with sudden onset, and other characteristic features, there must be a continued concern for the possibility of PCP in any patient who has a low CD4 cell count, substantial reduction in oxygenation, lack of PCP prophylaxis, and/or characteristic features on a chest X-ray. In these cases, it is important that the diagnostic evaluation include this consideration with bronchoscopy or induced sputum, or, if the probability is sufficiently great, empiric treatment that may or may not include agents active against common bacterial pathogens. The same vigilance applies to tuberculosis, particularly in countries where this is highly endemic. The expectorated sputum needs to be evaluated by stain and culture for AFB. Since the AFB smears show a sensitivity of only about 50%, it may be important to consider empiric treatment here as well.

Treatment

With regard to antibiotic selection for bacterial pneumonia, the standard practice in the USA for hospitalized patients is treatment with a fluoroquinolone or a cephalosporin (ceftriaxone or cefotaxime), combined with a macrolide (azithromycin or clarithromycin or erythromycin) (Table 30.3). This treatment should begin rapidly, preferably within 4 h of registration. Additional diagnostic tests to consider would be the urinary antigen assay for *S. pneumoniae* and Legionella.[23,24] Pathogen-directed treatment is always preferred but often unrealistic due to time delays in establishing the etiologic agent. Recommendations based on the pathogen are provided in Table 30.3.

Fungal Pneumonia (Tables 30.4, 30.5)[25,26,27]

Aspergillosis

Aspergillosis previously accounted for 1–4% of pneumonias in patients with AIDS.[28,29] This was a relatively late complication in patients usually with a CD4 cell count <50 cells/mm^3 and often combined with additional risk factors such as neutropenia and chronic administration of corticosteroids. There are two distinct clinical forms of pulmonary infection: invasive parenchymal aspergillosis in which the chest X-ray shows either a diffuse interstitial pneumonitis or the more characteristic pleural-based wedge-shaped infiltrate. These patients present with fever, cough, dyspnea, pleurisy, hypoxemia, hemoptysis and the X-ray features noted. The second form of pulmonary aspergillosis is tracheobronchial disease with ulcers or pseudomembranes, often with obstruction from mucus plugs.[30,31] The diagnosis is established by the presence of typical clinical features combined with demonstration of the organism in histopathology or a presumptive diagnosis can be made by positive cultures for aspergillus from respiratory secretions when accompanied by the characteristic clinical features.[32] The standard treatment is amphotericin B, usually in high dose of a lipid amphotericin. Itraconazole may also be used. In more recent years, preferred drugs often include voriconazole or caspofungin.[33,34,35] These agents have not had therapeutic trials with patients with HIV

Table 30.3 Treatment of bacterial pneumonia (based on guidelines of IDSA)

Outpatient
Empiric
  No abx × 3 months: Doxycycline or macrolide[a]
  Abx within 3 months: Fluoroquinolone[b], telithromycin, or Betalactam + macrolide
Hospitalized patient
Non-ICU: Fluoroquinolone[b] or betalactam[c] plus macrolide[a]
ICU Betalactam plus macrolide or betalactam plus fluoroquinolone[b]
Aspiration
  Betalactam-betalactamase inhibitor or clindamycin
  Alternative: Carhapenem[d]
Influenza + superinfection
  Betalactam[c] ± antiviral agent
Healthcare-associated
  Ceftriaxone, fluoroquinolone[b], ampicillin-sulbactam or ertapenem

Pathogen-specific
  S. pneumoniae
    Penicillin MIC <2 μg/mL: Penicillin or amoxicillin; alternatives-macrolide[a], telithromycin, cephalosporin-cefpodoxime,
      cefprozil, cefuroxime, cefdinir, cefditoren, ceftriaxone or cefotaxime, doxycycline, clindamycin, fluoroquinolone[b]
    Penicillin MIC ≥2 μg/mL: Cefotaxime, ceftriaxone, fluoroquinolone[b], telithromycin
    Alternatives: linezolid amoxicillin (3 g/day – if MIC ≤4 μg/mL)
  H. influenzae
    Non-betalactamase producing: Amoxicillin
    Betalactamase producing: Cephalosporin, amoxicillin-clavulanate
    Alternatives: fluoroquinolones[b], doxycycline, azithromycin, clarithromycin
  Mycoplasma pneumoniae
    Macrolide[a] or tetracycline
    Alternative: fluoroquinolone[b]
  Chlamydia pneumoniae
    Macrolide[a] or tetracycline
    Alternative: Fluoroquinolone[b]
  Legionella
    Fluoroquinolone[b], azithromycin, clarithromycin
    Alternative: Doxycycline
  Staph aureus
    MSSA: Nafcillin, oxacillin; Alternative: Clindamycin, cefazolin, trimethoprim-sulfamethiazole
    MRSA: Vancomycin or linezolid
  P. aeruginosa
    Anti-pseudomonad betalactam (ticarcillin, piperacillin, ceftazidime, cefepime, aztreonam, imipenem, meropenem)
      plus (ciprofloxacin or levofloxacin) or aminoglycoside
    Alternative: Aminoglycoside plus ciprofloxacin or levofloxacin

[a]Macrolide: Azithromycin or clarithromycin. [b]Fluoroquinolone: Levofloxacin (750 mg/day), gatifloxacin, moxifloxacin, gemifloxacin. [c]Betalactam: Ceftriaxone, cefotaxime. [d]Carbapenem: Imipenem, meropenem, ertapenem.

infection, but they appear superior to amphotericin B in other populations. Particularly important in the management is to reverse the predisposing factors as much as possible including increase in CD4 cell count with HAART, reversal of neutropenia, and discontinuation or reduction in dose of corticosteroids. The prognosis has been poor with a mortality rate exceeding 90% in the pre-HAART era.[28] The prognosis is presumably substantially better if the CD4 cell count can be reconstituted.

Cryptococcosis

Cryptococcosis is a relatively common complication in late-stage HIV infection. This was previously a common AIDS-defining diagnosis in the developed world and is well recognized as a major cause of severe disease throughout the developing world. This is best known as a cause of meningitis, but the lung is the portal of entry and many patients have pulmonary involvement concurrently or even

Table 30.4 Fungal infections

Agent	Course	Frequency, setting	Typical findings	Diagnosis	Treatment
Aspergillus	Acute or subacute	Up to 4% of AIDS patients; usually advanced HIV infection (median CD4 count 30 cells/mm²; about 60% have severe neutropenia (ANC <500 cells/mm³) ± chronic steroids; disseminated disease is uncommon	Focal infiltrate; cavity–often pleural-based, diffuse infiltrates or reticulonodular infiltrates	Sputum stain and culture; false-positive and false-negative cultures common. Best tests: Tissue pathology or sputum smear and typical CT and clinical features	Amphotericin B or itraconazole or caspofungin
Candida	Chronic or subacute	Common isolate, rare cause of pulmonary disease (median CD4 count 50 cells/mm³)	Bronchitis; rare cause of pneumonia (some say it does not exist)	Recovery in sputum or FOB specimen is meaningless (up to 30% of all expectorated sputum and FOB cultures in unselected patients yield *Candida* sp.); must have histologic evidence of invasion on biopsy	Fluconazole or amphotericin B
Coccidioides immitis±	Chronic or subacute	Up to 10% of AIDS patients in endemic area; usually advanced HIV infection (median CD4 count 50 cells/mm³); disseminated disease in 20–40%	Diffuse nodular infiltrates, focal infiltrate, cavity; hilar adenopathy[26]	Sputum, induced sputum, or FOB stain and culture; KOH of expectorated sputum is rarely positive; PAP stain or silver stain of BAL positive in 40%; culture of BAL usually positive; serology (CF) positive in 70%; skin test positive in <10%; blood cultures positive in 10%	Fluconazole, itraconazole, or amphotericin B
Cryptococcus	Chronic, subacute, or symptomatic	Up to 8–10% in AIDS patients; late-stage HIV infection (median CD4 count 50 cells/mm³); 80% have cryptococcal meningitis	Nodule, cavity, diffuse or nodular infiltrates	Sputum, induced sputum, or FOB stain and culture; serum cryptococcal antigen usually positive; CSF analysis indicated if antigen or organism found at any site	Fluconazole without CNS involvement amphotericin B
Histoplasma capsulatum±	Chronic or subacute	Up to 15% of AIDS patients in endemic area; usually advanced HIV infection with disseminated histoplasmosis (median CD4 count 50 cells/mm³); common features: fever, weight loss, hepatosplenomegaly, lymphadenopathy	Diffuse nodular infiltrates, nodule, focal infiltrate, cavity, hilar adenopathy[27,28]	Best test for diagnosis and follow-up of treatment is serum and urine polysaccharide antigen assay, with yield of 85% (blood) and 97% (urine). Available only through J. White (Indianapolis, IN) 800-HISTO-DG for US$70/assay; serology positive in 50–70%; yield with culture of sputum, 80%; marrow, 80%; blood cultures positive in 60–85%	Itraconazole or amphotericin B

Table 30.5 Treatment of fungal infection of the lung

Aspergillus

Preferred		Voriconazole 400 mg i.v. or p.o. q.12h × 2 days, then 200 mg q.12h
Duration		Based on clinical response
Alternative		Amphotericin B 1 mg/kg i.v. or lipid formulations of Amphotericin B 5 mg/kg per day
Maintenance		Inadequate data for recommendation

Cryptococcosis: disseminated disease

Preferred	Acute	Amphotericin B 0.7 mg/kg i.v. ± flucytosine 25 mg q.i.d. p.o. × 14 days, or liposomal Amphotericin × 14 days
	Consolidation	Fluconazole 400 mg/day p.o. × 8 weeks.
		Maintenance: Fluconazole 200 mg/day p.o. until CD4 count >100–200/mm^3 + asymptomatic × 6 months
Alternatives	Acute	Fluconazole 400–800 mg/day i.v. or p.o. ± flucytosine 25 mg q.i.d. p.o. × 14 days
	Consolidation	Itraconazole 200 mg/day p.o. × 8 weeks. Maintenance: Itraconazole 400 mg i.v. q.d.

Cryptococcosis: pulmonary without disseminated disease

Preferred		Fluconazole 200–400 mg/day p.o. lifelong or Itraconazole 200–400 mg/day or Amphotericin B 0.5–1.0 mg/kg per day i.v. (serious disease)
Duration		Until asymptomatic + CD4 count >100–200 cells/mm^3 × 6 months

Histoplasmosis: severe disseminated

Preferred	Acute	Amphotericin B 0.7 mg/kg per day i.v. or liposomal amphotericin B 4 mg/kg per day × 3–10 day
	Continuation	Itraconazole 200 mg caps b.i.d. p.o.
Alternative	Acute	Itraconazole 400 mg/day i.v.
	Continuation	Itraconazole oral solution 200 mg b.i.d. p.o. or fluconazole 800 mg/day p.o.
Maintenance		Itraconazole 200 mg/day p.o.

Histoplasmosis: mild disseminated disease

Preferred		Itraconazole 200 mg cap t.i.d. p.o. × 3 day, then 200 mg b.i.d. p.o. × 12 weeks, then 200 mg/day p.o.
Alternative		Fluconazole 800 mg/day p.o.

without meningitis. Prior to HAART there were reports that approximately 5–8% of all persons with late-stage HIV infection acquired disseminated cryptococcosis.[36] The usual symptoms with pulmonary involvement are fever, cough, and dyspnea that evolves over a period of weeks.[36,37,38] The chest X-ray usually shows interstitial infiltrates that may suggest PCP;[37,38,39] other changes on chest X-ray include focal infiltrates, cavities that may be clinically silent, hilar adenopathy, pleural effusions and/or reticulonodular infiltrates. The disease in the chest and in the CNS is often clinically silent so that the diagnosis of cryptococcal pulmonary infection should always prompt a lumbar puncture to detect cryptococcal meningitis as the most common recognized clinical form of the disease. About 90% of patients with cryptococcosis have a positive serum antigen assay for *C. neoformans*.[37] The organism can also often be found in respiratory secretions including sputum, or bronchoscopy aspirates.[38,39,40] The standard treatment for cryptococcal meningitis is amphotericin B, often combined with five fluorocytosine for 2 weeks fol-

lowed by the consolidation phase of fluconazole at 400 mg/day for 8 weeks and then fluconazole at 200 mg/day, until there is immune reconstitution.[41] For patients with pulmonary cryptococcosis, it is suspected but unproven, that fluconazole alone would be satisfactory if the pulmonary symptoms are not severe and cryptococcal meningitis has been excluded.

Histoplasmosis

Histoplasma capsulatum is endemic in the Mississippi, Ohio and St Lawrence River valleys; histoplasmosis was previously found in over 5% of persons living in this endemic area.[27,42,43] The frequency has become much less during the HAART era. The disease is acquired by inhalation of *H. capsulatum* microconidia. The disease generally remains localized in the lung in patients when the CD4 cell count is >300 cells/mm^3, but disseminated disease is often found when the CD4 cell count is <150 cells/mm^3. Common clinical features of pulmonary disease include cough, fever, and dyspnea that are usually indolent in onset. With disseminated disease, there are often typical lesions of the skin and mucosal surfaces, weight loss with wasting, bone marrow suppression with pancytopenia, hepatosplenomegaly with abnormal liver function tests with a cholangitic pattern, lymphadenopathy and/or diarrhea.[27,42,43] The chest X-ray usually shows a diffused interstitial infiltrate or a reticulonodular infiltrate; other less common findings are focal infiltrates, hilar adenopathy, and pleural effusions.[27,42,43] Some patients present with the septic shock syndrome, but this is found in <10% of patients. The diagnosis is based on detection of the *Histoplasma* antigen in blood or urine, excellent diagnostic tests for disseminated disease, but relatively insensitive when the infection are restricted to the lung.[43,44,45] The fungus can often be isolated from blood cultures, bone marrow or respiratory secretions, but recovery requires 2–4 weeks.[44]

Patients with severe disseminated disease should be treated with liposomal amphotericin B, which has proven superior to deoxycholate amphotericin B in terms of therapeutic response and reduced toxicity.[46] The amphotericin is usually given for 3–10 days and then treatment is changed to itraconazole at 200 mg capsules/day for 12 weeks and then maintenance treatment is given until there is immune reconstitution. Patients with acute pulmonary histoplasmosis and a CD4 cell count >500 may not require therapy and could be managed in a fashion similar to patients without HIV infection. For those on long-term maintenance, the usual dose of itraconazole is 200 mg twice daily until the CD4 cell count is >100 cells/mm^3.[47,48] The initial itraconazole is 200 mg/day intravenously.

References

1. Caiaffa WT, Graham NM, Vlahov D. Bacterial pneumonia in adult populations with human immunodeficiency virus (HIV) infection. Am J Epidemiol 1993; 138:909–922.
2. Wallace JM, Hao AV, Glassroth J, et al. Respiratory illness in persons with human immunodeficiency virus infection. Am Rev Respir Dis 1993; 148:1523–1529.
3. Mundy LM, Auwaerter PC, Oldach D, et al. Community-acquired pneumonia; Impact of immune status. Am J Respir Crit Care Med 1995; 152:1309.
4. Murray JF. Pulmonary complications of HIV-1 infection among adults living in Sub-Saharan Africa. J Tuberc Lung Dis 2005; 9:823.
5. Boyton RJ. Infectious lung complications in patients with HIV/AIDS. Curr Opin Pul Med 2005; 11:203–207.
6. Grau I, Pallares R, Tubau F, et al. Epidemiologic changes in bacteremic pneumococcal disease in patients with human immunodeficiency. Virus in the era of highly active antiretroviral therapy. Arch Intern Med 2005; 165:1533–1540.
7. Ishida T, Hashiomoto T, Arita M, et al. A 3-year prospective study of a urinary antigen-detection test for Streptococcus pneumoniae in community acquired pneumonia. J Infect Chemother 2004; 10:359.
8. Lopez-Palomo C, Martin-Zamorano M, Beitez E, et al. Pneumonia in HIV-infected patients in the HAART era: incidence, risk, and impact of the pneumococcal vaccination. J Med Virol 2004; 72:517–524.
9. Schuchat A, Broome CV, Hightower A, et al. Use of surveillance for invasive pneumococcal disease to estimate the size of the immunosuppressed HIV-infected population. JAMA 1991; 265:3275–3279.
10. Baddour LM, Klugman KP, Feldman C, et al. Combination antibiotic therapy lowers mortality among severely ill patients with pneumococcal bacteremia. Am J Resp Crit Care Med 2004; 170:440–444.
11. USPHS/IDSA Prevention of Opportunistic Infections Working Group. USPHS/IDSA guidelines for the prevention of opportunistic infections in persons infected with human immunodeficiency virus: Disease-specific recommendations. MMWR 1997; 51:RR-6.
12. Munoz P, Miranda ME, Llacaqueo A, et al. Haemophilus species bacteremia in adults. Arch Intern Med 1997; 157:1869.
13. Shepp DH, Tang IT, Ramundo MB, et al. Serious Pseudomonas aeruginosa infection in AIDS. J Acquir Immune Defic Syndr 1994; 7:823–831.
14. Thornsberry C, Ogilvie P, Kahn J, et al. Surveillance of antimicrobial resistance in Streptococcus pneumoniae, Haemophilus influenzae, and Moraxella catarrhalis in the United States in 1996–1997 respiratory season. Diagn Microbiol Infect Dis 1997; 29:249.
15. Fowler VG Jr, Miro JM, Hoen B, et al. Staphylococcus aureus endocarditis: a consequence of medical progress. JAMA 2005; 293:3012–3021.
16. Francis J, Doherty M, et al. Severe community-onset pneumonia in healthy adults caused by methicillin-resistant Staphylococcus aureus carrying the Panton-Valentine leukocidin genes. Clin Infect Dis 2005; 40:100–107.
17. Mendelson MH, Gurtman A, Szabo S, et al. Pseudomonas aeruginosa bacteria in patients with AIDS. Clin Infect Dis 1994; 18:886.
18. Hirschtick RE, Glassroth J, Jordan MC, et al. Bacterial pneumonia in persons infected with the human immunodeficiency virus. N Engl J Med 1995; 333:845.
19. Boschini A, Smacchia C, DiFine M, et al. Community-acquired pneumonia in a cohort of former injection drug users with and without human immunodeficiency virus infection: Incidence, etiologies, and clinical aspects. Clin Infect Dis 1996; 23:107.
20. Blatt SP, Dolan MJ, Hendrix CW, et al. Legionnaires' disease in human immunodeficiency virus-infected patients: Eight cases and review. Clin Infect Dis 1994; 18:227–232.
21. Marston BJ, Lipman HB, Breiman RF. Surveillance for Legionnaires' disease: Risk factors for morbidity and mortality. Arch Intern Med 1994; 154:2417–2422.
22. Rosen MJ, Clayton K, Schneider RF, et al. Intensive care of patients with HIV infection: utilization, critical illnesses and outcomes. Pulmonary complications of HIV Infection Study Group. Am J Resp Crit Care Med 1997; 155:67–71.
23. Stout JE, Yu VL. Legionellosis. N Engl J Med 1997; 337:682–687.
24. Mandell L, Bartlett JG, Dowell SF, et al. Update of practice guidelines for the management of community acquired pneumonia in immunocompetent adults. Clin Infect Dis 2003; 37:1405–1433.
25. Singh VR, Smith DK, Lawerence J, et al. Coccidioidomycosis in patients infected with human immunodeficiency virus: review of 91 cases at a single institution. Clin Infect Dis 1996; 23:563–568.
26. Wheat LJ, Kohler RB, Tewari RP. Diagnosis of disseminated histoplasmosis by detection of Histoplasma capsulatum antigen in serum and urine specimens. N Engl J Med 1986; 314:83–88.

27. Wheat LJ, Connolly-Stringfield PA, Baker RL, et al. Disseminated histoplasmosis in the acquired immune deficiency syndrome: clinical findings, diagnosis and treatment, and review of the literature. Medicine (Baltimore) 1990; 69:361–374.

28. Miller WT Jr, Sais GJ, Frank I, et al. Pulmonary aspergillosis in patients with AIDS: Clinical and radiographic correlations. Chest 1994; 105:37–44.

29. Denning DW, Follansbee SE, Scolaro M, et al. Pulmonary aspergillosis in the acquired immunodeficiency syndrome. N Engl J Med 1991; 324:654–662.

30. Pervex NK, Kleinerman J, Kattan M, et al. Pseudomembranous necrotizing bronchial aspergillosis: A variant of invasive aspergillosis in patients with hemophilia and acquired immune deficiency syndrome. Am Rev Respir Dis 1985; 131:961–963.

31. Kemper CA, Hostetler JS, Follansbee SE, et al. Ulcerative and plaque-like tracheobronchitis due to infection with Aspergillus in patients with AIDS. Clin Infect Dis 1993; 17:344–352.

32. Denning DW. Unusual manifestations of aspergillosis. Thorax 1995; 50:812–813.

33. Candoni A, Mestroni R, Damiani D, et al. Caspofungin as first line therapy of pulmonary invasive fungal infections in 32 immunocompromised patients with hematologic malignancies. Eur J Haematol 2005; 75:227–233.

34. Wieland T, Liebold A, Jagiello M, et al. Superiority of voriconazole over amphotericin B in the treatment of invasive aspergillosis after heart transplantation. J Heart Transplant 2005; 24:102–104.

35. Maertens J, Boogaerts M. Caspofungin in the treatment of candidosis and aspergillosis. Int J Infect Dis 2003; 7:94–101.

36. Mirza SA, Phelan M, Rimaldn D, et al. The changing epidemiology of cryptococcosis: an update from population-based active surveillance in 2 large metropolitan areas, 1992-2000. Clin Infect Dis 2003; 36:789–794.

37. Chuck SL, Sande MA. Infectious with Cryptococcus neoformans in the acquired immunodeficiency syndrome. N Engl J Med 1989; 321:794–799.

38. Clark RA, Greer D, Atkinson W, et al. Spectrum of Cryptococcus neoformans infection in 68 patients infected with human immunodeficiency virus. Rev Infect Dis 1990; 12:768–777.

39. Eng RH, Bishburg E, Smith SM, et al. Cryptococcal infections in patients with acquired immunodeficiency syndrome. Am J Med 1986; 81:19–23.

40. Malabonga VM, Basti J, Kamholz SL. Utility of bronchoscopic sampling techniques for cryptococcal disease in AIDS. Chest 1991; 99:370–372.

41. Saag MS, Graybill JR, Larsen R, et al. Practice guidelines for the management of cryptococcal meningitis. Clin Infect Dis 2000; 30:710–718.

42. Salzman SH, Smith RL, Aranda CL. Histoplasmosis in patients at risk for the acquired immunodeficiency syndrome in a nonendemic setting. Chest 1988; 93:916–921.

43. Wheat J, Sarosi G, McKinsey D, et al. Practice guidelines for the management of patients with histoplasmosis. Clin Infect Dis 2000; 30:688–695.

44. Wheat JL. Current diagnosis of histoplasmosis. Trends Microbiol 2003; 11:488–494.

45. Williams B, Fojtasek M, Connolly-Stringfield P, et al. Diagnosis of histoplasmosis by antigen detection during an outbreak in Indianapolis, Ind. Arch Pathol Lab Med 1994; 118:1205–1208.

46. Johnson P, Wheat LJ, Cloud G, et al. Safety and efficacy of liposomal amphotericin B compared with conventional amphotericin B for induction therapy of histoplasmosis in patients with AIDS. Ann Intern Med 2002; 137:105–109.

47. Wheat J, Hafner R, Korzun AH, et al. Itraconazole treatment of disseminated histoplasmosis in patients with the acquired immunodeficiency syndrome. Am J Med 1995; 98:336–342.

48. Hecht FM, Wheat J, Korzun AH, et al. Itraconazole maintenance treatment for histoplasmosis in AIDS: a prospective, multicenter trial. J Acquir Immune Defic Syndr Hum Retrovirol 1997; 16:100–107.

CHAPTER 31

HIV-associated Tuberculosis

Edward C. Jones-López
David J. Cennimo
Jerrold J. Ellner

Introduction

Throughout history, tuberculosis (TB) has ravaged the health of humans all over the world acquiring designations such as 'captain of death' and 'white plague'.[1] The geographic distribution and epidemiology of TB has changed over time[2] influenced by human migration and genetic susceptibility, environmental conditions, improved sanitation and air quality, medical advances and most recently, the emergence of the HIV pandemic.[3] The impact the human immunodeficiency virus (HIV) and *Mycobacterium tuberculosis* (Mtb) have had on each other cannot be over-emphasized. Together, they constitute an advancing and enormously deadly force. Although the interaction between these two pathogens is bidirectional,[4] this chapter will focus on how HIV has impacted on TB, modifying its epidemiology, natural history, clinical presentation, diagnosis, treatment, and prognosis.

Patients with TB and HIV infection sometimes differ from HIV-uninfected patients in their clinical and radiographic presentations. In particular, patients with advanced HIV disease are more likely to develop atypical radiographic findings and disseminated disease. The emergence and global distribution of TB drug resistance,[5] particularly among HIV-infected individuals, poses an additional threat to TB control. The burden of TB and HIV is increasingly impacting on resource-poor countries, where already frail health facilities are overwhelmed by their combined burden. Although this chapter presents a world view of the problem, most of the discussion is targeted to clinicians in low-income countries, where TB prevalence is highest.

Epidemiology

The burden of TB is increasingly concentrated in middle and low-income countries, with high or increasing HIV prevalence rates (sub-Saharan Africa) or countries with large populations (China, India). To help focus TB control efforts where they are most needed, the World Health Organization (WHO) has identified 22 high TB burden countries (HBC) that account for approximately 80% of all estimated new TB cases each year.[6] In 2004, the WHO estimates that more than 80% of all new TB patients occurred in three of the six geographically defined WHO regions: the South-East Asian region notified 35% of all cases; the African region 24%; and the Western Pacific region 22%. The HIV epidemic has concentrated the burden of TB disease even further. For example, 11 of the 15 countries with the highest estimated TB incidence rates *per capita* are in Africa.[6] Recognizing the enormous influence HIV plays in determining the incidence of TB within a country,[7] the WHO modified its previous geographically-based classification (six regions) to a more comprehensive breakdown of the world into eight TB epidemiological regions based on the estimated incidence of TB and the prevalence of HIV in TB cases (Fig. 31.1A–C).

When the HIV pandemic began in the early 1980s, TB control programs throughout the world were unprepared. Indeed, even in the USA, the

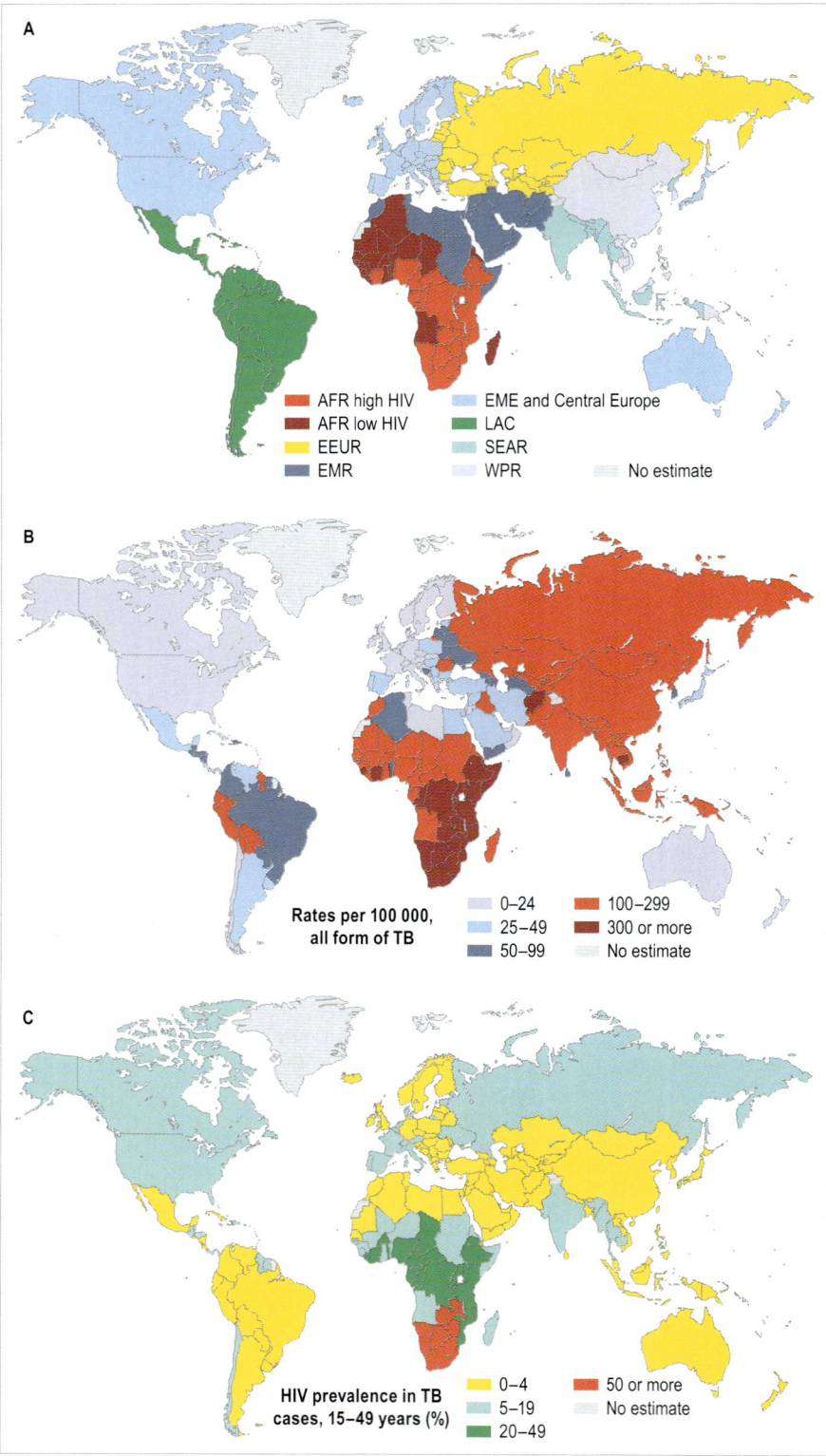

Figure 31.1 (A) (top): The eight TB epidemiological regions. (B) (middle): Estimated TB incidence rates (2003); (C) (bottom): Estimated prevalence of HIV infection in TB cases (2003). (Reproduced from The Global Plan to Stop TB 2006–2015; WHO 2006.)

A

AFR high HIV
AFR low HIV
EEUR
EMR
EME and Central Europe
LAC
SEAR
WPR
No estimate

B

Rates per 100 000, all form of TB

0–24
25–49
50–99
100–299
300 or more
No estimate

C

HIV prevalence in TB cases, 15–49 years (%)

0–4
5–19
20–49
50 or more
No estimate

infrastructure for TB control had deteriorated. Since HIV was first recognized 25 years ago, TB incidence and notification rates have remained tightly associated with HIV prevalence rates. In low-income countries, case fatality rates in TB disease has uncreased in parallel with HIV rates. The convergence of the two epidemics resulted in a sharp increase in TB notification rates throughout the world that evaporated decades of TB control efforts and prompted the unprecedented WHO declaration in 1993 that tuberculosis had become a public health world emergency. However, the impact of the HIV epidemic on the epidemiology of TB has not been homogeneous throughout the world. In WHO-defined Established Market Economies, where the pre-HIV TB incidence rate had been declining for decades, the HIV epidemic resulted in a transient increase in TB rates in the 1980s and early 1990s. In contrast, low and middle-income countries with high (5%) or rising HIV infection rates, many of whom had already high TB rates before the HIV epidemic began, suffered from a sharp increase in TB notification rates in the 1980s and continue to be overwhelmed by disturbingly high rates. The largest impact has been in sub-Saharan Africa where the number of TB cases has, on average, trebled since the mid-1980s. The HIV epidemic was directly responsible in reversing a slow but continuous decline in TB incidence throughout the world. In 2004, the *per capita* TB incidence rate was stable or falling in five out of six WHO regions, but growing at 0.6% per year globally.[6] The continuing increase is largely due to the increasing rate in Africa, fuelled by the HIV epidemic and the enormous pool of individuals with latent tuberculosis infection (LTBI). The African TB trend in 2004 was large enough to offset the global trend in decreasing or stable TB incidence rates. The current rate of growth is slower than in previous years, mainly because the HIV epidemic in Africa is slowing. In eastern Europe (mostly countries of the former Soviet Union), TB incidence increased during the 1990s, but peaked around 2001, and has since fallen.

The combined burden of disease caused by HIV and Mtb is daunting. In terms of numbers, 39 million people were living with HIV at the end of 2004 and the annual death toll from HIV/AIDS was about 3.1 million. It is estimated that one-third, or two billion, of the world population is infected with Mtb. About 13 million people are infected with both organisms. In 2004, there were 8.9 million (140/100 000) new cases of TB of which 3.9 (44%) million (62/100 000) were smear-positive and 741 000 (8%) were in adults infected with HIV.[6] In some African settings, over 50% of new TB cases are co-infected with HIV.

Although the global TB incidence rate is still slowly rising, prevalence is falling. WHO calculates that the expansion of the WHO-recommended DOTS strategy between 1990 and 2003 led to a fall in the global TB prevalence rate from 309 to 245 per 100 000 (including HIV-infected patients). In 2004, there were 14.6 million prevalent cases (229/100 000) of which 6.1 million were smear-positive (95/100 000).

The HIV epidemic has also resulted in increased TB-associated mortality, particularly in sub-Saharan Africa. An estimated 1.7 million people died from TB in 2004, 15% or 248 000 of whom were co-infected with HIV. The global death rate from TB peaked during the 1990s. Between 2002 and 2003, it fell by 2.5% overall, and by 3.5% among HIV-negative patients. If not for the strongly adverse trends in Africa, prevalence and death rates would be falling more rapidly worldwide. Death rates of HIV-positive TB patients on treatment have reached 20–30% compared with 5% achieved by adequate TB-control programs without HIV. When available, antiretroviral therapy (ART) drastically improves survival in HIV-associated TB. The WHO estimates that whereas the African Region alone accounts for 81% of the estimated 741 000 cases of TB among HIV-positive people in the world, only 4% were treated with ART in 2003. The Region of the Americas (mainly Brazil), on the other hand, accounts for 3% of the estimated cases but 96% of the 9388 TB cases with HIV infection were reported to have started on ART in 2003.[6] It is worth emphasizing that TB incidence and recurrence rates, even if reduced by ART, remain very high in HIV-infected patients accessing life prolonging ART.[8]

In addition to HIV, the other major obstacle to TB control in the world is the emergence of TB drug resistance, particularly multidrug resistant TB (MDR-TB) defined as resistance to at least isoniazid and rifampicin. More recently, the emergence of extensively drug resistant TB (XDR-TB), now defined as an MDR isolate that is also resistant to at least quinolones and an injectable second-line drug (aminoglycoside or capreomycin), in HIV-positive patients in South Africa has raised the specter of an epidemic of untreatable TB, rapidly spreading and with a high mortality rate.[9A] Most cases of drug resistance are secondary to non-compliance but primary MDR-TB is increasing in several countries in the world. Experience in eastern Europe has shown that if left unchecked, MDR-TB may propagate rapidly and become a major health threat and responsible for up to 15% of new TB cases. This epidemiological scenario is more likely in countries with poor TB control programs with high rates of HIV infection, where clusters of MDR-TB disease (hospital, prisons, military barracks) may rapidly extend to the general population. If and when this occurs, the cycle of infection with drug-resistant strains is extremely difficult to interrupt. Based on a combination of surveys and calculations in 2006, the WHO estimates 460 000 MDR-TB cases emerge every year, about one-half of them among new TB patients and the other half among patients that have been previously treated. China, India and the Russian Federation account for 68% of the estimated annual incidence of MDR-TB cases.[6]

Pathogenesis

Despite its public health importance, Mtb remains an elusive and poorly understood microorganism causing a complex and multifaceted disease, for which there are relatively few diagnostic tools and limited treatment options. A central constraint in controlling TB disease to date has been our incomplete understanding of the relative weight environment, host immunity and bacterial virulence factors play in determining the likelihood of infection and disease, following exposure to Mtb.

TB begins with the inhalation of Mtb-containing aerosols into the pulmonary alveoli. Here, the bacilli enter resident alveolar macrophages, dendritic cells and monocytes recruited from the bloodstream. Multiple distinct receptors, such as complement receptors (CR)1, (CR)3, (CR)4, the mannose receptor, CD14, surfactant protein A (Sp-A) receptors and scavenger receptors, all have the potential to recognize and bind Mtb *in vitro*.[9] Mtb can activate the alternative pathway of complement and become opsonized by complement products that facilitate uptake by complement receptors; Mtb also expresses surface polysaccharides that can directly interact with complement receptors. Besides expressing traditional phagocytic receptors for antibody and complement, macrophages and dendritic cells also express Toll-like receptors (TLRs) that recognize conserved antigens expressed on pathogens. Binding of TLRs to these pathogen-specific ligands initiates a signal transduction pathway in the host cell that culminates in the activation of NFκb and the induction of cytokines and chemokines that are crucial to eliciting the adaptive immune response against Mtb. The sequence of immune events following interaction of Mtb with TLRs and other receptors is only beginning to be understood. Nevertheless, it is clear that in the vast majority of individuals, the interaction culminates in the activation of a protective Th1 dominant immune response.[10] Clearly, the Th1 response is protective, but its role in host immunity is complicated by the following issues: (1) The Th1 immune response by the host, although sufficient to contain an initial infection, is incapable of achieving sterilizing immunity leaving the host vulnerable to disease reactivation; (2) Interferon (IFN)-γ production is enhanced in the lung of TB patients despite concomitant disease suggesting that this cytokine is not sufficient to protect from disease; (3) Despite an apparently robust Th1 immunity, individuals in high transmission areas may become re-infected with Mtb; (4) The Th1 response that controls Mtb replication also invokes immunopathology, such as lung cavitation, which increases infectivity and thereby maintains the cycle of transmission of Mtb to new hosts.

Several mechanisms including induction of Th2 and T-regulatory cells contribute to host susceptibility to TB. Th2 cells are characterized by secretion of IL-4 and IL-10. T-regulatory cells are a distinct subset of T cells that suppress Th1 responses and are characterized by the cell surface expression of CD25, cytoplasmic expression of FOXP3 and secretion of IL-10 and transforming growth factor-β. TB disease and particularly disease with a poor prognosis have been associated with increased production of IL-4 and IL-10. IL-10 secreting CD8 T cells have been described in anergic TB patients and increased levels of (CD4[+] D25) regulatory T cells have been reported in bronchoalveolar lavage of untreated TB patients. These studies imply that an imbalance in effector cell populations and modulation by regulatory T cells may determine progression from latent infection to disease.

Thus, there are several aspects of host immunity in TB that are not completely understood. First, the basis for innate resistance against Mtb infection is not known. Although individuals may have close exposure to a patient with infectious TB, some will develop Mtb infection and others will not. Mtb exposure leads to perturbations in the local and systemic immune response as suggested by the fact that exposed household contacts (HHCs) differ from unexposed controls in the greater frequency of IFN-γ-producing lymphocytes in bronchoalveolar lavage and circulating CD8 lymphocytes that inhibit the intracellular replication of Mtb.[11] Second, the basis for protective mechanisms that prevent progression from Mtb infection to disease is not known. Most Mtb-infected hosts contain the Mtb infection and enter a stage of clinical latency with the potential for delayed reactivation of disease. We now know that 'latency' is a misnomer. The efficacy of treatment of LTBI indicates that active bacterial metabolism is occurring at latent foci of infection. Further, the finding that HIV-infection promotes 'reactivation' of latent foci infection indicates that clinical latency must be continuously controlled by dynamic interactions between bacterial replication and host immunity. Certain medical conditions associated with immunosuppression upset this balance and lead to progressive disease. Lastly, we lack biomarkers that characterize Mtb-infected hosts with an increased risk of progressing to disease. In some cases, Mtb-infected persons may have medical risk factors (e.g. HIV infection, diabetes mellitus) predisposing them to progression from infection to disease; however in many cases, disease occurs in the absence of identifiable predisposing factors. Biomarkers to identify hosts with increased risk of progression would be extremely useful in targeting individuals for treatment of LTBI and other interventions such as trials of therapeutic vaccines.

In addition to host immunity, the risk of Mtb infection and disease may also be determined by mycobacterial virulence factors. There is a growing body of evidence suggesting mycobacteria are not homogenously virulent as shown by the fact that Mtb strains vary in their induction of cytokines, growth characteristics in liquid cultures, macrophages, and THP1 cells and growth kinetics in animal experiments.[12–15]

Clinical Aspects

TB is a complex, dynamic and multifaceted disease. The clinical spectrum of TB is best characterized as a disease continuum that begins after an individual is first exposed to aerosols containing Mtb. After the initial exposure occurs, the disease cycle may or may not initiate depending on environmental, immunological and bacterial factors that will determine the likelihood of Mtb transmission, the establishment of infection and the development of disease. It is worth discussing these three stages of the TB disease cycle separately, as they have epidemiological, pathophysiological and clinical relevance. *Transmission* and *infection* are frequently interchanged as though equivalent; there is however, a growing body of evidence suggesting otherwise.[16,17]

Mtb Transmission

In this discussion, transmission is defined as the capacity for Mtb to travel through the airspace separating an infectious case and a contact physically close enough to inhale cough-generated aerosols. As

defined here, transmission is probably determined by factors related to the infectiousness of the source case and environmental conditions. Although hypothetical at this time, it is conceivable that bacterial determinants also may play a role in the likelihood of transmission as not all mycobacterial strains may survive aerosolization equally. Host characteristics that influence the risk of transmission include the infectiousness of the source (as measured by smear AFB grade), the cough strength and, the proximity and intensity of the contact to the exposure.[16] Together these factors may determine the infecting inoculum and thus, the likelihood for the inhaled mycobacteria to attain the alveoli and initiate a host-bacterial interaction, that may or may not, result in Mtb infection.[17] Environmental conditions that may play a role in transmission include ambient air humidity, ventilation and exposure to UV light.[18] Thus, successful transmission is a necessary prelude to Mtb infection. Distinguishing successful from unsuccessful transmission is conceptually important particularly as regards to our understanding of innate immunity to Mtb infection. The effect HIV has on Mtb transmission has been studied extensively. Although there is still some disagreement because of contradictory results and methodological limitations, HIV does not seem to modify significantly the risk of Mtb transmission.[19] An exception may occur in advanced HIV disease in that a weakened cough decreases transmission.

Mtb Infection

The second stage of the disease cycle is the establishment of Mtb infection, an obligatory step before TB disease develops. This poorly understood yet pathophysiologically important phase is a necessary but not sufficient step leading to TB disease. Until recently, the only available tool to diagnose Mtb infection was the tuberculin skin test (TST) a well validated, but 100-year old test with multiple limitations.[20] Well-known limitations include the instability of TST over time,[21] its poor specificity due to cross reactivity with shared antigens present in both environmental mycobacteria and BCG vaccination strains and its poor sensitivity in certain clinical conditions such as advanced stages of HIV infection[22] due to depressed cell-mediated immunity leading to skin test anergy. In addition, the TST does not distinguish TB disease from LTBI.[23] Other potentially important limitations include that a single determination of TST does not indicate the time since Mtb infection occurred (recent TST converters are at higher risk of disease progression); in the case of multiple Mtb infections in a single individual, the TST does not provide information regarding the number or type[24] of infecting strains (this may be important if immunity is strain-specific). Finally, the TST is not able to discern if the infecting strain is viable or non-viable.[25] Despite its many limitations, TST remains the gold standard to detect Mtb infection and the basis for public health interventions to treat LTBI to prevent the development of TB disease.

The recent development of interferon-gamma releasing assays (IGRA, QuantiFeron Gold and T-spot) significantly improves the specificity of the diagnosis of Mtb infection because the assay is based on ESAT-6 and CFP-10 antigens which are specific to Mtb and not present in environmental mycobacteria or BCG strains. Although, the Centers for Disease Control and Prevention (CDC) have stated that the QuantiFeron-Gold assay can be used interchangeably with the TST there are several limitations. IGRAs have not been validated in large prospective studies for reliability of these tests over time (stability), the effect of repeated Mtb exposures on test results and their performance in programmatic conditions in high TB prevalence countries.[26] In addition, the high cost of these newer tests will surely limit their use to TB programs in high-income settings with a low annual risk of Mtb infection, where the intended goal is to eradicate Mtb infection with targeted LTBI treatment programs.[27]

By definition, LTBI refers to asymptomatic Mtb infection with no evidence of active disease. Thus, in the absence of symptoms, clinicians tend to consider patients with LTBI as a well-defined and stable population that will benefit from preventive treatment. However, for an individual moving in the clinical continuum from Mtb infection to disease, the line separating LTBI from early TB disease may be blurred as the detection of symptoms (or early pulmonary radiological findings with no accompanying symptoms) is almost entirely dependent on the timing of the medical evaluation. This is particularly the case with concurrent HIV infection. Typically, TB programs throughout the world detect new TB cases by passive ascertainment of symptomatic patients seeking attention at a health clinic for evaluation of symptoms that are present anytime from a few days to as long as years before the patient is evaluated. In contrast, the evaluation of an asymptomatic individual for Mtb infection is almost always performed proactively by health personnel and performed in the context of public health programs to guide treatment of LTBI in low TB prevalence settings (contact evaluation after a defined exposure, routine screen-ing programs for healthcare providers, immigrants from a high prevalence countries, etc). In such cases, the absence of symptoms may not be a reliable method to exclude active disease, particularly in settings with high TB and HIV prevalence rates where up to 10% of subjects evaluated for Mtb infection with little or no symptoms may have culture-confirmed TB disease at the time of the initial or repeat evaluations.[17,28] In a recent study, the duration of the latent period between exposure, infection, evidence of early disease and the onset of symptoms among Ugandan household contacts was as long as 22 months.[17] Our ability to distinguish LTBI from early TB disease is thus limited and requires a thorough evaluation before treatment for LTBI is initiated. The evaluation should include a careful clinical history, a complete physical exam and a chest radiograph. The history of recent Mtb exposure, HIV infection or the presence of clinical symptoms, however subtle, should trigger a more thorough evaluation that may include sputum (or gastric aspirate in children) examination for smear and culture. When available, it is useful to obtain a computed tomographic scan (CT) of the chest to visualize incipient changes not appreciated by simple radiography (intrathoracic adenopathy or early pulmonary changes). Lastly, the presence of any abnormalities in the above evaluation requires a re-evaluation after a period of observation to monitor the evolution of symptoms. The provision of treatment for LTBI is effective in both uninfected and HIV-infected individuals but not widely applied because of several obstacles discussed in the section of Mtb prevention below.

Once established, the initial infection with Mtb is frequently controlled, since only ~10% of HIV-negative infected individuals will progress to active disease during their lifetime. It is generally thought that those who are infected without disease manifestations may harbor a persistent dormant infection with the potential to reactivate after a long hiatus. Such reactivation of a latent infection contributes significantly to the pathogenesis of tuberculosis, and is believed to account for a substantial portion of TB cases in the HIV-infected[29]; however, recent evidence from Malawi shows that primary TB may account for a significant proportion of newly diagnosed cases in high HIV prevalence settings.[30] Although the precise immune mechanisms engendering protection in the acute or latent phase of TB remain incompletely defined, current evidence support the notion that effective acquired cellular immunity to Mtb is critically dependent on the activation of the Th1 subset of CD4$^+$ T cells. The risk of developing TB disease in those that are co-infected with HIV by reactivating a latent tuberculous infection increases to 5–15% annually, rising as immune deficiency worsens.[3] Contrary to what was believed for years, the risk of TB reactivation increases almost immediately after HIV infection is acquired and remains high for at least the first 4–5 years after HIV seroconversion.[29]

TB Disease

The third stage is the development of active TB disease, defined by the development of symptoms. The worldwide distribution of Mtb and its capacity to involve most body organs should remind practicing physicians to keep TB in the differential diagnosis for a long list of acute, sub-acute and chronic clinical syndromes. Pathophysiologically, TB disease may result from rapid progression shortly after the initial Mtb exposure (primary TB) or from reactivation of a latent Mtb infection acquired months, years or decades before disease develops (post-primary TB). Depending of the involved organ(s), the underlying immunological state and the age of a patient, TB may present as a myriad of clinical syndromes from fever of unknown origin to a fulminant presentation mimicking septic shock. The classic description of pulmonary TB presenting with cough, fever, weight loss, night sweats and hemoptysis reflects the fact that about 70% of all reported TB cases are pulmonary. Although the presence of cough for 2–3 weeks is non-specific, this duration of cough has traditionally served as the criterion for defining suspected TB and is used in most national and international guidelines. The likelihood of 'atypical' presentations, including the development of disseminated disease with positive blood cultures for mycobacteria, and pleural disease, increases in severely immunosuppressed patients such as those with advanced AIDS with low CD4+ lymphocytes. The most common sites of extra-pulmonary involvement are blood and extra-thoracic lymph nodes, followed by bone marrow, genitourinary tract, and the central nervous system.

The order of occurrence of Mtb and HIV infection is important to understanding the clinical manifestations of TB in those dually infected. In most high TB prevalence areas, Mtb infection is acquired in childhood from exposure to an active case in the household. HIV infections occur later with sexual activity. In this setting Mtb is likely to reactivate relatively early in the course of immunodeficiency and is typical in its manifestations (upper lobe, cavitary pulmonary opacities) as shown in Figures 31.2C and 31.2F. In areas of low TB prevalence, HIV-infected persons are likely to be exposed to TB in congregate settings (hospital ward, prisons, etc.). The TB may be atypical and often resembles and, in fact, represents primary TB with lower lobe, noncavitary opacities (Fig. 31.2D), pleural effusions (Fig. 31.2B), hilar or mediastinal adenopathy and concurrent or isolated extrapulmonary disease. In practice there is some overlap in presentation, however, both in high and in low prevalence areas.

In most low and middle income settings with high TB prevalence, diagnostic tools available to cli-

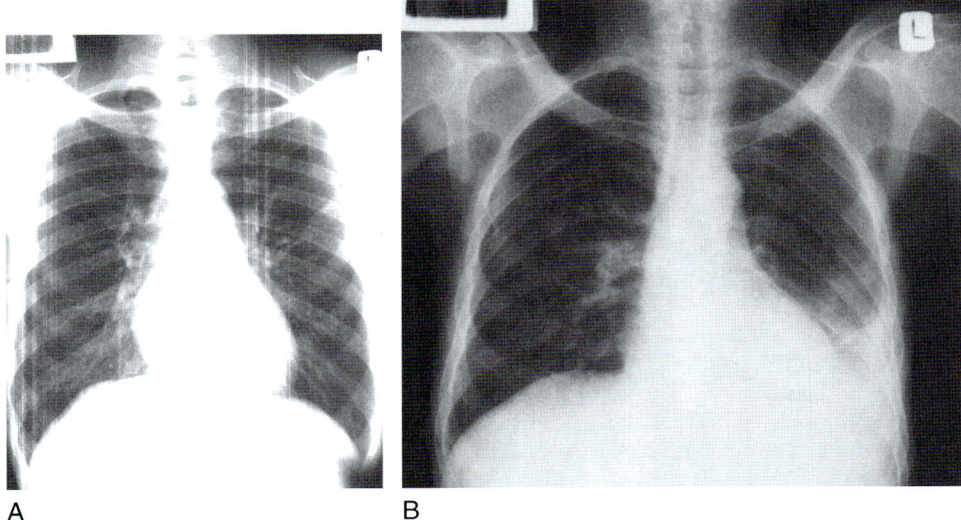

A   B

Figure 31.2 Representative chest radiographs from Ugandan HIV patients with culture-confirmed TB: (A) Normal; (B) Left pleural effusion.

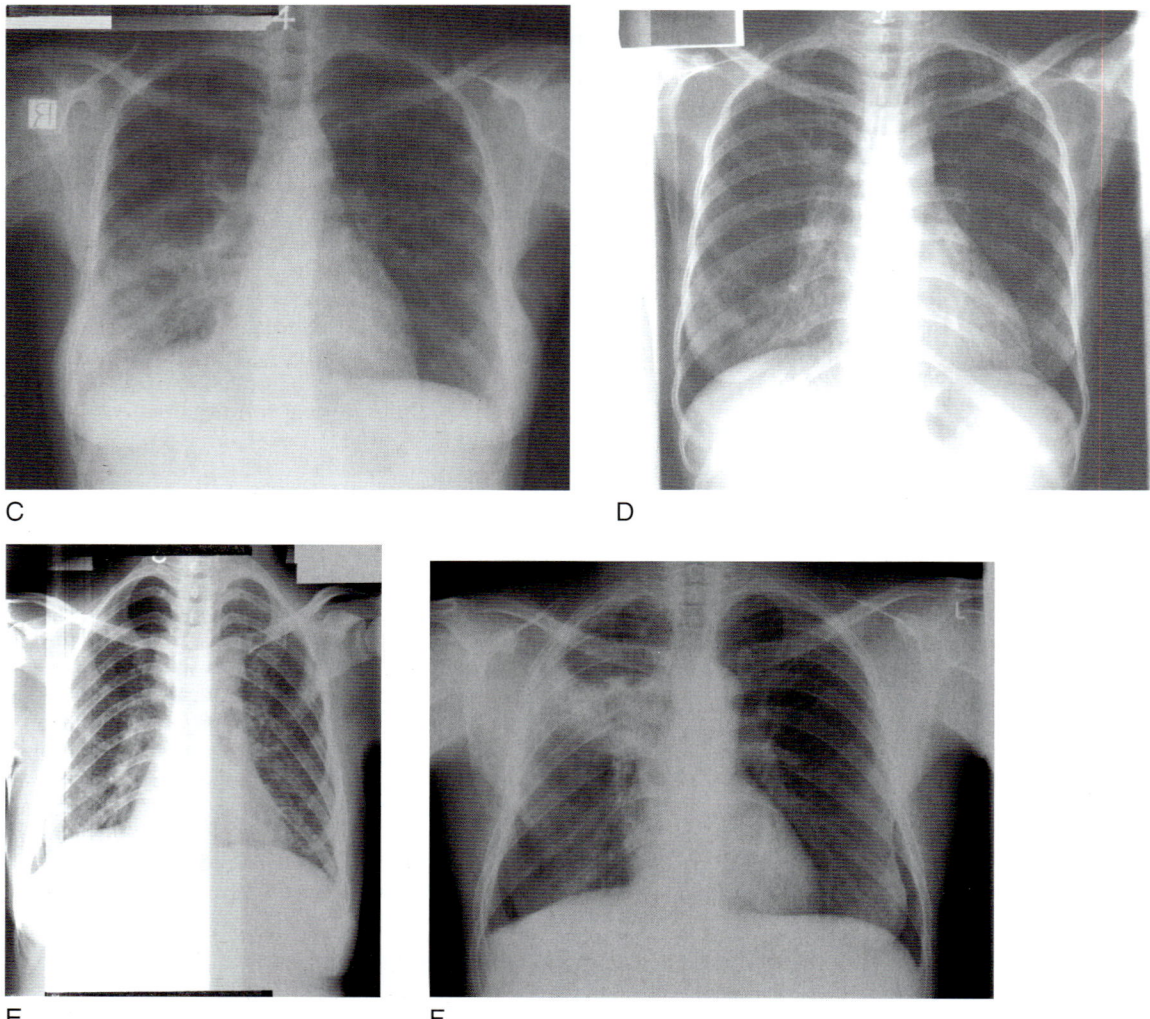

Figure 31.2, *cont'd* (C) Right cavitary disease; (D) Right lower lobe infiltrate; (E) Miliary infiltrate; (F) Right upper lobe infiltrate. (All images are from UMDNJ-Makerere University Research Collaboration archive.)

nicians are old, rudimentary and limited to detecting Mtb relatively late in the course of TB disease. Most TB programs in the world still heavily rely on three diagnostic tools for the diagnosis, treatment initiation and follow-up of TB in children and adults: the TST, sputum microscopy and chest X-ray. These methods are associated with multiple pitfalls including delays in diagnosis, empirical treatment and difficulties in monitoring treatment response. Together these limitations result in continued transmission, poor clinical outcomes and the development of drug resistance.

The microscopic examination of stained sputum is the most frequently relied upon diagnostic test as it is feasible in nearly all settings, and the diagnosis of TB can be strongly inferred by finding acid-fast bacilli by microscopic examination. In nearly all clinical circumstances in high prevalence areas, finding acid-fast bacilli in stained sputum is highly specific and, thus, is the equivalent of a confirmed diagnosis. In addition to being highly specific, identification of acid-fast bacilli by microscopic examination is particularly important for three reasons: it is the most rapid method for determining if a person has TB; it identifies persons who are at greatest risk of dying from the disease; and it identifies the most likely transmitters of infection. The main limitations of smear microscopy include its low sensitivity (50–60% in most studies), that no isolate is available for species identification and drug susceptibility testing and, that it does not distinguish viable from dead bacteria while monitoring response to treatment. Moreover, the prevalence of smear-negative TB may vary between 30–50% or higher in settings with high rates on HIV co-infection.[31]

A variety of strategies have been used to improve the performance of sputum smear microscopy.[32,33] Several studies have examined the optimum number of sputum specimens to establish a diagnosis of pulmonary TB. In a diagnostic evaluation for TB, at least two specimens should be obtained; a third specimen may be useful, but examination of more than three specimens adds minimally to the number of positive specimens obtained. The timing of specimen collection is also important. The yield appears to be greatest from early morning specimens. Although it is not practical to collect only early morning specimens, at least one specimen should be obtained from an early morning collection. The sensitivity of microscopy may increase 15–20% with concentration by centrifugation and/or sedimentation (usually after pretreatment with chemicals such as bleach, NaOH, and NaCl) or both, as compared with direct (unconcentrated) smear microscopy.[32] Fluorescence microscopy, in which auramine-based staining causes the acid-fast bacilli to fluoresce against a dark background, may be 10% more sensitive than conventional Ziehl-Neelsen (ZN) staining with light microscopy.[33] The specificity of fluorescence microscopy is comparable to Ziehl-Neelsen microscopy. The combination of increased sensitivity with little or no loss of specificity makes fluorescence microscopy a more accurate test, although the increased cost and complexity make it less applicable in many settings.

The probability of finding acid-fast bacilli in sputum smears by microscopy is directly proportional to the concentration of bacilli in the sputum. Sputum microscopy is likely to be positive when there are at least 10 000 organisms/mL of sputum. Some patients who are evaluated for pulmonary TB may have sputum smears which are described as scanty, defined as <10 organisms/100 high powered field (HPF). In some high TB prevalence areas, as many as 10% of the patients will have scanty sputum; until recently, a single scanty smear has not been accepted as diagnostic of pulmonary TB. In a recent study by Nigeria, 85% of scanty smears and 98% of

positive smears were culture positive for Mtb.[34] Smear negative pulmonary TB constitutes a significant public health problem leading to delays in diagnosis, over and under-treatment and may lead to increased Mtb transmission.[35,36] The diagnosis of sputum smear-negative pulmonary tuberculosis should be based on the following criteria: at least three negative sputum smears (including at least one early morning specimen); chest radiography findings consistent with TB; and lack of response to a trial of broad-spectrum antimicrobial agents. It is important to note that because the fluoroquinolones are active against the Mtb complex and thus, may cause transient improvement in persons with TB, they should be avoided in the initial treatment for possible bacterial pneumonia. At concentrations below 1000 organisms/mL of sputum, the chance of observing acid-fast bacilli in a smear is less than 10%. In contrast, properly performed culture can detect far lower numbers of acid-fast bacilli (detection limit is about 100 organisms/mL).

Traditional solid culture media (Lowenstein–Johnson or Ogawa) are more sensitive than AFB microscopy but require from 2–3 weeks to several months to grow and may have a high rate of contamination. Other solid media techniques (7H9, 7H10 and 7H11) have lower contaminations rates but are, in general, too onerous for low-income laboratory settings. Newer liquid culture methods such as the BACTEC 460 (detects radiolabeled CO_2 from replicating mycobacteria) and the simpler Mycobacterial Growth Indicator Tube (MGIT) systems can provide faster culture results (7–21 days) but remain too expensive and technologically demanding for low income settings. Lastly, nucleic acid amplification tests, introduced over the last decade and widely distributed in high-income settings, do not offer major advantages over culture at this time.[37] Although a positive result may be obtained faster than with any of the culture and DNA detection methods, these tests are expensive and not sufficiently sensitive for a negative result to exclude TB or to help in identifying Mtb in specimens from smear negative cases or extra pulmonary sites of disease. Cultures must be available if drug susceptibility testing is to be performed. Other approaches to establishing a diagnosis of TB such as serological tests are not of proven value and should not be used in routine practice at this time.

Chest radiography is a sensitive but non-specific test to detect TB.[38] Radiographic examination of the thorax may be useful to identify persons for further evaluation but a diagnosis of TB should never be established by radiography alone. Reliance on the chest radiograph as the only diagnostic test for TB will result in both over-diagnosis of TB and missed diagnoses of TB and other diseases. The radiological findings of HIV-associated TB are dependent on the level of CD4+ lymphocytes at the time of presentation. In patients with ≥350 cells/mL, most will present with classical radiographic findings of reactivation disease (apical/posterior consolidation of the upper lobes or consolidation of the superior segments of the lower lobes, cavitations, endobronchial spread or bronchiectasis), although some may resemble primary disease (pleural effusion, intrathoracic lymphadenopathy in mediastinum and hilum or, middle or lower lobe consolidation without cavitation), depending on the timing of Mtb infection and subsequent underlying pathogenic mechanism. Other radiographic presentations may include a miliary pattern, PCP-like diffuse infiltrates, spontaneous pneumothorax, minimal changes or a normal chest X-ray. Figures 31.2A–F show a representative samples of chest radiographs in HIV-infected patients from Uganda. In patients with lower CD4 cells with culture-confirmed TB, the likelihood of atypical radiographic findings increases and up to 20% of patients may have a normal or near-normal chest radiograph and thus the need to maintain a high index of suspicion and perform, when available, a chest CT. The inverse may also occur; HIV patients who present with an abnormal chest X-ray but no respiratory symptoms may still have significant pulmonary disease.[39] Because of the difficulties in diagnosing HIV-associated TB, all HIV-positive patients with pulmonary symptoms should be placed, if available, in respiratory isolation (or separated from non-TB patients) until TB is ruled out with serial AFB smears as discussed above.

Treatment

The treatment of TB focuses on both the patient and the community and should be designed to cure the patient without relapse, prevent transmission to others, and prevent the development of resistant organisms. The emphasis on preventing transmission and resistance underlies the early intensive treatment with multiple drugs. All patients with active TB disease must be treated with multiple drugs for a period of months. The decision to initiate anti-tuberculous therapy should be based on the clinical, radiological findings and epidemiological clues. It is sometimes necessary to initiate treatment before the results of smear and culture are known, particularly in high HIV prevalence settings where

the prevalence of smear negative tuberculosis is increased. The threshold for initiation must be low in patients with potentially life-threatening infections such as meningitis, pericarditis and miliary disease.[40]

Several national and international bodies have recommended treatment regimens for tuberculosis.[40–42] All recommendations are comprised of two phases, as shown in Table 31.1. An initial intensive phase is designed to kill the actively replicating organisms and sterilize the sputum. This phase has great individual and public health implications as this rapid killing is associated with decreased risk of transmission. After 2–3 months of treatment, 80–90% of patients should have negative sputum cultures. Rifampicin (R) and isoniazid (I) are both bactericidal drugs and constitute the backbone of the initial phase of treatment. Pyrazinamide (P) is added in the first 2 months as it allows the total regimen to be shortened from 9 to 6 months. Studies have shown no benefit to continuing pyrazinamide after the initial 2 months of treatment. Ethambutol (E) is added as a fourth drug if there is a possibility of resistance (recommended if the prevalence of primary isoniazid resistance ≥5%) or if the bacterial burden is thought high. Ethambutol may be discontinued when susceptibility to the other three drugs is confirmed. After the initial 2-month phase, the preferred regimen is to continue rifampicin and isoniazid for an additional 4 months. Patients who have cavitary disease at treatment initiation and continue to have positive cultures after 2 months of therapy are at high risk of relapse. Such patients should be initially evaluated for potential non-compliance or Mtb resistance. If neither is a factor, these patients should receive an additional 3 months of continuation therapy for a total of 9 months of treatment. The above standard treatment regimen is endorsed by CDC/ATS (USA) and WHO and recommended regardless of HIV status.[40–42] The doses, route of administration and mode of action of primary drugs are shown in Table 31.2.

In most low-income countries where budgetary constraints are paramount to policy decisions and there is limited access to timely drug susceptibility results, the use of rifampicin is usually more restricted. In such settings, TB treatment is often standardized based on a previous history of TB treatment (new versus re-treatment TB case), as recommended by WHO. In new TB cases, the 4-month RI continuation phase is replaced by a fixed 6-month treatment phase with IE. Recent evidence has shown regimens not containing rifampicin during the entire continuation phase are associated with a higher rate

Table 31.1 WHO-recommended treatment regimens

Treatment category	Patients	Tuberculosis treatment[a]	
		Initial phase (daily or three times per week)	Continuation phase (daily or three times per week)
I	New cases of smear-positive pulmonary tuberculosis or severe extrapulmonary tuberculosis or severe smear-negative pulmonary tuberculosis or severe concomitant HIV disease	2 months $H_3R_3Z_3E_3$ or 2 months $H_3R_3Z_3S_3$ 2 months HRZE or 2 months HRZS	4 months H_3R_3 4 months HR 6 months HE[b]
II[c]	Previously treated smear-positive pulmonary tuberculosis; relapse; treatment failure; treatment after default	2 months $H_3R_3Z_3E_3S_3$/1 month $H_3R_3Z_3E_3$ 2 months HRZES/1 month HRZE	5 months $H_3R_3E_3$ 5 months HRE
III[d]	New cases of smear-negative pulmonary tuberculosis or with less severe forms of extrapulmonary tuberculosis	2 months $H_3R_3Z_3E_3$ 2 months HRZE	4 months H_3R_3 4 months HR 6 months HE[b]

[a]Subscript after letters refers to the number of doses per week; daily has no subscript. H, isoniazid; R, rifampicin; Z, pyrazinamide; S, streptomycin; E, ethambutol. [b]A continuation phase of 6 months of HE has a higher failure and relapse rate than a continuation phase of 4 months of HR but can be used for mobile patients and those with limited access to health services; the HE regimen can also be used concomitantly with antiretroviral treatment of HIV-infected patients. [c]CDC/ATS and BTS recommend treatment for such patients based on susceptibility testing, with regimens tailored to the susceptibility profile. WHO recommends susceptibility testing whenever possible for patients with treatment failure. [d]WHO indicates that ethambutol need not be given in the initial phase of category III treatment if patients have non-cavitary, smear-negative pulmonary tuberculosis, or if patients are known to have a drug-susceptible organism, or for young children with primary tuberculosis.
Reproduced from Freiden et al. 2003.[41]

of failure and relapse.[43] However, these results should be carefully balanced against the risk of emerging drug resistance (particularly MDR-TB) that may result from the widespread use of rifampicin during a prolonged and unsupervised treatment period that frequently results in non-compliance. The WHO standardized re-treatment regimen consists of 2 months of streptomycin (S) + RIEP, 1 month of RIEP and 5 months of RIE.

Other drugs, listed in Table 31.3, can be used for the treatment of TB but the five 'first line' drugs should be employed preferentially and the use of 'second line' therapies should be restricted to patients with documented resistance or patients with limiting conditions (see below). The liberal use of fluoroquinolones in some parts of the world has already bred resistance in some organisms to this important class of drugs that play an essential role when drug resistance to first line drugs develops. The treatment of MDR-TB is quite complex and should be restricted to referral treatment centers and beyond the scope of this chapter.

The 6–9 month treatment period required for successful TB treatment is subject to patient non-compliance. Directly Observed Therapy (DOT) is the standard of care in many parts of the world for the treatment of TB. A trained observer monitors the patient, visualizing them taking each dose of the drug. Often this is coupled with social service support to form a holistic patient-centered approach to care.[41] The initial phase of TB treatment should always be administered, when possible, under DOT as this time represents the greatest potential risk for treatment failure and selection of resistant mutants if there are lapses in patient adherence to treatment. Various treatment regimens have been compiled and validated which allow for dosing 3 times per week,[40] providing some relief to DOT programs. Ideally, the entire course of treatment would be administered under DOT, particularly in treatment regimens other than daily dosing in HIV-infected individuals.[42] Response to treatment should be monitored by AFB smear and culture at least monthly until two consecutive specimens are negative. In settings with limited laboratory infrastructure, clinical progress may be the only measurable outcome. The culture sputum result at 2 months should be obtained as it has great significance in prognosticating relapse and determining duration of therapy, as explained above. In general, most cases of extrapulmonary tuberculosis can be successfully treated with the above regimens. Patients with extrapulmonary

Table 31.2 Doses, route of administration, and mode of action of primary TB drugs

Drug	Route	Mode of action	Daily dose			Twice-weekly dose			Thrice-weekly dose		
			Children	Adults	Maximum	Children	Adults	Maximum	Children	Adults	Maximum
Isoniazid	Oral or i.m[a]	Bactericidal	5–10 mg/kg[b]	5 mg/kg	300 mg	15 mg/kg	15 mg/kg (range 13–17)	900 mg	10 mg/kg	10 mg/kg (range 8–12)	900 mg
Rifampicin	Oral or i.v.	Bactericidal	10–20 mg/kg[c]	600 mg (range 8–12 mg/kg)	600 mg	10–20 mg/kg[c]	600 mg (range 8–12 mg/kg)	600 mg	10–20 mg/kg[c]	600 mg (range 8–12 mg/kg)	600 mg
Pyrazinamide[d]	Oral	Bactericidal	20–30 mg/kg	1.5 g (<50 kg) 2.0 g (51–74 kg) 2.5 g (>75 kg)	—	50 mg/kg (range 40–60 mg/kg)	2.5 g (<50 kg) 3.0 g (51–74 kg) 3.5 g (>75 kg)	—	35 mg/kg (range 30–40 mg/kg)	2.0 g (<50 kg) 2.5 g (51–74 kg) 3.0 g (>75 kg)	—
Ethambutol[e]	Oral	Bacteriostatic	15–25 mg/kg	15–25 mg/kg	2.5 g	30–50 mg/kg	45 mg/kg	—	30–50 mg/kg	30 mg/kg	—
Streptomycin	i.m, i.v.	Bactericidal	15–30 mg/kg	15 mg/kg	1000 mg	15 mg/kg	15 mg/kg	1000 mg	15 mg/kg	15 mg/kg	1000 mg
Thioacetazone	Oral	Bacteriostatic	2 mg/kg	150 mg	—	NR	NR	NR	NR	NR	NR

Adapted with permission from the New York City Department of Health. Tuberculosis treatment, 3rd edn. City Health Information: 1999, 18 (2) online. Available: www.nyc.gov/html/doh/pdf/chi/chi18-2.pdf. i.m, intramuscular; i.v, intravenous; NR, not recommended. [a]Intravenous and suppository forms are available in some countries. [b]WHO, IUATLD, and BTS recommend 5 mg/kg in children: CDC/ATS and the American Academy of Pediatrics recommend 10 mg/kg. [c]WHO, IUATLD, and BTS recommend 10 mg/kg in children: CDC/ATS and the American Academy of Pediatrics recommend 10–20 mg/kg. [d]WHO and CDC/ATS recommend dosing of pyrazinamide in adults on a weight basis, but dosing based on weight categories as recommended by BTS and by tuberculosis programmes is more useful in practice. Recommendations of dosing for this drug vary widely. Adults weighing <45 kg can have pediatric doses. The doses given here are based on the New York City Tuberculosis Control Program. [e]WHO, IUATLD, and BTS recommend 15 mg/kg ethambutol for daily administration in adults and children and 30 mg/kg for thrice-weekly dosing.
Reproduced from Freiden et al. 2003.[41]

Table 31.3 Second-line drugs used in the treatment of tuberculosis: Doses, major adverse reactions, and recommended regular monitoring

Drug	Route	Mode of action	Daily dose	Major adverse reaction[a]	Recommended regular monitoring	Comments
Capreomycin	i.v., i.m	Bactericidal	Children 15–30 mg/kg Adults 15 mg/kg Maximum 1000 mg	Auditory, vestibular, renal toxicity, eosinophilia; hypokalemia; hypomagnesemia	Audiometry, renal function, electrolytes	Ultrasound and warm compresses on injection site may reduce pain and induration.
Ciprofloxacin	Oral or i.v.	Bacteriostatic	Adults 750–1500 mg	Abdominal cramps; gastrointestinal upset; restlessness; insomnia; headache; interactions with warfarin and theophylline	—	Antacids containing aluminum, magnesium, or calcium, and sucralfate reduce absorption and should not be given within 2 h of dose. Caffeine effects may be increased. Not approved for use in children yet.
Cycloserine[b]	Oral	Bacteriostatic	Children 15–20 mg/kg Adults 500–1000 mg Divided doses	Psychosis; seizures; headache; depression; suicide; other CNS effects; rash; increased phenytoin concentrations	Assessment of mental status	Increase gradually, checking serum concentrations. Pyridoxine (vitamin B_6). 50 mg with each 250 mg may reduce CNS effects.
Ethionamide Protionamide[b]	Oral	Bacteriostatic	Children 15–20 mg/kg Adults 500–1000 mg Divided doses	Gastrointestinal upset; bloating; hepatotoxicity; hypothyroidism (especially with aminosalicylic acid); metallic taste	Hepatic function tests (if baseline abnormal); thyroid function	Antacids/antiemetics and lying flat for 20 min after doses may help tolerance. Start with 250 mg daily and increase as tolerated.
Kanamycin Amikacin	i.m, i.v.	Bactericidal	Children 15–30 mg/kg Adults 15 mg/kg Maximum 1000 mg	Auditory and renal toxicity; rare vestibular toxicity; hypokalemia; hypomagnesemia	Audiometry, renal function, electrolytes	Ultrasound and warm compresses on injection site may reduce pain and induration.
Levofloxacin	Oral or i.v.	Bacteriostatic, possibly bactericidal	Adults 500–1000 mg	Similar to ciprofloxacin but many fewer side-effects and drug interactions	—	Similar to ciprofloxacin. More active than ciprofloxacin and ofloxacin.

345

Table 31.3 Second-line drugs used in the treatment of tuberculosis: Doses, major adverse reactions, and recommended regular monitoring—cont'd

Drug	Route	Mode of action	Daily dose	Major adverse reaction[a]	Recommended regular monitoring	Comments
Moxifloxacin	Oral or i.v.	Bactericidal	Adults 400 mg	Similar to ciprofloxacin but fewer drug interactions	—	Similar to ciprofloxacin. Data on long-term use are limited at present. Avoid in patients with prolonged QT interval, and those receiving class Ia or III antiarrhythmic agents.
Ofloxacin	Oral or i.v.	Bacteriostatic	Adults 600–800 mg	Probably similar to ciprofloxacin; possibly fewer drug interactions	—	Similar to ciprofloxacin.
Aminosalicylic acid	Oral	Bacteriostatic	Children 150 mg/kg Adults 4 g every 12 h Maximum 12 g	Gastrointestinal upset; hypersensitivity; hepatotoxicity; hypothyroidism; low digoxin, high phenytoin concentrations; concentrations decreased by diphenhydramine	Thyroid function	Begin gradually and increase dose as tolerated. May cause hemolytic anemia in patients with deficiency of glucose-6-phosphate dehydrogenase.
Rifabutin	Oral	Bactericidal	Children 10–20 mg/kg Adults 5 mg/kg Maximum 300 mg	Rash; hepatitis; fever; neutropenia; thrombocytopenia; low concentrations of many drugs;[c] uveitis with high doses	Complete blood-cell count with platelets; hepatic function tests (if baseline abnormal)	Orange discoloration of secretions, urine, tears and contact lenses. Can be used in daily, twice-weekly, or thrice-weekly dosing. See text for dosing in HIV infection.[d] Methadone dose generally does not need to be increased. Patients should be advised to use barrier contraceptives during treatment.

Reproduced from Freiden et al. 2003.[41]

[a]Not all toxicities are listed here. Full prescribing information should be consulted from the package insert and pharmacology texts. [b]WHO recommends maximum doses of 750 mg for cycloserine, ethionamide and protinamide. [c]Including PIs NNRTIs, dapsone, ketoconazole, and oral contraceptives. [d]Twice weekly dosing not advised in AIDS patients. Contraindicated with delavirdine and saquinivir. Please see text for further details.

disease usually have a smaller Mtb bacterial burden. Infections in the CNS or spine, pericardial or bilateral pleural effusions, or multifocal joint/bone infection should be treated aggressively. Patients with meningitis or other CNS disease may benefit from extending therapy for 1 year.[44] The CNS penetration of anti-tuberculous drugs may be poor or unknown and may require individualizing treatment (see Table 31.5); some experts recommend ethionamide as a substitute for ethambutol in CNS disease.[44] Studies have conclusively proven the benefit of corticosteroids (prednisone 1 mg/kg or equivalent) in TB meningitis, pericarditis, and in patients with large pleural effusions.[44]

A list of major adverse reactions and recommended regular monitoring of primary drugs used in the treatment of tuberculosis are shown in Table 31.4. Baseline and monthly measurements of liver function are recommended for patients who are pregnant, within 3 months post partum, consume alcohol regularly or have chronic liver disease. Frequent measurements should also be performed for patients who have an increased risk of hepatotoxicity due to co-administered medications. Isoniazid and rifampicin should not be given in the symptomatic patient with liver enzymes >3 × normal or in the asymptomatic patient with liver enzymes >5 × normal.[40,42]

The use of antituberculous drugs in certain special conditions is shown in Table 31.5 and discussed below.

Pregnant or Breast-feeding

The WHO recommends the treatment of TB in pregnant women using I, R, P, E, whereas US guidelines do not recommend P unless there is no alternative. The risks of untreated TB in a pregnant woman far outweigh the risks of medications. Similarly, infants are at high risk of contracting TB from the close contact with their mothers, required by breast-feeding. Most anti-TB drugs are safe for breast-feeding and are not significantly concentrated in breast milk. If needed, the infant should be treated independently from the mother.[42]

Liver Disease

The presence of concomitant liver disease is particularly important to evaluate before TB treatment is initiated. Each TB drug has a particular toxicity profile. Whereas hepatotoxicity due to isoniazid is more likely as age increases, this should not preclude treatment of tuberculosis. There have been case reports of patients with fatal hepatotoxicity associated with the treatment of TB. Any signs of liver toxicity should be investigated promptly. The WHO does not recommend the use of pyrazinamide in patients who have known chronic liver disease. Guidelines do not currently recommend monitoring of liver enzymes in asymptomatic patients. Recent studies have shown elevation in transaminases especially in patients with Hepatitis B or C. When possible, it may be prudent to monitor liver function in patients who have a likelihood of preexisting liver disease (viral hepatitis, alcoholism, etc). If a patient with liver failure requires treatment for TB, ethambutol, streptomycin and a fluoroquinolone may be used. The most important risk factor for isoniazid-induced hepatotoxicity is alcohol consumption. Patients receiving isoniazid should be counseled to abstain from alcohol.[37,42]

Renal Disease

Isoniazid, rifampicin and pyrazinamide are all metabolized by the liver and thus safe to use in patients with renal disease. Ethambutol is excreted through urine and consideration should be given to replacing it with a second line drug. Patients should receive their medication via DOT after hemodialysis as dialysis eliminates most of these drugs. Patients with renal disease are at risk for neuropathy and should receive pyridoxine.[42]

Pyridoxine

All patients who are at risk for neuropathy (HIV, diabetes, renal failure and malnutrition), pregnant women, and persons with seizures should receive pyridoxine 50 mg/day while receiving isoniazid.[42]

Treatment in HIV-positive Individuals

The recommendations for TB treatment of HIV-infected patients are similar to those of HIV-uninfected patients. HIV patients have better outcomes when treated with short-course treatment with rifampicin. The response to treatment is similar in both HIV positive and HIV negative patients but the rate of TB recurrence is higher in HIV patients.[8] There is special concern for individuals who begin treatment with <100 CD4 cells as they have a higher rate of relapse when treated with non-daily treatment regimens. Twice-weekly rifamycin regimens should never be used in patients with CD4 <100.[41] Thiacetazone should never be given to HIV-infected patients because of its association with severe skin

Table 31.4 Major adverse reactions and recommended regular monitoring of primary drugs used in the treatment of tuberculosis

Drug	Major adverse reactions	Recommended regular monitoring	Comments
Isoniazid	Increases in hepatic enzymes; hepatitis; peripheral neuropathy; CNS effects; increased phenytoin concentrations; interaction with disulfiram	Hepatic function tests (if baseline abnormal)	Aluminum-containing antacids reduce absorption. Pyridoxine (vitamin B_6) can decrease peripheral neuritis and CNS effects, and should be used in alcoholic, pregnant, and malnourished patients.
Rifampicin	Hepatitis, fever, thrombocytopenia, flu-like syndrome. Lowers concentrations of many drugs, including methadone, warfarin, oral contraceptives, oral hypoglycemic agents, theophylline, dapsone, ketoconazole, protease inhibitors, and non-nucleoside reverse transcriptase inhibitors	Hepatic function tests (if baseline abnormal)	Orange discoloration of secretions, urine, tears, and contact lenses. Patients on methadone need a higher dose (average 50%) to avoid opioid withdrawal. Interaction with many drugs leads to low concentrations of one or both. May make glucose control more difficult in diabetes. Women should be advised to use barrier contraceptives during treatment. Contraindicated for patients taking most protease inhibitors and non-nucleoside reverse transcriptase inhibitors.
Pyrazinamide	Gastrointestinal upset; hepatotoxicity; hyperuricemia; arthralgias; gout, rarely; rash	Hepatic function tests (if baseline abnormal)	May complicate management of diabetes mellitus. Hyperuricemia can be used as indicator of compliance. Treat raised uric acid only if symptomatic.
Ethambutol	Diminished red-green color discrimination; decreased visual acuity; rash	Check color vision and visual acuity monthly	Optic neuritis may be unilateral; check each eye separately. If possible avoid in children too young to undergo vision testing.
Streptomycin	Auditory and renal toxicity; hypokalemia; hypomagnesemia	Audiometry, renal function, and electrolytes	Ultrasound and warm compresses on injection site may reduce pain and induration.
Thioacetazone	Rash and hypersensitivity reactions such as erythema multiforme and Steven–Johnson syndrome; gastrointestinal upset, hepatitis	Close observation for skin reactions	Do not use in HIV-infected patients. If rash develops, do not rechallenge.

Not all toxicities are listed here. Full prescribing information should be checked in the package insert or pharmacology texts.
Reproduced from Freiden et al. 2003.[41]

Table 31.5 TB treatment in special situations

Drug	Safety in pregnancy[a]	CNS penetration[b]	Dose in renal insufficiency[c]	Dose in hepatic insufficiency
Isoniazid	Has been used safely[d]	Good (20–100%)	No change	No change but use with caution
Rifampicin	Has been used safely (isolated reports of malformations)	Fair; inflamed meninges (10–20%)	No change	No change but use with caution
Rifabutin	Use with caution (limited data on safety)	Good (30–70%)	No change	No change but use with caution
Pyrazinamide	Recommended by WHO, not by US FDA (limited data on safety)	Good (75–10%)	Increase interval (use with caution)	No change but use with caution
Ethambutol	Has been used safely	Inflamed meninges only (4–64%)	Decrease dose/increase interval	No change
Aminoglycosides (streptomycin, kanamycin, amikacin)	Avoid[e] (associated with hearing impairment in fetus)	Poor[f]	Decrease dose/increase interval[g]	No change
Capreomycin	Avoid (limited data on safety)	Poor	Decrease dose/increase interval[g]	No change
Ciprofloxacin, levofloxacin, ofloxacin	Do not use (teratogenic in animals)	Fair (5–10%); inflamed meninges 50–90%	Decrease dose/increase interval	No change
Ethionamide, protionamide	Do not use (premature labour, congenital malformations)	Good (100%)	No change	No change, but use with caution
Cycloserine	Use with caution (limited data on safety)	Good (50–100%)	Decrease dose/increase interval	No change
Aminosalicylic acid	Has been used safely	Inflamed meninges only	Probably no change (limited data)	No change
Thioacetazone	Has been used safely	Unknown	Avoid	Avoid

[a]As with all medications given during pregnancy, antituberculosis medications should be used with extreme caution. The risk of tuberculosis to the fetus far outweighs the risk of most medications. Data are limited on the safety of antituberculosis medications during pregnancy. This table presents a consensus of published data and recommendations. [b]Steroid treatment seems to improve outcome in tuberculous meningitis, particularly in patients with altered mental status. [c]If possible, monitor serum drug concentrations of patients with renal insufficiency. [d]Supplement with pyridoxine (vitamin B₆). [e]If an injectable medication must be used during pregnancy, streptomycin is preferred. [f]Has been used intrathecally; efficacy not documented. [g]Avoid aminoglycosides and capreomycin in patients with reversible renal damage, if possible.
Reproduced from Freiden et al. 2003.[41]

reactions. Rifapentine, a long acting rifamycin, is not recommended in HIV-infected patients due to increased risks of resistance. Low serum concentrations of antimycobacterial drugs in HIV-infected patients may contribute to treatment failures. A study of 91 patients in Botswana (68% HIV positive) found low serum drug levels in a significant proportion of patients undergoing TB treatment including rifampicin (78%), isoniazid (30%), and ethambutol (41%). Only 1% of patients had low levels of pyrazinamide. Importantly, 26% had low plasma levels of both rifampicin and isoniazid, a factor that may contribute to poor outcomes and the emergence of resistance in a clinical setting.[45] Finally, it is important to maintain a high clinical suspicion for recurrence of TB disease after treatment is completed, as the risk of both relapse and reinfection is increased in HIV-positive patients. The risk of TB recurrence is not however, confined to HIV-positive individuals as shown by a recent study from South Africa where the rate of reinfection after successful treatment was four times that of new TB in mostly (>90%) HIV-negative subjects.[46]

Co-administration of TB and HIV Treatment

HIV infection significantly complicates the treatment of TB through multiple avenues including the high prevalence of drug side-effects and co-morbidities, the risk of drug–drug interactions, reduced drug absorption and the risk posed of developing an immune reconstitution inflammatory syndrome (IRIS) following the initiation of ART.[47] Also, the clinician must consider the effects of prophylaxis for opportunistic infections (OI) as a contributor to side-effects and drug–drug interactions. The significant overlap in toxicity between specific ART regimens and TB drugs, particularly as regards to hepatotoxicity, neuropathy and rash, make it difficult to attribute causality to a particular agent. For this reason, it is recommended to initiate one line of treatment at a time. An example of this problem is the development of rash in a patient with AIDS being treated for TB; in addition to the numerous other causes of HIV-associated rash that are beyond the scope of this discussion, the clinician would need to consider a drug reaction to TB drugs (I, R, and P), antiretroviral drugs (abacavir, didanosine and NNRTIs) or cotrimoxazole prophylaxis as a cause. If all of these drugs were started at the same time, it would be virtually impossible to determine the cause of the rash.

When determining an optimal treatment strategy for HIV-associated TB, it is important to consider the risk of drug interactions, the urgency to begin ART therapy and the presence of co-morbidities. The risk of intolerance and interaction should prompt vigilance in the clinician but should not discourage the treatment of co-infected patients, when initiation of antiretroviral therapy is indicated. The clinician must be mindful of the myriad of interactions between the rifamycins and many of the antiretroviral drugs (Table 31.6). Rifampicin, a potent stimulator of the cytochrome P450 3y system is prone to drug–drug interactions with several ARTs including zidovudine (AZT), non-nucleoside reverse transcriptase inhibitors (NNRTI) and protease inhibitors (PI). As a group, NRTI drugs are not metabolized by the cytochrome P450 system and are thus not susceptible to drug–drug interactions with the rifamycins. Standard anti-TB therapy can be administered safely with a minimum of side effects when combined with a triple NRTI regimen. However, this strategy has not been evaluated in a controlled study and should be considered empirical at this time and weighed against the risk of HIV drug resistance to NRTIs resulting from suboptimal virological suppression, as triple NRTI regimens have been shown to be inferior to NNRTI or PI-based regimens.

As shown in Table 31.6, most PIs and delavirdine should be avoided with rifampicin. It is generally safe to use efavirenz with rifampicin but the dose of efavirenz should be increased to 800 mg/day. However, it is important to note there have been reports of increased toxicity attributed to the higher levels of efavirenz and that the inducibility of the cytochrome P450 system is not universal and some individuals may not require a higher dose of efavirenz. If available, serum levels could help guide treatment. The information regarding the interaction between nevirapine and the rifamycins is less clear and some experts do not recommend the co-administration of rifampicin and nevirapine because of limited data and the risk of added hepatotoxicity. When used together, the nevirapine dose should be adjusted as indicated in Table 31.6. Rifabutin has similar *in vitro* antituberculous activity than rifampicin, with less potential for drug–drug interactions, and is currently recommended for the treatment of TB in HIV in the USA. If rifabutin is used with ritonavir boosted PIs, the dose of rifabutin should be decreased to 150 mg 2–3 times per week. If rifabutin is administered with efavirenz, the rifabutin dose is increased to 450–600 mg daily. The pharmacokinetics of the nevirapine/rifabutin interaction are favor-

Table 31.6 Recommendations for co-administering protease inhibitors (PI) and non-nucleoside reverse transcriptase inhibitors (NNRTI) with rifabutin and rifampin (USA 2003)

ARV class	ARV administered with rifabutin		ARV administered with rifampicin	
	ARV dose change	Rifabutin dose change	ARV dose change	Rifampicin dose change
NNRTI				
Efavirenz	None	↑ to 450–600 mg/day or 600 mg t.i.w.	↑ to 800 mg/day	None
Nevirapine	None	300 mg/day or 300 mg t.i.w.	consider ↑ to 300 mg b.i.d.	None
Delavirdine	Do not use	Do not use	Do not use	Do not use
PI				
Amprenavir	None	↓ to 150 mg/day or 300 mg t.i.w.	Do not use	Do not use
fos-Amprenavir	None	↓ to 150 mg/day or 300 mg t.i.w.	Do not use	Do not use
Atazanavir	None	↓ to 150 mg q.o.d. or 150 mg t.i.w.	Do not use	Do not use
Indinavir	↑ to 1000 mg t.i.d.	↓ to 150 mg/day or 300 mg t.i.w.	Do not use	Do not use
Nelfinavir	None	↓ to 150 mg/day or 300 mg t.i.w.	Do not use	Do not use
Saquinavir	Do not use	Do not use	Do not use	Do not use
DUAL PI				
Lopinavir/Ritonavir	None	↓ to 150 mg q.o.d. or 150 mg t.i.w.	Do not use	Do not use
Ritonavir added to any single PI	None	↓ to 150 mg q.o.d. or 150 mg t.i.w.	Do not use	Do not use

Information adapted from the CDC Guidelines (www.cdc.gov/nchstp/tb/tb_hiv_drugs/toc.htm
b.i.d., Twice daily; t.i.d., Thrice daily; q.o.d., Every other day; t.i.w., thrice weekly via DOT.

able and this would be the preferred combination. Although the multiple drug interactions with rifamycins make alternate regimens seem attractive, rifamycin-sparing regimens are clearly inferior in HIV patients with TB.[48]

Paradoxical worsening of tuberculosis disease has been described for decades and is referred to as the 'paradoxical reaction'.[49,50] The exact mechanism is not known, however, it is thought to be due to an increased recognition of mycobacterial antigens by a recovering immune system. This reaction is often more pronounced in HIV patients and is part of the spectrum of IRIS. Disease progression, non-compliance, drug failure and secondary infection must be ruled out before this diagnosis is entertained. The risk of IRIS has led to the recommendation to delay HAART until the initial 2 months of TB therapy has been completed.[49] Paradoxical reactions occur in 7–35% of patients with HIV and TB; mostly within the first 2 months of treatment with ARTs, but may occur up to 6 months after ART is initiated. Generally, patients who are receiving ART at the time of TB diagnosis should continue on their ART regimen. TB patients who have not started ART should have HIV treatment delayed for 2 months if their CD4 is >100 and they have evidence of stable immune status. If the patient has CD4 <100, it may be necessary to start ART earlier. In such cases, a delay of 2 weeks after the initiation of TB treatment is, however, acceptable.[50] These recommendations are empirical and may change once the results of ongoing clinical trials become available.

TB Prevention

Treatment of LTBI has been shown to be 60–90% effective in preventing progression to TB disease in both HIV-negative and HIV-positive individuals.[42] Treatment usually consists of 6–12 months of isoniazid. The CDC recommends a course of 9 months of isoniazid as the preferred regimen. A second line regimen of 4 months of rifampicin may be used in patients intolerant of isoniazid but this regimen is not as widely studied and may have an increased risk of relapse.[40,41] The British Thoracic Society recommends 6 months of isoniazid alone or 3 months of daily IR. A combination of rifampicin and pyrazinamide for 3 months had shown excellent results in preventing TB but was associated with significant hepatotoxicity, including several cases of acute liver failure leading to death and thus, no longer recommended. Several ongoing studies are evaluating other short-term LTBI regimens mostly involving HIV-negative subjects; these regimens cannot be recommended for HIV-positive patients before efficacy is established.

Current recommendations for the use of preventive therapy stress the importance of targeted screening for Mtb infection in groups at high risk for infection and disease. At this time, the widespread treatment of LTBI in resource constrained areas is not possible due to costs (mostly associated with excluding active TB before initiating LTBI treatment) and the concern of emerging drug resistance to isoniazid, a crucial drug in standardized WHO recommended regimens throughout the world. Special consideration should be given to children (≤5 years) exposed to an infectious case, individuals with TST conversion and HIV-infected patients with LTBI (TST ≥5 mm) as they have a high risk of progression to TB disease. In addition to treatment of latent TB infection, highly active antiretroviral therapy (HAART) is effective in preventing TB.[51] As explained above, the risk of TB recurrence after completion of treatment is high in HIV-positive patients. Secondary prevention with isoniazid is effective in preventing recurrence of TB in high transmission areas.[52,53]

BCG vaccination has been shown to protect against serious TB disease (miliary and CNS) in children. Its efficacy in this regard exceeds 70% in most studies. It is recommended for all infants at birth in areas with a high TB prevalence. The efficacy of BCG in preventing disease in adults is inconsistent, probably because of a confounding effect as a result of protection conferred from environmental mycobac-teria. As a result, the recommendations for BCG vaccination are country-specific.

References

1. Dubos J, Dubos R. The white plague. New Brunswick: Rutgers University Press; 1987.
2. Daniel T. The impact of tuberculosis on civilization. Infect Dis Clin North Am 2004; 18:157–165.
3. Nunn P, Williams B, Floyd K, et al. Tuberculosis control in the era of HIV. Nat Rev Immunol 2005; 5:819–826.
4. Toossi Z. Virological and immunological impact of tuberculosis on human immunodeficiency virus type 1 disease. J Infect Dis 2003; 188:1146–1155.
5. Centers for Disease Control and Prevention. (CDC). Emergence of mycobacterium tuberculosis with extensive resistance to second-line drugs – worldwide, 2000–2004. MMWR 2006; 24:301–305.
6. WHO. Global tuberculosis control: surveillance, planning, financing. Geneva, Switzerland: World Health Organization, 2006: WHO/HTM/TB/2006.362.
7. Stop TB Partnership and WHO. Global PLAN TO STOP TB 2006–2015. Geneva, Switzerland: World Health Organization, 2006: WHO/HTM/STB/2006.35.
8. Cock K De, Marston B. The sound of one hand clapping tuberculosis and antiretroviral therapy in Africa. Am J Respir Crit Care Med 2005; 172:3–4.
9A. Ghandhi NR, Moll A, Sturm AW, et al. Extensively drug-resistant tuberculosis as a couse of death in patients co-infected with tuberculosis and HIV in a rural area of Socith Africa. Lancet 2006; 368:1575–1580.
9. North RJ, Jung YJ. Immunity to tuberculosis. Annu Rev Immunol 2004; 22:599–623.
10. Flynn JL, Chan J. Immunology of tuberculosis. Annu Rev Immunol 2001; 19:93–129.
11. Carranza C, Juarez E, Torres M, et al. Mycobacterium tuberculosis growth control by lung macrophages and CD8 cells from patient contacts. Am J Respir Crit Care Med 2006; 173:238–245.
12. Lopez B, Aguilar D, Orozco H, et al. A marked difference in pathogenesis and immune response induced by different Mycobacterium tuberculosis genotypes. Clin Exp Immunol 2003; 133:30–37.
13. Manca C, Reed MB, Freeman S, et al. Differential monocyte activation underlies strain-specific Mycobacterium tuberculosis pathogenesis. Infect Immun 2004; 72:5511–5514.
14. Theus SA, Cave MD, Eisenach KD. Activated THP-1 cells: an attractive model for the assessment of intracellular growth rates of mycobacterium tuberculosis isolates. Infect Immun 2004; 72:1169–1173.
15. Reed MB, Domenech P, Manca C, et al. A glycolipid of hypervirulent tuberculosis strains that inhibits the innate immune response. Nature 2004; 431:84–87.
16. Fennelly KP, Martyny JW, Fulton KE, et al. Cough-generated aerosols of Mycobacterium tuberculosis: a new method to study infectiousness. Am J Respir Crit Care Med 2004; 169:604–609.
17. Guwatudde D, Nakakeeto M, Jones-Lopez EC, et al. Tuberculosis in household contacts of infectious cases in Kampala, Uganda. Am J Epidemiol 2003; 158:887–898.
18. Nardell EA. Environmental control of tuberculosis. Med Clin North Am 1993; 77:1315–1334.
19. Cruciani M, Malena M, Bosco O, et al. The impact of human immunodeficiency virus type 1 on infectiousness of tuberculosis: a meta-analysis. Clin Infect Dis 2001; 33:1922–1930.
20. Menzies D. Interpretation of repeated tuberculin tests. Boosting, conversion, and reversion. Am J Respir Crit Care Med 1999; 159:15–21.
21. Johnson JL, Nyole S, Okwera A, et al. Instability of tuberculin and Candida skin test reactivity in HIV-infected

Ugandans. The Uganda-Case Western Reserve University Research Collaboration. Am J Respir Crit Care Med 1998; 158:1790–1796.

22. Jones-Lopez EC, Okwera A, Mayanja-Kizza H, et al. Delayed-type hypersensitivity skin test reactivity and survival in HIV-infected patients in Uganda: should anergy be a criterion to start antiretroviral therapy in low-income countries? Am J Trop Med Hyg 2006; 74:154–161.

23. Ellner JJ. Immune dysregulation in human tuberculosis. J Lab Clin Med 1986; 108:142–149.

24. Anderson ST, Williams AJ, Brown JR, et al. Transmission of mycobacterium tuberculosis undetected by tuberculin skin testing. Am J Respir Crit Care Med 2006; 173:1038–1042.

25. Wilkinson KA, Kon OM, Newton SM, et al. Effect of treatment of latent tuberculosis infection on the T cell response to Mycobacterium tuberculosis antigens. J Infect Dis 2006; 193:354–359.

26. Pai M, Joshi R, Dogra S, et al. Serial testing of health care workers for tuberculosis using interferon-gamma assay. Am J Respir Crit Care Med 2006; 174:349–355.

27. Dewan PK, Grinsdale J, Liska S, et al. Feasibility, acceptability, and cost of tuberculosis testing by whole-blood interferon-gamma assay. BMC Infect Dis 2006; 6:47.

28. Mtei L, Matee M, Herfort O, et al. High rates of clinical and subclinical tuberculosis among HIV-infected ambulatory subjects in Tanzania. Clin Infect Dis 2005; 40:1500–1507.

29. Sonnenberg P, Glynn JR, Fielding K, et al. How soon after infection with HIV does the risk of tuberculosis start to increase? A retrospective cohort study in South African gold miners. J Infect Dis 2005; 191:150–158.

30. Glynn JR, Crampin AC, Yates MD, et al. The importance of recent infection with mycobacterium tuberculosis in an area with high HIV prevalence: A long-term molecular epidemiological study in Northern Malawi. J Infect Dis 2005; 192:480–487.

31. Elliott AM, Namaambo K, Allen BW, et al. Negative sputum smear results in HIV-positive patients with pulmonary tuberculosis in Lusaka, Zambia. Tuber Lung Dis 1993; 74:191–194.

32. Steingart KR, Ng V, Henry MC, et al. Sputum processing methods to improve the sensitivity and yield of smear microscopy for tuberculosis: a systematic review. Geneva: Special Programme for Research & Training in Tropical Diseases (TDR), World Health Organization, and Foundation for Innovative New Diagnostics (FIND), 2005: unpublished report.

33. Steingart KR, Ng V, Henry MC, et al. Fluorescence versus conventional sputum smear microscopy for tuberculosis: a systematic review. Geneva: Special Programme for Research & Training in Tropical Diseases (TDR), World Health Organization, and Foundation for Innovative New Diagnostics (FIND), 2005: unpublished report.

34. Lawson L, Yassin MA, Ramsay A, et al. Comparison of scanty AFB smears against culture in an area with high HIV prevalence. Int J Tuberc Lung Dis 2005; 9:933–935.

35. Samb B, Sow PS, Kony S, et al. Risk factors for negative sputum acid-fast bacilli smears in pulmonary tuberculosis: results from Dakar, Senegal, a city with low HIV seroprevalence. Int J Tuberc Lung Dis 1999; 3:330–336.

36. Behr MA, Warren SA, Salamon H, et al. Transmission of mycobacterium tuberculosis from patients smear-negative for acid-fast bacilli. Lancet 1999; 353:444–449. [erratum appears in Lancet 1999; 353:1714].

37. Flores LL, Pai M, Colford JM Jr, et al. In-house nucleic acid amplification tests for the detection of Mycobacterium tuberculosis in sputum specimens: meta-analysis and meta-regression. BMC Microbiol 2005; 5:55.

38. Koppaka R, Bock N. How reliable is chest radiography? In: Frieden TR, ed. Toman's tuberculosis. Case detection, treatment and monitoring. 2nd edn. Geneva: World Health Organization; 2004:51–60.

39. Gold JA, Rom WN, Harkin TJ. Significance of abnormal chest radiograph findings in patients with HIV-1 infection without respiratory symptoms. Chest 2002; 121:1472–1477.

40. Blumberg HM, Leonard MK, Jasmer RM. Update on the treatment of tuberculosis and latent tuberculosis infection. JAMA 2005; 293:2776–2784.

41. Frieden TR, Sterling TR, Munsiff SS, et al. Tuberculosis. Lancet 2003; 362:887–899.

42. Blumberg HM, Burman WJ, Chaisson RE, et al. American Thoracic Society/Centers for Disease Control and Prevention/Infectious Diseases Society of America: Treatment of tuberculosis. Am J Respir Crit Care Med 2003; 167:603–662.

43. Jindani A, Nunn A, Enarson D, et al. Two 8-month regimens of chemotherapy for treatment of newly diagnosed pulmonary tuberculosis: international multicenter randomized trial. Lancet 2004; 364:1244–1251.

44. Thwaites GE, Hien TT. Tuberculous meningitis: many questions, too few answers. Lancet Neurol 2005; 4:160–170.

45. Tappero JW, Bradford WZ, Agerton TB, et al. Serum concentrations of antimycobacterial drugs in patients with pulmonary tuberculosis in Botswana. Clin Infect Dis 2005; 41:461–469.

46. Verver S, Warren RM, Beyers N, et al. Rate of reinfection tuberculosis after successful treatment is higher than rate of new tuberculosis. Am J Respir Crit Care Med 2005; 171:1430–1435.

47. Dworkin MS, Adams MR, Cohn DL, et al. Factors that complicate the treatment of tuberculosis in HIV-infected patients. J Acquir Immune Defic Syndr 2005; 39:464–470.

48. Burman WJ. Issues in the management of HIV-related tuberculosis. Clin Chest Med 2005; 26:283–294.

49. Seyler C, Toure S, Messou E, et al. Risk factors for active tuberculosis after antiretroviral treatment initiation in Abidjan. Am J Respir Crit Care Med 2005; 172:123–127.

50. Breen RAM, Smith CJ, Cropley I, et al. Does immune reconstitution syndrome promote active tuberculosis in patients receiving highly active antiretroviral therapy? AIDS 2005; 19:1201–1206.

51. Badri M, Wilson D, Wood R. Effect of highly active antiretroviral therapy on incidence of tuberculosis in South Africa: a cohort study. Lancet 2002; 359:2059–2064.

52. Fitzgerald DW, Desvarieux M, Severe P, et al. Effect of post-treatment isoniazid on prevention of recurrent tuberculosis in HIV-1-infected individuals: a randomised trial. Lancet 2000; 356:1470–1474.

53. Churchyard GJ, Fielding K, Charalambous S, et al. Efficacy of secondary isoniazid preventive therapy among HIV-infected Southern Africans: time to change policy? AIDS 2003; 17:2063–2070.

CHAPTER 32

Disseminated *Mycobacterium avium* Complex and other Atypical Mycobacterial Infections

Mark A. Jacobson

Epidemiology

Although prior to the AIDS epidemic, disseminated *Mycobacterium avium* complex (MAC) infection had been reported only rarely, this infection became one of the most important opportunistic infections associated with the AIDS in many parts of the world. Disseminated MAC occurs almost exclusively in AIDS patients with an absolute CD4 T-cell count <50 cells/µL[1]; however, localized MAC infection can occur at higher CD4 counts, especially among patients with advanced AIDS who have been immune reconstituted by highly active antiretroviral therapy (HAART).[2]

Disseminated MAC in Industrialized Countries

In the era prior to the widespread availability of HAART in North America, Western Europe and Australia, one-third to one-half of AIDS patients in these regions developed disseminated MAC infection. In the USA, a study reported in 1986 that 53% of 79 autopsies showed evidence of disseminated MAC.[3] In another study in the late 1980s, conducted in patients with advanced HIV disease who had serial blood specimens cultured for mycobacteria over a median 1-year period, the 2-year actuarial

incidence of MAC mycobacteremia was 40%.[1] Also, in a sub-cohort analysis of 844 men with AIDS in the Multicenter AIDS Cohort Study followed during the same time period, 33.4% of those who received early *Pneumocystis carinii* prophylaxis subsequently developed disseminated MAC infection.[4] In Australia, during this same time period, 50% of AIDS patients developed disseminated MAC.[5] Similarly, an autopsy study conducted in Japan in the pre-HAART era reported that 40% of 43 autopsies had evidence of disseminated MAC.[6] Europe reported a more variable risk for AIDS patients developing disseminated MAC, with a similar risk to the USA and Northern Europe, but one-sixth that risk in south-Western Europe.[7]

Disseminated MAC in Resource-poor Countries

Disseminated MAC has been less common in parts of the world where tuberculosis is more prevalent, perhaps because of cross-reactive immunity or perhaps because end organ disease caused by tuberculosis tends to occur earlier in the course of HIV than disease caused by MAC. In the pre-HAART era, MAC was isolated from the blood of 18% of febrile AIDS patients in a study conducted in Brazil.[8] The point prevalence of disseminated MAC in hospitalized AIDS patients in South Africa has been reported to be only 10%,[9] and in Thailand, only 1%.[10]

Effect of Potent Antiretroviral Treatment Availability on MAC Incidence

With the advent of MAC prophylaxis in the early 1990s, the incidence of the infection began to decline in western industrialized countries. Between 1993 and 1994, a 40% decrease in the incidence of adult AIDS-defining disseminated *M. avium* complex (MAC) was noted by the United States Centers for Disease Control (CDC) that almost certainly resulted from the widespread introduction of rifabutin and macrolide MAC prophylaxis into clinical practice during this time period. After early 1996, when potent HIV protease inhibitor drugs became widely available in these countries, the incidence of new cases of disseminated MAC infection decreased by more than 80% compared with the period before 1994 in North American and Western Europe. More recently, a similar decrease in MAC bacteremia has been reported in Brazil after the widespread introduction of HAART into clinical practice in that country.[11]

Acquisition of MAC Infection

MAC is a ubiquitous soil and water saprophyte, and epidemiologic data suggests that disseminated MAC infection results from new environmental acquisition of the organism (rather than reactivation of quiescent, endogenous mycobacteria). For example, a common water source nosocomial outbreak of MAC disease was reported in an AIDS ward.[12] The route of MAC invasion in AIDS patients may be through the gastrointestinal or respiratory tract. The presence of large clusters of mycobacteria within macrophages of the small bowel lamina propria suggests that the bowel might be the portal of entry. However, respiratory isolation of MAC also frequently precedes disseminated infection, suggesting MAC infection may begin in the lungs as well.[13]

Pathogenesis

In AIDS, the key host defect allowing dissemination of MAC is macrophage dysfunction, specifically the failure of macrophages to kill phagocytized MAC. MAC is able to survive within macrophages unless intracellular killing mechanisms (which become defective in late stage AIDS) are activated. Defects in

the activity of cytokines that are essential for such intracellular killing of pathogens, such as interferon gamma, tumor necrosis factor, interleukin-12 and interleukin-2, have been implicated in the pathogenesis of disseminated MAC infection in certain rare heritable immune deficiency syndromes and probably have a role in the pathogenesis of this opportunistic infection in AIDS patients. However, to date, cytokine therapy has not been demonstrated to benefit AIDS patients with disseminated MAC.

In AIDS, MAC causes high-grade, widely disseminated infection. Nearly all AIDS patients with invasive MAC infection (as opposed to stool, urine, or respiratory secretion colonization) have positive mycobacterial blood cultures. In the majority of those cases autopsied, MAC also could be isolated from spleen, lymph nodes, liver, lung, adrenals, colon, kidney, and bone marrow. The magnitude of mycobacteremia can range from 1 to 10^4 colony-forming units per mL of blood. Tissue specimens from bone marrow, spleen, lymph nodes, and liver have yielded even higher microbial loads. Histopathologic studies of involved organs typically have shown absent or poorly formed granulomas and acid-fast bacteria within macrophages. In AIDS patients who have been immune reconstituted with HAART, there have been reports of localized, non-disseminated, MAC infection associated with granuloma formation, tissue destruction and abscess formation in lymph nodes or skin. These cases of MAC immune reconstitution disease have usually occurred soon after antiretroviral therapy was initiated, suggesting that reconstitution of either MAC-specific T-cell responses or of some innate, cytokine-related functions have occurred.

Clinical Manifestations

Effect of Disseminated MAC Infection on Survival in AIDS

Because most AIDS patients with disseminated MAC infection have other concomitant infections or neoplasms, and because MAC appears to result in little histopathologic evidence of inflammatory response or tissue destruction, the relationship between constitutional symptoms, organ dysfunction, and MAC infection was initially uncertain. Nevertheless, several large retrospective studies from the pre-HAART era strongly suggested a negative effect of disseminated MAC infection on mortality and morbidity in AIDS. Horsburgh and co-workers noted a median 4-month survival among 39 patients with untreated disseminated MAC infection compared with 11 months among 39 controls matched for absolute CD4 lymphocyte count, prior AIDS status, history of antiretroviral therapy, history of *Pneumocystis carinii* pneumonia (PCP) prophylaxis, and year of diagnosis (*P*<0.0001).[14] At San Francisco General Hospital, among 137 consecutive patients who had a sterile body site cultured for mycobacteria within 3 months of their first AIDS-defining episode of *Pneumocystis* pneumonia, median survival was significantly shorter in those with invasive MAC infection than in those with negative cultures (107 versus 275 days; *P*<0.01), even after controlling for age, absolute lymphocyte count, and hemoglobin concentration.[13]

Clinical Presentation of Disseminated MAC

The clinical presentation of disseminated MAC infection almost always includes fever and malaise. Weight loss is common, and often anemia or neutropenia is present. Diarrhea and malabsorption may occur as a result of MAC invasion of the gut wall. Abdominal pain may be present and can be severe as a result of bulky retroperitoneal adenopathy. Rarely, extrabiliary obstructive jaundice caused by periportal lymphadenopathy occurs. In a prospective natural history study of MAC bacteremia conducted at San Francisco General Hospital in the pre-HAART era, we observed, among patients with <50 CD4 T cells/µL, that a history of fever for >30 days, a hematocrit <30%, or a serum albumin level <3.0 g/dL were all sensitive predictors of MAC bacteremia.[15] However, neither severe fatigue, diarrhea, weight loss, neutropenia, nor thrombocytopenia discriminated between those who were subsequently found to be blood culture positive or negative for MAC.

MAC Immune Reconstitution Disease

As noted above, localized, non-disseminated MAC infection associated with granuloma formation, tissue destruction and abscess formation in lymph nodes or skin can occur in AIDS patients who have recently initiated antiretroviral therapy.[2] The clinical course is sometimes explosive with large abscess formation and very high fever. In general, these MAC immune reconstitution disease (IRD) cases have occurred in patients who had an absolute CD4 count <50 cells/µL before initiating HAART, and clinically appear soon after the absolute CD4 count rises to >100 cells/µL. MAC IRD sometimes involves the bone or lungs, with infiltrates apparent on chest X-ray. Blood mycobacterial cultures are usually negative at the time of MAC IRD presentation. MAC IRD can present either as worsening of a previously clinically resolved disseminated MAC infection or as a new clinical appearance of previously subclinical MAC infection. In some observational studies, IRD has occurred in up to one-third of patients who had a diagnosis of disseminated MAC prior to initiating HAART and in up to 4% of all patients who initiate HAART with a pre-treatment absolute CD4 count <100 cells/µL. Unlike disseminated infection (see below), these lesions have responded remarkably well to drainage and antimycobacterial therapy, although sometimes a short course of prednisone is needed before fever resolves. There is no need to discontinue HAART in such patients.

Diagnosis

Special blood culture techniques for isolating mycobacteria, such as the broth-based BACTEC system or agar-based Dupont Isolator system, appear to be the most sensitive methods for diagnosing disseminated MAC infection.[16] With these techniques, the sensitivity approaches 100%. Specific DNA probes for MAC have recently become available; these probes make it possible to differentiate MAC from other mycobacteria within hours when there is sufficient mycobacterial growth in broth or agar.[17] Time to culture positivity ranges from 5 to 51 days. It is uncommon for blood cultures to be negative when there is a positive histologic diagnosis from lymph node, liver, or bone marrow biopsies. However, one advantage of obtaining biopsied specimens is that stains may demonstrate acid-fast bacteria (AFB) or granuloma immediately, thus confirming a clinical suspicion of the diagnosis weeks before the blood cultures turn positive.

The clinical significance of MAC isolated from sputum or stool remains controversial. In our prospective natural history study, we found that only two-thirds of patients with negative blood cultures but positive stool or sputum cultures for MAC subsequently developed disseminated MAC infection.[18] Hence, neither stool nor sputum culture can be recommended as a screening test to identify patients likely to develop MAC bacteremia.

Therapy

MAC is not killed by standard antituberculous drugs at concentrations achievable in plasma. Yet, half or more of MAC strains can be inhibited by plasma achievable concentrations of rifabutin, rifampin, clofazimine, cycloserine, amikacin, ethionamide, ethambutol, azithromycin, clarithromycin, ciprofloxacin, or sparfloxacin . Unfortunately, drug levels necessary to kill MAC *in vitro* (minimum bactericidal concentration) have been 8 to >32 times that of inhibitory levels. While combinations of antimycobacterial agents have shown *in vitro* inhibitory synergism, bactericidal synergism has been more difficult to demonstrate. In addition, for *in vivo* killing, drugs must penetrate macrophages as well as the MAC cell wall. Nevertheless, in animal models of disseminated MAC infection, both single and combination antimycobacterial regimens have reduced mycobacterial colony counts by several logs and improved survival.

Results of several sequential trials reported by the California Collaborative Treatment Group (CCTG) highlight the caution needed when interpreting results of treatment trials that have no control arm. In 1990, this group reported striking microbiologic and clinical effects in previously untreated patients with disseminated MAC who were given a combination regimen that included intravenous amikacin and oral rifampin, ethambutol, and ciprofloxacin.[19] Given the modest results that had previously been reported with oral antimycobacterial agents used, many drew the conclusion from this uncontrolled trial that the amikacin was primarily responsible for the efficacy of this regimen. Subsequently, the CCTG reported similar microbiologic and clinical results in another similarly designed uncontrolled trial in which intravenous amikacin was replaced by oral clofazimine.[20] To address the question of amikacin's clinical utility, a randomized controlled trial was then conducted by the NIAID-sponsored AIDS Clinical Trials Group (ACTG) in which 72 patients with previously untreated disseminated MAC were all given a combination oral regimen of rifampin, ethambutol, ciprofloxacin, and clofazimine and were also randomly assigned to receive or not receive additional intravenous amikacin. In this controlled trial, there were no significant differences in microbiologic or clinical outcomes, demonstrating that the cost, inconvenience, and risk of toxicity of intravenous amikacin is unlikely to translate into a significant clinical benefit for patients with disseminated MAC.[21]

Macrolides: Clarithromycin and Azithromycin

Data on *in vivo* microbiologic efficacy against MAC have been most impressive with two macrolides, clarithromycin and azithromycin. A multicenter, randomized, placebo-controlled, dose-ranging trial of clarithromycin monotherapy in patients with previously untreated disseminated MAC reported a median decrease of >2 log in blood MAC colony-forming units-a more potent microbiologic effect than reported in any earlier treatment trials.[22] This microbiologic effect was accompanied by significant clinical improvement according to an analysis of symptoms and quality-of-life indices. However, an unusual dose-response effect was observed. Unacceptably high gastrointestinal toxicity occurred at the 2000 mg b.i.d. dose. Although the 1000 mg b.i.d. dose had greater microbiologic efficacy than the 500 mg b.i.d. dose, there was actually a trend toward increased mortality in the former group, which has subsequently been confirmed in other studies, indicating that the optimal dose for this drug is 500 mg b.i.d. Not surprisingly, drug resistance emerged after 2 months of monotherapy in this trial, affecting approximately half of patients in all dosing arms. Hence, one or more other antimycobacterial agents must be coadministered with the macrolide in an attempt to prevent or at least delay emergence of resistance, which is almost certain to be associated with clinical deterioration. On the other hand, this data should reassure clinicians that initiating MAC prophylaxis with clarithromycin in patients who already have subclinical disseminated MAC infection is very unlikely to lead to drug resistance, as long as blood cultures are obtained at the time that clarithromycin is started (i.e. blood cultures should turn positive and additional antimycobacterial medication can be added before macrolide resistance develops). Azithromycin is another effective macrolide for MAC treatment. The antimycobacterial efficacy of azithromycin or clarithromycin when combined with other agents for disseminated MAC has been compared in two randomized trials. In one study, 246 patients with disseminated MAC were randomized to an ethambutol-based regimen combined with either azithromycin 250 mg daily, azithromycin 600 mg daily or clarithromycin 500 mg b.i.d.[23] The lower-dose azithromycin arm was dropped early in the trial due to poor microbiologic efficacy. There was no significant difference in either microbiologic or survival outcomes between the high dose azithromycin and the clarithromycin arms; however, there were non-significant trends toward better survival, greater mycobacteremia clearance and lower relapse rates with clarithromycin in this trial. In another trial, 59 patients with disseminated MAC were randomized to receive an ethambutol-based regimen with either clarithromycin 500 mg b.i.d. or azithromycin 600 mg daily. Mycobacteremia clearance occurred in 86% of subjects assigned to clarithromycin versus 38% assigned to azithromycin ($P = 0.007$).[24] However, only 37 of the 59 patients were evaluable microbiologically, and only two deaths occurred during the short follow-up period, making generalizability of these results difficult.

Ethambutol

Non-macrolide antimycobacterial agents also have been evaluated in several randomized, controlled trials. In order to determine which of the orally bioavailable non-macrolide antimycobacterial agents might be the most potent *in vivo*, a randomized, controlled trial was conducted in which patients with previously untreated disseminated MAC were assigned to receive a 4-week regimen of rifampin, ethambutol, or clofazimine monotherapy.[25] In this trial, only ethambutol resulted in a statistically significant reduction in blood MAC colony-forming units, suggesting that ethambutol might be the most potent of these three antimycobacterial agents. A subsequent trial confirmed the clinical benefit of ethambutol when combined with clarithromycin.[26] A total of 80 patients with newly diagnosed disseminated MAC infection were all assigned to receive clarithromycin and clofazimine and randomized to receive or not receive ethambutol 800 mg q.d. Although 69% of patients in both groups initially responded microbiologically, the subsequent mycobacteremia relapse rate at 36 weeks was 50% with ethambutol and 91% without ethambutol ($P = 0.014$).

Rifabutin

Data regarding rifabutin treatment for disseminated MAC have also been promising. Interestingly, when rifabutin was evaluated in the 1980s as a treatment for MAC at doses of 100–300 mg/day, it was found to be ineffective. In a subsequent randomized, placebo-controlled trial in which patients with newly diagnosed disseminated MAC were assigned to receive clofazimine/ethambutol or clofazimine/ethambutol/rifabutin (600 mg/day), approximately half of the patients receiving the rifabutin-containing regimen had a >2-log decrease in blood

MAC colony-forming units or sterilization of the blood compared with none of those receiving only clofazimine/ethambutol.[27]

Clofazimine

Clofazimine appears to add no clinical efficacy and may actually be harmful when used in macrolide-based combination regimens. A trial assigned 106 patients with MAC bacteremia to clarithromycin and ethambutol and randomized these patients also to receive or not receive clofazimine 100 mg q.d. In this trial, clofazimine was not associated with any benefit in microbiologic response. In fact, patients assigned clofazimine had a significantly higher mortality, indicating that clofazimine should not be used in the initial treatment of disseminated MAC.

Optimal Combination Treatment Regimens

The long-term clinical benefit of combination regimens that include both macrolide and non-macrolide agents for treatment of disseminated MAC were confirmed in a randomized multicenter trial conducted by the Canadian MAC Study Group in which 187 evaluable patients with MAC mycobacteremia were randomized to receive a regimen of clarithromycin 1000 mg b.i.d., rifabutin 600 mg q.d., and ethambutol 15 mg/kg per day versus ciprofloxacin 750 mg b.i.d., rifampin 600 mg q.d., clofazimine 100 mg q.d., and ethambutol 15 mg/kg per day. The *in vivo* quantitative antimycobacterial effect was significantly better with the macrolide-containing regimen, as was median survival (8.6 versus 5.2 months; $P = 0.001$).[28]

Currently, the best options for the treatment of disseminated MAC appears to be a macrolide such as clarithromycin 500 mg b.i.d. or azithromycin 500–600 mg p.o. daily combined with either ethambutol 15 mg/kg p.o. daily, or rifabutin 300 mg daily, or perhaps both agents (Table 32.1). However, the issue of whether it is more effective to use a macrolide with one or both of these two drugs has not been fully resolved. There has been only one trial conducted that has addressed this issue. Benson and co-workers recently reported that 160 evaluable patients were randomized to receive either clarithromycin and ethambutol, clarithromycin and rifabutin, or all three drugs.[29] A complete microbiologic response, as defined by sterile blood cultures at 12 weeks, was seen in similar proportions in all three arms: 40%, 42%, and 51%, respectively ($P = 0.45$). However, a significant improvement in survival was

Table 32.1 Treatment regimen for disseminated *M. avium* complex infection

For patients likely to initiate effective, potent antiretroviral therapy within the next 6 months	For patients unlikely to initiate effective, potent antiretroviral therapy within the next 6 months
Clarithromycin 500 mg p.o. b.i.d. (or clarithromycin extended release formulation 1000 mg p.o. daily)[a]	Clarithromycin 500 mg p.o. b.i.d. (or clarithromycin extended release formulation 1000 mg p.o. daily)[a]
plus	*plus*
Ethambutol 15 mg/kg p.o. daily[b]	Ethambutol 15 mg/kg p.o. daily and rifabutin 300 mg p.o. daily[c]

[a]For patients intolerant of clarithromycin, azithromycin 500 or 600 mg p.o. daily can be substituted. [b]For patients intolerant of ethambutol, rifabutin 300 mg p.o. daily can be substituted (450–600 mg daily if co-administered with azithromycin rather than clarithromycin; 450 mg daily if co-administered with efavirenz; 150 mg daily if co-administered with indinavir or nelfinavir; 150 mg every other day if co-administered with ritonavir as part of a boosted protease-inhibitor regimen, see Ch. 13). [c]Rifabutin dose should be 450 to 600 mg daily if co-administered with azithromycin rather than clarithromycin, 450 mg daily if co-administered with efavirenz, 150 mg daily if co-administered with indinavir or nelfinavir, 150 mg every other day if co-administered with ritonavir as part of a boosted protease-inhibitor regimen, see Ch. 13.

observed in the three-drug arm (hazard ratio of death approximately halved). There was no significant difference in dose limiting toxicity between the three arms. This difference in survival has not been confirmed in any other trials, and it is not clear if it would be clinically relevant in the HAART era for patients who initiate effective antiretroviral therapy within the first few months after starting antimycobacterial therapy for disseminated MAC.

Drug Interactions between Anti-MAC and Antiretroviral Medications

Azithromycin and ethambutol do not have clinically important drug interactions with antiretroviral medications. Ritonavir can increase clarithromycin plasma levels enough that clarithromycin dosing should be reduced to 500 mg/day in patients on ritonavir-boosted protease inhibitor regimens who also have moderate renal insufficiency (estimated creatinine clearance <60 mL/min). Rifabutin has clinically significant drug interactions with some antiretroviral protease inhibitors and non-nucleoside reverse transcriptase inhibitors that do require dosage adjustment (Table 32.2).

Stopping Treatment after Immune Restoration

During the pre-HAART era, relapse of disseminated MAC typically occurred rapidly when chronic suppressive antimycobacterial therapy was discontinued. However, since the widespread availability of HAART in North America, there have been several reports describing series of patients who had under-

Table 32.2 Drug interactions between rifabutin and antiretroviral medications that require dosing adjustments. Recommended dosing adjustments when rifabutin is combined with antiretroviral drug

Antiretroviral drug	Antiretroviral dose	Rifabutin dose
Amprenavir	No change	150 mg daily
Nelfinavir	No change	150 mg daily
Indinavir	1000 mg t.i.d.	150 mg daily
Atazanavir	No change	150 mg every other day
Any Ritonavir-boosted protease inhibitor	No change	150 mg every other day
Efavirenz	No change	450 mg daily
Saquinavir	Contraindicated	Contraindicated

gone prolonged therapy for disseminated MAC infection, then initiated potent combination antiretroviral regimens and had subsequent absolute CD4 counts rise to >100 cells/μL with resolution of all MAC-related symptoms. After blood culture negativity was documented, these individuals discontinued antimycobacterial therapy and have had no relapse during long-term follow-up. It now appears to be safe for such HAART-immunorestored patients with a history of disseminated MAC who have completed at least 1 year of an appropriated antimycobacterial regimen to discontinue chronic suppressive therapy for MAC disease.

Empiric Treatment for Disseminated MAC and Tuberculosis

Finally, it is important for clinicians to remember that it may be difficult to distinguish tuberculosis from MAC disease in patients with advanced HIV disease. Therefore, an antituberculous regimen should be instituted whenever acid-fast bacteria are demonstrated (and cannot yet be differentiated between MAC and *M. tuberculosis*) in a specimen from a patient with HIV infection and clinical evidence of mycobacterial disease.

Prophylaxis

Since 40% of patients with advanced HIV disease (i.e. CD4 counts <50 cells/µL) are likely to develop disseminated MAC, it makes sense to develop a strategy for preventing this disease in patients at risk. There are few defined risk factors for predicting disseminated MAC disease, other than a low CD4[+] T cell count. Thus any prophylactic strategy has to be applied to the entire population at risk (i.e. all patients with <50 CD4[+] T cells/µL).

Clarithromycin

The most convincing data regarding the efficacy of MAC prophylaxis have been obtained with clarithromycin in a placebo-controlled study in which 667 patients with advanced HIV disease were randomized to receive either clarithromycin 500 mg or placebo b.i.d. During a median 10-month follow-up, only 6% of clarithromycin-assigned patients versus 16% of placebo-assigned patients developed mycobacteremia ($P<0.001$).[30] More importantly, median survival was significantly longer for clarithromycin- than for placebo-assigned patients (32% versus 41% mortality, $P = 0.026$). However, among the clarithromycin-assigned patients who did develop disseminated MAC infection, 58% had mycobacteremia with MAC isolates that were highly resistant to clarithromycin (minimum inhibitory concentration (MIC) >512 µg/mL). Clarithromycin at this same dose has also been compared with rifabutin and to the combination of clarithromycin and rifabutin in a large randomized trial involving 1216 patients with absolute CD4[+] T-cell counts <100 cells/µL. In this trial, clarithromycin was significantly more effective than rifabutin in preventing mycobacteremia (9% versus 15% of patients, $P<0.01$), but the addition of rifabutin to clarithromycin provided no significant increase in efficacy compared with clarithromycin alone.[31]

Azithromycin

A regimen of weekly azithromycin prophylaxis has been evaluated in a placebo-controlled, double blind trial in which 10.6% of 85 azithromycin recipients and 24.7% of 89 placebo recipients developed MAC infection (hazard ratio, 0.34; $P = 0.004$).[32] There was no difference between the groups in survival or in the macrolide susceptibility of breakthrough MAC bacteremia isolates. In another trial, 693 patients with <100 CD4[+] T cells/µL were randomized to azithromycin 1200 mg once weekly, daily rifabutin or the combination of both. Azithromycin was more effective than rifabutin in preventing mycobacteremia (7.6% versus 15.3%, $P = 0.008$), and the combination of both agents was more effective than either one alone (2.8% incidence of mycobacteremia, $P = 0.03$).[33] Among the patients in whom azithromycin prophylaxis was not successful, only 11% of MAC isolates were resistant to azithromycin. Both clarithromycin and azithromycin prophylaxis are well-tolerated. The main adverse effects of clarithromycin are nausea and altered taste and of azithromycin is diarrhea.

Rifabutin

Rifabutin alone at a dose of 300 mg/day also has been compared with placebo for MAC prophylaxis in two randomized trials conducted in over 1000 patients with advanced HIV disease. Rifabutin demonstrated efficacy by reducing the incidence of mycobacteremia by half. Patients who received rifabutin and subsequently developed mycobacteremia had blood MAC isolates that retained susceptibility to rifabutin. However, neither trial alone, nor the combined analysis, demonstrated that rifabutin significantly reduced mortality. In addition, rifabutin is problematic in terms of drug interactions with several classes of antiretroviral drugs (Table 32.2).

Prophylaxis recommendations

Therefore, the US Public Health Service recommends prophylaxis with clarithromycin or azithromycin (or rifabutin for macrolide-intolerant patients) for all HIV-infected patients with <50 CD4 cells/µL. Two randomized, placebo-controlled trials have addressed the question of whether chronic antimycobacterial prophylaxis is needed for patients who at one time had an absolute CD4 count <50 cells/μL but now, due to potent combination antiretroviral therapy, have absolute CD4 counts that have been sustained above 100 cells/μL.[34,35] Among the 583 patients who were assigned to receive placebo in these combined trials, there were only two cases of MAC infection, both localized to the vertebral spine. Thus, it is clear that MAC prophylaxis can be safely discontinued in HAART immunorestored patients who sustain absolute CD4 counts >100 cells/μL.

Other Atypical Mycobacterial Infections in Aids

Disseminated and localized infections caused by *M. kansasii, M. celatum, M. xenopi, M. simiae, M. haemophilum, M. marinum, M. scrofulaceum, M. gordonae, M. genavense, M. fortuitum, M. chelonae, M. malmoense, M. abscessus, M. triplex,* and *M. terrae* also have been reported in patients with AIDS. Those cases with disseminated disease generally have had clinical presentations similar to that of disseminated MAC infection, although pulmonary involvement is more common with disseminated *M. kansasii* infection. *In vitro* sensitivity of isolates to standard antituberculous drugs has been variable. Of note, cases of disseminated *M. simiae-avium* infection have been reported in Thailand and Malawi.

M. kansasii

M. kansasii has been the most frequently reported of these other atypical mycobacteria. A trend toward increased incidence of HIV-related *M. kansasii* was noted in Northern California in the mid-1990s. *M. kansasii* lung infection is also an emerging problem among HIV-infected people in South Africa, especially miners, and has been reported to occur at high CD4+ T-cell counts.[36] This organism, like MAC, is acquired from the environment, and no cases of human-human transmission have been documented. In three published series from New Orleans, Kansas City, and Miami, the clinical features of 119 cases of AIDS-related *M. kansasii* infection have been reported.[37-39] A total of 91% of these cases involved pulmonary disease; 32% had disseminated disease. The median absolute CD4+ T-cell count at diagnosis was <50 cells/μL in all three series. Fever, cough, weight loss were common in all three series. While cavitation was common in patients with disease limited to the lungs, it was rare in patients with dis-

seminated infection. Patients with AIDS-related *M. kansasii* infection have been reported to respond to therapy with combinations of agents including: isoniazid, rifampin, ethambutol, clarithromycin, ciprofloxacin. Although the American Thoracic Society recommends a combination of INH, rifampin, and ethambutol as therapy for this disease, clinicians must substitute clarithromycin and/or rifabutin for rifampin in patients receiving protease inhibitors. The recommended duration of therapy is a minimum of 18 months. *In vitro*, isoniazid resistance and clarithromycin sensitivity is commonly observed. Rifampin resistance is also an emerging problem. Thus, multidrug therapy should be tailored to the results of *in vitro* sensitivities of a culture isolate.

M. genavense

M. genavense is a more recently described pathogen that causes disseminated infection, clinically similar to disseminated MAC, in patients with CD4 counts <50 cells/μL.[40] This fastidious organism is difficult to detect and does not grow on conventional solid media. Small colonies can be detected in specially supplemented Middlebrook media, and low growth index can be observed in BACTEC broth. Since susceptibilities to drugs cannot be reliably determined, an empiric treatment choice must be made. Clinical reports indicate that clarithromycin-containing combination regimens may be effective therapy.

M. haemophilum

M. haemophilum is an atypical mycobacteria with a particular propensity to cause joint, bone, and ulcerative skin lesions (perhaps related to the lower temperature it requires for optimal growth) in addition to disseminated infection in patients with AIDS. A cluster of cases was reported in the New York City area. Clarithromycin and rifabutin appear to be the most active therapeutic agents.

References

1. Nightingale SD, Byrd LT, Southern PM, et al. Incidence of *Mycobacterium avium-intracellulare* complex bacteremia in human immunodeficiency virus-positive patients. J Infect Dis 1992; 165:1082–1085.
2. Race EM, Adelson-Mitty J, Kriegel GR, et al. Focal mycobacterial lymphadenitis following initiation of protease inhibitor therapy in patients with advanced HIV-1 disease. Lancet 1998; 351:252–255.
3. Hawkins CC, Gold JWM, Whimbey E, et al. *Mycobacterium avium* complex infections in patients with the acquired

immunodeficiency syndrome. Ann Intern Med 1986; 105:184–188.

4. Hoover DR, Saah A, Bacellar H, et al. Clinical manifestations of AIDS in the era of Pneumocystis prophylaxis. N Engl J Med 1993; 329:1922–1926.

5. Dore GJ, Hoy JF, Mallal SA, et al. Trends in incidence of AIDS illnesses in Australia from 1983 to 1994: the Australian AIDS cohort. J AIDS 1997; 16:39–43.

6. Ohtomo K, Wang S, Masunaga A, et al. Secondary infections of AIDS autopsy cases in Japan with special emphasis on *Mycobacterium avium*-intracellulare complex infection. Tohoku J Exp Med 2000; 192:99–109.

7. Blaxhult A, Fox Z, Colebunders R, et al. Regional and temporal changes in AIDS in Europe before HAART. Epidemiol Infect 2002; 129:565–576.

8. Barreto JA, Palaci M, Ferrazoli L, et al. Isolation of *Mycobacterium avium* complex from bone marrow aspirates of AIDS patients in Brazil. J Infect Dis 1993; 168:777–779.

9. Pettipher CA, Karstaedt AS, Hopley M. Prevalence and clinical manifestations of disseminated *Mycobacterium avium* complex infection in South Africans with acquired immunodeficiency syndrome. Clin Infect Dis 2001; 33:2068–2071.

10. Anekthananon T, Ratanasuwan W, Techasathit W, et al. HIV infection/acquired immunodeficiency syndrome at Siriraj Hospital, 2002: time for secondary prevention. J Med Assoc Thai 2004; 87:173–179.

11. Hadad DJ, Palaci M, Pignatari AC, et al. Mycobacteraemia among HIV-1-infected patients in Sao Paulo, Brazil: 1995 to 1998. Epidemiol Infect 2004; 132:151–155.

12. Reyn CF Von, Maslow JN, Barber TW, et al. Persistent colonisation of potable water as a source of *Mycobacterium avium* infection in AIDS. Lancet 1994; 343:1137–1141.

13. Jacobson MA, Hopewell PC, Yajko DM, et al. Natural history of disseminated *Mycobacterium avium* complex infection in AIDS. J Infect Dis 1991; 164:994–998.

14. Horsburgh CE, Havlik JA, Ellis DA, et al. Survival of patients with acquired immune deficiency syndrome and disseminated *Mycobacterium avium* complex infection with and without antimycobacterial chemotherapy. Am Rev Respir Dis 1991; 144:557–559.

15. Chin DP, Reingold AL, Horsburgh CR Jr, et al. Predicting *Mycobacterium avium* complex bacteremia in patients with the human immunodeficiency virus: A prospectively validated model. Clin Infect Dis 1994; 19:668–674.

16. Young LS. *Mycobacterium avium* complex infection. J Infect Dis 1988; 157:863–867.

17. Evans KD, Nakasone AS, Sutherland PA, et al. Identification of *Mycobacterium tuberculosis* and *Mycobacterium avium-M. intracellulare* directly from primary BACTEC cultures by using acridinium-ester labelled DNA probes. J Clin Microbiol 1992; 30:2427–2431.

18. Chin DP, Hopewell PC, Yajko DM, et al. *Mycobacterium avium* complex in the respiratory or gastrointestinal tract and the risk of M. avium complex bacteremia in patients with the human immunodeficiency virus. J Infect Dis 1994; 169:289–295.

19. Chiu J, Nussbaum J, Bozzette S, et al. Treatment of disseminated *Mycobacterium avium* complex infection in AIDS with amikacin, ethambutol, rifampin, and ciprofloxacin. Ann Intern Med 1990; 113:358–361.

20. Kemper CA, Meng TC, Nussbaum J, et al. Treatment of *Mycobacterium avium* complex bacteremia in AIDS with a four-drug oral regimen. Ann Intern Med 1992; 116: 466–472.

21. Parenti D, Williams PL, Hafner R, et al. A phase II/III trial of antimicrobial therapy with or without amikacin in the treatment of disseminated *Mycobacterium avium* infection in HIV-infected individuals. AIDS Clinical Trials Group Protocol 135 Study Team. AIDS 1998; 12:2439–2446.

22. Chaisson RE, Benson C, Dube M, et al. Clarithromycin therapy for bacteremic *Mycobacterium avium* complex disease. Ann Intern Med 1994; 121:905–911.

23. Dunne M, Fessel J, Kumar P, et al. A randomized, double-blind trial comparing azithromycin and clarithromycin in the treatment of disseminated *Mycobacterium avium* infection in patients with human immunodeficiency virus. Clin Infect Dis 2000; 31:1245–1252.

24. Ward TT, Rimland D, Kauffman C, et al. Randomized, open-label trial of azithromycin plus ethambutol vs. clarithromycin plus ethambutol as therapy for *Mycobacterium avium* complex bacteremia in patients with human immunodeficiency virus infection. Veterans Aff HIV Res Consortium Clin Infect Dis 1998; 27: 1278–1285.

25. Kemper C, Havlir D, Haghighat D, et al. The individual microbiologic effect of three antimycobacterial agents, clofazimine, ethambutol, and rifampin, on *Mycobacterium avium* complex bacteremia in patients with AIDS. J Infect Dis 1994; 170:157–164.

26. Dube MP, Sattler FR, Torriani FJ, et al. A randomized evaluation of ethambutol for prevention of relapse and drug resistance during treatment of *Mycobacterium avium* complex bacteremia with clarithromycin-based combination therapy. Calif Collab Treat Group J Infect Dis 1997; 176:1225–1232.

27. Sullam P, Gordin F. Wynne B, the Rifabutin Treatment Group: Efficacy of rifabutin in the treatment of disseminated infection due to *Mycobacterium avium* complex. Clin Infect Dis 1994; 19:84–86.

28. Shafran SD, Singer J, Zarowny DP, et al. A comparison of two regimens for the treatment of *Mycobacterium avium* complex bacteremia in AIDS: rifabutin, ethambutol, and clarithromycin versus rifampin, ethambutol, clofazimine, and ciprofloxacin. N Engl J Med 1996; 335:377–383.

29. Benson CA, Williams PL, Currier JS, et al. A prospective, randomized trial examining the efficacy and safety of clarithromycin in combination with ethambutol, rifabutin, or both for the treatment of disseminated *Mycobacterium avium* complex disease in persons with acquired immunodeficiency syndrome. Clin Infect Dis 2003; 37:1234–1243.

30. Pearce M, Crampton S, Henry D, et al. A randomized trial of clarithromycin as prophylaxis against disseminated *Mycobacterium avium* complex infection in patients with advanced acquired immunodeficiency syndrome. N Engl J Med 1995; 335:384–391.

31. Benson CA, Williams PL, Cohn DL, et al. Clarithromycin or rifabutin alone or in combination for primary prophylaxis of *Mycobacterium avium* complex disease in patients with AIDS: A randomized, double-blind, placebo-controlled trial. The AIDS Clinical Trials Group 196/Terry Beirn Community Programs for Clinical Research on AIDS 009 Protocol Team. J Infect Dis 2000; 181:1289–1297.

32. Oldfield EC, Fessel WJ, Dunne MW, et al. Once weekly azithromycin therapy for prevention of *Mycobacterium avium* complex infection in patients with AIDS: a randomized, double-blind, placebo-controlled multicenter trial. Clin Infect Dis 1998; 26:611–619.

33. Havlir DV, Dube MP, Sattler FR, et al. Prophylaxis against disseminated *Mycobacterium avium* complex with weekly azithromycin, daily rifabutin or both. N Engl J Med 1996; 335:392–398.

34. Currier JS, Williams PL, Koletar SL, et al. Discontinuation of *Mycobacterium avium* complex prophylaxis in patients with antiretroviral therapy-induced increases in CD4+ cell count. A randomized, double-blind, placebo-controlled trial. AIDS Clinical Trials Group 362 Study Team. Ann Intern Med 2000; 133:493–503.

35. El-Sadr WM, Burman WJ, Grant LB, et al. Discontinuation of prophylaxis for mycobacterium avium complex disease in HIV-infected patients who have a response to antiretroviral therapy. Terry Beirn Community Programs for Clinical Research on AIDS. N Engl J Med 2000; 342:1085–1092.

36. Corbett EL, Churchyard GJ, Hay M, et al. The impact of HIV infection on Mycobacterium kansasii disease in South African gold miners. Am J Respir Crit Care Med 1999; 160:10–14.

37. Campo RE, Carlos CE. *Mycobacterium kansasii* disease in patients infected with human immunodeficiency virus. Clin Infect Dis 1997; 24:1233–1238.

38. Bamberger DM, Driks MR, Gupta MR, et al. *Mycobacterium kansasii* among patients infected with human immunodeficiency virus in Kansas City. Clin Infect Dis 1994; 18:395–400.

39. Witzig RS, Fazal BA, Mera RM, et al. Clinical manifestations and implications of coinfection with *Mycobacterium kansasii*

and human immunodeficiency virus type 1. Clin Infect Dis 1995; 21:77–85.

40. Bessesen MT, Shlay J, Stone-Venohr B, et al. Disseminated *Mycobacterium genavense* infection: clinical and microbiological features and response to therapy. AIDS 1993; 7:1357–1361.

CHAPTER 33

Candida in HIV Infection

Emma Devitt
William G. Powderly

Epidemiology

Candidiasis is caused by fungi of the *Candida* species, which are yeasts that are ubiquitous in the environment. *Candida* species represent a common human commensal on skin and mucous membranes and between 30% and 80% of adults and children are colonized with *Candida* species.[1,2] The point prevalence of carriage is higher in at-risk groups, such as cancer patients and HIV-positive persons.[3-5] In general, such colonization with *Candida* does not cause infection. The primary defence mechanisms involved in protection against local infection with *Candida* involve the cell-mediated immune system. Progressive loss of T-cell function associated with HIV disease leads to an increased risk of direct local invasion of *Candida* and localized infection. Other host factors important in the defence against *Candida* infections include blood group secretor status, salivary flow rates, epithelial barrier, antimicrobial constituents of saliva, and presence of normal bacterial flora. Several studies suggest that HIV infection is associated with impairment in a number of these local mucosal defence mechanisms.

Mucosal candidiasis is a common opportunistic infection in HIV positive individuals. Oropharyngeal candidiasis usually occurs with low CD4 counts, but tends to be one of the earliest opportunistic infections and may be seen in patients with CD4+ T-lymphocyte counts >200/mm^3. The finding of oropharyngeal candidiasis should never be dismissed in an HIV-infected patient; it indicates progressive immune deficiency and should prompt the institution of effective antiretroviral therapy.

Prior to the era of highly active antiretroviral therapy (HAART), between 50 and 75% of HIV infected individuals developed at least one episode of mucosal candidiasis. Recurrent episodes are frequent with progressive immune deficiency. The incidence has declined since the introduction of HAART in the late 1990s. Higher HIV viral load is significantly associated with increased oral or vaginal colonization and candidiasis, an association that has been reduced by HAART.[6] However, in parts of the world where antiretrovirals are not widely available, mucosal candidiasis continues to represent a significant cause of morbidity. Esophageal candidiasis affects between 10% and 20% of patients with AIDS. *Candida* infection is the most common cause of esophageal disease in persons with HIV infection.

The epidemiology of mucocutaneous candidiasis has changed in the last 10 years primarily because of two factors. The first is the widespread use of antifungal agents, particularly the azoles. Continuous use of azoles has led to a decline in the prevalence of mucosal candidiasis but also has led to the emergence of refractory infections that tend to be resistant to azole drugs. The second factor influencing *Candida* epidemiology in AIDS has been the introduction of HAART, which has resulted in a significant decline in the incidence of all opportunistic illnesses including mucosal candidiasis and it is reasonable to expect that the incidence of mucocutaneous candidiasis in HIV-infected patients will continue to decline as more patients receive HAART.

The majority of cases of candidiasis in the setting of HIV infection are confined to mucosal surfaces i.e. oro-pharyngeal, esophageal and vulvovaginal; systemic candidiasis is rare and usually occurs in the setting of advanced HIV/AIDS (often in the setting of neutropenia) or represents nosocomial acquisition. While oropharyngeal and esophageal candidiasis are clearly HIV-associated illnesses, it is likely that vulvovaginal candidiasis is not. HIV-seropositive women have a higher prevalence of vaginal colonization with *Candida* when compared with seronegative women. However, the incidence of vulvovaginal candidiasis is unrelated to HIV serostatus and tends to reflect other risk factors for vulvovaginal candida infection such as sexual activity and socioeconomic status. The prevalence of vulvovaginal disease is also independent of CD4 count and does not increase with advancing immunodeficiency. However, the severity and frequency of recurrence of vulvovaginal candidiasis may be linked to progressive HIV infection, and as a consequence, this remains an important source of morbidity in infected women. This may indicate a difference in pathogenesis of candidal infection at the two sites.[7]

The most common causative organism of mucosal candidiasis is *Candida albicans*,[8] and this species is found in over 90% of isolates from patients with their first episode of oropharyngeal candidiasis. In patients with recurrent disease, it is often the same strain causing the relapses (about 50%) but other strains or other species may be implicated. The majority of disease is caused by organisms that are part of the normal flora of an individual, although rare cases of person-to-person transmission have been documented. With increasing antifungal use, non-*albicans* species with different antimicrobial susceptibilities become more commonly found e.g. *C. glabrata*, *C. tropicalis*, *C. krusei*, *C. dubliniensis*.[9,10] These species assume some greater importance, as they may be more likely to be associated with decreased susceptibility to azole antifungals.[11]

Clinical Manifestations

Oropharyngeal Candidiasis (OPC)

Almost all patients with OPC are symptomatic, complaining of a sore mouth or pain with swallowing. Usually on inspection, OPC is associated with visible creamy white plaques on the tongue, hard or soft palate. If scraped, these plaques have an erythematous base (this is the pseudomembranous form of OPC, often referred to as thrush). Other clinical manifestations include angular cheilitis, which is a non-specific inflammation of the angles of the mouth and acute or chronic atrophic candidiasis, which can present as erythematous tongue and/or thinning of the mucous membranes. Although usually associated with slight morbidity, OPC can be clinically significant. Severe OPC can interfere with the administration of medications and adequate nutritional intake, and may spread to the esophagus.

The differential diagnosis of oropharyngeal candidiasis includes:

1. *Oral hairy leukoplakia (OHL)* which is characterized as a raised white lesion of the oral mucosa usually found on the side of the tongue. It is associated with herpes viruses in the epithelial cells, particularly Epstein–Barr virus (EBV). It can be differentiated from candidiasis by failure to scrape off the plaque, or failure to respond to anti-fungal therapy. Antiviral therapy with acyclovir can be used for treatment.

2. *Mouth ulcers/aphthous ulcers.* Extensive oral ulceration can be seen in the setting of HIV. It has many different causes, examples include herpes simplex virus type I and II, cytomegalovirus (CMV), drug toxicities (e.g. Stevens–Johnson syndrome due to cotrimoxazole or anti-retrovirals) or idiopathic aphthous ulceration. These present as single or multiple discrete ulcers that are usually painful and may coalesce or become secondarily infected. Treatment involves identifying the cause and discontinuing the causative agent if relevant. In the case of viral ulceration, systemic antivirals such as acyclovir may be useful. In aphthous ulceration, topical steroids or analgesic mouthwashes are helpful and oral thalidomide therapy has been shown to be effective in severe cases.[12]

3. *Gingivitis and periodontitis.* Severe oral cavity disease has been seen in HIV infection. It usually presents with painful bleeding gums, halitosis and dental loosening. There may be ulceration of gums. It is caused by mixed aerobic and anaerobic infection and responds to topical agents, systemic therapy with metronidazole may be required.

4. *Kaposi sarcoma.* The typical purple lesions of KS can be found in the oral cavity usually on the palate. If large, the lesions may ulcerate due to local trauma. Biopsy will prove the diagnosis.

5. *Non-Hodgkin's Lymphoma* can cause oral cavity disease in HIV patients. It may present as a mass lesion, tonsillar in origin, or as ulceration of the mucosa. Again, biopsy will give a definitive diagnosis.

Oesophageal Candidiasis

Patients are usually symptomatic with dysphagia and odynophagia. Retrosternal pain or discomfort may be present. There may or may not be concurrent oral cavity involvement. Severe symptoms can lead to considerable difficulty in eating or swallowing liquids, which can interfere with nutrition. In a patient who complains of swallowing difficulty or retrosternal symptoms alone the presence of OPC is enough to give a high clinical suspicion of esophageal involvement and to institute definitive therapy. In atypical cases or those where initial antifungal therapy does not relive symptoms, direct visualization of the esophagus by endoscopy is the best way to make the diagnosis. The epithelial lining of the esophagus is coated in a pseudomembrane consisting of yeasts, epithelial cells, leukocytes and necrotic debris. Erosions or ulcers may be seen. An experienced endoscopist will often make the diagnosis on macroscopic appearance. Definitive diagnosis is made by brushings or biopsy of the mucosa. The differential diagnosis includes viral esophagitis as caused by cytomegalovirus (CMV) or herpes simplex (HSV) types I and II. Severe aphthous ulceration can also but less commonly affect the oesophagus. A helpful clinical clue in differentiating the different infectious causes of esophagitis in HIV-positive patients is that esophagitis due to *C. albicans* often results in complaints of food 'sticking in the throat,' whereas esophagitis due to HSV or CMV more often produces complaints of actual pain with swallowing.

Vulvovaginal Candidiasis (VVC)

As noted previously, this is a common clinical syndrome in women irrespective of HIV status or immune function. There are many additional predisposing factors to the development of genital candida infection – diabetes, oral contraceptive use, pregnancy, and systemic antibiotic therapy.

Vulvovaginal candidiasis generally presents with itching, a vaginal discharge (which may be watery or thick), vaginal erythema with adherent white discharge, dyspareunia, dysuria, and erythema and swelling of the labia and vulva. The cervix usually appears normal. Initial episodes tend to be uncomplicated, mild to moderate in severity, and sporadic, usually caused by *C. albicans*. More complicated VVC tends to occur in more immunocompromised hosts, are often recurrent and increasingly caused by non-*albicans* species.

Unprotected intercourse with a partner with vulvovaginal candidiasis may lead to the male partner developing candida balanitis. This manifests as itchy erythematous patches on the glans penis.

Disseminated Candidiasis and Candidemia

In HIV-positive individuals, this is a rare and usually late event usually in patients with advanced immunosuppression. It is most often a hospital-acquired infection, with non-*albicans* candida playing a significant role in pathogenesis. There has been a significant reduction in the incidence of nosocomial candidemia in HIV patients in the post-HAART era.[13] Risk factors are those of nosocomial acquisition including presence of a central venous catheter, gastric acid suppressants, nasogastric tubes, antibiotics, ITU admission[14] severe esophageal mucosal disease, advanced AIDS, concomitant opportunistic infections, non-*albicans* species and neutropenia. Virtually every body organ can be affected by candida infection. Involvement of eyes (endophthalmitis), central nervous system (meningitis,[15] encephalitis), and heart (endocarditis) are well described but rare in the setting of HIV infection.

Community acquired candidemia and disseminated candidiasis in HIV is occasionally seen in countries where IVDUs make up a significant proportion of the HIV population. This can present as end organ disease such as endocarditis, endophthalmitis or skin lesions.[16–18]

Diagnosis

The diagnosis of mucosal candidiasis is usually a clinical one. The presence of characteristic symptoms with or without clinical findings in an HIV-infected patient is often enough to institute treatment. In many ways, this constitutes a therapeutic trial, wherein if symptoms fail to settle on first line antifungal agents the diagnosis must be revisited – perhaps prompting invasive diagnostic tests. Oropharyngeal cultures often demonstrate *Candida* species, but are not diagnostic because colonization is common. The diagnosis of OPC can be confirmed by examining a 10% potassium hydroxide (KOH) slide preparation of a scraping of an active lesion. Pseudohyphae and budding yeast are characteristic findings. Culture is usually not necessary with initial episodes of OPC unless the lesions fail to clear with appropriate antifungal therapy. In patients with poorly responsive OPC, a culture should be obtained to look for drug-resistant yeast or those that respond poorly to certain azoles (e.g. *C. krusei* or *C. glabrata*).

The diagnosis of *Candida* vaginitis is made by the presence of a characteristic clinical appearance and observation of yeast forms on microscopic examination. A KOH preparation from vaginal lesions can confirm the diagnosis of candidiasis and differentiate it from other conditions that can be similar in appearance (e.g. trichomoniasis). Routine fungal cultures are rarely helpful in the absence of KOH-positive lesions because yeasts are normal inhabitants of the vaginal mucosa. A fungal culture should be obtained if a patient fails to respond to standard antifungal therapy to determine if resistance is contributing to the therapeutic failure.

In the microbiology laboratory *Candida* spp. are relatively easy to culture. They grow rapidly on simple media at 25–37°C. *Candida* colonies are smooth creamy white in color on agar plates. Specialized media can differentiate between species by colony color (CHROMagar *Candida*) and are very useful. Germ tube testing is a relatively quick method of determining if the organism is *Candida albicans* versus non-*albicans*. Many microbiology laboratories report yeast cultures as either *C. albicans* or non-*albicans* species based upon the germ tube test; if specific identification is required further discussion with the microbiologist is often necessary.

Efforts to develop a standardized reproducible and clinically relevant method of susceptibility testing for yeasts have yielded the NCCLS M27-A2 methodology.[19] This has data driven interpretive breakpoints for susceptibility of *Candida* spp. to antifungal agents (Table 33.1). Data relating to fluconazole and itraconazole is more readily available than for other antifungals. Susceptibility testing

of *Candida* spp. is not routinely used in most laboratories. The identification of the species is often enough to predict likely anti-fungal susceptibility and further testing is not required. However, in the setting of recurrent infection, failure to respond to initial therapy or systemic infection with non-*albicans* species, susceptibility testing may contribute to clinical decision making and can also be used to support a decision to switch from a parenteral to oral agent. The dose and delivery of the antifungal agent are very important in interpreting the data and host factors play a significant role in the clinical response to a particular agent irrespective of laboratory susceptibility data.[20]

Treatment

Many antifungal agents with activity against *Candida* spp. are now available. In general, therapy for mucosal candidiasis can be given as local preparations (usually as mouthwashes or suspensions for oropharyngeal disease or as creams or suppositories for vaginal disease), or as systemic preparations for more severe infections (Table 33.2).

Azoles

The azoles are the most commonly used drugs and are available as local (topical) and systemic products. The act as inhibitors of the demethylase enzyme involved in ergosterol synthesis – ergosterol being the essential sterol on the fungal cell membrane.

Fluconazole

Fluconazole is a triazole antifungal and is the most widely available and commonly used agent against *Candida* infection. It is available in oral and intravenous forms. It has very good bioavailability with the same doses being administered both orally and i.v. (200–800 mg/day usually). It is generally well tolerated but may cause headache (up to 13%), GI upset (≈10%) or liver blood test abnormalities especially at higher doses. It requires dose adjustment in severe renal impairment. It is a CYP450 inhibitor and can interact with other drugs metabolized by these enzymes, but there are few important interactions described for drugs used in HIV infection. Rifampin can decrease the concentrations of fluconazole and may lead to treatment failure. Nevirapine can also reduce fluconazole levels, but the clinical significance is unknown. Fluconazole is FDA category C

Table 33.1 Definition of *in vitro* resistance for *Candida* species. Range of MICs (μg/mL)

Antifungal agent	Susceptible	Susceptible – dose dependent	Resistant
Itraconazole	≤0.125	0.25–0.5	≥1.0
Fluconazole	≤8.0	16–32	>64
Amphotericin B	≤1.0	–	≥2.0

Adapted from NCCLS standard definitions for antifungal susceptibilities using microbroth or macrotube dilution methodology.

Table 33.2 Treatment guide

Clinical syndrome	Drugs	Mode of delivery	Preparation	Dose	Duration
Vulvovaginal Candidiasis	Clotrimazole; Miconazole; Butoconazole; Ticonazole	Topical	Cream, Pessary		3–5 days
	Boric acid	p.v.	Gelatin capsules	600 mg q.d.	14 days
	Fluconazole	p.o.	Capsule	150 mg	Single dose
Oropharyngeal Candidiasis	Clotrimazole	Topical	Troche	10 mg 5/day	7–14 days
	Nystatin	Topical	Suspension or pastilles	4–6 ml q.i.d 1–2 pastilles 4–5 times/day	7–14 days
	Amphotericin B	Topical	Suspension	1 ml==100 mg q.i.d.	7–14 days
	Fluconazole	p.o.	Capsule	100–400 mg q.d.	7–14 days
	Itraconazole	p.o.	Capsule or solution	200 mg q.d.	7–14 days
Esophageal Candidiasis	Fluconazole	p.o./i.v.	Capsule or infusion	200 mg q.d.	14–21 days
	Itraconazole	p.o.	Solution	200 mg q.d.	14–21 days
	Caspofungin	i.v.	Infusion	70 mg loading then 50 mg q.d.	14–21 days
	Amphotericin B deoxycholate; Lipid associated AmB	i.v.	Infusion	06–1 mg/kg per day; 3–5 mg/kg per day	14–21 days
	Voriconazole	p.o./i.v.	Tablet or infusion	100–200 mg b.i.d.	14–21 days
Candidemia	Fluconazole[a]	i.v.	Infusion	400–800 mg q.d.	14–21 days; # from negative cultures
	Amphotericin B deoxycholate	i.v.	Infusion	0.5–0.6 mg/kg per day	
	Lipid associated AmB	i.v.	Infusion	3–5 mg/kg per day	
	Caspofungin	i.v.	Infusion	70 mg loading then 50 mg q.d.	

[a]Consider p.o. switch towards end of Tx.

for use in pregnancy and it should be used with caution. It can be used for treatment of mucosal and disseminated candidiasis and for prophylaxis. Resistance to fluconazole has been shown to develop in patients who receive continuous or intermittent fluconazole.[21] It is active against most C. albicans strains; primary resistance is rare but strains with decreased susceptibility emerge over time at rates varying between 5–30% in patients with prolonged exposure to fluconazole.[22] C. glabrata and C. krusei often have decreased susceptibility to fluconazole.[23]

Itraconazole

Itraconazole is another triazole agent. It is available in oral capsules, pastilles, suspension and intravenous infusion (100–200 mg/day). It does not have as good oral bioavailability as fluconazole and requires gastric acidity for absorption. It has a similar side effect profile to fluconazole but drug interactions are more frequent. It is also category C for use in pregnancy. It is active against mucosal candidiasis. There is cross-resistance with fluconazole particularly in non-albicans species,[24-26] but there are strains of C. albicans with reduced susceptibility to fluconazole that may respond to itraconazole.

Voriconazole

Voriconazole is a newer azole agent available in oral and parenteral forms (100–200 mg q.12). It is as active as fluconazole in oesophageal candidiasis but was associated with more side-effects, especially reversible visual disturbances (23%).[27] It has significant interactions with efavirenz, ritonavir, and rifampin and concurrent use is not recommended. Voriconazole is rarely indicated as initial therapy but may be effective in patients with fluconazole-resistant disease, including infection caused by C. krusei.[28]

Cell Wall Synthesis Inhibitors (Caspofungin, Anidulafungin, and Micafungin)

These are a new class of antifungal agents of which caspofungin is the first to become readily available. They are only available in i.v. formulation. For caspofungin the dosage is 70 mg as a loading dose, and then 50 mg/day. A dosage increase of caspofungin to 70 mg/day is required with concomitant use of enzyme inducers such as rifampin, NNRTIs, phenytoin etc. Caspofungin has been shown to be as effective and as well tolerated as fluconazole in the treatment of oesophageal candidiasis,[29] including fluconazole-resistant infection. Similar data are emerging on the other two echinocandin agents (micafungin and anidulafungin).

Polyenes

Previously the mainstay of antifungal therapy, the polyenes are increasingly regarded as second-line therapies because of issues of toxicity and bioavailability. Polyenes are not well-absorbed after oral administration. This characteristic makes them potentially useful in the management of mucosal disease and oral suspensions of nystatin and amphotericin B are available. However, they must be administered frequently (4–5 times daily) and in relatively large volumes to be most effective, and these characteristics, in addition to their bitter taste, has made them less popular than the azoles for local therapy. Several formulations of amphotericin B are available for systemic use, including amphotericin B deoxycholate (dose 0.6–1 mg/kg per day), amphotericin B lipid complex (ABLC) (5 mg/kg per day), amphotericin B colloidal dispersion (3–6 mg/kg per day) and liposomal amphotericin B (3–5 mg/kg per day). Most experience in the treatment of systemic candidiasis is with the traditional form of amphotericin B. The three newer lipid associated formulations have not been shown to be superior to traditional amphotericin but have been shown to have less nephrotoxicity and are better tolerated. With the advent of better tolerated agents such as fluconazole and caspofungin, amphotericin B is now regarded as second-line therapy in proven candidiasis; the lipid formulations are preferred in patients felt to be at high risk of toxicities (renal, infusion reactions) from the traditional formulation.

Treatment of Oropharyngeal and Oesophageal Candidiasis

Initial episodes of oropharyngeal candidiasis usually respond well to any antifungal agent – topical azoles (clotrimazole troches one 10 mg troche 5 times/day); oral azoles (fluconazole 100 mg/day for 7–14 days; itraconazole solution 100 mg/day 7–14 days or ketoconazole) or oral polyenes (nystatin suspension/pastilles or oral amphotericin B). Patients with mild OPC, especially those with less advanced immunosuppression can be treated with topical agents, as these are less likely to have systemic side-effects.

Of the systemic agents, fluconazole has been well studied and is as effective or superior to topical therapy. Doses can range from 50–200 mg daily for uncomplicated OPC but higher doses should be used if there is a suspicion of esophageal involvement or if the patient has more advanced HIV disease. In general, the first episode of OPC will resolve within 2–3 days of starting fluconazole. Recurrent episodes often require higher doses and a more prolonged therapy. Itraconazole and ketoconazole have less reliable absorption when compared with fluconazole and are generally not preferred for uncomplicated episodes. If itraconazole is used, the oral suspension is preferable to the capsule formulation.

Recurrent episodes may prompt the need for suppressive therapy in select patients. Fluconazole, 200 mg once weekly, has been shown to decrease oropharyngeal and mucosal candidiasis by up to 50% with a low incidence of the evolution of fluconazole resistance (<5%).[30] However other studies of patients with advanced HIV showed lower CD4 count and oral azole exposure as important risk factors for development of resistance.[31] A large study examining the epidemiology of fluconazole resistance in AIDS patients linked continuous fluconazole use and trimethoprim-sulfamethoxazole prophylaxis with the onset of fluconazole-resistance mucosal disease. That study also showed that the emergence of fluconazole resistance was associated with poor survival, reflecting (as does the use of trimethoprim-sulfamethoxazole prophylaxis) the advanced immunodeficiency in these patients. Once resistance develops, higher doses of fluconazole up to 800 mg/day may be effective. Fluconazole resistance is often (but not *always*) associated with cross-resistance to the other azole antifungal agents. About half of patients with fluconazole-unresponsive esophageal candidiasis respond to itraconazole cyclodextrin solution at 100 mg b.i.d.

If antifungal resistance seems likely, a variety of alternative strategies can be employed. First, as noted, azole cross-resistance is not universal and a trial of itraconazole at 200 mg b.i.d. is warranted. Use of the itraconazole solution is preferred: due perhaps both to its local effects and its better absorption. Second, data from individuals with refractory esophageal candidiasis have shown response rates of >50% for voriconazole at its standard dosage of 200 mg twice daily. Third, topical solutions of polyenes may be used. Fourth, caspofungin (70 mg loading dose followed by 50 mg daily) has been shown to have response rates of 70–80% for esophageal candidiasis including that associated with fluconazole resistance. The potential utility of echinocandins in this

setting is further supported by positive findings in trials comparing anidulafungin with fluconazole and micafungin with fluconazole.

Oesophageal candidiasis requires systemic treatment. Oral fluconazole at 200 mg/day for 14–21 days will resolve symptoms in over 80% of patients within a week. Intravenous preparations may be needed in patients who have difficulty swallowing oral formulations. Again azoles, caspofungin, and amphotericin B are the agents of choice in descending order. Itraconazole solution and voriconazole have been shown to be as effective as fluconazole but are generally reserved for refractory cases. Advanced AIDS patients without HAART are likely to suffer from recurrent infections and long-term suppressive therapy with fluconazole 200 mg daily may be required.

Treatment of Vulvovaginal Candidiasis

Symptomatic relief is the aim of treatment. Often, topical agents are most effective with systemic therapy needed for severe or recurrent cases. Uncomplicated VVC usually respond well to topical agents such as clotrimazole, miconazole, butoconazole, tioconazole creams, and pessaries or boric acid 600 mg gelatin capsules administered intra-vaginally daily for 2 weeks. Oral fluconazole 150 mg as a single dose orally is very effective. Alternatively, itraconazole (200 mg b.i.d. for 1 day or 200 mg/day for 3 days) or ketoconazole (400 mg b.i.d. for 5 days) can be used.

More complicated vaginitis requires longer duration of therapy, either topical treatment >7 days or oral therapy with two doses of fluconazole 150 mg 72 h apart. Non-*albicans* candida may not respond as well to azole therapy but is an infrequent cause of vulvovaginal candidiasis.

Recurrent disease is usually due to azole-susceptible *C. albicans* and may require prolonged therapy or even long-term prophylaxis with weekly fluconazole. This may select for non-*albicans* strains but the significance of this is not certain.[32]

Treatment of Candidemia

This is a serious infection with a significant mortality and propensity to disseminate and cause end organ disease. Along with definitive anti-fungal therapy, removal of a causative intravascular catheter and evaluation for metastatic disease (i.e. ophthalmologic evaluation, echocardiography) are advised. Parenteral therapy is usually indicated initially with i.v. fluconazole, caspofungin or amphotericin B. The choice of agent should be based on the individual patients' status, prior antifungal exposure, likely causative organism or definitive microbiological data. Most patients can be switched to high doses of oral fluconazole (800 mg/day) when clinically stable. Therapy for candidemia should be given for at least 14 days after sterilization of the blood cultures.

Candida and HAART

Since the introduction of highly active antiretroviral therapy (HAART) in the late 1990s, the incidence and prevalence of opportunistic infections (OIs) in HIV-positive individuals on therapy has declined. This is true not only for initial episodes of mucosal or esophageal candidiasis but also for more advanced disease – for example, fluconazole resistant candidiasis had declined from 45% in 1994 to 10% in 2000 (P<0.0001) in one cohort.[33] However, in the resource limited setting where HAART is not widely available, OIs such as candida still constitute a large disease burden.

A large number of studies published after the availability of HAART showed a decline in the incidence and prevalence of mucosal candidiasis. Although, this can largely be attributed to the restoration of cell-mediated immunity, as reflected in the rise in CD4[+] lymphocyte count, there has been some interesting data suggesting a direct anti-candidal effect exhibited by HIV protease inhibitors both *in vitro*[34,35] and *in vivo*.[36] This has been attributed to inhibition of secreted aspartic proteinases (Saps) by HIV protease inhibitors.[37] Saps are key virulence factors of *C. albicans*. Inhibition of Sap expression is not seen with other antiretrovirals including the NNRTIs;[38,39] however there is little data to suggest that PIs are associated with better control of mucosal candidiasis than other antiretrovirals.

One manifestation of the successful treatment of HIV-infected persons with HAART is a risk of developing immune reconstitution disease (IRD). This manifests as the development of an acute inflammatory reaction to opportunistic pathogens as the immune system recovers. This is most commonly seen with mycobacterial disease; however, cases describing IRD with candidiasis (OPC)[40] have been reported.

Prevention of *Candida* Infections

As previously noted, several studies have shown that fluconazole, given daily or even weekly, could sig-

nificantly reduce the incidence of mucosal candidiasis in advanced HIV disease. Fluconazole has also been shown to be effective in reducing the prevalence of other invasive fungal infections. However, in the developed world, routine prophylaxis for candida infection has not been routinely recommended, largely because of cost and fears of resistance. Prophylaxis can be used in certain recurrent cases,[41] especially with esophageal disease. However, the availability of potent antiretroviral therapy has eliminated the need for any specific antimicrobial prophylaxis – an observation that is as true for candida infection as it is for other opportunistic diseases.

References

1. Schmidt-Westhausen AM, Bendick C, Reichart PA, et al. Oral candidosis and associated *Candida* species in HIV-infected Cambodians exposed to anti-mycotics. Mycoses 2004; 47:435–441.
2. Tekeli A, Dolapci I, Emral R, et al. *Candida* carriage and *Candida* dubliniensis in oropharyngeal samples of type 1 diabetes mellitus patients. Mycoses 2004; 47:315–318.
3. Al-Abeid HM, Abu-Elteen KH, Elkarmi AZ, et al. Isolation and characterization of *Candida* spp. In Jordanian cancer patients: prevalence, pathogenic determinants and antifungal sensitivity. Jpn J Infect Dis 2004; 57:279–284.
4. Gugnani HC, Becker K, Fegeler W, et al. Oropharyngeal carriage of *Candida* species in HIV-infected patients in India. Mycoses 2003; 46:299–306.
5. Pongsiriwet S, Iamaroon A, Sributee P, et al. Oral colonization of *Candida* species in perinatally HIV-infected children in northern Thailand. J Oral Sci 2004; 46:101–105.
6. Schuman P, Sobel JD, Ohmit SE, et al. Mucosal candidal colonization and candidiasis in women with or at risk for human immunodeficiency virus infection. HIV Epidemiology Research Study (HERS) Group. Clin Infect Dis 1998; 27:1161–1167.
7. Ohmit SE, Sobel JD, Schuman P, et al. Longitudinal study of mucosal *Candida* species colonization and candidiasis among human immunodeficiency virus (HIV)-seropositive and at-risk HIV-seronegative women. J Infect Dis 2003; 188:118–127.
8. Powderly WG, Mayer K, Perfect J. Diagnosis and treatment of oropharyngeal candidiasis in patients infected with HIV: a critical reassessment. AIDS Res Hum Retroviruses 1999; 15:1405–1412.
9. Cartledge JD, Midgley J, Gazzard BG. Non-albicans oral candidosis in HIV-positive patients. J Antimicrob Chemother 1999; 43:419–422.
10. Melo NR, Taguchi H, Jorge J, et al. Oral candida flora from Brazilian human immunodeficiency virus-infected patients in the highly active antiretroviral therapy era. Mem Inst Oswaldo Cruz 2004; 99:425–431.
11. Martinez M, Lopez-Ribot JL, Kirkpatrick WR, et al. Replacement of *Candida* albicans with C. dubliniensis in human immunodeficiency virus-infected patients with oropharyngeal candidiasis treated with fluconazole. J Clin Microbiol 2002; 40:3135–3139.
12. Paterson DL, Georghiou PR, Allworth AM, et al. Thalidomide as treatment of refractory aphthous ulceration related to human immunodeficiency virus infection. Clin Infect Dis 1995; 20:250–254.
13. Bertagnolio S, de Gaetano Donati K, Tacconelli E, et al. Hospital-acquired candidemia in HIV-infected patients.

Incidence, risk factors and predictors of outcome. J Chemother 2004; 16:172–178.

14. Puzniak L, Teutsch S, Powderly W, et al. Has the epidemiology of nosocomial candidemia changed? Infect Control Hosp Epidemiol 2004; 25:628–633.

15. Casado JL, Quereda C, Corral I. Candidal meningitis in HIV-infected patients. AIDS Patient Care STDS 1998; 12:681–686.

16. Bisbe J, Miro JM, Latorre X, et al. Disseminated candidiasis in addicts who use brown heroin: report of 83 cases and review. Clin Infect Dis 1992; 15:910–923.

17. Miro JM, del Rio A, Mestres CA. Infective endocarditis in intravenous drug abusers and HIV-1 infected patients. Infect Dis North Am 2002; 16:vii–viii, 273–295.

18. Kim RW, Juzych MS. Eliott D. Ocular manifestations of intravenous drug use. Infect Dis Clin North Am 2002; 16:607–622.

19. Pappas PG, Rex JH, Sobel JD, et al. Guidelines for the Treatment of Candidiasis. Clin Infect Dis 2004; 38:161–189.

20. Rex JH, Pfaller MA. Has antifungal susceptibility testing come of age? Clin Infect Dis 2002; 35:982–989.

21. Revankar SG, Kirkpatrick WR, McAtee RK, et al. A randomized trial of continuous or intermittent therapy with fluconazole for oropharyngeal candidiasis in HIV-infected patients: clinical outcomes and development of fluconazole resistance. Am J Med 1998; 105:7–11.

22. Martins MD, Lozano-Chiu M, Rex JH. Point prevalence of oropharyngeal carriage of fluconazole resistant candida in human immunodeficiency virus-infected patients. Clin Infect Dis 1997; 25:843–846.

23. Ostrosky-Zeichner L, Rex JH, Pappas PG, et al. Antifungal susceptibility survey of 2,000 blood stream *Candida* isolates in the United States. Antimicrob Agents Chemother 2003; 47:3149–3154.

24. Goldman M, Cloud GA, Smedema M, et al. Does long-term itraconazole prophylaxis result in in vitro azole resistance in mucosal *Candida albicans* isolates from persons with advanced human immunodeficiency virus infection? The national institute of Allergy and Infectious Diseases Mycoses study group. Antimicrob Agents Chemother 2000; 44:1585–1587.

25. Vazquez JA, Peng G, Sobel JD, et al. Evolution of anti-fungal susceptibility among *Candida* species isolates recovered from human immunodeficiency virus-infected women receiving fluconazole prophylaxis. Clin Infect Dis 2001; 33:1069–1075.

26. Barchiesi F, Colombo AL, McGough DA, et al. In vitro activity of itraconazole against fluconazole-susceptible and -resistant *Candida* albicans isolates from oral cavities of patients infected with human immunodeficiency virus. Antimicrob Agents Chemother 1994; 38:1530–1533.

27. Ally R, Schurmann D, Kreisel W, et al. Esophageal Candidiasis Study Group. A randomized, double blind, double dummy, multi-center trial of voriconazole and fluconazole in the treatment of esophageal candidiasis in immunocompromised patients. Clin Infect Dis 2001; 33:1447–1454.

28. Ostrosky-Zeichner L, Oude Lashof AM, Kullberg BJ, et al. Voriconazole salvage treatment of invasive candidiasis. Eur J Clin Microbiol Infect Dis 2003; 22:651–655.

29. Villanueva A, Gotuzzo E, Arathoon EG, et al. A randomized double-blind study of caspofungin versus fluconazole for the treatment of esophageal candidiasis. Am J Med 2002; 113:294–299.

30. Schuman P, Capps L, Peng G, et al. Weekly fluconazole for the prevention of mucosal candidiasis in women with HIV infection. Ann Int Med 1997; 126:689–698.

31. Maenza JR, Keruly JC, Moore RD, et al. Risk factors for fluconazole-resistant candidiasis in human immunodeficiency virus-infected patients. J Infect Dis 1996; 173:219–225.

32. Vazquez JA, Sobel JD, Peng G, et al. Evolution of vaginal candida species recovered from human immunodeficiency virus-infected women receiving fluconazole prophylaxis: the emergence of candida glabrata? Clin Infect Dis 1999; 28:1025–1031.

33. Tacconelli E, Bertagnolio S, Posteraro B, et al. Azole susceptibility patterns and genetic relationship among oral candida strains isolated in the era of highly active antiretroviral therapy. J Acquir Defic Syndr 2002; 31:38–44.

34. Cassone A, De Bernardis F, Torosantucci A, et al. In vitro and in vivo anticandidal activity of human immunodeficiency virus protease inhibitors. J Infect Dis 1999; 180:448–453.

35. Mata-Essayag S, Magaldi S, Hartung de Capriles C, et al. 'In vitro' antifungal activity of protease inhibitors. Mycopathologica 2001; 152:135–142.

36. Cauda R, Tacconelli E, Tumbarello M, et al. Role of protease inhibitors in preventing recurrent oral candidosis in patients with HIV infection: a prospective case-control study. J Acquir Immune Defic Syndr 1999; 21:20–25.

37. Bektic J, Lell CP, Fuchs A, et al. HIV protease inhibitors attenuate adherence of candida albicans to epithelial cells in vitro. FEMS Immunol Med Microbiol 2001; 31:65–71.

38. De Bernardis F, Tacconelli E, Mondello F, et al. Anti-retroviral therapy with protease inhibitors decreases virulence enzyme expression in vivo by *Candida* albicans without selection of avirulent strains or decreasing their anti-mycotic susceptibility. FEMS Immunol Med Microbiol 2004; 41:27–34.

39. Cassone A, Tacconelli E, De Bernardis F, et al. Antiretroviral therapy with protease inhibitors has an early, immune reconstitution-independent beneficial effect on *Candida* virulence and oral candidiasis in human immunodeficiency virus-infected subjects. J Infect Dis 2002; 185:188–195.

40. Jevtovic DJ, Salemovic D, Ranin J, et al. The prevalence and risk of immune restoration disease in HIV-infected patients treated with highly active antiretroviral therapy. HIV Med 2005; 6:140–143.

41. USPHS/IDSA. 1999 Guidelines for Prevention of Opportunistic Infections in persons Infected with Human Immunodeficiency Virus. Clin Infect Dis 2000; 30: S29–S65.

Cryptococcosis and other Fungal Infections (Histoplasmosis and Coccidioidomycosis) in HIV-infected Patients

Kathleen R. Page
Richard Chaisson
Merle Sande

Introduction

Systemic fungal infections are generally late manifestations of HIV disease. Overall, cryptococcal infection is the most common systemic fungal infection in HIV-infected patients. However, in certain endemic regions, histoplasmosis or coccidioidomycosis are more prevalent. These diseases can affect patients without HIV, but among HIV-infected patients, they tend to occur when the CD4 count is <200 cells/mm^3. Recent advances in the treatment of systemic fungal infections have substantially reduced the morbidity and mortality from these disorders. Immune reconstitution with antiretroviral therapy has led to significant declines in the incidence of fungal disease among HIV-infected individuals. However, among patients with limited access to HAART, opportunistic infection with fungal pathogens remain a major cause of death. This chapter reviews the approach to diagnosis (Table 34.1) and management of the most commonly occurring systemic mycosis in HIV-infected patients: cryptococcosis, histoplasmosis, and coccidioidomycosis.

Cryptococcus

Microbiology

Cryptococcus neoformans is a round or oval yeast (4–6 μm in diameter), surrounded by a capsule that can be up to 30 μm thick. The organism grows quite readily on fungal or bacterial culture media and usually is detectable within 1 week after inoculation, although in some circumstances up to 4 weeks are required for growth. Therefore, when *C. neoformans* is suspected, clinical cultures should be maintained for a minimum of 2 weeks, and preferably 4 weeks. The organism is differentiated from other pathogenic yeasts based on its growth characteristics. It grows well at 37°C, does not form pseudomycelin on cornmeal or rice-Tween agar, and hydrolyzes urea, a property that allows rapid presumptive identification.[1]

On the basis of antigenic differences in the capsule, biochemical use of nutrients, and distinct DNA base sequences, four serotypes (A, B, C, and D) of *Cryptococcus* have been delineated. Serotypes A and D are

Table 34.1 Sensitivity of commercially-available non-culture based diagnostic methods

Disease	Serology		Antigen detection			
Cryptococcosis						
Disseminated	N/A		Serum:	99%[49]		
Pulmonary	N/A		Serum:	96%[59]		
Meningeal	N/A		Serum:	99%[a,54]		
			CSF:	93–100%[49]		
Histoplasmosis						
Disseminated	Serum:	67–70%[b,108]	Serum:	80%;	Urine:	90%[108,112]
Pulmonary	Serum:	90–100%[108]			Urine:	15%[108]
Meningeal	CSF:	70–88%[98,107–109]	CSF:	40–70%[108,109]		
Coccidioidomycosis						
Disseminated	Serum:	75–94%[134,136,146,150]	N/A			
Pulmonary	Serum:	<10%[134]	N/A			
Meningeal	CSF:	50%[148]	N/A			

[a]Not specific for meningitis, must evaluate CSF. [b]Does not distinguish active disease from prior infection.

classified as *C. neoformans* var. *neoformans*, and serotypes B and C are classified as *C. neoformans* var. *gatii*.[2] *Cryptococcus neoformans* var. *neoformans* is the major cause of cryptococcal disease worldwide. Serotype A is the most common serotype infecting AIDS patients.[3,4] For reasons that are not clearly understood, *C. neofromans* var. *gatii* tends to infect immunocompetent hosts.[5] This subtype is found in certain geographic areas, including southern California, Africa, Australia, and Southeast Asia. Interestingly, even within these geographic areas, *C. neoformans* var. *gatii* does not appear to cause much disease in HIV-infected patients.[5–7]

Epidemiology and Pathogenesis

Before the onset of the AIDS epidemic, cryptococcal infection occurred in a small number of immunocompetent individuals, but most often in patients with a compromised immune system, such as diabetics, transplant recipients, patients with lymphoma, or patients requiring chronic steroid therapy.[5] In the AIDS era, cryptococcal disease became a leading opportunistic infections, affecting 6–10% of HIV-infected patients.[8–12] Among individuals who develop cryptococcal disease, it is the initial AIDS-defining illness in approximately 40%,[8,13–17] and the third most common central nervous system (CNS) disorder in AIDS patients, behind toxoplasmosis and HIV dementia.[18]

In the last decade, the incidence of disease caused by *C. neoformans* in developed countries has decreased dramatically. Although some decrease can be attrib-

uted to the more widespread use of azole therapy,[19] as with other opportunistic infections, highly active antiretroviral therapy (HAART) has played a predominant role in the declining rates of cryptococcal disease. Surveillance and clinical studies in the USA and Europe have shown a 2- to 10-fold decrease in the incidence of cryptococcosis since the introduction of HAART.[18,20-22] Demographic characteristics of patients with cryptococcus show that poor access to medical care is a major risk factor for developing cryptococcal disease in the HAART era.[7,20,22,23]

In areas of the world with limited access to antiretroviral therapy, cryptococcosis remains a major cause of morbidity and mortality. Studies from sub-Saharan Africa and Southeast Asia show that up to one-third of patients infected with HIV develop cryptococcal disease,[24–26] which is a major cause of death among HIV-infected patients.[27] Despite antifungal therapy, mortality from cryptococcal disease in these settings is exceedingly high,[27,28] with an average survival of <6 months after diagnosis.[29] In a prospective study of 92 patients hospitalized with cryptococcal meningitis at the national referral hospital in Kampala, Uganda, the mortality rate in the first 2 weeks of presentation was 42% despite therapy with amphotericin B.[30] Poor outcomes may be related to the late presentation of disease and suboptimal management of raised intracranial pressure.

Cryptococcus neoformans infection is acquired from the environment. Because it is ubiquitous in soil and dust, exposure to the organisms is practically unavoidable. The organism, most likely in an encapsulated form, is inhaled into the lungs and deposited in the small airways. Once there, yeast multiply and compress the surrounding tissue but, remarkably, cause little damage. The pulmonary infection is often asymptomatic. Indeed, in 85–95% of patients with cryptococcal meningitis, no evidence of pneumonitis is present.[8,13] The organism has a strong propensity for dissemination to the CNS but also may infect skin, bone, and the genitourinary tract.

Clinical Manifestations

The onset of cryptococcal disease usually is insidious. The most common symptoms are headache, malaise, and a prolonged febrile prodrome that may be indistinguishable from symptoms caused by other opportunistic infections.[8,13,14,31] The median time between the onset of symptoms and the diagnosis of cryptococcal disease is 30 days.[8,13,14] Diagnosis often is delayed by the waxing and waning course of the disease and the absence of specific symptoms.

CNS involvement is the most serious manifestation of cryptococcal disease. Over 75% of HIV-associated cryptococcal meningitis occurs in patients with CD4 counts <50 cells/µL. In general, CNS disease presents as a chronic meningitis, with headaches, nausea, and photophobia, but occasional can present with focal neurologic signs associated with mass lesions (cryptococcomas). In a prospective study conducted in Uganda, 20% of HIV-infected patients presenting with headaches were diagnosed with cryptococcal meningitis.[32] Classic signs of meningeal irritation are uncommon. HIV-infected patients presenting with seizures, altered mental status, psychosis, and dementia should be evaluated for cryptococcal meningitis. Pulmonary or disseminated disease may be associated, but usually CNS disease presents in isolation.

The incidence of extraneural cryptococcal disease in AIDS patients ranges between 20% and 60%.[8,13,15,16] Despite entry through the lung, evidence of pulmonary symptoms is present in only 20–30% of cases. Other sites of extraneural involvement include the joints, oral cavity, pericardium, myocardium, skin, mediastinum, and genitourinary tract, which is believed to be a sanctuary for C. neoformans that may lead to recurrent disease.[33]

Patients receiving HAART often present with atypical manifestations, such as isolated lymphadenopathy, and are more likely to have repeatedly negative initial fungal cultures, which can lead to diagnostic delays.[34] There have been several reports of immune reconstitution syndrome (IRIS) in patients with cryptococcosis and a rapid rise in CD4 count and decline in viral load after initiation of antiretro-

viral therapy. 10–30% of patients co-infected with C. neoformans and HIV develop IRIS while on HAART, usually within the first 2 months of therapy.[35,36] The syndrome is characterized by a paradoxical clinical deterioration resulting from an exuberant inflammatory response which may manifest itself as worsening or new lymphadenopathy, mediastinitis, new headache and stiff neck, CNS lesions, or subcutaneous abscesses.[35-43] Usually C. neoformans cultures are negative. Therapeutically, HAART is generally continued and antifungal therapy may be added to the regimen. There are no specific guidelines regarding the use of anti-inflammatory agents, although NSAIDS are often recommended, and thalidomide or steroids have been occasionally used for severe cases.[35]

The physical examination in patients with cryptococcal disease is also non-specific. In the series reported by Chuck and Sande, 56% of patients were febrile, although less than one-third had nuchal rigidity or other neurologic deficits.[8] Altered mental status, which is the most important predictor of poor outcome, is present in 20–30% of patients with cryptococcal disease. Papilledema is seen in <10% of patients. Raised, sometimes umbilicated, typical skin lesions that resemble those caused by Molluscum contagiosum or Penicillium marneffei are reported in 3–10% of patients with cryptococcal meningitis.

Diagnosis

Meningitis

The gold standard diagnostic test for cryptococcal meningitis is a positive CSF culture for C. neoformans. Therefore, a lumbar puncture is important in any individual with suspected cryptococcal meningitis. Most clinicians perform an imaging study before performing a lumbar puncture to exclude a space-occupying CNS lesion. Although cryptococcomas are rare, patients with CNS toxoplasmosis or lymphoma could present with symptoms similar to those caused by cryptococcal meningitis.[44,45] The most common findings noted on brain imaging studies are cerebral atrophy and ventricular enlargement.[8,14,45]

After an occult mass lesion has been ruled out, a lumbar puncture should be performed. In non-HIV associated cryptococcal meningitis, the CSF usually has a leukocytosis, hypoglycorrhachia, elevated protein, and a negative India ink preparation. In contrast, the CSF profile of HIV-infected patients with cryptococcal meningitis is normal in 25–50% of patients.[8,13,17,46,47] Over 50% of patients have a low CSF white blood count (≤20/mm³), and the India ink preparation is positive in 74–88% of HIV-infected patients with cryptococcal meningitis.[8,13,31,46,48] The differences in CSF profile between HIV and non-HIV-infected patients with cryptococcal meningitis probably reflect an impaired inflammatory response and higher fungal burden in immunocompromised patients.

Interpretation of the India ink stain should be performed by an experienced technician since false positive tests have been reported as a result of artifact. After staining, *C. neoformans* is visible as round cells 4–6 μm in diameter surrounded by a characteristic thick polysaccharide capsule (Fig. 34.1). Budding forms can usually be detected with viable *C. neoformans*. A positive India ink stain should be confirmed

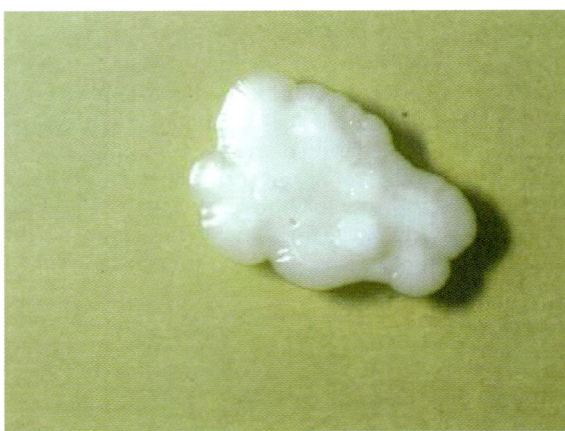

A

B

Figure 34.1 (A) Mature *C. neoformans* colony.
(B) Microscopic appearance of *C. neoformans*.
(Photographs courtesy of Dr William Merz, Department of Pathology, Johns Hopkins University School of Medicine.)

with a CSF cryptococcal antigen (CRAG) test or, ideally, with a CSF fungal culture.

CRAG testing of the CSF is a reliable and rapid diagnostic technique. Sensitivity of the CSF CRAG test is 93–99% and specificity 93–98%.[8,13,49] In non-HIV-infected patients, the median CSF titer is between 1:16 and 1:32, whereas in HIV-infected patients the median titer is 1:1024, and on occasion can exceed 1:1 million. An adequate number of dilutions should be performed to avoid false-negative tests due to a prozone phenomenon with high organism burden.[50] False-positive CRAG tests have been noted occasionally in patients with *Trichosporon beigelii* infections; however false-positive titers rarely exceed 1:8.[51–53]

Serum CRAG tests are positive in over 99% of patients with cryptococcosis and can be used to rule out cryptococcal meningitis in HIV-infected patients with a fever and a headache.[54] The serum CRAG is not useful for assess the response to therapy of predict relapses.[55,56] In the USA, a lumbar puncture is recommended if the serum CRAG is positive to evaluate for the presence of CNS involvement and to measure intracranial pressure. However, in resource-limited settings lumbar punctures may only be practically available for patients with advanced disease. In such scenarios, it is appropriate to screen ambulatory HIV-infected patients presenting with headaches with a serum CRAG and a chest radiograph to rule out tuberculosis. Patients with a positive CRAG, negative chest radiograph, and no focal neurologic signs or altered consciousness can be successfully treated with oral fluconazole.[57] In a study conducted in Entebbe, Uganda, screening with serum CRAG detected cryptococcal infection 20 days before the onset of frank meningitis, and early therapy with fluconazole reduced mortality rates.[32] However, patients with altered mental status or focal neurologic signs must have a lumbar puncture performed to confirm the diagnosis and to appropriately manage elevated intracranial pressure.

A definitive diagnosis of cryptococcal disease requires culturing the organisms from body fluids or tissue. CSF fungal cultures require a minimum of 2 mL to obtain maximum sensitivity. By definition, 100% of cases of cryptococcal meningitis have positive CSF fungal cultures. Approximately 66–80% of HIV-infected patients with cryptococcal meningitis have positive blood cultures for *C. neoformans*.[14,48]

Extraneural Cryptococcosis

The serum CRAG test has excellent sensitivity and specificity for the diagnosis of disseminated cryptococcosis without CNS involvement. Serum CRAF ≥1:8 should always be treated regardless of symptoms. Fungal blood cultures are often positive and bone marrow examination does not increase the diagnostic yield.[58] In contrast to immunocompetent patients with cryptococcal pneumonia, where the serum CRAG is often negative, HIV-infected patients with pulmonary cryptococcus usually have a positive test.[59] HIV-infected patients with pneumonia and a CD4 count ≤100 cell/μL should also have fungal cultures of sputum performed. *C. neoformans* can be readily identified using methenamine silver, mucicarmine, and periodic acid-Schiff stains, but cannot be detected with regular Gram's stain of tissue.

Prognosis

Left untreated, cryptococcal meningitis is uniformly fatal. With improved therapeutic interventions, mortality rates for cryptococcal meningitis in HIV-infected patients have improved from approximately 20%[48] to around 6%.[31] However, in areas with limited medical resources, mortality rates are significantly higher.[27-30] Even with amphotericin B therapy, patients with CSF-confirmed cryptococcal meningitis hospitalized in Uganda had a mortality rate of 42% within the first two weeks of therapy.[30] The most important baseline prognostic factor is mental status at the time of presentation. Individuals with altered sensorium have a much worse prognosis that those who are awake and alert.[14,48,60] High fungal burden, a positive India ink test, elevated intracranial pressure, and lack of inflammatory cells in the CSF are also associated with poor outcomes.[14,30,31,48,60] Early detection of cryptococcal infection with serum CRAG testing and treatment with fluconazole can decrease the rate of progression and mortality from cryptococcal disease in resource-limited settings.

Treatment

Antifungal Agents

Amphotericin B is a polyene antimicrobial agent that possesses a broad range of antifungal activity. Its fungicidal activity is due principally to the binding of ergosterol in the fungal membrane, resulting in increased membrane permeability, leakage of cellular components, and resultant cell death. The drug is very poorly absorbed when administered orally

(necessitating intravenous administration), has a very high volume of distribution, and is believed to be deposited in fatty tissues throughout the body. However, the penetration of amphotericin B into the CSF is poor.

The principal limitation of amphotericin is its toxicity profile. Virtually all patients who receive this therapy for more than 4 weeks will experience some degree of reversible renal insufficiency. During acute administration, fever, rigors, headache, and thrombophlebitis have been reported. Chronic administration results in electrolyte abnormalities, most notably hypokalemia and hypomagnesemia. Strategies to reduce the toxicity of amphotericin include slow administration of drug (over 4–6 h), the addition of heparin (1000 U/500 mL) to reduce the incidence of thrombophlebitis, premedication with antipyretics, premedication with meperidine in patients who have experienced severe rigors, and aggressive replacement of electrolytes. Lipid formulations of amphotericin are an acceptable alternative for patients who cannot tolerate regular amphotericin B.[61,62] These formulations allow higher doses (4 mg/kg) to be administered with less toxicity.

Flucytosine is a pyrimidine derivative similar in structure to 5-fluorouracil. When administered to susceptible fungi, flucytosine is converted to 5-fluorouracil and inhibits thymidylate synthetase, a vital enzyme needed for DNA synthesis. Flucytosine has a very favorable pharmacokinetic profile, including complete absorption from the gastrointestinal tract when administered orally, a satisfactory half-life of 3–4 h, and very little hepatic metabolism (the drug is excreted virtually unchanged by the kidney). Most importantly, flucytosine reaches high concentrations in the CSF, usually on the order of 70–90% of the serum levels. The principal toxicities of flucytosine occur primarily in organ systems that have rapidly dividing cells, such as the bone marrow (leucopenia), gastrointestinal tract (nausea, vomiting, diarrhea), and skin (rash). Optimally, drug levels should be obtained whenever flucytosine is used to minimize toxicity and maximize effectiveness. The levels should be above 50 μg/mL and below 100 μg/mL.

Fluconazole, a bistriazole, was the second oral azole agent approved for use in the USA. Fluconazole is well absorbed from the gastrointestinal tract (oral bioavailability 70–80%) and is able to achieve adequate serum levels even when exposed to an alkaline gastric environment. The drug is excreted predominantly via the kidneys and undergoes minimal metabolism by the liver. Most importantly, it penetrates well into the CSF, achieving concentrations of 60–80% of serum levels. The most common side effects are gastrointestinal in nature, although skin rash has been reported in up to 3% of patients taking the drug. Rare instances of Stevens–Johnson syndrome have been reported.

Itraconazole is a triazole with *in vitro* activity against *H. capsulatum, B. dermatitidis, C. neoformans,* and *Candida* species. It requires gastric acidity for absorption, is metabolized by the liver, and penetrates the CSF poorly. Concomitant administration with rifampin, Dilantin, carbamazepine, and antiacids significantly reduces drug levels. An oral suspension of the drug has improved absorption in the absence of gastric acidity.

Voriconazole is a recently approved oral antifungal agent in the USA. It has a very wide spectrum of antifungal activity, including *Aspergillus, Fusarium, Candida* species, *Cryptococcus, Trichosporum, Histoplasma, Blastomyces,* and *Coccidioides*. It well absorbed orally and has good bioavailability.[63] CSF concentrations range from 29% to 68% of concurrent serum levels.[63] The most commonly associated toxicities include reversible visual alterations and elevation of liver function tests. To date, no clinical trial has evaluated this drug for the treatment of cryptococcosis.

Non-meningeal Cryptococcal Disease

In immunocompetent patients, asymptomatic pulmonary cryptococcosis often resolves spontaneously and does not require antifungal therapy. In HIV-infected patients, however, pulmonary cryptococcosis should always be treated to prevent disseminated disease.[57] Isolated cryptococcemia indicates deep tissue invasion and should also be treated. In any presentation of extraneural disease, a lumbar puncture should be performed to rule out CNS involvement.

The treatment of non-meningeal cryptococcosis does not usually require parenteral therapy except in cases of severe pneumonia where amphotericin B may be given until there is clinical improvement and the patient can be switched to an oral azole. Most cases of mild to moderate disease are treated with daily oral fluconazole (200–400 mg/day).[57] The length of therapy has not been well established in clinical trials, though most experts advocate continuing lifelong therapy. In patients on HAART, therapy may be discontinued once the CD4 count rises over 200 cells/µL for at least 6 months.[64] Patients intolerant to fluconazole can be treated with itraconazole (200–400 mg/day), although variable itraconazole absorption often limits its efficacy.[57]

Table 34.2 Therapy of HIV-associated cryptococcal meningitis

Therapy	Duration
Induction therapy	
Amphotericin B 0.7 mg/kg q.d.[a] ± Flucytosine 25 mg/kg q.i.d. ± Daily LP if intracranial pressure is ↑	2 weeks
Fluconazole 400 mg p.o. q.d.b	8 weeks
Acceptable alternative for patients without neurologic complications[c]	
Fluconazole 400 mg p.o. q.d.	10 weeks
Maintenance therapy	
Fluconazole 200 mg p.o. q.d.[b]	Until CD4 count ≥200 cells/µL for 6 months
Primary prophylaxis	Not recommended

[a]Alternative: Liposomal amphotericin B (4 mg/kg per day).
[b]Alternative: Itraconazole (200 mg p.o. b.i.d.). [c]Authors' personal opinion.

Cryptococcal Meningitis

The treatment of cryptococcal meningitis in AIDS patients requires an initial induction therapy, followed by lifelong maintenance therapy (Table 34.2). Amphotericin B is more effective than azole therapy during the initial phase of treatment, leading to faster sterilization of the CSF, and fewer relapses.[48,65,66] The addition of flucytosine slightly increases the efficacy of amphotericin.[31,57,65] A recent study comparing amphotericin B monotherapy, amphotericin B plus flucytosine, amphotericin B and fluconazole, or triple therapy with amphotericin B, flucytosine and fluconazole, showed that amphotericin B and flucytosine is the most rapidly sterilizing regimen for cryptococcal meningitis but does not impact survival.[67] Amphotericin and flucytosine combination therapy is recommended in the USA. However, flucytosine causes significant hematologic toxicity and levels should be monitored closely. Patients who develop amphotericin-related nephrotoxicity or infusion reactions can be treated with the lipid formulations of amphotericin which, although more costly, are associated with less toxicity and similar efficacy.[61,62] Intrathecal amphotericin B should be reserved only for salvage therapy which do not respond to systemic antifungal therapy.[68] Following the 2-week induction phase with parenteral therapy, patients can be switched to oral fluconazole (400 mg/day) for

8 weeks. It is commonly recommended to evaluate the CSF for sterility after this period. The cryptococcal CSF antigen may remain positive for up to 1 year after successful therapy, so fungal cultures of the CSF should be performed.

In resource-limited settings, oral fluconazole is an attractive alternative for the treatment of cryptococcal meningitis in patients with mild symptoms and normal sensorium. Amphotericin and flucytosine may cause significant adverse reactions without adequate follow-up and patients in resource-limited areas may be at higher risk for experiencing toxicity. For example, in an African setting where underlying anemia was common and HIV patients were treated with the myelosuppressive antiretroviral AZT, one dose of flucytosine caused severe cytopenia in 50% of patients. Furthermore, early treatment with oral fluconazole reduced mortality in HIV-infected patients with headaches and a positive CRAG. Therefore, it is the authors' opinion that patients with cryptococcal meningitis without neurologic complications may be appropriately treated with 10 weeks of oral high dose (400 mg daily) fluconazole induction, followed by lower dose maintenance therapy (200 mg daily).

Over one-third of patients successfully treated for cryptococcal meningitis will relapse without maintenance therapy.[69] Typically, relapses are associated with the same strain of C. neoformans that caused the initial infection.[70,71] Therefore, following the 8 weeks of 400 mg/day fluconazole, patients must be placed on suppressive antifungal therapy.[69] Lower doses of fluconazole (200 mg/day) is the preferred maintenance regimen. In a large randomized trial, 18% of patients receiving amphotericin relapses compared to 2% assigned fluconazole.[72] Fluconazole maintenance therapy is also superior to itraconazole for preventing relapses.[73] Another major strategy to prevent relapses is the initiation of HAART. Several small studies in patients with a history of cryptococcal meningitis have shown that maintenance therapy can be safely discontinued in patients on HAART with sustained immunologic and virologic responses (CD4 counts >100–150 cell/μL).[64,74–76]

Management of Elevated Intracranial Pressure

Elevated intracranial pressure is a common and potentially life-threatening complication of cryptococcal meningitis.[77] In contrast to the usual pathophysiology of chronic meningitis in which proinflammatory responses play an important role, cryptococcal meningitis in HIV-infected patients is notable for a lack of inflammatory cells and seems to be directly related to high fungal titers which cause

an outflow obstruction. It is postulated that capsular polysaccharide and other fungal by-products impair CSF absorption through the arachnoid microvilli.[77]

In a retrospective study of 211 HIV-infected patients with cryptococcal meningitis, 60% were found to have initial opening pressures of ≥250 mm H_2O and 30% had a pressure ≥350 mm H_2O.[60] Those with opening pressures ≥350 mm H_2O had a significantly higher fungal burden and were more likely to have papilledema, hearing loss and meningismus.[60] Interestingly, this group was less likely to have fever and night sweats, perhaps reflecting an impaired ability to mount an inflammatory response. However, clinical findings were not sensitive or specific predictors of intracranial pressure elevation, and opening pressures should be measure in all patients with cryptococcal meningitis without contraindication to a lumbar puncture. Radiologic imaging of the brain is recommended prior to lumbar puncture since space-occupying lesions (cryptococcomas) can occur.[77]

The best therapeutic intervention for elevated intracranial pressure associated with cryptococcal meningitis is drainage of the CSF. This can usually be accomplished by large volume lumbar punctures removing up to 30 cc of CSF at one time, which should be repeated daily until the intracranial normalizes. Patients who require frequent lumbar punctures or whose opening pressure is ≥400 mm H_2O may benefit from a lumbar drain. Ventriculoperitoneal shunting may be indicated for persistently elevated pressures or progressive neurologic deficits.[57] Patients with rising intracranial pressure while on treatment are at high risk of adverse outcomes and death.[60] Perhaps due to the sparse cellular infiltrate and limited host response, corticosteroids do not improve clinical outcomes in HIV-associated cryptococcal meningitis.[60]

Investigational Therapies

Voriconazole is a recently developed derivative of fluconazole with wide-spectrum antifungal activity. It is a more potent inhibitor of fungal 14α-demethylase, resulting in the depletion of ergosterol.[63] Voriconazole has greater activity against C. neoformans than either itraconazole or fluconazole, with an MIC90 <0.5 μg/mL and is also active against fluconazole resistant isolates.[78–80] Although some studies have shown increased resistance against fluconazole, itraconazole and amphotericin,[81,82] a study of 1811 clinical isolated obtained from five continents showed that resistance to antifungal agents clinically used for the treatment of C. neoformans was uncommon and susceptibility patterns have remained stable over the last 15 years.[83] Therefore, the role of the more expensive voriconazole may be limited to rare cases refractory to standard antifungal therapy.[84]

Immunomodulatory therapy has also been evaluated as an adjuvant to standard antifungal regimens. A phase I evaluation of a murine-derived anticryptococcal antibody (MAb 18B7) showed that the antibody was well tolerated and reduced serum cryptococcal antigen titers.[85] In another study, addition of recombinant IFN-γ to the standard regimen of amphotericin B and flucytosine for the treatment of cryptococcal meningitis in HIV-infected patients did not cause significant toxicity and was associated with a trend towards improved mycologic and clinical success.[86] Although these findings are conceptually interesting, such therapies are unlikely to be available soon for widespread clinical use.

Histoplasmosis

Microbiology

Histoplasma capsulatum (Fig. 34.2) is a dimorphic fungus which exists as a mold in soil and as a yeast in humans. There are two varieties of *Histoplasma* which cause disease in humans: *H. capsulatum* var. *capsulatum* and *H. capsulatum* var. *duboisii*. The former is smaller (1–4 μm) and is found in the Americas, parts of Africa, Asia, and Australia. The latter measures 10–12 μm, is found only in Africa, and is the cause of African histoplasmosis.[87]

Epidemiology and Pathogenesis

Histoplasmosis is endemic in the central and south regions of the USA.[87] The endemic area extends along the river basins north into the Canadian provinces of Quebec and Ontario and south into Mexico, Central and South America. In the southern region of the USA, the endemic area extends to Alabama in the east and southwest Texas in the west. Certain cities, most notably Indianapolis and Kansas City are high incidence areas of histoplasmosis.

HIV-infected patients often serve as sentinel markers for histoplasmosis outbreaks.[88] Prior to the advent of HAART, approximately 5% of AIDS patients developed histoplasmosis in endemic areas.[87] In hyperendemic areas, histoplasmosis was reported to be the second or third most common opportunistic infection in HIV-infected patients.[87–90]

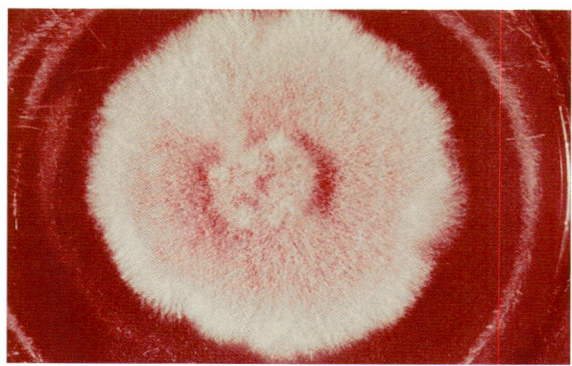

A

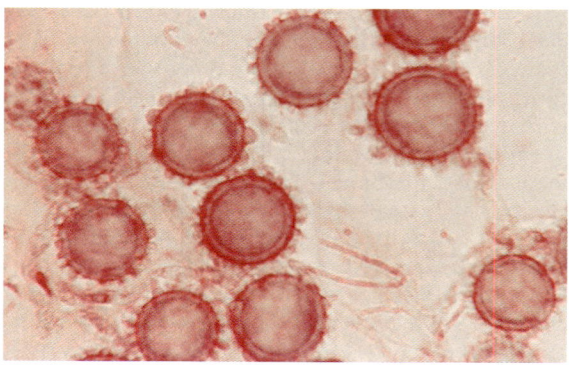

B

Figure 34.2 (A) *H. capsulatum* colonies on Saboraud's dextrose agar. (B) Microscopic appearance of *H. capsulatum* showing tuberculate chlamydospores. (Photographs courtesy of Dr William Merz, Department of Pathology, Johns Hopkins University School of Medicine.)

During an outbreak in Indianapolis, the incidence of histoplasmosis in HIV-infected individuals was 27%, and among those afflicted, histoplasmosis was the initial AIDS-defining illness in 50%.[88] The incidence of disseminated histoplasmosis has declined with the introduction of HAART.[91]

H. capsulatum prefers moderate, human climates and is found in soil and droppings from birds and bats.[92] The organism has never been cultured from birds, but it can infect bats, and rarely dogs, cats, horses, cats, swine, and a variety of rodents.[87] Certain areas, such as caves, chicken coops, bird roosts, and old buildings, are notorious for having high burdens of *H. capsulatum*, and histoplasmosis can be an occupational hazard.[87,92]

As with other systemic fungal infections, initial primary infection occurs in the lung after inhalation of arthroconidia (spores), which are rapidly converted into yeast at body temperature. The yeasts are phagocytosed by the reticuloendothelial cells in the lung. Dissemination probably occurs within the first 2 weeks of infection, prior to the onset of adaptive cell-mediated immunity. In immunocompetent individuals, the infection is often controlled by the host response and the patient may minimally symptomatic. Reactivation disease is a common form of disseminated histoplasmosis, especially in patients with defective T-cell immunity. In HIV-infected patients, histoplasmosis usually occurs when the CD4 count is ≤100 cells/µL.[93,94] In New York City, the prevalence of histoplasmosis is much higher in Hispanic men from endemic countries, and DNA fingerprinting has shown that strains originating from Panama are common in this population, underscoring the importance of reactivation disease.[87,95]

Clinical Manifestations

In contrast to immunocompetent individuals, in whom infection with *H. capsulatum* is usually self-limited, most HIV-infected patients exposed to the organism develop disseminated disease.[88] The median CD4 cell count at the time of diagnosis is 50 cells/µL.[88] Fever, weight loss, and other constitutional symptoms are present in over 95% of patients with disseminated disease.[88,90,93] Pulmonary symptoms are present in 50–60% of cases. On physical examination, approximately 30% have hepatosplenomegaly, 20% have lymphadenopathy, and 5–15% develop a rash.[88,90,93] Neurologic manifestations are reported in 10% of disseminated histoplasmosis cases.[96,97] Most patients develop a subacute meningitis, which may be basilar, one-third present with focal brain lesions.[96] Up to 18% of HIV-infected patients with disseminated histoplasmosis present with septic shock and acute respiratory distress syndrome (ARDS).[88,98] Renal insufficiency and low albumin at presentation are associated with a worse prognosis, and the mortality for patients with severe symptoms is 70%.[98] On rare occasions, histoplasmosis may present as retinitis, pericarditis, endocarditis, prostatitis, pancreatitis, adrenal insufficiency, or nephritis.[93,96,99,100] Immune reconstitution syndrome associated with histoplasmosis appears to be infrequent.[101]

Routine laboratory test results are generally nonspecific. Approximately one-third of patients present with leukopenia and anemia.[102] Occasionally, the organism can be seen on peripheral blood mononuclear cells. Liver function test abnormalities are common in HIV-infected patients, but lactate dehydrogenase (LDH) levels ≥600 may suggest histoplasmosis in patients presenting with fevers.[103] Chest radiographs are abnormal in approximately 50% of patients.[88,102,104] The most common abnormalities include diffuse interstitial or reticulonodular infiltrates. Mediastinal lymphadenopathy is evident in 20% of cases and cavitation is rare.

Diagnosis

Owing to the non-specific symptoms of disseminated histoplasmosis, the disease may be difficult to diagnose. This is especially true in non-endemic areas, where clinicians may not consider the diagnosis, or pathologists may be unaccustomed to identifying *H. capsulatum* in tissue specimens. Clinicians should remember that very transient exposures in an endemic area can lead to infection, so that a history of previous residence is not particularly useful in excluding histoplasmosis. Fortunately, there are several good rapid tests to aid in the diagnosis.

The gold standard is a positive culture of the organism from peripheral blood or tissue specimens. Blood cultures are positive in 50–70% of cases of disseminated histoplasmosis.[88,102,105] Lysis-centrifugation systems and BACTEC cultures have similar sensitivity, but the latter may take longer to become positive (10 days versus 18 days, respectively).[105] Culture of lymph nodes, liver, skin, and bronchioalveolar lavage is less sensitive, but may be useful in establishing the diagnosis. CSF cultures are positive in 65% of patients with histoplasma meningitis.[96,106]

Histopathologic examination of tissues is more rapid than culture and establishes the diagnosis in 50% of patients. The most accessible site to biopsy is the bone marrow. The organism can be identified within macrophages with methenamine silver stains or periodic acid Schiff stains. Characteristic macronidia with finger-like projections may not be observed in primary isolates, but are often detected after subculture. An experienced pathologist should review the samples since the organism may be confused with *Cryptococcus, Blastomycosis, Penicillium, Toxoplasma, Leishmania,* or *Pneumocystic jirovencii.*[92]

Serodiagnostic studies, which detect the presence of antibodies against *Histoplasma* antigens, are positive in over 80% of all patients with disseminated disease and 90% of those with pulmonary disease, but the sensitivity may decrease with profound immunosuppression.[102,107,108] However, the presence of antibody does not differentiate active from past infection and in endemic areas, over 50% of the total population may have positive serology against *Histoplasma.*[109] Furthermore, the antibody may cross-react with *Blastomycosis, Coccidiomycosis,* or *Paracoccidiomycosis* antigens.[107,110] Nonetheless, a negative antibody test in a patient with histoplasmosis is rare and should prompt further diagnostic work-up.

A rapid and sensitive test for histoplasmosis is antigen detection.[111] The urine antigen test is more sensitive than the serum antigen test for disseminated histoplasmosis (70% versus 90% sensitivity, respectively).[107] The overall specificity of the test is good, but the antigen test may cross-react with *Penicillium, Paracoccidiomycosis,* and *Blastomycosis* antigens.[112] Importantly, the test is useful in following the response to therapy.[88,113-115] Persistent antigenuria implies ongoing infection and increased titers (≥2-fold) suggest relapse and should be treated.[113]

Treatment

Untreated disseminated histoplasmosis has a mortality of 80%. Amphotericin B is the antifungal of choice for HIV-infected patients with moderate to severe disease, but treatment failure occurs in approximately 20–35% of patients.[88,116] In a randomized study of 81 HIV-infected patients with disseminated histoplasmosis, treatment with liposomal amphotericin resulted in higher success rates (88%) compared with regular amphotericin B (64%) and was associated with less toxicity.[116] However, there was no difference between the two groups in serious drug toxicity resulting in discontinuation of therapy, or in overall survival after completion of consolidation therapy. For mild disease, itraconazole therapy is successful in 85% of cases.[117,118] Fluconazole is less effective than itraconazole with 74% response rate at a dose of 800 mg per day, but relapses occur frequently and are associated with fluconazole resistance.[115,119,120] In experimental models, the new azoles posaconazole and voriconazole have good activity against *H. capsulatum*, but the role of these agents in human histoplasmosis has not been established.[121-123]

Current practice guidelines for HIV-infected patients with histoplasmosis recommend an initial 12-week intensive phase of therapy to induce remission, followed by chronic maintenance therapy to prevent relapse (Table 34.3).[124] Amphotericin B should be used for induction in hospitalized patients, and itraconazole (200 mg b.i.d.) can be used upon discharge or in ambulatory patients. Itraconazole is also effective against severe disease and is commonly used in patients who cannot tolerate amphotericin B due to renal insufficiency or other toxicities. Fluconazole (800 mg q.d.) can be used cautiously in patients who cannot tolerate itraconazole, but clinical response should be closely monitored. Patients with CNS involvement should be treated with 3–4 months of amphotericin B, followed by fluconazole (800 mg) daily, which has better blood–brain-barrier penetration than itraconazole. Liposomal amphotericin B may lead to improved outcomes in HIV-infected individuals and is recommended as primary therapy for *H. capsulatum* meningitis by some authorities.[97,116]

As with other systemic mycoses, the relapse rate in HIV-infected patients treated for histoplasmosis is high. Therefore, itraconazole maintenance therapy should be prescribed following induction therapy.[125] In an observational study of 32 patients with a history of histoplasmosis on HAART with CD4 cell counts ≥150 cell/μL, there were no relapses after discontinuation of therapy over a 2-year follow-up period, suggesting that itraconazole may be discontinued with immune restoration.[126] Primary prophylaxis with itraconazole for patients with low CD4 cell counts is not routinely recommended, but should be considered in endemic areas where the risk of histoplasmosis is >5–10/100 patient years.[124,127]

Table 34.3 Therapy for HIV-associated histoplasmosis

Phase of therapy	Severity of disease	Preferred drug	Duration of therapy
Induction	Mild	Itraconazole (200 mg b.i.d.)	12 weeks
	Moderate to severe	Amphotericin B[a] (0.7 mg/kg per day)	1–2 weeks
	Meningitis	Itraconazole (200 mg b.i.d.)	10–12 weeks
		Liposomal amphotericin B (4 mg/kg per day)	12 weeks
Maintenance		Itraconazole (200 mg q.d.)	until CD4 ≥200 for ≥6 months
Primary prophylaxis		Itraconazole (200 mg q.d.)	Consider in endemic area if CD4 ≤100

[a]Alternative: Liposomal Amphotericin B (4 mg/kg per day) or itraconazole (200 mg b.i.d.) for patients with renal insufficiency.

Coccidioidomycosis

Microbiology

Coccidioides immitis is a soil-dwelling dimorphic fungi, which is inhaled as arthroconidia (spores). The organism lives in the soil in the mycelial phase, and, when inhaled, aerosolized infections particles are inhaled into the lungs of potential hosts. Once in the alveolar space, the organism multiplies, resulting in a giant spherule (Fig. 34.3). Before the development of adaptive T-cell immunity, macrophages may ingest the organism but are unable to kill it. Dissemination of the organism can occur prior to the onset of adaptive immunity or in people with impaired cellular immune responses.

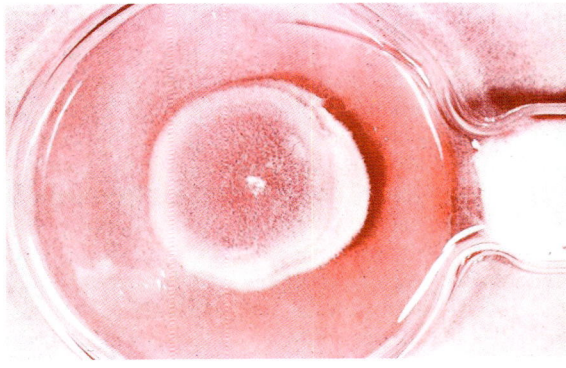

A

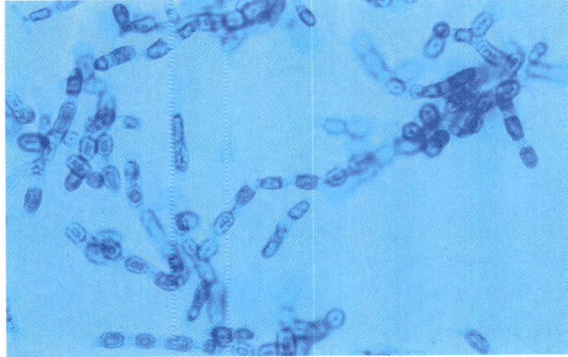

B

Figure 34.3 (A) *C. immitis* colony. (B) Arthrospores in colonies from a patient with *C. immitis* infection. (Photographs courtesy of Dr William Merz, Department of Pathology, Johns Hopkins University School of Medicine.)

Epidemiology

C. immitis is endemic in the southwestern USA, northern Mexico, and portions of Central and South America. HIV-associated coccidioidal disease is more common in these areas, but can occur in non-endemic regions, presumably due to reactivation disease.[128,129] From 1987 to 1992, 46% of coccidial cases in HIV-infected individuals occurred in non-endemic areas.[128] In endemic regions, coccidioidomycosis is an important opportunistic infection among HIV-infected patients.[130] Coincident with the rise of the HIV epidemic in Arizona, the number of reported cases of coccidioidomycosis increased significantly from 1990–1995.[131] Of all cases of coccidioidomycosis, 44% occurred in HIV-infected individuals, and 10% of hospitalized HIV-infected patients were diagnosed with coccidioidomycosis.[131] In a prospective study of 170 HIV-infected patients in Arizona, the estimated cumulative incidence of coccidioidomycosis over 41 months was 24.6%.[132] The major risk factor for developing HIV-associated coccidioidomycosis is a CD4 cell count ≤250 cells/μL.[132–136] The incidence of coccidioidal disease may be decreasing with the widespread use of HAART, but data from large epidemiologic studies is not available.[137,138]

Clinical Manifestations

Coccidioidal infection may occur in a wide variety of forms, ranging from positive serologic tests to life-threatening pneumonitis and meningitis.[133,135] Patients usually present with fevers, chills and night sweats.[135] Pulmonary involvement occurs in 66–80% of all HIV-associated cases.[133,135] The most common radiologic finding is diffuse reticulonodular infiltrates which may mimic PCP pneumonia[133,135,139] and is associated with a mortality rate of 68%.[135] Focal pulmonary disease has a better prognosis and usually occurs at higher CD4 cell counts. Histopathologically, HIV-associated pulmonary coccidioidomycosis is characterized by poor granuloma formation and high organism burden.[140]

Following pulmonary infection, *C. immitis* can disseminate to skin, bone, and CNS. Unique manifestations in HIV-infected patients include liver, intestinal, genitourinary, and extrathoracic lymph node involvement.[133] For unclear reasons, skeletal coccidioidomycosis is distinctly unusual in HIV-infected individuals. A subacute meningitis occurs in approximately 15% of HIV-infected patients with coccidioidomycosis.[135] CSF findings include hypoglycorrhachia, high protein, and a moderate

385

leukocytosis (<1500 cells/μL), which may have a polymorphonuclear predominance, or less commonly, can be eosinophilic.[141,142] Imaging studies may reveal hydrocephalus, basilar enhancement, or cerebral infarction.[143]

Diagnosis

Definitive evidence of *C. immitis* infection is obtained through direct visualization or culture of the organism from respiratory or other tissues. The organism grows easily on nearly any laboratory media, and a nucleic acid probe is available to rapidly identify *C. immitis* once isolated in culture.[144] However, the sensitivity of cultures is low, with <30% of blood culture positivity for disseminated disease, and <15% recovery from the CSF in cases of meningitis. Since *C. immitis* can be an occupational hazard and is listed by the Centers for Disease Control and Prevention (CDC) as a potential agent of bioterrorism appropriate biohazard precautions should be followed when hyphal growth becomes evident in culture and the laboratory should be notified if coccidioidomycosis is suspected. In tissue, *Coccidioides* can be easily identified by its characteristic large (20–70 μm) spherules which can be seen at ×100–400 magnification. Spherules are best identified with methenamine silver or Papanicolaou stain.

Serologic tests are commonly used to diagnose coccidioidomycosis.[145] Anti-coccidioidal antibodies are quite specific and tend to reflect active disease.[146] IgM antibodies are detectable 1 or 2 weeks after infection and persist up to 6 months. IgG antibodies appear later and persist until the infection is resolved. In patients with suspected coccidiomycosis, an immunodiffusion assay is used to screen for IgM or IgG antibodies. If the test is positive, a quantitative complement fixation test is performed to determine IgG titers. Quantitation of coccidioidal IgG titers is useful to assess prognosis and response to therapy.[145]

Complement fixation serologic tests can be performed on CSF samples, with high specificity and moderate sensitivity.[147] Asymptomatic HIV-infected patients with positive serologies have a high risk (~40%) of developing coccidioidomycosis within 2 years.[148] Serology may be negative during acute infection and has decreased sensitivity in HIV-infected patients. In fact, serology can be negative in 20–40% of HIV-infected patients with coccidioidomycosis, especially in those with diffuse pulmonary disease.[133,135,149] Therefore, a positive test can be diagnostic, but a negative test does not exclude coccidial disease. Concentration of serum can increase the sensitivity of serologic tests in HIV-infected patients with disseminated coccidioidomycosis to >90% (Pappagianis, personal communication).[150] Nucleic acid techniques can detect *C. immitis* in serum samples but are not commercially available.[151]

Treatment

In immunocompetent individuals, infection with *C. immitis* often resolves spontaneously and does not require therapy. HIV-infected patients, however, have a high risk of dissemination and should always be treated if infected with *C. immitis*.[148,152] Even with therapy (Table 34.4), coccidioidomycosis has a poor prognosis in HIV-infected patients, with a mortality rate ranging from 42% to 63%.[128,133,135] Diffuse pulmonary disease can be particularly severe and should be treated with amphotericin B (0.7 mg/kg per day) until there is significant clinical improvement.

Other manifestations of coccidioidomycosis, including focal pneumonia, disseminated disease, and meningitis, can be treated with azole antifungals. Several clinical trials have evaluated the efficacy of various azoles, but none have specifically addressed outcomes in HIV-infected patients. Fluconazole (400–800 mg q.d.) is the first-line recommended azole for the treatment of

Table 34.4 Therapy for HIV-associated coccidioidomycosis

Type of disease	Preferred drug	Duration of therapy
Diffuse pneumonia	Amphotericin B[a] (0.7 mg/kg per day)	Until clinical improvement
	Fluconazole[b] (400 mg/day)	Lifelong
Meningitis	Fluconazole (400 mg/day)	Lifelong
Other (focal pulmonary, skin, disseminated)	Fluconazole[b] (400 mg/day)	Lifelong

[a]Alternative: Liposomal amphotericin B (4 mg/kg per day). [b]Alternative: Itraconazole (400–600 mg/day). *Note*: Maintenance therapy should be continued even in patients with CD4 counts ≥200. Primary prophylaxis is controversial; consider in endemic area with CD4 count ≤100.

cocciodioidomycosis.[130] In HIV-negative individuals, the efficacy of fluconazole ranges from 55% in patients with chronic pulmonary disease to 86% in those with skeletal involvement.[153] The overall efficacy of itraconazole (200 mg b.i.d.) and ketoconazole (400 mg q.d.) is approximately 50%.[154–156] In a randomized study comparing fluconazole with itraconazole for progressive, non-meningeal cryptococcidioidomycosis, there was not a statistically significant difference between the two regimens.[157]

Fluconazole is the preferred antifungal for the treatment of coccidioidal meningitis.[60] In a study of 49 patients with coccidioidal meningitis, 79% responded to fluconazole (400 mg/day).[147] Therapy was continued for 37 months (mean) and clinical response was apparent after 4–8 months of therapy. HIV infection was present in nine of the 49 individuals and did not affect clinical outcomes. In a small study ($n = 10$), itraconazole was reported to have comparable efficacy.[158] For refractory cases, some authorities recommend intrathecal amphotericin B.[60,159] Hydrocephalus usually requires ventricular shunt placement.[60] Voriconazole is active against *C. immitis in vitro* and has been successfully used in a few cases of coccidioidal meningitis.[160]

Response to therapy should be monitored by serial coccidioidal IgG titers. Antibody levels become undetectable or very low in patients who resolve their infection. The risk of relapse after therapy for coccidioidomycosis is high even in immunocompetent patients, ranging from 20% to 39%.[153,157] Lifelong therapy is generally recommended for all patients with progressive pulmonary, disseminated, or meningeal disease.[152,161] HIV-infected patients on HAART can relapse despite immune reconstitution, and therefore discontinuation of secondary prophylaxis is not recommended even in patients with a CD4 cell count ≥250 cells/μL.[162]

Primary Fungal Prophylaxis

Three studies have evaluated the role of primary prophylactic antifungal therapy for HIV-infected patients with low CD4 counts.[127,163,164] Two studies conducted in the USA showed that fluconazole prophylaxis decreased the incidence of cryptococcosis, and itraconazole prophylaxis decreased the incidence of both cryptococcosis and histoplasmosis, especially in patients with CD4 counts ≤50 cells/μL, but there was no survival benefit.[127,163] Given the relatively low prevalence of systemic fungal infections in the USA, the widespread use of HAART, and the

risk of promoting drug resistance, routine antifungal primary prophylaxis is not routinely advocated. However, it may be considered in HIV-infected patients with CD4 cell counts ≤100 cells/μL who live in areas endemic for histoplasmosis or coccidioidomycosis.

In parts of Southeast Asia, where antiretroviral therapy may not be widely available and systemic mycoses are endemic, primary fungal prophylaxis may be warranted. A randomized-controlled trial of 127 patients in Thailand followed for 2 years showed a significant benefit of primary prophylaxis, with only 1 out of 63 (1.6%) of the patients receiving itraconazole (200 mg/day) developing a systemic fungal infection (*P. marneffei*), compared with 11/66 (16.7%) of patients receiving placebo (7/66 *Cryptococcus*, 4/66 *P. marneffei*).[164] Primary fungal prophylaxis is used in some areas of Thailand, but widespread implementation may be limited by a lack of adequate resources.

References

1. Sabetta JR, Andriole VT. Cryptococcal infection of the central nervous system. Med Clin North Am 1985; 69:333–344.
2. Wilson DE, Bennett JE, Bailey JW. Serologic grouping of Cryptococcus neoformans. Proc Soc Exp Biol Med 1968; 127:820–823.
3. Rinaldi MG, Drutz DJ, Howell A, et al. Serotypes of Cryptococcus neoformans in patients with AIDS. J Infect Dis 1986; 153:642.
4. Shimizu RY, Howard DH, Clancy MN. The variety of Cryptococcus neoformans in patients with AIDS. J Infect Dis 1986; 154:1042.
5. Speed B, Dunt D. Clinical and host differences between infections with the two varieties of Cryptococcus neoformans. Clin Infect Dis 1995; 21:28–36.
6. Swinne D, Nkurikiyinfura JB, Muyembe TL. Clinical isolates of Cryptococcus neoformans from Zaire. Eur J Clin Microbiol 1986; 5:50–51.
7. Tintelnot K, Lemmer K, Losert H, et al. Follow-up of epidemiological data of cryptococcosis in Austria, Germany and Switzerland with special focus on the characterization of clinical isolates. Mycoses 2004; 47:455–464.
8. Chuck SL, Sande MA. Infections with Cryptococcus neoformans in the acquired immunodeficiency syndrome. N Engl J Med 1989; 321:794–799.
9. Selik RM, Karon JM, Ward JW. Effect of the human immunodeficiency virus epidemic on mortality from opportunistic infections in the United States in 1993. J Infect Dis 1997; 176:632–636.
10. Dromer F, Mathoulin S, Dupont B, et al. Epidemiology of cryptococcosis in France: a 9-year survey (1985–1993). French Cryptococcosis Study Group. Clin Infect Dis 1996; 23:82–90.
11. Centers for Disease Control and Prevention (CDC). HIV/AIDS Surveillance report. Atlanta: CDC; 1991.
12. Currie BP, Casadevall A. Estimation of the prevalence of cryptococcal infection among patients infected with the human immunodeficiency virus in New York City. Clin Infect Dis 1994; 19:1029–1033.
13. Clark RA, Greer D, Atkinson W, et al. Spectrum of Cryptococcus neoformans infection in 68 patients infected

with human immunodeficiency virus. Rev Infect Dis 1990; 12:768–777.

14. Dismukes WE. Cryptococcal meningitis in patients with AIDS. J Infect Dis 1988; 157:624–628.

15. Eng RH, Bishburg E, Smith SM, et al. Cryptococcal infections in patients with acquired immune deficiency syndrome. Am J Med 1986; 81:19–23.

16. Kovacs JA, Kovacs AA, Polis M, et al. Cryptococcosis in the acquired immunodeficiency syndrome. Ann Intern Med 1985; 103:533–538.

17. Zuger A, Louie E, Holzman RS, et al. Cryptococcal disease in patients with the acquired immunodeficiency syndrome. Diagnostic features and outcome of treatment. Ann Intern Med 1986; 104:234–240.

18. Sacktor N, Lyles RH, Skolasky R, et al. HIV-associated neurologic disease incidence changes:: Multicenter AIDS Cohort Study, 1990–1998. Neurology 2001; 56:257–260.

19. Hajjeh RA, Conn LA, Stephens DS, et al. Cryptococcosis: population-based multistate active surveillance and risk factors in human immunodeficiency virus-infected persons. Cryptococcal Act Surveillance Group J Infect Dis 1999; 179:449–454.

20. Mirza SA, Phelan M, Rimland D, et al. The changing epidemiology of cryptococcosis: an update from population-based active surveillance in 2 large metropolitan areas, 1992–2000. Clin Infect Dis 2003; 36:789–794.

21. Kaplan JE, Hanson D, Dworkin MS, et al. Epidemiology of human immunodeficiency virus-associated opportunistic infections in the United States in the era of highly active antiretroviral therapy. Clin Infect Dis 2000; 30(Suppl):5–14.

22. Dromer F, Mathoulin-Pelissier S, Fontanet A, et al. Epidemiology of HIV-associated cryptococcosis in France (1985–2001): comparison of the pre- and post-HAART eras. AIDS 2004; 18:555–562.

23. Adeyemi OM, Pulvirenti J, Perumal S, et al. Cryptococcosis in HIV-infected individuals. AIDS 2004; 18:2218–2219.

24. Tansuphasawadikul S, Amornkul PN, Tanchanpong C, et al. Clinical presentation of hospitalized adult patients with HIV infection and AIDS in Bangkok, Thailand. J Acquir Immune Defic Syndr 1999; 21:326–332.

25. Hakim JG, Gangaidzo IT, Heyderman RS, et al. Impact of HIV infection on meningitis in Harare, Zimbabwe: a prospective study of 406 predominantly adult patients. AIDS 2000; 14:1401–1407.

26. Bogaerts J, Rouvroy D, Taelman H, et al. AIDS-associated cryptococcal meningitis in Rwanda (1983–1992): epidemiologic and diagnostic features. J Infect 1999; 39:32–37.

27. Corbett EL, Churchyard GJ, Charalambos S, et al. Morbidity and mortality in South African gold miners: impact of untreated disease due to human immunodeficiency virus. Clin Infect Dis 2002; 34:1251–1258.

28. Moosa MY, Coovadia YM. Cryptococcal meningitis in Durban, South Africa: a comparison of clinical features, laboratory findings, and outcome for human immunodeficiency virus (HIV)-positive and HIV-negative patients. Clin Infect Dis 1997; 24:131–134.

29. Mwaba P, Mwansa J, Chintu C, et al. Clinical presentation, natural history, and cumulative death rates of 230 adults with primary cryptococcal meningitis in Zambian AIDS patients treated under local conditions. Postgrad Med J 2001; 77:769–773.

30. Kambugu AKM, Mayanja-Kizza H, O'Brien M, et al. The high mortality of HIV associated Cryptococcal meningitis despite high dose amphotericin B therapy in Uganda. 41st Annual Meeting of IDSA, San Diego: 9–12 October 2003.

31. Horst CM van der, Saag MS, Cloud GA, et al. Treatment of cryptococcal meningitis associated with the acquired immunodeficiency syndrome. National Institute of Allergy and Infectious Diseases Mycoses Study Group and AIDS Clinical Trials Group. N Engl J Med 1997; 337:15–21.

32. French N, Gray K, Watera C, et al. Cryptococcal infection in a cohort of HIV-1-infected Ugandan adults. AIDS 2002; 16:1031–1038.

33. Larsen RA, Bozzette S, McCutchan JA, et al. Persistent Cryptococcus neoformans infection of the prostate after successful treatment of meningitis. Calif Collab Treat Group Ann Intern Med 1989; 111:125–128.

34. Manfredi R, Calza L, Chiodo F. AIDS-associated Cryptococcus infection before and after the highly active antiretroviral therapy era: emerging management problems. Int J Antimicrob Agents 2003; 22:449–452.

35. Lortholary O, Fontanet A, Memain N, et al. Incidence and risk factors of immune reconstitution inflammatory syndrome complicating HIV-associated cryptococcosis in France. AIDS 2005; 19:1043–1049.

36. Shelburne SA, Visnegarwala F, Darcourt J, et al. Incidence and risk factors for immune reconstitution inflammatory syndrome during highly active antiretroviral therapy. AIDS 2005; 19:399–406.

37. Woods ML. 2nd, MacGinley R, Eisen DP and Allworth AM. HIV combination therapy: partial immune restitution unmasking latent cryptococcal infection. AIDS 1998; 12:1491–1494.

38. Breton G, Seilhean D, Cherin P, et al. Paradoxical intracranial cryptococcoma in a human immunodeficiency virus-infected man being treated with combination antiretroviral therapy. Am J Med 2002; 113:155–157.

39. Blanche P, Gombert B, Ginsburg C, et al. HIV combination therapy: immune restitution causing cryptococcal lymphadenitis dramatically improved by anti-inflammatory therapy. Scand J Infect Dis 1998; 30:615–616.

40. Trevenzoli M, Cattelan AM, Rea F, et al. Mediastinitis due to cryptococcal infection: a new clinical entity in the HAART era. J Infect 2002; 45:173–179.

41. King MD, Perlino CA, Cinnamon J, et al. Paradoxical recurrent meningitis following therapy of cryptococcal meningitis: an immune reconstitution syndrome after initiation of highly active antiretroviral therapy. Int J STD AIDS 2002; 13:724–726.

42. Cattelan AM, Trevenzoli M, Sasset L, et al. Multiple cerebral cryptococcomas associated with immune reconstitution in HIV-1 infection. AIDS 2004; 18:349–351.

43. Boelaert JR, Goddeeris KH, Vanopdenbosch LJ, et al. Relapsing meningitis caused by persistent cryptococcal antigens and immune reconstitution after the initiation of highly active antiretroviral therapy. AIDS 2004; 18:1223–1224.

44. Sanchez-Portocarrero J, Perez-Cecilia E. Intracerebral mass lesions in patients with human immunodeficiency virus infection and cryptococcal meningitis. Diagn Microbiol Infect Dis 1997; 29:193–198.

45. Popovich MJ, Arthur RH, Helmer E. CT of intracranial cryptococcosis. AJR Am J Roentgenol 1990; 154:603–606.

46. Darras-Joly C, Chevret S, Wolff M, et al. Cryptococcus neoformans infection in France: epidemiologic features of and early prognostic parameters for 76 patients who were infected with human immunodeficiency virus. Clin Infect Dis 1996; 23:369–376.

47. Garlipp CR, Rossi CL, Bottini PV. Cerebrospinal fluid profiles in acquired immunodeficiency syndrome with and without neurocryptococcosis. Rev Inst Med Trop Sao Paulo 1997; 39:323–325.

48. Saag MS, Powderly WG, Cloud GA, et al. Comparison of amphotericin B with fluconazole in the treatment of acute AIDS-associated cryptococcal meningitis. The NIAID Mycoses Study Group and the AIDS Clinical Trials Group. N Engl J Med 1992; 326:83–89.

49. Tanner DC, Weinstein MP, Fedorciw B, et al. Comparison of commercial kits for detection of cryptococcal antigen. J Clin Microbiol 1994; 32:1680–1684.

50. Hamilton JR, Noble A, Denning DW, et al. Performance of cryptococcus antigen latex agglutination kits on serum and cerebrospinal fluid specimens of AIDS patients before and after pronase treatment. J Clin Microbiol 1991; 29:333–339.

51. Chanock SJ, Toltzis P, Wilson C. Cross-reactivity between Stomatococcus mucilaginosus and latex agglutination for cryptococcal antigen. Lancet 1993; 342:1119–1120.

52. Westerink MA, Amsterdam D, Petell RJ, et al. Septicemia due to DF-2. Cause of a false-positive cryptococcal latex agglutination result. Am J Med 1987; 83:155–158.

53. McManus EJ, Jones JM. Detection of a Trichosporon beigelii antigen cross-reactive with Cryptococcus neoformans capsular polysaccharide in serum from a patient with disseminated Trichosporon infection. J Clin Microbiol 1985; 21:681–685.

54. Asawavichienjinda T, Sitthi-Amorn C, Tanyanont V. Serum cryptococcal antigen: diagnostic value in the diagnosis of AIDS-related cryptococcal meningitis. J Med Assoc Thai 1999; 82:65–71.

55. Powderly WG, Cloud GA, Dismukes WE, et al. Measurement of cryptococcal antigen in serum and cerebrospinal fluid: value in the management of AIDS-associated cryptococcal meningitis. Clin Infect Dis 1994; 18:789–792.

56. Aberg JA, Watson J, Segal M, et al. Clinical utility of monitoring serum cryptococcal antigen (sCRAG) titers in patients with AIDS-related cryptococcal disease. HIV Clin Trials 2000; 1 1–6.

57. Saag MS, Graybill RJ, Larsen RA, et al. Practice guidelines for the management of cryptococcal disease. Infectious Diseases Society of America. Clin Infect Dis 2000; 30:710–718.

58. Ker CC, Hung CC, Huang SY, et al. Comparison of bone marrow studies with blood culture for etiological diagnosis of disseminated mycobacterial and fungal infection in patients with acquired immunodeficiency syndrome. J Microbiol Immunol Infect 2002; 35:89–93.

59. Meyohas MC, Roux P, Bollens D, et al. Pulmonary cryptococcosis: localized and disseminated infections in 27 patients with AIDS. Clin Infect Dis 1995; 21:628–633.

60. Graybill JR, Sobel J, Saag M, et al. Diagnosis and management of increased intracranial pressure in patients with AIDS and cryptococcal meningitis. The NIAID Mycoses Study Group and AIDS Cooperative Treatment Groups. Clin Infect Dis 2000; 30:47–54.

61. Leenders AC, Reiss P, Portegies P, et al. Liposomal amphotericin B (AmBisome) compared with amphotericin B both followed by oral fluconazole in the treatment of AIDS-associated cryptococcal meningitis. AIDS 1997; 11:1463–1471.

62. Coker RJ, Viviani M, Gazzard BG, et al. Treatment of cryptococcosis with liposomal amphotericin B (AmBisome) in 23 patients with AIDS. AIDS 1993; 7:829–835.

63. Pearson MM, Rogers PD, Cleary JD, et al. Voriconazole: a new triazole antifungal agent. Ann Pharmacother 2003; 37:420–432.

64. CDC. Guidelines for preventing opportunistic infections among HIV-infected persons–2002. Recommendations of the U.S. Public Health Service and the Infectious Diseases Society of America. MMWR 2002; 14:1–52.

65. Larsen RA, Leal MA, Chan LS. Fluconazole compared with amphotericin B plus flucytosine for cryptococcal meningitis in AIDS. A randomized trial. Ann Intern Med 1990; 113:183–187.

66. Gans J de, Portegies P, Tiessens G, et al. Itraconazole compared with amphotericin B plus flucytosine in AIDS patients with cryptococcal meningitis. AIDS 1992; 6:185–190.

67. Brouwer AE, Rajanuwong A, Chierakul W, et al. Combination antifungal therapies for HIV-associated cryptococcal meningitis: a randomised trial. Lancet 2004; 363:1764–1767.

68. Polsky B, Depman MR, Gold JW, et al. Intraventricular therapy of cryptococcal meningitis via a subcutaneous reservoir. Am J Med 1986; 81:24–28.

69. Bozzette SA, Larsen RA, Chiu J, et al. A placebo-controlled trial of maintenance therapy with fluconazole after treatment of cryptococcal meningitis in the acquired immunodeficiency syndrome. Calif Collab Treat Group. N Engl J Med 1991; 324:580–584.

70. Spitzer ED, Spitzer SG, Freundlich LF, et al. Persistence of initial infection in recurrent Cryptococcus neoformans meningitis. Lancet 1993; 341:595–596.

71. Brandt ME, Pfaller MA, Hajjeh RA, et al. Molecular subtypes and antifungal susceptibilities of serial Cryptococcus neoformans isolates in human immunodeficiency virus-associated Cryptococcosis. Cryptococcal Dis Act Surveillance Group J Infect Dis 1996; 174:812–820.

72. Powderly WG, Saag MS, Cloud GA, et al. A controlled trial of fluconazole or amphotericin B to prevent relapse of cryptococcal meningitis in patients with the acquired immunodeficiency syndrome. The NIAID AIDS Clinical Trials Group and Mycoses Study Group. N Engl J Med 1992; 326:793–798.

73. Saag MS, Cloud GA, Graybill JR, et al. A comparison of itraconazole versus fluconazole as maintenance therapy for AIDS-associated cryptococcal meningitis. National Institute of Allergy and Infectious Diseases Mycoses Study Group. Clin Infect Dis 1999; 28:291–296.

74. Vibhagool A, Sungkanuparph S, Mootsikapun P, et al. Discontinuation of secondary prophylaxis for cryptococcal meningitis in human immunodeficiency virus-infected patients treated with highly active antiretroviral therapy: a prospective, multicenter, randomized study. Clin Infect Dis 2003; 36:1329–1331.

75. Mussini C, Pezzotti P, Miro JM, et al. Discontinuation of maintenance therapy for cryptococcal meningitis in patients with AIDS treated with highly active antiretroviral therapy: an international observational study. Clin Infect Dis 2004; 38:565–571.

76. Aberg JA, Price RW, Heeren DM, et al. A pilot study of the discontinuation of antifungal therapy for disseminated cryptococcal disease in patients with acquired immunodeficiency syndrome, following immunologic response to antiretroviral therapy. J Infect Dis 2002; 185:1179–1182.

77. Denning DW, Armstrong RW, Lewis BH, et al. Elevated cerebrospinal fluid pressures in patients with cryptococcal meningitis and acquired immunodeficiency syndrome. Am J Med 1991; 91:267–272.

78. Espinel-Ingroff A. In vitro activity of the new triazole voriconazole (UK-109,496) against opportunistic filamentous and dimorphic fungi and common and emerging yeast pathogens. J Clin Microbiol 1998; 36:198–202.

79. Duin D van, Cleare W, Zaragoza O, et al. Effects of voriconazole on Cryptococcus neoformans. Antimicrob Agents Chemother 2004; 48:2014–2020.

80. Pfaller MA, Zhang J, Messer SA, et al. In vitro activities of voriconazole, fluconazole, and itraconazole against 566 clinical isolates of Cryptococcus neoformans from the United States and Africa. Antimicrob Agents Chemother 1999; 43:169–171.

81. Datta K, Jain N, Sethi S, et al. Fluconazole and itraconazole susceptibility of clinical isolates of Cryptococcus neoformans at a tertiary care centre in India: a need for care. J Antimicrob Chemother 2003; 52:683–686.

82. Hsueh PR, Lau YJ, Chuang YC, et al. Antifungal susceptibilities of clinical isolates of Candida species, Cryptococcus neoformans, and Aspergillus species from Taiwan: surveillance of multicenter antimicrobial resistance in Taiwan program data from 2003. Antimicrob Agents Chemother 2005; 49:512–517.

83. Pfaller MA, Messer SA, Boyken L, et al. Global trends in the antifungal susceptibility of Cryptococcus neoformans (1990 to 2004). J Clin Microbiol 2005; 43:2163–2167.

84. Perfect JR, Marr KA, Walsh TJ, et al. Voriconazole treatment for less-common, emerging, or refractory fungal infections. Clin Infect Dis 2003; 36:1122–1131.

85. Larsen RA, Pappas PG, Perfect J, et al. Phase I evaluation of the safety and pharmacokinetics of murine-derived anticryptococcal antibody 18B7 in subjects with treated cryptococcal meningitis. Antimicrob Agents Chemother 2005; 49:952–958.

86. Pappas PG, Bustamante B, Ticona E, et al. Recombinant interferon- gamma 1b as adjunctive therapy for AIDS-

related acute cryptococcal meningitis. J Infect Dis 2004; 189:2185–2191.

87. Cano MV, Hajjeh RA. The epidemiology of histoplasmosis: a review. Semin Respir Infect 2001; 16:109–118.

88. Wheat LJ, Connolly-Stringfield PA, Baker RL, et al. Disseminated histoplasmosis in the acquired immune deficiency syndrome: clinical findings, diagnosis and treatment, and review of the literature. Medicine (Baltimore) 1990; 69:361–374.

89. Graybill JR. Histoplasmosis and AIDS. J Infect Dis 1988; 158:623–626.

90. Sarosi GA, Johnson PC. Disseminated histoplasmosis in patients infected with human immunodeficiency virus. Clin Infect Dis 1992; 14(Suppl):60–67.

91. Jones JL, Hanson DL, Dworkin MS, et al. Trends in AIDS-related opportunistic infections among men who have sex with men and among injecting drug users, 1991–1996. J Infect Dis 1998; 178:114–120.

92. Wheat LJ, Kauffman CA. Histoplasmosis. Infect Dis Clin North Am 2003; 17:1–19.

93. Gutierrez ME, Canton A, Sosa N, et al. Disseminated histoplasmosis in patients with AIDS in Panama: a review of 104 cases. Clin Infect Dis 2005; 40:1199–1202.

94. Hajjeh RA. Disseminated histoplasmosis in persons infected with human immunodeficiency virus. Clin Infect Dis 1995; 21(Suppl):108–110.

95. Keath EJ, Kobayashi GS, Medoff G. Typing of Histoplasma capsulatum by restriction fragment length polymorphisms in a nuclear gene. J Clin Microbiol 1992; 30:2104–2107.

96. Wheat LJ, Batteiger BE, Sathapatayavongs B. Histoplasma capsulatum infections of the central nervous system. A clinical review. Medicine (Baltimore) 1990; 69:244–260.

97. Wheat LJ, Musial CE, Jenny-Avital E. Diagnosis and management of central nervous system histoplasmosis. Clin Infect Dis 2005; 40:844–852.

98. Wheat LJ, Chetchotisakd P, Williams B, et al. Factors associated with severe manifestations of histoplasmosis in AIDS. Clin Infect Dis 2000; 30:877–881.

99. Goodwin RA Jr., Shapiro JL, Thurman GH, et al. Disseminated histoplasmosis: clinical and pathologic correlations. Medicine (Baltimore) 1980; 59:1–33.

100. Burke DG, Emancipator SN, Smith MC, et al. Histoplasmosis and kidney disease in patients with AIDS. Clin Infect Dis 1997; 25:281–284.

101. Thompson GR 3rd, LaValle CE, 3rd, Everett ED. Unusual manifestations of histoplasmosis. Diagn Microbiol Infect Dis 2004; 50:33–41.

102. Sathapatayavongs B, Batteiger BE, Wheat J, et al. Clinical and laboratory features of disseminated histoplasmosis during two large urban outbreaks. Medicine (Baltimore) 1983; 62:263–270.

103. Corcoran GR, Al-Abdely H, Flanders CD, et al. Markedly elevated serum lactate dehydrogenase levels are a clue to the diagnosis of disseminated histoplasmosis in patients with AIDS. Clin Infect Dis 1997; 24:942–944.

104. Conces DJ Jr, Stockberger SM, Tarver RD. Disseminated histoplasmosis in AIDS: findings on chest radiographs. Am J Roentgenol 1993; 160:15–19.

105. Fuller DD, Davis TE Jr, Denys GA, et al. Evaluation of BACTEC MYCO/F Lytic medium for recovery of mycobacteria, fungi, and bacteria from blood. J Clin Microbiol 2001; 39:2933–2936.

106. Wheat J, French M, Batteiger B, et al. Cerebrospinal fluid Histoplasma antibodies in central nervous system histoplasmosis. Arch Intern Med 1985; 145:1237–1240.

107. Wheat LJ. Laboratory diagnosis of histoplasmosis: update 2000. Semin Respir Infect 2001; 16:131–140.

108. Wheat LJ, Kohler RB, Tewari RP, et al. Significance of Histoplasma antigen in the cerebrospinal fluid of patients with meningitis. Arch Intern Med 1989; 149:302–304.

109. Diercks FH, Kelly HB Jr, Klite PD, et al. Prevalence of histoplasmin sensitivity among school children in Panama City, Republic of Panama, 1962–1963. Arch Med Panamenos 1965; 14:53–59.

110. Wheat J, French ML, Kohler RB, et al. The diagnostic laboratory tests for histoplasmosis: analysis of experience in a large urban outbreak. Ann Intern Med 1982; 97:680–685.

111. Wheat LJ, Kohler RB, Tewari RP. Diagnosis of disseminated histoplasmosis by detection of Histoplasma capsulatum antigen in serum and urine specimens. N Engl J Med 1986; 314:83–88.

112. Wheat J, Wheat H, Connolly P, et al. Cross-reactivity in Histoplasma capsulatum variety capsulatum antigen assays of urine samples from patients with endemic mycoses. Clin Infect Dis 1997; 24:1169–1171.

113. Wheat LJ, Connolly-Stringfield P, Kohler RB, et al. Histoplasma capsulatum polysaccharide antigen detection in diagnosis and management of disseminated histoplasmosis in patients with acquired immunodeficiency syndrome. Am J Med 1989; 87:396–400.

114. Wheat LJ, Connolly-Stringfield P, Blair R, et al. Effect of successful treatment with amphotericin B on Histoplasma capsulatum variety capsulatum polysaccharide antigen levels in patients with AIDS and histoplasmosis. Am J Med 1992; 92:153–160.

115. Wheat LJ, Connolly P, Haddad N, et al. Antigen clearance during treatment of disseminated histoplasmosis with itraconazole versus fluconazole in patients with AIDS. Antimicrob Agents Chemother 2002; 46:248–250.

116. Johnson PC, Wheat LJ, Cloud GA, et al. Safety and efficacy of liposomal amphotericin B compared with conventional amphotericin B for induction therapy of histoplasmosis in patients with AIDS. Ann Intern Med 2002; 137:105–109.

117. Wheat J, Hafner R, Korzun AH, et al. Itraconazole treatment of disseminated histoplasmosis in patients with the acquired immunodeficiency syndrome. AIDS Clin Trial Group Am J Med 1995; 98:336–342.

118. Wheat LJ, Cloud G, Johnson PC, et al. Clearance of fungal burden during treatment of disseminated histoplasmosis with liposomal amphotericin B versus itraconazole. Antimicrob Agents Chemother 2001; 45:2354–2357.

119. Wheat J, MaWhinney S, Hafner R, et al. Treatment of histoplasmosis with fluconazole in patients with acquired immunodeficiency syndrome. National Institute of Allergy and Infectious Diseases Acquired Immunodeficiency Syndrome Clinical Trials Group and Mycoses Study Group. Am J Med 1997; 103:223–232.

120. Wheat LJ, Connolly P, Smedema M, et al. Emergence of resistance to fluconazole as a cause of failure during treatment of histoplasmosis in patients with acquired immunodeficiency disease syndrome. Clin Infect Dis 2001; 33:1910–1913.

121. Connolly P, Wheat LJ, Schnizlein-Bick C, et al. Comparison of a new triazole, posaconazole, with itraconazole and amphotericin B for treatment of histoplasmosis following pulmonary challenge in immunocompromised mice. Antimicrob Agents Chemother 2000; 44:2604–2608.

122. Connolly P, Wheat J, Schnizlein-Bick C, et al. Comparison of a new triazole antifungal agent, Schering 56592, with itraconazole and amphotericin B for treatment of histoplasmosis in immunocompetent mice. Antimicrob Agents Chemother 1999; 43:322–328.

123. Li RK, Ciblak MA, Nordoff N, et al. In vitro activities of voriconazole, itraconazole, and amphotericin B against Blastomyces dermatitidis, Coccidioides immitis, and Histoplasma capsulatum. Antimicrob Agents Chemother 2000; 44:1734–1736.

124. Wheat J, Sarosi G, McKinsey D, et al. Practice guidelines for the management of patients with histoplasmosis. Infectious Diseases Society of America. Clin Infect Dis 2000; 30:688–695.

125. Wheat J, Hafner R, Wulfsohn M, et al. Prevention of relapse of histoplasmosis with itraconazole in patients with the acquired immunodeficiency syndrome. Ann Intern Med 1993; 118:610–616.

126. Goldman M, Zackin R, Fichtenbaum CJ, et al. Safety of discontinuation of maintenance therapy for disseminated

histoplasmosis after immunologic response to antiretroviral therapy. Clin Infect Dis 2004; 38:1485–1489.

127. McKinsey DS, Wheat LJ, Cloud GA, et al. Itraconazole prophylaxis for fungal infections in patients with advanced human immunodeficiency virus infection: randomized, placebo-controlled, double-blind study. National Institute of Allergy and Infectious Diseases Mycoses Study Group. Clin Infect Dis 1999; 28:1049–1056.

128. Jones JL, Fleming PL, Ciesielski CA, et al. Coccidioidomycosis among persons with AIDS in the United States J Infect Dis 1995; 171:961–966.

129. Hernandez JL, Echevarria S, Garcia-Valtuille A, et al. Atypical coccidioidomycosis in an AIDS patient successfully treated with fluconazole. Eur J Clin Microbiol Infect Dis 1997; 16:592–594.

130. Galgiani JN, Ampel NM. Coccidioidomycosis in human immunodeficiency virus-infected patients. J Infect Dis 1990; 162:1165–1169.

131. CDC. Coccidioidomycosis – Arizona, 1990–1995. MMWR 1996; 45:1069–1073.

132. Ampel NM, Dols CL, Galgiani JN. Coccidioidomycosis during human immunodeficiency virus infection: results of a prospective study in a coccidioidal endemic area. Am J Med 1993; 94:235–240.

133. Fish DG, Ampel NM, Galgiani JN, et al. Coccidioidomycosis during human immunodeficiency virus infection. A review of 77 patients. Medicine (Baltimore) 1990; 69:384–391.

134. Ampel NM. Delayed-type hypersensitivity, in vitro T-cell responsiveness and risk of active coccidioidomycosis among HIV-infected patients living in the coccidioidal endemic area. Med Mycol 1999; 37:245–250.

135. Singh VR, Smith DK, Lawerence J, et al. Coccidioidomycosis in patients infected with human immunodeficiency virus: review of 91 cases at a single institution. Clin Infect Dis 1996; 23:563–568.

136. McKinsey DS, Spiegel RA, Hutwagner L, et al. Prospective study of histoplasmosis in patients infected with human immunodeficiency virus: incidence, risk factors, and pathophysiology. Clin Infect Dis 1997; 24:1195–1203.

137. Woods CW, McRill C, Plikaytis BD, et al. Coccidioidomycosis in human immunodeficiency virus-infected persons in Arizona, 1994–1997: incidence, risk factors, and prevention. J Infect Dis 2000; 181:1428–1434.

138. Ampel NM. Coccidioidomycosis among persons with human immunodeficiency virus infection in the era of highly active antiretroviral therapy (HAART). Semin Respir Infect 2001; 16:257–262.

139. Bronnimann DA, Adam RD, Galgiani JN, et al. Coccidioidomycosis in the acquired immunodeficiency syndrome. Ann Intern Med 1987; 106:372–379.

140. Graham AR, Sobonya RE, Bronnimann DA, et al. Quantitative pathology of coccidioidomycosis in acquired immunodeficiency syndrome. Hum Pathol 1988; 19:800–806.

141. Ismail Y, Arsura EL. Eosinophilic meningitis associated with coccidioidomycosis. West J Med 1993; 158:300–301.

142. Lo Re V. 3rd, Gluckman SJ. Eosinophilic meningitis. Am J Med 2003; 114:217–223.

143. Arsura EL, Johnson R, Penrose J, et al. Neuroimaging as a guide to predict outcomes for patients with coccidioidal meningitis. Clin Infect Dis 2005; 40:624–627.

144. Sandhu GS, Kine BC, Stockman L, et al. Molecular probes for diagnosis of fungal infections. J Clin Microbiol 1995; 33:2913–2919.

145. Pappagianis D. Serologic studies in coccidioidomycosis. Semin Respir Infect 2001; 16:242–250.

146. Pappagianis D, Zimmer BL. Serology of coccidioidomycosis. Clin Microbiol Rev 1990; 3:247–268.

147. Galgiani JN, Catanzaro A, Cloud GA, et al. Fluconazole therapy for coccidioidal meningitis. The NIAID-Mycoses Study Group. Ann Intern Med 1993; 119:28–35.

148. Sobonya RE, Barbee RA, Wiens J, et al. Detection of fungi and other pathogens in immunocompromised patients by bronchoalveolar lavage in an area endemic for coccidioidomycosis. Chest 1990; 97:1349–1355.

149. Antoniskis D, Larsen RA, Akil B, et al. Seronegative disseminated coccidioidomycosis in patients with HIV infection. AIDS 1990; 4:691–693.

150. Wolf JE, Little JR, Pappagianis D, et al. Disseminated coccidioidomycosis in a patient with the acquired immune deficiency syndrome. Diagn Microbiol Infect Dis 1986; 5:331–336.

151. Johnson SM, Simmons KA, Pappagianis D. Amplification of coccidioidal DNA in clinical specimens by PCR. J Clin Microbiol 2004; 42:1982–1985.

152. Galgiani JN, Ampel NM, Catanzaro A, et al. Practice guideline for the treatment of coccidioidomycosis. Infectious Diseases Society of America. Clin Infect Dis 2000; 30:658–661.

153. Catanzaro A, Galgiani JN, Levine BE, et al. Fluconazole in the treatment of chronic pulmonary and nonmeningeal disseminated coccidioidomycosis. NIAID Mycoses Study Group Am J Med 1995; 98:249–256.

154. Diaz M, Puente R, Hoyos LA de, et al. Itraconazole in the treatment of coccidioidomycosis. Chest 1991; 100:682–684.

155. Graybill JR, Stevens DA, Galgiani JN, et al. Itraconazole treatment of coccidioidomycosis. NAIAD Mycoses Study Group. Am J Med 1990; 89:282–290.

156. Brass C, Galgiani JN, Campbell SC, et al. Therapy of disseminated or pulmonary coccidioidomycosis with ketoconazole. Rev Infect Dis 1980; 2:656–660.

157. Galgiani JN, Catanzaro A, Cloud GA, et al. Comparison of oral fluconazole and itraconazole for progressive, nonmeningeal coccidioidomycosis. A randomized, double-blind trial. Mycoses Study Group Ann Intern Med 2000; 133:676–686.

158. Tucker RM, Denning DW, Dupont B, et al. Itraconazole therapy for chronic coccidioidal meningitis. Ann Intern Med 1990; 112:108–112.

159. Chiller TM, Galgiani JN, Stevens DA. Coccidioidomycosis. Infect Dis Clin North Am 2003; 17:41–57.

160. Proia LA, Tenorio AR. Successful use of voriconazole for treatment of Coccidioides meningitis. Antimicrob Agents Chemother 2004; 48:2341.

161. Dewsnup DH, Galgiani JN, Graybill JR, et al. Is it ever safe to stop azole therapy for Coccidioides immitis meningitis? Ann Intern Med 1996; 124:305–310.

162. Mathew G, Smedema M, Wheat LJ, et al. Relapse of coccidioidomycosis despite immune reconstitution after fluconazole secondary prophylaxis in a patient with AIDS. Mycoses 2003; 46:42–44.

163. Powderly WG, Finkelstein D, Feinberg J, et al. A randomized trial comparing fluconazole with clotrimazole troches for the prevention of fungal infections in patients with advanced human immunodeficiency virus infection. NIAID AIDS Clin Trials Group. N Engl J Med 1995; 332:700–705.

164. Chariyalertsak S, Supparatpinyo K, Sirisanthana T, et al. A controlled trial of itraconazole as primary prophylaxis for systemic fungal infections in patients with advanced human immunodeficiency virus infection in Thailand. Clin Infect Dis 2002; 34:277–284.

CHAPTER 35

Infection due to
Penicillium marneffei

Khuanchai Supparatpinyo
Thira Sirisanthana

Introduction

Penicillium marneffei infection is one of the most common opportunistic infection in persons with late human immunodeficiency virus (HIV) infection in southeast Asia, northeastern India, southern China, Hong Kong, and Taiwan. In northern Thailand, it is one of the four most common opportunistic infections which include tuberculosis, cryptococcal infection, and pneumocystic pneumonia.[1] Cases have also been reported in HIV-infected patients from the USA, Europe, Japan, and Australia following visits to the endemic area.[2] Diagnosis depends on familiarity with the clinical syndrome and a high index of suspicion. As in other systemic fungal infections, confirmation of the diagnosis requires demonstration of the fungus in the infected organ and culturing the organism from clinical specimens. The response to antifungal treatment is good if the treatment is started early. After the initial treatment, the patients need prolonged suppressive therapy to prevent relapse.

History

P. marneffei was first isolated from a bamboo rat in Vietnam in 1956.[2] The first naturally infected case was an American missionary with Hodgkin's disease who had been living in southeast Asia. The second reported case was in 1984 and was also from the USA. He had recurrent episodes of hemoptysis, thought to be caused by bronchiectasis. A pneumonectomy revealed granuloma. Tissue sections showed yeast cells of *P. marneffei*, and the culture grew the fungus. Also in 1984, five cases were reported from Thailand. In 1985, the first eight Chinese cases were reported from the Guangxi province of China that had occurred between 1964 and 1983. Additional cases were subsequently reported from southern China and Hong Kong. All cases had occurred prior to the AIDS epidemic in southeast Asia and China. The first case of *P. marneffei* infection in an HIV-infected native of southeast Asia was reported in 1989 from Bangkok, coinciding with the beginning of the AIDS epidemic in the region. The number of cases had markedly increased since then. At one tertiary hospital in Chiang Mai, northern Thailand, a total of 1180 patients with *P. marneffei* infection were seen between January 1991 and December 1997; almost all of these patients were also infected with HIV. Between 1991 and 2004, more than 6000 cases of *P. marneffei* infection in HIV-infected patients were reported to the Thai Ministry of Public Health. The prevalence of *P. marneffei* infection had also increased in other countries in the region as the HIV/AIDS epidemic spread. In a period of 5 months, 12 cases were diagnosed in one hospital in Ho Chi Minh City, Vietnam, among the 273 HIV-infected patients studied.[3] Of the 198 HIV-infected patients who attended one hospital in Manipur, northeastern India, during a 19-month period, 46 had *P. marneffei* infection.[4] Additional cases were reported from Hong Kong, Taiwan, Malaysia, Cambodia, and the provinces of Guangxi and Guangdong of China.

Mycology

Infection caused by *Penicillium* spp. due to species other than *P. marneffei* is rare. Only about 30 cases have been reported in the literature.[5] Whereas the other *Penicillium* spp. grow as monomorphic moulds bearing typical asexual propagules (conidia), *P. marneffei* is thermally dimorphic. It was originally classified among *Penicillium* species in the section Asymmetrica, subsection Divaricata in Raper and Thom's taxonomy. Pitt later assigned *P. marneffei* to the subgenus *Biverticillium*. Phylogenic analysis of nucleotide sequences of nuclear and mitochondrial ribosomal DNA regions revealed that *P. marneffei* is closely related to the species of *Penicillium* subgenus *Biverticillium* and sexual *Talaromyces* species with asexual biverticillate *Penicillium* state. Analysis of the complete sequence of the mitochondrial genome of *P. marneffei* revealed that it is more closely related to those of moulds, especially to that of *Aspergillus nidulans*, than to the mitochondrial genomes of yeasts.[6]

P. marneffei grows in a mycelial phase at 25°C on Sabouraud dextrose agar. The colony is grayish white and downy. The color of more mature colonies may vary. They may become yellow, or yellowish green; and then turn to gray, green or brown. Aged colonies are deep red, as a soluble red pigment diffuse into the agar. Microscopic examination of the mycelia shows typical structures of *Penicillium* species. They are septate hyphae with lateral and terminal conidiophores or penicilli. Penicilli are monoverticillate and/or biverticillate, with either symmetrical or asymmetrical branches. Metulae bear 3–16 phialides, each of which produces long basipetal unbranched chains of conidia. The conidia are oval, smooth-walled, measuring approximately $2\,\mu m \times 3\,\mu m$. Spiral hyphae are sometimes present. When transferred to brain-heart infusion agar and incubated at 37°C, white to tan-colored colonies of the yeast form develop within a few days. Microscopically, yeast cells of *P. marneffei* are globose to oval, measuring $2–3\,\mu m \times 2–6\,\mu m$ with a single septum.

Ecology, Mode of Transmission, and Natural History

Many important features of the ecology, mode of transmission and natural history of *P. marneffei* and *P. marneffei* infection remain unknown. A number of studies have surveyed rodent species and established that *P. marneffei* can infect four species of bamboo rats, namely *Rhyzomys sinensis, R. pruinosus, R. sumatranensis,* and the reddish-brown subspecies of *Cannomys badius*.[7] These infected animals showed no signs of illness. Gugnani and colleagues surveyed six species of sympatric rodents in northeastern India, namely *Bandicota bengalensis, Rattus norvegicus, R. rattus, R. niditus, Mus musculus,* and *C. badius.* Only *C. badius* was found to harbor *P. marneffei*.[7] Also, the geographic ranges of bamboo rats (*Cannomy* spp. and *Rhizomys* spp.) broadly follow the distribution of human cases of *P. marneffei* infection, namely southeast Asia, northeastern India, and southern China.[8] These studies suggested that bamboo rats may be an obligate stage in the life-cycle of the fungus. However, an attempt to epidemiologically link bamboo rats and human infection was not successful. Chariyalertsak and colleagues compared 80 patients with AIDS who had *P. marneffei* infection with 160 AIDS patients who did not have *P. marneffei* infection, in a case-control study.[9] The main risk factor found was a recent history of occupational or other exposures to soil, especially during the rainy season. Both cases and controls were often familiar with and had seen bamboo rats; 31.3% of cases and 28.1% of controls had eaten bamboo rats but this difference was not statistically significant. Reported cases of *P. marneffei* in HIV-infected infants also suggest that human and bamboo rat infection are not connected.[10] Bamboo rats live in the wild and have limited or no contact with these infants. In another study from Chiang Mai, it was found that disseminated *P. marneffei* infections have been markedly seasonal with a doubling of cases during the rainy season.[11] This suggested that there might be an expansion of the environmental reservoir with favorable conditions for growth during these rainy seasons and that both humans and bamboo rats are infected with *P. marneffei* from this common reservoir. It should be noted that attempts to isolate the fungus from 67 soil samples from the residential areas of patients with *P. marneffei* infection yielded negative results.[12] In addition, the same authors cultured many samples of bamboo and vegetation from the environment where human cases had occurred; all were negative.[12] Thus, definite proof of an environmental reservoir for *P. marneffei* within the soil, or other substrates, is also lacking.

The mode of transmission of *P. marneffei* to humans is not known. By analogy to other endemic fungal pathogens, such as *Coccidioides immitis* and *Histoplasma capsulatum*, it is likely that *P. marneffei* conidia are inhaled from an environmental reservoir. One case report from France suggested the airborne route of infection.[13] The patient was an

HIV-infected Congolese physician who had *P. marneffei* infection shortly after attending a 4-month course in tropical microbiology at the Institut Pasteur. The patient had never visited Asia. In the building where he attended class, a mycology course was being taught. Part of the course involved the morphologic identification of *P. marneffei*. The patient entered the mycology classroom on two occasions to see a friend. However, air samples taken in the building after the case was diagnosed did not yield any *P. marneffei*.[13] Also, it should be noted that attempts to culture the fungus from air from the patient's home in Chiang Mai, Thailand, using high-volume air samplers have repeatedly yielded negative results.

By analogy to histoplasmosis, it is likely that subclinical infections with *P. marneffei* may occur commonly in persons living in endemic areas who are exposed to the fungus in nature. By using Western immunoblot assay, Vanittanakom and colleagues found that this proportion of the population with latent asymptomatic infection was about 10% in northern Thailand.[14] It has already been mentioned that all infected bamboo rats studied in China, Thailand, and India did not show any signs of illness. The existence of subclinical infection in humans is also supported by a case report from Australia of an HIV-infected patient who had a latent period of more than a decade between exposure in an endemic area and the subsequent onset of clinical infection in Australia.[15] However, in many other instances, the clinical appearance of disseminated infection occurred within a few weeks of exposure to the organism. The seasonal variation of cases with disseminated *P. marneffei* infection as well as cases of *P. marneffei* in HIV-infected infants reported from northern Thailand also suggest that progress from infection to clinical dissemination is usually brisk.

Clinical Features

P. marneffei infection occurs late in the course of HIV infection. The CD4 cell count at the time of the diagnosis of *P. marneffei* infection is usually less than 50 cells/μL. Cases were reported in which *P. marneffei* infection occurred with other late HIV-related infections, such as cryptococcal meningitis, pneumocystic pneumonia, and cerebral toxoplasmosis. Patients commonly present with symptoms and signs of infection of the reticuloendothelial system. These include fever, generalized lymphadenopathy, hepatomegaly, and splenomegaly (Table 35.1).[4,16] Clinical manifestations associated with late HIV infection such as anorexia, asthenia, anemia, weight loss, and

Table 35.1 Clinical manifestations in 80 HIV-infected patients with disseminated *Penicillium marneffei* infection in northern Thailand[16]

	n	(%)
Symptoms		
Fever	74	92.5
Skin lesions	54	67.5
Cough	39	48.7
Diarrhea	25	31.2
Signs		
Body temperature ≥38.3°C	79	95.0
Pronounced weight loss	61	76.2
Anemia	62	77.5
Skin lesions	57	71.2
Generalized lymphadenopathy	46	57.5
Hepatomegaly	41	51.2
Splenomegaly	13	16.2
Genital ulcer	5	6.2

cachexia are seen in the majority of the patients. Symptoms and signs of infection of the respiratory system, e.g. cough, dyspnea, thoracic pain, and pulmonary infiltrates may also be present, reflecting the probable route of acquisition of the organism. Other presentations, such as skin lesions, arthritis, and osteomyelitis,[17] are secondary to dissemination of the fungus via the blood stream. Skin lesions are seen in >70% of the patients and, when present, are the best clues to the diagnosis. They are usually found as papules on the face, chest, and extremities. The center of the papule subsequently becomes necrotic, giving the appearance of an umbilicated papule (also called papulonecrotic skin lesion). Biochemical and hematologic laboratory values are nonspecific and may include elevation of liver enzymes and bilirubin, anemia, and leukocytosis or leucopenia. Roentgenograms of the chest may show diffuse reticulonodular, localized alveolar, or diffuse alveolar infiltrates. Clinical features in children are identical to those seen in adults.[10]

As the HIV epidemic spread in Asia and more patients were encountered, other clinical presentations of *P. marneffei* infection in HIV-infected patients were encountered. Cases with chest roentgenograms showing lung mass or single or multiple cavitary lesions had been reported.[18,19] Ukarapol and colleagues reported three children who presented with fever, mesenteric lymphadenitis, and abdominal pain. Two of the patients had had unnecessary abdominal operations for the diagnosis of peritonitis and acute appendicitis, respectively. All three cases had positive blood and bone marrow cultures for *P.*

marneffei.[20] Kantipong and colleagues reported six patients who presented with fever, hepatomegaly, and markedly elevated serum alkaline phosphatase levels. *P. marneffei* was demonstrated in the liver and cultured from the blood.[21] Mucosal lesions in the oral cavity, oropharynx, hypopharynx, stomach, colon, and genitalia had been reported.[16,22-24] *P. marneffei* could be demonstrated in or cultured from these lesions.

Diagnosis

The diagnosis of *P. marneffei* infection rests on the microscopic demonstration of the fungus in the tissues and/or isolation of the fungus from clinical specimens. *P. marneffei* can be readily cultured from various clinical specimens. Bone marrow culture is the most sensitive, followed by culture of the specimen obtained from skin biopsy, and blood culture (Table 35.2). At 25–30°C on Sabouraud dextrose agar, the fungus grows as a mould with typical filamentous reproductive structures of the genus *Penicillium*. Mould-to-yeast conversion is achieved by subculturing the fungus on to brain-heart-infusion agar and incubating at 35–37°C. Demonstration of this conversion is required before concluding that the isolate is *P. marneffei*. Alternatively, an exoantigen test[25] and a polymerase chain reaction (PCR)-hybridization assay[26] have been described, which can be used to rapidly identify cultures of the organism.

A simple bedside technique has been described that allows physicians to make a rapid presumptive diagnosis of the infection.[16] Microscopic examination of the Wright's-stained samples of the touch smears of skin, or lymph-node biopsy specimens, or bone-marrow aspirate demonstrate many intracellular and extracellular basophilic, spherical, oval, and elliptical yeast cells. Some of these cells have clear central septation, which is a characteristic feature of *P. marneffei*. This technique can be used with the small amount of tissue obtained by fine needle aspiration of the lymph node. It is particularly helpful in cases where there is no skin lesion and the lymphadenopathy is confined to the deep intra-abdominal nodes.[27] In addition, in patients with fulminant infection, *P. marneffei* can be seen in the peripheral blood smear.[28]

P. marneffei can be seen in histopathological sections stained with Grocott methenamine silver or periodic-acid Schiff. The organisms appear as unicellular round to oval cells which divide by cross-wall formation in macrophages or histiocytes. Extracellular elongated or sausage-shaped cells with one of two septa may also be seen. Neither the cell wall nor the cytoplasm of *P. marneffei* cells take up the hematoxylin-eosin stain well. Immunohistochemical techniques have been described for the identification tissue form of *P. marneffei*. In addition, *P. marneffei* had been identified from a skin biopsy specimen by PCR using a set of primers specific for the fungus.[29] Yousukh and colleagues described the histopathological findings in the liver biopsy from 30 HIV-infected patients with disseminated *P. marneffei* infection.[30] Hepatic lesions could be classified into one of three patterns, probably reflecting the level of host's immunity: diffuse, granulomatous, and mixed. The first pattern showed a diffuse infiltration of foamy macrophages that contained numerous *P. marneffei*. The granulomatous pattern showed a formation of multiple granulomata with various degrees of inflammatory cell infiltration. The mixed pattern showed features intermediate between the first two. The histopathological findings in other organs are similar to those described in the liver.[31]

Several tests have been described that detect antibody to *P. marneffei* in infected patients.[2] These include the immunodiffusion test,[25] the indirect fluorescent antibody test, the enzyme-linked immunosorbent assay (ELISA) of a purified recombinant mannoprotein of *P. marneffei*,[32] and the Western immunoblot test.[14] Similarly, several investigators have described methods to detect *P. marneffei* antigens in serum or urine of infected patients.[2] These include the immunodiffusion test, the latex agglutination test,[33] the ELISA tests,[33,34] and the PCR test.[26,35,36] However, these tests are not widely used because commercial reagents are not available. Also, large clinical trials are needed to show the usefulness of these tests in the diagnosis of active *P. marneffei* infection or to predict relapses, as well as to identify individuals who are infected with *P. marnef-*

Table 35.2 Sources of isolation of *Penicillium marneffei* in 80 HIV-infected patients with disseminated *Penicillium marneffei* infection in northern Thailand[16]

Specimen type	Number of specimens	
	Total	Positive (%)
Blood	78	59 (76)
Skin biopsy	52	47 (90)
Bone marrow	26	26 (100)
Sputum	41	14 (34)
Lymph node biopsy	9	9 (100)

fei but who are still asymptomatic. These persons may then benefit from preemptive treatment with antifungal agent similar to isoniazid treatment in asymptomatic persons with a positive tuberculin skin test.

Treatment

The mortality rate of patients with disseminated *P. marneffei* infection had been high, mostly because of a lack of timely diagnosis.[16] The outcome was much better in the hospital where physicians were aware of the clinical features of the infection and the diagnosis was made early. A study of 30 clinical isolates from northern Thailand revealed that all were susceptible to amphotericin B, itraconazole, ketoconazole, and miconazole. Clinical response to treatment correlated with *in vitro* susceptibility.[37] Sirisanthana and colleagues conducted an open-label non-comparative study to evaluate the combination of 0.6 mg/ kg per day of amphotericin B given intravenously for 2 weeks followed by 400 mg/day of itraconazole taken orally for 10 weeks.[38] Of the 74 patients treated, 72 (97.3%) responded. No serious adverse drug effects were observed. This regimen is recommended as the treatment of choice in HIV-infected patients with disseminated *P. marneffei* infection. However, in a report of 46 patients from northeastern India treatment with oral itraconazole alone was effective in all but one patient.[4] Thus, oral treatment with 400 mg/ day of itraconazole for 12 weeks is an alternative recommendation in patients with less severe disease.

Relapses of *P. marneffei* infection are common. In one study, 12 out of 40 patients who responded to initial treatment relapsed within 6 months.[37] Suppressive therapy is required for as long as significant immunocompromise persists. Supparatpinyo and colleagues conducted a controlled trial of 71 patients in northern Thailand.[39] A total of 20 of the 35 patients (57%) assigned to the placebo group relapsed, whereas none of the 36 patients given itraconazole 200 mg orally once daily relapsed. The drug was well tolerated.

Primary prophylaxis with antifungal agent should be considered in areas where fungal infections are common AIDS-associated opportunistic infections. In northern Thailand, disseminated fungal infection due to *P. marneffei, Cryptococcus neoformans,* and *Histoplasma capsulatum* as well as other fungal infection, such as Candidiasis are common, accounting for over one-third of the reported AIDS-defining illnesses.[1] Chariyalertsak and colleagues evaluated the

efficacy of primary prophylaxis with 200 mg/day of itraconazole given orally in a controlled study.[40] The trial was conducted in 129 HIV-infected patients who had CD4 cell count <200 cells/μL and had not experienced a systemic fungal infection. In the intention-to-treat analysis, disseminated *P. marneffei* infection developed in 1 of 63 patients (1.6%) assigned to receive itraconazole and a systemic fungal infection developed in 11 of 66 patients (16.7%) given placebo (seven patients had cryptococcal meningitis, and four patients had disseminated *P. marneffei* infection).

Conclusion

P. marneffei infection is one of the most common opportunistic infections in HIV-infected persons in southeast Asia, northeastern India, southern China, Hong Kong, and Taiwan. Many cases have also been reported in HIV-infected patients from the USA, Europe, Japan, and Australia, following visits to the endemic area. The response to antifungal treatment is good if the diagnosis is made and the treatment started early. Much remains to be learned about the ecology, mode of transmission, and natural history of *P. marneffei* infection. With improved access to highly active antiretroviral therapy for HIV-infected patients in the endemic area, additional research questions about when to stop secondary prophylaxis for *P. marneffei* infection and the incidence and management of immune restoration syndrome caused by the fungus have to be addressed.

References

1. Chariyalertsak S, Sirisanthana T, Saengwonloey O, et al. Clinical presentation and risk behaviors of patients with acquired immunodeficiency syndrome in Thailand, 1994-1998: regional variation and temporal trends. Clin Infect Dis 2001; 32:955–962.
2. Vanittanakom N, Sirisanthana T. *Penicillium marneffei* infection in patients infected with human immunodeficiency virus. Curr Top Med Mycol 1997; 8:35–42.
3. Huynh TX, Nguyen HC, Dinh Nguyen HM, et al. Penicillium and AIDS: a review of 12 cases reported in the Tropical Diseases Centre, Ho Chi Minh City (Vietnam). Sante 2003; 13:149–153.
4. Ranjana KH, Priyokumar K, Singh TJ, et al. Disseminated *Penicillium marneffei* infection among HIV-infected patients in Manipur state, India. J Infect 2002; 45:268–271.
5. Lyratzopoulos G, Ellis M, Nerringer R, et al. Invasive infection due to penicillium species other than *P. marneffei.* J Infect 2002; 45:184–195.
6. Woo PC, Zhen H, Cai JJ, et al. The mitochondrial genome of the thermal dimorphic fungus *Penicillium marneffei* is more closely related to those of molds than yeasts. FEBS Lett 2003; 555:469–477.

7. Gugnani HC, Fisher MC, Paliwal-Johsi A, et al. *Cannomys badius* as a natural animal host of Penicillium marneffei in India. J Clin Microbiol 2004; 42:5070–5075.

8. Corbet GB, Hill JE, eds. Subfamily Rhizomyinae: bamboo rats. In: The mammals of the Indo Malaya region: a systematic review. Oxford: Oxford University Press; 1992:404–407.

9. Chariyalertsak S, Sirisanthana T, Supparatpinyo K, et al. Case-control study of risk factors for *Penicillium marneffei* infection in human immunodeficiency virus-infected patients in northern Thailand. Clin Infect Dis 1997; 24:1080–1086.

10. Sirisanthana V, Sirisanthana T. Disseminated *Penicillium marneffei* infection in human immunodeficiency virus-infected children. Pediatr Infect Dis J 1995; 14:935–940.

11. Chariyalertsak S, Sirisanthana T, Supparatpinyo K, et al. Seasonal variation of disseminated *Penicillium marneffei* infections in northern Thailand: a clue to the reservoir? J Infect Dis 1996; 173:1490–1493.

12. Chariyalertsak S, Vanittanakom P, Nelson KE, et al. *Rhizomys sumatrensis* and *Cannomys badius*, new natural animal hosts of *Penicillium marneffei*. J Med Vet Mycol 1996; 34:105–110.

13. Hilmarsdottir I, Coutellier A, Elbaz J, et al. A French case of laboratory-acquired disseminated *Penicillium marneffei* infection in a patient with AIDS (correspondence). Clin Infect Dis 1994; 2:357–358.

14. Vanittanakom N, Mekaprateep M, Sittisombut N, et al. Western immunoblot analysis of protein antigens of *Penicillium marneffei*. J Med Vet Mycol 1997; 35:123–131.

15. Jones PD, See J. *Penicillium marneffei* infection in patients infected with human immunodeficiency virus: late presentation in an area of nonendemicity (letter). Clin Infect Dis 1992; 15:744.

16. Supparatpinyo K, Khamwan C, Baosoung V, et al. Disseminated *Penicillium marneffei* infection in southeast Asia. Lancet 1994; 344:110–113.

17. Louthrenoo W, Thamprasert K, Sirisanthana T. Osteoarticular penicilliosis marneffei. A report of eight cases and review of the literature. Br J Rheumatol 1994; 33:1145–1150.

18. McShane H, Tang CM, Conlon CP. Disseminated *Penicillium marneffei* infection presenting as a right upper lobe mass in an HIV positive patient. Thorax 1998; 53:905–906.

19. Cheng NC, Wong WW, Fung CP, et al. Unusual pulmonary manifestations of disseminated *Penicillium marneffei* infection in three AIDS patients. Med Mycol 1998; 36:429–432.

20. Ukarapol N, Sirisanthana V, Wongsawasdi L. *Penicillium marneffei* mesenteric lymphadenitis in human immunodeficiency virus-infected children. J Med Assoc Thai 1998; 81:637–640.

21. Kantipong P, Panich V, Pongsurachet V, et al. Hepatic penicilliosis in patients without skin lesions. Clin Infect Dis 1998; 26:1215–1217.

22. Tong AC, Wong M, Smith NJ. *Penicillium marneffei* infection presenting as oral ulcerations in a patient infected with human immunodeficiency virus. J Oral Maxillofac Surg 2001; 59:953–956.

23. Kronauer CM, Schar G, Barben M, et al. HIV-associated *Penicillium marneffei* infection. Schweiz Med Wochenschr 1993; 123:385–390.

24. Leung R, Sung JY, Chow J, et al. Unusual cause of fever and diarrhea in a patient with AIDS: *Penicillium marneffei* infection. Dig Dis Sci 1996; 41:1212–1215.

25. Sekhon AS, Li JSK, Garg AK. Penicilliosis marneffei: serological and exoantigen studies. Mycopathology 1982; 77:51–57.

26. Vanittanakom N, Vanittanakom P, Hay RJ. Rapid identification of *Penicillium marneffei* by PCR-based detection of specific sequences on the rRNA gene. J Clin Microbiol 2002; 40:1739–1742.

27. Chaiwun B, Khunamornpong S, Sirivanichai C, et al. Lymphadenopathy due to *Penicillium marneffei* infection: diagnosis by fine needle aspiration cytology. Mod Pathol 2002; 15:939–943.

28. Supparatpinyo K, Sirisanthana T. Disseminated *Penicillium marneffei* infection diagnosed on examination of a peripheral blood smear of a patient with human immunodeficiency virus infection. Clin Infect Dis 1994; 18:246–247.

29. Tsunemi Y, Takahashi T, Tamaki T. *Penicillium marneffei* infection diagnosed by polymerase chain reaction from the skin specimen. J Am Acad Derm 2003; 49:344–346.

30. Yousukh A, Jutavijittum P, Pisetpongsa P, et al. Clinicopathologic study of hepatic *Penicillium marneffei* in Northern Thailand. Arch Pathol Lab Med 2004; 128:191–194.

31. Drouhet E. Penicilliosis due to *Penicillium marneffei*: a new emerging systematic mycosis in AIDS patients traveling or living in Southeast Asia. J Mycol Med (Paris) 1993; 4:195–224.

32. Cao L, Chan KM, Chen D, et al. Detection of cell wall mannoprotein mp1p in culture supernatants of *Penicillium marneffei* and in sera of penicilliosis patients. J Clin Microbiol 1999; 37:981–986.

33. Desakorn V, Simpson AJH, Wuthiekanun V, et al. Development and evaluation of rapid urinary antigen detection tests for diagnosis of penicilliosis marneffei. J Clin Microbiol 2002; 40:3179–3183.

34. Chaiyaroj SC, Chawengkirttikul R, Sirisinha S, et al. Antigen detection assay for identification of *Penicillium marneffei* infection. J Clin Microbiol 2003; 41:432–434.

35. Vanittanakom N, Merz WG, Sittisombut N, et al. Specific identification of *Penicillium marneffei* by a polymerase chain reaction/hybridization technique. Med Mycol 1998; 36:169–175.

36. Prariyachatigul C, Chaiprasert A, Geenkajorn K, et al. Development and evaluation of a one-tube seminested PCR assay for the detection and identification of *Penicillium marneffei*. Mucoses 2003; 46:447–454.

37. Supparatpinyo K, Nelson KE, Merz WG, et al. Response to antifungal therapy by human immunodeficiency virus-infected patients with disseminated *Penicillium marneffei* infections and *in vitro* susceptibilities of isolates from clinical specimens. Antimicrob Agents Chemother 1993; 37:2407–2411.

38. Sirisanthana T, Supparatpinyo K, Perriens J, et al. Amphotericin B and itraconazole for treatment of disseminated *Penicillium marneffei* infection in human immunodeficiency virus-infected patients. Clin Infect Dis 1998; 26:1107–1110.

39. Supparatpinyo K, Perriens J, Nelson KE, et al. A controlled trial of itraconazole to prevent relapse of *Penicillium marneffei* infection in patients infected with the human immunodeficiency virus. N Engl J Med 1998; 339:1739–1743.

40. Chariyalertsak S, Supparatpinyo K, Sirisanthana T, et al. A controlled trial of itraconazole as primary prophylaxis for systemic fungal infections in patients with advanced human immunodeficiency virus infection in Thailand. Clin Infect Dis 2002; 34:277–284.

CHAPTER 36

AIDS-associated Toxoplasmosis

Carlos S. Subauste

Jose G. Montoya

Jack S. Remington

Introduction

Toxoplasma gondii is among the most prevalent causes of latent infection of the central nervous system (CNS) throughout the world. After an acute infection, cysts of *T. gondii* persist in the CNS and in multiple extra-neural tissues. Although normal human hosts maintain infection in a quiescent state, immunocompromised individuals may be at risk for reactivation and dissemination of chronic (latent) infection. Defective cellular immunity in HIV-infected patients results in loss of the primary arm of host defense against this parasite. Re-activation of latent infection in patients with AIDS may lead to clinically apparent disease (toxoplasmosis), which most frequently manifests as life-threatening encephalitis.

Because AIDS patients who develop toxoplasmic encephalitis (TE) are almost always chronically infected with the protozoan,[1] HIV-infected patients who are known to have antibodies to *T. gondii* should be considered at risk for development of TE. Seroprevalence varies between geographic locales and even within subpopulations of the same locale.[2,3] Studies performed in our laboratory have found a prevalence of *T. gondii* antibodies among HIV-positive adults of 8–16% in major urban areas of the USA. The prevalence is higher (=25%) among certain ethnic groups. Early studies indicated that 20–47% of *T. gondii*-seropositive AIDS patients ultimately developed TE.[4,5] More recently, the risk of toxoplasmosis has significantly decreased after introduction of primary prophylaxis against *T. gondii* and highly active antiretroviral therapy (HAART). The incidence in the USA, of TE among patients who had developed AIDS, declined from 2.1/100 person-years (PY) in 1992 to 0.7/100 PY in 1997.[6] However, TE remains a prevalent opportunistic infection in patients with signs and symptoms of central nervous system involvement, even in the late HAART era, particularly among severely immunosuppressed patients and especially in the absence of prophylaxis.[7]

Clinical Presentation

In the USA, AIDS patients who develop TE generally do so after the diagnosis of AIDS has been made.[8–11] Ingestion of undercooked or raw meat containing tissue cysts and of vegetables or other food products contaminated with oocysts is a major means of transmission of the parasite, as is direct contact with cat feces. Although cats are the definitive host for *T. gondii*, toxoplasma antibody seroconversion in adult HIV-infected individuals appears unrelated to cat ownership or exposure. Recently, unfiltered drinking water has been also implicated as a source of *T. gondii* infection.[12]

Because multi-focal involvement of the CNS frequently occurs in TE in AIDS patients, there may be a wide spectrum of clinical findings, including alteration of mental status, seizures, motor weakness, sensory abnormalities, cerebellar dysfunction, meningismus, movement disorders, and neuropsychiatric manifestations.[9,13-18] The characteristic presentation is usually one of the subacute onset with focal neurologic abnormalities in 58–89% of patients. Altered mental status, manifested by confusion, lethargy, delusional behavior, frank psychosis, global cognitive impairment, anomia, or coma, may be present initially in as many as 60% of patients.[9,13-15,19] Seizures are the reason for seeking medical attention in approximately one-third of AIDS patients with TE.[9,13-16,19] Focal neurologic deficits are evident on neurologic examination in approximately 60%.[9,13,14,19] Although hemiparesis is the most common focal neurologic finding, patients may have evidence of aphasia, ataxia, visual field loss, cranial nerve palsies dysmetria, hemichorea-hemiballismus, tremor, parkinsonism, akathisia, or focal dystonia.[9,20-23] In addition, infection of the spinal cord with *T. gondii* has been described in cases of transverse myelitis and conus medullaris syndrome.[24,25] A rapidly fatal panencephalitis form of diffuse cerebral toxoplasmosis also has been described.[26] Unfortunately, computed tomography (CT) of the head was unrevealing in these cases.[4,26]

Extracerebral sites with or without concomitant TE may be involved in HIV-infected individuals.[27-30] As is true for TE, extracerebral toxoplasmosis usually occurs in patients with CD4 counts of <100/mm³.[27,29] In patients with extracerebral toxoplasmosis, ocular and pulmonary sites are most commonly involved (50% and 26% of patients, respectively).[29]

Significant pulmonary disease including acute respiratory distress syndrome caused by toxoplasmosis has been reported.[28,31-33] Mortality, even in the presence of treatment for toxoplasmosis, is high in these patients. The most common clinical syndrome is prolonged febrile illness with cough, hypoxemia and dyspnea that is clinically indistinguishable from *Pneumocystis carinii* pneumonia. Associated extrapulmonary disease caused by *T. gondii* has been reported in approximately 50% of the patients at the time of clinical presentation. TE may precede or follow pulmonary toxoplasmosis if maintenance therapy is not instituted. A highly lethal syndrome of disseminated toxoplasmosis has been described in AIDS patients that consists of fever and sepsis-like syndrome with hypotension, disseminated intravascular coagulation, elevated lactate dehydrogenase, and pulmonary infiltrates.[27-29] This syndrome is usually not associated with clinical or radiologic evidence of TE.[27,28]

Ocular disease caused by toxoplasmosis occurs relatively infrequently in AIDS patients (when compared with the incidence of cytomegalovirus retinitis).[34-37] Ocular pain and loss of visual acuity are common complaints, and funduscopic examination typically reveals findings consistent with necrotizing retinochoroiditis. The lesions are yellow-white areas of retinitis with fluffy borders. In reported series, the lesions were multifocal in 17–50%,[34,37] bilateral in 18–40%,[34,35,37] and accompanied by optic neuritis in approximately 10%. Scant retinal inflammation is frequently observed in AIDS-associated toxoplasmic retinochoroiditis.[37] Thus the features of toxoplasmic retinochoroiditis commonly observed in the immunocompetent host may be absent in patients with AIDS. Vitreal inflammation may vary from mild localized vitreal haze to extensive vitreous inflammation.[34,35] Vasculitis and hemorrhage are uncommon. In most patients, the ocular lesions are located away from areas of pre-existing scars. This suggests that the pathogenesis of these lesions may be secondary to hematogenous seeding rather than local reactivation of infection. The presence of concurrent TE in AIDS patients with ocular toxoplasmosis has varied from 29% to 63%.[34,35,37]

Most AIDS patients with TE (80–95%) have CD4 T-lymphocyte counts of <100/mm³.[38-42] Cerebrospinal fluid (CSF) may be normal or reveal mild pleocytosis (predominantly lymphocytes and monocytes) and an elevated protein level, whereas the glucose content usually is normal.[9,11]

Congenital Toxoplasmosis and the HIV-infected Woman

Women infected with HIV are at risk for transmission of *T. gondii* infection to their fetuses if they are seronegative for *T. gondii* antibodies and acquire *T. gondii* infection during pregnancy. Maternal–fetal transmission of *T. gondii* can also occur in HIV-infected pregnant women who are chronically infected with *T. gondii* although the risk of transmission is low (less than 4%).[43,44] Studies that addressed this problem were conducted in cohorts of primarily asymptomatic women, most of whom had a CD4 T-lymphocyte count >200/mm³.[43,44] The risk of transmission may be higher in severely immunocompromised HIV-infected women, although there are insufficient data to accurately estimate this risk. In one study, one of the three dually infected mothers with CD4 T-lymphocyte counts <100/mm³ transmitted *T. gondii* infection to her baby.[43] When dually infected women developed toxoplasmosis during pregnancy, 75% of their infants were born with congenital toxoplasmosis and HIV infection.[45] All infants with congenital toxoplasmosis born to mothers who were HIV infected also were infected with HIV. The initial clinical presentation of congenital toxoplasmosis in the HIV-infected infant is similar to that in the non-HIV-infected but appears to run a more rapid and progressive course. The infants often appear normal at birth. In the ensuing months, they fail to gain weight or develop appropriately. The majority develop multisystem organ involvement, including the CNS, heart, and lungs.[46]

Diagnosis

At present, the definitive diagnosis of toxoplasmosis in AIDS patients can only be made by demonstration of the organism in tissues or amplification of *T. gondii* DNA from body fluids (i.e. CSF, BAL, vitreous fluid) (Box 36.1). In cases where TE is highly likely (see Management), brain biopsy can be deferred while awaiting results of empiric anti-*T. gondii* therapy and a lumbar puncture, if safe and feasible, can be performed for examination by PCR. The morbidity associated with obtaining a brain biopsy for the evaluation of focal brain lesions in HIV-infected patients is less than that from an erroneous diagnosis.[47] Thus, a brain biopsy should be strongly considered in cases where the likelihood of TE is low and only after the possibility of performing a lumbar puncture for testing by PCR has been considered. In addition to TE, examination of the CSF by PCR can also be diagnostic for progressive multifocal leukoencephalopathy (PML), EBV-associated central nervous system lymphoma, and CMV ventriculitis.[12,48]

Serology

Because TE in patients with AIDS almost always represents reactivation of chronic (latent) infection, the presence of immunoglobulin (Ig)G *T. gondii*-specific antibodies in an HIV-infected patient must be regarded as a marker for the potential development of toxoplasmosis. If the serologic status of an HIV-infected patient with suspected TE is unknown, IgG antibody status should be determined.

Although almost all AIDS patients with TE have detectable IgG *T. gondii* in their serum, published series have reported a 0–3% seronegativity rate.[19,49]

Although measurement of intrathecal production of antibody to *T. gondii* has been reported as a useful ancillary test by some investigators for the diagnosis of TE[50,51] and toxoplasmic chorioretinitis.[52] Others have found it to be of little use for the diagnosis of these clinical entities.[53,54]

Box 36.1

Methods for definitive or presumptive diagnosis of toxoplasmosis in patients with AIDS

- Histologic evaluation, including immunoperoxidase staining of tissue biopsies
- Visual demonstration of *T. gondii* in body fluids (CSF, BAL) by microscopic examination (i.e. using Wright-Giemsa stain)
- Isolation of *T. gondii* from tissue biopsies or body fluids (i.e. CSF, blood, BAL)
- Amplification of *T. gondii* DNA by PCR examination of body fluids (i.e CSF, blood, BAL, vitreous fluid) or tissue biopsies
- CT scans and/or MR images of the head
- Serology (including titer in differential agglutination assay, IgG, IgM[a])
- Intrathecal production of *T. gondii*-specific antibodies (rarely used).

BAL, bronchoalveolar lavage; CSF, cerebrospinal fluid; CT, computerized tomography; Ig, immunoglobulin; MR, magnetic resonance; PCR, polymerase chain reaction.
[a]Useful, mainly in areas of high seroprevalence. When feasible, IgM positive results should undergo confirmatory testing at a reference laboratory (i.e. the Toxoplasma Serology Laboratory at the Palo Alto Medical Foundation (PAMF-TSL), Palo Alto, CA. Available: www.pamf.org/serology/; Tel: 650 853 4848).

IgM *T. gondii* antibodies, routinely measured to diagnose acute toxoplasmosis in non-AIDS patients, are rarely demonstrable in AIDS patients with TE In HIV-infected patients whose toxoplasma serologies are unknown both IgG and IgM should be measured initially. Positive results in both tests should suggest (but it is not diagnostic) recently acquired infection.[4] All equivocal or positive toxoplasma IgM results in HIV-infected individuals should, whenever feasible, undergo confirmatory testing at a reference laboratory (i.e. the Toxoplasma Serology Laboratory at the Palo Alto Medical Foundation, see Box 36.1). Positive or equivocal IgM results are not necessarily diagnostic of an acute infection; in fact these may be false positive or observed in chronically infected individuals. IgA *T. gondii* antibodies are rarely elevated in AIDS patients with acute TE.[55] *Toxoplasma gondii* IgE antibodies measured by enzyme-linked immunosorbent assay and ISAGA have been detected in serum in a limited number of patients with TE.[56,57]

Isolations Studies

Isolation of *T. gondii* from body fluids or, in the appropriate clinical setting, from tissue obtained from a patient with AIDS should be considered diagnostic of active infection. Because isolation of the organism may not be evident for 6 days to 6 weeks after mice or tissue cultures are inoculated, the results often are not helpful in initial management of the patient. Nevertheless, isolation of the organism may obviate the future need for brain biopsy.

Toxoplasma gondii readily forms plaques in tissue cultures of human foreskin fibroblasts and most other cultured cells.[58,59] *Toxoplasma gondii* has been isolated from the blood in 14–38% of AIDS patients with toxoplasmosis.[14,60] *Toxoplasma gondii* also may be isolated from bronchoalveolar lavage (BAL) fluid in patients with toxoplasmic pneumonitis.[61]

DNA Detection

The high specificity of PCR testing for *T. gondii* DNA makes this method of diagnosis useful if a positive result is generated. The use of the polymerase chain reaction (PCR) has enabled detection of *T. gondii* DNA in brain tissue,[62,63] CSF (approximately 50–70%),[64-66] BAL fluid,[53,67] blood (generally between 10% and 30%),[64,68-70] aqueous humor[53,62] and vitreous fluid[71] of AIDS patients with toxoplasmosis. Because *T. gondii* cysts persist in certain organs (i.e. brain, skeletal and heart muscle and eyes) for years after infection, a positive PCR in these tissues does not necessarily reflect active infection.

Of note, attempts to perform prenatal diagnosis of congenital infection using PCR in amniotic fluid of pregnant women dually infected with HIV and *T. gondii* are hampered by the fact that amniocentesis is contraindicated in HIV-infected mothers because of the potential of transmission of HIV to the fetus during the procedure.

Neuroradiologic Studies

Imaging studies of the brain are essential for diagnosis and management of patients with toxoplasmic encephalitis.[72-75] Typically, multiple, bilateral, hypodense, enhancing mass lesions are found on CT scan.[9,76,77] Lesions have a predilection for, but are not limited to, the basal ganglia and hemispheric corticomedullary junction. A significant degree of enhancement of intracerebral lesions generally is present on CT scan.[9,13,72,75,76] *Toxoplasma gondii* abscesses may, however, fail to enhance or be solitary and located anywhere in the brain.[77-80]

Magnetic resonance imaging (MRI) is more sensitive than CT scan for detection of brain lesions of TE. Masses demonstrated by MRI may be absent on CT scan,[80,81] whereas the converse apparently is not true. In a review of AIDS patients with focal neurologic symptoms, a CT scan was as good as an MRI in detecting focal brain lesions (70% versus 74%). However, in AIDS patients with non-focal neurological symptoms, only 22% had CT scans that revealed focal lesions, compared with 42% found by MRI. As in CT scans, lesions found on MRI of AIDS patients with TE frequently are bilateral and located in the basal ganglia or cerebral corticomedullary junction.[80,82] Deep lesions, which generally range from 1 to 3 cm in diameter, may show central patterns of both low and high signal intensity, suggestive of necrosis.[79] Unlike CT scans, MRI reveals multiple lesions in more than 80% of patients with TE.[77,78,80,82] In fact, a single lesion seen on an MRI should alert the clinician to other possible causes of the focal neuroradiologic findings (e.g. lymphoma, progressive multifocal leukoencephalopathy (PML) fungal abscesses, tuberculoma, or Kaposi's sarcoma).[77] When a single lesion is present on an MRI, the probability of CNS lymphoma is at least equal to or higher than the probability of TE.[77]

The neuroradiologic response of TE to specific treatment is seen on CT as a reduction in mass effect, number and extent of lesions, and enhancement.[79] Although the time to resolution of lesions may vary from 20 days to 6 months, the vast majority of patients who respond clinically will show radiologic improvement (>50%) by the 3rd week of treatment.[83,84] The response of abnormalities as seen on MRI to specific therapy also varies with the location and complexity of the mass lesion. Persistent enhancement on CT scans or MRI after treatment for TE has been associated with a higher incidence of subsequent relapse of the encephalitis.[85] Findings on MRI and CT scans are not pathognomonic for TE. Primary CNS lymphoma cannot be distinguished from toxoplasmosis solely on the basis of neuroradiologic criteria (both present as contrast enhancing lesions with mass effect). However, the presence of hyperattenuation on non-enhanced CT scans and subependymal location suggest the possibility of lymphoma.[86] Other imaging techniques appear to be useful for distinction between CNS lymphoma and infectious processes in HIV-infected patients with focal brain lesions. Increased uptake on Thallium-201 single-photon emission computer tomography (^{201}Tl SPECT) is highly sensitive (96% sensitivity) for malignancy (CNS lymphoma) in HIV-infected patients.[87-89] Delayed imaging to detect persistent increased uptake (retention index) increases the specificity for CNS lymphoma from 76 to 100%.[89] ^{18}F-fluoro-2-deoxyglucose positron emission tomography (FDG-PET) is another imaging technique reported to accurately differentiate between CNS lymphoma and nonmalignant brain lesions in AIDS patients.[90,91] Whereas areas of decreased glucose metabolism were seen in all patients with TE, areas with increased glucose metabolism were observed in all patients with CNS lymphoma.[90,91] However, the real value of these imaging techniques based on metabolic and vascular differences between infection and neoplasia has not been established in AIDS patients.

Histopathology

Definitive diagnosis of TE often requires demonstration of the organism on histopathologic section of brain tissue obtained at biopsy. Some evidence suggests the superiority of open excisional biopsy compared to needle biopsy in making the histopathologic diagnosis of TE. The response of the brain to *T. gondii* infection can vary from a granulomatous reaction with gliosis and microglial nodule formation to a severe focal or generalized necrotizing encephalitis.[9,73,75,92] Perivascular and intimal inflammatory cell infiltrates can lead to fibrosis necrosis, which can result in hemorrhage[93] or thrombosis, accounting for neurologic signs and symptoms.

The presence of numerous *T. gondii* tachyzoites or cysts surrounded by an inflammatory reaction is diagnostic.[3] Cysts or free organisms not demonstrable on routine histopathologic examination can be identified using the peroxidase-antiperoxidase method.[94] A rapid, sensitive, and specific method for diagnosis of TE by electron microscopy has been described.[95] Thus, when routine histopathologic studies fail to provide a definitive diagnosis, appropriately fixed brain tissue should be stained by the immunoperoxidase technique or analyzed by electron microscopy in an attempt to identify *T. gondii* antigens or organisms.

Wright–Giemsa-stained smears or touch preparations should be made as immediately as is feasible from tissue obtained at surgery. Similarly, Wright–Giemsa stain of a cytocentrifuge preparation of CSF or BAL may reveal the presence of tachyzoites.[96,97]

Differential Diagnosis

The main differential diagnosis of focal brain lesions in HIV-infected patients is between CNS lymphoma and TE. In *T. gondii*-seropositive HIV-infected patients with a CD4 T-lymphocyte count of <100/mm^3, who are not receiving anti-*T. gondii* prophylaxis, the presence of multiple enhancing lesions is strongly suggestive of TE. In patients on prophylaxis, or those with a single brain lesion, the differential diagnosis includes CNS lymphoma, PML, fungal abscess, mycobacterial or cytomegaloviral disease, Kaposi's sarcoma in addition to TE. Because therapy is available for most of these disorders, brain biopsy for histopathologic diagnosis may be necessary for successful management of the patient. The characteristic appearance of progressive multifocal leukoencephalopathy on neuroimaging studies often facilitates differentiation of this disorder from other causes of intracerebral mass lesions.

Management

General Principles

Because TE generally reflects reactivation of a latent infection, all HIV-positive individuals should be tested for *T. gondii*-specific IgG antibody. Patients with positive titers are at risk for development of TE (Fig. 36.1).

MRI is more sensitive than a CT scan and thus is the preferred imaging technique, especially in patients without focal neurologic abnormalities. Patients with only one lesion or no lesions on CT scan should get a MRI to determine if more than one lesion is present. Because a single lesion on MRI is uncharacteristic of TE, CNS lymphoma and other causes of focal brain lesions should be suspected.[77,78] Early brain biopsy should be considered in this situation. CSF examination by PCR for *T. gondii*, EBV, JC and CMV viruses should also be entertained if lumbar puncture is deemed safe.

TE used to be the most common cause of focal brain lesions in AIDS patients.[72,73] Therefore, empiric anti-*T. gondii* therapy was considered appropriate for all *T. gondii*-seropositive HIV-infected patients with multiple focal brain lesions, *Toxoplasma* IgG antibodies, and CD4 counts <200. Brain biopsy was recommended in those who did not improve clinically within 7–10 days of initiation of specific anti-Toxo-

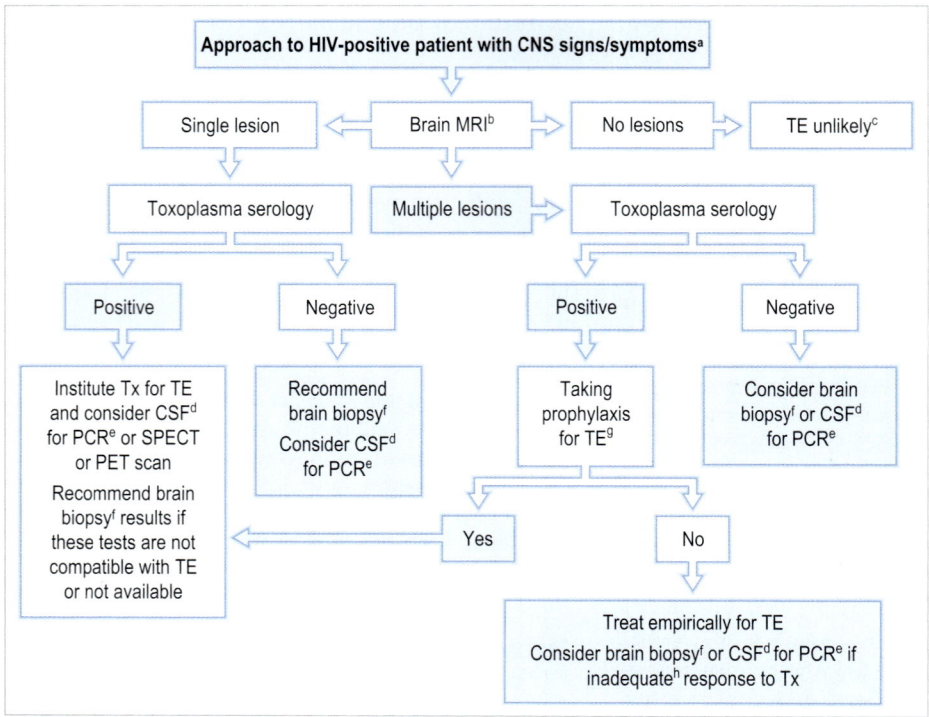

Figure 36.1 Guidelines for the evaluation and management of patients with suspected toxoplasmic encephalitis (TE). [a] Patients with TE may present with a non-focal neurological examination. [b] MRI is superior to CT scan. [c] Cases of diffuse non-focal TE have been rarely reported. [d] CSF should be obtained only if safe to perform a lumbar puncture. [e] In addition to PCR for *T. gondii*, consider PCR for EBV (PCNSL), JCV (PML) and CMV. [f] *T. gondii*-specific immunoperoxidase stain is both highly sensitive and specific for the diagnosis of TE. [g] For regimens considered to be effective for TE prophylaxis see Table 36-6. [h] Inadequate response to therapy is defined as deterioration of the neurological findings within 3 to 5 days of institution of an appropriate anti-*T. gondii* regimen or no significant clinical response (less than 50% improvement in neurological examination) within 7 to 10 days anti-*T. gondii* treatment.

CMV, cytomegalovirus; CSF, cerebrospinal fluid; CT, computed tomography; EBV, Epstein Barr virus; JCV, JCV virus; MRI, magnetic resonance imaging; PCNLS, primary central nervous system lymphoma; PCR, polymerase chain reaction; PET, positron emission tomography; PML, progressive multifocal leukoencephalopathy; SPECT, single-photon emission computed tomography; Tx, treatment.

plasma therapy. However, the incidence of TE in AIDS patients has decreased in recent years, owing to the use of primary anti-*T. gondii* prophylaxis and highly active anti-retroviral therapy.[6,98–102] In contrast, the frequency of CNS lymphoma has increased in patients with focal brain lesions.[100] Therefore, empiric anti-*T. gondii* therapy for all patients with a focal brain lesion without an aggressive diagnostic work-up may delay initiation of appropriate therapy and expose patients to potentially unnecessary and toxic regimens.

CSF for PCR studies, and/or ^{201}Tl SPECT, FDG-PET studies (Fig. 36.1) should be obtained in patients with a low likelihood of TE, provided that these tests are available and it is safe to perform a lumbar puncture. Patients who may benefit from these studies include those with: negative *T. gondii* IgG antibodies, CD4 T-lymphocyte count of >100/mm³, single lesion on MRI, or multiple lesions on MRI/CT scan while receiving primary *T. gondii* prophylaxis. If these tests are not available, early brain biopsy without awaiting response to anti-*T. gondii* therapy should be considered in these patients. The presence of multiple brain lesions in a *T. gondii* seropositive HIV-infected patient with a CD4 T-lymphocyte count <100/mm³ who is not receiving anti-*T. gondii* prophylaxis, is still considered highly predictive of TE.[103,104] Thus, awaiting clinical response to empiric anti-*T. gondii* therapy still appears to be an appropriate approach in this setting.[103]

Diffuse TE is rare but it frequently goes under-diagnosed and should be suspected when a patient with severe CD4 cell depletion and positive *T. gondii* serology experiences unexplained fever and neurologic disease. When diagnostic investigations fail to disclose a specific cause in these cases, a trial of empiric anti-*T. gondii* treatment should be considered.

In regard to what can be expected in relation to clinical and radiologic responses to therapy, a prospective study demonstrated that 71% of the patients had a complete or partial response.[83] The neurologic response was rapid, with 51% of patients showing signs of improvement by day 3 and 91% by day 14.[83] Thus, brain biopsy with or without change of therapy should be considered in patients whose condition worsens early in the course of therapy or in patients who do not show clinical improvement by 10–14 days of therapy.[83] Repeat neuroradiologic study by the same modality as originally selected should be performed 2–4 weeks after initiation of therapy in patients who demonstrate a satisfactory clinical response (or earlier if response is poor). Lesions should have diminished in size and possibly in number. Patients with extra-neurologic toxoplasmosis should be evaluated for CNS disease, because a significant number of them will also have intracerebral involvement.[105]

Corticosteroids should frequently be entertained for management of patients with intracranial hypertension caused by the mass effect from *T. gondii* abscesses. A recent study reported that there was no difference in the response rate and the time to response in patients who received corticosteroids when compared with those who did not.[83] At present, AIDS patients with TE should receive corticosteroids only when it is absolutely necessary. (If possible, no more than 2 weeks of therapy should be given.) Whether administration of anticonvulsant agents is necessary for prevention of seizures has not been determined.

It is important to distinguish between two forms of therapy for TE in patients with AIDS: primary therapy and maintenance therapy. Primary therapy is administered during the acute disease. Maintenance therapy is administered after an adequate clinical and neuroradiologic response has been observed. Unless HAART-induced immune reconstitution takes place, maintenance therapy should be continued for life, because the rate of relapse is prohibitively high when treatment is discontinued. Once the CD4 T-lymphocyte count has increased to >200/mm³ and the HIV viral load has been nondetectable for 6 months or longer, maintenance therapy can be safely discontinued in clinically stable patients.

Primary Therapy

Pyrimethamine, a potent dihydrofolate reductase inhibitor, is the cornerstone of current treatment of AIDS-associated TE. It is standard practice to administer the combination of pyrimethamine plus sulfadiazine or pyrimethamine plus clindamycin (Table 36.1).

Prospective, randomized studies of treatment of TE showed that pyrimethamine plus clindamycin and pyrimethamine plus sulfadiazine were equally efficacious during the acute phase of therapy.[14,106,107] When choosing a regimen that includes clindamycin, a panel of experts recommend administration of 600 mg of clindamycin orally (or intravenously) every 6 h.

Studies have revealed that trimethoprim-sulfamethoxazole (TMP-SMX) may be effective for acute therapy of TE.[108–110] A randomized, prospective study revealed that the clinical response rate to TMP-SMX (10 mg/kg per day of the trimethoprim component) was similar to that of pyrimethamine (50 mg/day) plus sulfadiazine (60 mg/kg per day).[110]

Standard therapy is limited by the high incidence of toxicity associated with both drugs in combination. The most notable toxicity of pyrimethamine is dose-related bone marrow suppression, resulting in thrombocytopenia, granulocytopenia, or megaloblastic anemia.[111–113] At doses of 75–100 mg/day, hematologic abnormalities should be anticipated but may be difficult to distinguish from those associated with HIV infection *per se*. Complete blood counts of patients receiving pyrimethamine should be monitored frequently for the development of drug-associated bone marrow toxicity.

Folinic acid (leucovorin calcium) may prevent marrow toxicity or be used to treat patients with marrow toxicity caused by pyrimethamine[3,111] and is not antagonistic to the activity of pyrimethamine or sulfadiazine against *T. gondii*.[114] The oral dose of folinic acid administered to these patients is usually 10–20 mg/day in divided doses (Table 36.1).[115] If hematologic abnormalities develop and malabsorption of the folinic acid is suspected, folinic acid may be administered parenterally. Some investigators increase folinic acid up to 50 mg/day for suspected pyrimethamine-associated hematologic toxicity.[13] Folic acid must not be used, because it may inhibit the anti-*T. gondii* activity of pyrimethamine.[114] Although 65–90% of patients with TE will have an initial favorable response to pyrimethamine plus sulfadiazine therapy,[9,13,14] untoward reactions to this combination, most frequently rash,[14] may limit duration of therapy. When treating a patient who devel-

Table 36.1 Guidelines for acute or primary treatment of AIDS patients with TE

Drugs	Dosage
Recommended regimens	
Pyrimethamine	p.o.: 200 mg loading followed by 50 (<60 kg) to 75 (≥60 kg) mg q.24 h
Folinic acid	p.o., o.v., or i.m.: 10–20 mg q.24 h (up to 50 mg q.d.)
plus sulfadiazine	p.o.: 1000 (<60 kg) to 1500 (≥60 kg) mg q.6 h
or clindamycin	o.v. or p.o.: 600 mg q.6 h (up to o.v. 1200 mg q.6 h)
Alternative regimens	
Trimethoprim-sulfamethoxazole	p.o. or o.v.: 5 mg (trimethoprim component)/kg q.6 h–q.12 h
Pyrimethamine plus folinic acid	As in recommended regimen
plus one of the following:	
Atovaquone	p.o.: 1500 mg q.12 h
Clarithromycin	p.o.: 500 mg q.12 h
Azithromycin	p.o.: 900–1200 mg q.24 h
Dapsone	p.o.: 100 mg q.24 h

ops skin rash it is important to keep in mind that not only sulfadiazine but also pyrimethamine can cause this side-effect.[116] Studies reveal that as many as 40% of AIDS patients who receive sulfadiazine and pyrimethamine for TE manifest signs of toxicity sufficiently severe to prompt discontinuation of the drug(s) during the primary phase of treatment.[13,117]

It is likely that sulfonamide is discontinued prematurely in many cases which, if it were continued, the rash would lessen or disappear. A number of investigators have stated that the majority of patients with AIDS who experience sulfonamide-associated cutaneous reactions can be successfully desensitized to these agents.[118] Crystal-induced nephrotoxicity is another well-recognized adverse reaction to sulfadiazine.[119] The most frequent adverse reactions seen in patients treated with pyrimethamine-clindamycin-skin rash and gastrointestinal and hematologic toxicities[14,106] are similar to those seen with pyrimethamine plus sulfadiazine.[14] The substantial toxicities associated with standard anti-*T. gondii* treatment underscore the urgent need to develop safe and effective alternative drug regimens.

In the search for such regimens, most studies have evaluated the safety and efficacy of a non-sulfonamide agent in combination with pyrimethamine.[106,120–122]

A study of the combination of atovaquone (administered orally as a suspension) plus either pyrimethamine or sulfadiazine as treatment for acute disease reported a 6-week response rates of 75% and 82%, respectively.[123] Thus, atovaquone/pyrimethamine can be used as an alternative treatment for patients

intolerant to sulfonamides, and atovaquone/sulfadiazine for patients who are intolerant to pyrimethamine. Promising results were observed using the combination of pyrimethamine 75 mg/day and clarithromycin 1 g every 12 h.[121] Although azithromycin plus pyrimethamine is effective for the treatment of some cases of TE in AIDS patients, its use should be approached with caution based on results of a recent study demonstrating an inferior response rate, especially during maintenance therapy.[124,125] In view of the dramatic immune reconstitution that is observed in AIDS patients as a result of HAART, it becomes central to the treatment of TE to add anti-retroviral drug regimens as soon as feasible. Immune reconstitution mediated TE has not been proven to occur but it has been suspected in several clinical settings among experienced clinicians.

Almost all the studies on the use of antimicrobial agents that have been described for the treatment of toxoplasmosis in AIDS patients have focused on patients with TE. Limited data suggest that patients with extracerebral toxoplasmosis also respond to therapy with pyrimethamine-sulfadiazine or pyrimethamine-clindamycin but that the mortality rate in patients with pulmonary or disseminated toxoplasmosis may be much higher than in patients with TE alone.[126]

Maintenance Treatment (Second Prophylaxis)

Whereas the combination of pyrimethamine plus sulfadiazine is highly active against the proliferative form, neither it, nor any of the currently used drugs is effective in eradicating the cyst form of *T. gondii*. It is believed that persistence of the cyst form accounts for relapse of TE after therapy is discontinued. The relapse rate of TE in patients who are not receiving HAART and maintenance therapy for toxoplasmosis is 50–80% at 12 months.[15,19] The CT scans or MR images of patients who relapse often demonstrate mass lesions in the same location as at initial presentation.[127] Thus it is essential that AIDS patients who complete a primary course of therapy and who have had a favorable clinical and radiologic response to therapy for TE receive lifelong anti-*T. gondii* agents unless they experience HAART-induced immune reconstitution (e.g. CD4 T-lymphocyte count >200/mm^3 and non-detectable HIV viral load for 6 months or longer).

After successful primary therapy, drug dosages are generally decreased for maintenance therapy (Table 36.2). There is no single regimen that both is effective and has an acceptable safety profile. Although TE can recur during maintenance therapy,[19,128] it is important to be aware that some of these failures are due to noncompliance.[127]

The regimen of pyrimethamine plus sulfadiazine appears to have a lower rate of relapse than other regimens and is recommended.[18,128,129] Patients on maintenance therapy with pyrimethamine-sulfadiazine do not require further prophylaxis for *P. carinii*.[129,130] Although most investigators favor the daily use of pyrimethamine-sulfadiazine, many patients are unable to continue this regimen because of drug toxicity, and alternative regimens will have to be considered (Table 36.2).[128,131,132]

A prospective, randomized study showed no significant differences in clinical outcome of patients who received pyrimethamine plus clindamycin versus pyrimethamine plus sulfadiazine.[106] However, another prospective, randomized study reported that, during maintenance therapy, the rate of relapse was double in patients treated with pyrimethamine plus clindamycin (22% versus 11%).[107] Whether the high relapse rate was due to the low dose of clindamycin (1.2 g/day) used remains to be determined. In addition, it is important to be aware that pyrimethamine-clindamycin does not prevent *P. carinii* pneumonia.[128,153]

Pyrimethamine-sulfadoxine (Fansidar) administered as one tablet twice weekly has been reported to be effective as maintenance therapy. Side-effects were relatively common (40%), with 7% of patients discontinuing therapy because of adverse effects.[134] Atovaquone may be an alternative for secondary prophylaxis in patients with intolerance to standard therapy or for whom such therapy failed.[135,136]

Table 36.2 Guidelines for maintenance treatment of AIDS patients with TE

	Oral dose	Frequency
Recommended regimens		
Pyrimethamine[a]	25–50 mg	q.24 h
plus sulfadiazine	1.0 mg	b.i.d.
Pyrimethamine	25–50 mg	q.24 h
plus clindamycin	300–600 mg	q.6 h
Alternative regimens		
Pyrimethamine	25–50 mg	q.24 h
plus one of the following:		
Dapsone	100 mg	b.i.w.
Atovaquone	750 mg	q.12 h
Clarithromycin	500 mg	q.12 h
Azithromycin	1200–1500 mg	q.24 h

[a]Folinic acid (leucovorin calcium) 10–20 mg q.24 h is recommended for all patients receiving pyrimethamine to help ameliorate the hematologic side-effects associated with pyrimethamine. The dose of folinic acid is titrated against the patient's hematologic indices, and up to 50 mg of folinic acid has been used.

Prevention (Primary Prophylaxis)

Serologic testing for *T. gondii* antibodies will distinguish those HIV-infected individuals who are at risk for reactivation of infection from those at risk for acquisition of infection. All patients who are seronegative for *T. gondii* antibodies and who have evidence of deficient cellular immunity, should be educated about appropriate precautions to take to prevent acquisition of *T. gondii* infection (Box 36.2). Seroconversion to *T. gondii* positivity in HIV-infected individuals has been reported to occur in 2% after a mean follow-up of 2 years.

Despite the availability of effective antimicrobial regimens, toxoplasmosis in AIDS patients is associated with a mortality rate of 70% by 12 months after the diagnosis of TE if HAART is not instituted.[42] Among AIDS patients taking failing regimens of HAART, the 1-year probability of that infection with human immunodeficiency virus (HIV) would progress or that death would occur after TE has been reported at 40% and 23%, respectively.[7] Thus the morbidity and mortality associated with toxoplasmosis in AIDS patients strongly support the use of prophylaxis in HIV-infected patients with CD4 T-lymphocyte counts of less than 200/mm^3.[125,137,138] Given that absolute CD4 T-lymphocyte counts and symptomatic HIV infection (Centers for Disease Control and Prevention Stage IV), appear to be independent risk factors for development of TE, primary

Table 36.3 Regimens used for primary prophylaxis against toxoplasmosis

Drug	Dosage schedule
TMP-SMX	p.o.: 1 DS tab q.d. p.o.: 1 SS tab q.d.
Pyrimethamine-dapsonea	p.o.: pyrimethamine 50 mg once a week; dapsone 50 mg q.d. p.o.: pyrimethamine 50 mg b.i.w.; dapsone 100 mg b.i.w. p.o.: pyrimethamine 75 mg once a week; dapsone 200 mg once a week p.o.: pyrimethamine 25 mg once a week; dapsone 100 mg once a week
Pyrimethamine-sulfadoxine (Fansidar)[a,b]	p.o.: 3 tabs every 2 weeks p.o.: 1 tab b.i.w.

DS, double strength; SS, single strength. [a]Folinic acid (Leucovorin) 25 mg q.w. is recommended for all patients receiving pyrimethamine to help ameliorate the hematologic side-effects associated with pyrimethamine. The dose of folinic acid is titrated against the patient's hematologic indices. [b]Each tablet contains pyrimethamine 25 mg, sulfadoxine 500 mg.

Box 36.2

Methods for preventing toxoplasmosis in patients with HIV infection

Individuals should take the following precautions:

- Cook meat to ≈116°C (well done, not pink)
- Avoid touching mucous membranes of mouth and eyes while handling raw meat
- Wash hands thoroughly after handling raw meat
- Wash kitchen surfaces that come into contact with raw meat
- Wash fruits and vegetables before consumption
- Prevent access of flies, cockroaches, and the like to fruits and vegetables
- Avoid contact with materials that are potentially contaminated with cat feces (e.g. cat litter boxes or wear gloves when handling such materials or when gardening)
- Disinfect cat litter box for 5 min with nearly boiling water
- Avoid drinking unfiltered water.

prophylaxis is considered appropriate in patients with CD4 T-lymphocyte counts <100/mm^3 regardless of clinical status and in patients with CD4 T-lymphocyte counts <200/mm^3 if they develop AIDS defining opportunistic infections or malignancies.[139] Numerous studies have reported the efficacy of TMP-SMX,[102,137,140–146] pyrimethamine-dapsone[143,147,148] or pyrimethamine-sulfadoxine,[149] in the prevention of TE in HIV-infected patients (Table 36.3). It must be emphasized that, among patients receiving primary prophylaxis with TMP-SMX,[144] pyrimethamine-dapsone,[150] or pyrimethamine-sulfadoxine, 40–60% will have untoward side-effects, and in 2–12% of the

total number of patients will require discontinuation of therapy.

Pyrimethamine alone is currently not considered a first-line regimen for primary prophylaxis against TE in patients who can tolerate TMP-SMX.[139]

Although there are no data available on the use of prophylaxis against congenital toxoplasmosis in HIV-infected women who are seropositive for *T. gondii* antibodies and whose *T. gondii* infection was acquired prior to pregnancy and in the distant past, administration of TMP/SMX SS 1 tablet q.d. throughout pregnancy for women with CD4 lymphocyte counts <200/mm^3 has been recommended.[151] Pyrimethamine-sulfadiazine after the 17th week of pregnancy should be considered for those who are more severely immunosuppressed and in whom fetal infection is highly suspected.

Discontinuation of primary and secondary prophylaxis

Although *in vitro* studies indicate that HAART does not fully restore cell-mediated immunity against *T. gondii* in all HIV-infected patients,[152] the use of HAART has been associated with a decline in mortality and incidence of opportunistic infections (including TE) in HIV-infected patients[6,98,99,101,102] These findings prompted studies that explored the safety of discontinuing prophylaxis against opportunistic pathogens in patients receiving HAART.

Observational and randomized studies indicate that it is safe to discontinue primary prophylaxis against *T. gondii* in adult and adolescent patients whose CD4 T-lymphocyte counts increase to more than 200/mm^3 for at least 3 months in response to HAART.[102,153–157] It is important to note that the majority of these patients were on protease inhibitor-containing regimens, had CD4 T-lymphocyte counts more than 200/mm^3 for an average of 8 months, their median CD4 T-lymphocyte count at study entry was more than 300/mm^3, and had undetectable plasma viral load.[153]

It appears reasonable to consider stopping maintenance therapy in patients who have completed acute phase treatment for TE, are free of signs and symptoms attributable to this disease, and have experienced sustained (= 6 months) increase in CD4 T-lymphocyte count to >200/mm^3.[125,138,155,157,158] Although no studies have directly addressed criteria for re-starting prophylaxis, it would be prudent to re-initiate primary and secondary prophylaxis in patients whose CD4 T-lymphocyte count decrease to <200/mm^3.[138]

Acknowledgments

The work discussed in this chapter was supported in part from grants AI48406, AI04717, and AI30230 from the National Institutes of Health, Bethesda, MD.

References

1. Luft BJ, Brooks RG, Conley FK, et al. TE in patients with acquired immune deficiency syndrome. JAMA 1984; 252:913–917.
2. Luft BJ, Castro KG. An overview of the problem of toxoplasmosis and pneumocystosis in AIDS in the USA: Implication for future therapeutic trials. Eur J Clin Microbiol Infect Dis 1991; 10:178–181.
3. Remington JS, McLeod R, Desmonts G. *Toxoplasmosis*. In: Remington JS, Klein JO, eds. Infectious diseases of the fetus and newborn infant. 4th edn. Philadelphia: W.B. Saunders; 1995:140–267.
4. Grant IH, Gold JWM, Rosenblum M, et al. *Toxoplasma gondii* serology in HIV-infected patients: the development of central nervous system toxoplasmosis. AIDS 1990; 4:519–521.
5. Israelski DM, Chmiel JS, Poggensee L, et al. Prevalence of toxoplasma infection in a cohort of homosexual men at risk of AIDS and TE. J AIDS 1993; 6:414–418.
6. Jones JL, Hanson DL, Dworkin MS, et al. Surveillance for AIDS-defining opportunistic illnesses, 1992-1997. MMWR CDC Surveill Summ 1999; 48:1–22.
7. Antinori A, Larussa D, Cingolani A, et al. Prevalence, associated factors, and prognostic determinants of AIDS-related TE in the era of advanced highly active antiretroviral therapy. Clin Infect Dis 2004; 39:1681–1691.
8. Luft BJ, Conley F, Remington JS, et al. Outbreak of central-nervous-system toxoplasmosis in western Europe and North America. Lancet 1983; 1:781–784.
9. Navia BA, Petito CK, Gold JW, et al. Cerebral toxoplasmosis complicating the acquired immune deficiency syndrome: clinical and neuropathological findings in 27 patients. Ann Neurol 1986; 19:224–238.
10. Selik RM, Starcher ET, Curran JW. Opportunistic diseases reported in AIDS patients: frequencies, associations, and trends. AIDS 1987; 1:175–182.
11. Wong B, Gold JWM, Brown AE, et al. Central-nervous-system toxoplasmosis in homosexual men and parenteral drug abusers. Ann Intern Med 1984; 100:36–42.

12. Montoya JG, Kovacs JA, Remington J. Toxoplasmosis. In: Mandell GL, Bennett JE, Dolin R, eds. Principles and practice of infectious diseases. 6th edn. Vol 2. Edinburgh: Churchill Livingstone; 2005:3170–3198.
13. Leport C, Raffi F, Matheron S, et al. Treatment of central nervous system toxoplasmosis with pyrimethamine-sulfadiazine combination in 35 patients with the acquired immunodeficiency syndrome. Efficacy of long-term continuous therapy. Am J Med 1988; 84:94–100.
14. Dannemann BR, McCutchan JA, Israelski DA, et al. Treatment of TE in patients with AIDS: A randomized trial comparing pyrimethamine plus clindamycin to pyrimethamine plus sulfadiazine. Ann Intern Med 1992; 116:33–43.
15. Haverkos HW, Remington JS, Chan JC. Assessment of *Toxoplasma* encephalitis (TE) therapy; A cooperative study. Am J Med 1987; 82:907–914.
16. Levy RM, Bredesen DE. Central nervous system dysfunction in acquired immunodeficiency syndrome. J AIDS 1988; 1:41–64.
17. Porter SB, Sande M. Toxoplasmosis of the central nervous system in the Acquired Immunodeficiency Syndrome. N Engl J Med 1992; 327:1643–1648.
18. Renold C, Sugar A, Chave J-P, et al. Toxoplasma encephalitis in patients with the acquired immunodeficiency syndrome. Medicine 1992; 71:224–239.
19. Pedrol E, Gonzales-Clemente JM, Gatell JM, et al. Central nervous system toxoplasmosis in AIDS patients: efficacy of an intermittent maintenance therapy. AIDS 1990; 4:511–517.
20. Carrazana E, Rossitch E, Martinez J. Unilateral 'akathisia' in a patient with AIDS and a toxoplasmosis subthalamic abscess. Neurology 1989; 39:449–450.
21. Carrazana EJ, Rossitch EJ, Samuels MA. Parkinsonian symptoms in a patient with AIDS and cerebral toxoplasmosis. J Neurol Neurosurg Psychiatry 1989; 52:1445–1446.
22. Koppel BS. Daras M. 'Rubrual' tremor due to midbrain Toxoplasmosis abscess. Mov Disord 1990; 5:254–256.
23. Tolge CF, Factor SA. Focal dystonia secondary to cerebral toxoplasmosis in a patient with acquired immune deficiency syndrome. Mov Disord 1991; 6:69–72.
24. Herskovitz S, Siegel SE, Schneider AT, et al. Spinal cord toxoplasmosis in AIDS. Neurol 1989; 39:1552–1553.
25. Mehren M, Burns PJ, Mamani F, et al. Toxoplasmic myelitis mimicking intramedullary spinal cord tumor. Neurology 1988; 38:1648–1650.
26. Gray F, Gherardi R, Wingate E, et al. Diffuse 'encephalitic' cerebral toxoplasmosis in AIDS: Report of four cases. J Neurol 1989; 236:273–277.
27. Lucet J-C, Bailly M-P, Bedos J-P, et al. Septic shock due to Toxoplasmosis in patients infected with the human immunodeficiency virus. Chest 1993; 104:1054–1058.
28. Oksenhendler E, Cadranel J, Sarfati C, et al. *Toxoplasma gondii* pneumonia in patients with the acquired immunodeficiency syndrome. Am J Med 1990; 88:18N–21N.
29. Rabaud C, May T, Amiel C, et al. Extracerebral toxoplasmosis in patients infected with HIV. Medicine 1994; 73:306–314.
30. Tschirhart D, Klatt E. Disseminated toxoplasmosis in the acquired immunodeficiency syndrome. Arch Pathol Lab Med 1988; 112:1237–1241.
31. Derouin F, Sarfati C, Beauvais B, et al. Prevalence of pulmonary toxoplasmosis in HIV-infected patients. AIDS 1990; 4:1036.
32. Schnapp L, Geaghan S, Campagna A, et al. *Toxoplasma gondii* pneumonitis in Patients Infected with the Human Immunodeficiency Virus. Arch Intern Med 1992; 152:1073–1076.
33. Charles PE, Doise JM, Quenot JP, et al. An unusual cause of acute respiratory distress in a patient with AIDS: primary infection with Toxoplasma gondii. Scand J Infect Dis 2003; 35:901–902.

34. Cochereau-Massin I, LeHoang P, Lautier-Frau M, et al. Ocular *Toxoplasmosis* in human immunodeficiency virus-infected patients. Am J Ophth 1992; 114:130–135.

35. Friedman DI. Neuro-ophthalmic manifestations of human immunodeficiency virus infection. Neurol Clin 1991; 9:55–72.

36. Gagliuso D, Teich S, Friedman A, et al. Ocular toxoplasmosis in AIDS patients. Trans Am Ophth Soc 1990; 88:63–88.

37. Holland G, Engstrom R Jr, Glasgow B, et al. Ocular toxoplasmosis in patients with acquired immunodeficiency syndrome. Am J Opthalmol 1988; 106:653–667.

38. Eliaszewicz M, Lecomte I, De Sa M. Relation between decreasing serial CD4 lymphocyte count and outcome of toxoplasmosis in AIDS patients: a basis for primary prophylaxis. 6th International Conference on AIDS, San Francisco, CA: 1990.

39. Araujo FG, Guptill DR, Remington JS. *In vivo* activity of piritrexim against *Toxoplasma gondii*. J Infect Dis 1987; 156:828–830.

40. Matheron S, Dournon E, Garakhanian S, et al. Prevalence of toxoplasmosis in 365 AIDS and ARC patients before and during zidovudine treatment. 6th International Conference on AIDS, San Francisco, CA: 1990.

41. Miro JM, Buira E, Mallolas J, et al. Relation between CD4+ lymphocyte counts, tuberculosis, other opportunistic infections(OI) or Kaposi's sarcoma (KS) in Spanish AIDS Patients. VIIth International Conference on AIDS, Florence, Italy: 1991.

42. Oksenhendler E, Charreau I, Tournerie C, et al. *Toxoplasma gondii* in advanced HIV infection. AIDS 1994; 8:483–487.

43. Minkoff H, Remington JS, Holman S, et al. Vertical transmission of toxoplasma by human immunodeficiency virus-infected women. Am J Obstet Gynecol 1997; 176:555–559.

44. Anon. Low incidence of congenital toxoplasmosis in children born to women infected with human immunodeficiency virus. European Collaborative Study and Research Network on Congenital Toxoplasmosis. Eur J Obstet Gynecol Reprod Biol 1996; 68:93–96.

45. Mitchell CD, Lewis L, McLellan S, et al. Increased risk of congential toxoplasmosis (Ct) among infants born to mothers infected with HIV-1 and *Toxoplasma gondii*. 3rd Conference on Retroviruses and Opportunistic Infections, Washington, DC: 28 January–1 February 1996.

46. Mitchell CD, Erlich SS, Mastrucci MT, et al. Congenital toxoplasmosis occurring in infants perinatally infected with human immunodeficiency virus 1. Pediatr Infect Dis J 1990; 9:512–518.

47. Cimino C, Lipton RB, Williams A, et al. The evaluation of patients with human immunodeficiency virus-related disorders and brain mass lesions. Arch Intern Med 1991; 151:1381–1384.

48. Tachikawa N, Goto M, Hoshino Y, et al. Detection of Toxoplasma gondii, Epstein-Barr virus, and JC virus DNAs in the cerebrospinal fluid in acquired immunodeficiency syndrome patients with focal central nervous system complications. Intern Med 1999; 38:556–562.

49. Suzuki Y, Israelski DM, Dannemann BR, et al. Diagnosis of TE in patients with acquired immunodeficiency syndrome by using a new serologic method. J Clin Microbiol 1988; 26:2541–2543.

50. Orefice G, Carrieri PB, de Marinis T, et al. Use of the intrathecal synthesis of antitoxoplasma antibodies in the diagnostic assessment and in the follow-up of AIDS patients with cerebral toxoplasmosis. Acta Neurol (Napoli) 1990; 12:79–81.

51. Potasman I, Resnick L, Luft BJ, et al. Intrathecal production of antibodies against *Toxoplasma gondii* in patients with TE and the acquired immunodeficiency syndrome (AIDS). Ann Intern Med 1988; 108:49–51.

52. Verbraak FD, Galema M, van den Hans Horn G, et al. Serological and polymerase chain reaction-based analysis of aqueous humour samples in patients with AIDS and necrotizing retinitis. AIDS 1996; 10:1091–1099.

53. Chakroun M, Meyohas MC, Pelosse B, et al. Émergence de la toxoplasmose oculaire au cours du SIDA. [Emergence of ocular toxoplasmosis in AIDS.] Ann Med Interne (Paris) 1990; 141:472–474.

54. Borges AS, Figueiredo JF. [Detection of anti-*Toxoplasma gondii* IgG, IgM and IgA immunoglobulins in the serum, cerebrospinal fluid and saliva of patients with acquired immunodeficiency syndrome and neurotoxoplasmosis]. Arq Neuropsiquiatr 2004; 62:1033–1037.

55. Stepick-Biek P, Thulliez P, Araujo FG, et al. IgA antibodies for diagnosis of acute congenital and acquired toxoplasmosis. J Infect Dis 1990; 162:270–273.

56. Pinon JM, Toubas D, Marx C, et al. Detection of specific immunoglobulin E in Patients with toxoplasmosis. J Clin Microbiol 1990; 28:1739–1743.

57. Wong SY, Hadju M-P, Ramirez R, et al. The role of specific immunoglobulin E in diagnosis of acute toxoplasma infection and toxoplasmosis. J Clin Microbiol 1993; 31:2952–2959.

58. Derouin F, Mazeron MC, Garin YJ. Comparative study of tissue culture and mouse inoculation methods for demonstration of Toxoplasma gondii. J Clin Microbiol 1987; 25:1597–1600.

59. Hofflin JM, Remington JS. Tissue culture isolation of Toxoplasma from blood of a patient with AIDS. Arch Intern Med 1985; 145:925–926.

60. Tirard V, Niel G, Rosenheim M, et al. Diagnosis of toxoplasmosis in patients with AIDS by isolation of the parasite from the blood. N Engl J Med 1991; 324:632.

61. Derouin F, Sarfati C, Beauvais B, et al. Laboratory diagnosis of pulmonary toxoplasmosis in patients with acquired immunodeficiency syndrome. J Clin Microbiol 1989; 27:1661–1663.

62. van de Ven E, Melchers W, Galama J, et al. Identification of *Toxoplasma gondii* infections by BI gene amplification. J Clin Microbiol 1991; 19:2120–2124.

63. Burg J, Grover C, Pouletty P, et al. Direct and sensitive detection of a pathogenic protozoan, *Toxoplasma gondii*, by polymerase chain reaction. J Clin Microbiol 1989; 27:1787–1792.

64. Dupon M, Cazenave J, Pellegrin J-L, et al. Detection of *Toxoplasma gondii* by PCR and tissue culture in cerebrospinal fluid and blood of human immunodeficiency virus-seropositive patients. J Clin Microbiol 1995; 33:2421–2426.

65. Ostergaard L, Nielsen AK, Black FT. DNA amplification on cerebrospinal fluid for diagnosis of cerebral toxoplasmosis among HIV-positive patients with signs or symptoms of neurological disease. Scand J Infect Dis 1993; 25:227–237.

66. Parmley SF, Goebel FD, Remington JS. Detection of *Toxoplasma gondii* DNA in cerebrospinal fluid from AIDS patients by polymerase chain reaction. J Clin Microbiol 1992; 30:3000–3002.

67. Bretagne S, Costa J-M, Fleury-Feith J, et al. Quantitative competitive PCR with bronchoalveolar lavage fluid for diagnosis of toxoplasmosis in AIDS patients. J Clin Microbiol 1995; 33:1662–1664.

68. Dupouy-Camet J, de Lavareda Souza L, Maslo C, et al. Detection of Toxoplasma gondii in venous blood from AIDS patients by polymerase chain reaction. J Clin Microb 1993; 31:1866–1869.

69. Filice G, Hitt J, Mitchell C, et al. Diagnosis of toxoplasma parasitemia in patients with AIDS by gene detection after amplification with polymerase chain reaction. J Clin Microb 1993; 31:2327–2331.

70. Pelloux H, Dupouy-Camet J, Derouin F, et al. A multicentre prospective study for the polymerase chain reaction detection of *Toxoplasma gondii* DNA in blood samples from 186 AIDS patients with suspected TE. Bio-Toxo Study Group. AIDS 1997; 11:1888–1890.

71. Montoya JG, Parmley S, Liesenfeld O, et al. Use of the polymerase chain reaction for diagnosis of ocular toxoplasmosis. Ophthalmology 1999; 106:1554–1563.

72. Post MJ, Kursunoglu SJ, Hensley GT, et al. Cranial CT in acquired immunodeficiency syndrome: spectrum of diseases and optimal contrast enhancement technique. AJR Am J Roentgenol 1985; 145:929–940.

73. Strittmatter C, Lang W, Wiestler OD, et al. The changing pattern of human immunodeficiency virus associated cerebral *toxoplasmosis*: a study of 46 postmortem cases. Acta Neuropathol 1992; 83:475–481.

74. Levy RM, Breit R, Russell E, et al. MRI-guided stereotaxic brain biopsy in neurologically symptomatic AIDS patients. J Acquir Immune Defic Syndr 1991; 4:254–260.

75. Post MJ, Chan JC, Hensley GT, et al. Toxoplasma encephalitis in Haitian adults with acquired immunodeficiency syndrome: a clinical-pathologic-CT correlation. AJR Am J Roentgenol 1983; 140:861–868.

76. Bursztyn EM, Lee BC, Bauman J. CT of acquired immunodeficiency syndrome. AJNR Am J Neuroradiol 1984; 5:711–714.

77. Ciricillo SF, Rosenblum ML. Imaging of solitary lesions in AIDS. J Neurosurg 1991; 74:1029.

78. Ciricillo SF, Rosenblum ML. Use of CT and MR imaging to distinguish intracranial lesions and to define the need for biopsy in AIDS patients. J Neurosurg 1990; 73:720–724.

79. De La Paz R. Enzmann D. Neuroradiology of acquired immunodeficiency syndrome. In: Rosenblum ML, ed. AIDS and the nervous system. New York: Raven Press; 1988:121–154.

80. Kupfer MC, Zee C-S, Colletti PM, et al. MRI evaluation of AIDS-related encephalopathy: Toxoplasmosis vs lymphoma. Mag Res Imag 1990; 8:51–57.

81. Levy RM, Mills CM, Posin JP, et al. The efficacy and clinical impact of brain imaging in neurologically symptomatic AIDS patients: A prospective CT/MRI study. J Acquir Immune Defic Syndr 1990; 3:461–471.

82. Post MJ, Sheldon JJ, Hensley GT, et al. Central nervous system disease in acquired immunodeficiency syndrome: prospective correlation using CT, MR imaging, and pathologic studies. Radiology 1986; 158:141–148.

83. Luft BJ, Hafner R, Korzun AH, et al. TE in patients with the acquired immunodeficiency syndrome. N Engl J Med 1993; 329:995–1000.

84. Levy RM, Rosenbloom S, Perrett LV. Neuroradiologic findings in AIDS: a review of 200 cases. AJR Am J Roentgenol 1986; 147:977–983.

85. Laissy J, Soyer P, Parlier C, et al. Persistent enhancement after treatment for cerebral toxoplasmosis in patients with AIDS: predictive value for subsequent recurrence. AJNR Am J Neuroradiol 1994; 15:1773–1778.

86. Dina TS. Primary central nervous system lymphoma versus toxoplasmosis in AIDS. Radiology 1991; 179:823–828.

87. O'Malley J, Ziessman H, Kumar P, et al. Diagnosis of intracranial lymphoma in patients with AIDS: value of ^{201}Tl single-photon emission computed tomography. AJR Am J Roentgenol 1994; 163:417–421.

88. Lorberboym M, Estok L, Machac J, et al. Rapid differential diagnosis of cerebral toxoplasmosis and primary central nervous system lymphoma by Thallium-201 SPECT. J Nucl Med 1996; 37:1150–1154.

89. Lorberboym M, Wallach F, Estok L, et al. Thallium-201 retention in focal intracranial lesions for differential diagnosis of primary lymphoma and nonmalignant lesions in AIDS patients. J Nucl Med 1998; 39:1366–1369.

90. Hoffman J, Waskin H, Schifter T, et al. FDG-PET in differentiating lymphoma from nonmaliganant central nervous system lesions in patients with AIDS. J Nucl Med 1993; 34:567–575.

91. Pierce M, Johnson M, Maciunas R, et al. Evaluating contrast-enhancing brain lesions in patients with AIDS by using positron emission tomography. Ann Intern Med 1995; 123:594–598.

92. Luft BJ, Remington JS. Toxoplasmosis of the central nervous system. In: Remington JS, Swartz MN, eds. Current clinical topics in infectious diseases. 6 edn. New York: McGraw-Hill; 1985:315–358.

93. Wijdicks EFM, Borleffs JCC, Hoepelman AIM, et al. Fatal disseminated hemorrhagic TE as the initial manifestation of AIDS. Ann Neurol 1991; 29:683–686.

94. Conley FK, Jenkins KA, Remington JS. *Toxoplasma gondii* infection of the central nervous system. Use of the peroxidase-antiperoxidase method to demonstrate toxoplasma in formalin fixed, paraffin embedded tissue sections. Hum Pathol 1981; 12:690–698.

95. Cerezo L, Alvarez M, Price G. Electron microscopic diagnosis of cerebral toxoplasmosis. Case report. J Neurosurg 1985; 63:470–472.

96. DeMent SH, Cox MC, Gupta PK. Diagnosis of central nervous system Toxoplasma gondii from the cerebrospinal fluid in a patient with acquired immunodeficiency syndrome. Diagn Cytopathol 1987; 3:148–151.

97. Bottone EJ. Diagnosis of acute pulmonary toxoplasmosis by visualization of invasive and intracellular tachyzoites in Giemsa-stained smears of bronchoalveolar lavage fluid. J Clin Microbiol 1991; 29:2626–2627.

98. Palella FJ Jr, Delaney KM, Moorman AC, et al. Declining morbidity and mortality among patients with advanced human immunodeficiency virus infection. HIV Outpatient Study Invest N Engl J Med 1998; 338:853–860.

99. Brodt HR, Kamps BS, Gute P, et al. Changing incidence of AIDS-defining illnesses in the era of antiretroviral combination therapy. AIDS 1997; 11:1731–1738.

100. Ammassari A, Scoppettuolo G, Murri R, et al. Changing disease patterns in focal brain lesion-causing disorders in AIDS. J Acquir Immune Defic Syndr Hum Retrovirol 1998; 18:365–371.

101. Belanger F, Derouin F, Grangeot-Keros L, et al. Incidence and risk factors of toxoplasmosis in a cohort of human immunodeficiency virus-infected patients: 1988-1995. HEMOCO and SEROCO Study Groups. Clin Infect Dis 1999; 28:575–581.

102. Abgrall S, Rabaud C, Costagliola D. Incidence and risk factors for TE in human immunodeficiency virus-infected patients before and during the highly active antiretroviral therapy era. Clin Infect Dis 2001; 33:1747–1755.

103. Antinori A, Ammassari A, De Luca A, et al. Diagnosis of AIDS-related focal brain lesions: A decision-making analysis based on clinical and neuroradiologic characteristics combined with polymerase chain reaction assays in CSF. Neurol 1997; 48:687–694.

104. Raffi F, Aboulker JP, Michelet C, et al. A prospective study of criteria for the diagnosis of TE in 186 AIDS patients. AIDS 1997; 11:177–184.

105. Leport C, Remington JS. *Toxoplasmose* au cours du SIDA. Presse Med 1992; 21:1165–1171.

106. Katlama C. Evaluation of the efficacy and safety of clindamycin plus pyrimethamine for induction and maintenance therapy of TE in AIDS. Eur J Clin Microbiol Infect Dis 1991; 10:189–191.

107. Katlama C, De Wit S, O'Doherty E, et al. Pyrimethamine-clindamycin vs. pyrimethamine-sulfadiazine as acute and long-term therapy for TE in patients with aids. Clin Infect Dis 1996; 22:268–275.

108. Canessa A, Del Bono V, De Leo P, et al. Cotrimoxazole therapy of *Toxoplasma gondii* encephalitis in AIDS patients. Eur J Clin Microbiol Inf Dis 1992; 11:125–130.

109. Solbreux P, Sonnet J, Zech F. A retrospective study about the use of cotrimoxazole as diagnostic support and treatment of suspected cerebral toxoplasmosis in AIDS. Acta Clin Belg 1990; 45:85–96.

110. Torre D, Casari S, Speranza F, et al. Randomized trial of trimethoprim-sulfamethoxazole versus pyrimethamine-sulfadiazine for therapy of TE in patients with AIDS. Ital Collab Study Group Antimicrob Agents Chemother 1998; 42:1346–1349.

111. Kaufman HE, Geisler PH. The hematologic toxicity of pyrimethamine (Daraprim) in man. Arch Ophthalmol 1960; 64:140–146.

112. Myatt AV, Coatney GR, Hernandez T, et al. A further study of the toxicity of pyrimethamine (Daraprim) in man. Am J Trop Med Hyg 1953; 2:1000–1001.

113. Myatt AV, Hernandez T, Coatney GR. Studies in human malaria. XXXIII. The toxicity of pyrimethamine (Daraprim) in man. Am J Trop Med Hyg 1953; 2:788–794.

114. Frenkel JK, Hitchings GH. Relative reversal by vitamins (p-Aminobenzoic, folic and folinic acids) of the effects of sulfadiazine and pyrimethamine on toxoplasma, mouse and man. Antibiot Chemother 1957; 7:630–638.

115. Nixon PF, Bertino JR. Effective absorption and utilization of oral formyltetrahydrofolate in man. N Engl J Med 1972; 286:175–179.

116. Rousseau F, Pueyo S, Morlat P, et al. Increased risk of TE in human immunodeficiency virus-infected patients with pyrimethamine-related rash. Clin Infect Dis 1997; 24:396–402.

117. Guichard A, Zamora L, Calmes E, et al. Cutaneous Side Effects: A Major Problem In The Treatment of Toxoplasmosis Encephalitis (TE). VII International Conference on AIDS, Florence, Italy: 1991.

118. Gluckstein D, Ruskin J. Rapid oral desensitization to trimethoprim-sulfamethoxazole (TMP-SMZ): use in prophylaxis for *Pneumocystis carinii* pneumonia in patients with AIDS who were previously intolerant to TMP-SMZ. Clin Infect Dis 1995; 20:849–853.

119. Molina J, Belenfant X, Doco-Lecompte T, et al. Sulfadiazine-induced crystalluria in AIDS patients with toxoplasma encephalitis. AIDS 1991; 5:587–589.

120. Dannemann BR, Israelski DM, Remington JS. Treatment of TE with intravenous clindamycin. Arch Intern Med 1988; 148:2477–2482.

121. Fernandez-Martin J, Leport C, Morlat P, et al. Pyrimethamine-clarithromycin combination for therapy of acute Toxoplasma encephalitis in patients with AIDS. Antimicrob Agents Chemother 1991; 35:2049–2052.

122. Leport C, Bastuji-Garin S, Perronne C, et al. (Letter to the editor) An open study of the pyrimethamine-clindamycin combination in AIDS patients with brain toxoplasmosis. J Infect Dis 1989; 160:557–558.

123. Chirgwin K, Hafner R, Leport C, et al. Randomized phase II trial of atovaquone with pyrimethamine or sulfadiazine for treatment of TE in patients with acquired immunodeficiency syndrome: ACTG 237/ANRS 039 Study. AIDS Clinical Trials Group 237/Agence Nationale de Recherche sur le SIDA, Essai 039. Clin Infect Dis 2002; 34:1243–1250.

124. Saba J, Morlat P, Raffi F, et al. Pyrimethamine plus azithromycin for treatment of acute TE in patients with AIDS. Eur J Clin Microbiol Infect Dis 1993; 12:853–856.

125. Jacobson JM, Hafner R, Remington J, et al. Dose-escalation, phase I/II study of azithromycin and pyrimethamine for the treatment of TE in AIDS. AIDS 2001; 15:583–589.

126. Rabaud C, May T, Lucet JC, et al. Pulmonary toxoplasmosis in patients infected with human immunodeficiency virus: a French national study. Clin Infect Dis 1996; 23:1249–1254.

127. Walckenaer G, Leport C, Longuet P, et al. Relapses of brain toxoplasmosis (BT) in 15 AIDS patients. 31st Interscience Conference on Antimicrobial Agents and Chemotherapy, Chicago, Illinois: 1991.

128. Leport C, Tournerie C, Raguin G, et al. Long-term follow-up of patients with AIDS on maintenance therapy for toxoplasmosis. Eur J Clin Microbiol Infect Dis 1991; 10:191–193.

129. Podzamczer D, Miró J, Bolao F, et al. Twice-weekly maintenance therapy with sulfadiazine-pyrimethamine to prevent recurrent TE in patients with AIDS. Ann Intern Med 1995; 123:175–180.

130. Heald A, Flepp M, Chave J-P, et al. Treatment for cerebral toxoplasmosis protects against *Pneumocystis carinii* pneumonia in patients with AIDS. Ann Intern Med 1991; 115:760–763.

131. de Gans J, Portegies P, Reiss P, et al. Pyrimethamine alone as maintenance therapy for central nervous system toxoplasmosis in 38 patients with AIDS. J AIDS 1992; 5:137–142.

132. Foppa CU, Bini T, Gregis G, et al. A retrospective study of primary and maintenance therapy of TE with oral clindamycin and pyrimethamine. Eur J Clin Microbiol Infect Dis 1991; 10:187–189.

133. Girard P, Lepretre A, Detruchis P, et al. Failure of pyrimethamine-clindamycin combinations for prophylaxis of *Pneumocystis carinii* pneumonia. Lancet 1989; 8652:1459.

134. Ruf B, Schurmann D, Bergmann F, et al. Efficacy of pyrimethamine/sulfadoxine in the prevention of TE relapses and Pneumocystis carinii pneumonia in HIV-infected patients. Eur J Clin Microbiol Infect Dis 1993; 12:325–329.

135. Katlama C, Mouthon B, Gourdon D, et al. Atovaquone as long-term suppressive therapy for TE in patients with AIDS and multiple drug intolerance. AIDS 1996; 10:1107–1112.

136. Torres R, Weinberg W, Stansell J, et al. Atovaquone for salvage treatment and suppression of TE in patients with AIDS. Clin Infect Dis 1997; 24:422–429.

137. Mallolas J, Zamora L, Gatell JM, et al. Primary prophylaxis for Pneumocystis carinii pneumonia: a randomized trial comparing cotrimoxazole, aerosolized pentamidine and dapsone plus pyrimethamine. AIDS 1993; 7:59–64.

138. Benson CA, Kaplan JE, Masur H, et al. Treating opportunistic infections among HIV-infected adults and adolescents: recommendations from CDC, the National Institutes of Health, and the HIV Medicine Association/ Infectious Diseases Society of America. Clin Infect Dis 2005; 40:138–140.

139. Leport C, Chêne G, Morlat P, et al. Pyrimethamine for primary prophylaxis of TE in patients with human immunodeficiency virus infection: A double-blind, randomized trial. J Infect Dis 1996; 173:91–97.

140. Carr A, Tindall B, Brew BJ, et al. Low-dose trimethoprim-sulfamethoxazole prophylaxis for TE in patients with AIDS. Ann Intern Med 1992; 117:106–111.

141. Nicholas P, Pierone G, Lin J, et al. Trimethoprim-sulfamethoxazole in the prevention of cerebral toxoplasmosis. 6th International Conference on AIDS, San Francisco, CA: 1990.

142. O'Farrell N, Bradbeer C, Fitt S, et al. Cerebral toxoplasmosis and co-trimoxazole prophylaxis. Lancet 1991; 337:986.

143. Podzamczer D, Salazar A, Jiménez J, et al. Intermittent trimethoprim-sulfamethoxazole compared with dapsone-pyrimethamine for the simultaneous primary prophylaxis of Pneumocystis pneumonia and toxoplasmosis in patients infected with HIV. Ann Intern Med 1995; 122:755–761.

144. Podzamczer D, Santin M, Jimenez J, et al. Thrice-weekly cotrimoxazole is better than weekly dapsone-pyrimethamine for the primary prevention of *Pneumocystis carinii* pneumonia in HIV-infected patients. Aids 1993; 7:501–506.

145. Ruskin J, LaRiviere M. Low-dose co-trimoxazole for prevention of *Pneumocystis carinii* pneumonia in human immunodeficiency virus disease. Lancet 1991; 337:468–471.

146. Ribera E, Fernandez-Sola A, Juste C, et al. Comparison of high and low doses of trimethoprim-sulfamethoxazole for primary prevention of TE in human immunodeficiency virus-infected patients. Clinical Infect Dis 1999; 29:1461–1466.

147. Clumeck N. Some aspects of the epidemiology of toxoplasmosis and pneumocystosis in AIDS in Europe. Eur J Clin Microbiol Infect Dis 1991; 10:177–178.

148. Clotet B, Sirera G, Romeu J, et al. Twice-weekly dapsone-pyrimethamine for preventing PCP and cerebral toxoplasmosis. AIDS 1991; 5:601–602.

149. Köppen S, Grunewald T, Jautzke G, et al. Prevention of Pneumocystis carinii pneumonia and *TE* in human immunodeficiency virus infected patients: a clinical approach comparing aerosolized pentamidine and pyrimethamine/sulfadoxine. Clin Investig 1992; 70:508–512.

150. Girard P-M, Landman R, Gaudebout C, et al. Dapsone-pyrimethamine compared with aerosolized pentamidine as

a primary prophylaxis against *Pneumocystis carinii* pneumonia and toxoplasmosis in HIV infection. N Engl J Med 1993; 328:1514–1520.

151. Liesenfeld O, Wong SY, Remington JS. Toxoplasmosis in the setting of AIDS. In: Bartlett JG, Merigan TC, Bolognesi D, eds. Textbook of AIDS medicine. 2nd edn. Baltimore: Williams & Wilkins; 1999:225–259.

152. Subauste CS, Wessendarp M, Smulian AG, et al. Role of CD40 ligand signaling in defective type 1 cytokine response in human immunodeficiency virus infection. J Infect Dis 2001; 183:1722–1731.

153. Mussini C, Pezzotti P, Govoni A, et al. Discontinuation of Primary Prophylaxis for *Pneumocystis carinii*, pneumonia and TE in human immunodeficiency virus Type I-infected patients: The changes in opportunistic prophylaxis study. J Infect Dis 2000; 181:1635–1642.

154. Furrer H, Egger M, Opravil M, et al. Discontinuation of primary prophylaxis against Pneumocystis carinii pneumonia in HIV-1-infected adults treated with combination antiretroviral therapy. Swiss HIV Cohort Study. N Engl J Med 1999; 340:1301–1306.

155. Kirk O, Lundgren JD, Pedersen C, et al. Can chemoprophylaxis against opportunistic infections be discontinued after an increase in CD4 cells induced by highly active antiretroviral therapy? AIDS 1999; 13:1647–1651.

156. Furrer H, Opravil M, Bernasconi E, et al. Stopping primary prophylaxis in HIV-1-infected patients at high risk of toxoplasma encephalitis. Swiss HIV Cohort Study Lancet 2000; 355:2217–2218.

157. Miro JM, Podzamczer D, Pena JM, et al. Discontinuation of primary and secondary *Toxoplasma gondii* prophylaxis is safe in HIV-1 infected patients after immunological recovery with HAART. Final results of the GESIDA 94/98 study. Abstracts of the 39th Interscience Conference on Antimicrobial Agents and Chemotherapy, San Francisco, CA: 1998.

158. Soriano V, Dona C, Rodriguez-Rosado R, et al. Discontinuation of secondary prophylaxis for opportunistic infections in HIV-infected patients receiving highly active antiretroviral therapy. AIDS 2000; 14:383–386.

CHAPTER 37

Hepatitis Virus Infections

Marion Peters
Oren K. Fix

Introduction

Viral hepatitis has become one of the major causes of morbidity and mortality in HIV-infected individuals. For those on highly active antiretroviral therapy (HAART), co-infection with either hepatitis B virus (HBV) or hepatitis C virus (HCV) leads to accelerated progression to chronic hepatitis, cirrhosis, and hepatocellular carcinoma.[1] For those initiating HAART, co-infection is associated with higher rates of hepatotoxicity and immune recovery may be associated with reactivation of viral hepatitis, especially with HBV. For these reasons, understanding the basic epidemiology, natural history and therapy of viral hepatitis is essential in HIV-infected individuals. Since the introduction of HAART, immune restoration has prolonged the lives of HIV-infected patients. As a result, morbidity and mortality associated with chronic liver disease has emerged as a significant problem facing HCV-HIV-co-infected patients and their caregivers. Hepatotoxicity associated with HAART complicates the treatment of HBV/HCV-HIV co-infected patients, and anti-HCV treatment is complicated by lower response rates and toxic drug interactions. More studies are emerging that focus on the population of HCV-HIV co-infected persons, and our understanding of the natural history of co-infection in the current HAART era and the response to anti-HCV and HIV treatment has improved significantly.

Epidemiology

Hepatitis B is a partially double stranded DNA virus and a member of the hepadnavirus family. Worldwide, over 400 million individuals are infected with HBV, approximately two-thirds of cases in Asia and 25% in Africa.[2] The majority of individuals in these areas acquire HBV infection vertically at birth or in infancy, but infections can also be acquired by parenteral or sexual routes in adults. After exposure, the risk of development of chronic disease varies with age and immune status. Over 95% of neonates compared with <5% of adults exposed develop chronic hepatitis and approximately 20% of HIV-infected individuals who are exposed as adults develop chronic HBV.[3] The eight known genotypes vary in distribution geographically: predominantly genotypes B and C in Asia; genotype A in Northern Europe; genotype D in the Mediterranean and Middle East; genotype F in South America; and genotypes A and E in Africa.[2] Because of the diversity of the population in the USA, genotypes A through D are commonly found. Co-infection with HBV is seen in two different settings: in countries of high endemicity (Asia and Africa), HIV may affect those with a high background incidence of HBV; or both HIV and HBV infection may be acquired in adulthood through similar modes of transmission (USA, Europe). Thus co-infection with HBV and HIV varies geographically with up to 25.9% of HIV subjects in Nigeria being HBsAg positive compared with 6–10% of HIV subjects in the USA.[4]

Hepatitis C is an RNA flavivirus that infects approximately 2.7 million persons in the USA and an estimated 170 million persons worldwide. HCV is transmitted parenterally with the highest prevalence of HCV infection found among injection drug users, hemophiliacs who received pooled clotting factor concentrates, and recipients of multiple blood transfusions prior to testing. Due to the shared modes of transmission, co-infection with HCV and HIV is common and there are an estimated 150 000–300 000 co-infected with HCV and HIV in the USA.[5] A total of 25–30% of HIV-infected persons in the USA and Europe are infected with HCV, while 5–10% of HCV-infected persons are also infected with HIV.[6] The prevalence of HCV-HIV co-infection differs by the population studied: 50–90% of HIV-infected injection drug users; the majority of HIV-infected hemophiliacs; but 4–8% of HIV-infected homosexual men, which is similar to the prevalence found in HIV-negative homosexuals.[5,7] Sexual and vertical transmission of HCV is, at best, inefficient but co-infection with HIV and HCV increases the risk of perinatal transmission of either virus. Percutaneous exposure to infected blood carries a 30% risk of HBV transmission and a 3% risk of HCV transmission, compared with a 0.3% risk of HIV transmission. HCV-HIV co-infection is associated with higher HCV RNA levels and an accelerated rate of progression to cirrhosis.[6] In the USA, HIV individuals usually are infected with genotype 1 but in Europe other genotypes (2 and 3) are also found in HIV and genotype 4 is frequent in some IVDU populations.[6,8]

Natural History

Hepatitis B

Since the introduction of HAART in 1996, there has been a significant reduction in the occurrence of opportunistic infections, and liver disease has emerged as one of the leading causes of death in HIV patients. In a retrospective review, 50% of deaths in a cohort of HIV-infected patients in 1998 were due to end-stage liver disease.[1] Co-infection with hepatitis B and HIV leads to increased chronicity[3] and accelerated progression of liver disease to end-stage liver disease.[9] In the US HIV MACS cohort subjects with both HIV and HBV had a higher mortality from liver disease, especially if associated with a low CD4 nadir count.[9] In addition, HIV infection can lead to reactivation of HBV, higher HBV DNA levels and higher incidence of chronicity, likely associated with immunosuppression, as is seen after organ transplantation and chemotherapy.[4] Serum aminotransferases are usually lower in HIV co-infected individuals and are less useful in determining the need for therapy.

Hepatitis C

Co-infection with HIV is also associated with increased levels of HCV RNA and accelerated pro-

gression of HCV-related liver disease.[10] HIV seropositivity, alcohol consumption, older age at the time of HCV infection, and CD4 cell count <200 cells per μL have been shown to be associated with a higher rate of fibrosis progression.[11] Prior to the widespread use of HAART, HCV-HIV co-infection was associated with more rapid progression to cirrhosis: in one study, 7 years compared with 23 years in HCV-mono-infected patients;[12] and in another French study, from 26 years in HIV-infected subjects to 38 years in HCV mono-infected subjects.[13]

The effect of HCV infection on the natural history of HIV is controversial. The Swiss HIV Cohort Study,[14] a prospective cohort study of 3111 HIV-infected subjects receiving HAART, demonstrated an increased risk of progression to AIDS and death, as well as decreased CD4 cell recovery, in subjects co-infected with HCV compared with HCV-uninfected subjects. Even among subjects with well-controlled HIV replication, this study found that HCV-positive subjects had over three times the risk of developing AIDS-defining opportunistic illnesses and death compared with HCV-negative subjects.[14] Though the study initially reported delayed CD4 cell recovery 1 year after the start of HAART among HCV-positive subjects as compared with HCV-negative subjects, further data showed no difference in recovery of CD4 cells after 4 years of follow-up.[15] A prospective cohort study of 1955 subjects in an urban HIV clinic in Baltimore, Maryland, however, did not find differences in the progression to AIDS, death, or decline in CD4 cell count <200 cells/μL when comparing HCV-infected with HCV-uninfected subjects, even after controlling for the administration of HAART and well-controlled HIV replication.[16] In the subset of subjects receiving HAART, HCV-infected subjects had rates of well-controlled HIV replication that were similar to HCV-uninfected subjects, and in the subset of subjects receiving effective HAART, no difference was detected in the increase in absolute CD4 cell count and CD4 cell percentage up to 3 years after the start of HAART. From these and other data, the current consensus appears to be that HCV does not have a significant effect on the natural history of HIV disease nor does HCV alter the response to effective antiretroviral therapy in HCV and HIV co-infected patients.

Hepatitis A Virus

Hepatitis A virus (HAV) is an RNA virus that occurs worldwide in sporadic or epidemic forms. It is transmitted almost exclusively by the fecal-oral route, but can also be transmitted from person to person as a sexually transmitted disease, described primarily among homosexual men.[17] Risk factors for HAV infection in homosexual men include high numbers of sexual partners and sexual practices that involve oroanal contact.[18] A case-control study involving homosexual men with HIV-infection during a single, prolonged outbreak of acute HAV found that, at the onset of symptoms, HAV viral load was higher and the duration of HAV viremia was longer in HIV-infected subjects compared to HIV-uninfected subjects.[17] In this study, the ALT level in the HIV-infected subjects was lower than in HIV-uninfected subjects, corresponding to a less severe illness in HIV-infected subjects. Since hepatic injury in HAV is the result of the host immune response, immunosuppression in HIV can be predicted to result in a less severe and more prolonged HAV infection. Though this study was done after the introduction of HAART, no information on HAART use was provided and no correlation between duration or severity of HAV infection and CD4 cell counts was noted.

Diagnosis

Given the high prevalence of co-infection in certain populations, all HIV-infected persons should be screened for HCV and HBV infection. For diagnosis of acute HBV infection, hepatitis B surface antigen (HBsAg) and IgM antibody to hepatitis B core antigen (anti-HBc) are used. For chronic HBV infection, both HBsAg and total anti-HBc should be tested. If either is positive, then serum HBV DNA should be tested as atypical serologies occur with HBV and HIV co-infection. Some studies have shown HBV viremia in subjects whose only marker for HBV in the serum was total anti-HBc for over 2 years.[19] The prevalence of serum HBV DNA in individuals whose sole marker for HBV is total anti-HBc varies from 2–45% depending on the study, but viremia is rare in HBV mono-infected individuals.[20,21]

For chronic HCV infection, serum HCV antibody should be tested using an enzyme immunoassay (EIA). Positive EIA results should be confirmed by quantitative testing for HCV RNA. There is a 4–6% false negative rate with EIA in HIV infection, especially in those with low CD4 counts.[6] HIV-infected patients with undetectable HCV antibody should undergo HCV RNA testing if there is unexplained liver disease, such as elevated liver enzymes.

Evaluation and Management

Patients with viral hepatitis and HIV co-infection should be evaluated for the presence of chronic liver disease (Table 37.1). This should include history and physical examination for signs of chronic liver disease, as well as measurement of serum albumin, aminotransferases (AST and ALT), bilirubin, prothrombin time, and platelet count. Histologic evaluation by liver biopsy is at present the most reliable method to determine disease activity and fibrosis stage. Although there is great interest in serum markers of fibrosis, at present they are optimal in determining inactive disease and cirrhosis but relatively poor in differentiating intermediate fibrosis stages.[22] Screening for hepatocellular carcinoma with α-fetoprotein and imaging is recommended for HBV patients over 40 years or with family history and for those HCV patients with cirrhosis.

Patients should be vaccinated against hepatitis A and hepatitis B if they are susceptible.[23] Vaccination against HAV is safe and well-tolerated and confers protective immunity in virtually all healthy recipients. However, lower responses are noted in older subjects, patients with liver disease and immune suppressed individuals.[23] Prior to the introduction of HAART, vaccination with two double-doses of HAV vaccine, given either 1 or 6 months apart, resulted in a protective serologic response in 88% of HIV-infected homosexual men compared with 100% response in HIV-uninfected homosexual men.[18] A CD4 cell count >200 cells/μL correlated with an increased chance of seroconversion and a higher titer of anti-HAV antibody, but those initiating HAART after a nadir CD4 cell count of <50 cells/μL demonstrated even lower response rates to HAV vaccination, with 46% seroconverting after two vaccinations. For HBV vaccine, the responses are low (47%):

Table 37.1 Monitoring clinical status of patients with liver disease

Synthetic function	Prothrombin time, serum albumin
Inflammation	AST, ALT, liver biopsy
Fibrosis	Liver biopsy, serum markers
Hepatocellular carcinoma	α-fetoprotein, imaging studies
Check HAV and HBV status	Vaccinate to HAV and HBV if not immune

HAV, hepatitis A virus; HBV, hepatitis B virus; AST, aspartate aminotransferase; ALT, alanine transferase.

even using double dose (40 µg), in those with CD4 cell counts ≥350, only 64% of individuals responded.[24] This suggests that, even with HAART-induced restoration of immune function, HIV-infected patients may have an inadequate response to HAV and HBV vaccinations.

Treatment

The goal of treatment of viral hepatitis is to decrease viral replication, to lessen symptoms, to improve histology with decrease in inflammation and fibrosis, and thus to decrease progression to cirrhosis and hepatocellular carcinoma and ultimately to improve life-time survival.

HBV Therapy

The first critical question in HBV and HIV co-infected individuals is whether the patient requires HIV or HBV therapy, or both. If HIV therapy is also indicated, then an anti-HBV drug must be included as part of the antiretroviral (ART) regimen. If however HIV therapy is not indicated, then a drug with HBV but no HIV efficacy should be used to treat the HBV infection (Table 37.2). The majority of patients with HBV worldwide have immune controlled and inactive disease with HBsAg positivity but normal liver enzymes and low titer HBV DNA in serum. Activation of HBV can occur at any time and is manifest by the presence of HBeAg in serum, elevated serum aminotransferases and elevated serum HBV DNA ($>10^5$ copies/mL). In addition to the goals of therapy noted above, goals specific for the management of HBV infection are seroconversion from HBeAg to anti-HBe and ultimately loss of HBsAg with seroconversion to anti-HBs.[2] Mutations in the core gene can lead to inability to produce HBeAg in the presence of active viral replication (elevated HBV DNA and serum aminotransferases with no HBeAg in serum) so called 'precore mutant' HBV infection. This type of infection is increasing worldwide particularly in those infected since birth with genotypes B and C (Asia) and D (Mediterranean). HBeAg seroconversion is not an endpoint for these pre-core mutants and long-term therapy is the rule. In immune suppressed patients, serum HBV DNA is higher and reactivation of HBV infection occurs with recovery of immune control, usually 8–12 weeks after starting ART therapy. In addition, seroconversion to anti-HBe and anti-HBs are less commonly achieved with HIV co-infection and long-term therapy is the rule. Caution should be used in comparing measurements of HBV DNA, which vary between studies and laboratories with multiple different assays using different lower limits of detection.

Currently licensed therapies for the treatment of HBV infection are interferon alpha, an immunomodulatory agent, and nucleos(t)ide analogs lamivudine (3TC, Epivir), adefovir dipivoxil (Hepsera) and entecavir (Baraclude). In addition, tenofovir disoproxil (Viread) and emtricitabine (FTC) are licensed for HIV but have activity against HBV (Table 37.2).

Recombinant α-interferons were the first drugs approved for the treatment of hepatitis B infection. However, their use in HIV co-infection is limited as response rates have generally been poor. Studies of newer pegylated interferons in HBV are limited to those without HIV infection and show benefit of pegylated forms over standard conventional IFN in both HBV HBeAg positive and negative disease, with control of HBV DNA in 41–73%.[25] Predictors of response were female gender, low serum HBV DNA levels and high serum ALT. The latter two are uncommonly found in HBV-HIV co-infection and thus interferon is rarely used at this time.

Nucleos(t)ides are competitive inhibitors of HBV DNA polymerase (reverse transcriptase) causing premature termination of DNA chain elongation,

Table 37.2 Therapies for HBV

Drug	Dose/day	Treats wild type HBV	Treats YMDD	Treats HIV
LAM/3TC	100 mg	Yes	No	Yes
ADV	10 mg	Yes	Yes	No
TDF	300 mg	Yes	Yes	Yes
FTC	200 mg	Yes	Yes	Yes
Entecavir	0.5 mg	Yes	Yes (1 mg/day)	No
Telbivudine	600 mg	Yes	No	No

LAM, lamivudine; ADV, adefovir dipivoxil; TDF, tenofovir disoproxil; FTC, emtricitabine.

resulting in inhibition of viral replication. However, the inhibition of polymerases is non-specific, and can also bind to human DNA polymerase. Thus, there is a potential to induce mitochondrial toxicity and multi-organ failure and mitochondrial toxicity has been implicated in the etiology of some of the dose-limiting adverse effects such as peripheral neuropathy, lactic acidosis, and steatosis associated with nucleoside analogs. For the management of HBV infection there are now an increasing number of nucleotide and nucleoside analogs which are active against wild type HBV and some against HBV with YMDD and other compensatory mutations with choices for treatment of HBV and HIV or for HBV alone (Table 37.2). Lamivudine was the first oral drug licensed for HBV with few side-effects and daily therapy. In HBV-HIV individuals, it decreases HBV DNA by 4 logs after 48 weeks of therapy.[26] However, resistance to lamivudine increases with time on therapy and is more rapid in patients co-infected with HIV, with 90% of subjects who have HIV and HBV developing HBV resistance to lamivudine by 4 years.[27] Adefovir has been used successfully in co-infected individuals for up to 4 years with no reports as yet of resistance.[28] However, resistance up to 18% after 4 years has been reported in mono-infected HBV individuals who have HBeAg negative disease (Locarnini EASL 2005, abstract). Other drugs with HBV activity are emtricitabine and tenofovir disoproxil, which have activity against HBV and HIV and are approved for the treatment of HIV infection. They are being studied for the treatment of HBV infection and early data suggests that they will be useful in the treatment of co-infected individuals.[29,30] Entecavir has no HIV activity but good HBV activity and is also being studied in HBV-HIV co-infected individuals.[30]

HCV Therapy

Initial treatment trials of HCV-HIV co-infection using standard interferon and ribavirin had disappointingly low rates of sustained viral response and high rates of side effects. Three important multicenter, randomized trials investigating the use of pegylated interferon and ribavirin in HCV-HIV co-infected patients were recently published, and reported more favorable response rates. The AIDS Clinical Trials Group (ACTG) A5071 study compared treatment of HCV-HIV co-infected subjects with pegylated interferon α-2a plus ribavirin (in escalating doses) with standard interferon α-2a plus ribavirin.[31] Treatment with pegylated interferon and

ribavirin was associated with a significantly higher rate of sustained viral response (SVR: undetectable HCV RNA 24 weeks after cessation of therapy) compared with standard interferon and ribavirin (27% versus 12%). The APRICOT study randomized subjects to pegylated interferon α-2a plus ribavirin, pegylated interferon alfa-2a plus placebo, or standard interferon α-2a plus ribavirin.[32] Again, the overall rate of sustained viral response was significantly higher in the pegylated interferon plus ribavirin group (40%), compared with pegylated interferon plus placebo (12%), or standard interferon plus ribavirin (20%). Despite high CD4 cell counts in both these trials, the rate of sustained viral response with pegylated interferon and ribavirin was lower than the rates observed in HCV-mono-infection using similar therapy (54–63%).[33] A third multicenter, randomized trial (RIBAVIC) similarly compared the response to pegylated interferon α-2b plus ribavirin with standard interferon α-2b plus ribavirin in HCV-HIV co-infected subjects.[34] The overall sustained viral response rate was 27% in the pegylated interferon group, >20% in the standard interferon group. Possible reasons for the lower response rates in these trials compared with similar treatment regimens in HCV-mono-infection include insufficient early ribavirin dosage, higher prevalence of cirrhosis (in the ACTG A5071 and RIBAVIC trials), and higher HCV RNA levels seen in HCV-HIV co-infection. Antiviral therapy in both trials was well tolerated and did not adversely affect control of HIV disease. Despite reduced CD4 cell counts, the percentage of CD4 cells increased, and HIV RNA levels did not increase during the study periods. All three trials showed a significantly lower sustained viral response rate for subjects with HCV genotype 1 compared with genotypes 2 and 3, a phenomenon that is also seen with treatment in HCV-mono-infection. These trials also demonstrated lower response rates in genotypes 2 and 3 compared with similar treatment regimens for HCV-mono-infection. Therefore, 48 weeks of therapy is recommended in HCV-HIV co-infected patients with genotypes 2 and 3 compared with only 24 weeks in patients who are not infected with HIV (Table 37.3).

In the ACTG A5071 trial, improvement in liver histology was seen in 35% of a subset of subjects who did not have a virologic response.[31] This finding suggests a role for interferon maintenance therapy to slow the progression of liver fibrosis in HCV-HIV co-infected patients. For genotype 1 subjects, studies are underway to evaluate the use of long-term low-dose therapy to decrease progression of fibrosis in those who fail to respond with clearance of virus.

Table 37.3 Monitor therapy in HIV patients co-infected with HCV or HBV

	Therapy	Monitor
HBV	Nucleos(t)ide analogs Long-term therapy the rule Always add anti-HBV drug to ART	Chose drug depending upon need for concomitant HIV therapy AST, ALT for inflammation HBV DNA 3-monthly Monitor for resistance
HCV	Pegylated IFN and ribavirin 48 weeks for all genotypes Decision: HCV RNA at 12 weeks Cytokine support for cytopenias	CBC closely for pancytopenia AST, ALT monthly TSH 3-monthly If ≥2 log drop in HCV RNA from baseline, continue for 48 weeks

HBV, hepatitis B virus; HCV, hepatitis C virus; AST, aspartate aminotransferase; ALT, alanine transferase; CBC, complete blood count.

Therapy should be monitored closely for side-effects of interferon and ribavirin therapy, including flu-like symptoms; interferon-associated thyroid dysfunction; neuropsychiatric disorders such as depression, irritability, and insomnia; and cytopenias, such as neutropenia, lymphopenia, anemia, and thrombocytopenia. The frequency of these side-effects in the treatment of HCV-HIV co-infected subjects did not differ significantly from what was observed in the treatment of HCV-mono-infected subjects.[31,32] As seen in the major pegylated interferon treatment trials, lymphopenia may be associated with a decrease in absolute CD4 cell count; however, CD4 cell percentage is typically unchanged or increased, with no observed additional risk for infection.[5,31] Another concern in the treatment of HCV-HIV co-infected patients is the potential for drug interactions between ribavirin and nucleoside reverse transcriptase inhibitors. Ribavirin, a guanosine nucleoside analog, interferes with the intracellular phosphorylation of pyrimidine 2′, 3′-dideoxynucleosides, including zidovudine, zalcitabine, and stavudine. Ribavirin also increases the phosphorylation of didanosine and may lead to increased toxicity, including pancreatitis and mitochondrial dysfunction.[35,36] The combination of didanosine and ribavirin should be avoided, and the combination of zidovudine or stavudine with ribavirin should be used with caution.

Guidelines for the treatment of HCV in co-infected patients suggest the optimization of HAART before initiating HCV therapy, particularly when the CD4 cell count is <350 cells/μL.[6] Ideal candidates for HCV treatment have CD4 cell counts >350 cells/μL and HIV RNA <50 000 copies/mL. Similar to the treatment of HCV-mono-infection, lack of an early virologic response (EVR: a decrease in HCV RNA by at least 2 log after 12 weeks of therapy) predicts non-response and treatment should be discontinued (Table 37.3).[31] In those with EVR, 50% will have a sustained virologic response, with clearance of HCV noted 6 months after stopping therapy, but half will relapse. In contrast to treatment of HCV-mono-infection, treatment duration in HCV-HIV co-infection should be 48 weeks in all HCV genotypes. Whether long-term therapy in non-responders will lead to histologic benefit is presently being evaluated.

Antiretroviral-associated Hepatotoxicity

All classes of antiretroviral drugs have been associated with the development of hepatotoxicity, defined by significant elevations in liver enzymes.[37] Hepatotoxicity may be dose-dependent or idiosyncratic (unpredictable due to hypersensitivity or a metabolic abnormality). In recent studies of hepatotoxicity associated with HAART, the risk of hepatotoxicity has been consistently associated with elevated baseline transaminases and the presence of HBV or HCV co-infection.[38–46] Proposed mechanisms of hepatotoxicity include decreased drug metabolism, immune restoration, and mitochondrial dysfunction.[5] Despite the increased risk of hepatotoxicity in the setting of HCV or HBV co-infection, most (80–90%) co-infected patients do not develop hepatotoxicity.[40]

Studies that have followed subjects after the onset of biochemical hepatotoxicity have demonstrated that significant clinical hepatotoxicity is rare, and transaminases return to baseline in the majority of cases even if the offending medication is continued (adaptation).[39,47] Therefore, it is probably not necessary to discontinue HAART if hepatotoxicity develops, unless the patient is symptomatic, hypersensitivity associated (fever, lymphadenopathy, rash) or there are significant elevations in the aminotransferases.

Although the incidence of antiretroviral-associated hepatotoxicity increased with the introduction of protease inhibitors (PI), establishing a direct link between PI and liver impairment has been difficult. High-dose ritonavir is associated with increased hepatotoxicity compared to boosted ritonavir[40] and other PI.[41,48,49] Other studies report an association between indinavir use and liver toxicity.[50,51] The risk of developing severe liver impairment with saquinavir, nelfinavir, lopinavir, and amprenavir is reportedly low.[51,52]

Of the non-nucleoside reverse transcriptase inhibitors (NNRTI), nevirapine (NVP) is consistently associated with an increased risk of hepatotoxicity in several studies.[42,53,54] Several reported cases of severe liver toxicity, some fatal, are associated with NVP use for post-exposure prophylaxis.[55] Risk factors proposed for NVP-induced hepatotoxicity are conflicting but have included higher baseline CD4 count, female sex, HBV or HCV co-infection, alcohol consumption, wasting, concomitant use of stavudine, and abnormal baseline liver function abnormalities. Nevirapine hepatotoxicity commonly occurs early in treatment suggesting an idiosyncratic mechanism. However, in other reports, the hepatotoxicity of NVP-containing regimens had a later onset of >120 days, with the risk increasing with an increasing duration of treatment and in cirrhotics.[43,56] An exposure-toxicity relationship has been established in a single study showing a direct correlation between plasma NVP concentrations and hepatotoxicity independent of the presence of HCV co-infection, which contrasts with other findings.[57] One study[58] showed higher NVP levels in subjects with higher aminotransferase levels and in HBV or HCV co-infected subjects, while another study[59] showed no correlation between high NVP levels and high aminotransferase levels.

Efavirenz (EFV) has been associated with a lower risk of hepatotoxicity compared with NVP in two studies, where the rate of severe toxicity was 16% and 12% for NVP and 8% and 4% for EFV, respectively.[60,61] However, at least one study found an increased risk associated with EFV compared with NVP.[44] Others reported low rates of 1.4% and 1.1% for NVP and EFV, respectively.[62] There is clearly an increased risk of hepatotoxicity with the use of both NVP and EFV compared with the use of either drug alone.[53,54] The NNRTI are substrates for cytochrome P450 metabolic pathways, so variability in drug metabolism between individuals may explain hepatotoxicity. It remains unclear whether NNRTI-associated hepatotoxicity is dose-dependent or idiosyncratic.

The majority of nucleoside reverse transcriptase inhibitors (NRTI) can cause mitochondrial toxicity and have the potential to cause liver injury. NRTI inhibit γ-DNA polymerase, the enzyme responsible for mitochondrial DNA replication. Cases of lactic acidosis and steatosis are more frequently reported with didanosine, stavudine, or zidovudine. It is believed that cumulative exposure to NRTI is a factor in the development of lactic acidosis.

Liver Transplantation

Prior to the widespread use of HAART, HIV infection was considered an absolute contraindication to solid organ transplantation, including orthotopic liver transplantation, because of the high mortality rate of opportunistic infection associated with HIV and anti-rejection immunosuppression.[6,63] With restoration of immune function using HAART, post-transplant survival appears to be comparable with that seen among HIV-negative liver transplant recipients. Many transplantation centers in the USA and Europe have begun to investigate the outcomes related to solid organ transplants in HIV-positive recipients. A study of orthotopic liver transplantation in HIV-positive patients at several centers found no difference in post-transplant survival compared with age- and race-comparable HIV-negative patients.[63] While subjects in the cohort with HCV-HIV co-infection had shorter post-transplantation survival compared with HCV-negative subjects, survival was similar to that of comparable HCV mono-infected recipients. Survival in this cohort was also poorer among subjects with post-transplant antiretroviral intolerance, post-transplant CD4 cell count <200 cells/μL, and post-transplant HIV viral load >400 copies/mL. In contrast, pre-transplant antiretroviral intolerance, CD4 cell count, and HIV viral load were not associated with decreased survival.

Conclusion

Viral hepatitis is increasingly being recognized in HIV-infected individuals and has become one of the major causes of morbidity and mortality. Co-infection with either hepatitis B or hepatitis C leads to accelerated progression to chronic hepatitis, cirrhosis, and hepatocellular carcinoma. In addition, co-infection with either HBV or HCV is associated with higher rates of hepatotoxicity and immune recovery may be associated with reactivation of viral hepatitis, especially with HBV. Selection of therapy for HIV mandates understanding the HBV and HCV status of the individual. All individuals should be evaluated for co-infections and vaccinations for HAV and HBV performed if needed. Our understanding of the natural history of viral hepatitis and HIV in the current ART era and the response to anti-HCV and HIV treatment has improved significantly over recent years.

References

1. Bica I, McGovern B, Dhar R, et al. Increasing mortality due to end-stage liver disease in patients with human immunodeficiency virus infection. Clin Infect Dis 2001; 32:492–497.
2. Lai CL, Ratziu V, Yuen MF, et al. Viral hepatitis B. Lancet 2003; 362:2089–2094.
3. Hadler SC, Judson FN, O'Malley PM, et al. Outcome of hepatitis B virus infection in homosexual men and its relation to prior human immunodeficiency virus infection. J Infect Dis 1991; 163:454–459.
4. Thio CL. Hepatitis B in the human immunodeficiency virus-infected patient: epidemiology, natural history, and treatment. Semin Liver Dis 2003; 23:125–136.
5. Sulkowski MS, Thomas DL. Hepatitis C in the HIV-infected person. Ann Intern Med 2003; 138:197–207.
6. Rockstroh JK, Spengler U. HIV and hepatitis C virus co-infection. Lancet Infect Dis 2004; 4:437–444.
7. Goedert JJ, Brown DL, Hoots K, et al. Human immunodeficiency and hepatitis virus infections and their associated conditions and treatments among people with haemophilia. Haemophilia 2004; 10(Suppl):205–210.
8. Soriano V, Nunez M, Sanchez-Conde M, et al. Response to interferon-based therapies in HIV-infected patients with chronic hepatitis C due to genotype 4. Antivir Ther 2005; 10:167–170.
9. Thio CL, Seaberg EC, Skolasky R, Jr, et al. HIV-1, hepatitis B virus, and risk of liver-related mortality in the Multicenter Cohort Study (MACS). Lancet 2002; 360:1921–1926.
10. Sherman KE, Rouster SD, Chung RT, et al. Hepatitis C Virus prevalence among patients infected with Human Immunodeficiency Virus: a cross-sectional analysis of the US adult AIDS Clinical Trials Group. Clin Infect Dis 2002; 34:831–837.
11. Benhamou Y, Di MV, Bochet M, et al. Factors affecting liver fibrosis in human immunodeficiency virus-and hepatitis C virus-coinfected patients: impact of protease inhibitor therapy. Hepatology 2001; 34:283–287.
12. Soto B, Sanchez-Quijano A, Rodrigo L, et al. Human immunodeficiency virus infection modifies the natural history of chronic parenterally-acquired hepatitis C with an unusually rapid progression to cirrhosis [see comments]. J Hepatol 1997; 26:1–5.
13. Benhamou Y, Bochet M, Di Martino V, et al. Liver fibrosis progression in human immunodeficiency virus and hepatitis C virus coinfected patients. The Multivirc Group. Hepatol 1999; 30:1054–1058.
14. Greub G, Ledergerber B, Battegay M, et al. Clinical progression, survival, and immune recovery during antiretroviral therapy in patients with HIV-1 and hepatitis C virus coinfection: the Swiss HIV Cohort Study. Lancet 2000; 356:1800–1805.
15. Kaufmann GR, Perrin L, Pantaleo G, et al. CD4 T-lymphocyte recovery in individuals with advanced HIV-1 infection receiving potent antiretroviral therapy for 4 years: the Swiss HIV Cohort Study. Arch Intern Med 2003; 163:2187–2195.
16. Sulkowski MS, Moore RD, Mehta SH, et al. Hepatitis C and progression of HIV disease. JAMA 2002; 288:199–206.
17. Ida S, Tachikawa N, Nakajima A, et al. Influence of human immunodeficiency virus type 1 infection on acute hepatitis A virus infection. Clin Infect Dis 2002; 34:379–385.
18. Neilsen GA, Bodsworth NJ, Watts N. Response to hepatitis A vaccination in human immunodeficiency virus-infected and -uninfected homosexual men. J Infect Dis 1997; 176:1064–1067.
19. Hofer M, Joller-Jemelka HI, Grob PJ, et al. Swiss HIV Cohort Study. Frequent chronic hepatitis B virus infection in HIV-infected patients positive for antibody to hepatitis B core antigen only. Eur J Clin Microbiol Infect Dis 1998; 17:6–13.
20. Mphahlele MJ, Lukhwareni A, Burnett RJ, et al. High risk of occult hepatitis B virus infection in HIV-positive patients from South Africa. J Clin Virol 2006; 35:14–20.
21. Shire NJ, Rouster SD, Rajicic N, et al. Occult hepatitis B in HIV-infected patients. J Acquir Immune Defic Syndr 2004; 36:869–875.
22. Bissell DM. Assessing fibrosis without a liver biopsy: are we there yet? Gastroenterology 2004; 127:1847–1849.
23. Murdoch DL, Goa K, Figgitt DP. Combined hepatitis A and B vaccines: a review of their immunogenicity and tolerability. Drugs 2003; 63:2625–2649.
24. Fonseca MO, Pang LW, de Paula CN, et al. Randomized trial of recombinant hepatitis B vaccine in HIV-infected adult patients comparing a standard dose to a double dose. Vaccine 2005; 23:2902–2908.
25. Marcellin P, Lau GK, Bonino F, et al. Peginterferon alfa-2a alone, lamivudine alone, and the two in combination in patients with HBeAg-negative chronic hepatitis B. N Engl J Med 2004; 351:1206–1217.
26. Benhamou Y, Katlama C, Lunel F, et al. Effects of lamivudine on replication of hepatitis B virus in HIV-infected men. Ann Intern Med 1996; 125:705–712.
27. Benhamou Y, Bochet M, Thibault V, et al. Long-term incidence of hepatitis B virus resistance to lamivudine in human immunodeficiency virus-infected patients. Hepatology 1999; 30:1302–1306.
28. Benhamou Y, Bochet M, Thibault V, et al. Safety and efficacy of adefovir dipivoxil in patients co-infected with HIV-1 and lamivudine-resistant hepatitis B virus: an open-label pilot study. Lancet 2001; 358:718–723.
29. Peters M, Anderson J, Lynch P, et al. Randomized controlled study of tenofovir and adefovir in chronic hepatitis B virus and HIV infection: ACTG AS127. Hepatology 2006; 44:1110–1116.
30. Quan DJ, Peters MG. Antiviral therapy: nucleotide and nucleoside analogs. Clin Liver Dis 2004; 8:371–385.
31. Chung RT, Andersen J, Volberding P, et al. Peginterferon Alfa-2a plus ribavirin versus interferon alfa-2a plus ribavirin for chronic hepatitis C in HIV-coinfected persons. N Engl J Med 2004; 351:451–459.
32. Torriani FJ, Rodriguez-Torres M, Rockstroh JK, et al. Peginterferon alfa-2a plus ribavirin for chronic hepatitis C virus infection in HIV-infected patients. N Engl J Med 2004; 351:438–450.
33. Hadziyannis SJ, Sette H Jr, Morgan TR, et al. Peginterferon-alpha2a and ribavirin combination therapy in chronic hepatitis C: a randomized study of treatment duration and ribavirin dose. Ann Intern Med 2004; 140:346–355.
34. Carrat F, Bani-Sadr F, Pol S, et al. Pegylated interferon alfa-2b vs standard interferon alfa-2b, plus ribavirin, for chronic hepatitis C in HIV-infected patients: a randomized controlled trial. JAMA 2004; 292:2839–2848.
35. Moreno A, Quereda C, Moreno L, et al. High rate of didanosine-related mitochondrial toxicity in HIV/HCV-coinfected patients receiving ribavirin. Antivir Ther 2004; 9:133–138.
36. Rockstroh JK, Reichel C, Hille H, et al. Pharmacokinetics of azidothymidine and its major metabolite glucuronylazidothymidine in hemophiliacs coinfected with human immunodeficiency virus and chronic hepatitis C. Am J Ther 1998; 5:387–391.

37. Pol S, Lebray P, Vallet-Pichard A. HIV infection and hepatic enzyme abnormalities: intricacies of the pathogenic mechanisms. Clin Infect Dis 2004; 38(Suppl):65–72.

38. Kontorinis N, Dieterich DT. Toxicity of non-nucleoside analogue reverse transcriptase inhibitors. Semin Liver Dis 2003; 23:173–182.

39. Stern JO, Robinson PA, Love J, et al. A comprehensive hepatic safety analysis of nevirapine in different populations of HIV-infected patients. J Acquir Immune Defic Syndr 2003; 34:S21–S33.

40. Sulkowski MS, Mehta SH, Chaisson RE, et al. Hepatotoxicity associated with protease inhibitor-based antiretroviral regimens with or without concurrent ritonavir. AIDS 2004; 18:2277–2284.

41. Sulkowski MS, Thomas DL, Chaisson RE, et al. Hepatotoxicity associated with antiretroviral therapy in adults infected with human immunodeficiency virus and the role of hepatitis C or B virus infection. JAMA 2000; 283:74–80.

42. Torti C, Lapadula G, Casari S, et al. Incidence and risk factors for liver enzyme elevation during highly active antiretroviral therapy in HIV-HCV co-infected patients: results from the Italian EPOKA-MASTER Cohort. BMC Infect Dis 2005; 5:58.

43. Martinez E, Blanco JL, Arnaiz JA, et al. Hepatotoxicity in HIV-1-infected patients receiving nevirapine-containing antiretroviral therapy. AIDS 2001; 15:1261–1268.

44. Meraviglia P, Schiavini M, Castagna A, et al. Lopinavir/ritonavir treatment in HIV antiretroviral-experienced patients: evaluation of risk factors for liver enzyme elevation. HIV Med 2004; 5:334–343.

45. Saves M, Vandentorren S, Daucourt V, et al. Severe hepatic cytolysis: incidence and risk factors in patients treated by antiretroviral combinations. Aquitaine Cohort, France, 1996–1998. Groupe d'Epidemiologie Clinique de Sida en Aquitaine (GECSA). AIDS 1999; 13:115–121.

46. Monforte AA, Bugarini R, Pezzotti P, et al. Low frequency of severe hepatotoxicity and association with HCV coinfection in HIV-positive patients treated with HAART. J Acquir Immune Defic Syndr 2001; 28:114–123.

47. Sherman KE, Shire NJ, Cernohous P, et al. Liver injury and changes in hepatitis C Virus (HCV) RNA load associated with protease inhibitor-based antiretroviral therapy for treatment-naive HCV-HIV-coinfected patients: lopinavir-ritonavir versus nelfinavir. Clin Infect Dis 2005; 41:1186–1195.

48. Bonfanti P, Landonio S, Ricci E, et al. Risk factors for hepatotoxicity in patients treated with highly active antiretroviral therapy. J Acquir Immune Defic Syndr 2001; 27:316–318.

49. Aceti A, Pasquazzi C, Zechini B, et al. Hepatotoxicity development during antiretroviral therapy containing protease inhibitors in patients with HIV: the role of hepatitis B and C virus infection. J Acquir Immune Defic Syndr 2002; 29:41–48.

50. Matsuda J, Gohchi K. Severe hepatitis in patients with AIDS and haemophilia B treated with indinavir. Lancet 1997; 350:364.

51. Kontorinis N, Dieterich D. Hepatotoxicity of antiretroviral therapy. AIDS Rev 2003; 5:36–43.

52. Gonzalez-Requena D, Nunez M, Jimenez-Nacher I, et al. Short communication: liver toxicity of lopinavir-containing regimens in HIV-infected patients with or without hepatitis C coinfection. AIDS Res Hum Retroviruses 2004; 20:698–700.

53. Law WP, Dore GJ, Duncombe CJ, et al. Risk of severe hepatotoxicity associated with antiretroviral therapy in the HIV-NAT Cohort, Thailand, 1996–2001. AIDS 2003; 17:2191–2199.

54. van Leth F, Phanuphak P, Ruxrungtham K, et al. Comparison of first-line antiretroviral therapy with regimens including nevirapine, efavirenz, or both drugs, plus stavudine and lamivudine: a randomised open-label trial, the 2NN Study. Lancet 2004; 363:1253–1263.

55. Benn PD, Mercey DE, Brink N, et al. Prophylaxis with a nevirapine-containing triple regimen after exposure to HIV-1. Lancet 2001; 357:687–688.

56. Bonnet F, Lawson-Ayayi S, Thiebaut R, et al. A cohort study of nevirapine tolerance in clinical practice: French Aquitaine Cohort, 1997-1999. Clin Infect Dis 2002; 35:1231–1237.

57. Nunez M, Gonzalez-Requena D, Gonzalez-Lahoz J, et al. Short communication: interactions between nevirapine plasma levels, chronic hepatitis C, and the development of liver toxicity in HIV-infected patients. AIDS Res Hum Retroviruses 2003; 19:187–188.

58. Almond LM, Boffito M, Hoggard PG, et al. The relationship between nevirapine plasma concentrations and abnormal liver function tests. AIDS Res Hum Retroviruses 2004; 20:716–722.

59. Dailly E, Billaud E, Reliquet V, et al. No relationship between high nevirapine plasma concentration and hepatotoxicity in HIV-1-infected patients naive of antiretroviral treatment or switched from protease inhibitors. Eur J Clin Pharmacol 2004; 60:343–348.

60. Martin-Carbonero L, Nunez M, Gonzalez-Lahoz J, et al. Incidence of liver injury after beginning antiretroviral therapy with efavirenz or nevirapine. HIV Clin Trials 2003; 4:115–120.

61. Sulkowski MS, Thomas DL, Mehta SH, et al. Hepatotoxicity associated with nevirapine or efavirenz-containing antiretroviral therapy: role of hepatitis C and B infections. Hepatology 2002; 35:182–189.

62. Palmon R, Koo BC, Shoultz DA, et al. Lack of hepatotoxicity associated with nonnucleoside reverse transcriptase inhibitors. J Acquir Immune Defic Syndr 2002; 29:340–345.

63. Ragni MV, Belle SH, Im K, et al. Survival of human immunodeficiency virus-infected liver transplant recipients. J Infect Dis 2003; 188:1412–1420.

CHAPTER 38

Bartonella Infections in HIV-infected Individuals

Jane E. Koehler

Historical Perspective

Bacillary angiomatosis (BA) was first described by Stoler and colleagues in 1983[1] in an HIV-infected patient with multiple subcutaneous nodules. Numerous bacilli were observed by Warthin–Starry staining of the biopsied nodules, and the subcutaneous masses resolved during erythromycin therapy. Subsequently, the BA bacilli visualized using the Warthin–Starry silver stain were noted to have an appearance similar to that of the cat scratch disease (CSD) bacillus.[2,3] The BA bacillus remained refractory to isolation attempts for many years, impeding identification efforts. Studies of bacterial DNA extracted from BA lesions subsequently identified the bacillus as closely related to *Bartonella* (*Rochalimaea*) *quintana*,[4] and after isolation of the bacillus from the blood of two HIV-infected patients without BA,[5] the organism was further characterized and named *B. henselae* in 1992.[6,7] The *Bartonella* genus has expanded from a single species in 1993 to >20 species. The BA bacillus was directly cultivated from cutaneous BA lesions for the first time in 1992, which led to the identification of two species of the genus *Bartonella* as causative agents of BA: *B. henselae* or *B. quintana*.[8] To date, the *Bartonella* species causing BA has been identified in more than 60 AIDS patients; in all these cases, only two species have been found to cause BA or bacillary peliosis hepatis.[8,9] Interestingly, the two different species differ in the predilection to form a specific type of lesion. *Bartonella henselae*, but never *B. quintana*, has been associated with peliosis of the liver or spleen, or both.[9] *Bartonella henselae* also is associated with lymphadenopathy, and *B. quintana* with subcutaneous nodules in late stage HIV infection.[9]

Clinical Presentation of *Bartonella* Infections

In patients with severe immunosuppression due to HIV infection, organ transplantation or chemotherapy, infection with *B. henselae* or *B. quintana* can produce unique vascular proliferative lesions known as BA.[10,11] BA occurs as a late manifestation of HIV infection; in a study of 42 patients with BA, the median CD4 lymphocyte count was 21 cells/mm[3].[12] These vascular proliferative lesions can form in many different organs, including skin, bone, brain parenchyma, lymph nodes, bone marrow and gastrointestinal and respiratory tract. A histopathologically different vascular proliferative response to *Bartonella* infection, known as bacillary peliosis hepatis (BP), is seen in the liver and spleen.[13] One notable aspect of focal *Bartonella* infection, especially cutaneous BA, is the chronic, indolent nature of the disease: lesions may be present for as long as 1 year before a diagnosis is made.[8,12]

HIV-infected individuals also can develop manifestations of *Bartonella* infection other than vascular proliferation. Bacteremia with[14] or without[5,6] endocarditis has been reported in HIV-infected individuals, in the absence of focal BA or BP involvement. Patients with higher CD4 cell counts can develop focal necrotizing infections due to *B. henselae* in lymph nodes, liver or spleen that have an appearance similar to that of CSD in immunocompetent individuals. Rarely, HIV-infected individuals with CD4 cell counts <50 can manifest this necrotizing lymphadenitis without vascular proliferation.[15]

A case-control study comparing clinical findings of 42 patients with BA and/or BP compared with 84 control patients found that case-patients were significantly more likely than controls to have fever, abdominal pain, lymphadenopathy, hepatomegaly, splenomegaly, a low CD4 cell count, anemia and/or an elevated serum alkaline phosphatase.[12] With the exception of cutaneous lesions, many of the clinical findings are not specific, and the major obstacle to diagnosis of *Bartonella* infection in the presence of concomitant HIV infection is recognition of the disease by the physician. Bacillary peliosis and all forms of BA can be indistinguishable from a number of other infectious or malignant conditions, and the diagnosis can usually be made only after biopsy and careful histopathological evaluation of tissue, or by direct culture of *Bartonella* species from blood or the affected organ.[16]

Cutaneous Bacillary Angiomatosis

The most frequently-diagnosed BA lesions are those affecting the skin.[16] Cutaneous BA lesions can have myriad presentations, including vascular proliferative lesions with a smooth red or eroded surface (Fig. 38.1, groin BA lesion) or papules that enlarge to form friable, exophytic lesions (Fig. 38.1, finger BA lesion). These vascular lesions of cutaneous BA are particularly difficult to distinguish clinically from Kaposi sarcoma (KS) and thus histopathological examination of biopsied tissue is essential. Bacillary angiomatosis may appear as a cellulitic plaque, usually overlying an osteolytic lesion (Fig. 38.2A). Less vascular-appearing lesions can be dry and scaly (Fig. 38.3) and some lesions are subcutaneous, with or without overlying erythema (Fig. 38.4). BA lesions

also can develop as very deep, highly vascular soft tissue masses (Fig. 38.5).[8]

Osseous Bacillary Angiomatosis

Bartonella infection of the bone causes osteolytic lesions that are extremely painful. The long bones including tibia, fibula and radius are most commonly involved[16,17] although osseous BA has occurred in a rib[17] and vertebra.[18,19] A roentgenogram usually demonstrates well-circumscribed osteolysis (Fig. 38.2B), and these lytic lesions are always detected by technetium-99m methylene diphosphonate bone scans.[17] Osseous BA should be a primary consideration in the differential diagnosis of a lytic bone lesion in HIV-infected patients.

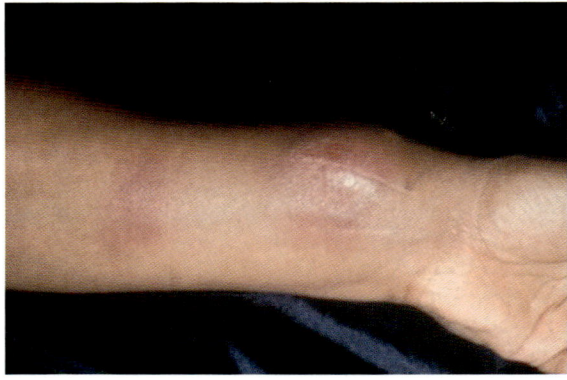

A

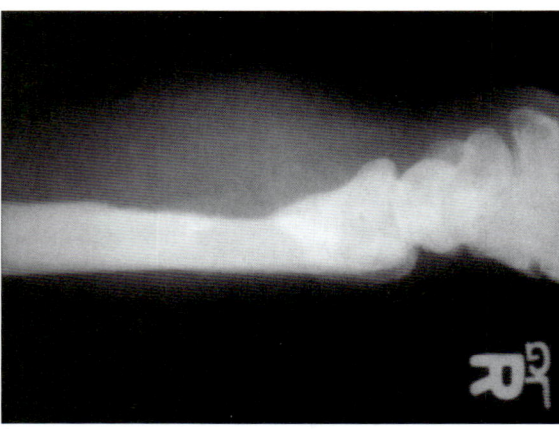

B

Figure 38.2 (A) A tense, firm, erythematous wrist mass due to BA. (B) A roentgenogram of the wrist of the same patient, demonstrating cortical bone erosion of the radius, with active periostitis, adjacent to the vascular soft tissue mass. (Reproduced with permission from Koehler, et al.[2])

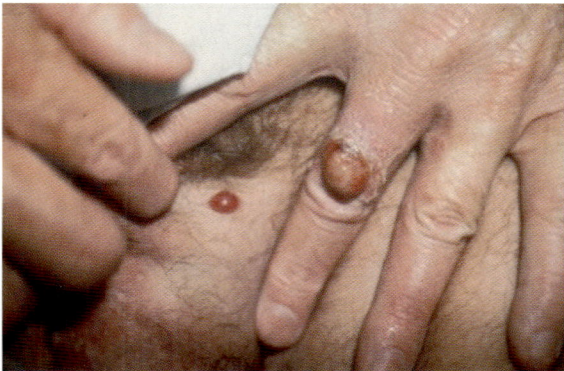

Figure 38.1 A friable, exophytic angiomatous BA nodule of the finger and an evolving dome-shaped vascular papule in the same patient. (Reproduced with permission from Koehler, et al.[2])

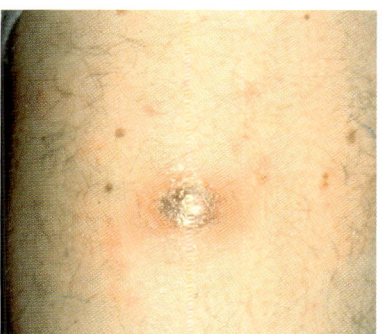

Figure 38.3 Unusual appearing erythematous, dry, scaling plaque of cutaneous BA mimicking staphylococcal pyoderma. *Bartonella quintana* was cultured from this lesion. (Reproduced with permission from Koehler and Tappero.[16])

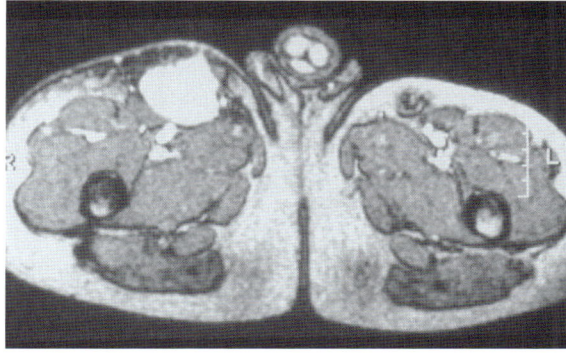

Figure 38.5 Magnetic resonance imaging showing a deep, highly vascular subcutaneous soft-tissue mass of BA in the anterior right thigh. (Reproduced with permission from Koehler and Tappero.[16])

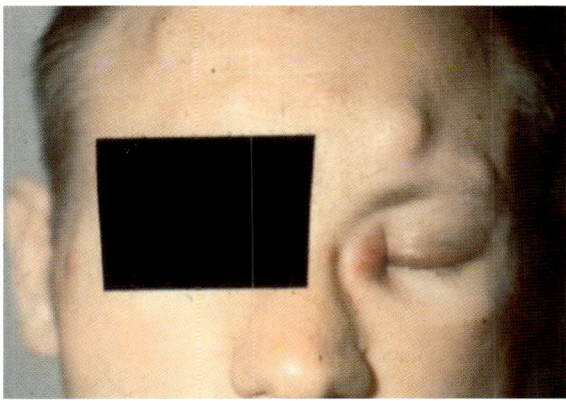

Figure 38.4 Multiple subcutaneous BA nodules in a patient with concomitant KS of the medial left eye canthus. (Reproduced with permission from Koehler and Tappero.[16])

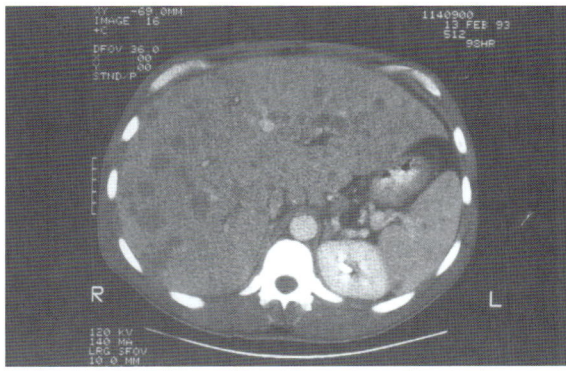

Figure 38.6 Computed tomography of the abdomen, showing hepatosplenomegaly with numerous low density hepatic parenchymal lesions, in addition to pelvic ascites and pulmonary effusions. Percutaneous biopsy of the liver demonstrated peliosis hepatis by histopathology. (Reproduced with permission from Koehler and Tappero.[16])

Splenic and Hepatic Bacillary Peliosis

Bacillary peliosis hepatis, a vascular lesion of the liver associated with infiltration of small bacilli, was first described in eight HIV-infected individuals by Perkocha and co-workers.[13] The symptoms of patients with BP hepatis usually include abdominal pain and fever. All eight patients had hepatomegaly, and six also had splenomegaly.[13] Two of the patients had a splenectomy, and histopathological examination revealed BP of the spleen. One-quarter of the patients also had cutaneous BA lesions. The serum alkaline phosphatase was more prominently elevated than the hepatic transaminases in these patients with BP hepatitis. Abdominal CT of the peliotic liver usually reveals numerous hypodense lesions,[16,20] as shown in Figure 38.6, but this appearance is not specific for BP,

and thus the diagnosis of *Bartonella* infection must be confirmed by histopathological evaluation. Additionally, some HIV-infected patients with hepatic *Bartonella* infection develop inflammatory nodules in the liver but not peliosis hepatis.[21] Patients with splenic BP may have thrombocytopenia or pancytopenia, and abdominal ascites may be present.[22,23]

Gastrointestinal and Respiratory Tract Bacillary Angiomatosis

Histopathologically-proven BA of the gastrointestinal tract has been described by several groups.[24-26] The lesions can involve oral, anal, peritoneal and gastrointestinal tissue appearing as raised, nodular, ulcerated intraluminal mucosal abnormalities of the stomach, large and small intestine during endoscopy.[25] Extraluminal, intra-abdominal BA presenting with massive upper gastrointestinal hemorrhage also has been described.[26] Hemorrhage occurred when the highly vascular mass eroded through small intestine; *B. quintana* was cultured from tissue obtained by transabdominal needle biopsy of the mass.

Bacillary angiomatosis lesions of the respiratory tract have been observed in the larynx;[24,27] in one of these patients, the BA lesions enlarged to cause an asphyxiative death.[24] Endobronchial BA lesions have been visualized during bronchoscopy, and described as polypoid lesions located in the segmental bronchi and the trachea.[28,29] Several of these patients also had cutaneous BA. *Bartonella* infection also can cause pulmonary nodules in the immunocompromised patient: a renal transplant patient with chemotherapy-induced immunocompromise developed high fever (41°C) and bilateral pulmonary nodules.[30] *Bartonella henselae* DNA was demonstrated in parenchymal lung nodule biopsy specimens.

Lymph Node Bacillary Angiomatosis

Lymph node involvement has been described frequently in association with cutaneous lesions or peliosis of the liver or spleen.[16] In these cases, the lymph nodes most commonly affected are those draining the BA lesion, and histopathological examination may reveal angiomatous changes within the lymph node. In other cases, however, BA may involve only a single or several lymph nodes, in the absence of cutaneous or other organ involvement.

Central Nervous System Manifestations of *Bartonella* Infection

Bartonella infection has been associated with aseptic meningitis[15] or parenchymal brain masses,[31] in HIV-infected individuals. A left temporal lobe mass due to BA developed in an HIV-infected patient with new onset of seizures and facial nerve deficit.[31] The etiology of the mass remained undetermined for 8 months until the patient developed a cutaneous BA lesion. Treatment with erythromycin led to resolution of the cutaneous lesion and neurologic deficit; the parenchymal mass decreased in size during antibiotic treatment. Another patient developed fever, headache, diabetes insipidus and altered mental status with multiple, small contrast-enhancing brain

lesions, including a single suprasellar lesion.[32] Examination of biopsied brain tissue revealed an inflammatory infiltrate primarily involving the leptomeninges, and clumps of bacillary organisms by Warthin–Starry staining. *B. henselae* DNA was amplified from the biopsy material. The lesions and symptoms resolved after treatment with doxycycline and rifampin.

Retinal disease can occur in patients with AIDS and infection with *B. henselae*. The manifestations are often more severe than those seen in immunocompetent patients and can include neuroretinitis and retinochoroiditis.[33] Warren and co-workers[34] described an HIV-infected patient who developed severe and progressive retinal disease that did not respond to treatment for *Toxoplasma* or CMV. Retinal biopsy was performed, revealing vascular proliferation consistent with BA. Sequencing of amplified DNA extracted from the biopsy specimen identified *B. henselae* DNA. The patient was treated with minocycline or doxycycline with resolution of the retinitis and improvement in his visual acuity.

Unusual Bacillary Angiomatosis Presentations

Several cases of BA involving the bone marrow have been reported.[4,22,35] Hepatosplenomegaly and thrombocytopenia were noted in both of these patients, and both resolved after antibiotic treatment. Venous thrombosis of the left upper extremity occurred in an AIDS patient with *B. quintana* bacteremia during relapse.[8] This was characterized by multiple noncontiguous, erythematous, tender superficial thromboses in the absence of trauma or intravenous drug use, and all rapidly resolved after institution of antibiotic therapy.

Cutaneous BA complicating pregnancy in an HIV-infected woman was reported by Riley and co-workers.[36] Cutaneous lesions resolved after antibiotic treatment, and the subsequent pregnancy and delivery were uneventful. BA lesions have been described in several pediatric patients: one patient was immunocompromised due to chemotherapy[37]; the other was 3.5 years old and had been infected with HIV-1 perinatally.[38]

Bacteremia with *Bartonella* Species and Fever of Unknown Origin

Many patients with BA and BP also have *Bartonella* bacteremia. One half of our patients with culture-positive focal BA or BP also had the corresponding *Bartonella* species simultaneously isolated from the blood.[9] *Bartonella* bacteremia in the absence of focal BA disease has been reported by a number of groups,[5,6,39] and may be more common than focal *Bartonella* disease. In a study of 382 patients with fever of undetermined etiology, 68 patients (18%) had evidence of *Bartonella* infection by serology and/or culture. A total 12 patients had bacteremia with *B. henselae* or *B. quintana* (six each).[39] When examined carefully by a health care provider experienced in the recognition of BA, six of the 12 bacteremic patients were found to have lesions suspicious for BA, and the other six had isolated bacteremia without focal *Bartonella* disease. The median CD4 cell count was 33 cells/mm[3] for the case patients in this study, indicating that both BA and *Bartonella*-related fever with bacteremia are usually identified in late stage HIV infection. Also of note, endocarditis was described in one patient with HIV infection and culture-proven *B. quintana*.[14]

Diagnosis of *Bartonella* Infections

Histopathological Diagnosis

Obtaining tissue for diagnosis

Biopsy is the principal procedure available for the diagnosis of cutaneous BA. Because KS lesions can be clinically indistinguishable from those of BA, any new vascular lesion should be biopsied. In patients with previously-diagnosed KS, any vascular lesion that has a different appearance or rate of growth also should be biopsied, because KS and cutaneous BA can occur simultaneously in the same patient.[40] Pedunculated lesions can be biopsied by shave excision, and smaller, papular or subcutaneous lesions should be examined by punch biopsy. Biopsy of the cellulitic plaque that frequently overlies osteolytic lesions may be sufficient to yield a diagnosis of BA, but in some patients, open excisional bone biopsy is necessary.[8] Fine needle aspiration of BA lymph nodes has not been useful in diagnosis of BA in our center, thus open excisional or incisional biopsy remains the optimal technique for diagnosis. For BP of the liver or spleen, the diagnostic procedure with greatest yield appears to be excisional wedge biopsy of the liver or splenectomy, however, peliosis hepatis has been diagnosed by either transvenous liver biopsy[41] or percutaneous liver biopsy.[23] As with cutaneous lesions, several opportunistic infections and malignancies can have a similar appearance on computed tomography of the abdomen, and thus biopsy is extremely important to direct specific treatment. No case of hemorrhage following percutaneous biopsy of a peliotic liver has been reported, however, this remains a theoretical concern.

Histopathological characteristics

A characteristic vascular proliferation is seen on routine hematoxylin and eosin staining of BA or BP tissue (Fig. 38.7A). Numerous bacilli also can be demonstrated in these lesions by modified silver staining (e.g. Warthin–Starry, Steiner, Dieterle) or electron microscopy (Fig. 38.7B).[11,13] Other stains, such as those for tissue gram-staining, fungi or acid-fast mycobacteria do not stain *Bartonella* bacilli.

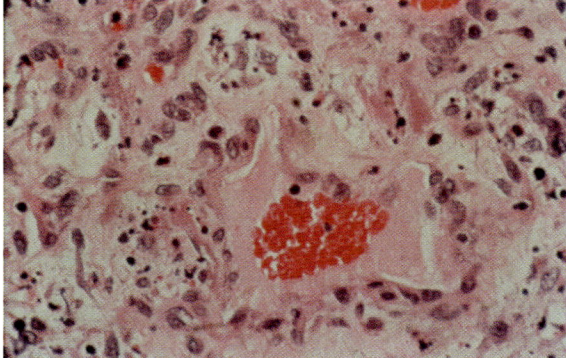

A

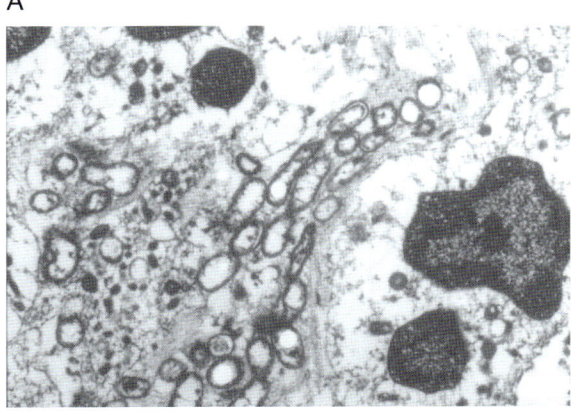

B

Figure 38.7 (A) Hematoxylin and eosin staining of a biopsied cutaneous BA lesion demonstrating a dermal vessel. The vessel is lined with protuberant endothelial cells surrounded by myxoid connective tissue containing neutrophils and amphophilic granular material in close proximity to the vascular lumen. (B) Transmission electron micrograph of cutaneous tissue showing multiple trilaminar cell-walled bacillary organisms. (Reproduced with permission from Koehler, et al.[2])

Cutaneous BA lesions may be misdiagnosed histopathologically, most often as KS,[2,3,28,42] angiosarcoma[18,19,24,42] and pyogenic granuloma.[27,43] The histopathological appearance of cutaneous BA lesions may be indistinguishable from pyogenic granuloma (lobular capillary hemangioma) and verruga peruana, the late, chronic phase of infection with *B. bacilliformis*.[3] A histopathological diagnosis of pyogenic granuloma, angiosarcoma or peliosis of the liver or spleen in an HIV-infected patient should prompt further evaluation of the tissue for bacilli, to determine whether the lesion may actually be due to *Bartonella* infection. The presence of bacillary organisms is the diagnostic feature that distinguishes cutaneous BA, extracutaneous BA, and parenchymal BP from these other diagnoses (with the exception of the cutaneous lesions of verruga peruana, which are associated with *B. bacilliformis* bacilli).

Serological Diagnosis

Bartonella antibodies can be detected in patients with cat scratch disease by an indirect fluorescence antibody (IFA) test developed at the Centers for Disease Control and Prevention.[44] This test also detects *Bartonella* antibodies in serum from patients with BA.[45] Antibodies to *Bartonella* were detected in seven HIV-infected patients with biopsy-confirmed cutaneous BA, and no antibodies were detected in seven HIV-infected patients without BA. For three of the patients with *Bartonella* antibodies, examination of banked serum revealed the presence of *Bartonella* antibodies as long as 7 years prior to the development of BA disease, suggesting infection with this bacterium occurred years before the diagnosis of BA. Prior to the diagnosis of BA in these three patients, a four-fold rise in titer occurred, raising the possibility of either relapse or reinfection. Culture-proven relapse in another BA patient[8] also was predicted by a rising serum antibody titer.[45] This IFA is useful for the diagnosis of BA and other *Bartonella*-associated infections in HIV-infected patients, as well as in following the response to antibiotic treatment.

Culture of *Bartonella* Species from Blood and Tissue of Patients with BA

Slater and co-workers[5] first reported isolation of *Bartonella* species from blood using lysis-centrifugation tubes (Isostat; Wampole, Cranbury, New Jersey) and plating onto chocolate agar or fresh heart infusion agar with 5% rabbit blood without antibiotics. Blood collection tubes containing EDTA also can be used to isolate *B. henselae* from the blood of an HIV-infected patient;[6] this standard CBC collection tube is much less expensive and more readily available. *Bartonella* bacteremia can be detected using acridine orange staining of aliquots removed from Bactec blood culture bottles.[46] The use of semi-quantitative cultures demonstrates that immunocompromised patients may have a high-grade bacteremia with *Bartonella*, with blood cultures yielding >1000 colony-forming units/mL of blood.[8]

Isolation of *Bartonella* species directly from cutaneous BA lesions is difficult due to the fastidious growth characteristics of this genus. Either *B. quintana* or *B. henselae* can be isolated by mincing a sterilely-obtained skin,[8] lymph node,[47] splenic[23] or hepatic biopsy specimen in inoculation media,[8] then spreading onto fresh heart infusion agar with 5% rabbit blood or onto chocolate agar and incubating for at least three weeks in a humid, 5% CO_2 environment.[8] The highest recovery rate of *Bartonella* species from cutaneous BA lesions has been accomplished using an endothelial cell monolayer co-cultivation system,[8] or shell vial culture assay[48] but these systems are not readily available to most microbiology labs. Because culture of *Bartonella* species from biopsied cutaneous or hepatic tissue remains difficult, culture from blood represents the most accessible method of isolating *Bartonella* species; however, bacteremia is not always present in patients with cutaneous BA or BP.

Treatment of *Bartonella* Infections

Choice of Antibiotics

There have been no controlled trials for antibiotic treatment of BA. The first patient diagnosed with BA was treated empirically with erythromycin, with complete resolution of subcutaneous nodules.[1] From subsequent reports, and our experience at San Francisco General Hospital, it is evident that erythromycin or doxycycline is the drug of first choice for patients with BA and BP (Fig. 38.8). Oral erythromycin therapy of 500 mg four times a day or oral doxycycline therapy with 100 mg twice a day is standard, but intravenous therapy should be given to patients with severe disease or those unable to tolerate oral medication. Resolution of BA due to *B. henselae* was reported in one HIV-infected patient following oral tetracycline treatment[8] and two immunocompetent patients with *B. henselae* bacteremia[5]; an immuno-

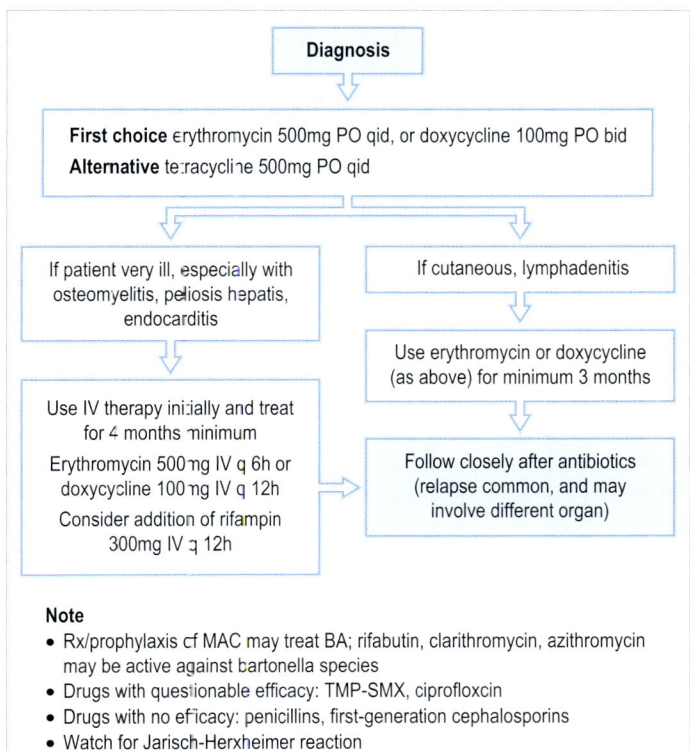

Figure 38.8 Algorithm for treatment of *Bartonella* infections in HIV-infected individuals. MAC, *Mycobacterium avium* complex; TMP-SMX, trimethoprim-sulfamethoxazole.

competent patient with cutaneous BA was successfully treated with minocycline.[49] In several retrospective descriptions of patients with cutaneous BA, resolution of lesions was noted to be temporally related to institution of antimycobacterial therapy[2,3,50-52] presumably due to the rifampin component.

A summary of recommended treatment for patients with *Bartonella* infection, in the presence or absence of immunocompromise, was published recently.[53] Although immunocompetent patients with *B. henselae* infection (cat scratch disease) usually do not need to be treated with antibiotics, all immunocompromised patients with *Bartonella* infection should be treated with an appropriate antibiotic for at least 3 months, regardless of the degree of immunosuppression. Note that some patients develop a Jarisch-Herxheimer reaction after the first several doses of antibiotic, with exacerbation of systemic symptoms and fever.[8] This response may be attenuated by pretreatment with an antipyretic, but severely ill AIDS patients should be monitored closely after the first several doses.

The clinical response of patients with BA to treatment with erythromycin, doxycycline and tetracycline usually corresponds to the *in vitro* susceptibilities of *B. quintana* and *B. henselae* to these antibiotics.[5,54-56] However, there is little correlation between the *in vivo* and *in vitro* antibiotic susceptibilities for other antibiotics, especially those that target steps in cell-wall synthesis, e.g. penicillins. It is obvious from numerous reports that penicillin, penicillinase-resistant penicillins, aminopenicillins and first generation cephalosporins have no activity against the *B. quintana* and *B. henselae* bacilli in BA lesions.[2,3,8,27,40,43,57] An apparent initial response to some antibiotics, e.g. vancomycin[27] or a first generation cephalosporin[43] likely represents the treatment of superinfecting skin flora. We pretreated one patient who had superinfected cutaneous BA lesions with cephradine to improve selective recovery of *Bartonella* organisms from the lesions,[8] and *B. quintana* was isolated from the BA lesions of another patient who had received nafcillin and gentamicin for several days prior to biopsy.[9] The discrepancies between *in vitro* and *in vivo* sensitivities may occur because the bacilli present in BA lesions have different cell wall characteristics from those grown on agar; changes that alter susceptibility to cell wall-active antibiotics. Additionally, the fastidious nature

Table 38.1 Clinical efficacy of antibiotics in the treatment of BA and BP

Definite	Possible	Inconclusive	None
Erythromycin	Rifampin	Ceftriaxone	Penicillin
Doxycycline	Gentamicin	Ceftizoxime	Ceph¹
Tetracycline		Ciprofloxacin	PCN-D
Minocycline		TMP/SMX	

Ceph¹, first-generation cephalosporins; PCN-D, penicillin derivatives (PCNase-resistant penicillins and aminopenicillins); TMP-SMX, trimethoprim-sulfamethoxazole.

of *Bartonella* species makes accurate susceptibility testing difficult to perform.

Rifampin may have clinical efficacy in treating *Bartonella* infections (Table 38.1), but use of this drug alone is not recommended due to the rapid development of resistance to rifampin. For severely ill patients, we administer rifampin in addition to a first line drug (erythromycin or doxycycline) during the initial several weeks of therapy. For some other antibiotics listed in Table 38.1 with possible clinical efficacy, single case reports have been associated with improvement in lesions or symptoms, but the response to these antibiotics is not consistent enough to warrant their recommendation at present. It also is difficult to directly attribute improvement of symptoms to treatment with a specific antibiotic when many patients have concomitant infection with other pathogens. The clinical efficacy of ciprofloxacin, trimethoprim/sulfamethoxazole and third generation cephalosporins remains inconclusive. One pregnant patient received 2 weeks of ceftizoxime treatment for cutaneous BA and had complete resolution of lesions.[36] In our study of patients with BA, we have observed progression of BA lesions in patients treated with ciprofloxacin.[58] Although one patient improved with trimethoprim/sulfamethoxazole,[28] most patients demonstrated no improvement or had progression of lesions,[12,14,36,38,57] and we have isolated *B. henselae* from the tissue of two patients taking prophylactic oral trimethoprim/sulfamethoxazole.[9] In contrast, no *Bartonella* isolate was recovered from any BA patient treated with a tetracycline or erythromycin (even after a single dose)[59] and prior treatment with a macrolide has been found to be significantly protective against development of BA.[9]

Relapse

Both *B. quintana*[60] and *B. henselae*[61] produce relapsing illness in immunocompetent hosts; it is thus not sur-

prising that immunocompromised patients with BA or BP frequently experience relapse, despite prolonged antibiotic therapy.[5,6,8,27,40,43,57,62] It should be noted that reinfection remains a possibility in these patients, but the majority of these cases probably represent relapse. The frequency of relapse appears to be increased when patients are treated with antibiotics for a shorter duration. Over the years, we have increased the duration of treatment for all presentations of BA, as the result of our increased experience, and we currently recommend that all patients with BA be treated for a minimum of 3 months, and those with peliosis hepatis be treated for a minimum of 4 months.[53] If relapse occurs after a first or second full course of an appropriate antibiotic, prophylactic treatment with a macrolide or doxycycline should be administered as long as the CD4 count remains <200 cells/mm³.

Treatment of Cutaneous Bacillary Angiomatosis Lesions

Immunocompromised patients with cutaneous BA should be evaluated for parenchymal and osseous disease before beginning treatment, because presence of either of these requires treatment for a longer duration. For cutaneous disease alone, antibiotic therapy can be given orally. Response of cutaneous lesions is usually rapid, with improvement in 1 week and complete resolution by 1 month, although hyperpigmentation may persist at the site of the lesion. As a result of our experience, we treat patients with cutaneous lesions for 3 months, and if relapse occurs, we extend treatment for an additional 4 months and occasionally, treat indefinitely.

Treatment of Osseous Bacillary Angiomatosis Lesions

Duration of antibiotic therapy for patients with *Bartonella* osteomyelitis is not well-established. We treated one patient (Fig. 38.2) with erythromycin, which the patient self-administered at a dose of 500 mg orally six times a day for 2 months, followed by 500 mg four times a day for an additional 2 months.[2] This patient had complete resolution of the osteolytic lesion and no relapse of BA during the subsequent 24 months, when he died of another opportunistic infection. Relapse occurred in another patient with osseous BA,[8] despite 4 months of oral treatment with 500–1000 mg erythromycin four times a day; the osseous BA healed but relapse with *B. quintana* bacteremia occurred 1 month after stopping erythromycin. For patients with osseous BA, it may be most appropriate to treat initially with several weeks of intravenous antibiotics (erythromycin or doxycycline), followed by prolonged, and perhaps indefinite, oral antimicrobial therapy. Serial technetium-99m methylene diphosphonate bone scans or roentgenograms can be used to monitor treatment efficacy, although resolution of osseous lesions is delayed, as seen with other causes of osteomyelitis.

Treatment of Hepatic and Splenic Bacillary Peliosis

Most patients with BP have severe systemic symptoms, including nausea and vomiting that may substantially decrease absorption of oral antibiotics. Additionally, oral erythromycin or doxycycline may not be tolerated by these patients, and thus initial treatment should be with intravenous antibiotics for several weeks, followed by oral therapy for at least 4 months, and possibly, indefinitely. Treatment progress can be monitored by following liver function tests and by serial computed tomography, if peliotic lesions are visualized at the time of diagnosis (Fig. 38.6).

Treatment of *Bartonella* Bacteremia

If possible, *Bartonella* blood cultures should be performed for patients with all forms of BA, prior to antibiotic treatment. Because endocarditis can develop during infection with *B. quintana*,[14,63] *B. henselae*[64] and rarely, other *Bartonella* species, all patients with *Bartonella* bacteremia and a cardiac murmur should be evaluated further with echocardiography. Within 1 week after institution of antibiotic treatment, immunocompromised patients with isolated *Bartonella* bacteremia usually note resolution of fever and most other constitutional symptoms, although one patient did not have permanent remission of fever until he had received 8 weeks of treatment.[5] An initial period of intravenous antibiotic therapy is probably appropriate for bacteremia, followed by at least 3 months of oral antibiotic therapy. If endocarditis is documented, 6 weeks of intravenous antibiotic therapy should be administered, followed by 3 months of oral antibiotic treatment.

Epidemiology and Prevention of *Bartonella* Infections

Arthropods serve as vectors of *Bartonella* species: e.g. *B. quintana* is known to be transmitted from the human reservoir to other humans via the body louse,[60] and the cat flea is the vector that transmits *B. henselae* from cat to cat. Ticks also are possible vectors of *Bartonella* species: two patients reported tick bites preceding the diagnosis of *B. henselae* bacteremia.[7,61] However, at present the vector most strongly implicated in transmission of *B. henselae* to humans is the domestic cat.

Serological studies initially revealed that *B. henselae* is the principal bacterial agent causing CSD in immunocompetent individuals.[44] Subsequent, corroborating data included the direct culture of *B. henselae* from lymph nodes with histopathological characteristics suggestive of CSD[47] and the demonstration of *Bartonella* DNA (but not *A. felis* DNA) in the CSD skin test antigen.[65] Similarly, an association between cat exposure and the development of BA was noted in many case reports,[16] and the first systematic evaluation of the relationship between cat contact, numerous other environmental exposures and development of BA was conducted by Tappero and co-workers[58] This case-control study found a significant epidemiological association between development of BA and traumatic cat exposure (cat bite or cat scratch). Both CSD and BA due to *B. henselae* have been statistically associated with cat exposure.[9,58,66] The association between *B. henselae*-infected cats and development of BA in the cat owners was demonstrated in 1994, when bacteremia was detected in all seven cat contacts of four patients with BA due to *B. henselae*.[67] It was further found that about 40% of the domestic cat population sampled in the greater San Francisco Bay Area was bacteremic with *B. henselae*,[67,68] providing compelling evidence that the domestic cat is the major reservoir for *B. henselae*.

The cat flea has been established as a vector of *B. henselae* among cats.[69] Initially, an epidemiological association between owning a kitten with fleas and development of CSD was described.[66] Also, a seroprevalence survey of *B. henselae* antibodies in pet cats throughout regions of North America revealed that the regions with the highest average prevalences of antibodies coincided with the geographic areas predicted to have the highest prevalence of the cat flea (e.g. Hawaii, coastal California, the Pacific Northwest and south central plains).[70] Viable *B. henselae* bacilli were isolated from several fleas combed from a bacteremic cat,[67] and *B. henselae* transmission from cat to cat via the cat flea was demonstrated in 1996.[69] Finally, Foil and co-workers[71] demonstrated that the feces of fleas fed on bacteremic cats are infectious and capable of transmitting *B. henselae* to uninfected cats.

According to the Humane Society, there are 77.6 million owned cats in the USA. Despite this large number, and the high percentage of cats with *B. henselae* infection, transmission of *B. henselae* to humans is relatively rare, and thus the benefit of these companion animals far outweighs the risk of *B. henselae* infection.[72] We suggest that several practical measures be followed to reduce the risk of *B. henselae* infection in HIV-infected individuals: (1) wash hands after petting and handling pets; (2) wash bites and scratches immediately with soap and water; (3) never allow any pet to lick an open wound; and (4) minimize flea infestation of pets (keep pets indoors and use flea protection products).

Although the domestic cat has been identified as the major reservoir and vector for *B. henselae*, it is quite evident that *B. quintana*, which causes nearly half of the BA infections in San Francisco, is not associated with cat contact. In a study of 49 patients and 96 matched controls, patients with BA caused by *B. quintana* infection were significantly more likely than controls to be homeless, have low socioeconomic status and have had recent infestation with head or body lice.[9] Physicians should consider *B. quintana* infection as a cause of fever in homeless patients, whether cutaneous lesions are present or absent. Strategies to prevent infection with *B. quintana* are currently limited to reducing homelessness and exposure to body lice.

Acknowledgments

Dr Koehler is supported by funds from NIH grant R01 AI52813 and from a Burroughs Wellcome Fund Award in Translational Research.

References

1. Stoler MH, Bonfiglio TA, Steigbigel RT, Pereira M. An atypical subcutaneous infection associated with acquired immune deficiency syndrome. Am J Clin Pathol 1983; 80:714–718.
2. Koehler JE, Leboit PE, Egbert BM, et al. Cutaneous vascular lesions and disseminated cat-scratch disease in patients with the acquired immunodeficiency syndrome (AIDS) and AIDS-related complex. Ann Intern Med 1988; 109:449–455.
3. Leboit PE, Berger TG, Egbert BM, et al. Epithelioid haemangioma-like vascular proliferation in AIDS: Manifestation of cat-scratch disease bacillus infection? Lancet 1988; i:960–963.
4. Relman DA, Loutit JS, Schmidt TM, et al. The agent of bacillary angiomatosis: An approach to the identification of uncultured pathogens. N Engl J Med 1990; 323:1573–1580.
5. Slater LN, Welch DF, Hensel D, et al. A newly recognized fastidious gram-negative pathogen as a cause of fever and bacteremia. N Engl J Med 1990; 323:1587–1593.
6. Regnery RL, Anderson BE, Clarridge JE, et al. Characterization of a novel *Rochalimaea* species, *R. henselae* sp. nov., isolated from blood of a febrile, human immunodeficiency virus-positive patient. J Clin Microbiol 1992; 30:265–274.
7. Welch DF, Pickett DA, Slater LN, et al. *Rochalimaea henselae* sp. nov., a cause of septicemia, bacillary angiomatosis, and parenchymal bacillary peliosis. J Clin Microbiol 1992; 30:275–280.
8. Koehler JE, Quinn FD, Berger TG, et al. Isolation of *Rochalimaea* species from cutaneous and osseous lesions of bacillary angiomatosis. N Engl J Med 1992; 327:1625–1631.
9. Koehler JE, Sanchez MA, Garrido CS, et al. Molecular epidemiology of *Bartonella* infections in patients with bacillary angiomatosis-peliosis. N Engl J Med 1997; 337:1876–1883.
10. Cockerell CJ, Leboit PE. Bacillary angiomatosis: A newly characterized, pseudoneoplastic, infectious, cutaneous vascular disorder. J Am Acad Derm 1990; 22:501–512.
11. Leboit PE, Berger TG, Egbert BM, et al. Bacillary angiomatosis: The histopathology and differential diagnosis of a pseudoneoplastic infection in patients with human immunodeficiency virus disease. Am J Surg Pathol 1989; 13:909–920.
12. Mohle-Boetani JC, Koehler JE, Berger TG, et al. Bacillary angiomatosis and bacillary peliosis in patients infected with human immunodeficiency virus: Clinical characteristics in a case-control study. Clin Infect Dis 1996; 22:794–800.
13. Perkocha LA, Geaghan SM, Yen TSB, et al. Clinical and pathological features of bacillary peliosis hepatis in association with human immunodeficiency virus infection. N Engl J Med 1990; 323:1581–1586.
14. Spach DH, Callis KP, Paauw DS, et al. Endocarditis caused by *Rochalimaea quintana* in a patient infected with human immunodeficiency virus. J Clin Microbiol 1993; 31:692–694.
15. Wong MT, Dolan MJ, Lattuada CP Jr, et al. Neuroretinitis, aseptic meningitis, and lymphadenitis associated with *Bartonella* (*Rochalimaea*) *henselae* infection in immunocompetent patients and patients infected with human immunodeficiency virus type 1. Clin Infect Dis 1995; 21:352–360.
16. Koehler JE, Tappero JW. Bacillary angiomatosis and bacillary peliosis in patients infected with human immunodeficiency virus. Clin Infect Dis 1993; 17:612–624.
17. Baron AL, Steinbach LS, Leboit PE, et al. Osteolytic lesions and bacillary angiomatosis in HIV infection: Radiologic differentiation from AIDS-related Kaposi sarcoma. Radiology 1990; 177:77–81.
18. Herts BR, Rafii M, Spiegel G. Soft-tissue and osseous lesions caused by bacillary angiomatosis: Unusual manifestations of cat-scratch fever in patients with AIDS. Am J Radiol 1991; 157:1249–1251.
19. Schinella RA, Greco MA. Bacillary angiomatosis presenting as a soft-tissue tumor without skin involvement. Hum Pathol 1990; 21:567–569.
20. Wyatt SH, Fishman EK. Hepatic bacillary angiomatosis in a patient with AIDS. Abdom Imaging 1993; 18:336–338.
21. Slater LN, Pitha JV, Herrera L, et al. *Rochalimaea henselae* infection in acquired immunodeficiency syndrome causing inflammatory disease without angiomatosis or peliosis. Demonstration by immunocytochemistry and corroboration by DNA amplification. Arch Pathol Lab Med 1994; 118:33–38.
22. Milam M, Balerdi MJ, Toney JF. Epithelioid angiomatosis secondary to disseminated cat scratch disease involving the bone marrow and skin in a patient with acquired immune

deficiency syndrome: A case report. Am J Med 1990; 88:180–183.

23. Slater LN, Welch DF, Min KW. *Rochalimaea henselae* causes bacillary angiomatosis and peliosis hepatis. Arch Intern Med 1992; 152:602–606.

24. Cockerell CJ, Whitlow MA, Webster GF, et al. Epithelioid angiomatosis: A distinct vascular disorder in patients with the acquired immunodeficiency syndrome or AIDS-related complex. Lancet 1987: 2:654–656.

25. Tuur SM, Macher AM, Angritt P, et al. AIDS case for diagnosis series. Milit Med 1988; 153:M57–M64.

26. Koehler JE, Cederberg L. Intra-abdominal mass associated with gastrointestinal hemorrhage: A new manifestation of bacillary angiomatosis. Gastroenterology 1995; 109:2011–2014.

27. Van Der Wouw PA, Hadderingh RJ, Reiss P, et al. Disseminated cat-scratch disease in a patient with AIDS. AIDS 1989; 3:751–753.

28. Slater LN, Min KW. Polypoid endobronchial lesions. A manifestation of bacillary angiomatosis. Chest 1992; 102:972–974.

29. Foltzer MA, Guiney WB Jr, Wager GC, et al. Bronchopulmonary bacillary angiomatosis. Chest 1993; 104:973–975.

30. Caniza MA, Granger DL, Wilson KH, et al. *Bartonella henselae*: Etiology of pulmonary nodules in a patient with depressed cell-mediated immunity. Clin Infect Dis 1995; 20:1505–1511.

31. Spach DH, Panther LA, Thorning DR, et al. Intracerebral bacillary angiomatosis in a patient infected with human immunodeficiency virus. Ann Intern Med 1992; 116: 740–742.

32. George TI, Manley G, Koehler JE, et al. Detection of *Bartonella henselae* by polymerase chain reaction in brain tissue of an immunocompromised patient with multiple enhancing lesions. Case report and review of the literature. J Neurosurg 1998; 89:640–644.

33. Cunningham ET Jr, Koehler JE. Ocular bartonellosis. Am J Ophthalmol 2000; 130:340–349.

34. Warren K, Goldstein E, Hung VS, et al. Use of retinal biopsy to diagnose *Bartonella* (formerly *Rochalimaea*) *henselae* retinitis in an HIV-infected patient. Arch Ophthalmol 1998; 116:937–940.

35. Kemper CA, Lombard CM, Deresinski SC, et al. Visceral bacillary epithelioid angiomatosis: Possible manifestations of disseminated cat scratch disease in the immunocompromised host: A report of two cases. Am J Med 1990; 89:216–222.

36. Riley LE, Tuomala RE. Bacillary angiomatosis in a pregnant patient with acquired immunodeficiency syndrome. Obstet Gynecol 1992; 79:818–819.

37. Myers SA, Prose NS, Garcia JA, et al. Bacillary angiomatosis in a child undergoing chemotherapy. J Pediatr 1992; 121:574–578.

38. Malane MS, Laube TA, Chen CK, Fikrig S. An HIV-1-positive child with fever and a scalp nodule. Lancet 1995; 346:1466.

39. Koehler J, Sanchez M, Tye S, et al. Prevalence of *Bartonella* infection among human immunodeficiency virus-infected patients with fever. Clin Infect Dis 2003; 37:559–566.

40. Berger TG, Tappero JW, Kaymen A. Leboit PE. Bacillary (epithelioid) angiomatosis and concurrent Kaposi's sarcoma in acquired immunodeficiency syndrome. Arch Derm 1989; 125:1543–1547.

41. Marullo S, Jaccard A, Roulot D, et al. Identification of the Rochalimaea henselae 16S rRNA sequence in the liver of a french patient with bacillary peliosis hepatis. J Infect Dis 1992; 166:1462.

42. Angritt P, Tuur SM, Macher AM, et al. Epithelioid angiomatosis in HIV infection: Neoplasm or cat-scratch disease? Lancet 1988; 1:996.

43. Marasco WA, Lester S, Parsonnet J. Unusual presentation of cat scratch disease in a patient positive for antibody to the human immunodeficiency virus. Rev Infect Dis 1989; 11:793–803.

44. Regnery RL, Olson JG, Perkins BA, Bibb W. Serological response to Rochalimaea henselae antigen in suspected cat-scratch disease. Lancet 1992; 339:1443–1445.

45. Tappero J, Regnery R, Koehler J. Detection of serologic response to *Rochalimaea henselae* in patients with bacillary angiomatosis (BA) by immunofluorescent antibody (IFA) testing. 32nd Interscience Conference on Antimicrobial Agents and Chemotherapy; 1992: American Society for Microbiology.

46. Larson AM, Dougherty MJ, Nowowiejski DJ, et al. Detection of *Bartonella* (*Rochalimaea*) *quintana* by routine acridine orange staining of broth blood cultures. J Clin Microbiol 1994; 32:1492–1496.

47. Dolan MJ, Wong MT, Regnery RL, et al. Syndrome of *Rochalimaea henselae* adenitis suggesting cat scratch disease. Ann Intern Med 1993; 118:331–336.

48. Scola B La, Raoult D. Culture of *Bartonella quintana* and *Bartonella henselae* from human samples: A 5-year experience (1993 to 1998). J Clin Microbiol 1999; 37:1899–1905.

49. Tappero JW, Koehler JE, Berger TG, et al. Bacillary angiomatosis and bacillary splenitis in immunocompetent adults. Ann Intern Med 1993; 118:363–365.

50. Knobler EH, Silvers DN, Fine KC, et al. Unique vascular skin lesions associated with human immunodeficiency virus. J Am Med Assoc 1988; 260:524–527.

51. Hall AV, Roberts CM, Maurice PD, et al. Cat-scratch disease in patient with AIDS: Atypical skin manifestation. Lancet 1988; 2:453–454.

52. Lopez-Elzaurdia C, Fraga J, Sols M, et al. Bacillary angiomatosis associated with cytomegalovirus infection in a patient with AIDS. Br J Derm 1991; 125:175–177.

53. Rolain JM, Brouqui P, Koehler JE, et al. Recommendations for treatment of human infections caused by *Bartonella* species. Antimicrob Agents Chemother 2004; 48:1921–1933.

54. Daly JS, Worthington MG, Brenner DJ, et al. *Rochalimaea elizabethae sp. nov.* Isolated from a patient with endocarditis. J Clin Microbiol 1993; 31:872–881.

55. Myers WF, Grossman DM, Wisseman CLJ. Antibiotic susceptibility patterns in *Rochalimaea quintana*, the agent of trench fever. Antimicrob Agents Chemother 1984; 25:690–693.

56. Maurin M, Gasquet S, Ducco C, et al. MICs of 28 antibiotic compounds for 14 *Bartonella* (formerly *Rochalimaea*) isolates. Antimicrob Agents Chemother 1995; 39:2387–2391.

57. Szaniawski WK, Don PC, Bitterman SR, et al. Epithelioid angiomatosis in patients with AIDS. J Am Acad Derm 1990; 23:41–48.

58. Tappero JW, Koehler JE. *Rochalimaea* infections. Ann Intern Med 1993; 119:535–536.

59. Whitfeld MJ, Kaveh S, Koehler JE, et al. Bacillary angiomatosis associated with myositis in a patient infected with human immunodeficiency virus. Clin Infect Dis 1997; 24:562–564.

60. Strong RPL. Trench fever: Report of commission, medical research committee, American Red Cross. Oxford: Oxford University Press; 1918.

61. Lucey D, Dolan MJ, Moss CW, et al. Relapsing illness due to *Rochalimaea henselae* in immunocompetent hosts: Implication for therapy and new epidemiological associations. Clin Infect Dis 1992; 14:683–688.

62. Krekorian TD, Radner AB, Alcorn JM, et al. Biliary obstruction caused by epithelioid angiomatosis in a patient with AIDS. Am J Med 1990; 89:820–822.

63. Drancourt M, Mainardi JL, Brouqui P, et al. *Bartonella* (*Rochalimaea*) *quintana* endocarditis in three homeless men. N Engl J Med 1995; 332:419–423.

64. Holmes AH, Greenough TC, Balady GJ, et al. *Bartonella henselae* endocarditis in an immunocompetent adult. Clin Infect Dis 1995; 21:1004–1007.

65. Perkins BA, Swaminathan B, Jackson LA, et al. Case 22-1992–pathogenesis of cat scratch disease. N Engl J Med 1992; 327:1599–1601.

66. Zangwill KM, Hamilton DH, Perkins BA, et al. Cat scratch disease in Connecticut. Epidemiology, risk factors, and

evaluation of a new diagnostic test. N Engl J Med 1993; 329:8–13.

67. Koehler JE, Glaser CA, Tappero JW. *Rochalimaea henselae* infection. A new zoonosis with the domestic cat as reservoir. JAMA 1994; 271:531–535.

68. Chomel BB, Abbott RC, Kasten RW, et al. *Bartonella henselae* prevalence in domestic cats in California: Risk factors and association between bacteremia and antibody titers. J Clin Microbiol 1995; 33:2445–2450.

69. Chomel BB, Kasten RW, Floyd-Hawkins K, et al. Experimental transmission of *Bartonella henselae* by the cat flea. J Clin Microbiol 1996; 34:1952–1956.

70. Jameson P, Greene C, Regnery R, et al. Prevalence of *Bartonella henselae* antibodies in pet cats throughout regions of North America. J Infect Dis 1995; 172: 1145–1149.

71. Foil L, Andress E, Freeland RL, et al. Experimental infection of domestic cats with *Bartonella henselae* by inoculation of *Ctenocephalides felis* (Siphonaptera: Pulicidae) feces. J Med Entomol 1998; 35:625–628.

72. Regnery RL, Childs JE, Koehler JE. Infections associated with *Bartonella* species in persons infected with human immunodeficiency virus. Clin Infect Dis 1995; 21 (Suppl):94–98.

CHAPTER 39

Management of Herpesvirus Infections (Cytomegalovirus, Herpes Simplex Virus, and Varicella-Zoster Virus)

W. Lawrence Drew

Kim S. Erlich

Cytomegalovirus

General Comments

With the advent of highly active antiretroviral therapy (HAART), there has been a marked decline in cytomegalovirus (CMV) disease. The syndromes discussed below still occur in the early months of HAART, because the CD4 lymphocytes require weeks to months to become fully functional.[1] CMV disease is also seen in those patients who have eluded medical care and in those who fail or are intolerant of HAART.

Infection with CMV is extremely common in patients with AIDS and can result in several clinical illnesses, including chorioretinitis, esophagitis, colitis, pneumonia, and several neurologic disorders. Not all patients with blood, urine, or tissue cultures positive for CMV will develop clinical illness related to the infection. In patients with advanced AIDS (CD4 lymphocyte counts of <50 cells/mm^3), the risk of developing CMV disease and death is directly related to the quantity of CMV nucleic acid in plasma. In a study of over 600 advanced AIDS patients, each log$_{10}$ increase in baseline CMV, DNA load was associated with an approximate 3-fold increase in CMV disease and 2-fold increase in mortality at 1 year.[2]

Diagnosis of disease caused by CMV may require tissue biopsy with histologic evidence of viral inclusions and inflammatory response. Detection of CMV antigen or nucleic acid in tissue is an alternative method for establishing that CMV is actually present in tissue. Viral culture is useful only if no other pathogen is identified in tissue. This section reviews the most common clinical manifestations of CMV and their management (Table 39.1).

Chorioretinitis

Ocular disease caused by CMV occurs only in patients with severe immunodeficiency and was especially common in patients with AIDS prior to the advent of HIV protease inhibitors. Clinical evidence of CMV retinitis (Fig. 39.1) occurred in as many as 40% of AIDS patients, and autopsy series revealed that CMV retinitis was present in up to 30% of patients. With the routine use of prophylaxis against *Pneumocystis*, retinitis became a common presenting manifestation of AIDS, but it more often

Table 39.1 Treatment of cytomegalovirus (CMV) infection in AIDS patients

	Preferred therapy	Alternative therapy
CMV retinitis[a,b,c]		
Sight-threatening lesions	GCV implant + valganciclovir 900 mg q.d. p.o. or valganciclovir 900 mg b.i.d. p.o.	GCV i.v.; Foscarnet i.v.; Cidofovir i.v.
Peripheral lesions	Valganciclovir 900 mg b.i.d. p.o.	Same as above ($\approx^1/_2$ induction dose)
Maintenance therapy	Valganciclovir 900 mg o.d. p.o.	Same as above ($\approx^1/_2$ induction dose)
Relapsing and/or	Re-induction with GCV/VCV GCV implant;	Cidofovir (if only UL97 mutation); Fomivirsen
GCV resistant	Ganciclovir i.v. + Foscarnet i.v.	
CMV gastrointestinal disease	Ganciclovir i.v. for 3–6 weeks or Foscarnet i.v. for 3–6 weeks or Valganciclovir (if absorbing) for 3–6 weeks	
CMV neurological disease	Ganciclovir i.v. + Foscarnet i.v.	

[a]If not already begun, antiretroviral therapy should be initiated concurrent with anti-CMV therapy, except possibly when treating CNS disease. [b]For retinitis, anti-CMV therapy should be continued until CD4 count has exceeded 100–150 cells/mm³ for ≥6 months and the retinitis is inactive. If anti-CMV therapy is discontinued, regular monthly eye exams should be continued. [c]Early relapses of CMV retinitis in patients treated systemically are usually due to inadequate drug penetration; re-induction with the same drug is often effective. Drug resistance may occur in patients treated for ≥3 months. Therapy of these patients may be guided by antiviral susceptibility testing.

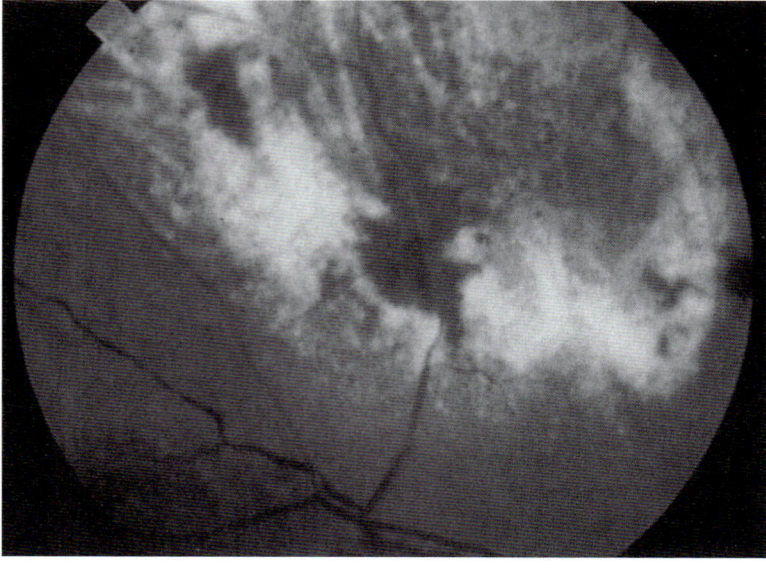

Figure 39.1 Funduscopic appearance of CMV retinitis, illustrating 'cottage cheese and catsup' appearance resulting from perivascular exudates and hemorrhages. (Courtesy of Dr L. Schwartz, San Francisco, California.)

occurred months to years after the diagnosis of AIDS had been established. The incidence of CMV disease is currently low primarily because of the efficacy of protease inhibitors in controlling primary HIV disease.

Decreased visual acuity, the presence of floaters, or unilateral visual field loss is often the presenting complaint of a patient with retinitis. Ophthalmologic examination typically reveals large creamy to yel-lowish white granular areas with perivascular exu-dates and hemorrhages (Fig. 39.1). These lesions initially occur more often at the periphery of the fundus and, if left untreated, progress centrally within 2–3 weeks. Retinitis usually begins unilater-ally, but progression to bilateral involvement is common because of an associated viremia. Systemic CMV infection involving other viscera is frequently present.

CMV accounts for at least 90% of HIV-related infectious retinopathies. Differentiating suspected CMV retinitis lesions from cotton-wool spots is essential. Cotton-wool spots appear as small, fluffy, white lesions with indistinct margins and are not associated with exudates or hemorrhages. They are common in AIDS patients, are usually asymptomatic, and represent areas of focal ischemia. These lesions do not progress and often undergo spontaneous regression. Toxoplasmosis is the second most common opportunistic infection of the eye but is characterized by little if any hemorrhage. It is associated with cerebral toxoplasmosis in the majority of patients. Syphilis, herpes simplex virus (HSV), varicella-zoster virus (VZV), and tuberculosis are other infections that may rarely involve the retina.

Virtually all patients with CMV retinitis have CD4 lymphocyte counts of <50 cells/mm^3, and routine ophthalmologic screening of patients with pupillary dilation, as well as indirect ophthalmoscopy, may be valuable when cell counts decline to this level. It is also important to inquire about visual abnormalities, especially increased floaters, and to examine the fundus carefully when there are visual complaints. Patients with confirmed CMV chorioretinitis should be treated with ganciclovir, foscarnet, or cidofovir.[3–5] These agents are equally effective in the initial treatment of CMV chorioretinitis, although disease usually progresses despite continued treatment.[6] The toxic effects of these agents vary widely but the usual drug of choice is ganciclovir.

Nervous System

CMV commonly involves the central nervous system (CNS) in AIDS patients. About 20–40% of AIDS patients have been identified with CMV CNS involvement in different autopsy series.[7–9] CMV causes a spectrum of neurologic syndromes in AIDS patients, ranging from polyradiculopathy, encephalitis with dementia, and ventriculoencephalitis to mononeuritis multiplex and painful neuropathy.

Polyradiculopathy and myelitis

The clinical syndrome of CMV polyradiculopathy and myelitis usually has an insidious onset with low back pain radiating to the perianal area and progressive lower extremity weakness, hypo- or areflexia, and variable sensory deficit with usually preserved proprioception and vibratory sensation. In association with bladder and/or anal sphincter dysfunction, most patients develop urinary retention and fecal incontinence. The disease clinically resembles Guillain–Barré syndrome but may be differentiated by lack of sphincter and upper extremity involvement in the latter.

Diagnosis of CMV polyradiculopathy is based on the characteristic neurologic features described above. The cerebrospinal fluid (CSF) abnormalities are very unusual for a viral infection: pleocytosis with predominant polymorphonuclear leukocytosis and hypoglycorrhachia. Culture of CSF is usually positive but antigen or DNA assays are more sensitive methods of diagnosis. Magnetic resonance imaging (MRI) may reveal enhancement of leptomeninges and clumping of lumbosacral roots. Characteristic pathologic changes seen in CMV polyradiculopathy are demyelination and destruction of axons.

Acute CMV polyradiculopathy should be differentiated from idiopathic lumbosacral polyradiculopathy, in which CSF pleocytosis is predominantly mononuclear and clinical improvement is seen without CMV treatment. Lymphoma, tuberculosis, syphilis, and toxoplasmosis also cause similar clinical syndromes.

Encephalitis with dementia and ventriculoencephalitis

Cytomegalovirus encephalitis (CMVE) with a distinct clinical syndrome of dementia and CMV ventriculoencephalitis are the two syndromes of CMVE described in AIDS patients. CMVE with dementia, the more common of the two syndromes, is well described neuropathologically[10] as a multifocal, scattered micronodular encephalitis that resembles HIV encephalitis, which causes HIV-associated dementia (HIVD). CMV ventriculoencephalitis is a late and terminal event with acute onset of encephalitis often associated with cranial nerve involvement and nystagmus. CMVE-associated dementia has been described and compared with HIVD.[11] The significance of differentiating CMVE and HIVD lies in the different drugs available for treatment.

CMVE is seen more commonly among homosexual men, which may reflect the increased CMV seroprevalence in homosexual men.[12] CMVE always occurs in patients with CD4 counts of <100/mm^3 and should be suspected in homosexual men presenting with a subacute encephalopathy who have had AIDS for more than 1 year. Clinicians should suspect a diagnosis of CMVE in patients who have a history of systemic CMV infection, especially those with CMV retinitis who develop encephalopathic features and change in mental status.

Patients with dementia caused by CMVE usually have a more acute onset and rapid progression than patients with HIVD. The encephalopathic symptoms include delirium and confusion, lethargy and somnolence, apathy and withdrawal, personality changes, and focal neurologic signs with cranial nerve involvement. During the course of illness, recurrent fever episodes may occur that may be attributed to other opportunistic infections (e.g. *Mycobacterium avium-intracellulare*). Psychomotor slowing, primitive reflexes, and peripheral neuropathy may also be seen in CMVE. Distal sensory polyneuropathy usually antedates the onset of CMVE.[13]

The course of encephalopathic illness in both CMVE and HIVD includes progressive worsening in mental status until death. The median survival of CMVE patients is significantly shorter (weeks) compared with that of HIVD patients (months). Autopsies reveal a range of neuropathology including ependymal and subependymal necrosis, areas of demyelination, and microglial nodules that are more frequently encountered than typical nuclear and cytoplasmic CMV inclusions.[14] Neuropathologic evaluations of CMVE and HIV co-infection of single cells suggests that CMV and HIV mutually help each other's replication in the brain.[15]

It is difficult to make a definitive diagnosis of CMVE, and laboratory investigations are not very helpful in distinguishing CMV from HIVD. Electrolyte abnormality, especially hyponatremia, is more commonly present in CMVE patients.[16] There are insufficient data to determine whether CMV antigen or DNA is regularly detected in CSF. Imaging study with MRI brain scans showing meningeal enhancement consistent with ventriculitis and periventricular enhancement are helpful in differentiating CMVE from HIVD. However, periventricular enhancement may also be seen in lymphoma, toxoplasmosis, and pyogenic brain abscesses. Progressive ventriculomegaly, if seen in serial computed tomography scans, is highly suspicious of CMVE.[17,18]

Combination therapy with ganciclovir and foscarnet is recommended, especially when disease progression is noted with single-agent therapy. Comparative trials of simple versus combined therapy have not been performed.

Mononeuritis multiplex

This is the least common of all the neurologic syndromes attributed to CMV. Clinical characteristics of CMV mononeuritis are more varied than the polyradiculopathy/myelitis. Patients may present with multifocal, patchy and/or asymmetrical sensory and motor deficits. Cranial nerve palsies caused by CMV, especially in the recurrent laryngeal nerve in the setting of severe immunosuppression, have been reported.[19] This symptom may occur with other neurologic manifestations of CMV (e.g. polyradiculopathy, encephalitis, or retinitis). Pathologic findings in peripheral nerve biopsies have shown endoneurial necrosis with cellular infiltrates and Schwann cells showing CMV inclusions.

Painful distal neuropathy

This syndrome of painful distal symmetrical neuropathy of subacute onset limited to the feet and associated with some numbness and weakness has been reported with CMV infection.[20]

Gastrointestinal System

CMV colitis previously occurred in at least 5–10% of AIDS patients but is now uncommon due to the efficacy of HAART. Diarrhea, weight loss, anorexia, and fever frequently are present. The differential diagnosis includes infection by other gastrointestinal pathogens, including *Cryptosporidium*, *Giardia*, *Entamoeba*, *Mycobacterium*, *Shigella*, *Campylobacter*, and *Strongyloides stercoralis*, and involvement by lymphoma or Kaposi's sarcoma. Endoscopy usually reveals diffuse submucosal hemorrhages and mucosal ulcerations, although a grossly normal-appearing mucosa may be encountered in up to 10% of those with histologic evidence of CMV colitis (Fig. 39.2). Biopsy reveals vasculitis, neutrophilic infiltration, and nonspecific inflammation, but the diagnosis is confirmed by the presence of characteristic CMV inclusions, antigen, or nucleic acid and the absence of other pathogens.

Clinically evident esophagitis in AIDS patients most commonly is due to either *Candida albicans* or HSV, but may also be caused by CMV. Patients with CMV esophagitis are apt to have pain on swallowing and distal ulceration on endoscopy. As in colitis, diagnosis should be established through endoscopic examination and biopsy.

Patients with symptomatic esophagitis or enterocolitis who have CMV (and not other pathogens) detected by endoscopy, histology, or culture should benefit from anti-CMV treatment for 3–6 weeks and should be considered for continued maintenance treatment in part as a means of preventing retinitis.[21]

The efficacy of anti-CMV treatment in patients with enterocolitis is not dramatic.[22] When compared with placebo, a significant antiviral effect was

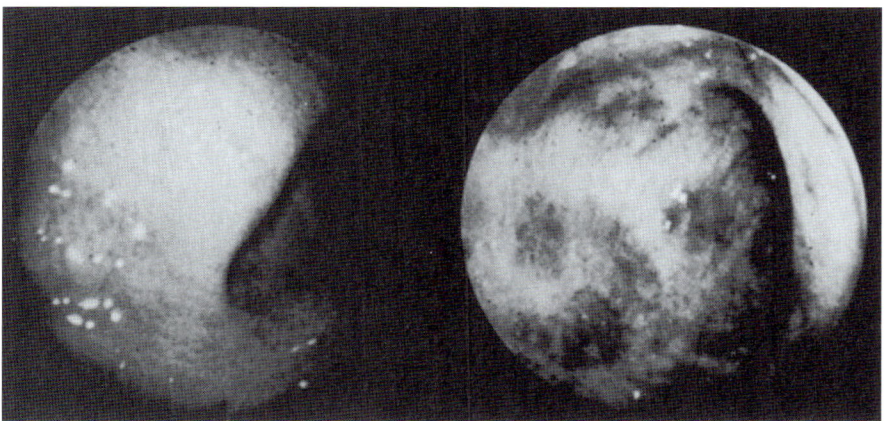

Figure 39.2 Sigmoidoscopic appearance of CMV colitis (two views), demonstrating diffuse submucosal hemorrhages and mucosal ulcerations. (Courtesy of Dr D. Dieterich, New York, New York.)

observed but a clinical benefit was less apparent. Diarrhea and abdominal discomfort were not relieved, but, in general, patients seemed to improve with this therapy.[22]

Pulmonary System

Pulmonary manifestations

Isolation of CMV from pulmonary secretions or lung tissue in AIDS patients with pneumonia who undergo bronchoscopy is common, but a true pathogenic role of the virus in the disease process is not readily established. Many patients with pulmonary disease and CMV isolation from the lung have concomitant infection with other pathogens, especially *Pneumocystis jiroveci*. Many of the patients respond to therapy directed at *P. jiroveci* pneumonia alone, raising the question of whether CMV is a true pulmonary pathogen in AIDS patients. However, patients with positive CMV cultures and histologic findings from lung tissue and no other pathogens identified on diagnostic bronchoscopy may truly have invasive CMV pneumonia.

When CMV causes pulmonary disease in AIDS patients, the syndrome is that of an interstitial pneumonitis. Patients often complain of gradually worsening shortness of breath, dyspnea on exertion, and a dry, nonproductive cough. The heart and respiratory rates are elevated, but auscultation of the lungs often reveals minimal findings with no evidence of consolidation. Chest radiographs show diffuse interstitial infiltrates similar to those in patients with *P. jiroveci* pneumonia. Hypoxemia is invariably present.

Anti-CMV therapy should be considered when a patient has documented CMV pulmonary infection as the only pathogen identified and a progressive, deteriorating clinical course.[23-25]

Treatment of CMV Infection

Ganciclovir

Structure and mechanism of action Ganciclovir (DHPG, Cytovene) is a nucleoside analog that differs from acyclovir (Zovirax) by a single carboxyl side chain. This structural change confers on the drug approximately 50 times greater activity than acyclovir against CMV. Acyclovir has low activity against CMV because it is not well phosphorylated in CMV-infected cells. This is due to the absence of the gene for thymidine kinase (TK) in CMV. Ganciclovir, however, is active against CMV because it does not require TK for phosphorylation. Instead another viral-encoded phosphorylating enzyme (UL 97) is present in CMV-infected cells.[26] It is capable of phosphorylating ganciclovir and converting it to the monophosphate. Cellular enzymes then convert the monophosphate to the active compound, ganciclovir triphosphate. Ganciclovir triphosphate acts to inhibit the viral DNA polymerase.

Pharmacology and dosage Ganciclovir is available for clinical use in intravenous and oral formulations, as well as a sustained release intraocular implant. Intravenous ganciclovir is used for initial induction therapy, followed by either intravenous or oral ganciclovir for maintenance therapy. A more recently studied highly effective treatment alternative is the combination of oral ganciclovir and the intraocular ganciclovir implant.[27] Oral ganciclovir is also used for prevention.

Initial intravenous induction treatment for CMV disease consists of 5 mg/kg twice daily for 14–21 days or until there is an adequate clinical response. The standard intravenous dosage for maintenance therapy is approximately one-half the induction dose (i.e. 5 mg/kg per day, 7 days/week) or, if given orally, 1000 mg three times daily, with food.

When administered by intravenous infusion over 1 h in the usual dosage of 5 mg/kg, peak ganciclovir blood levels are approximately 8–9 µg/mL, and the serum half-life is 3.5 h. The absolute bioavailability of oral ganciclovir capsules is 6–9%. When administered orally as 1000 mg three times daily with food, peak serum levels are approximately 1 µg/mL, and the serum half-life is approximately 5 h. Because ganciclovir is excreted unchanged through the kidneys, dosage for intravenous ganciclovir must be reduced in patients with renal impairment. Dosage adjustments should also be considered for oral ganciclovir. The appropriate dose reductions are presented in Table 39.2. Initial response in retinitis (improvement or stabilisation in vision or ophthalmoscopic appearance) occurs in approximately 75% of treated patients.[5] By comparison, the disease is relentlessly progressive in 90% of patients if left untreated. Visual-field defects present at the onset of therapy do not reverse, but a decrease in visual acuity caused by edema of the macula may improve with treatment. Retinal detachment may occur in later stages as the necrotic retina scars and thins.

Prior to the availability of HAART, maintenance therapy throughout the life of the patient was critical for CMV retinitis because the virus is only suppressed by ganciclovir and is not eliminated. Even with continued maintenance therapy, CMV retinitis eventually progressed. Why this occurred is not clearly understood, but it is likely related to suboptimal drug delivery to the retina. This hypothesis is supported by the longer times to progression achieved with the ganciclovir intraocular implant, which delivers greater concentrations of ganciclovir to the vitreous.[28] Viral resistance does not appear to be involved in most progressions of CMV retinitis.[29]

With successful HAART, it is possible for selected patients with CMV retinitis to discontinue maintenance therapy. Oral valganciclovir is equivalent to intravenous ganciclovir and is the drug of choice for maintenance therapy.[30]

Oral ganciclovir maintenance therapy is associated with a risk of more rapid rate of retinitis progression compared with intravenous therapy (mean of 5–12 days' earlier progression in three studies).[31]

Intravitreal injection of ganciclovir has been used in certain special situations, such as in patients in whom neutropenia limited the systemic use of the drug, and in one series[32] appeared effective and relatively safe. Sustained intravitreal release of ganciclovir has been accomplished using a surgical implantable device.[16,33,34] This implant, which is designed to deliver ganciclovir into the vitreous over several months, has been shown to be highly efficacious for local control of retinitis. In addition, in a large controlled study that evaluated combined oral ganciclovir (4500 mg/day) and the implant for treatment of CMV retinitis, the combination not only delayed progression of retinitis but reduced the risk

Table 39.2 Ganciclovir dosage adjustment in patients with impaired renal function

Creatinine clearance (mL/min)[a]	i.v. induction dose (mg/kg)	Induction dosing interval (h)	Maintenance dose (mg/kg)	Maintenance dosing interval (h)	Oral dose
>70	5.0	12	5.0	24	1000 mg t.i.d.
50–69	2.5	1	2.5	24	1500 mg q.d.
25–49	2.5	24	1.25	24	1000 mg q.d.
10–24	1.25	24	0.625	24	500 mg q.d.
<10	1.25	3 t.i.w. following hemodialysis		3 t.i.w. following hemodialysis	500 mg 3 t.i.w. following hemodialysis

[a]Creatinine clearance can be related to serum creatinine by the following formulas:

For males: $\dfrac{140 - \text{age (years)} \times \text{weight (kg)}}{72 \times \text{serum creatinine (mg/dL)}}$

For females: 0.85 × male value.

of developing contralateral retinitis or extraocular CMV disease. The incidence of Kaposi's sarcoma was also reduced.[27] The implant delivers approximately five times as much ganciclovir compared with i.v. and may be useful in treating low-level GCV-resistant CMV retinitis.

Clinical use Administration of ganciclovir or valganciclovir is indicated for the treatment of acute CMV infection, but other herpesvirus, including HSV-1, HSV-2, VZV, and human herpesvirus (HHV)-6, are also susceptible to the drug *in vitro*. Because AIDS patients with severe CMV infection frequently have illnesses caused by other herpesviruses, a bonus of ganciclovir therapy may be an associated prevention or improvement of these infections. Ganciclovir is probably also active against Epstein–Barr virus.

Virologic response to ganciclovir CMV cultures of blood and urine rapidly become negative in patients treated with ganciclovir[35] (Fig. 39.3). Most of these patients had CMV retinitis, although AIDS patients with CMV infections of other organ systems are included. Of these patients, 87% had a complete virologic response (conversions of culture from positive to negative or a more than 100-fold reduction in CMV titer) in urine, and 83% had a complete response in blood culture. The median time until response was 8 days for both blood and urine cultures.

Resistance Erice and co-workers[36] reported three patients whose clinical course suggested the emergence of resistance and whose CMV isolates exhibited increases in the concentration of ganciclovir required to inhibit the virus in tissue culture over baseline determinations. In a separate report, after 3 months of continuous intravenous ganciclovir therapy, approximately 10% of patients were excreting resistant strains of CMV (arbitrarily defined as strains that are only inhibited by four times or more the median concentration of ganciclovir required to inhibit a group of pretherapy isolates).[37] In virtually all isolates, there was a mutation in the phosphorylating gene.[38] These strains remain sensitive to foscarnet, which may be used as an alternative therapy. As treatment continues, a polymerase mutation conferring further ganciclovir resistance may occur. Many strains with this mutation are cross resistant to cidofovir but usually remain sensitive to foscarnet.[39,40]

In another investigation of CMV resistance in 38 retinitis patients treated with intravenous or oral ganciclovir, the *in vitro* 50% inhibitory concentration

(IC_{50}) increased with duration of ganciclovir exposure in strains isolated during treatment.[41]

Resistant strains (defined as having an IC50 >6 µmol/L) were first identified after 50 days of treatment, and resistance was infrequent, occurring in about 6% of patients treated with oral ganciclovir and about 3% of patients treated with intravenous ganciclovir. Most patients did not shed CMV at the time of retinitis progression, but a patient with 'breakthrough' shedding of virus during treatment as more likely to demonstrate resistance.

In another report of 76 retinitis patients initially treated with ganciclovir, 11.4% had a resistant strain of CMV (IC50 >6 µmol/L) by 6 months.[42]

Toxicity Toxicity may limit therapy with ganciclovir. The following adverse effects may occur. CBCs, electrolytes and renal function should be monitored weekly while on therapy.

Effects of hematopoiesis Leukopenia and anemia may affect up to 40 and 25%, respectively, of patients receiving intravenous ganciclovir for treatment of CMV disease. The incidence of both is lower during administration of oral ganciclovir (3000 mg daily) for either maintenance treatment of retinitis or primary prevention of CMV disease (Table 39.3). Many AIDS patients have low white blood cell counts before therapy, so the contribution of ganciclovir to leucopenia is not always clear. Neutropenia may develop at any time and is usually reversible, although at least five patients are known to have had irreversible suppression. Cytokines, such as granulocyte colony-stimulating factor (G-CSF; filgrastim), are effective in reversing ganciclovir-induced neutropenia. Severe neutropenia (absolute neutrophil count <500/mm^3) requires a ganciclovir dose interruption until evidence of marrow recovery is observed and neutrophil counts have risen, preferably to >1000/mm^3. Thrombocytopenia occurs in up to 6% of ganciclovir-treated patients. Valganciclovir has a toxicity profile similar to that of oral ganciclovir. For example, patients receiving maintenance treatment for CMV retinitis at a dose of 900 mg/day experienced neutropenia of <500/µL (19%) and thrombocytopenia <25 000/µL (4%).

Toxicities in other organ systems Gastrointestinal adverse events, most commonly diarrhea, nausea, anorexia, and vomiting, affect a substantial number of patients treated with intravenous or oral ganciclovir. Data from a large double-blind safety comparison of oral ganciclovir (3000 mg daily) to placebo, however, suggest that the rates of these

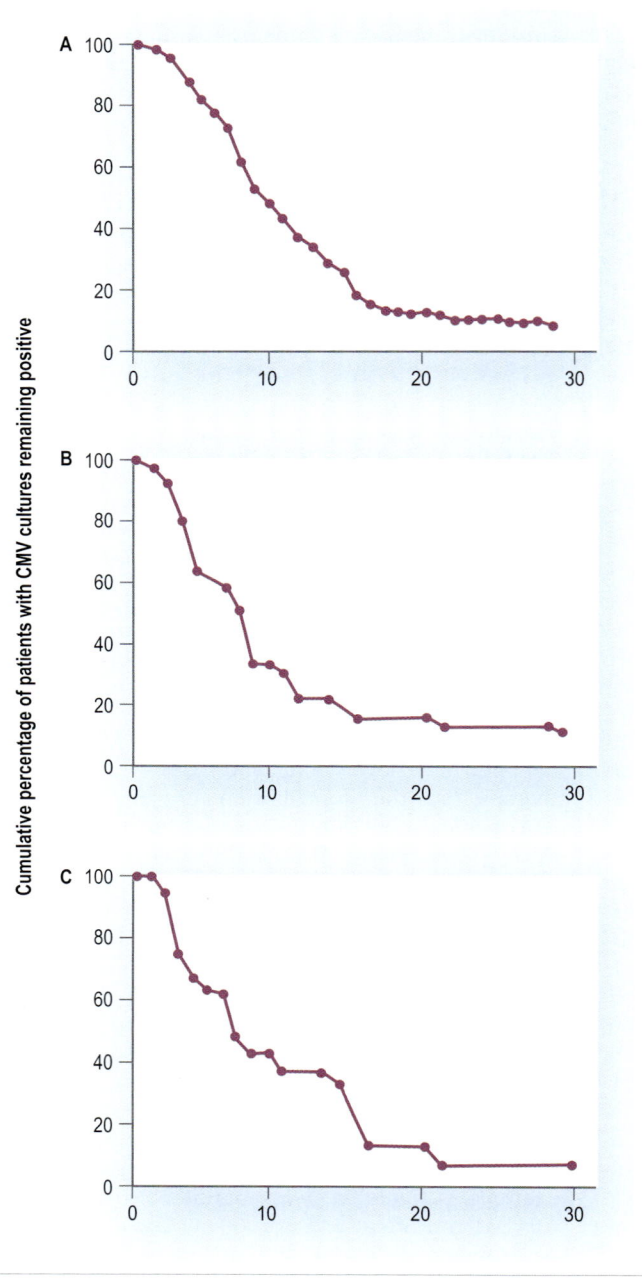

Figure 39.3 Time course of conversion of CMV cultures of specimens of (A) urine (*n*=107), (B) blood (*n* = 41), or (C) throat (*n* = 21) washings from positive (before treatment) to negative (after treatment with ganciclovir). Cultures from individual patients were performed at various times after start of treatment. Numbers in parentheses are the number of patients in whom the particular body fluid or site was sequentially cultured. (Reprinted from Buhles, et al.[35])

events are only modestly higher among ganciclovir-treated patients; 48% developed diarrhea (versus 42% of placebo-treated patients, 19% developed anorexia (placebo, 16%) and 14% developed vomiting (placebo, 11%).[43] In patients receiving valganciclovir, diarrhea occurred in 41%, nausea in 30%, and vomiting in 24%. Neuropathy and paresthesia are the most frequent adverse events involving the nervous system, affecting up to 21% and 10% of patients, respectively, but only neuropathy occurred more often in ganciclovir-versus placebo-treated patients (21% versus 15%, respectively). Neuropathy occurred in 9% of patients receiving valganciclovir. A minority of ganciclovir-treated patients will

Table 39.3 Selected laboratory abnormalities in patients receiving ganciclovir for treatment of CMV retinitis and prevention of CMV disease

CMV retinitis treatment	CMV disease prevention Oral (3000 mg/dL)	i.v. (5 mg/kg per day)	Oral (3000 mg/dL)	Placebo
Number of patients	320	175	478	234
Neutropenia (ANC/L)				
<500	18	25	10	6
500–749	17	14	16	7
750–1000	19	26	22	16
Anemia (high, g/dL)				
<6.5	2	5	1	<1
6.5–7.9	10	16	5	3
8.0–9.5	25	26	15	16

Data are percentages of patients. ANC; absolute neutrophil count; high, hemoglobin.

experience modest elevations in serum creatinine (maximum levels of at least 1.5 mg/dL, or >25% increases over pretreatment levels).

Gonadal toxicity In pre-clinical animal studies, ganciclovir and therefore valganciclovir is a potent inhibitor of spermatogenesis and may also suppress female fertility. Sperm counts in humans before and during ganciclovir therapy, however, have been performed too infrequently to provide meaningful information on spermatogenesis. Patients wishing to have children should use ganciclovir only for the strongest indications.

Teratogenesis Because ganciclovir and also valganciclovir is a mutagen and teratogen in animals, effective contraception should be practiced by men and women with childbearing potential during treatment. Ganciclovir should be used during pregnancy only if the potential benefit justifies the potential risk to the fetus.

Foscarnet

Foscarnet, also known as phosphonoformate or phosphonoformic acid, is a pyrophosphate that inhibits the DNA polymerase of CMV. Specifically, the drug blocks the pyrophosphate-binding site of the viral DNA polymerase, preventing cleavage of pyrophosphate from deoxyadenosine triphosphate.[44] This action is relatively selective in that CMV DNA polymerase is inhibited at concentrations <1% of that required to inhibit cellular DNA polymerase. Unlike such nucleosides as acyclovir and ganciclovir, foscarnet does not require phosphorylation intracellularly to be an active inhibitor of viral DNA

polymerases. This biochemical fact becomes especially important with regard to viral resistance, because the principal mode of viral resistance to nucleoside analogs is a mutation that eliminates phosphorylation of the drug in virus-infected cells. Foscarnet can be used to treat patients with ganciclovir-resistant CMV; cross-resistant to foscarnet is very rare. However, patients treated with foscarnet may develop foscarnet resistance due to mutations in the viral polymerase UL54.[40]

Pharmacology The recommended initial therapy is foscarnet administered intravenously as 60 mg/kg every 8 h or as 90 mg/kg every 12 h. A dose of 120 mg/kg per day may be superior in efficacy to 90 mg/kg per day,[45] but this dose may also be more toxic.

CSF concentrations of foscarnet are approximately 40% of serum levels. Excretion is entirely renal, without a hepatic component. Oral bioavailability is estimated at 12–22%, but it is poorly tolerated.

Adverse effects include renal impairment, anemia, hypocalcemia (especially ionized calcium), hypomagnesemia, and hypophosphatemia. It is important to measure renal function frequently and adjust dosage accordingly to minimize toxicity. Daily pre-infusion of 1 L of saline may reduce nephrotoxicity during maintenance therapy.

Palestine and co-workers[4] reported a randomized control trial of foscarnet in the treatment of CMV retinitis in AIDS patients. Patients were assigned to receive either no therapy or immediate treatment with intravenous foscarnet. The justification for the design was that the lesions were peripheral and not threatening visual acuity. The mean time to progression of retinitis was 3 weeks in the control group versus 13 weeks in the treatment group, thereby proving that foscarnet is effective therapy. Also, an excellent antiviral effect was achieved in the treatment group (i.e. 9 of 13 patients had positive blood cultures for CMV at entry, and all nine had CMV cleared from their blood by the end of the 3-week induction period). Adverse effects were seizures, hypomagnesemia, hypocalcemia, and elevated serum creatinine levels.

A study comparing foscarnet with ganciclovir in the treatment of sight-threatening CMV retinitis was reported.[6] The two drugs were equivalently effective in treating retinitis. The mean time to progression of retinitis was approximately 56 days in both groups. The notable difference in the study was that patients treated with foscarnet had a 4-month longer survival time than those receiving ganciclovir. The explanation for the difference in survival time is not clear and does not seem entirely attributable to differences in the ability to take concurrent antiretroviral medications. However, this analysis was based on tabulating whether a patient had ever received any antiretroviral therapy (e.g. zidovudine, dideoxycytidine (ddC), or ddI) and did not assess the quantitative ability of patients to take these medications. Presumably, it was more difficult for the patient to be on concurrent zidovudine therapy while taking ganciclovir because of additive myelosuppression. Thus, whether the survival benefit of foscarnet was due to these other medications or was an inherent effect of foscarnet therapy itself remains unclear. Now that cytokines (e.g. granulocyte-macrophage colony-stimulating factor and G-CSF) and other antiretrovirals (ddI, ddC) without extreme myelosuppressive toxicity are available, it should be possible for patients to continue receiving antiretroviral medications while taking ganciclovir.[46]

Ganciclovir and foscarnet

The results of a Studies of Ocular Complications of AIDS trial of combination therapy versus monotherapy for relapsed CMV retinitis were published in early 1996.[47] Combination therapy (5 mg/kg per day ganciclovir and 90 mg/kg per day foscarnet) was significantly superior in delaying progression than either ganciclovir alone (10 mg/day) or foscarnet alone (120 mg/kg per day). This study also showed no advantage in switching monotherapy. That is, patients in whom monotherapy failed with ganciclovir and then switched to high-dose foscarnet did not do better than patients who continued ganciclovir at the higher dose. The median times to progression

were: foscarnet group, 1.3 months; ganciclovir group, 2.0 months; and combination group, 4.3 months ($P <0.001$). Side-effects were not statistically significantly different in any group, but the quality of life was poorest in the combination group as a result of the prolonged daily infusion time of 3.1 h.

Cidofovir, or HPMPC, represents a departure from previous nucleoside analogs because it appears to the cell as a nucleotide. It has a phosphonate moiety attached to a cytosine analog and does not require phosphorylation by viral-encoded enzyme. It is therefore active against the majority of ganciclovir-resistant CMV strains that only have resistance mutations in UL97, the phosphorylating gene. When polymerase, UL54, mutations occur in ganciclovir treated patients, cross-resistance to cidofovir is frequent. These resistance mutations also occur in patients treated with cidofovir de novo.[40] The drug also has an extremely long half-life, permitting intravenous administration as infrequently as every 2 weeks during maintenance treatment.[48]

Cidofovir is nephrotoxic, especially to the proximal renal tubule, but this can apparently be diminished by prehydration and concomitant probenecid therapy. Renal function and toxicity must be monitored carefully, and proteinuria or a rising creatinine level are reasons for dosage reduction, interruption, or discontinuation. Concurrent administration of other nephrotoxic drugs must be avoided and there must be at least a 7-day period of 'washout' of these drugs if their use precedes administration of cidofovir. Despite its potential for toxicity, the drug is effective and convenient and it may find an important niche in anti-CMV therapy.

Immune recovery uveitis is an immunologic reaction to CMV characterized by inflammation in the anterior chamber or vitreous. It occurs after the initiation of HAART and is most frequent in patients with a substantial rise in CD4 counts in the 4–12 weeks after initiation of therapy. Treatment consists of periocular corticosteroids or a short course of systemic steroids.

Prevention of CMV Infection

Ganciclovir

The oral form of ganciclovir is approved by the Food and Drug Administration (FDA) for prevention of CMV disease in patients with advanced HIV infection. The approval was based on a placebo-controlled study of 725 patients known to be CMV sero- or culture-positive, the majority of whom had CD4 lymphocyte cell counts under 50 cells/mm^3. Ganciclovir taken prophylactically as 1000 mg orally three times daily decreased the cumulative risk of developing CMV disease over 12 months from 26–14% (an overall risk reduction of nearly 50%).[43] Ganciclovir also effectively decreased and suppressed CMV excretion throughout the treatment period as measured by prevalence of CMV-positive urine cultures.

Herpes Simplex Virus

Herpes simplex virus types 1 and 2 (HSV-1, HSV-2) cause disease in both normal and immunocompromised hosts and are responsible for substantial morbidity in patients with AIDS. Most adult patients with AIDS have been infected with one or both HSV types before the development of AIDS, and are not susceptible to primary HSV infection following new exposure. During initial HSV infection, viral latency develops in the nerve root ganglia corresponding to the site of mucccutaneous inoculation. Latent virus can then reactivate at any time throughout the life of the host, and all infected persons are at risk for virus shedding and recurrent symptomatic disease. Recurrent HSV mucocutaneous eruptions are common in patients with HIV infection and can be severe, with extensive tissue destruction and prolonged viral shedding.[49–51]

Recent studies confirm the high prevalence of both HSV-1 and HSV-2 in the general population.[52–54] Type-specific serologic studies conclude that up to 70% of the population are infected with HSV-1, and up to 21.9% are infected with HSV-2. HSV-2 infection rates are higher in women than in men and higher in African-Americans and Mexican-Americans than in Caucasians.[52–54] The presence of underlying HSV infection may increase the risk of acquiring HIV infection following exposure to HIV. This increased risk for HIV may occur as a result of the presence of susceptible CD4 T cells present in HSV ulcerations.[55,56] Recent data suggests that antiviral suppression of HSV may reduce the risk of acquiring HIV.[56a] The prevalence of HSV infection in homosexual AIDS patients exceeds that of the general population and likely reflects the common risk factor for transmission of both HSV and HIV (sexual contact). Serologic studies have revealed that up to 77% of HIV-infected patients have been previously infected with HSV. AIDS subgroups who did not acquire HIV infection through sexual contact, such as hemophiliacs and transfusion recipients, have rates of HSV infection that are lower than the incidence in AIDS as a whole, and are likely comparable with those in the general population. The presence

of latent HSV infection in this high percentage of patients with HIV infection explains the frequency of clinical disease in this population. Clinical observations suggest that the frequency and severity of HSV recurrences may increase with advancing immunosuppressions.[54,57-60]

Clinical Presentation

Because most HIV-infected patients have been infected with HSV before acquiring HIV, recurrent HSV is much more common than primary HSV infection in this population. HSV infection in AIDS patients may appear similar to the typical HSV lesions observed in the normal host or, alternatively, lesions may appear quite atypical and unusual because of the immunosuppressed state associated with HIV infection. The severity of clinical illness depends on several factors, including the anatomic site of initial infection, the degree of immunosuppression, and whether the clinical episode represents initial primary infection (no previous exposure to either HSV type), initial non-primary infection (previous exposure to the heterologous HSV type), or recurrent infection.[49-51]

Localized mucocutaneous ulcerative lesions, without visceral or cutaneous dissemination, is the most frequent presentation of HSV infection in HIV-infected patients. Because the lesions may appear atypical, a high index of suspicion is required by the clinician in evaluating any mucocutaneous lesion in a patient with HIV infection. Chronic or persistent HSV infection may lead to an initial diagnosis of AIDS; an individual with confirmed HIV infection and no other cause of immunodeficiency who has ulcerative HSV infection present for longer than 1 month has sufficient criteria for a diagnosis of AIDS.

Orolabial infection

Orolabial infection in adults with AIDS is usually due to recurrent disease from previously latent infection. Primary infection of the mouth or nose may occur, however, in a seronegative individual who acquires infection at this site for the first time. Primary infection is more likely to occur in children with AIDS than in adults, because HIV infection in children (especially those infected prenatally) is more likely to precede initial exposure to HSV.

The incubation period of primary HSV infection ranges between 2 and 12 days. In the normal host, primary orolabial infection may be asymptomatic or result in clinically apparent gingivostomatitis.[51-54,61] Immunocompromised patients are at greater risk than normal hosts of developing a severe clinical illness during primary HSV-1 infection, with a painful vesicular eruption occurring along the lips, tongue, pharynx, or buccal mucosa. The vesicles rapidly coalesce and rupture to form large ulcers covered by a whitish yellow necrotic film.[61,62] Fever, pharyngitis, and cervical lymphadenopathy are often present in adults, whereas infants may display poor feeding and persistent drooling.

Following initial or primary infection, all infected patients remain at risk for virus reactivation and recurrent disease. Recurrent HSV gingivostomatitis ('fever blisters') may occur spontaneously or as a result of external stimuli, such as a febrile illness, excessive wind or ultraviolet light exposure to the lips, surgical manipulation of the trigeminal nerve, or stress. Prodromal symptoms, consisting of tingling or numbness at the site of the impending recurrence, may be present from 12 to 24 h before the onset of an HSV recurrence. Instituting antiviral chemotherapy during the prodrome may have a beneficial effect on the illness and may abort the development of visible cutaneous lesions (see Treatment of HSV Infection, below). Recurrences may increase in frequency and severity as immunosuppression worsens, although many AIDS patients will have only infrequent, mild, self-limiting recurrences throughout their disease.[57,61]

In the normal host, orolabial herpes lesions usually heal in 7–10 days. By comparison, AIDS patients often have a prolonged illness with markedly delayed healing of mucocutaneous lesions. If left untreated, chronic ulcerative lesions with persistent viral shedding may last for several weeks.[62]

Genital infection

After a 2- to 12-day incubation period, many individuals with primary genital herpes develop local symptoms.[49-51] Symptoms will be most apparent in patients with primary genital infection (no prior infection with the heterologous HSV type) as compared with patients with non-primary initial infection (prior infection with the heterologous HSV type). When present, signs and symptoms include small papules that rapidly evolve into fluid-filled vesicles. These lesions are usually painful and tender to palpation. The vesicles ulcerate rapidly and, in the normal host, heal over 3–4 weeks by crusting and re-epithelialization. Tender inguinal adenopathy is common, and dysuria may be present even if the urethra is not infected. Systemic symptoms, such as fever, headache, myalgias, malaise, and meningismus, may be present during primary infection.[49-51]

In the normal host, recurrent genital herpes is less severe than primary infection. Compared with primary infection, recurrent herpes typically results in fewer external lesions, a shorter duration of illness, and the absence of systemic symptoms.[49-51] As with primary infection, recurrent genital herpes in patients with AIDS may be more severe and prolonged as compared with that seen in the normal host. Prolonged new lesion formation, continued tissue destruction, persistent virus shedding, and severe local pain are not uncommon findings in this setting. As with orolabial herpes, the frequency and severity of genital recurrences may increase with advancing immunosuppression, and symptoms may last for several weeks if left untreated.[57,63]

Asymptomatic genital HSV shedding in non-immunocompromised patients occurs on between 1% and 6% of the days on which cultures are obtained.[64,65] HIV-infected patients infected with HSV shed HSV at even higher rates, and asymptomatic shedding may increase with advancing immunosuppression.[66] All HSV-infected individuals (whether HIV infected or not) should be counseled about asymptomatic HSV shedding and the risk of transmission to sexual partners despite the absence of symptoms or visible lesions.[67]

Anorectal infection

Chronic perianal herpes was among the first reported opportunistic infections associated with AIDS. HSV is the most frequent cause of non-gonococcal proctitis in sexually active homosexual men.[68,69] HSV proctitis usually results from primary HSV-2 infection but may also occur as a result of HSV-1 infection or recurrent disease caused by either viral type. Severe anorectal pain, perianal ulcerations, constipation, tenesmus, and neurologic symptoms in the distribution of the sacral plexus (sacral radiculopathy, impotence, and neurogenic bladder) are common findings of HSV proctitis. These signs and symptoms help differentiate HSV proctitis from proctitis from other causes (Fig. 39.4).[68] Anorectal or sigmoidoscopic examination in patients with HSV proctitis typically reveals a friable mucosa, diffuse ulcerations, and occasional intact vesicular or pustular lesions.[68]

Recurrent perianal lesions caused by HSV in the absence of true proctitis is a common finding in patients with AIDS. Local pain, tenderness, itching, and pain on defecation are prominent symptoms of these lesions. Shallow ulcers in the perianal region are often visible on external examination, and ulcerative lesions frequently coalesce and extend along the gluteal crease to involve the area overlying the

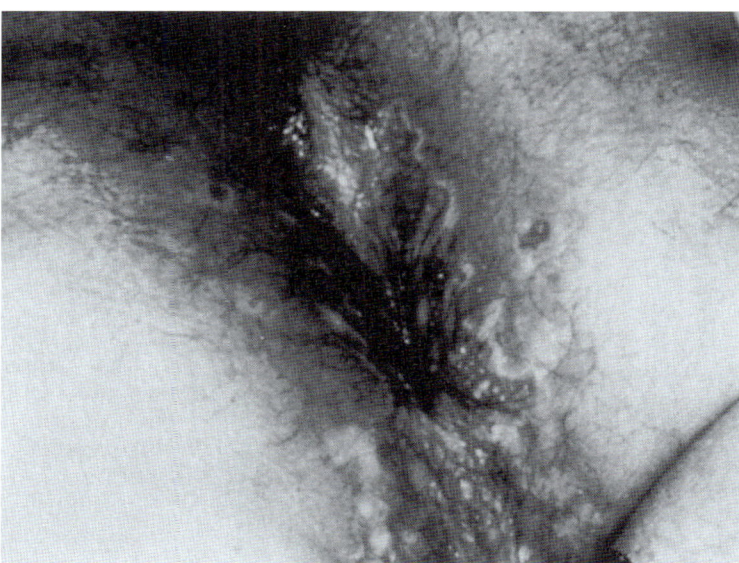

Figure 39.4 Perianal ulcerations typical of herpes simplex.

sacrum. These lesions are often atypical in appearance and may be confused with pressure decubiti (Fig. 39.4). To prevent misdiagnosis, all perianal ulcerations and anal fissures in patients with AIDS should be examined for the presence of HSV by culture or direct antigen detection.

Esophagitis

Symptoms of HSV esophagitis typically include retrosternal pain and odynophagia. Patients may present with acute onset of dysphagia or with chronic swallowing complaints, and symptoms may be severe enough to interfere with eating and adequate nutrition. Visible herpetic lesions in the oropharynx may not be present, and the clinical picture may be confused with *Candida* or CMV esophagitis. Radiographic contrast studies typically reveal a cobblestone appearance of the esophageal mucosa, but this finding is nonspecific and is also present with esophagitis from other causes (Fig. 39.5).[70] Definitive diagnosis of HSV esophagitis should be made by direct endoscopic visualization of the esophageal mucosa with positive viral studies and histopathologic evidence of invasive viral infection.[71]

Encephalitis

HSV encephalitis occurs rarely in AIDS but is the most life-threatening complication of HSV infection. Both HSV-1 and HSV-2 have been identified in brain tissue of AIDS patients, and simultaneous brain infections with HSV and CMV have been reported.[72-74] In adults with AIDS, HSV encephalitis usually occurs as a complication of primary or reactivated orolabial HSV infection. In neonates, the disease may occur as a result of primary HSV infection at the time of birth.[51]

The presentation of HSV encephalitis in adults with AIDS is often highly atypical. A subacute illness with subtle neurologic abnormalities is common in AIDS patients with HSV encephalitis, suggesting that host immune responses contribute to the clinical manifestations of the disease.[61,74] Headache, meningismus, and personality changes may develop gradually as the illness progresses. Alternatively, however, some AIDS patients with HSV encephalitis present with acute onset of symptoms. Abrupt onset of fever, headache, nausea, lethargy, and confusion may occur with temporal lobe abnormalities, cranial nerve defects, and focal seizures. Grand mal seizures, obtundation, coma, and death may eventually ensue.

The clinical diagnosis of HSV encephalitis may be extremely difficult, because other central nervous system infections (including HIV encephalopathy, *Cryptococcus neoformans,* and *Toxoplasma gondii*) may present with similar features. Studies have demonstrated the utility of detecting HSV DNA in CSF by the polymerase chain reaction technique as a method of non-invasive diagnosis of HSV encephalitis, although false-positive and false-negative results do occur.[75,76] CSF usually reveals nonspecific findings, including elevated protein and a lymphocytic pleocytosis. Viral CSF cultures are usually negative.[76]

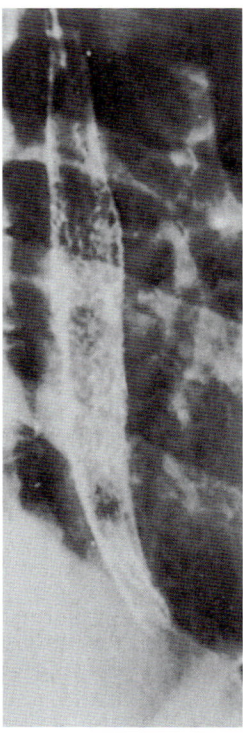

Figure 39.5 Barium esophagram revealing a cobblestone appearance of the esophageal mucosa. These findings are typical in both HSV esophagitis and *Candida* esophagitis. (Reprinted with permission from Farthing, et al.[70])

Other non-invasive diagnostic studies (such as computed tomography scan, radionuclide brain scan, or electroencephalography) are rarely diagnostic but may reveal localized abnormalities (often in the temporal lobes) to guide diagnostic brain biopsy. Definitive diagnosis may require brain biopsy and the recovery of virus or demonstration of viral antigens from tissue specimens.[77] The histopathologic abnormalities typically observed in normal hosts (hemorrhagic cortical necrosis and lymphocytic infiltration) may be absent in AIDS patients.[72-74,77] AIDS patients with suspected HSV encephalitis should be treated with high-dose intravenous acyclovir pending results of diagnostic studies.

Drug-resistant HSV infection

Since the initial description of acyclovir-resistant HSV infection in patients with AIDS, numerous additional reports have appeared in the literature.[79,80] The incidence of acyclovir-resistant HSV infections in immunocompromised hosts had been estimated as 4–5%,[79] but the incidence of AIDS has decreased

since the success of HAART therapies. The most common mechanism of acyclovir resistance in patients with AIDS is the selection and overgrowth of HSV strains deficient in the enzyme thymidine kinase. These mutated TK-deficient strains do not phosphorylate acyclovir or penciclovir to the active antiviral compounds, and these viruses are resistant to standard dosages of acyclovir, valacyclovir and famciclovir. Although these strains have reduced virulence in animal models[81] and only rarely cause clinical disease in non-immunocompromised hosts,[82] they are capable of causing severe clinical illness in patients with advanced HIV diseas.[81] Other mechanisms of drug resistance, including alteration of TK and DNA polymerase specificity, have been described but occur much less frequently. Most reports of drug-resistant HSV have cited localized chronic mucocutaneous infection, but cases of disseminated mucocutaneous disease,[80] meningoencephalitis,[83] and esophagitis[79] caused by these strains have been described.

Treatment of HSV Infection

Mucocutaneous HSV infections in patients with AIDS are often symptomatic and can be a source of great discomfort. Visceral involvement or disseminated HSV disease can be life threatening, and all symptomatic HSV infections should be treated aggressively even if they are reactivations. The prompt administration of antiviral chemotherapy in patients with acute HSV infection reduces morbidity and the risk of serious complications. Currently, several effective antiviral drugs are available, and the clinician must choose the appropriate medication and the optimal route of administration (topical, oral, or intravenous).

Acyclovir

Acyclovir, a synthetic purine nucleoside analog, was the first antiviral agent approved by the FDA for treatment of mucocutaneous HSV infection. Acyclovir has been available and widely used since the early 1980s and, until recently, has been the undisputed antiviral agent of choice for HSV infections in patients with AIDS and for other immunocompromised and non-immunocompromised hosts.[84] The drug has significant activity against HSV-1, HSV-2, and VZV. Despite excellent *in vitro* activity against these viruses, the bioavailability of oral acyclovir is only about 20%, resulting in relatively low serum drug levels following oral administration as compared with levels achieved with intravenous therapy.

Despite these findings, the serum levels of acyclovir achieved with standard acyclovir dosing (200 mg five times daily or 400 mg t.i.d.) exceed the levels required to inhibit the growth of HSV-1 and HSV-2, although higher oral doses (800 mg five times daily) are needed to achieve inhibitory serum drug levels to treat the more resistant VZV (see below).[84] Acyclovir has a high therapeutic-to-toxic ratio because it undergoes selective activation and phosphorylation by virus-induced TK only in HSV- and VZV-infected cells. Acyclovir triphosphate selectively inhibits HSV DNA polymerase and results in early termination of DNA chain synthesis. The drug has slightly higher activity against HSV-1 than HSV-2.

Acyclovir distributes into all tissues, including the brain and CSF, and is cleared by renal mechanisms. The serum half-life in patients with normal renal function is 2.5–3.3 h. The dose of intravenous acyclovir is 15 mg/kg per day in three divided doses for treatment of mucocutaneous infection and 30 mg/kg per day for HSV encephalitis. Although oral dosage adjustment is not required because of poor bioavailability, the intravenous dose should be reduced in patients with impaired renal function (Table 39.4). High-dose intravenous therapy can be associated with crystalluria, and adequate hydration should be maintained in patients on intravenous acyclovir to prevent this complication.[84]

Numerous studies have shown acyclovir to be effective for treatment of primary as well as recurrent HSV infection, and as suppressive therapy for patients with frequently recurring HSV. In the immunocompromised patient treatment of recurrence is only marginally beneficial, but in AIDS patients with more severe recurrence treatment is more likely to impact the disease. The drug has an excellent safety record and is usually well tolerated, although some patients may complain of headache or nausea. Acyclovir can be administered orally,[85-91] intravenously,[92,93] or topically,[63,88] and the optimal route of administration, dosage, and duration of therapy depend on the site and severity of the HSV infection. Oral acyclovir is usually appropriate for outpatients with localized, non-life-threatening mucocutaneous HSV infection. Intravenous therapy should be prescribed for patients with disseminated disease, HSV encephalitis, or visceral organ involvement. Additionally, intravenous therapy is indicated for those patients who do not respond adequately to oral treatment, raising concern over issues such as poor drug absorption, poor compliance with oral therapy, or the development of drug-resistant infection. Topical acyclovir ointment is only minimally effective and should not be prescribed in the place of systemic antiviral therapy.

Valacyclovir

Valacyclovir hydrochloride is the L-valyl ester of acyclovir, and is available and effective in the treatment of HSV[94] and VZV[95] infections. Following oral administration, valacyclovir is rapidly absorbed from the gastrointestinal tract. The drug is rapidly and extensively converted to acyclovir *in vivo*, and the resulting acyclovir serum levels are much higher than those achieved with oral acyclovir. Pharmacokinetic studies reveal that a therapeutic drug level equivalent to acyclovir 800 mg five times daily can be achieved with 1000 mg valacyclovir given every 8 h.[94-96]

Because of the improved bioavailability of valacyclovir as compared with acyclovir, studies have evaluated less frequent dosing for patients with HSV infection. Valacyclovir is effective in the treatment of first-episode HSV infection at a dose of 500 mg to 1 g twice daily, and in the treatment of recurrent HSV infection at a dose of 500 mg twice daily if initiated within the first 24 h of signs or symptoms. Therapy should be continued until all lesions are dry and crusted. Additionally, valacyclovir is effective as suppressive therapy at a dose of 250 mg twice daily, 500 mg once daily (for patients with fewer than 10 recurrences per year), and 1 g once daily (for patients with 10 or more recurrences per year).[96] Dosage reduction is recommended in patients with a creatinine clearance <50 mL/min (Table 39.5).

A study evaluating very high valacyclovir dosing (8 g/day) for suppression of CMV in patients with advanced HIV disease suggested a possible association between valacyclovir and the syndromes of thrombotic thrombocytopenic purpura and hemolytic-uremic syndrome (TIP/HUS). A cause-and-effect relationship has not been firmly established, however, and these findings have not been observed

Table 39.4 Dosage adjustment of intravenous acyclovir in patients with renal dysfunction

Creatinine clearance (mL/min per 1.73 m²)	Standard dose (%)	Dosing interval (h)
>50	100	8
25–50	100	12
10–25	100	12
0–10	50	24

Usually 5 mg/kg; 10 mg/kg is used for HSV CNS infections and in some instances for VZV infections.

Table 39.5 Dosage adjustment of valacyclovir in patients with renal dysfunction

Creatinine clearance (mL/min)	Dosage for herpes zoster	Dosage for genital herpes Initial treatment	Recurrent episodes
≥50	1 g every 8 h	1 g every 12 h	500 mg every 12 h
30–49	1 g every 12 h	1 g every 12 h	500 mg every 12 h
10–29	1 g every 24 h	1 g every 24 h	500 mg every 24 h
<10	500 mg every 24 h	500 mg every 24 h	500 mg every 24 h

in patients receiving standard dosages of valacyclovir. In view of these observations, caution should be used when prescribing valacyclovir in HIV-infected patients, and the standard recommended dosages should not be exceeded.[96]

Famciclovir

Famciclovir is the diacetyl 6-deoxy analog of the active antiviral compound penciclovir. When taken orally, famciclovir is readily absorbed from the upper gastrointestinal tract, and is rapidly converted into penciclovir. In a manner similar to acyclovir, penciclovir undergoes phosphorylation to the triphosphate compound by viral-induced TK and cellular enzymes. Penciclovir triphosphate acts as a competitive inhibitor of the natural substrate required for viral DNA replication, but does not irreversibly terminate DNA replication. The drug has a very long half-life (10–20 h) in HSV-infected cells, ensuring prolonged antiviral activity.[97–101]

Clinical studies have shown that oral famciclovir is effective in the treatment of first episode HSV infections at a dose of 250 mg three times daily and is effective in the treatment of recurrent HSV infection at a dose of 125 mg twice daily if given within the first 6 h of symptoms or signs. Therapy should be continued until all lesions are dry and crusted. Additionally, famciclovir is effective as suppressive therapy at a dose of 250 mg twice daily.[96,98,99,101] Dosage reduction is recommended in patients with creatinine clearance less than 60 mL/min (Table 39.6).

Topical penciclovir has been approved by the FDA for the treatment of recurrent HSV gingivostomatitis. Unlike topical acyclovir, penciclovir appears to have a beneficial effect on recurrent mucocutaneous HSV infection when compared with placebo.[102] Topical penciclovir has not been extensively evaluated in patients with HIV infection, however, and

Table 39.6 Dosage adjustment of famciclovir in patients with zoster and renal dysfunction

Creatinine clearance (mL/min)	Dosage regimen
≥60	500 mg every 8 h
40–59	500 mg every 12 h
20–39	500 mg every 24 h

There are insufficient data to recommend a dosage for patients with creatinine clearance <20 mL/min. Famvir is supplied as 50 mg white, oval, film-coated tablets debossed with FAMVIR on one side and 500 on the other, in bottles of 30 and in single unit packages (blister packs) of 50 (intended for institutional use only). 500 mg 30s: NDC 0007-4117-13; 500 mg SUP 50s: NDC 0007-4117-19. Store at controlled room temperature (15–30°C; 59–86°F). ©Smith Klein Beecham, 1998. Manufactured by SmithKline Beecham Pharmaceuticals, Crawley, UK, for SmithKline Beecham Pharmaceuticals, Philadelphia, PA 19101.

may not be as effective as systemic therapy in this immunocompromised population.

Foscarnet

Foscarnet (phosphonoformic acid) is an inorganic pyrophosphate with a broad range of antiviral activities against herpesviruses as well as HIV.[44] Studies have demonstrated foscarnet to be effective in the treatment of CMV disease and in the treatment of drug-resistant HSV and VZV infections. Unlike acyclovir and famciclovir, foscarnet does not require viral enzyme-mediated phosphorylation for activity. Hence, foscarnet remains an effective antiviral agent for treatment of TK-deficient, drug-resistant HSV.[38,103,104] Foscarnet is superior to vidarabine in the treatment of acyclovir-resistant HSV infections in patients with AIDS, and remains a treatment of choice for this illness at a dose of 40 mg/kg three times daily.[38]

Foscarnet must be given intravenously, and side-effects (including nausea, fever, headache, anemia, and renal failure) are common. Because of the potential for nephrotoxic effects and electrolyte imbalances, close monitoring of renal function and serum levels of potassium, calcium, phosphate, and magnesium is required. Variable penetration into the CSF has been reported. Dosage adjustments are required in patients with renal dysfunction.

Other antiviral drugs

Cidofovir is a long-acting antiviral drug approved by the FDA for the treatment of CMV retinitis, and also appears to be effective in the treatment of drug-resistant HSv.[105,106] Cidofovir has a prolonged serum half-life, allowing for once-weekly intravenous administration. Nephrotoxicity can occur with therapy, however, and pretreatment with intravenous fluids and probenecid is recommended. A gel form of cidofovir for topical use is effective for mucocutaneous drug-resistant HSV infections.[107]

Management of patients with HSV infection

Most AIDS patients with primary or recurrent mucocutaneous HSV infections are not ill enough to require hospitalization and are suitable candidates for outpatient treatment. The treatment of choice for most HSV infections in AIDS is either oral acyclovir, oral valacyclovir, or oral famciclovir (Table 39.7). Because therapy with valacyclovir or famciclovir results in serum antiviral levels comparable to those with intravenous acyclovir, many AIDS patients with severe HSV infections who can tolerate oral therapy can be treated as outpatients.

Although the bioavailability and resultant serum drug levels with oral acyclovir are not as favorable

as those with valacyclovir or famciclovir, acyclovir remains a safe, effective, and well-tolerated treatment regimen in HIV-infected patients with HSV infection. Most HIV-infected patients respond well to oral acyclovir, although many clinicians use higher doses of acyclovir in HIV-infected patients than those recommended in non-immunocompromised.

Patients with symptomatic HSV disease should be treated as early as possible with acyclovir 400 mg three to five times daily, valacyclovir 500–1000 mg twice daily, or famciclovir 125–500 mg twice daily until all lesions are healed.

Patients requiring suppressive therapy because of frequent or exceptionally severe recurrence can be treated with acyclovir 400 mg–800 mg 2–3 times daily valacyclovir 500 mg twice daily or famciclovir 500 mg twice daily. These doses are higher than those used for non-HIV infected patients with HSV, but are endorsed by the Centres for Disease Control and Prevention.[107a] As mentioned above, FDA-approved doses of valacyclovir should be used cautiously in patients with HIV infection because of the observation of TTP/HUS with high-dose (8 g/day) therapy.

Intravenous acyclovir should be reserved for patients with severe or extensive mucocutaneous HSV infection and for patients with viral dissemination, visceral organ infection (e.g. brain, esophagus, eye), or neurologic complications (atonic bladder, transverse myelitis). Intravenous therapy may also be indicated for AIDS patients who require antiviral chemotherapy but are unable to tolerate or absorb oral antiviral therapy because of nausea, dysphagia, or protracted diarrhea. The dose of intravenous acyclovir for patients with mucocutaneous HSV infection and normal renal function is 15 mg/kg per day in three divided doses.[92] Patients with life-threatening HSV infection (encephalitis, neonatal infection, disseminated infection) or visceral organ involvement (esophagitis, proctitis), should receive intravenous acyclovir 30 mg/kg per day in three divided doses.[93] Treatment should last for a minimum of 10 days, but longer therapy may be necessary if response to therapy is slow. As noted above, the dose of intravenous acyclovir should be adjusted in patients with impaired renal function (Table 39.4). Oral treatment with acyclovir, valacyclovir, or famciclovir can be substituted for i.v. acyclovir once the patient is ready for hospital discharge.

Because of their limited absorption, topical acyclovir and topical penciclovir are probably much less effective than either oral or intravenous therapy in the treatment of HSV infections in AIDS. Although topical therapy slightly decreases the duration of

---

Table 39.7 Management of HSV infections in AIDS

Mucocutaneous infection, mild	Acyclovir 400 mg t.i.d., Famciclovir 500 mg b.i.d. or Valacyclovir 1000 mg b.i.d.
Mucocutaneous infection, severe	Acyclovir 5 mg/kg i.v. t.i.d., Famciclovir 500 mg b.i.d. or Valacyclovir 1000 mg b.i.d.
Suppression of mucocutaneous lesions	Acyclovir 400 mg–800 mg 2–3 times a day Famciclovir 500 mg b.i.d. or Valacyclovir 500 mg b.i.d.
Acyclovir-resistant infection	Foscarnet 40 mg/kg i.v. t.i.d.

viral shedding in immunocompromised hosts with mucocutaneous HSV infection, these non-systemic therapies do not reduce new lesion formation or the risk of dissemination. There is no added benefit to combining topical therapy with either oral or intravenous antiviral therapy. Topical therapy has little, if any, usefulness in the clinical setting.[88]

Systemic antiviral therapy should be continued until all mucocutaneous lesions have crusted or re-epithelialized. This may require longer treatment than the usual duration of therapy prescribed in the non-immunocompromised host, because HSV lesions may heal slowly in AIDS patients even with optimal antiviral chemotherapy. If lesions do not heal while the patient is receiving antiviral therapy, repeat viral cultures should be obtained, high-dose oral therapy (e.g. acyclovir 800 mg 5 times daily, famciclovir 500 mg t.i.d., valacyclovir 1 g t.i.d., or intravenous acyclovir 30 mg/kg per day) may be given, and the possibility of drug-resistant HSV infection should be considered. If available, antiviral susceptibility testing should be performed in this setting to determine whether drug-resistant HSV infection is present. If antiviral testing is not available, patients who continue to have positive cultures for HSV and no evidence of clinical response despite high-dose intravenous acyclovir should be treated presumptively for drug-resistant infection with intravenous foscarnet.

Suppressive acyclovir therapy for HSV infection

Many AIDS patients suffer from frequently recurring HSV infection or develop new HSV recurrences shortly after antiherpes chemotherapy is discontinued. These patients can often be managed with suppressive antiviral therapy.[85–87,90,91,96,98,101,108a] AIDS patients requiring suppressive therapy should initially be treated with a regimen of oral acyclovir 400 mg–800 mg 2–3 times daily, valacyclovir 500 mg twice daily, valacyclovir 500–1000 mg once or twice daily or famciclovir 500 mg twice daily. Increased daily dosage may be necessary to control recurrences, but gastrointestinal intolerance may limit the amount of drug that can be taken, Breakthrough recurrences that develop while the patient is receiving suppressive therapy may be controlled by increasing the daily suppressive dose. Breakthrough recurrences may or may not represent the emergence of drug-resistant strains.[109] Patients who demonstrate a good response to suppressive therapy at high doses may attempt a reduction in the daily suppressive dose.[87,108] Some clinicians and patients choose to continue suppressive therapy longer than FDA recommendations,

in order to avoid re-development of symptomatic recurrences. Recurrences which occur after discontinuing antiviral suppression may be more severe than those experienced before starting suppression. Suppression therapy has been used continuously for over 15 years without evidence of adverse reactions or cumulative toxicity. Studies have shown that the incidence of asymptomatic virus shedding is decreased while a patient is on acyclovir suppression.[110] Individuals maintained on long-term suppressive therapy should be cautioned, however, that recurrences will likely develop after discontinuation of therapy and that the first recurrence may be more severe than those previously experienced.[85,86,90,91] In a study which evaluated immunocompetent, heterosexual, HSV discordant couples, the use of daily valacyclovir 500 mg suppression reduced the risk of HSV transmission from the infected individual to the susceptible partner.[111] This study did not include patients with HIV to prevent transmission or acquisition of HSV. Acyclovir suppression has also been shown to reduce asymptomatic HSV shedding and may also play a role in preventing transmission to sexual contacts.[112] Many HIV-positive patients receiving acyclovir may also be taking zidovudine or other antiretroviral agents. Recent studies suggest that suppressive therapy for HSV results in a reduction in HIV RNA. This data is suggestive that HSV may play a role in recognition of HIV, and that suppressive therapy against HSV may be a useful adjunctive therapy in patients co-infected with both HSV and HIV.[56a,112a,112b,112c]

Management of drug-resistant HSV infection

With the increased incidence of drug-resistant HSV infections observed in patients with AIDS, several studies have examined the utility of alternate antiviral agents and treatment regimens. Standard doses of intravenous or oral acyclovir have no clinical benefit if the HSV isolate is resistant to acyclovir (ID50 >3.0 µg/mL) *in vitro*. Most acyclovir-resistant strains isolated from patients with AIDS have been TK-deficient and are therefore also resistant to valacyclovir and famciclovir. These strains remain susceptible to foscarnet, which does not require phosphorylation for activity. Studies have confirmed that foscarnet is effective in the treatment of these TK-deficient, drug-resistant HSV infections, and foscarnet remains the treatment of choice in this setting.[38,103,104] The dosage of foscarnet used for the treatment of acyclovir-resistant HSV infections in AIDS patients is 40 mg/kg every 8 h (with reduction in dose for renal dysfunction).

Continuous-infusion acyclovir therapy has been effective in a few AIDS patients with severe acyclovir-resistant HSV infection. Acyclovir has been administered at a dosage of 1.5–2.0 mg/kg per h for 6 weeks, and complete resolution of acyclovir-resistant HSV proctitis has been reported.[113] Other investigational agents for possible treatment of drug-resistant HSV infections include topical trifluridine,[114] topical cidofovir gel,[107] and intravenous cidofovir.[105]

As with many opportunistic infections in AIDS patients, there is a high incidence of recurrent HSV disease after successful treatment for drug-resistant HSV. Some (but not all) relapses in this setting have been due to drug-resistant strains, suggesting that these mutant viruses are capable of causing latency in the immunocompromised host. Chronic prophylaxis with daily acyclovir, valacyclovir, famciclovir, or foscarnet can be considered in patients who are treated successfully for drug-resistant HSV, although there are no data to confirm efficacy in this setting. Foscarnet-resistant strains of HSV have been reported, raising concerns over the possible selection for multi-drug-resistant HSV with suppressive therapy.[106,115]

Varicella-Zoster Virus

Primary VZV infection is usually a childhood illness, with attack rates exceeding 90% in susceptible household contacts.[116] Most adults with AIDS have been previously infected with VZV and (as with HSV) are not susceptible to primary infection.

AIDS patients develop recurrent VZV infection (zoster) more frequently than do age-matched immunocompetent hosts. A retrospective review of 300 AIDS patients with Kaposi's sarcoma revealed that 8% of patients had at least one prior attack of zoster, an incidence seven times greater than expected by the age of the study group. Zoster also occurs with a higher-than-expected frequency in HIV-infected individuals who appear otherwise healthy. Additionally, some HIV-infected patients develop more than one episode of zoster in a relatively short period of time; an uncommon occurrence in immunocompetent hosts.[117-121]

Primary Infection-Varicella

Varicella in immunocompetent children is usually a benign illness. Adults, however, are more likely to develop complications during primary VZV infec-

tion. Viral dissemination to visceral organs occurs in up to one-third of immunocompetent adults with primary infection.[116] Although most adults with AIDS have been previously infected with VZV and are not susceptible to primary infection,[122] for those who are, a protracted and potentially life-threatening illness could follow.[117]

Recurrent Infection-Zoster

Unlike primary VZV infection, recurrent VZV infection (zoster) is common in patients with AIDS. The illness usually begins with radicular pain and is followed by a localized or segmental erythematous rash covering 1–3 dermatomes. Maculopapules develop in the dermatomal area, and the patient experiences increasing pain. The maculopapules progress to fluid-filled vesicles, and contiguous vesicles may become confluent, with true bullae formation. In most HIV-infected patients, the lesions remain confined to a dermatomal distribution and heal by crusting and re-epithelialization. Occasionally, however, widespread cutaneous or visceral dissemination may occur. Extensive cutaneous dissemination may appear identical to primary varicella. Visceral dissemination to lung, liver, or the CNS may produce a life-threatening illness.[117-120,123]

Reactivated infection involving the ophthalmic division of the trigeminal nerve often results in infection of the cornea (zoster ophthalmicus). The presence of vesicles on the tip of the nose is often associated with involvement of the eye. Although healing without sequelae may occur, untreated patients are at increased risk to develop anterior uveitis, corneal scarring, and permanent visual loss.[109] Acyclovir-resistant zoster is a rare complication, and has a peculiar dermatomal wart-like, nonhealing appearance.[124]

Complications

Complications of VZV infection are common in immunocompromised patients and may cause prolonged morbidity and death. Dissemination of virus to the lung, liver, and CNS has been associated with a mortality rate of 6–17%. Varicella pneumonia may occur during primary VZV infection or during reactivated infection with visceral dissemination in immunocompromised patients. Symptoms are variable. Many patients develop only mild respiratory symptoms, whereas others suffer from severe hypoxemia and succumb to respiratory failure. Radiographic abnormalities are usually out of proportion to the clinical findings, with diffuse nodular densities on chest radiograph and occasional pleural effusions.[116,125]

Encephalitis is a rare complication of VZV infection in AIDS patients but may occur with or without visceral dissemination. The illness begins 3–8 days after the onset of varicella or 1–2 weeks after the development of zoster, although occasional AIDS patients have developed progressive neurologic disease caused by VZV up to 3 months after the onset of localized zoster.[123] Headache, vomiting, lethargy, and cerebellar symptoms (ataxia, tremors, dizziness) are prominent findings. Diagnosis based on clinical criteria alone can be difficult, because other CNS infections can present in a similar fashion. The diagnosis of VZV encephalitis is documented by finding VZV DNA by polymerase chain reaction or VZV antibody in CSF. Postherpetic neuralgia, defined as prolonged pain following resolution of the cutaneous lesions from zoster, can be severe and disabling.[116,126,127]

Although post-herpetic neuralgia is a more common occurrence in elderly individuals with zoster, AIDS patients also may be at risk for this complication. Polyradiculopathy similar to that caused by CMV may rarely be due to VZV. In these cases, VZV may be isolated from CSF.

Management of VZV Infection

HIV-infected patients who develop primary or recurrent VZV infection should be treated promptly with an effective antiviral regimen (Table 39.8).[128] Acyclovir, valacyclovir, and famciclovir are safe and effective in the treatment of patients with primary or recurrent VZV infection. Treatment should be started as soon as the diagnosis is made (preferably within 72 h of rash onset), and should be continued until all the external lesions are dry and crusted (usually 7–10 days).

Because VZV is less susceptible than is HSV to acyclovir, valacyclovir, and famciclovir, the dosages of antiviral therapy used for treatment of VZV infections must be higher than those recommended for HSV. Oral acyclovir in the dosage used to treat HSV does not produce serum drug levels high enough to inhibit VZV in tissue culture, and is unlikely to be effective in patients with active VZV infection. To treat VZV with oral acyclovir, a dose of 800 mg five times daily should be prescribed.[125,129-131] This higher dose does produce serum drug levels high enough to inhibit the growth of VZV *in vitro*, and this regimen has been shown to modestly decrease the incidence and severity of postherpetic neuralgia in non-immunocompromised patients.[127,132]

Valacyclovir and famciclovir (discussed in detail above) are also effective agents against VZV and are suitable for oral treatment of acute VZV infections. Because of their improved bioavailability, these drugs have the advantage of producing higher serum drug levels than that achieved with oral acyclovir. Treatment with valacyclovir 1 g t.i.d.[95] or famciclovir 500 mg t.i.d.[100,133] reduces the severity of acute VZV infection and appears to reduce the severity and duration of postherpetic neuralgia.[97,126] Although the favorable pharmacokinetics and higher serum drug levels achieved with these agents could be expected to offer a therapeutic advantage as compared with oral acyclovir, no comparative trials evaluating clinical outcome in HIV-infected patients have been reported.

As mentioned in the section on treatment of HSV, the possible association between valacyclovir and TTP/HUS in patients with advanced HIV disease must be kept in mind when prescribing valacyclovir. Although a cause-and-effect relationship has not been firmly established, caution should be used when prescribing valacyclovir in HIV-infected patients, and the standard FDA-recommended dosages should not be exceeded.[96]

Most AIDS patients with localized zoster are not ill enough to require hospitalization, and are suit-

Table 39.8 Management of VZV infections in AIDS

Clinical presentation	Treatment
Primary infection (varicella)	Acyclovir, 30 mg/kg per day i.v., or acyclovir, 800 mg p.o. 5 times daily, or valacyclovir 1g p.o. t.i.d., or famciclovir 500 mg p.o. t.i.d.
Recurrent infection (localized zoster)	Acyclovir, 30 mg/kg per day i.v., or acyclovir, 800 mg p.o. 5 times daily, or valacyclovir 1g p.o. t.i.d., or famciclovir 500 mg p.o. t.i.d.
Recurrent infection, disseminated	Acyclovir, 30 mg/kg per day i.v.
Severe infection caused by acyclovir-resistant VZV	Foscarnet, 40 mg/kg t.i.d. i.v. (not FDA approved)

Modified with permission from Drew, et al.[128]

able for outpatient therapy with oral acyclovir, oral valacyclovir, or oral famciclovir. Intravenous acyclovir remains an available option, however, and has been shown to be effective in the treatment of patients with VZV infection. Treatment with intravenous acyclovir reduces the duration of viral shedding, new lesion formation, the incidence of dissemination, and mortality rates in immunocompromised hosts with VZV infection.[129,134] Intravenous acyclovir should be prescribed for those patients with disseminated disease or visceral organ involvement, and for those patients who are unable to tolerate oral therapy. The dosage of intravenous acyclovir for patients with VZV infection is 30 mg/kg per day in three divided doses (with dosage adjustments for renal dysfunction; see Table 39.4). Treatment should be continued for at least 7 days or until all external lesions are crusted. The decision whether to hospitalize an individual patient for intravenous acyclovir must be based on several factors, including the severity of the infection, the immune status of the host, and whether visceral or cutaneous dissemination has occurred.

Treatment with steroids to prevent post-herpetic neuralgia remains a controversial topic with regard to the non-immunocompromised population, but recent studies have failed to document the efficacy of this practice,[135,136] although the general quality of life may be improved. Because of the potential for further immunosuppression and increasing the risk of VZV dissemination in patients with AIDS, however, steroids should not be routinely prescribed for this indication in this population.

Treatment of Drug-resistant VZV Infection

Drug-resistant VZV has been identified in patients with AIDS, these patients may present with atypical-appearing cutaneous lesions that shed VZV intermittently despite ongoing high-dose antiviral therapy. All strains have been isolated from patients previously treated with acyclovir for recurrent VZV or HSV infection, and these strains may be resistant to acyclovir, valacyclovir, and famciclovir by deficiency of the enzyme thymidine kinase.[137] Foscarnet has been shown to be effective in small studies, but remains investigational for this purpose.[124] The intravenous dosage used has been 40 µg/kg three times daily.

Prevention of VZV Infection

Varicella-zoster immune globulin (VZIG) is effective in preventing severe primary VZV infection in susceptible (i.e. seronegative) immunocompromised hosts if administered within 96 h from the time of a significant exposure. Care should be taken to ensure that an exposed individual is truly susceptible to infection (by serologic testing if there is no history of chickenpox) prior to administration of VZIG, VZIG is contraindicated in individuals with a history of prior chickenpox and in those who have serologic evidence of previous VZV infection. VZIG is not effective as treatment in individuals who present with acute VZV infection.

Two attenuated, live VZV vaccines are licensed in the USA for prevention of primary VZV infection (varicella) and recurrent disease (zoster) in non-immunocompromised hosts.[138,139,139a] Both vaccines contain the live, attenuated OKA strain of VZV, although the zoster vaccine contains higher titers of virus than that found in the varicella vaccine. The efficacy and safety of these vaccines in HIV infected patients has not been well studied, and caution should be used in this population since the vaccine contains a live virus and there is the theoretical risk of dissemination in immunocompromised hosts. A small number of patients receiving the varicella vaccine have developed a varicella-like rash after administration,[141] and this rash contains live virus that is transmissible. HIV infected patients who receive the vaccine and develop a varicella-like rash following vaccination should be treated with one of the effective antiviral drugs discussed above. Because the vaccine strain produces latency after administration, vaccinated individuals renmain at risk to devleop zoster later in life.[138,139,142]

Conclusion

Herpesvirus (CMV, HSV, VZV) infections are common in AIDS patients and often exist in a chronic or progressive form. Oral ganciclovir prophylaxis can reduce the risk of developing CMV disease. CMV retinitis occurs in up to 40% of AIDS patients and can be treated effectively with ganciclovir or foscarnet. Perianal ulcers, proctitis, and other clinical syndromes caused by HSV can be treated effectively with acyclovir, valacyclovir, or famciclovir. These drugs can be administered daily to prevent HSV recurrences. Herpes zoster in a young adult may be the first indication of immune deficiency resulting from HIV. Because VZV is less susceptible to antiviral drugs than HSV, higher doses of acyclovir, valacyclovir, or famciclovir are required to achieve inhibitory blood levels. HSV and VZV resistant to acyclovir and related drugs are usually susceptible to foscarnet.

References

1. O'Sullivan C, Drew WL, McMullen D, et al. Decrease of cytomegalovirus replication in human immunodeficiency virus infected patients after treatment with highly active antiretroviral therapy. J Infect Dis 1999; 180:847–849.
2. Spector SA, Wong R, Hsia K, et al. Plasma cytomegalovirus (CMV) DNA load predicts CMV disease and survival in AIDS patients. J Clin Invest 1998; 101:497.
3. Felsenstein D, D'Amico DJ, Hirsch MS, et al. Treatment of cytomegalovirus retinitis with 9-[2-hydroxy1-(hydroxymethyl)ethoxymethyl]guanine. Ann Intern Med 1985; 103:377.
4. Palestine AG, Polis MA, DeSmet MD, et al. A randomized, controlled trial of foscarnet in the treatment of cytomegalovirus retinitis in patients with AIDS. Ann Intern Med 1991; 115:665.
5. Spector SA, Weingeist T, Pollard RB, et al. A randomized, controlled study of intravenous ganciclovir therapy for cytomegalovirus peripheral retinitis in patients with AIDS. J Infect Dis 1993; 168:557.
6. Jabs D, and the Studies of Ocular Complications of AIDS Research Group, in collaboration with the AIDS Clinical Trials Group. Mortality in patients with the acquired immunodeficiency syndrome treated with either foscarnet or ganciclovir for cytomegalovirus retinitis. N Engl J Med 1992; 326:213.
7. Budka H, Costanzi G, Cristina S, et al. Brain pathology induced by infection with the human immunodeficiency virus (HIV): A histological, immunocytochemical and electron microscopical study of 100 autopsy cases. Acta Neuropathol (Berl) 1987; 75:185.
8. Petito CK, Cho E-S, Lehman W, et al. Neuropathology of acquired immunodeficiency syndrome (AIDS): An autopsy review. J Neuropathol Exp Neurol 1986; 45:635.
9. Snider WD, Simpson DM, Nielsen S, et al. Neurological complications of acquired immune deficiency syndrome: Analysis of 50 patients. Ann Neurol 1983; 14:403.
10. Morgello S, Cho E, Nielsen S, et al. Cytomegalovirus encephalitis in patients with acquired immunodeficiency syndrome: An autopsy study of 30 cases and review of literature. Hum Pathol 1987; 18:289.
11. Holland NR, Power C, Mathews VP, et al. Cytomegalovirus encephalitis in AIDS. Neurology 1994; 44:507.
12. Drew WL, Mintz L, Miner RC, et al. Prevalence of cytomegalovirus infection in homosexual men. J Infect Dis 1981; 143:188.
13. Fiala M, Singer EJ, Graves MC, et al. AIDS dementia complex complicated by cytomegalovirus encephalopathy. J Neurol 1993; 240:223.
14. Vinters HV, Kwok MK, Ho HW, et al. Cytomegalovirus in the nervous system of patients with the acquired immune deficiency syndrome. Brain 1989; 112:245.
15. Casareale D, Fiala M, Chang CM, et al. Cytomegalovirus enhances lysis of HIV infected T lymphoblasts. Int J Cancer 1989; 44:124.
16. Anand R, Nightingale D, Fish RH, et al. Control of cytomegalovirus retinitis using sustained release of intraocular ganciclovir. Arch Ophthalmol 1993; 111:223.
17. Walot I, Miller BL, Chang L, et al. Neuroimaging findings in patients with AIDS. Clin Infect Dis 1996; 22:906.
18. Clough LA, Clough JA, Maciunsas RJ, et al. Diagnosing CNS mass lesions in patients with AIDS. AIDS Reader 1997; 7:83.
19. Small PM, McPhaul LW, Sooy CD, et al. Cytomegalovirus infection of the laryngeal nerve presenting as hoarseness in patients with acquired immunodeficiency syndrome. Am J Med 1989; 86:108.
20. Fuller GN, Jacobs JM, Guiloff RJ. Axonal atrophy in the painful peripheral neuropathy in AIDS. Acta Neuropathol 1990; 81:198.
21. Whitley RJ, Jacobson MA, Friedberg DN, et al. Guidelines for the treatment of cytomegalovirus diseases in patients with AIDS in the era of potent antiretroviral therapy. Arch Intern Med 1998; 158:957.
22. Dieterich DT, Kotler DP, Busch DF. Ganciclovir treatment of cytomegalovirus colitis in AIDS: A randomized, double-blind, placebo-controlled multicenter study. J Infect Dis 1993; 167:278.
23. Emanuel D, Cunningham I, Jules-Elysee K, et al. Cytomegalovirus pneumonia after bone-marrow transplantation successfully treated with the combination of ganciclovir and high-dose intravenous immune globulin. Ann Intern Med 1988; 109:777.
24. Reed EC, Bowden RA, Dandliker PS, et al. Treatment of cytomegalovirus pneumonia with ganciclovir and intravenous cytomegalovirus immunoglobulin in patients with bone marrow transplants. Ann Intern Med 1988; 109:783.
25. Shepp DH, Dandliker PS, de Miranda P, et al. Activity of 9-[2-hydroxy-1-(hydroxymethyl)ethoxymethyl]guanine in the treatment of cytomegalovirus pneumonia. Ann Intern Med 1985; 103:368.
26. Sullivan V, Taliarico CL, Stanat SC, et al. A protein kinase homologue controls phosphorylation of ganciclovir in human cytomegalovirus-infected cells. Nature 1992; 358:162.
27. Martin D, Kuppermann B, Wolitz R, et al. Combined oral ganciclovir and intravitreal ganciclovir implant for treatment of patients with cytomegalovirus retinitis: A randomized, controlled study. 37th Interscience Conference on Antimicrobial Agents and Chemotherapy: 1997; Toronto.
28. Musch DC, Martin DF, Gordon JF, et al. Treatment of cytomegalovirus retinitis with a sustained-release ganciclovir implant. N Engl J Med 1997; 337:83.
29. Drew WL, Ives D, Lalezari JP, et al. Oral ganciclovir as maintenance treatment for cytomegalovirus retinitis in patients with AIDS. N Engl J Med 1995; 333:615.
30. Martin DF, Sierra-Madero J, Walmsley S, et al. for the Valganciclovir Study Group. A controlled trial of valganciclovir as induction therapy for cytomegalovirus. N Engl J Med 2002; 346:1119–1126.
31. The Oral Ganciclovir European and Australian Cooperative Study Group. Intravenous versus oral ganciclovir: European/Australian comparative study of efficacy and safety in the prevention of cytomegalovirus retinitis recurrence in patients with AIDS. AIDS 1995; 9:471.
32. Cantrill HL, Henry K, Melroe H, et al. Treatment of cytomegalovirus retinitis with intravitreal ganciclovir: Long-term results. Ophthalmology 1989; 96:367.
33. Martin DF, Parks DJ, Mellow D, et al. Treatment of cytomegalovirus retinitis with an intraocular sustained-release ganciclovir implant. Arch Ophthalmol 1994; 112:1531.
34. Sanborn GE, Anand R, Torti RE, et al. Sustained-release ganciclovir therapy for treatment of cytomegalovirus retinitis. Arch Ophthalmol 1992; 110:188.
35. Buhles WC Jr, Mastre BJ, Tinker AJ, et al. Ganciclovir treatment of life- or sight-threatening cytomegalovirus infection: Experience in 314 immunocompromised patients. Rev Infect Dis 1988; 10(Suppl):S495.
36. Erice A, Chou S, Biron K, et al. Progressive disease due to ganciclovir-resistant cytomegalovirus in immunocompromised patients. N Engl J Med 1989; 320:289.
37. Drew WL, Miner RC, Busch DF, et al. Prevalence of resistance in patients receiving ganciclovir for serious cytomegalovirus infection. J Infect Dis 1991; 163:716.
38. Safrin S, Crumpacker C, Chatis P, et al. A controlled trial comparing foscarnet with vidarabine for acyclovir-resistant mucocutaneous herpes simplex in the acquired immunodeficiency syndrome. N Engl J Med 1991; 325:551.

39. Jacobson MA, Drew WL, Feinberg J, et al. Foscarnet therapy for ganciclovir-resistant cytomegalovirus retinitis in patients with AIDS. J Infect Dis 1991; 163:1348.

40. Chou S, Lurain NS, Thompson KD, et al. Viral DNA polymerase mutations associated with drug resistance in human cytomegalovirus. J Infect Dis 2003; 188:32–39.

41. Drew WL, Stempien MJ, Andres J, et al. Cytomegalovirus resistance in patients with CMV retinitis and AIDS treated with oral or intravenous ganciclovir. J Infect Dis 1999; 179:1352–1355.

42. Jabs DA, Enger C, Dunn JP, et al. Cytomegalovirus retinitis and viral resistance: Ganciclovir resistance. J Infect Dis 1998; 177:770.

43. Spector SA, McKinley GF, Lalezari JP, et al. Oral ganciclovir for the prevention of cytomegalovirus disease in persons with AIDS. N Engl J Med 1996; 334:1491.

44. Chrisp P, Clissold SP. Foscarnet: A review of its antiviral activity, pharmacokinetic properties and therapeutic use in immunocompromised patients with cytomegalovirus retinitis. Drugs 1991; 41:104.

45. Jacobson MA, Causey D, Polsky B. A dose-ranging study of daily maintenance intravenous foscarnet therapy for cytomegalovirus retinitis in AIDS. J Infect Dis 1993; 168:444.

46. Cimoch PJ, Lavelle J, Pollard R, et al. Pharmacokinetics of oral ganciclovir alone and in combination with zidovudine, didanosine, and probenecid in HIV-infected subjects. J AIDS Acquir Immune Defic Syndr Hum Retrovirol 1998; 17:227.

47. Studies of Ocular Complications of AIDS Research Group in Collaboration with the AIDS Clinical Trials Group. Combination foscarnet and ganciclovir therapy vs monotherapy for the treatment of relapsed cytomegalovirus retinitis in patients with AIDS: The cytomegalovirus Retreatment Trial. Arch Ophthalmol 1996; 114:23.

48. Lalezari JP, Drew WL, Glutzer E, et al. (S)-1-[3hydroxy- 2-(ph osphonylmethoxy)propyl]- cytosine (cidofovir): Results of a Phase I/II study of a novel antiviral nucleotide analogue. J Infect Dis 1995; 171:788.

49. Corey L, Adams HG, Brown ZA, et al. Genital herpes simplex virus infections: Clinical manifestations, course, and complications. Ann Intern Med 1983; 98:958.

50. Corey L, Homes KK. Genital herpes simplex virus infections: Current concepts in diagnosis, therapy, and prevention. Ann Intern Med 1983; 98:973.

51. Corey L, Spear PG. Infections with herpes simplex viruses (parts 1 and 2). N Engl J Med 1986; 314:686, 749.

52. Fleming DT, McQuillan GM, Johnson RE, et al. Herpes simplex virus type 2 in the United States, 1976 to 1995. N Engl J Med 1997; 337:1105.

53. Johnson RE, Nahmias AJ, Magder LS, et al. A seroepidemiologic survey of the prevalence of herpes simplex virus type 2 infection in the United States. N Engl J Med 1989; 321:7.

54. Nahmias AJ, Keyserling H, Lee FK. Herpes simplex viruses 1 and 2. In: Evans A, ed. Viral Infections of Humans: Epidemiology and Control. 3rd edn. New York: Plenum Press; 1989:393.

55. Reynolds SJ, Risbud AR, Shepherd ME, et al. Recent herpes simplex virus type 2 infection and the risk of human immunodeficiency virus type 1 acquisition in India. J Infect Dis 2003; 187:1509–1512.

56. Bartlett JG. Recent developments in the management of Herpes Simplex Virus Infection in HIV-infected persons. Clin Infect Dis 2004; 39:237–239.

56a. Nagot N, Ouedraogo A, Foulongne V, et al. Reduction of HIV-1 RNA levels with therapy to suppress herpes simplex virus. N Engl J Med 2007; 356:790–799.

57. Quinnan GV, Masur H, Rook AH, et al. Herpes simplex infections in the acquired immune deficiency syndrome. JAMA 1984; 252:72.

58. Safrin S, Arvin A, Mills J, et al. Comparison of the Western immunoblot assay and a glycoprotein G enzyme immunoassay for detection of serum antibodies to herpes

simplex virus type 2 in patients with AIDS. J Clin Microbiol 1992; 30:1312.

59. Siegel D, Golden E, Washington E, et al. Prevalence and correlates of herpes simplex infections: The population-based AIDS in Multiethnic Neighborhoods study. JAMA 1992; 268:1702.

60. Stewart JA, Reef SE, Pellett PE, et al. Herpesvirus infections in persons infected with human immunodeficiency virus. Clin Infect Dis 1995; 21(Suppl):S114.

61. Spruance SL, Overall JC, Kern ER, et al. The natural history of recurrent herpes simplex labialis: Implications for antiviral therapy. N Engl J Med 1977; 297:68.

62. Straus SE, Smith HA, Brickman C, et al. Acyclovir for chronic mucocutaneous herpes simplex virus infection in immunosuppressed patients. Ann Intern Med 1982; 96:270.

63. Whitley RJ, Levin M, Barton N, et al. Infections caused by herpes simplex virus in the immunocompromised host: Natural history and topical acyclovir therapy. J Infect Dis 1984; 150:323.

64. Brock BV, Selke S, Benedetti J, et al. Frequency of asymptomatic shedding of herpes simplex virus in women with genital herpes. JAMA 1990; 263:418.

65. Koelle DM, Benedetti J, Langenberg A, et al. Asymptomatic reactivation of herpes simplex virus in women after the first episode of genital herpes. Ann Intern Med 1992; 116:433.

66. Augenbraun M, Feldman J, Chirgwin K, et al. Increased genital shedding of herpes simplex virus type 2 in HIV-seropositive women. Ann Intern Med 1995; 123:845.

67. Wald A, Zeh J, Selke S, et al. Virologic characteristics of subclinical and symptomatic genital herpes infections. N Engl J Med 1995; 333:770.

68. Goodell SE, Quinn TC, Mkrtichian F, et al. Herpes simplex proctitis in homosexual men: Clinical, sigmoidoscopic, and histopathologic features. N Engl J Med 1983; 308:868.

69. Siegel FP, Lopez C, Hammer BS, et al. Severe acquired immunodeficiency in male homosexuals, manifested by chronic perianal ulcerative herpes simplex lesions. N Engl J Med 1981; 305:1439.

70. Farthing CF, Brown SE, Staughton RCD. A Colour Atlas of AIDS and HIV Disease Slide Set. 2nd edn. London: Mosby; 1989.

71. Genereau T, Lortholary O, Bouchaud O, et al. Herpes simplex esophagitis in patients with AIDS: Report of 34 cases. Clin Infect Dis 1996; 22:926.

72. Dix RD, Bredesen DE, Davis RL, et al. Herpesvirus neurological diseases associated with AIDS: Recovery of viruses from central nervous system (CNS) tissues, peripheral nerve, and cerebrospinal fluid (CSF). International Conference on AIDS; 1985; Atlanta.

73. Dix RD, Bredesen DE, Erlich KS, et al. Recovery of herpes-viruses from cerebrospinal fluid of immunodeficient homosexual men. Ann Neurol 1985; 18:611.

74. Dix RD, Waitzman DM, Follansbee S, et al. Herpes simplex virus type 2 encephalitis in two homosexual men with persistent adenopathy. Ann Neurol 1985; 17:203.

75. Lakeman FD. Whitley RJ, and the National Institute of Allergy and Infectious Diseases Collaborative Antiviral Study Group: Diagnosis of herpes simplex encephalitis: Application of polymerase chain reaction to cerebrospinal fluid from brain-biopsied patients and correlation with disease. J Infect Dis 1995; 171:857.

76. Landry ML. False-positive polymerase chain reaction results in the diagnosis of herpes simplex encephalitis. J Infect Dis 1995; 172:1641.

77. Nahmias AJ, Whitley RD, Visintine AN, et al. Herpes simplex virus type 2 encephalitis: Laboratory evaluations and their diagnostic significance. J Infect Dis 1982; 146:829.

78. Kahlon J, Chatterjee S, Lakeman FD, et al. Detection of antibodies to herpes simplex virus in the cerebrospinal fluid of patients with herpes simplex encephalitis. J Infect Dis 1987; 155:38.

79. Englund JA, Zimmerman ME, Swierkosz EM, et al. Herpes simplex virus resistant to acyclovir: A study in a tertiary care center. Ann Intern Med 1990; 112:416.

80. Marks GL, Nolan PE, Erlich KS, et al. Mucocutaneous dissemination of acyclovir-resistant herpes simplex virus in a patient with AIDS. Rev Infect Dis 1989; 11:474.

81. Erlich KS, Mills J, Chatis P, et al. Acyclovir-resistant herpes simplex virus infections in patients with the acquired immunodeficiency syndrome. N Engl J Med 1989; 320:293.

82. Kost RG, Hill EL, Tigges M, et al. Recurrent acyclovir-resistant genital herpes in an immunocompetent patient. N Engl J Med 1993; 329:1777.

83. Gateley A, Gander RM, Johnson PC, et al. Herpes simplex type 2 meningoencephalitis resistant to acyclovir in a patient with AIDS. J Infect Dis 1990; 161:711.

84. Whitley RJ. Gnann JW. Acyclovir: A decade later. N Engl J Med 1993; 327:782.

85. Douglas JM, Critchlow C, Benedetti J, et al. Double blind study of oral acyclovir for suppression of recurrences of genital herpes simplex virus infection. N Engl J Med 1984; 310:1551.

86. Fife KH, Crumpacker CS, Mertz CJ, et al. Recurrence and resistance patterns of herpes simplex virus following cessation of >6 years of chronic suppression with acyclovir. J Infect Dis 1994; 169:1338.

87. Kaplowitz LG, Baker D, Gelb L, et al. Prolonged continuous acyclovir treatment of normal adults with frequently recurring genital herpes simplex virus infection. JAMA 1991; 265:747.

88. Kinghorn GR, Abeywickreme I, Jeavons M, et al. Efficacy of combined treatment with oral and topical acyclovir in first episode genital herpes. Genitourin Med 1986; 62:186.

89. Shepp DH, Newton BA, Dandliker PS, et al. Oral acyclovir therapy for mucocutaneous herpes simplex virus infections in immunocompromised marrow transplant recipients. Ann Intern Med 1985; 102:783.

90. Straus SE, Seidlin M, Takiff H, et al. Oral acyclovir to suppress recurring herpes simplex virus infections in immunodeficient patients. Ann Intern Med 1984; 100:522.

91. Wade JC, Newton B, Flournoy N, et al. Oral acyclovir for prevention of herpes simplex virus reactivation after marrow transplantation. Ann Intern Med 1984; 100:823.

92. Wade JC, Newton B, McLaren C, et al. Intravenous acyclovir to treat mucocutaneous herpes simplex virus infection after marrow transplantation. Ann Intern Med 1982; 96:265.

93. Whitley RJ, Alford CA, Hirsch MS, et al. Vidarabine versus acyclovir therapy in herpes simplex encephalitis. N Engl J Med 1986; 314:144.

94. Spruance SL, Tyring SK, DeGregorio B, et al. A large-scale, placebo-controlled, dose-ranging trial of peroral valacyclovir for episodic treatment of recurrent herpes genitalis. Arch Intern Med 1996; 156:1729.

95. Beutner KR, Friedman DJ, Forszpaniak C, et al. Valaciclovir compared with acyclovir for improved therapy for herpes zoster in immunocompetent adults. Antimicrob Agents Chemother 1995; 39:1546.

96. Centers for Disease Control and Prevention. guidelines for treatment of sexually transmitted diseases. MMWR 1998; 47:20.

97. Gnann JW. New antivirals with activity against varicella-zoster virus. Ann Neurol 1994; 34:S69.

98. Mertz GJ, Loveless MO, Levin MJ, et al. Oral famciclovir for suppression of recurrent genital herpes simplex virus infection in women: A multicenter, double-blind, placebo-controlled trial. Arch Intern Med 1997; 157:343.

99. Sacks SL, Aoki FY, Diaz-Mitoma F, et al. Patient-initiated, twice-daily oral famciclovir for early recurrent genital herpes: A randomized, double-blind multicenter trial. JAMA 1996; 276:44.

100. Saltzman R, Jurewicz R, Boon R. Safety of famciclovir in patients with herpes zoster and genital herpes. Antimicrob Agents Chemother 1994; 38:2454.

101. Schacker T, Hu H, Koelle DM, et al. Famciclovir for the suppression of symptomatic and asymptomatic herpes simplex virus reactivation in HIV-infected persons: A double-blind, placebo-controlled trial. Ann Intern Med 1998; 128:21.

102. Spruance SL, Rea TL, Thoming C, et al. Penciclovir cream for the treatment of herpes simplex labialis: A randomized, multicenter, double-blind, placebo controlled trial. JAMA 1997; 277:1374.

103. Chatis PA, Miller CH, Schrager LE, et al. Successful treatment with foscarnet of an acyclovir resistant mucocutaneous infection with herpes simplex virus in a patient with acquired immunodeficiency syndrome. N Engl J Med 1989; 320:297.

104. Erlich KS, Jacobson MA, Koehler JE, et al. Foscarnet therapy for severe acyclovir-resistant herpes simplex virus type-2 infections in patients with the acquired immunodeficiency syndrome (AIDS): An uncontrolled trial. Ann Intern Med 1989; 110:710.

105. Lalezari JP, Drew WL, Glutzer E, et al. Treatment with intravenous (s)-1[3-hydroxy-2-(phosphonylmethoxy)propyl)-cytosine of acyclovir-resistant mucocutaneous infection with herpes simplex virus in a patient with AIDS. J Infect Dis 1994; 170:570.

106. Snoeck R, Andrei G, Gerard M, et al. Successful treatment of progressive mucocutaneous infection due to acyclovir- and foscarnet-resistant herpes simplex virus with (S)-1-(3-hydroxy-2-phosphonylmethoxypropyl)cytosine (HPMPC). J Infect Dis 1994; 18:570.

107. Lalezari J, Schacker T, Feinberg J, et al. A randomized, double-blind placebo-controlled trial of cidofovir gel for the treatment of acyclovir-unresponsive mucocutaneous herpes simplex virus infection in patients with AIDS. J Infect Dis 1997; 176:892.

107a. Centers for Disease Control and Prevention. Sexually Transmitted Disease Treatment Guidelines 2006. MMWR Morb Mortal Wkly Rep 2006; 55.

108. Goldberg LH, Kaufman R, Kurtz TO, et al. Long-term suppression of recurrent genital herpes with acyclovir: A 5-year benchmark study. Arch Derm 1993; 129:582.

108a. DeJesus E, Wald A, Warren T, et al. Valacyclovir for the suppression of recurrent genital herpes in human immunodeficiency virus-infected subjects. J Infect Dis 2003; 188:1009–1016.

109. Nusinoff-Lehrman S, Douglas JM, Corey L, et al. Recurrent genital herpes and suppressive oral acyclovir therapy: Relation between clinical outcome and in vitro sensitivity. Ann Intern Med 1986; 104:786.

110. Wald A, Zeh J, Barnum G, et al. Suppression of subclinical shedding of herpes simplex virus type 2 with acyclovir. Ann Intern Med 1996; 124:8.

111. Corey L, Wald AA, Patel R, et al. Once daily valacyclovir to reduce the risk of Transmission of Genital Herpes. N Engl J Med 2004; 350:11–20.

112. Gupta R, Wald A, Krantz E, et al. Valacyclovir and acyclovir for suppression of shedding of herpes simplex virus in the genital tract. J Infect Dis 2004; 190:1374–1381.

112a. Corey L. Herpes Simplex Virus Type 2 and HIV-1: The Dialogue between the 2 Organisms Continues J Infect Dis 2007; 195:1242–1244.

112b. Corey L, Wald A, Celum C, Quinn TC. The effects of herpes simplex virus-2 on HIV-1 acquistition and transmission: a review of two overlapping epidemics, J Acquir Immun Defic Syndr 2004; 35:435–445.

112c. Kapiga SH, Sam NE, Bang H, et al. The role of herpes simplex virus type 2 and other genital infections in the acquisition of HIV-1 among high-risk women in northern Tanzania. J Infect Dis 2007; 195:1260–1269.

113. Engel JP, Englund JA, Fletcher CV, et al. Treatment of resistant herpes simplex virus with continuous-infusion acyclovir. JAMA 1990; 263:1662.

114. Kessler HA, Hurwitz S, Farthing C, et al. Pilot study of topical trifluridine for the treatment of acyclovir resistant mucocutaneous herpes simplex disease in patients with

AIDS (ACTG 172). J Acquir Immune Defic Syndr Hum Retrovirol 1996; 12:147.

115. Safrin S, Kemmerly S, Plotkin B, et al. Foscarnet resistant herpes simplex virus infection in patients with AIDS. J Infect Dis 1994; 169:193.

116. Weller TH. Varicella and herpes zoster: Changing concepts of the natural history, control, and importance of a not-so-benign virus (parts 1 and 2). N Engl J Med 1983; 309:1362, 1434.

117. Buchbinder SP, Katz MH, Hessol NA, et al. Herpes zoster and human immunodeficiency virus infection. J Infect Dis 1992; 166:1153.

118. Cole EL, Meisler DM, Calabrese LH, et al. Herpes zoster ophthalmicus and acquired immune deficiency syndrome. Arch Ophthalmol 1984; 102:1027.

119. Cone LA, Schiffman HA. Herpes zoster and the acquired immunodeficiency syndrome. Ann Intern Med 1984; 100:462.

120. Friedman-Kien AE, Lafleur FL, Gendler E, et al. Herpes zoster: A possible early clinical sign for development of acquired immunodeficiency syndrome in high-risk individuals. J Am Acad Derm 1986; 14:1023.

121. Gershon AA, Mervish N, LaRussa P, et al. Varicella-zoster virus infection in children with underlying human immunodeficiency virus infection. J Infect Dis 1997; 176:1496.

122. Rogers MF, Morens DM, Stewart JA, et al. National case-control study of Kaposi's sarcoma and Pneumocystis carinii pneumonia in homosexual men: Part 2, Laboratory results. Ann Intern Med 1983; 99:151.

123. Ryder JW, Croen K, Kleinschmidt-DeMasters BK, et al. Progressive encephalitis three months after resolution of cutaneous zoster in a patient with AIDS. Ann Neurol 1986; 19:182.

124. Safrin S, Berger TG, Gilson I, et al. Foscarnet therapy in five patients with AIDS and acyclovir-resistant varicella-zoster virus infection. Ann Intern Med 1991; 115:19.

125. Wallace MR, Katz MH, Hessol NA, et al. Treatment of adult varicella with oral acyclovir: A randomized, placebo-controlled trial. Ann Intern Med 1992; 117:358.

126. Gilden DH. Herpes zoster with postherpetic neuralgia-persisting pain and frustration. N Engl J Med 1994; 330:932.

127. Huff JC, Drucker LL, Clemmer A, et al. Effect of oral acyclovir on pain resolution in herpes zoster: A reanalysis. J Med Virol 1993; 1(Suppl):93.

128. Drew WL, Buhles W, Erlich KS. Herpesvirus infections (cytomegalovirus, herpes simplex virus, varicella-zoster virus). How to use ganciclovir (DHPG) and acyclovir. Infect Dis Clin North Am 1988; 2:495–509.

129. Balfour HH, Bean B, Laskin OL, et al. Acyclovir halts progression of herpes zoster in immunocompromised patients. N Engl J Med 1983; 308:1448.

130. Laskin O. Acyclovir: Pharmacology and clinical experience. Arch Intern Med 1984; 144:1241.

131. Haake DA, Zakowski PC, Haake DL, et al. Early treatment with acyclovir for varicella pneumonia in otherwise healthy adults: Retrospective controlled study and review. Rev Infect Dis 1990; 12:788.

132. Huff JC, Bean B, Balfour HH, et al. Therapy of herpes zoster with oral acyclovir. Am J Med 1988; 85 (Suppl):84.

133. Tyring S, Barbarash RA, Nahlik JE, et al. Famciclovir for the treatment of acute herpes zoster: Effects on acute disease and postherpetic neuralgia. A randomized, double blind, placebo controlled trial. Ann Intern Med 1995; 123:89.

134. Shepp DH, Dandliker PS, Meyers JD. Treatment of varicella zoster virus infection in severely immunocompromised patients. N Engl J Med 1986; 314:208.

135. Whitley RJ, Weiss H, Gnann JW, et al. Acyclovir with and without prednisone for the treatment of herpes zoster: A randomized, placebo controlled trial. Ann Intern Med 1996; 125:376.

136. Wood MJ, Johnson RW, McKendrick MW, et al. A randomized trial of acyclovir for 7 days or 21 days with and without prednisolone for treatment of acute herpes zoster. N Engl J Med 1994; 330:896.

137. Jacobson MA, Berger TG, Fikrig S, et al. Acyclovir (ACV)-resistant varicella zoster virus (VZV) infection following chronic oral ACV therapy in patients with AIDS. Ann Intern Med 1990; 112:187.

138. Gershon AA, Steinberg SP, LaRussa P, et al. Immunization of healthy adults with live attenuated varicella vaccine. J Infect Dis 1988; 158:132.

139. White CJ, Kuter BJ, Hidebrand CS, et al. Varicella vaccine (VARIVAX) in healthy children and adolescents: Results from clinical trials, 1987 to 1989. Pediatrics 1991; 87:604.

140. Oxman MN, Levin MJ, Johnson GR, et al. A Vaccine to Prevent Herpes Zoster and Postherpetic Neuralgia in Older Adults, New Eng J Med 2005; 352:2271–2284.

141. LaRussa P, Steinberg S, Meurice F, et al. Transmission of vaccine strain varicella-zoster virus from a healthy adult with vaccine-associated rash to susceptible household contacts. J Infect Dis 1997; 176:1072.

142. Hardy I, Gershon AA, Steinberg SP, et al. The incidence of zoster after immunization with live attenuated varicella vaccine. N Engl J Med 1991; 325:1545.

CHAPTER 40

HIV-associated Neoplasia

Lawrence D. Kaplan

Introduction

The increased risk of neoplastic disease in the setting of immunodeficiency is well established, and has been observed in individuals with primary immunodeficiency disorders, iatrogenic immunodeficiency occurring in the setting of solid organ or hematopoietic stem cell transplant, and in the setting of human immunodeficiency virus infection (HIV).

The fact that the incidence of aggressive B-cell non-Hodgkin's lymphoma and Kaposi's sarcoma was markedly increased in the setting of HIV infection was recognized very early in the AIDS epidemic. Those neoplasms which are considered to be AIDS-defining based upon Centers for Disease Control recommendations are listed in Table 40.1, and include Kaposi's sarcoma, aggressive B-cell lymphoma, and invasive squamous carcinoma of the cervix. The relative risks of these neoplasms are listed along with several other malignancies for which a causal relationship with HIV disease is strongly implied based upon the relative risk of these malignancies in the HIV seropositive population. However, it is important to recognize that although immunodeficiency clearly plays a role in some of these, others such as cervical and anal carcinomas arise from sexually acquired HPV infection and appear to be unrelated to level of immune function.[1] Some, such as squamous conjunctival cancer and leiomyosarcoma, are less commonly seen in Western countries than are Kaposi's sarcoma and B-cell lymphoma; and others such as Hodgkin's disease have a less significant increase in incidence in the risk population.

It has been suggested that 'immune surveillance' is most effective against those neoplasms with viral etiologies. The listing in Table 40.1 of suspected viral pathogens associated with each of these neoplasms would suggest that this is correct, although the exact mechanism by which these viruses may give rise to each of these neoplasms is not always clear.

It is important to recognize that the changes that have occurred in both the epidemiology of these neoplasms and their natural history with respect to clinical outcome has been markedly altered since the widespread introduction in 1996 of highly active antiretroviral therapies (HAART) for the treatment of HIV disease. In general, the incidence of many of these neoplasms has declined, while at the same time, the likelihood of successful treatment has significantly improved. In many cases, treatment options that were previously considered impractical or inappropriate for this patient population due to safety concerns are now routinely used with good success.

This chapter will focus on the clinical management of lymphoproliferative disease and Kaposi's sarcoma in the setting of HIV infection, with a special focus on the impact of HAART on the management of these illnesses.

Epidemiology of HIV-associated Malignancies

The introduction of highly active antiretroviral combinations in 1996 has not only resulted in a dramatic change in the epidemiology and natural history of HIV disease, but clearly has also influenced the spectrum of HIV-associated malignancies. In one of the largest epidemiologic studies to date, patient records were linked between the Swiss HIV cohort study and the Swiss National Cancer Registries.[2] Relative risks for cancer in this group of 7304 HIV-infected individuals followed for 28 836 person years (PY) were determined based upon standardized

Table 40.1 Relative risks and viral associations for neoplasms associated with HIV infection

Neoplasm	Relative risk	Viral association
Kaposi's sarcoma	>10 000	KSHV
B-cell NHL	100–400	EBV, KSHV
Cervical carcinoma	2.9–4	HPV
Anal carcinoma	14	HPV
Hodgkin lymphoma	7–11	EBV
Leiomyosarcoma	10 000	EBV
Squamous conjunctival CA	13	HPV

KSHV, Kaposi's sarcoma-associated herpes virus; EBV, Epstein–Barr virus; HPV, human papilloma virus.

incidence ratios (SIRs). SIRs for Kaposi's sarcoma of 192 and for non-Hodgkin's lymphoma of 76.4 confirmed the very high incidence of these neoplasms in the seropositive population. Significantly elevated SIRs were also observed for anal cancer (SIR = 33.4) and Hodgkin's lymphoma (SIR = 17.3). Other neoplasms with elevated incidence ratios, albeit significantly lower than for the above neoplasms, included cervical, head/neck, lung, and non-melanomatous skin cancers. In HAART users, SIRs for KS (25.3) and non-Hodgkin's lymphoma (24.2) were lower than those for non-users (KS SIR 239, and non-Hodgkin's lymphoma SIR 99.3). No clear impact of HAART on SIRs was noted for cervical cancer or other non-acquired immunodeficiency syndrome-defining cancers, and the increased risk of head/neck and lung cancers was primarily associated with tobacco use. The risk for Kaposi's sarcoma and non-Hodgkin's lymphoma increased steadily as CD4 cell counts declined. These observations confirm those from prior studies demonstrating a significant decline in the incidence of Kaposi's sarcoma and non-Hodgkin's lymphoma since the introduction of HAART.[3,4] The decrease in incidence of non-Hodgkin's lymphoma overall has been significantly less dramatic than that for Kaposi's sarcoma. For the lymphomas, the most dramatic decline has been for primary central nervous system lymphoma.[5] In sub-Saharan Africa, where the use of antiretroviral therapy is not widespread, the incidence of Kaposi's sarcoma and non-Hodgkin's lymphoma remains high, although the excess risk due to HIV infection is more difficult to ascertain due to the fact that malignancies such as Kaposi's sarcoma and Burkitt's lymphoma are endemic in this geographic region.[6]

Lymphoproliferative Disease

Non-Hodgkin's Lymphoma

The non-Hodgkin's lymphomas (NHL) observed in HIV seropositive individuals include systemic NHL, primary central nervous system NHL, and primary effusion lymphomas. Each of these will be considered individually in the following sections.

Systemic NHL

Despite the dramatic effect of HAART on the survival of HIV-infected patients, systemic NHL continues to be a significant source of morbidity and mortality, accounting for 16% of deaths in the HIV seropositive population.[7]

Approximately two-thirds of HIV-associated lymphomas are categorized as diffuse large B-cell lymphomas, and approximately 25% as Burkitt's lymphomas (these are associated with higher CD4 counts). The remaining cases include small numbers of low-grade B-cell lymphomas, anaplastic large-cell lymphomas, plasmablastic lymphomas, and rare T-cell lymphomas.[8]

The pathogenesis of these lymphomas is not clearly understood, and potentially involves a variety of different mechanisms. Pathogenesis may involve interactions between host bacters, HIV infection, antigenic stimulation, and cytokine dysregulation. Between 40% and 60% of HIV-associated lymphomas are associated with the Epstein–Barr virus.[9] EBV is more commonly associated with the large-cell lymphomas and less commonly with Burkitt-type lymphomas. It is commonly believed that the excessive B-cell stimulation associated with HIV infection results in the proliferation of antigen-selected B-cell clones,[8,10] with subsequent genetic changes leading to the evolution of a transformed clonal lymphoma. The molecular pathogenesis of AIDS-NHL is characterized by distinct genetic pathways, including chromosomal rearrangements of c-MYC and BCL6 in AIDS-associated Burkitt's lymphoma and AIDS-associated diffuse large B-cell lymphoma, respectively.[8]

Clinical management

Most patients with HIV-associated lymphoma present with advanced-stage and extranodal disease. Two-thirds of patients have Stage IV disease at the time of presentation, and 90% have extranodal lymphoma at the time of diagnosis.[11,12] Meningeal involvement at the time of diagnosis has been observed in 3–20% of patients. Although the median

CD4 count at the time of diagnosis had been reported to be in the 100–180 cells/mL range, it has been suggested that the introduction of highly active antiretroviral therapy has resulted in individuals presenting with higher CD4 counts and fewer HIV-related complications prior to diagnosis of NHL.[7]

Studies of prognostic factors in this patient population have indicated that factors associated with the underlying immunodeficiency disease such as CD4 count, prior AIDS diagnosis, and performance score were more important predictors of clinical outcome than were features associated with lymphoma such as stage, LDH, bone marrow, or CNS involvement.[13] Since the introduction of HAART, the immune function as measured by CD4+ lymphocyte count remains consistently the most important predictor of clinical outcome.[14] However, the commonly used international prognostic index, which includes prognostic factors such as age, performance score, stage, extranodal disease, and serum LDH, clearly has utility as a predictive model in the patient population.[13]

In the pre-HAART era, treatment outcomes were poor regardless of treatment choice, with complete response rates of approximately 50%, and median survivals in the 5–8 month range.[11,15] A cooperative group study assessing the utility of standard-dose versus low-dose M-BACOD chemotherapy in this patient population demonstrated that the dose-reduced arm provided equivalently poor outcome compared with standard-dose therapy (35 versus 31 weeks, respectively; $P = 0.25$), but was associated with less toxicity.[15] Those receiving reduced-intensity therapy were more likely to recur and succumb to AIDS-related lymphoma, whereas the full-dose therapy was more frequently associated with infectious complications.

Since the introduction of HAART therapy in 1996, several studies have provided strong evidence of significant improvement in clinical outcome in patients receiving HAART relative to historical controls who were not receiving adequate antiretroviral therapy (Table 40.2).[7,16,17] Furthermore, there is evidence that those patients experiencing failure of virologic control on HAART have poorer outcomes after therapy of their disease. These findings have resulted in HAART therapy becoming an important component of management of patients with HIV-associated NHL. Unfortunately, there is little data available concerning potential pharmacokinetic interactions between the variety of antiretroviral agents commonly used today and cytotoxic agents. A single study evaluating potential pharmacokinetic interactions between cyclophosphamide, doxorubicin, vincristine, and a fixed protease inhibitor-containing antiretroviral regimen showed only a modest decline in cyclophosphamide clearance.[18] Others, however, have suggested an increased risk of neutropenia among patients receiving chemotherapy in combination with a protease inhibitor-containing antiviral regimen.[19] However, no effect on disease-free or

Table 40.2 Retrospective studies of treatment for HIV-associated non-Hodgkin's lymphoma pre- and post-HAART

Author	Type/comments	HAART (n)		CR (%): (HAART)			Median overall survival: HAART		
		No	Yes	No	Yes	P	No	Yes	P
Vaccher, et al. (2001)[17]	HAART: more neuropathy, anemia, fewer OIs	80	24	36	50	NS	7	NR	–
Navarro, et al. (2003)	CHOP regimen, all systemic ARL in this series; 2 year OS 60 versus 22%	54	39	39	60	0.019	22%	60%[a]	–
Hoffmann, et al. (2003)	CHOP regimen; HAART response associated with much better OS	142	61	48	71	0.006	9	NR	–
Besson, et al. (2001)	CHOP-like regimens	63	42	NR	NR		6.3	21.2	0.004
Gerard, et al. (2002)[5]	Higher-dose therapy more frequent post-HAART	131	115	55	69	0.04	9.5	NR	<0.0001

[a]Overall survival at 2 years. CHOP, cyclophosphamide, doxorubicin, vincristine, prednisone; HAART, highly active antiretroviral therapies; OIs, opportunistic infections; OS, overall survival; NR, not reported; NS, not significant.

overall survival was observed. It has been generally recommended that antiretroviral therapy be administered concurrently in patients receiving chemotherapy for HIV-NHL.

Infusional chemotherapy

The use of infusional combination chemotherapy regimens for the treatment of NHL both in the setting of HIV disease and the non-immunodeficient patient population has attracted significant interest in recent years. Three different infusional regimens have been studied in the HIV-NHL population, and the outcomes of these trials are indicated in Table 40.3. Sparano and co-workers. were the first to study the infusional regimen CDE, in which cyclophosphamide, doxorubicin and etoposide are infused over 96 h every 28 days.[16] This trial included patients who were treated both in the pre- and post-HAART eras, and demonstrated a 2-year overall survival in the post-HAART group of 47% with no treatment-related mortality, compared with the pre-HAART-era patients who had an overall 2-year survival of 30% with a 10% treatment-related mortality.

The regimen that has generated the greatest interest is the EPOCH regimen. In this regimen, doxorubicin, vincristine, and etoposide are administered as a continuous 96-h infusion and cyclophosphamide is administered as a bolus i.v. infusion on day 5. Patients enrolled on this Phase II National Cancer Institute trial did not receive antiretroviral therapy until chemotherapy was complete. Despite the fact that 59% of patients fell into the intermediate-high or high risk groups by the International Prognostic Index, and 41% had CD4 counts ≤100 cells/mL[3], the complete remission rate was 74%, and at 53 months of follow-up, the disease-free survival was 92% and

overall survival 60%.[20] The EPOCH regimen is currently being studied in a multi-center clinical trial through the NCI-sponsored AIDS Malignancies Consortium.

Use of rituximab

Rituximab is a humanized monoclonal anti-CD20 antibody currently in widespread use for treatment of a variety of B-cell non-Hodgkin's lymphomas. Its use in combination with CHOP chemotherapy for treatment of diffuse large B-cell lymphoma in HIV-negative patients became standard of care after publication of the randomized Groupe D'Etude de Lymphome de L'Adulte (GELA) study demonstrating a survival advantage for patients older than age 60 receiving CHOP plus Rituximab versus CHOP alone.[21] However, its role in therapy for HIV-NHL remains unclear. Spina and co-workers recently reported the pooled results of three prospective Phase II trials evaluating rituximab in combination with infusional CDE chemotherapy in 74 patients with HIV-associated aggressive B-cell lymphoma.[22] Most patients received concurrent HAART. These investigators reported a complete remission rate of 70% and estimated 2-year failure free and overall survival rates of 59% and 64%, respectively. A total of 14% of patients in this study had opportunistic infections during or within 3 months of the completion of chemotherapy. Six (8%) patients died due to infection, including two cases of bacterial sepsis during chemotherapy. Preliminary data from an AIDS Malignancies Consortium randomized Phase III trial of CHOP chemotherapy with or without rituximab raises similar concerns, as treatment-related infectious deaths occurred inn 14% of patients receiving R-CHOP compared with 2% in the chemo-

Table 40.3 Hematopoietic stem cell transplant for HIV-lymphoma

Author	Type/comments	n	Transplant rate (%)	CR	Median F/U	Overall survival
Gabarre, et al. (2004)	Relapsed/refractory NHL/HL CBV prep	14	NR	10/14	9 mos	50% at 9 months
Krishnan, et al. (2005)	Relapsed or high-risk first remission NHL	20	100	16/20	32 mos	85% at 32 months
Re, et al. (2003)	Refractory/relapsed NHL BEAM prep	20	65	8/9	12 mos	39% at 24 months
Serrano, et al. (2005)	Relapsed/refractory or high-risk first remission NHL, HD	14	79	8/14	30 mos	65% at 30 months

CBV, cyclophosphamide, carmustine, etoposide; BEAM, carmustine, etoposide, AraC, melphalan; HL, Hodgkin's lymphoma; HD, Hodgkin's disease NHL, non-Hodgkin's lymphoma; mos, median overall survival; NR, not reported.

therapy-alone group ($P = 0.035$). A majority of these deaths occurred in patients with baseline CD4 lymphocyte counts <50/mm³.[23] Although this study showed trends toward improvement of response rate and survival times with the addition of Rituximab, it is recommended that this agent be used cautiously in this patient population, particularly in those individuals with CD4 counts <50/mm³.

Hematopoietic cell transplantation for HIV-NHL

Recently, several reports have indicated the potential value of high-dose chemotherapy and autologous stem cell transplant (Table 40.3). In the largest of these studies, 20 patients with HIV-associated lymphoma who had either relapsed or refractory disease or high-risk first remission received high-dose chemotherapy with autologous stem cell infusion.[24] Mobilization and stem cell collection were successful in all patients. There was no engraftment failure, although one patient who was receiving zidovudine had delayed engraftment. Two patients who were not compliant with prophylaxis developed pneumocystic pneumonia. Two developed disseminated herpes zoster, one developed CMV retinitis, and two developed asymptomatic CMV viremia. All of these patients responded to therapy. With a 31.8-month median follow-up time, 17 of the patients remain in remission. Progression-free survival is 85%, and overall survival 85% for the entire group. Other small series of patients undergoing autologous transplant similarly have demonstrated effective stem cell mobilization and collection, lack of unexpected toxicities, and significant long-term disease-free survival times.[25-27] In view of this experience, high-dose chemotherapy with autologous stem cell transplant should be considered the best treatment option for individuals with refractory or relapsed HIV-NHL.

Primary CNS lymphoma

Primary central nervous system NHL (PCNSL) usually occurs in severely immunocompromised late-stage HIV-infected individuals, the vast majority of whom have CD4+ lymphocyte counts <50/mm³. Not surprisingly, the incidence of PCNSL has fallen significantly since the introduction of HAART.[28]

PCNSL in the setting of HIV infection is universally associated with Epstein–Barr virus,[10] and this observation may prove valuable in diagnosis of the disease. EBV is rarely detected in the spinal fluid of HIV patients without primary central nervous system lymphoma, but it is fairly consistently detected in the spinal fluid of patients with this tumor. In one study EBV DNA was detected by a nested polymerase chain reaction (PCR) in the CSF in seven of eight patients with PCNSL, diagnosed by brain biopsy (87.5% sensitivity), and in none of the 11 controls with non-lymphomatous mass lesions (100% specificity). A total of 21 AIDS patients with or without neurological disorders but without focal brain lesions were PCR-negative.[29] In another study, EBV DNA was detected in the CSF from 16/20 (80%) patients with PCNSL.[30] In combination with imaging studies, EBV PCR may obviate the need for brain biopsy.[31]

Most HIV-PCNSLs are characterized as diffuse large B-cell lymphomas, and tend to be multifocal in the brain. Confusion, memory loss, lethargy and focal neurologic findings are the most frequent presenting symptoms and signs.

Historically, prognosis for these individuals has been poor. Whole brain radiotherapy has been used palliatively, and survival has been in the 1–3 month range, with most patients dying from opportunistic infection. However, more recent trends towards the use of chemotherapy alone or in combination with radiotherapy in non-HIV patients with PCNSL, have carried over into the HIV population, especially with the advent of HAART, which seems to make such therapy more tolerable. A pre-HAART study in HIV-PCNSL patients with a median CD4 of 30/mm³ resulted in a 50% complete response rate and a median survival of 10 months.[32] More recent cohort data suggest that immune recovery associated with HAART can dramatically improve survival. A retrospective review of 111 patients with PCNSL found that the use of HAART and radiotherapy were each associated with significantly improved survival.[33]

It is recommended that patients with HIV-related PCNSL receive treatment as closely adherent to the institutional standard of care for non-HIV PCNSL as possible, while taking into account severity of immunodeficiency and performance status of each individual patient. At UCSF, this most commonly involves the use of a high-dose methotrexate-containing chemotherapy regimen without radiotherapy. HAART should be administered to all such patients as a component of the overall management of their lymphoma.

Hodgkin's Lymphoma

As described in an earlier section, Hodgkin's disease is not included in the Centers for Disease Control AIDS Case definition. However, multiple cohort studies have demonstrated an epidemiologic association with an approximately 10-fold increase in the risk of Hodgkin's lymphoma in the setting of HIV infection relative to the general population.[2] Hodgkin's lymphoma in the setting of HIV infection has largely been associated with a predominance of two unfavorable subtypes: lymphocyte-depleted and mixed-cellularity.[34,35] Clonal EBV is identified in approximately 80–100% of cases associated with HIV infection.[10]

Early clinical trials of standard chemotherapy regimens for HIV-associated Hodgkin's lymphoma showed poor long-term survival, with treatment being frequently complicated by severe and prolonged myelosuppression.[35] Significant improvement in tolerance and clinical outcome in patients with HIV-associated Hodgkin's lymphoma have been documented since the introduction of HAART. Retrospective evaluation of 108 patients from a single institution demonstrated improvement in complete response rate from 64.5 to 74.5% and improvement in 2-year disease-free survival from 45 to 62% ($P = 0.03$) in the years following introduction of HAART.[36] In the second study, 57 patients with HIV-HD diagnosed between 1990 and 2002 were evaluated retrospectively. In a Cox model, the only factors independently associated with OS were HAART response (relative hazard (RH) 0.19; 95% confidence interval (CI) 0.06–0.60), complete remission (RH 0.30, 95% CI 0.13–0.72), and age <45 years (RH 0.23; 95% CI 0.09–0.60). Median survival time in patients without HAART response was 18.6 months, whereas the median survival time in patients with HAART response was not reached (89% OS at 24 months).[37]

It is not clear that there is a best chemotherapy option for patients with HIV-HL, just as this is not entirely clear in the non-HIV population either. With the use of HAART, it does appear that standard full-dose chemotherapy regimens such as ABVD and Stanford V are well tolerated in this patient population. In a study of 59 patients, Spina and co-workers demonstrated a 69% relative dose intensity for the Stanford V regimen.[38] However, Grade III or IV neutropenia occurred in 78% despite growth factor support in all patients, and Grade II or III neuropathy occurred in 47%. Patients with an International Prognostic Score of ≤2 had 83% freedom from progression at 2 years, but those with IPS ≥2 had only 41% freedom from progression. This outcome is still significantly lower than that observed in the non-HIV population. Based on these experiences, it is recommended that the majority of individuals with HIV-HL receive the same standard approaches to therapy that are used in the general population, including chemo- or chemo-radiotherapy regimens

based upon the staging of disease and other prognostic factors. Both the standard ABVD and Stanford V regiments appear to be reasonably well-tolerated.

Other Lymphoproliferative Disease in HIV Infection

Primary effusion lymphoma (PEL)

Primary effusion lymphoma (PEL) accounts for <5% of all AIDS-related lymphomas. The disease is characterized by presentation as a body cavity effusion. Virtually 100% of these cases are associated with Kaposi's sarcoma-associated herpes virus (KSHV, HHV-8), and Epstein–Barr Virus (EBV) has been identified in the vast majority of cases. These lymphomas are generally associated with absence of B- or T-cell markers, although the presence of immunoglobulin gene rearrangements in most cases suggests a B-cell origin. Most of these individuals present with advanced HIV disease and severe immunodeficiency.[39] As a result, complete response rates have been <50%, and overall survival is in the 3–6 month range.[39] CHOP-like regimens were generally utilized and most of the reported experience was prior to the introduction of HAART. Whether the introduction of HAART has resulted in a decline in the incidence of these lymphoproliferative disorders or might result in improvement in therapeutic outcome remains unknown. Recently, immunophenotypic analysis and gene expression studies have suggested that PEL will be a variant of plasmablastic lymphoma based upon features of both immunoblasts and plasma cells. This could potentially result in future changes in the therapeutic approach.

Plasmablastic lymphoma

Although this lymphoproliferative disorder has been observed in non-immunodeficient individuals, it has been reported predominately in patients with HIV disease.[40,41] These lymphomas are typically negative for B- and T-cell markers, generally carry a phenotype more typical of mature plasma cells, and are associated with HHV8.[42] Morphologically, the malignant cells appear most like plasmablasts but carry a phenotype most typical of mature plasma cells. Monoclonal gammopathy is not commonly noted, helping to distinguish this entity from solitary plasmacytoma. Historically, these lymphomas have been associated with a poor prognosis, and a median survival of approximately 9 months.[43] Recent reports suggest that the prognosis may have improved since the introduction of HAART.[44]

Multicentric Castleman's disease

This lymphoproliferative disorder characteristically presents with polyclonal hypergammaglobulinemia, generalized lymphadenopathy, hepatosplenomegaly, constitutional symptoms and often, autoimmune hemolytic anemia.[45] Lymph node histologic findings are characteristic with perifollicular vascular proliferation, and germinal center angiosclerosis. Overexpression of IL6 appears to be the hallmark of this disease.[46] The disease has been associated with HHV-8 infection of the B-cells in the mantle zone of the lymph node.[47] The clinical course of this lymphoproliferative disorder can vary from an indolent, waxing and waning course, to one that is extremely aggressive and may in some cases transform to non-Hodgkin's lymphoma. Based on anecdotal reports, there may be some benefit to the use of HAART,[48] rituximab, interferon-α,[49] splenectomy.[50] Although some transient responses to anti-herpes virus agents have been reported, overall results with these agents have been disappointing.[51] Rituximab appears to be a more promising therapeutic modality. In one study, three of five patients remained in complete remission, with follow-up between 4 and 14 months.[52] The other two patients died rapidly without response. Other anecdotal reports have reported similar outcomes. Chemotherapy has generally been associated with relatively transient responses and poor long-term outcome.[45]

Kaposi's Sarcoma

Pathogenesis

The epidemic form of Kaposi's Sarcoma (KS) was identified very early in the AIDS epidemic, and was one of the first opportunistic disorders recognized as an AIDS-defining condition. HIV seropositive homosexual males have the greatest risk of developing KS.[1] Cases in heterosexual injection drug users are significantly less common and are rare in HIV-infected women, where the disease is usually associated with a bisexual male partner.

The epidemiology of KS has always suggested a sexually transmissible etiology and Kaposi's Sarcoma Herpesvirus (KSHV, HHV8) has been identified in virtually all tissue specimens from individuals with KS, whether HIV-infected or not. Its seroprevalence and association with number of homosexual partners strongly suggests its sexual transmission.[53]

The pathogenesis of KS, although not clearly understood, involves interactions between Kaposi's

sarcoma herpesvirus (KSHV, HHV8), HIV and immune dysregulation.[54] KSHV is a lymphotropic gamma-2 herpesvirus whose seroprevalence correlates with the incidence rates of clinical KS in various subpopulations. The latent form of viral infection predominates in individuals with KS. The viral genome encodes a variety of genes that are homologs of normal human cell cycle regulatory and angiogenesis factors such as vCyclin D, vbcl-2, basic fibroblast growth factor (bFGF), vascular endothelial growth factor (VEGF), and a G protein-coupled receptor that is capable of inducing angiogenesis *in vitro*.[54] HIV may directly influence development of KS production of Tat protein, which in combination with bFGF induces KS-like lesions in nude mice. There is also evidence that platelet-derived growth factor receptor (PDGFR) may play a role in inducing KS spindle cell growth and inducing angiogenesis by upregulating production of VEGF.[54]

The clear association of KS with immunodeficiency in this population as well as in transplant recipients indicates that HIV may play both a direct and indirect role in the pathogenesis of this disease.

Clinical Presentation

Epidemic KS typically presents at multiple mucocutaneous sites. Lymphatic and visceral sites of disease have been historically common, with 40% having gastrointestinal involvement at diagnosis. GI KS is usually asymptomatic but can occasionally cause vague abdominal pain, bleeding, or obstruction. Pleuropulmonary disease is seen in severely immunocompromised patients and is usually associated with cough, bronchospasm, dyspnea and eventually hypoxemia. The dramatic decline in the incidence of epidemic KS since the introduction of HAART has resulted in fewer individuals presenting with advanced, symptomatic disease.

Clinical Management

Management of KS is largely palliative. In the HAART era, this more often than not involves cosmetic treatment of unsightly cutaneous lesions. However, as the disease becomes more advanced, lesions may be associated with pain, extremity edema, soft-tissue infection, and GI or respiratory symptoms. These symptoms may warrant specific KS-directed therapy.

In addition to reducing the incidence of KS, there is strong evidence for an antitumor effect of HAART in those with established clinical disease. A total of 10 of 21 patients with KS reported by Gill and co-workers had objective KS response (six complete response; four partial response) with HAART alone.[55] Of the 20 subjects with detectable KSHV viremia prior to HAART, 60% had an undetectable KSHV load with antiretroviral therapy. There was no significant difference between subjects receiving protease inhibitor- or nonnucleoside reverse transcriptase inhibitor-based treatment combinations. Monfardini and co-workers reported complete responses in 19 and partial responses in three of 24 (91% response) patients treated with HAART alone.[56] The tumor stage of these patients was not reported. In this prospective trial, there was a statistically significant association between decrease in HIV viral load, increase in CD4+ lymphocytes, and response. An additional prospective study also demonstrated an association between response and restoration of immune function.[57] A prospective French trial evaluated clinical and virologic responses in 26 patients treated with protease inhibitor-containing HAART regimens. Clinical responses were observed in 85% of patients. Multivariate analysis demonstrated that reduction of KSHV viral load to undetectable levels and improvement in CD4 count were the only factors correlated with KS response.[58]

It is most important, however, to note that while HAART alone may be sufficient therapy for individuals with limited cutaneous or mucocutaneous disease, it is not adequate therapy for those with more advanced or symptomatic disease. In a recent study of 28 patients with moderate to advanced KS, those receiving liposomal doxorubicin in addition to HAART had a markedly better response rate at 48 months than did those on HAART alone (76% versus 20%).[59]

While HAART is recommended for virtually all patients with a KS diagnosis, individuals with advanced and/or symptomatic KS should receive some form of local or systemic therapy specific for KS. A variety of standard therapeutic approaches are summarized below.

Local Therapies

These are generally appropriate for treating unsightly or symptomatic lesions. They may be used in those individuals with limited disease as an adjunct to HAART or in those unresponsive to antivirals.

Radiotherapy

At one time radiotherapy was the mainstay of local therapy. Used as a single 80 Gy or equivalent frac-

tionated dose, it is an active treatment modality. It is less commonly used now due to long-term local toxicities when administered over large cutaneous surfaces, resulting in loss of skin elasticity, discomfort, and occasionally contractures. When used, it should be administered only to small fields for treating localized mucocutaneous lesions. Lower fractionated doses may be associated with less-significant long-term toxicities. Doses of 15 Gy for oral lesions, 20–Gy for lesions involving eyelids, conjunctiva, and genitals, and 30 Gy for cutaneous lesions have been shown to be sufficient to produce shrinkage of the tumor and good palliation of the symptoms.[60]

Alitretinoin gel

Alitretinoin gel (1%): A randomized phase III vehicle-controlled study of topical administration of this agent demonstrated a 37% response rate compared with 7% in vehicle control patients.[61] It was particularly useful for facial lesions, although often associated with excessive local irritation. This agent was just recently taken out of production, although it may still be available in some areas.

Intralesional vinblastine

Generally used as dilute injected solution, this cytotoxic agent is a vesicant useful for treating small cosmetically unsightly mucocutaneous lesions. There is pain associated with injection and several injections may be required. It often leaves some hyperpigmentation behind.

Cryotherapy

Liquid nitrogen cryotherapy is commonly used by dermatologists for local treatment of small lesions. Multiple therapies may also be required with this modality, which tends to leave a hypopigmented area following therapy.

Systemic Therapy

Chemotherapy

Cytotoxic therapy (Table 40.4) is still the most effective treatment for advanced, symptomatic disease. First-line standard of care is liposomal doxorubicin, which had a higher response rate than a standard three-drug combination (ABV) in a randomized phase III trial[62] and, other than myelosuppression, is a very well-tolerated agent with a low incidence of gastrointestinal toxicity and rare alopecia. For those individuals who are poorly responsive to or relapse after Doxil therapy, paclitaxel has been shown to have response rates as high as 70% in previously treated patients with advanced KS.[63] The use of oral etoposide has been recommended by some due to its ease of administration. In a recent Brazilian study, 21 patients received daily oral etoposide at a dose of 20 mg/m^2 every 8 h for 7 days every 21 days. This treatment was associated with an objective response rate of 83%.[64] This agent is associated with a 44% incidence of alopecia, making it less favorable than Doxil as first line therapy. It is also associated with significant myelosuppression. Finally, vinorelbine was associated with a 43% response rate in a group of 35 individuals with KS refractory to a variety of prior chemotherapy regimens.[65] Other chemotherapeutic regimens with activity in KS are listed in Table 40.4, but should only be considered if the above agents fail or are associated with excessive toxicity.

Interferon-α

IFN was documented to have activity in HIV-KS very early in the AIDS epidemic. Its use in high doses, often associated with potentially debilitating constitutional toxicities, has limited its use. However, more recent data suggest it may be effective at lower doses (1 million units daily, s.c.) when combined with antiretroviral therapy.[66] This may be an option for patients who have limited disease that is unresponsive to HAART and who do not require chemotherapy. Responses to this agent are strongly associated with CD4 count. Those with CD4 <100/mm^3 are unlikely to respond.

Investigational Agents

Several approaches to therapy based upon the pathogenesis of the disease have been studied in recent years.

Col-3

Col-3, a matrix metalloproteinase inhibitor, had a 44% response rate in a phase I AIDS Malignancies Consortium (AMC) trial,[67] and is currently being evaluated in a phase II study. MMPs are enzymes that exist within the extracellular matrix and play an important role in tumor invasion and angiogenesis.

Thalidomide

Thalidomide as a single agent at doses 200–1000 mg/m^2 had a 40% response rate in 20 patients with KS treated at the National Cancer Institute.[68] However, the usefulness of this agent may be limited by its toxicity profile, as 35% of these patients discontinued the drug prior to completion of therapy due to toxicity. These toxicities, including somnolence, neutropenia, depression and neuropathy, become more prevalent at the higher dose levels.

Imatinib mesylate

Imatinib mesylate (Gleevec), a PDGF receptor and c-kit inhibitor currently used in treatment of CML, showed a 50% response rate in 10 patients treated with 300 mg twice daily.[69] Follow-up biopsies demonstrated responses to be associated with inhibition of PDGF receptor activity. This agent was well-toler-

Table 40.4 Cytotoxic therapy for Kaposi's sarcoma

Agent	Dose	Response(%)	Toxicity
Liposomal Doxorubicin	20 mg/m^2 q. 21 days	46–59	Neutropenia; cardiomyopathy
Paclitaxel	100 mg/m^2 q. 14 days	59–79	Neutropenia; myalgias; neuropathy; alopecia
Vinorelbine	30 mg/m^2 q. 14 days	43	Neutropenia; neuropathy
Etoposide	20 mg/m^2 p.o.7 days, every 21 days	83	Neutropenia; alopecia
Bleomycin Vincristine	15 mg/m^2 } q.21 days 2 mg	23	Pulmonary fibrosis; peripheral neuropathy
Doxorubicin Bleomycin Vincristine	20 mg/m^2 10 mg/m^2 } q. 14 days 1 mg	25	Neutropenia; pulmonary neuropathy; cardiomyopathy

ated and is currently being studied in a phase II trial in the AMC.

Recommendations

Patients with a new diagnosis of KS should be started on HAART as first-line therapy. Whether it is important to use a protease-inhibitor (PI)-containing regimen is unclear, but for those patients whose KS does not respond to a non-PI-containing regimen, the addition of a PI might be considered. Patients with advanced, symptomatic disease should be started on cytotoxic therapy, preferably with liposomal doxorubicin, along with HAART. This will provide a more rapid and effective response than HAART alone. Topical therapies may be used as adjuncts to HAART for patients who desire additional cosmetic therapy. Clinical trials will continue to investigate the use of less-toxic, pathogenesis-based approaches to therapy.

The improvements in the management of this disease have been remarkable, most of all in terms of prevention, which as a result of effective anti-HIV therapies has provided a >80% decline in the incidence of this opportunistic malignancy since 1996. HAART alone may be effective management for the majority of patients with KS, reducing the need for toxic chemotherapeutic agents. As we move toward pathogenesis-directed therapies for KS itself, the future is indeed bright for control of this neoplasm.

References

1. Goedert JJ. The epidemiology of acquired immunodeficiency syndrome malignancies. Semin Oncol 2000; 27:390–401.
2. Clifford GM, Polesel J, Rickenbach M, et al. Cancer risk in the Swiss HIV Cohort Study: associations with immunodeficiency, smoking, and highly active antiretroviral therapy. J Natl Cancer Inst 2005; 97:425–432.
3. Babiker A, Darbyshire J, Pezzotti P, et al. Changes over calendar time in the risk of specific first AIDS-defining events following HIV seroconversion, adjusting for competing risks. Int J Epidemiol 2002; 31:951–958.
4. Jacobson LP, Yamashita TE, Detels R, et al. Impact of potent antiretroviral therapy on the incidence of Kaposi's sarcoma and non-Hodgkin's lymphomas among HIV-1-infected individuals. Multicenter AIDS Cohort Study J Acquir Immune Defic Syndr 1999; 21(Suppl):S34–S41.
5. Gerard L, Galicier L, Maillard A, et al. Systemic non-Hodgkin lymphoma in HIV-infected patients with effective suppression of HIV replication: persistent occurrence but improved survival. J Acquir Immune Defic Syndr 2002; 30:478–484.
6. Newton R, Ziegler J, Beral V, et al. A case-control study of human immunodeficiency virus infection and cancer in adults and children residing in Kampala, Uganda. Int J Cancer 2001; 92:622–627.
7. Matthews GV, Bower M, Mandalia S, et al. Changes in acquired immunodeficiency syndrome-related lymphoma since the introduction of highly active antiretroviral therapy. Blood 2000; 96:2730–2734.
8. Knowles DM. Etiology and pathogenesis of AIDS-related non-Hodgkin's lymphoma. Hematol Oncol Clin North Am 2003; 17:785–820.
9. Carbone A, Gaidano G, Gloghini A, et al. Differential expression of BCL-6, CD138/syndecan-1, and Epstein–Barr virus-encoded latent membrane protein-1 identifies distinct histogenetic subsets of acquired immunodeficiency syndrome-related non-Hodgkin's lymphomas. Blood 1998; 91:747–755.
10. Ambinder RF. Epstein–Barr virus associated lymphoproliferations in the AIDS setting. Eur J Cancer 2001; 37:1209–1216.
11. Kaplan LD, Abrams DI, Feigal E, et al. AIDS-associated non-Hodgkin's lymphoma in San Francisco. JAMA 1989; 261:719–724.
12. Kaplan LD, Kahn JO, Crowe S, et al. Clinical and virologic effects of recombinant human granulocyte-macrophage colony-stimulating factor in patients receiving chemotherapy for human immunodeficiency virus-associated non-Hodgkin's lymphoma: results of a randomized trial. J Clin Oncol 1991; 9:929–940.
13. Straus DJ, Huang J, Testa MA, et al. Prognostic factors in the treatment of human immunodeficiency virus-associated non-Hodgkin's lymphoma: analysis of AIDS Clinical Trials Group protocol 142–low-dose versus standard-dose m-BACOD plus granulocyte-macrophage colony-stimulating factor. National Institute of Allergy and Infectious Diseases. J Clin Oncol 1998; 16:3601–3606.
14. Little RF. AIDS-related non-Hodgkin's lymphoma: etiology, epidemiology, and impact of highly active antiretroviral therapy. Leuk Lymphoma 2003; 44(Suppl):S63–S68.
15. Kaplan LD, Straus DJ, Testa MA, et al. Low-dose compared with standard-dose m-BACOD chemotherapy for non-Hodgkin's lymphoma associated with human immunodeficiency virus infection. National Institute of Allergy and Infectious Diseases AIDS Clinical Trials Group. N Engl J Med 1997; 336:1641–1648.
16. Sparano JA, Lee S, Chen MG, et al. Phase II trial of infusional cyclophosphamide, doxorubicin, and etoposide in patients with HIV-associated non-Hodgkin's lymphoma: an Eastern Cooperative Oncology Group Trial (E1494). J Clin Oncol 2004; 22:1491–1500.
17. Vaccher E, Spina M, di Gennaro G, et al. Concomitant cyclophosphamide, doxorubicin, vincristine, and prednisone chemotherapy plus highly active antiretroviral therapy in patients with human immunodeficiency virus-related, non-Hodgkin lymphoma. Cancer 2001; 91:155–163.
18. Ratner L, Lee J, Tang S, et al. Chemotherapy for human immunodeficiency virus-associated non-Hodgkin's lymphoma in combination with highly active antiretroviral therapy. J Clin Oncol 2001; 19:2171–2178.
19. Bower M, McCall-Peat N, Ryan N, et al. Protease inhibitors potentiate chemotherapy-induced neutropenia. Blood 2004; 104:2943–2946.
20. Little RF, Pittaluga S, Grant N, et al. Highly effective treatment of acquired immunodeficiency syndrome-related lymphoma with dose-adjusted EPOCH: impact of antiretroviral therapy suspension and tumor biology. Blood 2003; 101:4653–4659.
21. Coiffier B, Lepage E, Briere J, et al. CHOP chemotherapy plus rituximab compared with CHOP alone in elderly patients with diffuse large-B-cell lymphoma. N Engl J Med 2002; 346:235–242.
22. Spina M, Jaeger U, Sparano JA, et al. Rituximab plus infusional cyclophosphamide, doxorubicin, and etoposide in HIV-associated non-Hodgkin lymphoma: pooled results from 3 phase 2 trials. Blood 2005; 105:1891–1897.
23. Kaplan LD, Lee J, Scadden D. No benefit from rituximab in a randomized phase III trial of CHOP with or without rituximab for patients with HIV-associated non-Hodgkins lymphoma: updated data from AIDS Malignancies Consortium (Abstract 1488). Blood 2003; 102:409a.

24. Krishnan A, Molina A, Zaia J, et al. Durable remissions with autologous stem cell transplantation for high-risk HIV-associated lymphomas. Blood 2005; 105:874–878.

25. Gabarre J, Marcelin AG, Azar N, et al. High-dose therapy plus autologous hematopoietic stem cell transplantation for human immunodeficiency virus (HIV)-related lymphoma: results and impact on HIV disease. Haematologica 2004; 89:1100–1108.

26. Re A, Cattaneo C, Michieli M, et al. High-dose therapy and autologous peripheral-blood stem-cell transplantation as salvage treatment for HIV-associated lymphoma in patients receiving highly active antiretroviral therapy. J Clin Oncol 2003; 21:4423–4427.

27. Serrano D, Carrion R, Balsalobre P, et al. HIV-associated lymphoma successfully treated with peripheral blood stem cell transplantation. Exp Hematol 2005; 33:487–494.

28. Kadan-Lottick NS, Skluzacek MC, Gurney JG. Decreasing incidence rates of primary central nervous system lymphoma. Cancer 2002; 95:193–202.

29. De Luca A, Antinori A, Cingolani A, et al. Evaluation of cerebrospinal fluid EBV-DNA and IL-10 as markers for in vivo diagnosis of AIDS-related primary central nervous system lymphoma. Br J Haematol 1995; 90:844–849.

30. Bossolasco S, Cinque P, Ponzoni M, et al. Epstein–Barr virus DNA load in cerebrospinal fluid and plasma of patients with AIDS-related lymphoma. J Neurovirol 2002; 8:432–438.

31. Antinori A, De Rossi G, Ammassari A, et al. Value of combined approach with thallium-201 single-photon emission computed tomography and Epstein–Barr virus DNA polymerase chain reaction in CSF for the diagnosis of AIDS-related primary CNS lymphoma. J Clin Oncol 1999; 17:554–560.

32. Jacomet C, Girard PM, Lebrette MG, et al. Intravenous methotrexate for primary central nervous system non-Hodgkin's lymphoma in AIDS. AIDS 1997; 11:1725–1730.

33. Newell ME, Hoy JF, Cooper SG, et al. Human immunodeficiency virus-related primary central nervous system lymphoma: factors influencing survival in 111 patients. Cancer 2004; 100:2627–2636.

34. Thompson LD, Fisher SI, Chu WS, et al. HIV-associated Hodgkin lymphoma: a clinicopathologic and immunophenotypic study of 45 cases. Am J Clin Pathol 2004; 121:727–738.

35. Spina M, Berretta M, Tirelli U. Hodgkin's disease in HIV. Hematol Oncol Clin North Am 2003; 17:843–858.

36. Gerard L, Galicier L, Boulanger E, et al. Improved survival in HIV-related Hodgkin's lymphoma since the introduction of highly active antiretroviral therapy. AIDS 2003; 17:81–87.

37. Hoffmann C, Chow KU, Wolf E, et al. Strong impact of highly active antiretroviral therapy on survival in patients with human immunodeficiency virus-associated Hodgkin's disease. Br J Haematol 2004; 125:455–462.

38. Spina M, Gabarre J, Rossi G, et al. Stanford V regimen and concomitant HAART in 59 patients with Hodgkin disease and HIV infection. Blood 2002; 100:1984–1988.

39. Simonelli C, Spina M, Cinelli R, et al. Clinical features and outcome of primary effusion lymphoma in HIV-infected patients: a single-institution study. J Clin Oncol 2003; 21:3948–3954.

40. Delecluse HJ, Anagnostopoulos I, Dallenbach F, et al. Plasmablastic lymphomas of the oral cavity: a new entity associated with the human immunodeficiency virus infection. Blood 1997; 89:1413–1420.

41. Flaitz CM, Nichols CM, Walling DM, et al. Plasmablastic lymphoma: an HIV-associated entity with primary oral manifestations. Oral Oncol 2002; 38:96–102.

42. Cioc AM, Allen C, Kalmar JR, et al. Oral plasmablastic lymphomas in AIDS patients are associated with human herpesvirus 8. Am J Surg Pathol 2004; 28:41–46.

43. Cattaneo C, Facchetti F, Re A, et al. Oral cavity lymphomas in immunocompetent and human immunodeficiency virus infected patients. Leuk Lymphoma 2005; 46:77–81.

44. Teruya-Feldstein J, Chiao E, Filippa DA, et al. CD20-negative large-cell lymphoma with plasmablastic features: a clinically heterogenous spectrum in both HIV-positive and -negative patients. Ann Oncol 2004; 15:1673–1679.

45. Waterston A, Bower M. Fifty years of multicentric Castleman's disease. Acta Oncol 2004; 43:698–704.

46. Oksenhendler E, Carcelain G, Aoki Y, et al. High levels of human herpesvirus 8 viral load, human interleukin-6, interleukin-10, and C reactive protein correlate with exacerbation of multicentric Castleman disease in HIV-infected patients. Blood 2000; 96:2069–2073.

47. Cesarman E. The role of Kaposi's sarcoma-associated herpesvirus (KSHV/HHV-8) in lymphoproliferative diseases. Recent Results Cancer Res 2002; 159:27–37.

48. Lanzafame M, Carretta G, Trevenzoli M, et al. Successful treatment of Castleman's disease with HAART in two HIV-infected patients. J Infect 2000; 40:90–91.

49. Andres E, Maloisel F. Interferon-alpha as first-line therapy for treatment of multicentric Castleman's disease. Ann Oncol 2000; 11:1613–1614.

50. Lerza R, Castello G, Truini M, et al. Splenectomy induced complete remission in a patient with multicentric Castleman's disease and autoimmune hemolytic anemia. Ann Hematol 1999; 78:193–196.

51. Berezne A, Agbalika F, Oksenhendler E. Failure of cidofovir in HIV-associated multicentric Castleman disease. Blood 2004; 103:4368–4369.

52. Marcelin AG, Aaron L, Mateus C, et al. Rituximab therapy for HIV-associated Castleman disease. Blood 2003; 102:2786–2788.

53. Martin JN, Ganem DE, Osmond DH, et al. Sexual transmission and the natural history of human herpesvirus 8 infection. N Engl J Med 1998; 338:948–954.

54. Bubman D, Cesarman E. Pathogenesis of Kaposi's sarcoma. Hematol Oncol Clin North Am 2003; 17:717–745.

55. Gill J, Bourboulia D, Wilkinson J, et al. Prospective study of the effects of antiretroviral therapy on Kaposi sarcoma–associated herpesvirus infection in patients with and without Kaposi sarcoma. J Acquir Immune Defic Syndr 2002; 31:384–390.

56. Monfardini S, Cattelan AM, De Rossi A, et al. Highly effective antiretroviral therapy (HAART) and clinical outcome of AIDS related Kaposi's sarcoma: A prospective study (Abstract 3295). Proc Am Soc Clin Oncol 2003; 22:820.

57. Dupont C, Vasseur E, Beauchet A, et al. Long-term efficacy on Kaposi's sarcoma of highly active antiretroviral therapy in a cohort of HIV-positive patients. CISIH 92. Centre d'information et de soins de l'immunodeficience humaine. Aids 2000; 14:987–993.

58. Pellet C, Chevret S, Blum L, et al. Virologic and immunologic parameters that predict clinical response of AIDS-associated Kaposi's sarcoma to highly active antiretroviral therapy. J Invest Derm 2001; 117:858–863.

59. Martin-Carbonero L, Barrios A, Saballs P, et al. Pegylated liposomal doxorubicin plus highly active antiretroviral therapy versus highly active antiretroviral therapy alone in HIV patients with Kaposi's sarcoma. Aids 2004; 18:1737–1740.

60. Kirova YM, Belembaogo E, Frikha H, et al. Radiotherapy in the management of epidemic Kaposi's sarcoma: a retrospective study of 643 cases. Radiother Oncol 1998; 46:19–22.

61. Bodsworth NJ, Bloch M, Bower M, et al. Phase III vehicle-controlled, multi-centered study of topical alitretinoin gel 0.1% in cutaneous AIDS-related Kaposi's sarcoma. Am J Clin Derm 2001; 2:77–87.

62. Northfelt DW, Dezube BJ, Thommes JA, et al. Pegylated-liposomal doxorubicin versus doxorubicin, bleomycin, and vincristine in the treatment of AIDS-related Kaposi's sarcoma: results of a randomized phase III clinical trial. J Clin Oncol 1998; 16:2445–2451.

63. Gill PS, Tulpule A, Espina BM, et al. Paclitaxel is safe and effective in the treatment of advanced AIDS-related Kaposi's sarcoma. J Clin Oncol 1999; 17:1876–1883.

64. Sprinz E, Caldas AP, Mans DR, et al. Fractionated doses of oral etoposide in the treatment of patients with aids-related

Kaposi sarcoma: a clinical and pharmacologic study to improve therapeutic index. Am J Clin Oncol 2001; 24:177–184.

65. Nasti G, Errante D, Talamini R, et al. Vinorelbine is an effective and safe drug for AIDS-related Kaposi's sarcoma: results of a phase II study. J Clin Oncol 2000; 18:1550–1557.

66. Krown SE, Li P, Von Roenn JH, et al. Efficacy of low-dose interferon with antiretroviral therapy in Kaposi's sarcoma: a randomized phase II AIDS clinical trials group study. J Interferon Cytokine Res 2002; 22:295–303.

67. Cianfrocca M, Cooley TP, Lee JY, et al. Matrix metalloproteinase inhibitor COL-3 in the treatment of AIDS-related Kaposi's sarcoma: a phase I AIDS malignancy consortium study. J Clin Oncol 2002; 20:153–159.

68. Little RF, Wyvill KM, Pluda JM, et al. Activity of thalidomide in AIDS-related Kaposi's sarcoma. J Clin Oncol 2000; 18:2593–2602.

69. Koon HB, Bubley GJ, Pantanowitz L, et al. Imatinib-induced regression of AIDS-related Kaposi's sarcoma. J Clin Oncol 2005; 23:982–989.

CHAPTER 41

Managing HIV Infection in Children and Adolescents

Andrew T. Pavia

Epidemiology

The epidemiology of HIV disease in children in developed countries has changed substantially. These changes have been driven by the evolving epidemiology of HIV infection in women, the ability to prevent mother to child transmission, the dramatic increases in survival for children treated with combination antiretroviral therapy,[1-3] and the evolution of drug resistance. Women make up an increasing proportion of AIDS cases and new HIV infections. Between 2000 and 2003, the proportion of new AIDS cases among women increased from 24–27%.[4] The number of new infections in women has increased somewhat, while the death rate dropped dramatically between 1995 and 2000 and has been relatively stable since then. Therefore, the number of women living with HIV/AIDS has increased steadily in developed countries. In 1996, the Centers for Disease Control (CDC) estimated that 6000–7000 infants were born to HIV-infected women each year in the USA. Accurate and current data on the number of pregnancies among HIV-infected women are not available, but it is likely that more children are born to HIV-infected women each year.

Since 1992, the number of children younger than 13 years diagnosed with AIDS in developed countries has decreased dramatically, representing one of the remarkable successes in the fight against HIV. In the USA, the estimated number of children younger than 13 diagnosed with AIDS fell from 952 in 1992, to 59 in 2003.[4] However, because of improved survival, the number of children living with HIV in developed countries has remained stable. By the end of 2003, an estimated 1957 children were living with

AIDS in the USA and its territories, and an additional 2968 children were reported to be living with HIV infection (not AIDS) from the 41 states with name-based reporting.

Thus, a large number of children are living with HIV/AIDS in the USA and other developed countries, but few new infections are occurring. Most children have been infected for many years, and usually have received prolonged antiretroviral therapy. Many are, or soon will be adolescents. The major challenges of treatment no longer revolve around when to start therapy and what initial therapy to use. Managing viral resistance, complications of therapy and the psychological and social impact of HIV infection have become increasingly important.

Natural History

Timing of Infection

HIV progresses more rapidly in children with perinatal infection than among children infected at an older age or among adults. It has long been recognized that there was a bimodal distribution of clinical progression.[5-7] About 20% of children had early onset of symptoms before the advent of effective therapy. These children have a rapid downhill course in the first 12 months of life, marked by rapid decline in CD4 count, development of category C disease, often including pneumonia due to *Pneumocystis jiroveci* (formerly *P. carinii pneumonia*), or death.

There appear to be a number of predictors of rapid progression, including severe maternal disease,[8] evidence of *in utero* transmission (positive PCR, culture or p24 assay at birth), early hepato-splenomegaly,[9] and higher viral loads after 1 month of life.[10,11] CD4 and CD8 counts below the 5th percentile in infancy were associated with rapid progression among babies infected *in utero* in one study,[12] perhaps reflecting early destruction of the thymus.

The natural history of HIV among adolescents who have acquired infection through adult behaviors in general parallels adults. However, younger age at infection is associated with significantly slower progression in the absence of highly active antiretroviral therapy (HAART).[13,14]

Declining CD4 count and CD4% are the hallmarks of HIV disease progression in children. CD4 count normally declines with age, making interpretation somewhat problematic. CD4% is less age dependent and is very useful in disease staging (Table 41.1). The revised CDC classification uses both immunologic status and clinical status and is useful for staging.

Predicting Progression

Quantitative measurement of plasma viral RNA revolutionized the management of HIV in adults; similar data in children required a few more years to accumulate.[10,15,16] The kinetics of plasma HIV RNA in children differs from adults in several ways, however. First, children tend to have higher viral loads, with median peak values between 100 000 copies and 1 000 000 copies. Second, after primary infection, the viral load slowly declines during the first year of life, in contrast to the rapid 2–3 log drop in adults. Third, although viral load is consistently associated with prognosis, it has been difficult to establish specific levels that are sensitive and specific for high risk.[17] These differences may reflect a greater number of target cells, and a limited ability to mount

an immune response by the immature immune system. Children infected *in utero* tend to have modest viral loads at birth, but the peak value at 1–2 months is higher than those with presumed intra-partum infection.

CD4 count and percentage are independent predictors of progression to category C disease or death. A pivotal meta-analysis of survival data on 3941 European and American children with HIV infection in the pre-HAART era demonstrated that CD4% and viral load were independent predictors of progression to AIDS or death over the next 12 months; CD4% was the strongest short-term predictor.[17] The risk of progression at a given CD4 level or viral load varied by age. Importantly, among children <12 months, the risk of progression remains moderately elevated even when the CD4% was high or the viral load was low. Growth failure is a sensitive indicator of disease activity and improved growth is a marker of successful antiviral therapy.

With the advent of three-drug combination antiretroviral therapy for children, survival has increased dramatically. In a cohort of 1000 children in the UK, there was an 80% decline in mortality and hospital admissions between 1994 and 1990, along with a 50% decline in progression to AIDS.[18]

Early Diagnosis and Management of the Exposed Infant

Diagnosis of HIV Infection

Currently, the diagnosis of HIV infection in children born to HIV-infected mothers can be made in most infants by 2–4 weeks of age using methods that directly detect virus. Detection of virus by peripheral blood mononuclear cell (PBMC) co-culture, DNA PCR of the infants PBMCs, or HIV RNA in

Table 41.1 1994 revised human immunodeficiency virus pediatric classification system: Immune categories based on age-specific CD4+ T-lymphocyte count and percentage

Immune category	<12 months No./mL (%)	1–5 years No./mL (%)	6–12 years No./mL (%)
Category 1: No suppression	>1500 (>25%)	>1,000 (>25%)	>500 (>25%)
Category 2: Moderate suppression	750–1499 (15–24%)	500–999 (15–24%)	200–499 (15–24%)
Category 3: Severe suppression	<750 (<15%)	<500 (<15%)	<200 (<15%)

From Centers for Disease Control and Prevention; 1994 revised classification system for human immunodeficiency virus infection in children less than 13 years of age. MMWR 1994; 43 (RR-12):1–10.

plasma is presumptive evidence of infection but *must* be confirmed by repeat testing.

Viral culture was considered the gold standard, but is slow, cumbersome and expensive. Currently, DNA PCR is the method of choice for diagnosis of HIV in infants. In a meta-analysis of data from 271 infected children, HIV DNA PCR was only moderately sensitive in the first 48 h of life (38%; 90% confidence interval (CI), 29–46%). Sensitivity rose rapidly during the second week; 93% of infected children (90% CI, 76–97%) were PCR positive by 14 days of age. Several studies suggests that quantitative RNA PCR is at least as sensitive and specific as DNA PCR, and offers the advantages of using smaller blood volumes and providing important prognostic data.[19-22] False positives can occur and levels <10 000 copies/mL should be considered suspect. Measurement of p24 antigen, either conventionally or with immune dissociation, is not recommended for the diagnosis of neonatal HIV infection because it is less sensitive than PCR or culture, and false positives may occasionally occur.

Most experts recommend obtaining a first sample for DNA PCR or culture during the first 48 h of life. Cord blood should not be used because of the possibility of contamination with maternal blood. A positive viral test in the first 48 h of life presumptively identifies children who were infected *in utero*, who may have a more rapid disease course. However, in another study, plasma RNA measurement after the first month of life appeared to be more prognostic than time of first positive test.

For infants with an initial negative test, testing should be repeated at 14–28 days of life. Testing at 14 days offers the potential to stop zidovudine monotherapy for patients with presumed infection and begin combination therapy during the period of acute infection. For infants with initial negative tests, testing should be repeated again at 1–2 months of age. If the initial tests are all negative, testing should be repeated at 3–6 months of age. Any positive test should be confirmed immediately by testing of a separate blood sample, and two positive tests should be considered diagnostic of infection. We recommend obtaining quantitative plasma RNA (viral load) as well as DNA PCR for confirmatory testing. This provides independent confirmation and important prognostic information. Two negative blood samples for DNA PCR or culture, one after at least 1 month of age, and another after 3 months of age, reasonably excludes HIV infection. HIV antibody should be checked at 12 months, and if still detectable, monitored until antibody becomes undetectable.

Use of PCP Prophylaxis

Pneumocystis jiroveci pneumonia occurs most often between 3 and 6 months of age in perinatally infected children. Disease may develop before HIV infection is confirmed or before a drop in CD4 counts has been documented. Because of continuing mortality with CD4-based guidelines for prophylaxis, the CDC published revised guidelines recommending that PCP prophylaxis be initiated at 4–6 weeks of life for all HIV-exposed infants. Prophylaxis should be continued until HIV-infection can be excluded (see above). It is reasonable to consider the pre-test likelihood of infection. A child born to a mother on combination therapy with an undetectable viral load who has had negative PCRs at 2–4 weeks of life and again at 6 weeks has a predictive value negative of >99.9%. Prophylaxis should be continued until 12 months of age in all infected infants. After that age, prophylaxis is recommended for all children with severe immunosuppression (CDC category 3). Trimethoprim sulfamethoxazole is the preferred drug. The recommended dose is 150 mg/m^2 per day in divided doses on three consecutive days each week, but there are several acceptable alternatives.[23]

Monitoring in the HIV-exposed or HIV-infected Infant

Infants born to HIV-infected women should receive oral AZT during the first 6 weeks of life based on the PACTG 076 protocol. Myelosuppression is common with both AZT and trimethoprim sulfamethoxazole, and the complete blood count should be monitored. Plasma viral RNA and CD4 count and percentage should be monitored once the diagnosis of HIV is established. These are measured at baseline, 1 and 2 months after starting antiretroviral therapy, and at least every 3 months. A suggested monitoring scheme is shown in Table 41.2.

Vaccination

Timely vaccination is important for HIV-infected children. Guidelines are available.[23] Inactivated vaccines (hepatitis B, *Haemophilus influenzae* type B, diphtheria-tetanus-pertussis, IPV) are given according to the schedule recommended for all children. Measles, mumps and rubella vaccine (MMR) is a live vaccine, which poses a theoretic risk to severely immunocompromised children and the vaccine should not be given to those in immunologic

Table 41.2 Suggested schedule for routine monitoring of HIV-exposed and infected infants

Intervention	Birth	2–4 weeks	1–2 months	3–6 months	1 year
AZT	X	X	Through week 6		
PCP prophylaxis[a]			X	X	
CBC with differential	X	X	X	X	
HIV DNA PCR	X	X	X	X	
HIV Plasma RNA[b]	b	b	b	b	
CD4 absolute and %[c]					
HIV antibody					X

[a]PCP prophylaxis is continued until HIV is excluded or for the first 12 months of life in children who are infected or whose infection status is unknown.
[b]See text for use of HIV Plasma RNA PCR as an alternative to HIV DNA PCR. HIV plasma RNA should be measured immediately if infection is suspected based on a positive HIV DNA PCR. If no treatment is initiated, plasma RNA should be monitored every 3 months. If treatment is initiated or changed, plasma RNA should be monitored 4 weeks and 8 weeks after changing therapy and every 3 months thereafter.
[c]CD4 counts should be repeated every 2–3 months in children who are infected.

category 3. HIV-infected children without imm-unosuppression should receive their first dose as soon as possible after the first birthday. The second dose need not be delayed until school entry; it can be given as soon as 1 month after the first dose. Varicella vaccine can be safely given to children with normal immunologic function (category 1). Annual immunization against influenza is recommended for all HIV-infected children. Initially, two doses are given, separated by at least 1 month. Since infections with encapsulated organisms are prominent among HIV-infected children, the potential benefit of pneumococcal vaccine is large. Unfortunately, children <2 years old respond poorly to polysaccharide vaccines; immunization with pneumococcal heptavalent conjugate vaccine (PCV-7) is recommended for all children younger than 60 months. After completion of the series, the 23-valent pneumococcal vaccine should also be given after 24 months of age. Re-vaccination should be offered after 3–5 years.

Vaccination is also important for HIV-infected adolescents. They should receive annual influenza vaccine and 23-valent pneumococcal polysaccharide vaccine. Their immunization status to hepatitis A, hepatitis B, and measles should be reviewed and updated. Recently, meningococcal conjugate vaccine and tetanus diphtheria acellular pertussis (Tdap) have been recommended for adolescents. Vaccines for human papillomavirus and herpes simplex are likely to be important for HIV-infected adolescents when available.

Antiviral Therapy

Principles of Therapy

The goal of antiviral therapy in children, as in adults, is to suppress viral replication to extremely low levels to prevent loss of CD4 cells and to allow immune reconstitution. If viral replication continues in the face of antiretroviral agents, ongoing mutation will lead to drug resistance. Combination therapy with three or more agents offers the greatest opportunity to achieve maximal suppression. The ability to adhere to a regimen is a key determinant of continued viral suppression. The complexity of HIV therapy in children and adolescents and the rapidly changing evidence base suggest that children with HIV should receive care from physicians with substantial expertise in HIV and in conjunction with multidisciplinary teams. Whenever possible, children should be offered the opportunity to participate in clinical trials.

It is important, however, to appreciate ways in which children differ from adults. The majority of HIV-infected children are infected around the time of delivery, and therapy can potentially be started during primary infection. Theoretically, this offers children an advantage that is rare in adults. Intact thymic architecture offers the potential for greater immune reconstitution, and in one study, thymic volume on CT scan correlated with completeness of immune reconstitution.

However, many of the differences lead to challenges. In general, clinical trial data in children are limited, and pharmacokinetic studies may be inadequate. The disposition of drugs changes during growth and development, changing from infancy into childhood, and again during adolescence. In general, volume of distribution is larger, and clearance is faster, which may require more frequent dosing. In general, rates of viral suppression to below the limits of quantification have been lower in trials among children and adolescents than among adults. The developing central nervous system of children appears to be more vulnerable to damage by HIV. Regimens therefore should be highly active in the CNS Young children usually require liquid formulations, which may be unpalatable or simply not available. Young children are dependent on the caregiver's ability to give medications consistently, on schedule and in spite of protests. Older children may be concerned about taking antiviral therapy in public or at school. The social problems that are common in families with HIV-infected children (poverty, homelessness, parents who may be ill or absent, substance abuse, mental illness, isolation, fear of disclosure) compound the problems of complex regimens, unpleasant tasting medicine, and sometimes resistance from the child or adolescent. Thus, problems with adherence can be daunting.

When to Start

Recommendations on starting therapy and preferred regimens have been formulated by the Working Group on Antiretroviral Therapy and Medical Management of HIV-Infected Children in the US and the Paediatric European Network for Treatment of AIDS (PENTA) (Table 41.3).[24,25] These guidelines are largely evidence-based, and are periodically updated but reflect a rapidly changing state of the art. The decision to start therapy balances the probability of developing severe clinical disease in the near term and the risk of irreversible damage to the immune system or developing organs with the known difficulties of maintaining suppression in children, short-term side-effects, the risk of developing drug resistance mutations and the possibility of running out of effective agents. In addition, we are just beginning to appreciate long-term toxicities in children, including abnormalities of lipid, glucose and bone metabolism.

Table 41.3 Recommendations for when to start antiviral therapy in children; USA, Europe and WHO

	DHHS	PENTA	WHO
Infants	<1 year with CDC category A, B or C disease <1 year with CD4% <25% (Recommended) All infants regardless of symptoms or CD4% (Consider)	<1 year with CDC category B or C disease (Recommended) <1 year with CD4% <25% (Recommended) Viral load >1 million copies/mL (Strongly consider) Younger than 1 year regardless of symptoms or CD4% (Consider)	<18 months, virologically confirmed infection with WHO Pediatric Stage III (Recommended) <18 month, virologically confirmed infection with WHO Pediatric Stage II (consider using CD4% <20%) (Recommended) <18 months, virologically confirmed infection with WHO Pediatric Stage I and CD4% <20% (Recommended) <18 months, HIV seropositive, but virologic confirmation not available, WHO Pediatric Stage III and CD4% <20% (Recommended)
Children	CDC category C disease or CD4% <15% (Recommended) CDC category A or B disease or CD4% 15–25% or Viral load >5 log (Consider)	CDC category C disease or Markedly decreased CD4% (1–3 years <20%; 4–13 years <15%) (Recommended) CD4% <20% or viral load >250 000 copies (Consider)	WHO Pediatric Stage III disease or CD4% <15% (Recommended) WHO Pediatric Stage II disease (Recommended) Consider using CD4% <15% as a criteria

DHHS, Department of Health and Human Services (US) Working Group (Working Group on Antiretroviral Therapy and Medical Management of HIV-infected Children, 2005 #287). Online. Available: http//AIDSinfo.nih.gov; PENTA, Paediatric European Network for the Treatment of AIDS 2004 (Sharland 2004 #657). Online. Available: www.ctu.mrc.ac.uk/penta/guidelines.htm; WHO, World Health Organization: Scaling up antiretroviral therapy in resource limited settings (Draft: 2003 revision). Online. Available: www.who.int/3by5/publications/documents/arv_guidelines/en

A meta-analysis of 3941 children from eight cohorts in the pre-treatment era showed that CD4% was the best predictor of the risk of AIDS over the next 12 months, but the ability of CD4% or viral load to predict outcome varied with age. Among infants, it was difficult to identify any level of markers at which the risk of progression is low (Fig. 41.1).[17] The high viral loads and poor host control of HIV replication in infants also argue for aggressive therapy. Among infants, therefore, treatment is recommended for infants with any level of symptoms or any level of immunosuppression (CD4% <25%). However, many experts would strongly consider starting treatment in any HIV infected infant, regardless of clinical status or surrogate markers. Preliminary studies of antiviral therapy in infants have demonstrated significant clinical benefit but relatively low rates of complete suppression.[26] On the other hand, prospective cohort studies have shown dramatic reductions in clinical progression before the age of three, associated with increased use of early potent antiretroviral therapy.[1]

In children with category C disease, treatment should always be started, as well as in those with severe immunosuppression (CD4% <15%). Treatment for children older than 1 year with limited or no symptoms is more problematic. For those with preserved immune function, one approach would be to treat all children. This approach is in contrast to the more conservative approach that has evolved for treating adults. The aggressive approach can be considered when the family or caregivers are committed to aggressive therapy, there is adequate medical and social support, and there is a high likelihood of good adherence.

A second approach is to defer therapy in older children who have limited symptoms, no evidence of immune dysfunction, and are at low risk of rapid progression based on HIV RNA. The risk of progression is intermediate when the CD4% is <20%, especially in younger children and therapy should be considered, but the decision is less clear. Viral loads >100 000 copies/mL are associated with higher rates of progression or death, and treatment should be considered. Patients in whom deferral of therapy might be preferred are older children, those with minimal symptoms, well preserved CD4 and low viral loads. Perhaps the most important consideration, and one which requires thoughtful clinical judgment, is whether to defer therapy in low and intermediate risk patients because of the risk of poor adherence and development of resistance outweighs the benefit of immediate therapy. If antiretroviral therapy is deferred, it is wise to consider starting therapy if new symptoms develop, if the CD4% is falling rapidly or if the viral load increases by more than 0.7 log (confirmed by repeated measures).

Initial Therapy

When therapy is begun for children, combination therapy with at least three drugs, including two nucleoside reverse transcriptase inhibitors and either a non-nucleoside reverse transcriptase inhibitor or a potent protease inhibitor, is preferred. Monotherapy

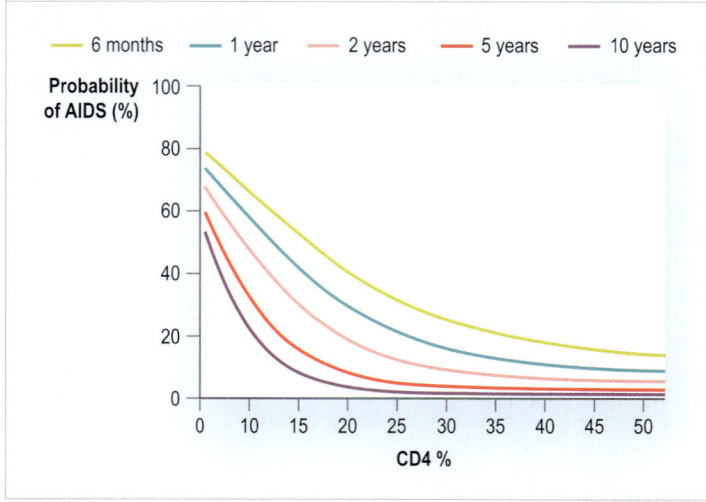

Figure 41.1 Probability of developing AIDS in the next 12 months among 3941 children by age and CD4%. (From the HIV Paediatric Prognostic Markers Collaborative Study, HPPMCS).[17]

and the use of two nucleoside analogs are no longer considered adequate therapy.

Selection of appropriate drugs is complicated by the limited availability of adequate pharmacokinetic data to allow appropriate drug exposure, the availability and palatability of liquid formulations, and the availability of clinical efficacy data. In the US Guidelines, the combination of two nucleoside analogs plus either lopinavir/ritonavir, efavirenz (or nevirapine for children <3 or who cannot swallow capsules are designated as strongly recommended (Table 41.4). Some regimens are designated as alternative regimens, either because data are limited or suggest lower efficacy or because of toxicity. Data

---

Table 41.4 Options for initial antiretroviral therapy in children with HIV infection

Protease inhibitor-based regimens	
Strongly recommended	Two NRTIs[a] *plus* Lopinavir/Ritonavir *or* Nelfinavir *or* Ritonavir
Alternative recommendation	Two NRTIs[a] *plus* Amprenavir (children >4 years old)[b] *or* Indinavir
Non-nucleoside reverse transcriptase inhibitor-based regimens	
Strongly recommended	Children >3 years: Two NRTIs1 *plus* Efavirenz[c] (with or without Nelfinavir)
	Children <3 years or who cannot swallow capsules: Two NRTIs1 *plus* Nevirapine[c]
Alternative recommendation	Two NRTIs1 *plus* Nevirapine[c] (children >3 years)
Nucleoside analog-based regimens	
Strongly recommended	None
Alternative recommendation	Zidovudine *plus* Lamivudine *plus* Abacavir
Use in special circumstances	Two NRTIs[a]
Regimens that are not recommended	Monotherapy[d]
	Certain two NRTI combinations[a]
	Two NRTIs *plus* Saquinavir as a sole protease inhibitor[e]
Insufficient data to recommend	Two NRTIs1 *plus* Delavirdine
	Dual protease inhibitors, including saquinavir soft or hardgel capsule with low dose ritonavir, with the exception of Lopinavir/Ritonavir[d]
	NRTI *plus* NNRTI *plus* protease inhibitor[f]
	Tenofovir-containing regimens
	Enfuvirtide (T-20)-containing regimens
	Emtricitabine (FTC)-containing regimens
	Atazanavir-containing regimens
	Fosamprenavir-containing regimens
	Tipranavir-containing regimens

[a]Dual NRTI combinations:
- Strongly recommended choices: Zidovudine plus didanosine or lamivudine; or stavudine plus lamivudine.
- Alternative choices: Abacavir plus zidovudine or lamivudine; or didanosine plus lamivudine.
- Use in special circumstances: Stavudine plus didanosine; or zalcitabine plus zidovudine.
- Insufficient data: Tenofovir- or emtricitabine-containing regimens.
- Not Recommended: Zalcitabine plus didanosine, stavudine or lamivudine; or zidovudine plus stavudine; or emtricitabine plus lamivudine.

[b]Amprenavir should not be given to children <4 years due to polypropylene glycol content.
[c]Efavirenz currently available only in capsule form, although liquid formulation is under study. Nevirapine is preferred NNRTI for children <3 years because of liquid formulation and well established PK.
[d]Except zidovudine chemoprophylaxis given to HIV-exposed infants during the first 6 weeks of life, provided there is no evidence of HIV infection. If an infant is confirmed to be HIV-infected, ZDV monotherapy should be stopped and replaced with combination therapy.
[e]With the exception of lopinavir/ritonavir, there are limited data on the safety and pharmacokinetics of protease inhibitors boosted with low dose ritonavir in children (e.g.: saquinavir/r, indinavir/r, fosamprenavir/r, atazanavir/r). Nonetheless, these combinations may be useful in second or third-line regimens.
[f]One study examined efavirenz plus nelfinavir plus one or two NNRTIs and showed efficacy.
(Adapted from Guidelines for the use of antiretroviral agents in pediatric HIV infection, 3 November 2005. Online. Available: http://aidsinfo. nih.gov; accessed 30 December 2005. (Working Group on Antiretroviral Therapy and Medical Management of HIV-infected Children, 2005 #287).

were insufficient to make recommendations for several drugs that have important potential roles, including tenofovir, emtricitabine, atazanavir, fosamprenavir, tipranavir, and the fusion inhibitor T-20. Some of these agents, along with lamivudine, abacavir, and didanosine are used in once daily regimens in adults. These agents and a variety of once daily regimens are under study.

Initial studies demonstrated rates of viral suppression to <400 copies/mL were substantially lower than among adults. However, in a study of 100 antiretroviral therapy-naive and pre-treated children treated with lopinavir/ritonavir with nucleoside analogs, 79% had viral loads below 400 copies at 48 weeks; 88% of antiretroviral-naive children were suppressed. Given the higher and more consistent drug exposure with this boosted protease inhibitor, it suggests that consistent drug exposures may be central to effective treatment.

When to Change

In children, even more than in adults, the decision to change therapy must balance the need to better control viral replication, and the higher likelihood of control with earlier switching against the limited number of active drugs and the problems of cross-resistance. In children, there is a real need not to exhaust the limited options. When there is major toxicity or if new data suggest that the current therapy is inadequate, the regimen must be changed. For minor clinical or laboratory toxicities, it is worth trying to manage the symptoms.

When therapy appears to be failing, the issues are more complex. When the initial regimen is failing, there may be several acceptable options. In children who have been exposed to many regimens and have many drug resistance mutations, there may be limited opportunities to design an effective regimen.

Before changing therapy, it is essential to carefully assess adherence and to try and solve adherence problems. Otherwise, the new regimen is doomed to fail.

There are three broad indicators of drug failure, as suggested by the Working Group on Antiretroviral Therapy in Children: virologic, immunologic, and clinical. Virologic indicators have the advantage of being easily quantifiable and often correlate with the emergence of drug-resistant virus. If a change is observed, RNA measurements should be repeated before deciding to change therapy. Failure to achieve a minimally acceptable response after 8–12 weeks

(1 log for protease inhibitor-containing regimens) should prompt a change. The repeated detection of viral RNA after a period falling below limits of quantification, or an increase of 0.7–1 log from the nadir indicate virologic failure. Failure to achieve a viral load <400–500 copies 4–6 months after beginning an aggressive initial regimen is an inadequate response. However, this goal may be difficult to achieve.

Virologic failure may not be an indicator of immediate clinical or immunologic failure, and the decision to change therapy should weigh the available options and the CD4 response. Stable or increasing CD4 counts in the face of continued viral replication among children who remain on therapy are common, as in adults.[27]

Immunologic progression is an indicator of increased risk of death. Therefore, therapy should be changed in the face of immunologic progression and detectable virus. CD4% is less affected by age and mild illness and is often a better indicator. A change to a new immunologic category, or, for those with CD4% <15%, a decrease of 5 percentiles, are clear indicators of immunologic progression. However, rate of change should also be considered. A 30% change in absolute CD4 count or CD4% in 6 months is worrying.

Certain types of clinical progression are ominous and should prompt changes in therapy. Growth failure or progressive neurodevelopmental decline are clear indicators of disease progression. Although definitive data are lacking on the clinical efficacy, agents which achieve good antiretroviral activity in the CSF should be used. These include AZT, d4T, 3TC, and nevirapine.

The choice of agents for 'salvage' therapy is difficult, and there are few clear guidelines. Strategies recommended in adults also make sense for children. Whenever possible, three to four new agents which the child has not seen, and which are not predicted to be cross-resistant should be used.

Resistance Testing

Limited data demonstrate that the prevalence of resistance among newly diagnosed HIV-infected children is similar to the 10–20% prevalence among recently infected adults. Resistance testing should be strongly considered before beginning therapy in children whose mothers have resistant virus or unknown resistance status or who have had treatment exposure. Resistance testing is appropriate to guide selection of new regimens for children who have experienced virologic failure.

Therapeutic Drug Monitoring

The patient-to-patient variability of bioavailability, drug metabolism and levels is generally larger for children than adults. Complex drug interactions may make it difficult to predict drug levels. To date, however, there are no prospective data to demonstrate that therapeutic drug monitoring will improve treatment outcomes. In the absence of prospective data, it is reasonable to consider therapeutic drug monitoring for children when available. Appropriate situations might include those on regimens for which dosing recommendations are based on limited data, children on unusual combinations or with complex drug-drug interactions, or those who might have difficulty with drug absorption.[28]

Prophylaxis of other Opportunistic Infections

Primary prevention of specific opportunistic infections is extremely important for children with advanced immunosuppression. Guidelines have been formulated by the Infectious Diseases Society of America with the Centers for Disease Control and Prevention which categorize the advisability of prophylaxis, the CD4 levels and the agents of choice.

At present, there are insufficient data to recommend stopping primary prophylaxis in children under most circumstances. However, the safety of stopping primary prophylaxis in adults is clearly established, and preliminary experience in children has been encouraging.[29,30] Many clinicians are comfortable stopping primary prophylaxis in children with prolonged and stable immune reconstitution.

Lifelong suppression (secondary prevention) has been the standard of care for children with PCP, *Toxoplasma gondii* infection, and *Mycobacterium avium* complex.[31] Secondary prevention to prevent recurrence can safely be stopped for many opportunistic infections in adults when immune reconstitution has been maintained for 6 months at levels above where the opportunistic infection occurs. This has not been adequately studied in children.

Management

Comprehensive management of the HIV-infected child is beyond the scope of this chapter. Optimal care requires a multidisciplinary approach, and if possible, a dedicated team. Careful attention must be given to nutrition, developmental assessment, psychosocial issues, and education. Teaching about HIV and multiple strategies to support adherence are critical. Medical care of the mother is important to the child's health as well as the mother's. If possible, HIV services for mother and child should be available at the same site and should be coordinated. Periodic case management meetings to coordinate issues among providers and agencies are extremely useful.

Adolescents

Adolescents infected with HIV pose unique challenges. The needs of children who were infected perinatally who have survived into adolescence are different from those who are infected during adolescence. Survivors of perinatal infection are an increasing population. They have demonstrated slow disease progression, but often have advanced disease and may have been extensively pre-treated. They have often outlived their parents. Most adolescents who are recently infected were infected through sexual activity. HIV infection through sexual abuse occurs, and can only be diagnosed if there is awareness and careful investigation. Adolescent behavior problems, including drug use or having run away are relatively common, and there is a high prevalence of mental illness among adolescents living with HIV.[32] Screening instruments for depression may be helpful. The clinical course of disease for adolescents infected sexually or through drug use is more similar to adults; adult treatment guidelines are appropriate.

Some issues are common among adolescents. Disclosure of infection status is a difficult and often overwhelming issue. Rapid growth, changes in metabolism and increases in muscle mass in males and in fat for women affect drug metabolism. Adolescents in early puberty (Tanner stage I and II) should be dosed as children. Those in late puberty (Tanner V) should be dosed as adults. There are no clear guidelines for those at intermediate stages. Puberty may be delayed in those with long-standing HIV infection and delayed growth may be an additional stress.

Adherence with medical care and with antiretroviral therapy is particularly difficult for adolescents. Autonomy, distrust of authority, embarrassment, lack of support, and low self esteem may be issues. Adolescents are often unable to grasp long-term risks and consequences. Some have chaotic lives. Medical care and medications may make the adolescent feel different and at times, vulnerable.

Multidisciplinary teams, including mental health, social work, educators, and peer to peer counseling, may be helpful. In some adolescents at moderate risk of progression, it may be wise to delay antiretroviral therapy until adherence is more likely.

Unanswered Questions

Despite the important gains in antiviral therapy and the promise of further improvement, there remain frustrating gaps in our knowledge and our ability to deliver antiviral therapy to children. Early diagnosis of HIV-infected children and early treatment with fully suppressive regimens holds enormous promise. However, we need to learn much more about the pharmacology of antiretroviral drugs in all stages of growth. All agents must be studied in infants and children during the early phase of development. As with adults, we do not yet know the optimal combinations and sequences of drugs, nor the best way to ensure adherence to difficult and complex regimens. The long-term consequences of changes in lipid, glucose and bone metabolism may be more complex and potentially more serious in children over decades of treatment.[33]

Once daily regimens and CD4-guided intermittent therapy are options that might improve adherence and decrease the emergence of resistance. Their use in children and adolescents must be evaluated.

The prevention of perinatal transmission is the ultimate answer to controlling pediatric AIDS. In developed countries, it should be possible to virtually eliminate perinatal transmission of HIV through universal screening of pregnant women, use of effective antiviral regimens during pregnancy and delivery, and optimal obstetrical management.

References

1. Berk DR, Falkovitz-Halpern MS, et al. Temporal trends in early clinical manifestations of perinatal HIV infection in a population-based cohort. JAMA 2005; 293:2221–2231.
2. de Martino M, Tovo PA, Balducci M, et al. Reduction in mortality with availability of antiretroviral therapy for children with perinatal HIV-1 infection. Italian Register for HIV Infection in Children and the Italian National AIDS Registry. JAMA 2000; 284:190–197.
3. McConnell MS, Byers RH, Frederick T, et al. Trends in antiretroviral therapy use and survival rates for a large cohort of HIV-infected children and adolescents in the United States, 1989–2001. J Acquir Immune Defic Syndr 2005; 38:488–494.
4. CDC. HIV/AIDS Surveillance Report, 2003. Atlanta, GA: Centers for Disease Control and Prevention; 2004.
5. Blanche S, Newell ML, Mayaux MJ, et al. Morbidity and mortality in European children vertically infected by HIV-1. The French Pediatric HIV Infection Study Group and European Collaborative Study. J Acquir Immune Defic Syndr Hum Retrovirol 1997; 14:442–450.
6. Barnhart HX, Caldwell MB, Thomas P, et al. Natural history of human immunodeficiency virus disease in perinatally infected children: an analysis from the Pediatric Spectrum of Disease Project. Pediatrics 1996; 97:710–716.
7. Anon. Natural history of vertically acquired human immunodeficiency virus-1 infection. The European Collaborative Study. Pediatrics 1994; 94:815–819.
8. Ioannidis J, Tatsioni A, Abrams EJ, et al. Maternal viral load and rate of disease progression among vertically HIV-1 infected children; an international meta-analysis. AIDS 2004; 18:99–108.
9. Mayaux MJ, Burgard M, Teglas JP, et al. Neonatal characteristics in rapidly progressive perinatally acquired HIV-1 disease. Fr Pediatr HIV Infect Study Group JAMA 1996; 275:606–610.
10. Shearer WT, Quinn TC, LaRussa P, et al. Viral load and disease progression in infants infected with human immunodeficiency virus type 1. Women and Infants Transmission Study Group. N Engl J Med 1997; 336:1337–1342.
11. Rich KC, Fowler MG, Mofenson LM, et al. Maternal and infant factors predicting disease progression in human immunodeficiency virus type 1-infected infants. Women and Infants Transmission Study Group. Pediatrics 2000; 105:e8.
12. Nahmias AJ, Clark WS, Kourtis AP, et al. Thymic dysfunction and time of infection predict mortality in human immunodeficiency virus-infected infants. J Infect Dis 1998; 178:680–685.
13. Carre N, Deveau C, Belanger F, et al. Effect of age and exposure group on the onset of AIDS in heterosexual and homosexual HIV-infected patients. SEROCO Study Group AIDS 1994; 8:797–802.
14. Rosenberg PS, Goedert JJ, Biggar RJ. Effect of age at seroconversion on the natural AIDS incubation distribution. Multicenter Hemophilia Cohort Study and the International Registry of Seroconverters. AIDS 1994; 8:803–810.
15. Dickover RE, Dillon M, Leung KM, et al. Early prognostic indicators in primary perinatal human immunodeficiency virus type 1 infection: importance of viral RNA and the timing of transmission on long-term outcome. J Infect Dis 1998; 178:375–387.
16. Palumbo PE, Raskino C, Fiscus S, et al. Predictive value of quantitative plasma HIV RNA and CD4+ lymphocyte count in HIV-infected infants and children. JAMA 1998; 279:756–761.
17. Dunn D. Short-term risk of disease progression in HIV-1-infected children receiving no antiretroviral therapy or zidovudine monotherapy: a meta-analysis. Lancet 2003; 362:1605–1611.
18. Gibb DM, Duong T, Tookey PA, et al. Decline in mortality, AIDS, and hospital admissions in perinatally HIV-1 infected children in the United Kingdom and Ireland. Br Med J 2003; 327:1019.
19. Nesheim S, Palumbo P, Sullivan K, et al. Quantitative RNA testing for diagnosis of HIV-infected infants. J Acquir Immune Defic Syndr 2003; 32:192–195.
20. Simonds RJ, Brown TM, Thea DM, et al. Sensitivity and specificity of a qualitative RNA detection assay to diagnose HIV infection in young infants. Perinatal AIDS Collab Transm Study AIDS 1998; 12:1545–1549.
21. Steketee RW, Abrams EJ, Thea DM, et al. Early detection of perinatal human immunodeficiency virus (HIV) type 1 infection using HIV RNA amplification and detection. N Y City Perinatal HIV Transm Collab Study J Infect Dis 1997; 175:707–711.
22. Young NL, Shaffer N, Chaowanachan T, et al. RNA and DNA PCR for early diagnosis of infants born to HIV-infected mothers, Thailand. Int Conf AIDS 1998; 12:(abstract 794).
23. Masur H, Kaplan JE, Holmes KK. Guidelines for preventing opportunistic infections among HIV-infected persons 2002.

Recommendations of the U.S. Public Health Service and the Infectious Diseases Society of America. Ann Intern Med 2002; 137:435–478.

24. NPHRC and HRSA. Guidelines for the use of antiretroviral agents in pediatric HIV infection. National Pediatric and Family HIV Resource Center (NPHRC), the Health Resources and Services Administration (HRSA), 2005.

25. Sharland M, Blanche S, Castelli G, et al. Committee PS. PENTA guidelines use antiretroviral therapy. HIV Med 2004; 5:61–86.

26. Aboulker JP, Babiker A, Chaix ML, et al. Highly active antiretroviral therapy started in infants under 3 months of age: 72-week follow-up for CD4 cell count, viral load and drug resistance outcome. AIDS 2004; 18:237–245.

27. Deeks SG, Barbour JD, Grant RM, et al. Duration and predictors of CD4 T-cell gains in patients who continue combination therapy despite detectable plasma viremia. AIDS 2002; 16:201–207.

28. Fraaij PL, van Kampen JJ, Burger DM, et al. Pharmacokinetics of antiretroviral therapy in HIV-1-infected children. Clin Pharm 2005; 44:935–956.

29. Nachman S, Gona P, Dankner W, et al. The rate of serious bacterial infections among HIV-infected children with immune reconstitution who have discontinued opportunistic infection prophylaxis. Pediatrics 2005; 115: e488–e494.

30. Urschel S, Ramos J, Mellado M, et al. Withdrawal of Pneumocystis jirovecii prophylaxis in HIV-infected children under highly active antiretroviral therapy. AIDS 2005; 19:2103–2108.

31. Mofenson LM, Oleske J, Serchuck L, et al. Treating opportunistic infections among HIV-exposed and infected children: recommendations from CDC, the National Institutes of Health, and the Infectious Diseases Society of America. Clin Infect Dis 2005; 40(Suppl):1–84.

32. Gaughan DM, Hughes MD, Oleske JM, et al. Psychiatric hospitalizations among children and youths with human immunodeficiency virus infection. Pediatrics 2004; 113: e544–e551.

33. McComsey GA, Leonard E. Metabolic complications of HIV therapy in children. AIDS 2004; 18:1753–1768.

CHAPTER 42

Special Issues Regarding Women with HIV Infection

Meg D. Newman

Epidemiology

In 1997, approximately 41% of adults living with HIV/AIDS were women; by 2002, this proportion had risen to 50%. Of the approximately 40 million adults worldwide living with HIV/AIDS in 2002, about 19.2 million were women. Every day, approximately 5500 women are newly infected with HIV, and more than 3000 die from AIDS-related illnesses.

In most parts of the world, HIV infection is increasing faster among women than men. Nowhere is the trend more apparent than in sub-Saharan Africa where women comprise 58% of existing HIV infections. Among young people aged 15–24, women are 2.5 times more likely than men to be HIV infected. In most southern African countries, more than one in five pregnant women are HIV infected. According to UNAIDS, a trend analysis of antenatal clinic sites in eight countries between 1997 and 2002 shows HIV prevalence among pregnant women, leveling off at almost 40% in Gaborone, Botswana and Manzini, Swaziland, and at almost 16% in Blantyre, Malawi, and 20% in Lusaka, Zambia. In the USA, women comprise the fastest growing population of persons with AIDS.[1] As of December 2004, there were 176 190 women who have been diagnosed with AIDS in the USA. In recent years and cumulatively, a significant trend in adult women has been the increased acquisition of HIV infection through heterosexual contact (43%) and the decreased acquisition of the virus through intravenous (IV) drug use (26%). Point estimates of cases diagnosed with AIDS as of 2004 by ethnicity reveal disproportionately high rates among African American women (48.2 per 100 000), Latina women (11.1 per 100 000), American Indian/Alaskan Native women (6.4 per 100 000), Asian/Pacific Islander women (1.6 per 100 000), compared with white women (2.1 per 100 000). In viewing these statistics, it is important to remember that African American and Latina women represent 25% of all US women, but comprise >76% of all the cases in US women.[2]

The AIDS Epidemic in Young Women

In industrialized countries, the IDU epidemic in men is reflected in the heterosexual epidemic in women, which is in turn reflected in the epidemic among children. The most alarming trends of heterosexual transmission are now occurring in young women both globally and nationally.

Cumulative data of AIDS cases in the USA as of December 2001 illustrate the preponderance of heterosexual sex as the mode of transmission for young women ages 13–25. In this age group, heterosexual contact dominates as a means of transmission for women, whereas it is a relatively uncommon mode of transmission in young men of this age group.[3] Most of these young women have not reported intravenous drug use and are likely to have partners an average of 5 years older than themselves. It is well documented that women of any age may have trouble negotiating with their male sexual partners for condom use, and one could speculate that the age gap between younger women and their sexual partners is likely to worsen this trend.[4] Finally, normal physiology in young women includes cervical ectopy, where the columnar cells of the endocervix are more exposed and allow more efficient transmission of HIV. Younger populations of women, particularly women of color, require urgent outreach, and intervention measures. The 2005 UN Development Fund for Women (UNIFEM) report narrates the ingredients of a global crisis among women and girls: women are much less likely to be financially independent and secure, are controlled by the violence of men or fear of violence, are often regarded as socially inferior, and often assume the responsibility of caring for the other family members and relatives with HIV. These realities often force girls out of education and job training, and push girls and women into commercial sex work in order to survive, where negotiating for condom use is often unsuccessful. Most women worldwide get their infection as a result of heterosexual transmission, often from partners who do not reveal their own HIV infection and risk factors.[5]

Heterosexual Transmission

Among HIV-discordant couples (those with only a single HIV-positive partner), heterosexual transmission from the male to the female partner is approximately eight times more efficient than female-to-male transmission. Most infections have occurred by the vaginal route, although participation in anal sex increases the risk.[6–8] The cumulative incidence of transmission within discordant couples suggests an approximate 20% risk of transmission from male to female from unprotected sex over a sustained period in a fixed partnership. A study from northern California, which began prospectively following patients in 1985, found that only two (2.4%) of the 82 male partners of HIV-infected females became infected, but 68 (19%) of the 360 female partners of infected men became infected.[6] Male-to-female transmission risk per sexual contact in this study was estimated to be 0.0009.[6]

In a more recent study from Rakai, Uganda, monogamous serodiscordant couples were followed prospectively. In this cohort of 97 seropositive men, 17 (17.5%) of their wives became infected with HIV. Among the 77 seropositive women, 21 (27.3%) of their husbands became infected.[9] Many factors may explain this difference in female-to-male transmission risk compared with US studies, including HIV viral load,[10] concurrent genital ulcer disease, and HIV subtype (see below).

Risk Factors Associated with Heterosexual Transmission

Factors associated with increased transmission include other sexually transmitted diseases (STDs),

lack of condom use, advanced disease state (measured by CD4, viral load, or AIDS diagnosis), anal intercourse, number of sexual contacts, genital ulcerative disease, and use of an intrauterine contraceptive device (IUD) (Box 42.1).[6,11] Cervical ectopy, discussed previously, is emerging as a risk in women for acquisition of HIV from infected men. It is possible that the increased levels of heterosexual transmission in adolescent women may be partially explained by the natural occurrence of cervical ectopy in this age group.[12,13]

Increased HIV viral load in the infected partner is associated with increased risk of transmission in heterosexual couples. In the Rakai study, each 10-fold increase in viral load was associated with an increase by a factor of 2.45 (95% confidence interval, CI: 1.85, 3.26) in the risk of transmission, and no cases of HIV transmission were reported within serodiscordant couples in which the seropositive partner had an HIV viral load of <1500 copies/mL.[10] It should be kept in mind that this study was conducted in a population without access to antiretroviral drugs. Infectious virus in genital secretions may persist despite undetectable serum viral load in individuals taking antiretroviral therapy,[14] and resistance mutations not seen in plasma virus may occur in the genital compartment.[15] Accordingly, for a given plasma viral load, the risk of transmission of HIV from an individual on antiretroviral treatment may be different from the risk observed in the Rakai study, and the resulting infection may be more difficult to treat because of pre-existing drug resistance.

Box 42.1

HIV gynecological care

- Cervical pap smears every 6 months for women with CD4 <200
- Abnormal findings including ASCUS, AGCUS or persistent inflammation go onto colposcopy
- Dysplasia is not limited to the cervix: Careful inspection of vulvar and perianal areas is equally as important
- Oral contraceptive can be used but a barrier method is also recommended
- Remember that Hepatitis C and B, Kaposi's sarcoma are also STIs
- Mammography recommendations do not differ for women with HIV
- PID often presents with fewer WBC but more tubo-ovarian abscesses.

Sexually transmitted infections, particularly those associated with symptoms or genital ulcerations, appear to increase the risk of HIV transmission. A study of heterosexual couples in Haiti found an increased risk of HIV acquisition when genital ulcers were reported in the initially seronegative partner.[16] The Rakai study also found an increased rate of HIV transmission within couples with a seropositive partner who experienced genital discharge or dysuria. In a study in Kenya, higher levels of cervical herpes simplex virus (HSV) type 2 were associated with higher levels of HIV and with more frequent detection of HIV-infected cells in cervical secretions.[17]

Increased Physiologic Risk of HIV Acquisition

Risk of HIV acquisition is not static in women over time but varies by physiological risk factors as well as the social factors discussed already.

Normal physiology in young women includes cervical ectopy, as well as pregnancy and the initial post-partum period also denotes a time of increased risk of acquisition of HIV infection that may be due to enhanced levels of progesterone. Progesterone has been considered to play a primary role in causing cervical ectopy in animal primate models and likely plays an important role as a risk factor for increased transmission. Other hormonal factors that may enhance transmission either by direct immunosuppression, or promote the activation of these target cells lining the genital tract are not well described at this juncture. Ongoing research will hopefully elucidate these critical issues.

HIV subtype C and circulating recombinant form (CRF) 01 (A/E) (formerly called subtype E) have been found to replicate more efficiently than subtype B in Langerhans cells, the antigen-presenting cells hypothesized to be responsible for vaginal transmission. In Thailand, where CRF01(A/E) predominates, and in India and southern Africa, where subtype C is common, heterosexual transmission is the major route of HIV infection, whereas in North America, where subtype B predominates, heterosexual transmission is less common. It has been speculated that the introduction of CRF01(A/E) or subtype C into North America might result in increased heterosexual transmission.[18]

Lack of circumcision has been associated with increased risk of HIV acquisition by men in Africa,[10] and Kreiss and colleagues found that uncircumcised homosexual men in the USA had a twofold increased risk of HIV infection.[19]

Transmission of HIV in Lesbians

Transmission of HIV between women was reported as early as 1984,[20] but documented cases are very rare. A number of small studies have been conducted but tend to include only small numbers of women having sex with women (WSW) who have no other HIV risk factors, such as injection drug use. Through September 1989, 79 women with AIDS had reported sex with a female only, but 95% were IDUs.[21] Sporadic cases of direct transmission have been reported, but analysis is hampered by lack of data regarding baseline serology or blood exposure during sex.

WSW may engage in sexual activity with men for pleasure, as commercial sex workers, or they may be victims of sexual assault. Some women IDUs who engage in sex with other women are associated with riskier injection drug use and sexual behaviors and therefore are at a higher risk of acquiring HIV than other women IDUs.[22] WSW who are also IDUs were more likely than other IDUs to share needles, to exchange sex for drugs or money, to be homeless, and to seroconvert. This more marginalized group and their sexual partners would likely benefit from specially targeted prevention programs.

Although the risk of sexual transmission of HIV between WSW appears to be low, women who are partners of women infected with HIV should observe principles of safer sexual activity and avoid mucous membrane contact with all potentially infectious secretions (Box 42.2).[23]

Box 42.2

Primary care of HIV-infected women

- Obtain CMV IgG for all women with HIV and avoid CMV+ blood products if IgG is negative
- Watch for mitochondrial toxicity *especially in obese women*
- Do not forget age-appropriate healthcare maintenance
- Smoking cessation is a modifiable risk factor that decreases dysplasia progression – make it part of the treatment goal
- If women have multiple risk factors for osteopenia or osteoporosis (steroids, smoking, low BMI, malnutrition, ethnicity) screen *before* they are postmenopausal.

Clinical Manifestations

Factors that may influence the presentation of HIV or response to therapy in women include altered pharmacokinetics of drugs, due either to gender or to interactions between commonly associated drugs (such as methadone or oral contraceptive pills), and possibly to differences in the immune system between men and women. Symptoms of middle-stage HIV in women, as in men, are extremely non-specific, including night sweats, diarrhea, fatigue, cough, and weight loss. There are no marked differences between the sexes in the presentation or natural history of such common AIDS-defining diseases as *Pneumocystis jiroveci* (formerly *carinii*) pneumonia (PCP), disseminated *Mycobacterium avium* complex, *Cryptococcus*, and toxoplasmosis.

Opportunistic Infections and HIV-associated Infections

AIDS-defining diagnoses seen frequently in data combined from a number of small cohorts of women include PCP, esophageal candidiasis, disseminated *Mycobacterium avium*, and mucocutaneous HSV.[24] Women are not protected from any of the other AIDS-defining opportunistic infections.[25] Bacterial infections, especially respiratory infections with such encapsulated organisms as *Streptococcus pneumoniae* and *Haemophilus influenzae*, occur more frequently in IDUs than in homosexual men and occur with equal frequency in heterosexual men and women.[26]

Opportunistic Infections: Prophylaxis and CMV Antibody Screening

Appropriate opportunistic infection (OI) prophylaxis is necessary for both women and men, and no gender-specific recommendations can be made. In the USA, immunoglobulin G (IgG) antibodies to CMV are almost always positive in homosexual men and healthcare providers sometimes overlook this screening among women. Yet, the prevalence of CMV antibodies in women are similar to rates in the general adult population. CMV IgG screening is warranted for all women and the CMV-negative patient in need of a transfusion should always receive CMV-negative blood to avoid future risk of CMV end-organ disease.[27]

Progression of Disease

It is well established that gender itself is not a predicator of increased morbidity and mortality for those living with HIV infection. Results of early studies from the beginning of the HIV epidemic analyzing progression and survival in HIV disease suggested a difference based on gender. Many early studies indicated that the prognosis for women was worse than for men regardless of risk group or race. These studies reflected late access to limited care – a common scenario for women early in the AIDS epidemic.[28] All of the work since the mid-1990s and continuing into the highly active antiretroviral therapy (HAART) era disputes that women have increased levels of morbidity and mortality as a result of gender and supports the contention that earlier results reflected poor access to care.[29]

Studies of disease progression in women are limited and, when available, are derived from three principal sources: large national databases, which usually include the diagnosis of AIDS and the date of death with little additional interval information; small- to moderate-sized cohort studies of 50–200 women in industrialized countries, often followed for <3 years; and larger cohort studies conducted in developing countries.[30] One report summarized a dozen studies that overall reveal that the survival and course of disease in men and women is not substantially different when patients are matched for socioeconomic status, risk group, and access to care.[31] Reports from the CDC suggest that survival time of women and heterosexual men is similar. A population-based rural cohort study in Uganda also found no difference in gender-specific mortality rates.[32]

A US study of 3779 men and 768 women, with median T-cell counts higher in the group of women (240 cells/μL, versus 137 cells/μL in the men), found that women were at increased risk of death (relative risk: 1.3) during a 15-month period. It is important to note that there was no increased risk of HIV disease progression in women, that increased risk of death was found primarily among IDUs, and that the deaths were secondary to bacterial pneumonia and endocarditis, both likely related to injection drug use. The study authors noted that these findings may represent differential access to care, treatments, or social support.[29] The most important predictors of survival or progression appear to be CD4 count, viral load, and the specific AIDS-defining diagnosis – not gender.

Multiple studies that followed seroincident cohorts of women and men after HAART was commonly available confirm that women and men benefit equally from HAART and that female gender is not a risk factor for accelerated disease. Although gender is not the basis for distinguishing morbidity and mortality risk, it is now well substantiated that viral loads are lower in woman than men at a specific CD4 count.[33] This interesting sex effect will be discussed in the following section.

It is important for medical providers to maintain a low threshold to counsel and test for HIV, remembering that women infected with HIV through heterosexual transmission may be unaware of their partners' HIV status and therefore may not perceive themselves at risk of infection. HIV and AIDS for women is an issue of access to healthcare, and the care system is not always well suited to their needs. Because women may access healthcare through sources other than a primary care provider, emergency departments, family planning clinics, STD clinics, youth guidance centers, jail clinic facilities, and drug treatment units, are important sites for targeting efforts at early diagnosis and use of early intervention with antiviral and prophylactic therapies.

Association between Gender and Viral Load

Multiple studies in North America, Europe and Africa have found that women have lower viral loads than men at a similar CD4 cell count.[34] The European Collaborative Study looked at the question of whether this phenomenon is limited to adults alone or relevant to children. They looked specifically at children who acquired their infection from vertical transmission and found that HIV RNA reached a peak at 3 months of age and at its peak was higher for girls than boys This changes by 4 years of age when boys' HIV RNA levels become higher and by age 5, girls are on average one half log 10 lower than boys.

Investigation of HIV viral load levels in 527 IDUs at baseline (using branched DNA [bDNA]) and from 285 of the 527 at follow-up, 3 years later (using polymerase chain reaction, PCR) found that women IDUs had lower median viral load measurements than men with similar CD4 counts. Using bDNA, initial viral load levels were 3365 copies/mL for women (median CD4 count 518/μL) and 8907 copies/mL for men (median CD4 count 518/μL). Using PCR at follow-up, viral load levels were 45 416 copies/mL for women (median CD4 count 417/μL) and 93 130 copies/mL for men (median CD4 count 390 cells/μL).

These results suggested that women had median viral load levels that were only about half the viral loads of men with a similar CD4 cell count, and that women with the same viral load as men had a 1.6-fold higher risk of AIDS (95% CI: 1.10, 2.32).[35]

A separate study found that HIV RNA was not different in women and men with CD4 counts below 200 cells/μL, but that at CD4 counts of 200–500 cells/μL, women demonstrated 40% lower HIV RNA levels than men, and that at CD4 counts above 500/μL, levels were 24% lower in women.[36]

These studies were further corroborated in a large CDC cohort of 3776 participants (2467 men and 1309 women). Women with CD4 counts of 0–199 cells/μL had viral loads that were 40% lower than men; women with CD4 counts 200–499 cells/μL had viral loads that were 48% lower; and those women with CD4 of >500 cells/μL had viral loads that were 57% lower. All of these results were statistically significant, indicating that women have lower viral loads on average than men with comparable CD4 counts.[37,38]

There is a paucity of data supporting the use of a specific viral load threshold as an independent factor for initiating antiretroviral therapy. The precise timing for initiating antiretrovirals in patients with >200 but <350 CD4+ cells/μL thus remains controversial in the patient without clinical illness related to HIV infection. Moreover, multiple studies over the last decade highlight that women and men who have equal access to care have similar rates of progression to AIDS and death.

Gynecologic Manifestations

Much attention has been given to disorders that may be more frequent, more severe, and less responsive to therapy in HIV-infected women (particularly those with advanced immunosuppression) than in women without HIV infection: human papillomavirus (HPV)-associated cervical disorders such as cervical intraepithelial neoplasia (CIN); *Candida* vaginitis; and pelvic inflammatory disease (PID). These disorders are recognized as HIV-associated conditions in the expanded CDC case definition.

Cervical Disorders

Human papilloma virus and cervical neoplasia

HPV is believed to be an etiologic factor in human cervical cancer and has been investigated since the 1970s. Approximately 95% of cervical condyloma, all grades of CIN, and invasive cervical cancer contain HPV DNA. HPV types 16 and 18 have been found most commonly in cervical cancer, and types 6 and 11 are most frequently associated with benign condylomas or low-grade squamous intraepithelial lesions (SILs).[39,40]

Immune suppression appears to make one particularly susceptible to infection by oncogenic strains of HPV. Reports indicate that autograft transplant recipients receiving immunosuppressive treatments have a ninefold increase in incidence of HPV anogenital infection and a 16-fold increase in incidence of CIN compared with the general population.

HPV prevalence, acquisition, and retention are higher in HIV-positive women than in matched controls. By DNA analysis, types 16, 18, and 33 are associated most frequently with CIN in HIV-positive women especially in women with CD4 counts of <200 cells/μL.[41-43]

A large, prospective, multicenter study conducted by the CDC in conjunction with investigators in Miami and New York compared HIV-positive and -negative women, all of whom had Pap smears, colposcopy, and evaluation for HPV by PCR. This controlled, prospective trial confirmed numerous prior uncontrolled studies of HIV-positive cohorts in finding that CIN is more frequent in HIV-positive women (20% in HIV-positive compared with 4% in HIV-negative women) and that more advanced CIN is more likely to be associated with a more advanced stage of immunosuppression. By multivariate analysis, HPV (odds ratio (OR) = 9.8), HIV infection (OR = 3.5) and CD4 count (OR = 2.7) were independently associated with CIN.[39] The Women's Interagency HIV Study (WIHS), a large natural history study of HIV-infected women, reported on a cohort of 2015 HIV-infected women and 577 HIV-seronegative controls. Those women who were HIV infected had the highest rates of HPV infection (58%), compared with seronegative controls (26%). HIV-infected women also demonstrated a 42% prevalence of infection with multiple types of HPV versus a 16% prevalence of multiple types in HIV uninfected women. Risk factors for CIN/SIL were CD4 lymphocytes <200 cells/μL, higher risk HPV types, and infection with multiple types of HPV. In a meta-analysis examining 19 studies incorporating 728 HIV-infected women, dysplasia was found to occur in 64% of those with AIDS and in 36% of HIV-positive women.[44,45]

HPV infection in uninfected women is also more transient than in HIV-infected women and this limited ability for spontaneous clearing of HPV infection plays a key role in development of CIN.

Immune restoration secondary to effective HAART plays an important role in regression of CIN in some HIV-infected women. Even in women with similar CD4+ cell counts, those that are on HAART have a significantly greater chance of regression. There are two studies which did not demonstrate a regression of CIN on HAART but those two studies did not address the length of time on HAART, which is likely to play an important role in regression.[46-48]

Although CIN is more common in HIV-infected women, invasive cervical cancer (ICC), has not been demonstrated to occur in HIV-infected women with access to appropriate screening and treatment.[49]

Treatment of CIN

As in HIV-uninfected women, CIN 1 appears to have a low rate of progression to CIN 2 or 3. It should also be noted that treatment of CIN 1 has a high failure rate in HIV-infected women. One strategy a woman with CIN 1 if she has a CD4 count of 200 cells/μL or higher and has demonstrated the willingness and ability to commit to follow-up appointments. Careful surveillance allows the clinician to treat any progression of CIN. Cryotherapy is appropriate for CIN 1 if a woman has a CD4 count <200 cells/μL or is likely to be lost to follow-up evaluations.

Appropriate treatment of CIN 2 or 3 requires use of an ablative or an excisional procedure. Cryotherapy is appropriate for CIN 2 or 3 if the following criteria are met; there is a satisfactory colposcopy and no prior cervical treatment, and if the lesion is completely visible, <2 cm in diameter, and is affecting no more than two quadrants.

Laser ablation can be useful for women who have lesions that are >2 cm or involve three or more quadrants. Laser ablation can also be used to treat vaginal lesions. Loop electrical excisional procedure (LEEP) is helpful when cryotherapy is not appropriate due to size of the lesion or if the location of the lesion is high in the endocervix. LEEP is not possible when cervical architecture is disrupted secondary to a prior LEEP or cone biopsy.

Cold knife cone biopsy cannot be done in the clinic and requires an operating room. It is best reserved for a high-grade lesion where malignancy is detected on Pap smear and microinvasive disease or a glandular lesion may be present. Cone biopsy may also be used for a diagnostic test if LEEP cannot be done for the reasons described above.

Topical application of the antineoplastic agent 5-fluorouracil (5-FU) appears to be a useful adjunctive modality after standard excisional or ablative treatment of CIN 2 or 3.[50]

The role of smoking and CIN should be explained to all patients, and smoking cessation should be recommended and supported in all patients.

In HIV-negative women, there is a small risk (5–10%) of CIN 2 or 3 recurring after therapy. All of the treatments for CIN 1, 2, and 3 appear less effective in HIV-positive women, especially those women with more advanced immunosuppression, and the risk of recurrence is much higher.[51] Careful surveillance with treatment of recurrences is necessary to prevent the development of invasive cervical cancer. Two small studies suggest that effective ART plays a beneficial role in decreasing recurrence and progression of CIN.[52]

Genital Warts

Genital warts (GW) may be large, multifocal, and more prone to recurrence in HIV-positive individuals than in those without HIV infection. Traditional topical treatments such as trichloroacetic acid (TCA), cryotherapy with liquid nitrogen, or cryoprobe are usually effective. Liquid nitrogen may be less painful at the time of application than TCA. In applying TCA, it may be difficult to prevent the compound from affecting adjacent healthy tissue. Liquid nitrogen may allow the clinician to apply the therapy to a more circumscribed area. Laser or surgical excision may be required in cases recalcitrant to these therapies or in lesions involving large surface areas.

Topical application of imiquimod analog 2% cream has been tested in women without HIV infection, in men in a number of small trials, and in one trial involving HIV-infected patients. A systematic review in 2001 demonstrated that complete clearance of warts occurred in only 51% of HIV-negative patients treated with imiquimod 2% or 5%; one trial in HIV-positive patients did not find imiquimod to be effective.[53]

Treatment success of imiquimod in HIV-uninfected patients is reasonable but not outstanding, and initial evidence suggests treatment in HIV-infected patients is not effective. Although imiquimod offers the HIV-infected patient the greater privacy of home administration, it has not replaced the traditional treatments of TCA and liquid nitrogen.

Vaginal Candidiasis

Vaginal candidiasis may cause more severe morbidity in HIV-infected women than in the general population.[54] The revised CDC case definition of 1993 designated severe vaginal candidiasis as an HIV-associated symptomatic disorder. Vaginal candidiasis may occur in early or late HIV disease, but, surprisingly, many women with severe immunosuppression do not have *Candida* vaginitis. Physicians who see women with recurrent or refractory vaginal candidiasis should offer HIV counseling and testing.[55,56]

Genital Ulcerative Disease

Genital ulcerative disease is a well-described risk factor for transmission of HIV. A wide array of conditions may present with genital ulcerations, including HSV, CMV, syphilis, chancroid, gonorrhea, acid-fast bacterial infections, other bacterial or fungal pathogens, malignancies, drug reactions, and idiopathic ulcers such as aphthous ulcers. Genital ulcers may be painful, disabling, difficult to treat, and merit a full diagnostic evaluation.

Giant Idiopathic Aphthous Genital Ulcers

Giant idiopathic aphthous genital ulcers occur infrequently but are painful, disabling, and difficult to treat. Such ulcers should be evaluated for the presence of HSV, CMV, syphilis, chancroid, gonorrhea, bacterial or fungal pathogens, and malignancies. The pathogenesis may be similar to giant esophageal aphthous ulcers. The mainstay of treatment of oral or genital aphthous ulcers is a 1–2-week course of topical steroids and, if unsuccessful, systemic steroids. Thalidomide may be effective for esophageal aphthous ulcers associated with HIV, but there is little published experience on the treatment of aphthous genital ulcers in women.[57]

In the acute retroviral syndrome of early HIV infection, genital ulcerations generally present only in those who have acquired HIV through sexual transmission. Because sexual exposure is the most common route of transmission in women, assessment of possible acute retroviral syndrome should include evaluation for genital aphthous ulcerations.[58]

Pelvic Inflammatory Disease

HIV-positive patients may present with lower white blood cell counts than their HIV-uninfected counterparts. Tubo-ovarian abscess formation has been reported to occur in as many as 25% of HIV-infected women with PID versus 12% of HIV-uninfected controls with PID. Therefore, more surgical intervention may be required, especially in patients with more advanced HIV disease. Standard antibiotic regimens that include anaerobic coverage (such as metronidazole plus a fluoroquinolone) can be used initially in the less complicated patient. Most clinicians maintain a low threshold to hospitalize, and treat with i.v. antibiotics if the HIV disease is advanced.[59]

Antiretroviral Treatment in Women

Gender and Antiretroviral Efficacy

Guidelines established for licensed antiretroviral therapies and prophylaxis against PCP and other opportunistic infections are derived from large studies conducted on men and women. Although men predominated in these studies, the results led to licensure and established recommendations for persons of both sexes. Data from two large studies by the ACTG,[60,61] comparing zidovudine and placebo in asymptomatic or mildly symptomatic HIV-infected patients suggested no difference in benefit from zidovudine for women versus men.

Although subsequent studies sought more participation from women, their representation in trials has remained low, resulting in an ongoing paucity of definitive data on efficacy and toxicity of antiretroviral drugs in women. Clinical experience suggests that combinations of antiretroviral medications are indeed effective in women. A study of the protease inhibitor ritonavir in combination with reverse transcriptase inhibitors in 90 women and 996 men found that women and men experienced similar toxicity, with women having more nausea (63% versus 56% in men), vomiting (49% versus 31%), malaise, and fatigue (47% versus 34%), and perioral numbness and tingling (37% versus 27%). Men were noted to experience more diarrhea (62% versus 49%).[62] A study of the efficacy and toxicity of the protease inhibitor nelfinavir in 78 women and 616 men found similar decreases in viral load among women and men following nelfinavir treatment. Increases in CD4 lymphocyte counts were greater in women (116 cells/µL versus 84 cells/µL in men). Diarrhea was more common in men, but women had more abdominal pain (6.7% in women versus 1.5% in men), itching (3% in women versus 0.3% in men), and skin rash (5% in women versus 2% in men). None of these toxicities

has a predictable or obvious gender-related predilection.[63]

An analysis of gender differences during treatment with the protease inhibitor combination lopinavir/ritonavir found that at 60 weeks of treatment, 65% of the men and 61% of the women had HIV RNA levels <50 copies/mL. Average gains in CD4 cells were also virtually identical: 257 cells/µL for the 66 women and 242 cells/µL for the 260 men. Discontinuation rates were very low for both genders (0% for women and 1% for men).

Moderate to severe nausea was identified more often by women (14%) than by men (6%); rates of dyspepsia demonstrated a similar trend (8% for women and 2% for men). It is notable that diarrhea was experienced equally by men and women (in approximately 15%). At week 60, women did have a statistically significant lower rate of triglyceride elevation above 750 mg/dL.[64]

A study of 33 subjects on a regimen of zidovudine, lamivudine, and indinavir found that the intracellular concentrations of the active triphosphate metabolites of zidovudine and lamivudine were elevated in women regardless of CD4 count. Compared with men, women had 2.3-fold higher intracellular zidovudine triphosphate concentration and 1.6-fold higher intracellular lamivudine triphosphate concentration. No differences in plasma levels were detected. Higher levels of intracellular triphosphates were also correlated with more rapid attainment and prolonged maintenance of viral loads 50 RNA copies/mL. In this small cohort, women reached viral loads of <50 copies/mL in half the time required by men. It is possible that higher intracellular levels may result in higher rates of nucleoside analog-associated toxicities in women.[65] Studies looking at carbovir triphosphate yielded similar results.[66] Further studies are needed to investigate the potential implications for safety and efficacy of antiretroviral therapy in women.

Antiretroviral Drug Interactions and Adverse Effects

Women who are using oral contraceptives containing ethinyl estradiol should be aware that protease inhibitors such as ritonavir, fosamprenavir, lopinavir-ritonavir, nelfinavir or the nonnucleoside reverse transcriptase inhibitor nevirapine may substantially reduce the bioavailability of ethinyl estradiol. It should be noted that atazanavir has the opposite effect and co-administration results in excessively high levels of ethinyl estradiol. For a variety of reasons, including protection from other STDs, and lowering risk of transmission to others, a barrier method of protection is always recommended for HIV-infected women as the primary means of contraception.[67] Potential issues affecting the toxicity of antiretroviral treatment in women include lower mean body weight, lower mean hemoglobin level (with the potentially complicating effect of zidovudine or dapsone in further inducing anemia), and absence of established controls and norms for CD4 counts in women compared to men.

Women are certainly not immune to the metabolic or morphologic alterations that affect HIV-infected men.

Conclusion

Globally, women represent the majority of HIV-infected individuals. Clinical management of HIV infection in women requires considerable further study about HIV pathogenesis, co-infections, and reproductive tract malignancies. The methods of enrolling women in epidemiologic and clinical trials need improvement to achieve statistically significant results in end points, mortality, and natural history.

References

1. UNAIDS/WHO. AIDS epidemic update 2003. 25 November: UNAIDS/WHO; 2003.
2. CDC. HIV/AIDS surveillance report 2004. Vol. 16. Atlanta: US Department of Health and Human Services, Centers for Disease Control and Prevention; 2005.
3. CDC. HIV/AIDS surveillance report 2002. Vol. 13. Atlanta: US Department of Health and Hyman Services, Centers for Disease Control and Prevention; 2002.
4. Shevitz A, Pagano M, Chiasson MA, et al. The association between youth, women, and acquired immunodeficiency syndrome. J Acquir Immune Defic Syndr Hum Retrovirol 1996; 13:427–433.
5. UNIFEM Report 2005.
6. Padian NS, Shiboski SC, Glass SO, et al. Heterosexual transmission of human immunodeficiency virus (HIV) in Northern California: results from a ten-year study. Am J Epidemiol 1997; 146:350–357.
7. Padian NS, Shiboski SC, Jewell NP. Female-to-male transmission of human immunodeficiency virus. JAMA 1991; 266:1664–1667.
8. Padian N, Marquis L, Francis DP, et al. Male-to-female transmission of human immunodeficiency virus. JAMA 1987; 258:788–790.
9. Gray RH, Wawer MJ, Brookmeyer R, et al; Rakai Project Team. Probability of HIV-1 transmission per coital act in monogamous, heterosexual, HIV-1-discordant couples in Rakai, Uganda. Lancet 2001; 357:1149–1153.
10. Quinn TC, Wawer MJ, Sewankambo N, et al. Viral load and heterosexual transmission of human immunodeficiency virus type 1. Rakai Proj Study Group. N Engl J Med 2000; 342:921–929.
11. Royce RA, Sena A, Cates W Jr, et al. Sexual transmission of HIV. N Engl J Med 1997; 336:1072–1078.
12. Klevens RM, Fleming PL, Mays M. Patterns of reporting multiple risks for HIV infection in the United States. 4th Conference on Retroviruses and Opportunistic Infections, Washington DC; 1997.
13. Marx PA, Spira AI, Gettie A, et al. Progesterone implants enhance SIV vaginal transmission and early virus load. Nat Med 1996; 2:1084–1089.
14. Zhang H, Dornadula G, Beumont M, et al. Human immunodeficiency virus type 1 in the semen of men receiving highly active antiretroviral therapy. N Engl J Med 1998; 339:1803–1809.
15. Si-Mohamed A, Kazatchkine MD, Heard I, et al. Selection of drug-resistant variants in the female genital tract of human immunodeficiency virus type 1-infected women receiving antiretroviral therapy. J Infect Dis 2000; 182:112–122.
16. Deschamps MM, Pape JW, Hafner A, et al. Heterosexual transmission of HIV in Haiti. Ann Intern Med 1996; 125:324–330.
17. McClelland RS, Wang CC, Overbaugh J, et al. Association between cervical shedding of herpes simplex virus and HIV-1. AIDS 2002; 16:2425–2430.
18. Soto-Ramirez LE, Renjifo B, McLane MF, et al. HIV-1 Langerhans' cell tropism associated with heterosexual transmission of HIV. Science 1996; 271:1291–1293.
19. Kreiss JK, Hopkins SG. The association between circumcision status and human immunodeficiency virus infection among homosexual men. J Infect Dis 1993; 168:1404–1408.
20. Marmor M, Weiss LR, Lyden M, et al. Possible female-to-female transmission of human immunodeficiency virus. Ann Intern Med 1986; 105:969.
21. Chu SY, Buehler JW, Fleming PL, et al. Epidemiology of reported cases of AIDS in lesbians, United States 1980-89. Am J Public Health 1990; 80:1380–1381.
22. Kennedy MB, Scarlett MI, Duerr AC, et al. Assessing HIV risk among women who have sex with women: scientific and communication issues. J Am Med Women's Assoc 1995; 50:103–107.
23. White JC. HIV risk assessment and prevention in lesbians and women who have sex with women: practical information for clinicians. Health Care Women Int 1997; 18:127–138.
24. Farizo KM, Buehler JW, Chamberland ME, et al. Spectrum of disease in persons with human immunodeficiency virus infection in the United States. JAMA 1992; 267:1798–1805.
25. Greenberg AE, Thomas PA, Landesman SH, et al. The spectrum of HIV-1-related disease among outpatients in New York City. AIDS 1992; 6:849–859.
26. Witt DJ, Craven DE, McCabe WR. Bacterial infections in adult patients with the acquired immune deficiency syndrome (AIDS) and AIDS-related complex. Am J Med 1987; 82:900–906.
27. Clarke LM, Duerr A, Feldman J, et al. Factors associated with cytomegalovirus infection among human immunodeficiency virus type 1-seronegative and -seropositive women from an urban minority community. J Infect Dis 1996; 173:77–82.
28. Bastian L, Bennett CL, Adams J, et al. Differences between men and women with HIV-related Pneumocystis carinii pneumonia: experience from 3, 070 cases in New York City in 1987. J Acquir Immune Defic Syndr 1993; 6:617–623.
29. Melnick SL, Sherer R, Louis TA, et al. Survival and disease progression according to gender of patients with HIV infection. The Terry Beirn Community Programs for Clinical Research on AIDS. JAMA 1994; 272:1915–1921.
30. Anastos K, Denenberg R, Solomon L. Human immunodeficiency virus infection in women. Med Clin North Am 1997; 81:533–553.
31. Hessol NA, Palacio H. Gender, ethnicity and transmission category variation in HVI disease progression. AIDS 1996; 10:69–74.

32. Morgan D, Malamba SS, Maude GH, et al. An HIV-1 natural history cohort and survival times in rural Uganda. AIDS 1997; 11:633–640.

33. Porter K, Babiker A, Bhaskaran K, et al. Determinants of survival following HIV-1 seroconversion after the introduction of HAART. Lancet 2003; 27:348–355.

34. Gandhi M, Bacchetti P, Miotti P, et al. Does patient sex affect human immunodeficiency virus levels? Clin Infect Dis 2002; 35:313–322.

35. Farzadegan H, Hoover DR, Astemborski J, et al. Sex differences in HIV-1 viral load and progression to AIDS. Lancet 1998; 352:1510–1514.

36. Anastos K, Gange SJ, Lau B, et al. Association of race and gender with HIV-1 RNA levels and immunologic progression. J Acquir Immune Defic Syndr 2000; 24:218–226.

37. Lee LM. No sex differences in improved AIDS survival in the treatment era United States 1993–1997. Abstract P9. National Conference on Women and HIV/AIDS, Los Angeles, CA: 9–12 October 1999.

38. Lee LM, Karon JM, Selik R, et al. Survival after AIDS diagnosis in adolescents and adults during the treatment era, United States, 1984–1997. JAMA 2001; 285:1308–1315.

39. Sun XW, Ellerbrock TV, Lungu O, et al. Human papillomavirus infection in human immunodeficiency virus-seropositive women. Obstet Gynecol 1995; 85:680–686.

40. Sun XW, Kuhn L, Ellerbrock TV, et al. Human papillomavirus infection in women infected with the human immunodeficiency virus. N Engl J Med 1997; 337:1343–1349.

41. Hillemanns P, Ellerbrock TV, McPhillips S, et al. Prevalence of anal human papillomavirus infection and anal cytologic abnormalities in HIV-seropositive women. AIDS 1996; 10:1641–1647.

42. Palefsky J. Human papillomavirus-associated malignancies in HIV-positive men and women. Curr Opin Oncol 1995; 7:437–441.

43. Wright TC Jr, Ellerbrock TV, Chiasson MA, et al. Cervical intraepithelial neoplasia in women infected with human immunodeficiency virus: prevalence, risk factors, and validity of Papanicolaou smears. NY Cervical Dis Study Obstet Gynecol 1994; 84:591–597.

44. Prins M, Hessol NA. Sex and the course of HIV Infection in the pre and highly active antiretroviral therapy eras. AIDS 2005; 19:357–370.

45. Korn AP, Landers DV. Gynecologic disease in women infected with human immunodeficiency virus type 1. J Acquir Immune Defic Syndr Hum Retrovirol 1995; 9:361–370.

46. Delmas MC, Larsen C, van Benthem B, et al. Cervical squamous intraepithelial lesions in HIV-infected women: prevalence, incidence and regression. European Study Group on Natural History of HIV Infection in Women. AIDS 2000; 12:1775–1784.

47. Schuman P, Ohmit SE, Klein RS, et al. Longitudinal study of cervical squamous intraepithelial lesions in human immunodeficiency virus (HIV)-seropositive and at risk seronegative women. J Infect Dis 2003; 188:128–136.

48. Uberti-Foppa C, Ferrari D, Lodini S, et al. Long-term effect of highly active antiretroviral therapy on cervical lesions in HIV-positive women. AIDS 2003; 17:2136–2138.

49. Massad LS. Seaberg EC, Watts DH, et al. Low incidence invasive cervical cancer among HIV-infected US women in a prevention program. AIDS 2004; 18:109–113.

50. Maiman M, Watts DH, Andersen J. A phase three randomized trial of topical vaginal 5-fluorouracil maintenance therapy versus observation after standard treatment for high grade cervical dysplasia in HIV-infected women: ACTG 200. Abstract 466. 6th Conference on Retroviruses and Opportunistic Infections, Chicago, IL: 1999.

51. Wright TC Jr, Koulos J, Schnoll F, et al. Cervical intraepithelial neoplasia in women infected with the human immunodeficiency virus: outcome after loop electrosurgical excision. Gynecol Oncol 1994; 55:253–258.

52. Robinson WR, Hamilton CA, Michaels SH, et al. Effect of excisional therapy and highly active antiretroviral therapy on cervical intraepithelial neoplasia in women infected with human immunodeficiency virus. Am J Obstet Gynecol 2001; 184:538–543.

53. Moore RA, Edwards JE, Hopwood J, et al. Imiquimod for the treatment of genital warts: a quantitative systematic review. BMC Infect Dis 2001; 1:3.

54. Boken DJ, Swindells S, Rinaldi MG. Fluconazole-resistant Candida albicans. Clin Infect Dis 1993; 17:1018–1021.

55. Spinillo A, Michelone G, Cavanna C, et al. Clinical and microbiological characteristics of symptomatic vulvovaginal candidiasis in HIV-seropositive women. Genitourin Med 1994; 70:268–272.

56. Spinillo A, Capuzzo E, Egbe TO, et al. Torulopsis glabrata vaginitis. Obstet Gynecol 1995; 85:993–998.

57. Schuman P, Christianen C, Sobel JD. Aphthous genital ulceration in three women with AIDS. A429. 3rd Conference on Retroviruses and Opportunistic Infections; 1996; Washington DC.

58. Vanhems P, Routy JP, Hirschel B, et al. Collaborative Group. Clinical features of acute retroviral syndrome differ by route of infection but not by gender and age. J Acquir Immune Defic Syndr 2002; 31:318–321.

59. Korn AP. Related pelvic inflammatory disease in women infected with HIV. AIDS Patient Care STDS 1998; 12:431–434.

60. Easterbrook PJ, Keruly JC, Creagh-Kirk T, et al. Racial and ethnic differences in outcome in zidovudine-treated patients with advanced HIV disease. Zidovudine Epidemiology Study Group. JAMA 1991; 266:2713–2718.

61. Lagakos S, Fischl MA, Stein DS, et al. Effects of zidovudine therapy in minority and other subpopulations with early HIV infection. JAMA 1991; 266:2709–2712.

62. Currier JS, Yetzer E, Potthoff A, et al. Gender differences in adverse events on ritonavir; An analysis from the Abbott 247 study. Proceedings of the National Conference on Women and HIV, Pasadena, CA: May 1997; 304.7.

63. Gersten M, Chapman S, Farnsworth A, et al. The safety and efficacy of Viracept (Nelfinavir mesylate) in female patients who participated in pivotal phase II/III double blind randomized controlled trials. Proceedings of the National Conference on Women and HIV, Pasadena, CA: May 1997; 304. 1.

64. Levin J. Kaletra in women. In: AIDS 2002 July 2002, Barcelona, Spain.

65. Anderson PL, Kakuda TN, Kawle S, et al. Antiviral dynamics and sex differences of zidovudine and lamivudine triphosphate concentrations in HIV-infected individuals. AIDS 2003; 17:2159–2168.

66. Harris M, Back D, Kewn S, et al. Intracellular carbovir triphosphate levels in patients taking abacavir once a day. AIDS 2002; 16:1196–1197.

67. Mildvan D, Yarrish R, Marshak A, et al. Pharmacokinetic interaction between nevirapine and ethinyl estradiol/norethindrone when administered concurrently to HIV-infected women. J Acquir Immune Defic Syndr 2002; 29:471–477.

CHAPTER 43

Prevention of Mother-to-Child Transmission of HIV-1

Lynne M. Mofenson

Introduction

On a global basis, it is estimated that approximately 700 000 children are newly infected with HIV-1 each year, nearly 2000 children each day; the majority of these infections occur in sub-Saharan Africa. The primary mode of acquisition of HIV-1 in children worldwide is through mother-to-child transmission (MTCT). Prior to the development of effective interventions to reduce MTCT, the estimated rates of transmission ranged from 15–25% in non-breast-feeding populations in the USA and Europe and 25–40% in breast-feeding populations in resource-constrained countries.

Although there has been dramatic progress in reducing HIV-1 MTCT since 1994, when Pediatric AIDS Clinical Trials Group (PACTG) 076 protocol demonstrated that a regimen of zidovudine (AZT) given during pregnancy, labor and to the newborn reduced transmission by 67%,[1] currently two perinatal HIV-1 epidemics exist.[2] In resource-rich countries like the USA, transmission has been reduced to less than 2%, and elimination of perinatal HIV-1 infection is within reach, since most HIV-1-infected women receive highly active antiretroviral therapy (HAART), operative delivery via elective cesarean section is safe, and formula feeding is available.

However, in resource-constrained countries, which are where most HIV-1-infected women reside, the perinatal epidemic continues unabated. Although clinical trials have identified simple, less expensive, effective antiretroviral prophylaxis regimens more relevant to such countries, implementation of these regimens has been slow, the existing limited maternal–child healthcare infrastructure has had difficulty in supporting the addition of antenatal HIV-1 counseling and testing and antiretroviral prophylaxis programs, and postnatal transmission of HIV-1 through breast-feeding remains a significant problem.

This chapter will discuss risk factors for MTCT; review progress in prevention of MTCT, concentrating on antiretroviral interventions; and discuss guidelines related to prevention of MTCT in resource-rich and constrained settings.

Risk Factors for HIV-1 MTCT

HIV-1 can be transmitted during pregnancy, labor, and through breast milk. While different risk factors may influence HIV-1 transmission during each of these time periods, maternal plasma HIV-1 viral load has consistently been a strong independent predictor of transmission risk regardless of timing of transmission.[3] Hence, interventions that reduce viral load might be expected to influence transmission risk during each of these periods.

In Utero and Intrapartum Transmission

In the absence breast-feeding and antiretroviral prophylaxis, *in utero* transmission proportionally accounts for 25–30% and intrapartum transmission 65–70% of MTCT. During pregnancy, the placenta provides an important physical and immune barrier between maternal and fetal circulations, and also apparently against *in utero* HIV-1 infection, as the absolute rate of *in utero* transmission is only 5–10%. Although the exact mechanisms of *in utero* transmission have not been elucidated, factors that disrupt placental integrity, such as chorioamnionitis, might be expected to play a role. Genetic factors (e.g. HLA type, CCR5 genotype) and viral characteristics, such as viral subtype, have been reported to influence *in utero* transmission.

Intrapartum transmission can occur through direct access of cell-free or cell-associated virus to the infant systemic circulation by maternal-fetal transfusions that occur during uterine contractions in labor, or indirectly through the infant swallowing HIV-1 present in genital tract fluids during delivery, with resultant viral passage through the gastrointestinal mucosa to underlying lymphoid cells, followed by systemic dissemination. The importance of the intrapartum period in transmission is demonstrated by the proven efficacy of interventions restricted to the intrapartum period, such as elective cesarean section performed prior to labor and rupture of membranes, to reduce MTCT.[4-8]

Risk factors for transmission during each of these time periods were examined in 1709 infants with known infection status born between 1990 and 2000 in the Women and Infants Transmission.[3] Maternal antenatal viral load and use of antiretroviral therapy were associated with risk of both *in utero* and intrapartum transmission. Controlling for viral load and antiretroviral therapy, low birth weight was significantly associated with *in utero* transmission, while maternal age, antenatal CD4+ count, year of birth, pre-term delivery, birth weight, and duration of membrane rupture were associated with intrapartum transmission.

Postnatal Transmission

Breast-feeding substantially increases the risk of HIV-1 MTCT. Postnatal infection can account for 30–50% of all transmission in breast-feeding populations.[9] There is a significant diminution of the efficacy of successful antiretroviral interventions preventing *in utero* and intrapartum transmission in breast-feeding populations. For example, short-course antepartum/intrapartum AZT reduced transmission by 50% in formula-fed Thai infants,[10] but use of the same regimen in breast-fed African infants resulted in an efficacy of 37% at age 3 months, decreasing to 28% at age 24 months.[11,12] Thus, to achieve optimal prevention of MTCT in a breast-

feeding setting, additional interventions will be needed to reduce postnatal transmission.

Determining the timing of breast-milk transmission has been complicated by the difficulty in distinguishing between intrapartum and early breast-milk transmission; thus, most studies have focused on postnatal transmission occurring after age 1 month. The Breast-feeding and HIV International Transmission Study was an individual patient meta-analysis of data from 4085 children in nine clinical trials in breast-feeding populations; 993 (24%) were definitively infected.[13] Of 539 children with known timing of infection, 225 (42%) had late postnatal transmission (occurring after age 1 month). The overall risk of late postnatal transmission was 8.9 infections per 100 child-years of breast-feeding, with the risk being generally constant throughout the breast-feeding period; the cumulative probability of late postnatal transmission at age 18 months was 9.3%.

Although the risk of HIV-1 transmission through breast milk persists for the duration of breast-feeding, the early breast-feeding period (first 1–2 months) may be the period of highest risk.[9] This is illustrated by the results of the SAINT trial, in which all women and infants received effective prophylaxis against intrapartum transmission (either AZT/3TC or single dose nevirapine).[14] The trial included formula and breast-fed infants; in this context, breast-feeding was the most significant risk factor for MTCT. By age 8 weeks, breast-feeding accounted for a 6% increase in the absolute risk of transmission; in multivariate analysis, the risk of HIV-1 infection was 2.2-fold higher among breast-fed than formula-fed infants during the first 4 weeks of life, and 7.9-fold higher between ages 4 and 8 weeks.

In addition to duration of infant breast-feeding, risk factors for breast-milk transmission include high maternal viral load, both in plasma and breast milk; low CD4+ count; breast-milk immunologic factors; breast pathology including clinical and subclinical mastitis, nipple bleeding, cracked nipples, or breast abscess; and infant pathology that disrupts mucosal integrity, such as thrush.[9,15] Several studies have suggested that exclusive breast-feeding is associated with lower risk of transmission than mixed feeding with both breast milk and non-human milk, fluids, or other foods.[15,16] In a study over 2700 HIV-infected mother/infant pairs in Zimbabwe, the rate of late postnatal transmission (after age 6 weeks) was 1.3% at age 6 months and 6.9% at age 18 months in exclusively breast-fed infants compared with 4.4% and 14.1%, respectively, in infants with mixed feeding.[16]

Antiretroviral Interventions to Prevent HIV-1 MTCT

The complexity and cost of the 3-part PACTG 076 regimen significantly limited its applicability and implementation within resource-constrained settings. Thus, researchers began to explore the development of shorter, less expensive prophylactic regimens more applicable to resource-constrained settings. Clinical trials initially focused on shortened AZT-alone prophylaxis regimens, and moved to evaluating whether combination antiretroviral regimens, such as short-course AZT combined with lamivudine (3TC), might have improved efficacy over AZT alone. Studies also evaluated whether even simpler, less expensive, single-drug regimens, such as single-dose intrapartum/neonatal nevirapine (NVP), would be effective, and whether combining such regimens with other short-course regimens might result in improved efficacy.

The overall results from these trials, as well as open-label and observational studies, demonstrate that a number of different regimens have efficacy in preventing *in utero* and intrapartum transmission, but that efficacy is diminished in breast-feeding populations due to the postnatal acquisition of HIV-1 infection through breast milk. Current studies are focused on whether antiretroviral prophylaxis of the lactating woman and/or her breast-feeding infant might be a safe and effective way to reduce postnatal transmission in settings where feeding with breast-milk alternatives is not safe, acceptable, feasible, affordable, and sustainable.

Mechanisms of Action of Antiretroviral Prophylaxis

Antiretroviral drugs can reduce *in utero* and intrapartum MTCT through a number of different mechanisms, including: decreasing maternal viral load in blood and genital secretions through antenatal drug administration to the mother; provision of pre-exposure prophylaxis to the infant through administration of drug to the mother during labor, resulting in systemic drug levels in the infant at a time of intensive exposure of the infant's skin and mucus membranes to HIV-1 in the mother's genital tract during labor and passage through the birth canal; and provision of post-exposure prophylaxis through administration of drug to the infant after birth to protect against cell-free or -associated virus that entered the circulation or had direct contact with the mucosa of the infant during delivery.

Efficacy is likely multifactorial. In women with high viral loads, it is likely that lowering the viral load by antenatal antiretroviral therapy is a critical component of protection. However, antiretroviral drugs have been shown to reduce the risk of transmission even among women with HIV-1 RNA levels <1000 copies/mL.[17] Additionally, the level of HIV-1 RNA at delivery and use of antenatal antiretroviral therapy are each independently associated with the risk of transmission, suggesting that antiretroviral prophylaxis does not work solely through reduction in viral load.[18]

Studies have demonstrated that the quantity of cell-free and -associated virus in cervico-vaginal secretions is associated with the risk of MTCT, independent of plasma viral load.[19,20] Thus, providing prophylaxis to the infant immediately before and after extensive viral exposure during labor and delivery is an additional important mechanism of efficacy; consistent with the importance of pre- and post-exposure prophylaxis, results of randomized, controlled clinical trials (discussed below) have demonstrated that intrapartum/postpartum antiretroviral regimens, without any maternal drug component, can significantly decrease MTCT.[6,7]

Clinical Trials for Prevention of HIV-1 MTCT

Table 43.1 summarizes the results of the major clinical trials of antiretroviral interventions for the prevention of MTCT. These trials have built sequentially on each other and have identified a number of simple regimens effective in reducing MTCT. Direct comparison between trials is difficult, as they enrolled patient populations from different geographic areas, infected with different viral subtypes, having different infant feeding practices, and the infant age at which efficacy was determined may differ. However, some general conclusions can be drawn.

Short-term efficacy has been demonstrated for regimens with AZT alone; AZT plus 3TC; single-dose NVP; and more recently, combining single-dose NVP with either short-course AZT or AZT/3TC. Combination regimens, such as short-course AZT plus single-dose NVP, are more effective than single-drug regimens in reducing MTCT, and when it is feasible and affordable, a longer antenatal/intrapartum/postpartum regimen is superior in preventing MTCT than a shorter 2-part antepartum/intrapartum or intrapartum/postpartum regimen.

Table 43.1 Clinical trials of antiretroviral drugs for prevention of mother-to-child HIV-1 transmission

Study (location/s)	Infant feeding	Regimen	Antenatal/ intrapartum	Postpartum	Efficacy
PACTG 076 (USA, France)	Formula	AZT versus placebo	Long (from 14 weeks) intravenous intrapartum	Long (6 weeks) (infant only)	MTCT at 18 months, 8.3% AZT versus 25.5% placebo (68% efficacy)
Bangkok short-course AZT Trial (Thailand)	Formula	AZT versus placebo	Short (from 36 weeks) oral intrapartum	None	MTCT at 6 months, 9.4% AZT versus 18.9% placebo (50.1% efficacy)
Thai Perinatal HIV Prevention Trial (PHPT-1) (Thailand)	Formula	AZT different length AP and infant PP regimens, no placebo	Long (from 28 weeks), Short (from 36 weeks) oral intrapartum	Long (for 6 weeks) Short (for 3 days) (infant only)	Short-Short stopped early due to significantly higher MTCT (10.5%). MTCT at 6 months, 6.5% Long-Long versus 4.7% Long-Short versus 8.6% Short-Long (statistical equivalence). However, in utero transmission significantly lower with Long versus Short maternal antenatal AZT (1.6% versus 5.1%)
Ivory Coast short-course AZT Trial (Ivory Coast)	Breast-feeding	AZT versus placebo	Short (from 36 weeks) oral intrapartum	None	MTCT at 3 months, 16.5% AZT versus 26.1% placebo (37% efficacy)
DITRAME/ANRS 049a (Ivory Coast, Burkina Faso)	Breast-feeding	AZT versus placebo	Short (from 36 weeks) oral intrapartum	Short (1 week) (mother only)	MTCT at 6 months, 18.0% AZT versus 27.5% placebo (38% efficacy); MTCT at 15 months, 21.5% versus 30.6% (30% efficacy). MTCT at 24 months (pooled analysis with other Ivory Coast trial), 22.5% versus 30.2% (26% efficacy)
PETRA (South Africa, Tanzania, Uganda)	Breast-feeding	AZT + 3TC in three regimens (3-part ante/intra/ postpartum; 2-part intra/ postpartum; intrapartum) versus placebo	Short (from 36 weeks) oral intrapartum	Short (7 days) (mother and infant)	MTCT at 6 weeks, 5.7% 3-part (63% efficacy) versus 8.9% 2-part (42% efficacy) versus 14.2% intrapartum versus 15.3% placebo. MTCT at 18 months, 14.9% 3-part versus 18.1% 2-part versus 20% intrapartum versus 22.2% placebo
HIVNET 012 (Uganda)	Breast-feeding	Intrapartum/ postpartum NVP versus AZT	No antenatal ARV oral intrapartum: Single dose NVP 200 mg versus AZT	Single-dose NVP 2 mg/kg within 72 h of birth versus short AZT (7 days) (infant only)	MTCT 15.7% in NVP arm versus 25.8% in AZT arm (41% efficacy) at 18 m

Study	Feeding	Intervention	Regimen	Dose	Results
PACTG 316 (USA, Europe, Brazil, Bahamas)	Formula	Intrapartum/postpartum NVP versus placebo in women already receiving AZT or AZT plus other ARV (77% on combination therapy)	Non-study antepartum ARV oral intrapartum: Single-dose NVP 200 mg + intravenous AZT	Single NVP dose 2 mg/kg within 72 h of birth + 6 weeks AZT (infant only)	Trial stopped early due to very low MTCT in both arms. MTCT at 6 months, 1.4% NVP versus 1.6% placebo
SAINT (South Africa)	Breast-feeding (42%) and formula feeding	Intrapartum/postpartum NVP versus AZT + 3TC	No antenatal ARV oral intrapartum: Single-dose NVP 200 mg versus AZT + 3TC	Single NVP dose within 48 h of birth versus short AZT + 3TC (7 days) (mother and infant)	MTCT at 8 weeks, 12.3% NVP versus 9.3% AZT + 3TC (p = 0.11)
Thai Perinatal HIV Prevention Trial-2 (PHPT-2) (Thailand)	Formula	AZT versus AZT + maternal/infant single-dose NVP versus AZT + maternal single-dose NVP only	Long (AZT from 28 weeks) oral intrapartum: AZT + single-dose NVP or placebo	1 week AZT alone versus 1 week AZT + single-dose NVP	AZT alone arm stopped early due to significantly higher MTCT: MTCT at 6 months, 6.3% AZT alone versus 1.1% with AZT plus maternal/infant NVP versus 2.1% with AZT plus maternal NVP alone. Final analysis, MTCT at 6 months, 2.8% with AZT plus maternal NVP only versus 1.9% with AZT plus maternal/infant NVP
DITRAME PLUS/ANRS 1201.0 (Abidjan, Cote d'Ivoire)	Breast-feeding (54%) and formula feeding	Open label, AZT boosted by intrapartum/postpartum NVP	Short (from 36 weeks) oral intrapartum: Single-dose NVP 200 mg + AZT	Single-dose NVP + 1 week AZT (infant only)	MTCT at 6 weeks, 6.5% (95% CI, 3.9–9.1%). Compared with MTCT in historical control AZT alone (1995–2000) 12.8% (in AZT alone group, breast-feeding rate was 97.6%)
DITRAME PLUS/ANRS 1201.1 (Abidjan, Cote d'Ivoire)	Breast-feeding (66%) and formula feeding	Open label, AZT + 3TC boosted by intrapartum/postpartum NVP	Short (from 32 weeks) oral intrapartum: Single-dose NVP 200 mg + AZT + 3TC	AZT + 3TC for 3 days (mother only) Single-dose NVP + 1 week AZT (infant only)	MTCT at 6 weeks, 4.7% (95% CI, 2.4–7.0%). MTCT not significantly different than observed with DITRAME 1201.0 regimen AZT + single dose NVP (P = 0.34).
SIMBA (Rwanda, Uganda)	Breast-feeding (median duration 3.3–3.5 months, upper intraquartile range, 4.9–5.3 months)	NVP versus 3TC for 6 months postnatally in breast-feeding neonates exposed antenatally to AZT + ddI	Short (AZT + ddI from 36 weeks) oral intrapartum: AZT + ddI	AZT + ddI for 1 week postpartum (mother only) NVP once then twice daily versus 3TC twice daily while breast-feeding (infant only)	MTCT at 6 months, 7.8%, no difference between the two infant arms. MTCT by age (note median duration of breastfeeding 3.3–3.5 months): MTCT birth (to 3 days), 5.3% MTCT 4–28 days, 1.6% MTCT 1–6 months, 0.9% Overall, postpartum to 6 months, 2.4%

Table 43.1 Clinical trials of antiretroviral drugs for prevention of mother-to-child HIV-1 transmission—cont'd

Study (location/s)	Infant feeding	Regimen	Antenatal/ intrapartum	Postpartum	Efficacy
NVAZ-1 (Malawi)	Breast-feeding	Neonatal single-dose NVP only versus NVP + AZT	No ARV antepartum or intrapartum (late presenters)	Single-dose NVP immediately after birth + AZT twice daily for 1 week (infant only)	Overall MTCT at 6–8 weeks, 15.3% NVP + AZT versus 20.9% NVP only. MTCT at 6–8 weeks in babies who were uninfected at birth, 7.7% NVP + AZT versus 12.1% NVP only (36s% efficacy)
NVAZ-2 (Malawi)	Breast-feeding	Neonatal single-dose NVP only versus NVP + AZT	No ARV antepartum oral intrapartum: Single-dose NVP to mother	Single-dose NVP immediately after birth + AZT twice daily for one week (infant only)	Overall MTCT at 6–8 weeks, 16.3% NVP + AZT versus 14.1% NVP only. MTCT at 6–8 weeks in babies who were uninfected at birth, 6.9% NVP + AZT versus 6.5% NVP only
MASHI (Botswana)	Breast-feeding and formula feeding (randomized)	Factorial design, randomized to mode of infant feeding and maternal/infant single-dose NVP versus placebo. Infant placebo discontinued 08/02 (after PHPT-2 results), study modified to maternal NVP versus placebo, with all infants receiving single-dose NVP.	Short (AZT from 34 weeks) oral intrapartum: AZT + single-dose NVP or placebo	Single-dose NVP + 1 month AZT if formula feeding Single-dose NVP + 6 months AZT if breast-feeding	Original study (maternal/infant NVP versus placebo): NVP provides added efficacy in formula-fed but not breast-fed infants. MTCT at 1 month, formula-fed infants, 2.4% NVP/NVP versus 8.3% PL/PL; breast-fed infants, 8.4% NVP/NVP versus 4.1% PL/PL. Revised study (maternal NVP versus placebo, all infant NVP): No added efficacy from maternal NVP regardless infant feeding mode. MTCT at 1 month, 4.3% NVP/NVP versus 3.7% PL/NVP. Infant feeding: Breast-feeding + AZT higher transmission than formula. MTCT at 7 months, 9.1% breast-feeding + AZT versus 5.6% formula. However, higher infant mortality with formula at 7 months, 9.3% formula versus 4.9% breast-feeding + AZT. Incremental risk of postnatal MTCT between 1–7 months, 4.5% (comparable with postnatal MTCT in BHITS meta-analysis between 1–6 months, 4.2%, with no infant prophylaxis). HIV-free survival at 18 months did not differ between arms. MTCT or death at 18 months, 14.2% formula (33 infected, 46 deaths) versus 15.6% breast-feed + AZT (54 infected, 34 deaths)

MTCT, Mother-to-child HIV-1 transmission; AZT, Zidovudine; 3TC, Lamivudine; NVP, Nevirapine; PL, Placebo; BHITS, Breastfeeding and HIV International Transmission Study

Almost all trials have included an oral intrapartum prophylaxis component, with varying durations of maternal antenatal and/or infant (and sometimes maternal) postpartum prophylaxis. Regimens with antenatal components starting as late as 36 weeks' gestation and lacking an infant prophylaxis component can reduce the risk of transmission;[10] however, longer duration of antenatal therapy (starting at 28 weeks' gestation) is more effective than shorter (starting at 36 weeks' gestation).[21] More prolonged post-exposure prophylaxis of the infant does not appear to substitute for longer duration of maternal therapy.[21]

Regimens that include no antenatal prophylaxis but include intrapartum and postpartum drug administration are also effective.[6,7] However, the PETRA study demonstrated that intrapartum pre-exposure prophylaxis alone, without continued post-exposure prophylaxis of the infant, is not effective.[6] The SAINT trial demonstrated that the two proven effective intrapartum/postpartum regimens (AZT/3TC or NVP) are similar in efficacy and safety.[14]

Although the short-course regimens identified as effective in non-breast-feeding populations are also effective in breast-feeding populations, efficacy is diminished over time.[6,7,12] The reduction in efficacy is greatest with AZT or AZT/3TC short-course regimens, and less with single-dose NVP. This is likely due to the prolonged half-life of NVP in pregnant women in labor and neonates, with detectable drug levels that can persist for 2 weeks or longer following a single dose, thereby providing a much longer period of prophylaxis than AZT and 3TC, which have much shorter half-lives.

In an attempt to improve the efficacy of short-course regimens but retain a regimen that remains appropriate to the cost limitations existing in resource-constrained countries, more recently, researchers have evaluated whether the addition of a potent intrapartum intervention – the single-dose NVP regimen – to short-course regimens might increase efficacy. In the setting of short-course AZT alone or AZT/3TC regimens, the PHPT-2 study in non-breast-feeding women in Thailand, the MASHI study in Botswana (in the formula-fed, but not the breast-fed, strata), and the DITRAME studies in a partly breast-feeding population in the Ivory Coast, demonstrated that the addition of single-dose NVP did significantly increase efficacy (Table 43.1).[22–24] However, a clinical trial conducted in resource-rich countries, PACTG 316, demonstrated that the addition of single-dose NVP did not appear to offer significant benefit in the setting of potent combination antiretroviral therapy throughout pregnancy and very low viral load at the time of delivery.[25] The relative importance of the maternal and infant components of single-dose NVP in the context of short-course AZT regimens remains unclear; the Thailand PHPT-2 study suggests that the infant NVP dose at day 2 of life may not add significant efficacy to the maternal NVP dose alone; however, the Botswana MASHI study suggests that maternal NVP may not be necessary when infant single-dose NVP is provided at birth.[22,24]

In some countries, a significant proportion of women may lack antenatal care and first present to the healthcare system during labor. A trial was conducted in a breast-feeding population in Malawi to define the optimal infant prophylaxis regimen in resource-constrained settings when no antenatal maternal therapy was received. The addition of one week of AZT therapy to infant single-dose NVP reduced the risk of transmission by 36% compared with infant single-dose NVP alone.[8] However, when maternal intrapartum NVP was received, thereby providing pre-exposure prophylaxis in addition to post-exposure prophylaxis, the infant single-dose NVP alone was as effective as the combined NVP/AZT infant post-exposure prophylaxis regimen.[26] In resource-rich countries, standard prophylaxis in the absence of maternal therapy is 6 weeks of infant AZT; to define the optimal infant prophylaxis regimen in these settings, an ongoing study in infants born to women who have not received antenatal therapy is comparing the standard 6-week infant AZT regimen to AZT combined with either three NVP doses during the first week of life or 2 weeks of nelfinavir and 3TC.

In breast-feeding populations, the impact of the current short-course antiretroviral prophylaxis regimens on the long-term risk of infant infection is diminished due to the continued risk of transmission during the breast-feeding period. Several ongoing and planned trials will assess the effect of antiretroviral prophylaxis provided to the mother during lactation or to the breast-feeding infant. Preliminary results from the SIMBA trial suggest that infant prophylaxis may provide some protection against transmission (Table 43.1).[27] However, this study, which compared infant prophylaxis with NVP versus 3TC in the context of maternal antepartum, intrapartum and 1-week postpartum AZT/ddI, lacked a control group, and had high rates of exclusive breast-feeding (85%) and a median duration of breast-feeding of only 3.5 months, making interpretation difficult. Additionally, in the MASHI trial, the incremental risk of postnatal transmission between age 1–7 months in infants who were breast-fed and received 6 months of AZT was 4.5%, very similar to the 4.2% rate of late postnatal transmission through 6 months in the breast-feeding meta-analysis in breast-fed infants who did not receive antiretroviral prophylaxis (Table 43.1).[13,23]

Short and Long-term Safety of Antiretroviral Exposure for Infants and Women

Infant

The short-course antiretroviral regimens studied in clinical trials and used in resource-constrained settings have been associated with minimal infant toxicity. Short-term data from these trials indicate that antiretroviral exposure may be associated with transient, mild hematologic abnormalities that resolve following completion of prophylaxis.[28–30]

In infants exposed to the more complex and prolonged maternal antiretroviral prophylaxis regimens used in resource-rich countries, while short-term toxicity appears to be minimal and generally transient, long-term infant outcome data are not yet available. The available data indicate no increased risk of congenital abnormalities among offspring of women with first trimester use of most antiretroviral drugs, and specifically with receipt of AZT, 3TC, abacavir, stavudine (d4T), NVP, and nelfinavir.[31] However, there are concerns related to efavirenz (EFV). Animal data indicate that prenatal EFV exposure may be associated with central nervous system defects in infant cynomolgus monkeys, and there have been four retrospective reports of severe central nervous system defects (e.g. meningomyelocele) in human infants after first trimester exposure to EFV-containing regimens.[32] The US Food and Drug Administration has classified EFV as Pregnancy Class D (positive evidence of human fetal risk); EFV use should be avoided in the first trimester of pregnancy and women of childbearing potential should undergo pregnancy testing before initiating EFV therapy, and be counseled about the risk to the fetus and need to avoid pregnancy.[32]

While receipt of AZT during pregnancy has not been associated with adverse pregnancy outcome, data are conflicting as to whether receipt of combination antiretroviral therapy during pregnancy is associated with pre-term delivery. A European study found an increased risk of pre-term delivery in women who received antenatal combination antiretroviral therapy, particularly those including prote-

ase inhibitors and started early in pregnancy, but a large meta-analysis of seven clinical studies in the USA did not find that combination antiretroviral therapy was associated with increased rates of pre-term labor.[33,34]

Pre-clinical data indicate that some antiretroviral drugs, particularly the nucleoside analogs, are carcinogenic *in vitro* and can be associated with mitochondrial toxicity. In follow-up for as long as 16 years, no malignancies have been reported in uninfected children with antiretroviral exposure. However, researchers in France have reported the rare occurrence of mitochondrial dysfunction in uninfected infants with *in utero* antiretroviral exposure to the standard long prophylaxis regimens used in resource-rich countries. In a cohort of 4392 uninfected HIV-1-exposed children, evidence of mitochondrial dysfunction was identified in 12 children (with two deaths), yielding an 18-month incidence of 0.26%.[35] All infants had perinatal antiretroviral exposure, and risk was higher among infants exposed to combination antiretroviral drugs (primarily AZT/3TC) than AZT alone. All children presented with neurologic symptoms, often with abnormal magnetic resonance imaging and/or a significant episode of hyperlactatemia, and all had an identified deficit in one of the mitochondrial respiratory chain complexes and/or abnormal muscle biopsy histology. In separate publications, the same group reported an increased risk of simple febrile seizures during the first 18 months of life and small but persistent, clinically insignificant decreases in neutrophil and platelet counts among uninfected infants with antiretroviral exposure.[36,37]

Investigators in the USA and Europe have evaluated other prospective cohorts. No deaths similar to those reported from France were identified in a large database that included >16 000 HIV-exposed children with and without perinatal antiretroviral drug exposure followed prospectively in several large cohorts in the USA.[38] In follow-up of 2414 uninfected children, about half of whom had perinatal antiretroviral exposure, for as long as 16 years (median 2.2 years), the European Collaborative Study reported uninfected children with antiretroviral exposure were no more likely to suffer from a serious adverse health event (including febrile seizures) in the short- to medium-term than those without antiretroviral drug exposure.[39] While continued follow-up of infants exposed to antiretroviral drugs for potential adverse long-term effects is critical, current data indicate that if such toxicity is observed, it is probably relatively rare, and the potential risks of antiretroviral exposure for the infant need to be placed in perspective with the proven benefit of anti-retroviral therapy for the health of the infected woman and in reducing the risk of HIV-1 MTCT by up to 70%.

Pregnant Women

Minimal toxicity has been seen in women receiving the short-course antiretroviral regimens studied in clinical trials and used in resource-constrained settings.[30] Toxicity issues have been primarily confined to women receiving longer, more complex, combination regimens; primary toxicity concerns include lactic acidosis with nucleoside analog drugs; rash and hepatic toxicity with NVP; and potential for hyperglycemia with protease inhibitors.[32]

It is unclear if pregnancy augments the incidence of the lactic acidosis/hepatic steatosis syndrome reported in non-pregnant individuals receiving nucleoside analog drugs. Cases of lactic acidosis, including maternal and fetal fatalities, have been reported in HIV-1-infected pregnant women receiving prolonged therapy with nucleoside analogs, particularly the combination of d4T and didanosine (ddI), with women presenting with symptoms in late pregnancy. Physicians caring for HIV-1-infected pregnant women receiving nucleoside analog drugs need to be alert for the early diagnosis of this syndrome, and combination d4T/ddI is not recommended for use in pregnant women unless no alternative is available.[32]

Severe symptomatic, and rarely fatal, hepatic toxicity associated with chronic NVP therapy is more frequent in females, particularly women with $CD4^+$ count >250/mm^3. Although deaths due to hepatic failure have been reported in HIV-infected pregnant women receiving NVP-containing HAART, it is unknown if pregnancy increases the risk of hepatotoxicity. Pregnant women who have $CD4^+$ count >250/mm^3 and are receiving antiretroviral drugs solely for prevention of MTCT should only use NVP as a component of a combination regimen if the benefit clearly outweighs the risk.[32] Hepatic toxicity has *not* been observed in women receiving single-dose NVP. Women who experience clinical hepatotoxicity or rash should while receiving NVP have the drug discontinued and should not receive NVP therapy in the future.

Protease inhibitors can be associated with metabolic abnormalities, including hyperglycemia and new onset diabetes. It is unknown if these complications are more frequent in HIV-1-infected pregnant women. In a study of 1407 women receiving antiret-rovirals for prevention of MTCT (23% AZT alone, 36% combination without protease inhibitors, 41% combination with protease inhibitors), moderate symptoms or laboratory abnormalities occurred in less than 5% of women.[40] However, although the overall rate of gestational diabetes was 2.1%, similar to the 2–3% expected in the general population, it was highest, 4.6%, in pregnant women receiving treatment with protease inhibitors starting in early pregnancy.

Antiretroviral Drugs in Breast-feeding Women

Passage of antiretroviral drugs into breast milk in humans has been evaluated for only a few antiretroviral drugs. However, in rodent studies, most antiretroviral drugs are excreted into the breast milk of lactating rats, and AZT, 3TC and NVP have all been detected in the breast milk of HIV-infected women.

The efficacy of potent antiretroviral therapy of the mother to prevent postnatal HIV-1 transmission through breast milk is unknown. Use of drugs that significantly lower maternal plasma viral load could also lower viral load in the breast milk, and reduce the risk of postnatal transmission. However, if anti-retroviral drugs penetrate the breast milk in subop-timal concentrations or some drugs of the regimen penetrate into the breast milk while others do not, drug levels in the milk may not be sufficient to decrease viral replication. The presence of inadequate drug levels or penetration of only a single drug into the milk could promote the development of drug-resistant virus in the milk, which could be transmitted to the infant. Additionally, the toxicity of chronic antiretroviral exposure of the infant via drugs that are present in breast milk are unknown; one study demonstrated high levels of antiretroviral drugs in breast-fed infants of women receiving HAART.[41]

A number of international clinical trials will evaluate the effect of using HAART in breast-feeding women who do not require therapy for their own health on the risk of postnatal MTCT; in this case, treatment would be provided solely for reducing breast-milk transmission and stopped after weaning.[42] At the present time there are no data to address the safety and efficacy of this approach.

Antiretroviral Drug Resistance

Short-course antiretroviral drug regimens that do not fully suppress viral replication that are used to prevent HIV-1 MTCT may be associated with the development of antiretroviral drug resistance. This is most likely to occur with prophylaxis regimens using antiretroviral drugs for which a single point mutation can confer drug resistance, such as NVP or 3TC.

In the Ugandan HIVNET 012 study of single-dose intrapartum/newborn NVP for prevention of MTCT, 25% of 279 women receiving single-dose NVP developed detectable NVP resistance mutations by 6 weeks postpartum, most commonly the K103N mutation. In follow-up samples from 12–18 months postpartum, resistance mutations were no longer detectable and wild-type virus again predominated.[43,44] Factors associated with development of NVP resistance following single-dose exposure include delivery maternal viral load and CD4+ cell count; viral subtype (rates are higher with subtypes D and C, than with A); time of sampling following exposure (rates are higher closer to time of exposure); number of maternal doses; and possibly body compartment (rates may be higher in breast milk than plasma).

Rapid development of genotypic resistance to 3TC has also been observed when 3TC has been given as part of a dual NRTI regimen with ZDV in pregnant women to prevent mother-to-child transmission. In a study in France, where 3TC was added to ZDV after 32 weeks' gestation, 39% of 132 women had detectable high-level resistance (M184V) to 3TC at 6 weeks' postpartum; resistance was only detected in women who had received 3TC for 4 weeks or longer during pregnancy.[45]

The transient presence of detectable resistance does not have any deleterious short-term clinical effect on infected women and infants, and despite the high prevalence of 3TC resistance in the French study, the transmission rate in this group was only 1.6%. Whether the presence of transient drug resistance may be associated with diminished virologic response to subsequent 3TC or NNRTI-based therapy is unknown. In a study in Thailand, response to NVP-based HAART was assessed in immunocompromised women with and without prior single-dose NVP exposure; for those with exposure, the median time following receipt of single-dose NVP to initiation of therapy was only 6 months. The rate of maximal viral suppression (HIV-1 RNA <50 copies/mL) after 6 months of NVP-based HAART was lower in women with recent prior single-dose NVP exposure, although clinical and immunologic responses were not different.[46] Further research is ongoing to more definitively address this issue, including whether duration of time between receipt

of single-dose NVP and initiation of HAART impacts response to therapy.

Research is also ongoing to develop interventions to prevent development of resistance following single-dose NVP. Preliminary data from a South African study suggest that combining single-dose NVP with AZT/3TC given intrapartum and for 4 or 7 days postpartum reduced the risk of resistance.[47] However, a final analysis of the data is needed before definitive conclusions can be drawn, and the optimal regimen and duration of time following single-dose NVP requires further study.

Non-antiretroviral Interventions

In general, with the exception of elective cesarean delivery, the results of non-antiretroviral interventions to prevent MTCT have been disappointing. Approaches have included treatment/prophylaxis of chorioamnionitis; vaginal virucidal cleansing; and nutritional supplementation. Studies are ongoing to evaluate immunogenicity and safety of HIV-1 vaccines in neonates in prelude to a trial to evaluate the efficacy of active or active/passive immunization to reduce MTCT.

Prevention of Chorioamnionitis

Clinical and/or histologic chorioamnionitis appears to be associated with MTCT in some, although not all, studies. Chorioamnionitis is associated with significant inflammation and activation of immune cells in the placenta, which could lead to breaks in the placental barrier, allowing passage of virus or infected lymphocytes from the mother to the fetus. However, preliminary data from a controlled clinical trial in Malawi and Zambia in which empiric therapy for chorioamnionitis was provided with a short course of antibiotics was given to infected pregnant at 20–24 weeks' gestation and again during delivery found that such therapy did not reduce HIV-1 MTCT or infant morbidity and mortality.

Vaginal Microbicides

Use of a microbicide to cleanse the birth canal before vaginal delivery could potentially reduce the amount of intrapartum viral exposure the infant receives, and hence intrapartum transmission. However, several African clinical trials using vaginal swabbing or lavage with 0.2–0.4% chlorhexidine, as well as a study of 1% benzalkonium chloride vaginal suppositories during the last month of pregnancy and intrapartum, did not find any reduction in MTCT. However, in one chlorhexidine study, there were improvements in maternal and infant morbidity and mortality.

Micronutrient Supplementation

Vitamin A and/or multinutrient supplementation was evaluated for prevention of MTCT in four randomized, placebo-controlled perinatal trials in Malawi, South Africa, Tanzania, and Zimbabwe. Unfortunately, final results from all trials did not demonstrate efficacy of supplementation to reduce *in utero*, intrapartum or early breast milk transmission of HIV. In one study that continued postnatal maternal supplementation during lactation reported that multivitamin supplementation may reduce late breast-feeding transmission but only among women with low baseline CD4+ cell counts. They also reported that postnatal vitamin A alone may paradoxically increase the risk of breast-milk transmission, although this was not observed in the other trials.

Elective Cesarean Delivery

Prolonged duration of membrane rupture is associated with the risk of MTCT; elective cesarean delivery (performed prior to labor and membrane rupture) has been shown to reduce the risk of MTCT in an individual patient data meta-analysis including 8533 non-breast-feeding mother-child pairs from 15 prospective US and international cohort studies, and a randomized clinical trial.[4,5] However, non-elective cesarean delivery (performed *after* onset of labor or rupture of membranes) did not reduce MTCT compared with vaginal delivery.

In these studies, elective cesarean delivery reduced transmission among women receiving antiretroviral drugs (primarily AZT alone). However, it is unclear if benefit would be observed in women on HAART with undetectable virus. The European Collaborative Study recently reported data from 4525 women that suggested MTCT was reduced with elective cesarean delivery among all women delivering in the HAART era; however, among the subset of 560 women with undetectable HIV-1 RNA levels, while on univariate analysis elective cesarean delivery was associated with a significant reduction in MTCT, this effect was no longer significant after adjusting for antiretroviral therapy.[48] In women with low risk of transmission, such as those on HAART with low viral load, the risk of operative delivery to the mother may outweigh the potential benefit in reducing MTCT. Additionally, postoperative complications are slightly more common after elective cesarean delivery among HIV-infected than uninfected women, with the difference greatest among women with immunologic suppression.[32]

Current Guidelines for Prevention of MTCT for the USA

Current guidelines for antiretroviral therapy and elective cesarean delivery for the USA[32] are shown in Table 43.2 (see Public Health Service Task Force guidelines online at: http://AIDSInfo.nih.gov for more detail). Based on studies indicating that MTCT rates are extremely low in women with HIV-1 RNA levels that are very low or undetectable, particularly when they have received antiretroviral therapy, HAART is recommended for pregnant women with HIV-1 RNA >1000 copies/mL. Additionally, elective cesarean delivery should be considered for such women if HIV RNA levels remain >1000 copies/mL near delivery. Because antiretroviral prophylaxis is beneficial in reducing perinatal transmission even among infected pregnant women with HIV-1 RNA <1000 copies/mL, use of prophylaxis is recommended for all pregnant women regardless of antenatal HIV RNA level. In this situation, use of the standard AZT prophylaxis alone or combination regimens can be considered. Use of AZT alone is reasonable in this situation, long-term follow-up of women from PACTG 076 have shown no adverse effects in terms of disease progression, mortality, HIV RNA levels or AZT resistance between those who received AZT alone compared to placebo. Women who do not require therapy for their own health can discontinue prophylaxis after delivery. When antenatal therapy has not been received, several effective regimens are available when intrapartum/postpartum therapy can be administered based on clinical trial data previously discussed (Table 43.1). When the mother has received no antiretroviral therapy during pregnancy or intrapartum, 6 weeks of AZT should be given to the infant.

Current Guidelines for Prevention of MTCT for Resource-constrained Settings

WHO guidelines for antiretroviral therapy for treating pregnant women and preventing MTCT were updated in July 2006 (Table 43.3).[49] For women who

Table 43.2 Recommendations for antiretroviral drug use by pregnant HIV-1-infected women and prevention of mother-to-child transmission in the USA

Clinical situation	Recommendation		
HIV-1-infected women of child-bearing potential and indications for initiating antiretroviral therapy	HAART as per US treatment guidelines. Avoid drugs with teratogenic potential in women of child-bearing age (efavirenz) unless adequate contraception can be ensured. Exclude pregnancy before starting treatment with efavirenz.		
HIV-1-infected women with indications for antiretroviral therapy, are receiving HAART, and become pregnant	Woman	Continue current HAART regimen except discontinue drugs with teratogenic potential (efavirenz) or with known adverse potential for the pregnant mother (combination d4T/ddI). Discontinuation of drugs during the first trimester is not recommended. If it is decided to discontinue antiretroviral drugs during the first trimester, stop all drugs (if regimen includes drug with long half-life such as NNRTI, consider stopping NRTIs 3–7 days after stopping NNRTI although limited data on utility). Continue HAART regimen during intrapartum period (AZT given as continuous infusion during labor) and postpartum. Elective cesarean delivery if plasma HIV-1 RNA remains >1000 copies/mL near delivery.	
	Infant	AZT for 6 weeks.	
HIV-1-infected pregnant women with antenatal plasma HIV-1 RNA >1000 copies/mL	Woman	HAART (ideally containing AZT when possible). Due to risk of severe hepatic toxicity with NVP in women with CD4 >250, use NVP in this situation only if benefit clearly outweighs risk and alternatives not available. Continue HAART regimen during intrapartum period (AZT given as continuous infusion during labor). Discontinue HAART postpartum unless has indications for continued therapy (if regimen includes drug with long half-life such as NNRTI, consider stopping NRTIs 3–7 days after stopping NNRTI although limited data on utility). Elective cesarean delivery if plasma HIV-1 RNA remains >1000 copies/mL near delivery.	
	Infant	AZT for 6 weeks.	
HIV-1-infected pregnant women with antenatal maternal plasma HIV-1 RNA <1000 copies/mL	Woman	AZT given antepartum after the first trimester and intravenously intrapartum. *or* HAART (ideally containing AZT after the first trimester), plus AZT given intravenously intrapartum. Discontinue HAART postpartum (if regimen includes drug with long half-life such as NNRTI, consider stopping NRTIs 3–7 days after stopping NNRTI although limited data on utility).	
	Infant	AZT for 6 weeks.	
HIV-1 infected women who have received no antiretroviral therapy prior to labor	Several effective regimens are available to choose from for women who have had no prior therapy: 1. AZT		
		Woman	AZT given intravenously during labor.
		Infant	AZT for 6 weeks.
	or 2. PETRA AZT + 3TC		
		Woman	AZT + 3TC during labor.
		Infant	AZT + 3TC for 1 week.

Table 43.2 Recommendations for antiretroviral drug use by pregnant HIV-1-infected women and prevention of mother-to-child transmission in the USA—cont'd

Clinical situation	Recommendation
	or 3. Single-dose NVP
	Woman Single-dose NVP (if delivery is imminent, do not give the maternal intrapartum NVP dose but follow the recommendations in next scenario). Intrapartum AZT+3TC plus one week postpartum AZT+3TC should be considered to reduce NVP resistance.
	Infant Single-dose NVP at 48–72 h of age.
	or 4. Combination AZT + NVP
	Woman AZT given intravenously during labor, plus single-dose NVP at onset labor. Intrapartum 3TC plus one week postpartum AZT+3TC should be considered to reduce NVP resistance.
	Infant Single-dose NVP plus AZT for 6 weeks.
Infant born to HIV-1-nfected women who has received no antiretroviral therapy prior to or during labor	AZT given for 6 weeks to the infant, started as soon as possible after delivery (preferably within 6–12 h of birth). *or* Some clinicians may choose to use AZT in combination with additional antiretroviral drugs, but appropriate dosing regimens for neonates are incompletely defined and the additional efficacy of this approach in reducing transmission is not known.

Adapted from Public Health Service Task Force recommendations for use of antiretroviral drugs in pregnant HIV-1-infected women for maternal health and interventions to reduce perinatal HIV-1 transmission in the USA. For most recent guidelines see online at: http://AIDSInfo.nih.gov (accessed 1 March 2005). HAART, highly active antiretroviral therapy; AZT, Zidovudine; 3TC, Lamivudine; NVP, Nevirapine.

Table 43.3 World Health Organization recommendations for antiretroviral drug use in HIV-1-infected pregnant women in resource-limited settings

Clinical situation	Recommendation
HIV-1-infected women with childbearing potential and indications for starting therapy.	HAART regimen choice should follow WHO recommendations. First line regimen for child-bearing age women: AZT + 3TC + NVP Avoid drugs with teratogenic potential in women of child-bearing age (efavirenz) unless adequate contraception can be ensured. Exclude pregnancy before starting treatment with efavirenz.
HIV-1-infected women on HAART who become pregnant	Woman Continue current regimen except discontinue drugs with known adverse potential for the pregnant mother (combination d4T/ddI) and discontinue drugs during the first trimester that have teratogenic potential (efavirenz) (women who are receiving efavirenz and are in the second or third trimester can continue the current regimen). Continue HAART regimen during intrapartum period and postpartum.
	Infant AZT for 1 week (four weeks of AZT if mother receives <4 weeks antepartum HAART).
Women first diagnosed with HIV-1 infection during pregnancy with clinical indications for HAART	Woman Follow guidelines for non-pregnant women except exclude drugs with teratogenic potential (efavirenz) during the first trimester and drugs with known adverse potential for the pregnant mother (combination of d4T/ddI).

Table 43.3 **World Health Organization recommendations for antiretroviral drug use in HIV-1-infected pregnant women in resource-limited settings—cont'd**

Clinical situation	Recommendation	
		First line regimen: AZT + 3TC + NVP. For severely ill woman, benefit of therapy during the first trimester exceeds theoretical risk of teratogenicity, and therapy should be initiated regardless of trimester of pregnancy. Continue HAART regimen during intrapartum period and postpartum.
	Infant	AZT for one week (four weeks of AZT if mother receives <4 weeks antepartum HAART).
Pregnant HIV-1-infected women without indication for HAART		Initiate ARV prophylaxis to reduce the risk of peripartum MTCT:
	Woman	AZT starting at 28 weeks' gestation or as soon as feasible after that; continue with oral AZT during labor plus single-dose NVP at the onset of labor. Intrapartum 3TC plus one week postpartum AZT+3TC should be given to mother reduce NVP resistance if possible.
	Infant	Single-dose NVP plus AZT for 1 week (4 weeks of AZT if mother receives <4 weeks antepartum AZT).
Pregnant women of unknown HIV-1 infection status at time of labor or HIV-1-infected pregnant women who have not received antepartum antiretroviral drugs		If there is time, counsel and offer HIV-1 rapid test; if positive, initiate intrapartum prophylaxis. If insufficient time to obtain HIV-1 test result while in labor, offer HIV-1 test as soon as possible after delivery, and follow the recommendations in next scenario. Recommended alternatives: 1. AZT plus single-dose NVP:
	Woman	AZT during labor plus signle-dose NVP. When possible, intrapartum 3TC plus one week postpartum AZT+3TC should be given to mother to reduce NVP resistance. If delivery is imminent, do not give the maternal intrapartum NVP dose but follow the recommendations in the next scenario.
	Infant	Single-dose NVP as soon as possible after birth plus AZT for four weeks.
		or 2. PETRA AZT + 3TC
	Woman	AZT + 3TC during labor and for one week postpartum
	Infant	AZT + 3TC for one week.
		or 3. Single-dose NVP (situations where AZT and 3TC not available):
	Woman	Single-dose nevirapine at noset of labor. If delivery is imminent, do not give the matrernal intrapartum NVP dose but follow the recommendations in the next scenario.
	Infant	Single-dose nevirapine at age 48–72 hours.
Infants born to HIV-1-infected women who have not received antepartum and intrapartum antiretroviral drugs		Single-dose NVP as soon as possible after birth plus AZT for four weeks. If regimen is started more than 2 days after birth, it is unlikely to be effective.
HIV-1-infected women who are breast-feeding		If indications for therapy, initiate or continue HAART as per non-pregnant scenario. If there are no indications for therapy, there are insufficient data regarding the safety and efficacy of use of ARVs solely to prevent breast-milk HIV-1 transmission to recommend use outside of clinical trial setting.

Adapted from the WHO: Antiretroviral drugs for treating pregnant women and preventing HIV infection in infants: guidelines on care, treatment and support for women living with HIV/AIDS and their children in resource-constrained settings (World Health Organization, Geneva, Switzerland 2004); guidelines were updated July 2006; URL: http://www.who.int/hiv/pub/guidelines/pmtct/en/index.html
HAART, highly active antiretroviral therapy; WHO, World Health Organization; D4T, Stavudine; AZT, Zidovudine; 3TC, Lamivudine; NVP, Nevirapine; ARV, antiretroviral; NNRTI, non-nucleoside reverse transcriptase inhibitor; NRTI, nucleoside analog reverse transcriptase inhibitor.

meet the WHO criteria for initiation of therapy for their own health (CD4$^+$ cell count <200/mm^3 or severe symptomatic HIV disease), a standard HAART regimen is recommended. For women who lack indications for therapy for their own health, several different short-course regimens that have been proven to reduce MTCT are available (Table 43.3); when resources permit, short course antenatal and intrapartum AZT combined with single-dose maternal NVP and single-dose infant NVP combined with 1 week of infant AZT is recommended (Table 43.3).

Conclusion

Although there has been dramatic progress in reducing HIV MTCT since 1994, two perinatal epidemics now exist. One epidemic is in resource-rich countries, where most HIV-infected women receive HAART, transmission has been reduced to less than 2%, and elimination of perinatal infection is within reach. The other is in resource-limited countries, where the majority of HIV-infected women live, and while effective prophylaxis regimens have been identified, antiretroviral treatment is generally not available, the limited maternal-child healthcare infrastructure has difficulty in supporting the addition of HIV counseling and testing and antiretroviral prophylaxis programs, and breast-feeding remains a necessity for most infants. A major challenge for the upcoming decade will be to bridge the gap in prevention of MTCT between resource-rich and resource-limited countries.

References

1. Connor EM, Sperling RS, Gelber R, et al. Reduction of maternal-infant transmission of human immunodeficiency virus type 1 with zidovudine treatment. N Engl J Med 1994; 3312:1173–1180.
2. Mofenson LM. Tale of two epidemics – the continuing challenge of preventing mother-to-child HIV transmission (editorial). J Infect Dis 2003; 187:721–724.
3. Magder LS, Mofenson L, Paul ME, et al. Risk factors for in utero and intrapartum transmission of HIV. J Acquir Immune Defic Syndr 2005; 38:87–95.
4. The International Perinatal HIV Group. The mode of delivery and the risk of vertical transmission of human immunodeficiency virus type 1: a meta-analysis of 15 prospective studies. N Engl J Med 1999; 340:977–987.
5. The European Mode of Delivery Collaboration. Elective caesarean-section versus vaginal delivery in prevention of vertical HIV-1 transmission: a randomized clinical trial. Lancet 1999; 353:1035–1039.
6. The PETRA Study Team. Efficacy of three short-course regimens of zidovudine and lamivudine in preventing early and late transmission of HIV-1 from mother to child in Tanzania, South Africa, and Uganda (PETRA study): a randomised, double-blind, placebo-controlled trial. Lancet 2002; 359:1178–1186.
7. Jackson JB, Musoke P, Fleming T, et al. Intrapartum and neonatal single-dose nevirapine compared with zidovudine for prevention of mother to child transmission of HIV-1 in Kampala, Uganda: 18 month follow-up of the HIVNET 012 randomised trial. Lancet 2003; 362:859–868.
8. Taha TE, Kumwenda NI, Gibbons A, et al. Short postexposure prophylaxis in newborn babies to reduce mother to child transmission of HIV-1: NVAZ randomized clinical trial. Lancet 2003; 362:1171–1177.
9. Fowler MG, Newell ML. Breast-feeding and HIV-1 transmission in resource-limited settings. J Acquir Immune Defic Syndr 2002; 30:230–239.
10. Shaffer N, Chuachoowong PA, Mock C, et al. Short-course zidovudine for perinatal HIV-1 transmission in Bangkok, Thailand: a randomized controlled trial. Lancet 1999; 353:773–780.
11. Wiktor S, Ekpini E, Karon J, et al. Short course oral zidovudine for prevention of mother-to-child transmission of HIV-1 in Abidjan, Cote d'Ivoire: a randomised trial. Lancet 1999; 353:781–785.
12. Leroy V, Karon JM, Alioum A, et al. Twenty-four month efficacy of a maternal short-course zidovudine regimen to prevent mother to child transmission of HIV-1 in West Africa. AIDS 2002; 16:631–641.
13. The Breast-feeding and HIV International Transmission Study Group. Late postnatal transmission of HIV-1 in breast-fed children: an independent patient data meta-analysis. J Infect Dis 2004; 189:2154–2166.
14. Moodley D, Moodley J, Coovadia H, et al. The South African intrapartum nevirapine trial (SAINT): a multicenter, randomized, controlled trial of nevirapine compared to a combination of zidovudine and lamivudine to reduce intrapartum and early postpartum mother to child transmission of human immunodeficiency virus type-1. J Infect Dis 2003; 187:725–735.
15. John-Stewart G, Mbori-Ngacha D, Ekpini R, et al. Breast-feeding and transmission of HIV-1. J Acquir Immune Defic Syndr 2004; 35:196–202.
16. Piwoz E, Iliff P, Tavengwa N, et al. Early introduction of non-human milk and solid foods increases the risk of postnatal HIV-1 transmission in Zimbabwe. Abstract MoPpB2008. XV International AIDS Conference, Bangkok, Thailand: 11–16 July 2004.
17. Ioannidis JPA, Abrams EJ, Ammann A, et al. Perinatal transmission of human immunodeficiency virus type 1 by pregnant women with RNA virus loads <1000 copies/mL. J Infect Dis 2001; 183:539–545.
18. Cooper ER, Charurat M, Mofenson L, et al. Combination antiretroviral strategies for treatment of pregnant HIV-1-infected women and prevention of perinatal HIV-1 transmission. J Acquir Immune Defic Syndr 2002; 29:484–494.
19. Chuachoowong R, Shaffer N, Siriwasin W, et al. Short-course antenatal zidovudine reduces both cervicovaginal human immunodeficiency virus type 1 RNA levels and risk of perinatal transmission. J Infect Dis 2000; 181:99–106.
20. Tuomala RE, O'Driscoll PT, Bremer JW, et al. Cell-associated genital tract virus and vertical transmission of human immunodeficiency virus type 1 in antiretroviral-experienced women. J Infect Dis 2003; 187:375–384.
21. Lallemant M, Jourdain G, Le Coeur S, et al. A trial of shortened zidovudine regimens to prevent mother-to-child transmission of human immunodeficiency virus type 1. N Engl J Med 2000; 343:982–991.
22. Lallemant M, Jourdain G, Le Coeur S, et al. Single-dose perinatal nevirapine plus standard zidovudine to prevent mother to child transmission of HIV-1 in Thailand. N Engl J Med 2004; 351:217–228.
23. Shapiro R, Thior I, Gilbert P, et al. Maternal single-dose nevirapine may not be needed to reduce mother to child HIV transmission in the setting of maternal and infant zidovudine and infant single-dose nevirapine: the results of

a randomized clinical trial in Botswana. Abstract 74B. 12th Conference on Retroviruses and Opportunistic Infections, Boston, MA: 22–25 February 2005.

24. ANRS 1201/1202 DITRAME PLUS Study Group. Field efficacy of zidovudine, lamivudine and single-dose nevirapine to prevent peripartum HIV transmission. AIDS 2005; 19:309–318.

25. Dorenbaum A, Cunningham CK, Gelber RD, et al. Two-dose intrapartum/newborn nevirapine and standard antiretroviral therapy to reduce perinatal HIV-1 transmission: a randomized trial. JAMA 2002; 288: 189–198.

26. Taha TE, Kumwenda NI, Hoover DR, et al. Nevirapine and zidovudine at birth to reduce perinatal transmission of HIV in an African setting: a randomized controlled trial. JAMA 2004; 292:202–209.

27. Vyankandondera J, Luchters S, Hassink E, et al. Reducing risk of HIV-1 transmission from mother to infant through breast-feeding using antiretroviral prophylaxis in infants (SIMBA). Abstract LB7. 2nd International AIDS Society Conference on HIV Pathogenesis and Treatment, Paris, France: 13–16 July 2003.

28. Taha TE, Kumwenda N, Gibbons A, et al. Effect of HIV-1 antiretroviral prophylaxis on hepatic and hematological parameters of African infants. AIDS 2002; 16:851–858.

29. Taha TE, Kumwenda N, Kafulafula G, et al. Haematological changes in African children who received short-term prophylaxis with nevirapine and zidovudine at birth. Ann Trop Paediatr 2004; 24:301–309.

30. Mofenson LM, Munderi P. Safety of antiretroviral prophylaxis of perinatal transmission for HIV-infected pregnant women and their infants. J Acquir Immune Defic Syndr 2002; 30:200–215.

31. Antiretroviral Pregnancy Registry Steering Committee. Antiretroviral Pregnancy Registry International Interim Report for 1 January 1989 through 31 January 2004. Wilmington, NC: Registry Coordinating Center; 2004. Online. Available: www.apregistry.com

32. Centers for Disease Control and Prevention. Recommendations for use of antiretroviral drugs in pregnant HIV-1-infected women for maternal health and interventions to reduce perinatal HIV-1 transmission in the United States. Online. Available: http://AIDSInfo.nih.gov (accessed 28 February 2005).

33. The European Collaborative Study prepared by C. Thorne D. Patel and M-L. Newell. Increased risk of adverse pregnancy outcomes in HIV-infected women treated with highly active antiretroviral therapy in Europe. AIDS 2004; 18:2337–2339.

34. Tuomala RE, Shapiro DE, Mofenson LM, et al. Antiretroviral therapy during pregnancy and the risk of an adverse outcome. N Engl J Med 2002; 346:1863–1870.

35. Barrett B, Tardieu M, Rustin P, et al. Persistent mitochondrial dysfunction in HIV-1-exposed but uninfected infants: clinical screening in a large prospective cohort. AIDS 2003; 17:1769–1785.

36. French Perinatal Cohort Study Group. Risk of early febrile seizure with perinatal exposure to nucleoside analogs. Lancet 2002; 359:583–584.

37. Le Chenadec J, Mayaux M-J, Guihenneuc-Jouyaux C, et al. Perinatal antiretroviral treatment and hematopoiesis in HIV-uninfected infants. AIDS 2003; 17:2053–2061.

38. Perinatal Safety Review Working Group. Nucleoside exposure in the children of HIV-infected women receiving antiretroviral drugs: absence of clear evidence for mitochondrial disease in children who died before 5 years of age in five United States cohorts. J Acquir Immune Defic Syndr 2000; 25:261–268.

39. European Collaborative Study. Exposure to antiretroviral therapy in utero or early life: the health of uninfected children born to HV-infected women. J Acquir Immune Defic Syndr 2003; 32:380–387.

40. Watts DH, Balasubramanian R, Maupin RT, et al. Maternal toxicity and pregnancy complications in human immunodeficiency virus-infected women receiving antiretroviral therapy: PACTG 316. Am J Obstet Gynecol 2004; 190:506–516.

41. Shapiro RL, Holland D, Capparelli EV, et al. HIV inhibitory plasma concentrations of antiretrovirals detected in breast-feeding infants of women receiving antiretroviral treatment in Botswana. 42nd Annual Meeting of the Infectious Disease Society of America, Boston, MA: October 2004.

42. Gaillard P, Fowler MG, Dabis F, et al. Use of antiretroviral drugs to prevent HIV-1 transmission through breast-feeding: from animal studies to randomized clinical trials. J Acquir Immune Defic Syndr 2004; 35:178–187.

43. Eshleman SH, Guay LA, Mwatha A, et al. Characterization of nevirapine resistance mutations in women with subtype A vs D HIV-1 6-8 weeks after single-dose nevirapine (HIVNET 012). J Acquir Immune Defic Syndr 2004; 35:126–130.

44. Eshleman SH, Mracna M, Guay L, et al. Selection and fading of resistance mutations in women and infants receiving nevirapine to prevent HIV-1 vertical transmission (HIVNET 012). AIDS 2001; 15:1951–1957.

45. Mandelbrot L, Landreau-Mascaro A, Rekacewicz C, et al. Lamivudine-zidovudine combination for prevention of maternal-infant transmission of HIV-1. JAMA 2001; 285:2083–2093.

46. Jourdain G. Ngo-Giang-Huong N, Le Coeur S, et al. Intrapartum exposure to nevirapine and subsequent maternal responses to nevirapine-based antiretroviral therapy. N Engl J Med 2004; 351:229–240.

47. McIntyre J, Martinson N, Investigators for the Trail 1413, et al. Addition to short course Combivir (CBV) to single dose Viramune (sdNVP) for prevention of mother-to-child transmission (MTCT) of HIV-1 can significantly decrease the subsequent development of maternal NNRTI-resistant virus. Abstract LbOrB09. XV International AIDS Conference, Bangkok, Thailand: 11–16 July 2004.

48. European Collaborative Study. Mother to child transmission of HIV infection in the era of highly active antiretroviral therapy. Clin Infect Dis 2005; 40:458–465.

49. WHO. Antiretroviral drugs for treatment pregnant women and preventing HIV infection in infants: guidelines on care, treatment, and support for women living with HIV/AIDS and their children in resource-constrained settings. Geneva: World Health Organization; 2004. Updated July 2006 guidlines can be accessed at http://www.who.int/hiv/pub/guidelines/pmtct/en/index.htm

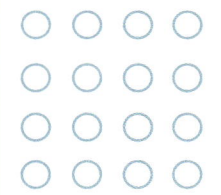

CHAPTER 44

HIV Disease Among Substance Users: Treatment Issues

R. Douglas Bruce
Frederick L. Altice
Gerald Friedland

Epidemiology

HIV/AIDS and illicit drug use adversely impact tens of millions of people, with explosive epidemics of both described worldwide. Injection drug use (IDU), largely of opiates, has been reported in 136 countries and 114 of these have reported HIV among this population (Fig. 44.1).[1] The link between drug use, particularly IDU, and HIV has been well described since the beginning of the HIV pandemic.[2] The world's most volatile and emerging HIV epidemics are in areas that are fueled by illicit drug use, particularly heroin. Such places include the former states of the Soviet Union,[3] other Eastern European countries,[4] Southeast Asia,[5] South America,[6] and China.[7] Particularly troubling is that many of these epidemics are among individuals younger than 30 and within the most densely populated regions of the world. Injection drug use is especially important in the HIV/AIDS epidemic among women and children. In many of these areas, a substantial proportion of illicit drug users are women or the sexual partners of male drug users, significantly contributing to perinatally acquired HIV infection. Not only does IDU provide a vector for transmission of HIV, but substance use is itself a barrier to obtaining prenatal care. Without prenatal care, interventions cannot be instituted to decrease the risk of mother-to-child transmission of HIV.

Substantial advances in the treatment of opiate dependence have been made in recent years, which can impact favorably on clinical and public health outcomes of both drug dependence and HIV/AIDS, but, as is the case with highly active antiretroviral therapy (HAART), these have been limited in their availability. The World Health Organization, the United Nations Office on Drugs and Crime and the Joint United Nations Programme on HIV/AIDS have each supported the expansion of opiate substitution therapies[8] – evidence-based therapies that have proven to be effective for both primary and secondary HIV prevention[9] and cost-effective to society.[10]

In light of the increasingly central role of injection drug use in the global HIV/AIDS epidemic, issues of HIV clinical care and therapeutics in this population are of great importance. Of particular relevance are the special clinical features of HIV disease in drug dependent patients, the treatment of HIV disease itself in this population, the special difficulties in providing care to drug users and the treatment of drug dependence.

HIV Disease in Drug Users

The natural history of HIV disease among drug users has been demonstrated to be similar to that in other transmission risk categories.[11] Drug users are, however, at an increased risk for a number of other infections compared with other risk categories. Although most of these infections and other compli-

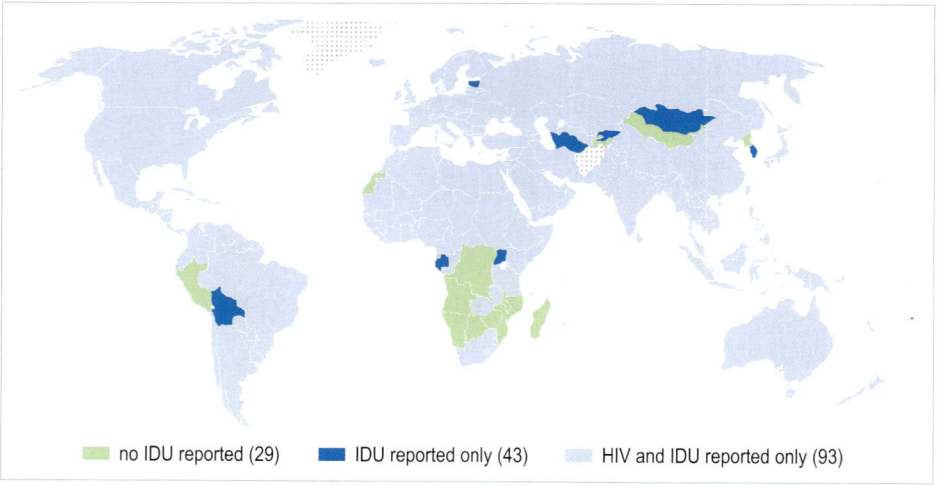

no IDU reported (29) ■ IDU reported only (43) ■ HIV and IDU reported only (93)

Figure 44.1 Worldwide distribution of HIV and injection drug use (IDU). Green, no IDU reported (29); Dark blue, IDU reported only (43); Light blue, HIV and IDU reported (93). (Adapted from WHO programme on substance abuse.)

cations were common among drug users prior to the HIV epidemic, their incidence and severity have been accentuated, and clinical presentation affected by HIV infection. In both inpatient and outpatient settings, these are more common than specific HIV-related complications and often confound both diagnosis and treatment.

Multiple features of injection drug use contribute to the increased risk of infection (Box 44.1): (1) increased rates of skin, mucous membrane, and nasopharyngeal carriage of pathogenic organisms; (2) unsterile injection techniques; (3) contamination of injection equipment or drugs with micro-organisms, which may be present in residual blood in shared injection equipment; (4) humoral, cell-mediated, and phagocyte defects induced by HIV infection and/or drug use; (5) poor dental hygiene; (6) impairment of gag and cough reflexes resulting in increased risk for aspiration and pneumonia; (7) alteration of the normal microbial flora by self-administered antibiotic use; (8) increased prevalence of exposure to certain pathogens (notably *Mycobacterium tuberculosis*); (9) concomitant behaviors such as cigarette smoking, alcohol use, or exchange of sex for drugs or money; and (10) decreased access to and/or lack of appropriate use of preventive and primary healthcare services.

A detailed discussion of these infections and their management is beyond the focus of this chapter. Table 44.1 offers a summary of substance misuse-related complications in HIV-infected injection drug users. This chapter will address specific issues for

---

Box 44.1

Features of injection drug use (IDU) contributing to the infectious diseases listed in Table 44.1

1. Increased rates of skin, mucous membrane, and nasopharyngeal carriage of pathogenic organisms.
2. Unsterile injection techniques.
3. Contamination of injection equipment or drugs with micro-organisms, which may be present in residual blood in shared injection equipment.
4. Humoral, cell-mediated, and phagocyte defects induced by HIV infection and/or drug use.
5. Poor dental hygiene.
6. Impairment of gag and cough reflexes due to intoxication resulting in increased risk for pneumonia.
7. Alteration of the normal microbial flora by self-administered antibiotic use.
8. Increased prevalence of exposure to certain pathogens (notably *Mycobacterium tuberculosis*).
9. Concomitant behaviors such as cigarette smoking (i.e. increased susceptibility to pulmonary infections), alcohol use (i.e. increased progression of hepatic fibrosis for HCV infected drug users), or exchange of sex for drugs or money (i.e. exposure to sexually transmitted infections).
10. Decreased access to and/or lack of appropriate use of preventive and primary healthcare services.

Table 44.1 A summary of drug use related complications in HIV-infected injection drug users

Location	Disease	Organisms	Treatment	Comments
Skin and soft tissue	Cellulitis	Group A and other streptococci, *Staphylococcus aureus*	Anti-staphylococcal agents	Consider hospitalization Consider MRSA
	Abscess Necrotizing fasciitis	Same as for cellulitis Polymicrobial	Same as for cellulitis Parenteral antibiotics to cover both Gram(+) and (−) organisms	Incision and drainage Consider if crepitus noted; immediate surgical consultation required
	Septic thrombophlebitis	*Staphylococcus aureus*	Antistaphylococcal agents	Surgical exploration and vein ligation
Cardiovascular	Endocarditis	*Staphylococcus aureus*, streptococci, enteric Gram(−) rods	Anti-staphylococcal agents until cultures grow Treat for 4–6 weeks	Consider if (a) regurgitant murmur, (b) presence of peripheral or pulmonary emboli (c) blood culture (+), (e) echocardiogram Consider MRSA
Pulmonary	Community acquired pneumonia	*S. Pneumonia, H. influenza*, atypical organisms Tuberculosis Opportunistic infection PCP	PCN, cephalosporin, macrolide Isoniazid, Rifampin, Pryzinamide, Ethambutol Bactrim	Consider even with normal chest X-ray Consider rifabutin due to PI interactions. Rifampin has strong methadone interaction
	Septic emboli	*Staphylococcus aureus*, streptococci, enteric Gram(−) rods	Anti-staphylococcal agents until cultures grow	Common complication, consider with pleuritic chest pain
Liver	Hepatitis	Hepatitis B Hepatitis C	Interferon, Lamivudine, Adefovir, Entecavir, Telbivudine Pegylated Interferon + Ribavirin	HBsAg positive HCV antibody positive with detectable RNA
Neurology	Altered mental status	Substance induced, dementia head trauma Metabolic, opportunistic infection		Consider urine toxicology Consider pattern and tempo of event (slowly progressive or sudden onset)
	Neuropathy Cerebrovascular accident	Substance induced (cocaine or amphetamines) Brain abscess Hemorrhage due to emboli	Amitriptyline, Gabapentin Same as for endocarditis	
Renal	Heroin or HIV nephropathy	Both present with nephrotic syndrome	Renal biopsy to establish diagnosis. Electron microscopy distinguishes diagnosis	Focal and segmental glomerular sclerosis (FSGS) with progression to renal failure in weeks to months

co-managing and treating HIV infection itself among users of illicit drugs.

Treatment of HIV Infection in Drug Users

Highly active antiretroviral therapy (HAART) has resulted in impressive benefit for people living with HIV/AIDS, including decreasing morbidity,[12] mortality,[13] hospitalization,[14] and has been demonstrated from a societal perspective to be cost-effective.[15] Despite the widespread availability of antiretroviral medications in resource-rich settings, IDUs have derived less benefit than other populations.[16] This disparity in benefit among IDUs is and will likely continue to be experienced in resource-limited settings even as antiretroviral medications (ARVs) become increasingly available for adults and children with HIV disease. The reasons for the disparity are multi-factorial.

In many societies worldwide, both HIV and illicit drug use are stigmatized such that either or both conditions are often cloaked in secrecy and may result in a lack of detection and treatment.[17,18] Drug users are among the most socially marginalized populations and often hidden by circumstances and/or choice from mainstream medical care. Even when available, healthcare services are often constructed in ways that are difficult for many drug users to access, either by their absence in communities with high prevalence of drug use or by their organization which does not accommodate the chaotic and sometimes unpredictable use of services characteristic of drug using populations. In addition, clinical care for drug users with HIV disease is often challenging and stressful for clinicians and other healthcare workers as a result of the complex array of substance misuse-related medical, psychological and social problems. The frequent co-morbid underlying psychiatric disease often contributes to these difficulties. Substance misusers may also have increased difficulties with adherence to medications[19] which may be compounded by their underlying co-morbid diseases, increased side-effects and drug interactions.

There is often mutual suspicion between drug users and healthcare providers. Clinicians tend to have stereotypic views of drug users and may harbor negative feelings about the social worth of injection drug users. As with other 'difficult' patients, physicians may come to view drug users as manipulative, unmotivated, and undeserving of care.[20] The chronic relapsing nature of chemical dependence as a medical disease is often not appreciated by clinicians nor is the fact that drug users may be quite diverse and heterogeneous. Many physicians assume that drug users' antisocial behavior and drug use indicate a lifelong lack of concern for others and indifference to their own well-being, rather than a consequence of chemical dependence. Conversely, drug users often are mistrustful of the healthcare system and harbor expectations that they will be treated punitively. Drug users often conceal their continuing drug use from healthcare professionals out of fear of rejection prompted by previous difficult encounters with the healthcare system. In turn, clinicians are sometimes reluctant to confront patients with their suspicions about ongoing drug use, fearing that the confrontation will compromise their relationship. The failure to acknowledge ongoing drug use itself, however, can compromise the clinician–patient relationship since one of the most important aspects of the patient's health is off limits for discussion.

Because the life of a chemically dependent patient is often chaotically organized around their substance use needs, successful programs for this population have developed some or all of the following characteristics: (1) pharmacologic (e.g. methadone and buprenorphine programs) and/or non-pharmacological treatment (e.g. 12 steps) for substance use;[21] (2) flexible outpatient and community care settings (e.g. walk-in clinics, mobile healthcare programs[22]); (3) low-threshold sites to engage active users (e.g. syringe exchange sites[20]); (4) modified directly observed therapy,[23] (5) intensive outreach and case management services;[24] or (6) treatment during incarceration.[25]

Clinicians involved in the care of drug users with HIV, should be aware of several key principles (Box 44.2), which include the following: (1) Become educated about substance abuse and its wide array of treatment options; (2) Establish a multidisciplinary team of individuals with expertise in managing HIV, substance abuse, and mental illness, and broadened to include social work, nursing, case management and community outreach. Identify a single provider to maximize consistency; (3) Obtain a thorough history of the patient's substance abuse history, practices, needle and syringe source, drug abuse complications, and treatment history. Non-judgmental, clinical assessment of this information is essential. Non-judgmental discussion of the adverse health and social consequences of drug use and the benefits of abstinence may increase the patient's understanding of his or her disease and interest in change; (4) Be aware of pharmacological drug interactions between HIV therapies and substance abuse therapies and provide simplified, low pill burden regi-

Box 44.2

Key principles for HIV clinicians involved in the care of drug users

1. *Become educated about substance abuse* and its wide array of treatment options.
2. *Establish a multidisciplinary team* of individuals with expertise in managing HIV, substance abuse, and mental illness, and broaden to include social work, nursing, case management and community outreach. Identify a single provider to maximize consistency.
3. *Obtain a thorough history of the patient's substance abuse* history, practices, needle and syringe source, drug abuse complications, and treatment history. Non-judgmental, clinical assessment of this information is essential. Non-judgmental discussion of the adverse health and social consequences of drug use and the benefits of abstinence may increase the patient's understanding of his or her disease and interest in change.
4. *Be aware of pharmacological drug interactions between HIV and substance abuse therapies* and provide simplified, low pill burden regimens to improve treatment adherence.
5. *Link HIV and substance abuse treatment goals* such that success in one arena is linked to improved outcomes in the other.
6. *Establish a relationship of mutual respect with the patient.* Avoid moral condemnation or attribution of addiction to moral or behavioral weakness. Acknowledge that addiction is a medical disease, compounded by psychological and social circumstances. As such, it should be treated using evidence-based guidelines with a combination of pharmacological and behavioral interventions. Reducing or stopping drug use is difficult, as is sustaining abstinence. Success may require several attempts and relapse is common. Complete abstinence may not be a realistic goal for many substance-misusing patients. Rather, increasing the proportion of days, weeks, and months free from mind-altering substances is an acceptable goal.
7. *Work closely with a drug treatment program.*
8. *Define and agree on the roles and responsibilities* of both the healthcare team and the patient. Establish a formal treatment contract that specifies the services to be provided to the patient, the care giver's expectations about the patient's behavior, and the consequences of behavior that violates the contract. Such a contract should be agreeable to both parties and not simply a contract of the physician's expectations.
9. *Set appropriate limits and respond consistently to behavior that violates those limits.* These should be imposed in a professional manner that reflects the aim of enhancing patients' well-being, and not in an atmosphere of blame or judgment.
10. *Carefully evaluate pain syndromes* and provide sufficient analgesia as medically indicated.
11. *Always consider acute substance ingestion when evaluating behavior change and neurologic disease.* Use urine toxicology testing to evaluate behavioral changes and to discourage illicit drug use by HIV-infected injection drug users during hospital stay.
12. *Work consistently as a team.* Do not make agreements about treatment decisions until the entire team has become involved. This will avoid 'splitting' behaviors that often unravel the fabric of a multidisciplinary team.
13. *Consider integrating drug treatment into the HIV clinical care settings.* While there are no specific recommendations for accomplishing this goal, a number of key approaches have been described. These include complete integration where all clinicians are stakeholders in the treatment of both conditions, the integration of a specialized addiction specialist team or a hybrid model where both are implemented.

mens to improve treatment adherence; (5) Link HIV and substance abuse treatment goals such that success in one arena is linked to improved outcomes in the other; (6) Establish a relationship of mutual respect. Avoid moral condemnation or attribution of addiction to moral or behavioral weakness. Acknowledge that addiction is a medical disease, compounded by psychological and social circumstances. As such, it should be treated using evidence-based guidelines with a combination of pharmacological and behavioral interventions. Reducing or stopping drug use is difficult, as is sustaining abstinence. Success may require several attempts and relapse is common. Complete abstinence may not be a realistic goal for many substance-misusing patients. Rather, increasing the proportion of days, weeks, and months free from mind-altering substances is an acceptable goal; (7) Work closely with a drug treatment program; (8) Define and agree on the roles and responsibilities of both the healthcare team and the patient. Establish a formal treatment contract that specifies the services to be provided to the patient, the care giver's expectations about the patient's behavior, and the consequences of behavior that violates the contract. Such a contract should be agreeable to both parties and not simply a contract of the physician's expectations; (9) Set appropriate limits and respond consistently to behavior that violates those limits. These should be imposed in a professional manner that reflects the aim of enhancing patients' well-being, and not in an atmosphere of blame or judgment; (10) Carefully evaluate pain syndromes and provide sufficient analgesia as medically indicated;[26] (11) Always consider acute substance ingestion when evaluating behavior change and neurologic disease. Use urine toxicology testing to evaluate behavioral changes and to discourage illicit drug use by HIV-infected injection-drug users during hospital stay; (12) Work consistently as a team. Do not make agreements about treatment decisions until the entire team has become involved. This will avoid 'splitting' behaviors that often unravel the fabric of a multidisciplinary team; and (13) Consider integrating drug treatment into the HIV clinical care settings. While there are no specific recommendations for accomplishing this goal, a number of key approaches have been described.[27] These include complete integration where all clinicians are stakeholders in the treatment of both conditions, the integration of a specialized addiction specialist team or a hybrid model where both are implemented.[28]

Commonly Used Illicit Drugs

The illicit drugs most closely associated with HIV infection globally are heroin and cocaine, but methamphetamine use is an evolving problem. Each of these can be administered by a variety of routes. Injection with shared contaminated needles and syringes or other injection paraphernalia carry the greatest risk for HIV transmission and other complications. Non-injection use of cocaine and methamphetamine, however, increasingly facilitates HIV transmission through its association with the exchange of drugs for sex or money or as a result of intoxication. It is important to be aware of local patterns of drug availability and routes of use.

Heroin

There are a number of opioid drugs and medications with abuse potential. Heroin is a short-acting, semi-synthetic opioid produced from opium. It may be smoked, inhaled, or injected; peak heroin euphoria begins shortly after injection and lasts approximately 1 h, followed by 1–4 h of sedation. Withdrawal symptoms commence several hours later. As a consequence, most heroin dependent individuals inject 2–4 times per day. Many heroin users will mediate the sedating effects of heroin by injecting a small amount of cocaine with heroin, a mixture known as a 'speedball.' The unsterile method of use, unpredictable concentrations in street samples, adulterants in the injection mixture and the lifestyle necessary to procure drugs, are responsible for most heroin-associated medical complications.

Cocaine

Cocaine is available as a water-soluble hydrochloride salt which is injected or taken by nasal inhalation, 'snorted'. Although cocaine hydrochloride is destroyed by heat, it may be chemically converted to a free-base ('crack') cocaine, which can be smoked. Pulmonary absorption of 'crack' is as rapid as intravenous injection. Cocaine's half-life is short, resulting in the need for frequent administration. Active cocaine users may inject or inhale cocaine as many as 20 times a day. Cocaine induces feelings of elation, omnipotence and invincibility and with rapid development of psychological dependence. The multiple psychological and physical effects of cocaine can markedly disrupt clinical care. As such, programs that are non-judgmental are essential to continue to engage these patients in care rather than risk losing them to follow-up and diminish the likelihood of risk reduction interventions.

Methamphetamine

Methamphetamine is a psychostimulant that is similar in chemical structure to amphetamine but has more profound effects on the central nervous system. It can be smoked, snorted, injected or administered rectally. Like cocaine, methamphetamine ingestion produces stimulation and similar feelings of euphoria; however, methamphetamine has a longer duration of action (6–8 h after a single dose). Tolerance develops rapidly and escalation of dose and frequency is required. As is the case with cocaine, methamphetamine use is associated with high-risk sexual behavior.[29]

Substance Abuse Treatment

Chemical dependence is a chronic, relapsing and treatable disease, characterized by compulsive drug-seeking and drug use. Although exposure to addictive substances is widespread in society, high vulnerability to addiction is more limited and is the product of biologic, psychological and environmental influences. Thus, identification of addictive disease and referral to appropriate treatment services is an essential part of the clinical care of HIV-infected patients. Indeed, successful treatment of HIV disease in drug users often requires attention to and treatment of substance abuse. There is a wide variety of treatment modalities. Selection of the appropriate program is an individual decision based in part upon the drug used, the length and pattern of the patient's drug use, personal psychosocial characteristics, and local availability (Table 44.2).[30] Resources are limited in many communities, substantially limiting options for referral.

The most effective treatment for opiate addiction for long-term opiate dependent patients, particularly injection drug users, is opiate substitution therapy.[31,32]

Medically Supervised Opiate Withdrawal

Withdrawal from opioids involves the gradual reduction of dosage over a period of time. Although patients can be withdrawn using the drug to which they are addicted, in most instances it is easier to substitute methadone or buprenorphine for the primary opioid of addiction. It is usually not possible to know with certainty how much drug the patient has been taking, though self-reports are often reliable. Regardless of the amount, myalgias, diarrhea, and insomnia and irritability associated with withdrawal can be reduced with a daily oral dose of 25–30 mg of methadone or 16 mg of buprenorphine. This dose of methadone, however, will not eliminate drug craving, whereas 16 mg of buprenorphine will often eliminate craving.[33] Decreasing the methadone dose by 10–20% every few days after the withdrawal syndrome is suppressed, should maintain patient comfort. Buprenorphine, due to its longer half-life, can be tapered off more rapidly. The decision to medically supervise opiate withdrawal or to recommend chronic opiate substitution therapy depends on a number of factors. In general, supervised opiate withdrawal should be reserved for short-term opiate users (<2 years), young adults and non-injectors. Otherwise, relapse to drug use among chronic opiate users exceeds 85% when patients undergo supervised opiate withdrawal without chronic opiate substitution therapy.[34]

Table 44.2 Modalities of substance abuse treatment

Treatment	Benefits	Limitations	Appropriate for whom?	Inappropriate for whom?	Location
Therapeutic community	Can address polysubstance abuse	Low retention rates	Highly motivated individuals	Individuals with family/work commitments	Community settings
Methadone	Reduces crime, transmission of infectious diseases, high retention rates	Does not address other drug use; potential for diversion	Heavy use of opiates	Non-opiate dependent patients; individuals abusing other sedatives (e.g. benzodiazepines)	May require more infrastructure
Buprenorphine	Reduces crime, transmission of infectious diseases, high retention rates	Does not address other drug use; possibly less potential for diversion than methadone	Opiate dependent patients. Improved safety profile compared with methadone	Non-opiate dependent patients; individuals abusing other sedatives (e.g. benzodiazepines)	Due to improved safety profile, may be more widely accessible
Naltrexone	Effective among very motivated individuals	Lacking high motivation, treatment is ineffective	Individuals with high levels of social support and motivation	Individuals with low social support and/or motivation	Not a narcotic and so less regulation

Adapted with permission from Smith-Rohrberg et al.[28]

Treatment of Opioid Dependence

The treatment of choice for the patient who is opioid-dependent and has HIV disease is chronic maintenance with an opiate agonist such as methadone or buprenorphine.[26] In addition to agonist therapy, the patient should be enrolled in a comprehensive drug treatment program designed to prevent the abuse of other drugs and promote rehabilitation. Agonist treatment of opioid dependence is particularly important for the patient with co-morbid HIV infection because effective treatment enhances HIV treatment and may decrease the risk taking behaviors.[35]

Methadone maintenance has been shown to be effective in decreasing psychosocial and medical morbidity associated with opioid dependence. Furthermore, it improves overall health status, is associated with decreased criminal activity and improved social functioning, in addition to its benefit in decreasing the spread of HIV among injection drug users. Methadone, a semisynthetic, long-acting opioid analgesic, is particularly valuable for its oral bioavailability, long half-life of 24–36 h, and the consistent plasma levels that are obtained with regular administration. A single daily dose is given to maintain stable plasma levels. As a result, tolerance develops and regular methadone users do not experience the euphoria of the heroin cycle. Drug-seeking behavior decreases, creating the possibility for the development of more constructive behaviors and relationships. In the first 6 months of treatment, however, some patients may experience side-effects common to other opiates, but tolerance to the majority of these effects develops rapidly. Persistent side-effects include diaphoresis, constipation, and amenorrhea (the majority of women experience the return of menses after 12–18 months of therapy).

There is no optimal dose of methadone for treatment of opioid dependent patients who must be assessed individually for treatment response. Generally, doses of 30–60 mg daily will block opioid withdrawal symptoms, but higher doses in the 80–120 mg daily range are needed to reduce opioid craving and decrease illicit drug use. These higher doses are also associated with greater retention in treatment.[36]

Buprenorphine, unlike methadone which is a full agonist, is a partial μ-receptor agonist. As a partial agonist, there is a plateau of its agonist effects at higher doses which improves its safety profile compared with methadone and may reduce its likelihood for medication diversion.[37] The plateau includes an upper limit on the severity of side-effects associated with overdose, such as respiratory depression.[38] Buprenorphine has a higher binding affinity for the μ-receptor than heroin or methadone.[39] Because buprenorphine dissociates slowly from the μ-receptor, alternate day dosing is possible.[40] Buprenorphine has been prescribed in France since 1996 and resulted in dramatic improvements in the treatment of opioid dependence there. Buprenorphine was approved for use in the USA in 2002 and population outcome data are still being collected. Worldwide, it is becoming increasingly more available.[41] Integration of buprenorphine is now being incorporated into HIV clinical care settings for HIV prevention and stabilization to initiate HAART and using various different models of care prevention.

Naltrexone, an opiate receptor antagonist, can also be used in the treatment of opioid dependence. Naltrexone has demonstrated efficacy in highly motivated populations.[42,43] Its use among HIV-infected drug users is discouraged as methadone and buprenorphine have higher retention rates and allow for engagement when less motivation for treatment exists.

HIV-infected drug users must have as their treatment plan an evidence-based approach to provide appropriate and adequate treatment for substance abuse in order to improve the psychological and physiological disruptions that perpetuate the often unstable life of a drug dependent person.

Treatment for Cocaine and Methamphetamine Dependence

Unlike the case for treatment of opiate dependence, effective and evidence-based treatments have not been developed for the management of stimulant use. The lack of successful, standardized treatment strategies for stimulant users is a significant problem as the epidemics of cocaine and methamphetamine use grow. In the absence of effective programs to treat stimulant use, HIV care providers may feel helpless and frustrated. Counseling is the only treatment modality shown to decrease use of cocaine and methamphetamine.[44] Referral to a substance abuse treatment program, if available, is essential.

Mental Illness and Illicit Drug Use

A thorough discussion of mental illness as it relates to substance misuse and HIV is outside the scope of this chapter. It must be noted, however, that substance misuse and mental illness are closely interrelated with HIV. Individuals with all three diagnoses are likely to engage in high-risk behaviors,[45] and when untreated, continue to fuel the HIV epidemic resulting in continuing transmission of HIV. These three diagnoses should be viewed as overlapping spheres of influence, with each diagnosis affecting the other. Conceptually, this is important because successful therapy requires screening, diagnosis and treatment of all three spheres of influence rather than ignoring any one single area.[46] For this reason, it is essential to ensure a comprehensive and integrated approach to managing these three co-morbid conditions.[47]

Drug Interactions with HIV Therapies

The WHO is committed to expanding access to antiretroviral therapies for HIV disease to resource-limited areas with a high prevalence of IDU.[48] As such, there will be increasing treatment opportunity for HIV-infected opiate dependent persons. In some areas, this will be accompanied by a parallel increase in the availability of evidence-based substance abuse treatment. Thus, it is essential to be familiar with the current state-of-the-art data on drug metabolism and expected or actual pharmacokinetic interactions between HIV therapeutics and opiate substitution therapy (Table 44.3).[49] This understanding is critical as opiate substitution therapy may alter metabolism of antiretroviral medications resulting in increased toxicity or reduced efficacy. Alternatively, antiretroviral medications may alter the levels of opiate substitution therapy resulting in clinical opiate withdrawal or overdose.

The currently approved nucleoside reverse transcriptase inhibitors (NRTIs) do not affect methadone levels in a clinically significant manner and therefore do not precipitate opiate withdrawal. Methadone, however, affects the pharmacokinetics of several of the NRTIs. Many of the currently available NRTIs have been examined for pharmacologic interactions with methadone. Detailed pharmacokinetic studies of the interaction between zidovudine and methadone have been conducted in human subjects.[50] Although zidovudine did not affect methadone concentrations, methadone increased zidovudine drug levels by approximately 40%. As a result, patients may experience symptoms associated with excessive zidovudine dosing that may be confused with symptoms of opiate withdrawal. Such symptoms may include headache, abdominal pain, myalgias, fatigue, and irritability, and may be attributed to reduced methadone levels and opiate with-

drawal or to zidovudine toxicity or both. In addition, increased zidovudine levels may result in laboratory abnormalities, such as anemia and hepatitis.

Zidovudine is the only NRTI studied in combination with buprenorphine. Buprenorphine did not alter the pharmacokinetics of zidovudine in a clinically meaningful manner. The administration of a co-formulated tablet of lamivudine/zidovudine did not significantly alter the pharmacokinetic parameters of methadone.[37] Abacavir[51] and tenofovir[52] have also been studied with methadone and do not appear to have a clinically significant interaction with methadone. Results from studies with stavudine and didanosine indicate neither drug affects methadone levels; however, methadone appeared to alter the disposition of both NRTIs. Methadone decreases drug levels of stavudine but at a level that is unlikely to be clinically significant. Methadone, however, decreases the levels of the buffered tablet formulation of didanosine by 66%; this level of decrease is of clinical concern. The newer, enteric-coated (EC) formulation appears to have corrected this problem and is the preferred formulation when methadone and didanosine are co-administered.[53]

Nevirapine, a non-nucleoside reverse transcriptase inhibitors (NNRTIs), was the first antiretroviral medication described that precipitated opiate withdrawal.[54] Another NNRTI, efavirenz, also markedly reduces methadone levels and precipitates clinical opiate withdrawal.[55] Both NNRTIs appear to exert their effect through marked induction of cytochrome P450 isoenzymes. While efavirenz significantly reduces buprenorphine levels, preliminary studies indicate that this reduction is not associated with symptoms of opiate withdrawal.[56] Delavirdine, an inhibitor of the CYP 3A4, modestly elevates methadone and buprenorphine levels but likely without clinical consequences of opiate overdose. Long-term studies, however, are lacking and providers should carefully observe for opiate intoxication.[57,58]

Most protease inhibitors (PIs) do not appear to have clinically meaningful effects upon methadone levels. Ritonavir,[59] indinavir,[60] nelfinavir,[61] amprenavir,[62] atazanavir,[63] and the combination of saquinavir/ritonavir (400/400 mg b.i.d.)[64] and (1600 mg/100 mg),[65] have been studied and changes in dosing of methadone do not appear to be needed with any of these agents. One study of the co-formulated capsule of lopinavir/ritonavir administration with methadone demonstrated a decrease in methadone levels without the clinical development of opiate withdrawal.[66] Another study using a standardized scale to measure opiate withdrawal, however, reported that 27% of subjects coadministered

Table 44.3 Interactions between antiretrovirals and methadone, and buprenorphine

Medication	Effect on methadone	Effect On BUP	ARV	Comments
NRTI				
Abacavir (ABC)	↑ clearance	Not studied	↓ C_{max}	Unclear if ↑ in M clearance is caused by ABC ↓ C_{max} not clinically relevant
Didanosine (ddI)	No clinical effect	Not studied	↓ ddI AUC by 57% for buffered tablet, partially corrected by EC capsule to within range in historical controls	EC capsule recommended for M patients
Entriva (FTC)	Not studied	Not studied	Not studied	
Lamivudine (3TC)	No clinical effect	Not studied	Not studied	AZT/3TC co-formulation studied only
Stavudine (d4T)	No clinical effect	Not studied	↓ d4T AUC_{12h} by 23% and C_{max} by 44%	Changes unlikely to be clinically significant
Tenofovir (TDF)	No clinical effect	Not studied	Not studied	
Zalcitabine (ddC)	Not studied	Not studied	Not studied	
Zidovudine (AZT)	No clinical effect	No clinical effect	↑ AZT AUC by 40%	Watch for AZT related toxicity (symptoms and laboratory)
NNRTI				
Delavirdine (DLV)	↑ AUC by 19%; ↑ C_{max} by 10%	Increases BUP AUC, but no clinical effect	No clinical effect	Likely not clinically relevant, but should be used with caution as long-term effects (>7 days) unknown.
Efavirenz (EFV)	Significant effect – mean ↓ methadone AUC by 57%	No clinical effect	Decreases BUP AUC, but no clinical effect	Opiate withdrawal form M common. M dose increase necessary
Nevirapine (NVP)	Significant effect – mean ↓ methadone AUC by 46%	Not studied	No clinical effect	Opiate withdrawal common. Methadone dose increase necessary.

PI				
Amprenavir (AMP)	↓ AUC of R-methadone by 13%	Not studied	↓ AUC by 30%	Decreases in AUC do not appear to be clinically significant
Atazanavir (ATV)	No effect	Clinically significant effect	No effect	30% develop oversedation. Slower titration upwards of buprenorphine dose advised
Fosamprenavir (fAMP)	Not studied	Not studied	Not studied	As a pro-drug of amprenavir, will likely have the same interactions noted above.
Indinavir (IND)	No effect	Not studied	↓ C_{max} between 16% and 28% and ↑ C_{min} between 50% and 100%	Differences do not appear to be clinically significant
Lopinavir/ritonavir (LPV/r)	↓ AUC by 26–36%	No clinical effect	Not studied	↓ AUC of M caused by lopinavir. One study reported opioid withdrawal symptoms in 27% of patients. M dose increase may be necessary in some patients.
Nelfinavir	↓ AUC by 40%	No clinical effect	↓ AUC of active M8 metabolite by 48%	Despite ↓ M AUC, clinical withdrawal is usually absent and a priori dosage adjustments are not needed. Decrease in AUC of M8 unlikely to be clinically significant. TDM may be useful in patients with good adherence and virologic failure.
Ritonavir (RTV)	↓ AUC by 37% in one study and no effect in another (see text)	Increases BUP AUC, but no clinical effect	Not studied	No dosage adjustment
Saquinavir (SQV)	↓ AUC by 20–32%	Not studied	Not studied	Saquinavir boosted with ritonavir studied. Despite ↓ M AUC, clinical withdrawal was not reported.
Tipranavir (TPV)	↓ M by 50%[a]	Not studied	Not reported	M may need to be increased

[a]Decrease in methadone not specified as AUC or C_{max}. NRTI, nucleoside reverse transcriptase inhibitors; NNRTI, non-nucleoside reverse transcriptase inhibitors; PI, protease inhibitor; AUC, area under curve; TDM, therapeutic drug monitoring; M, methadone; BUP, buprenorphine. (Adapted with permission from Bruce et al.[44])

lopinavir/ritonavir and methadone experienced clinical opiate withdrawal.[53] The package insert for tipranavir reports that standard dosing of tipranavir/ritonavir (500/200 mg b.i.d.) may result in a decrease in methadone levels requiring an increase in methadone dose.[67] However, atazanavir appears to have a potential pharmacodynamic interaction with buprenorphine that can lead to oversedation in some individuals. Buprenorphine can be used with atazanavir, but slower upward titration of dosing is advised with monitoring.[68,69] The protease inihibitors nelfinavir, ritonavir, and the co-formulation lopinavir/ritonavir have been studied with buprenorphine and found to be without clinically meaningful interaction.

Several medications used to treat or prevent opportunistic infections in HIV-infected individuals deserve brief comment. Rifampin, a potent inducer of cytochrome P450, produces rapid and profound reductions in methadone levels and development of opiate withdrawal; as such, rifampin should be changed to rifabutin or methadone doses increased rapidly and dramatically to avoid opiate withdrawal and discontinuation of all medications.[71] Fluconazole, a known inhibitor of cytochrome P450 metabolism, increases methadone exposure, and methadone dosage may need to be reduced.[72]

Special Issues in Prevention

Risk Reduction

The relapsing pattern of drug use and the wide array of serious infectious and other medical consequences require the development of preventive risk reduction strategies. Risk reduction does not promote injection drug use, but seeks to decrease the frequency of adverse events that are related to this practice. Risk reduction is based on the underlying principle that injection drug use is a chronic and relapsing disease which may not be cured in the individual or eliminated from society but can be conducted in a way that minimizes harm to the user and others. While complete cessation of drug use remains a laudable goal, reduction in drug use frequency and safer injection practices is more realistic for many drug users until abstinence can be achieved. Risk reduction strategies have been effectively incorporated into some drug treatment programs, syringe exchange programs and safe injection rooms.[73,74] There are several practical components inherent to risk reduction strategies. Education about and provision of drug use paraphernalia (e.g. needles and syringes) for more hygienic injection practices for the prevention of infectious complications of injection are essential. In addition to the distribution or exchange of injection equipment, these programs typically include HIVAIDS education, condom distribution, and referral or enrollment in a variety of drug treatment, medical, and social services.[75] Specifically, some programs provide onsite medical and drug treatment, resulting in reductions in emergency department use by IDUs.[76]

Provision of primary medical care services linked to drug-abuse treatment is a way to promote preventive therapies to enhance harm reduction. In this and all other clinical settings, in addition to the treatment of HIV disease and prevention of complications, injection drug users should be routinely screened for hepatitis B and C, latent *M. tuberculosis* infection, syphilis, and other sexually transmitted disease. They should be offered pneumococcal, influenza, tetanus, and hepatitis A and B immunization and (when appropriate) prophylaxis for tuberculosis.

The ultimate goal of risk-reduction strategies should be the reduction or prevention of illicit drug use itself, the development of strategies that will minimize the serious medical consequences of drug misuse, and the development of strategies that will eliminate drug misuse and its root causes. Until we are successful in this arena, we stand little chance of limiting the spread and consequences of HIV disease in this and related populations.

References

1. UNAIDS. Report on the Global HIV/AIDS Epidemic. Geneva: UNAIDS; 2002.
2. Anonymous. Risk behaviors for HIV transmission among intravenous-drug users not in drug treatment–United States, 1987–1989. MMWR 1990; 39:273–276.
3. Abdala N, Carney JM, Durante AJ, et al. Estimating the prevalence of syringe-borne and sexually transmitted diseases among injection drug users in St Petersburg, Russia. Int J Std AIDS October 2003; 14:697–703.
4. Kelly JA, Amirkhanian YA. The newest epidemic: a review of HIV/AIDS in Central and Eastern Europe. Int J Std AIDS June 2003; 14:361–371.
5. Saelim A, Geater A, Chongsuvivatwong V, et al. Needle sharing and high-risk sexual behaviors among IV drug users in Southern Thailand. AIDS Patient Care St 1998; 12:707–713.
6. Caiaffa WT, Proietti FA, Carneiro-Proietti AB, et al. Epidemiological Study of Injection Drug Users in Brazil (AjUDE-Brasil Project). The dynamics of the human immunodeficiency virus epidemics in the south of Brazil: increasing role of injection drug users. Clin Infect Dis 2003; 37(Suppl):376–381.
7. Zhang C, Yang R, Xia X, et al. High prevalence of HIV-1 and hepatitis C virus coinfection among injection drug users in the southeastern region of Yunnan, China. J Acquir Immune Defic Syndr 2002; 29:191–196.

8. World Health Organization, United Nations Office on Drugs and Crime, UNAIDS. Substitution maintenance therapy in the management of opioid dependence and HIV/AIDS prevention: position paper. World Health Organization, United Nations Office on Drugs and Crime, UNAIDS; 2004.

9. Kerr T, Wodak A, Elliott R, et al. Opioid substitution and HIV/AIDS treatment and prevention. Lancet 2004; 364:1918–1919.

10. Doran CM, Shanahan M, Mattick RP, et al. Buprenorphine versus methadone maintenance: a cost-effectiveness analysis. Drug Alcohol Depend 2003; 71:295–302.

11. Alcabes P, Friedland GH. Injection drug use and human immunodeficiency virus infection. Clin Infect Dis 1995; 20:1467–1479.

12. Dworkin MS, Williamson JM. Adult/Adolescent Spectrum of HIV Disease Project. AIDS wasting syndrome: trends, influence on opportunistic infections, and survival. J Acquir Immune Defic Syndr 2003; 33:267–273.

13. Mocroft A, Ledergerber B, Katlama C, et al. EuroSIDA study group. Decline in the AIDS and death rates in the EuroSIDA study: an observational study. Lancet 2003; 362:22–29.

14. Gebo KA, Diener-West M, Moore RD. Hospitalization rates in an urban cohort after the introduction of highly active antiretroviral therapy. J Acquir Immune Defic Syndr 2001; 27:143–152.

15. Anis AH, Guh D, Hogg RS, et al. The cost effectiveness of antiretroviral regimens for the treatment of HIV/AIDS. Pharmacoeconomics 2000; 18:393–404.

16. van Asten LC, Bourassa F, Schiffer V, et al. Limited effect of highly active antiretroviral therapy among HIV-positive injecting drug users on the population level. Eur J Public Health 2003; 13:347–349.

17. Kaplan AH, Scheyett A, Golin CE. HIV and stigma: analysis and research program. Curr HIV/AIDS Rep 2005; 2:184–188.

18. Mateu-Gelabert P, Maslow C, Flom PL, et al. Keeping it together: stigma, response, and perception of risk in relationships between drug injectors and crack smokers, and other community residents. AIDS Care 2005; 17:802–813.

19. Palepu A, Yip B, Miller C, et al. Factors associated with the response to antiretroviral therapy among HIV-infected patients with and without a history of injection drug use. AIDS 2001; 15:423–424.

20. Friedland GH. AIDS and compassion. JAMA 1998; 259:2898–2899.

21. Ball JC, Ross A. The effectiveness of methadone maintenance treatment. New York: Springer-Verlag; 1991.

22. Altice FL, Springer S, Buitrago M, et al. Pilot study to enhance HIV care using needle exchange-based health services for out-of-treatment injecting drug users. J Urban Health 2003; 80:416–427.

23. Altice FL, Mezger JA, Hodges J, et al. Developing a directly administered antiretroviral therapy intervention for HIV-infected drug users: Implications for program replication. Clin Infect Dis 2004; 38(Suppl):376–387.

24. Thompson AS, Blankenship KM, Selwyn PA, et al. Evaluation of an innovative program to address the health and social service needs of drug-using women with or at risk for HIV infection. J Community Health 1998; 23:419–440.

25. Springer SA, Pesanti E, Hodges J, et al. Effectiveness of antiretroviral therapy among HIV-infected prisoners: reincarceration and the lack of sustained benefit after release to the community. Clin Infect Dis 2004; 38:1754–1760.

26. Basu S, Bruce RD, Barry D, Altice FL. Pharmacological pain control for HIV-infected adults with a history of drug dependence. J Subs Abuse Treat 2007; in press.

27. Altice FL, Sullivan LE, Smith-Rohrberg D, et al. The potential role of buprenorphine in the treatment of opioid dependence in HIV-infected individuals and in HIV infection prevention. Clin Infect Dis 2006; 43(Suppl 4):S178–183.

28. Basu S, Smith-Rohrberg D, Bruce RD, et al. Models for integrating buprenorphine therapy into HIV care. Clin Infect Dis 2006; 42:716–721.

29. Urbina A, Jones K. Crystal methamphetamine, its analogues, and HIV infection: medical and psychiatric aspects of a new epidemic. Clin Infect Dis 2004; 38:890–894.

30. Smith-Rohrberg D, Bruce RD, Altice FL. Review of corrections based therapy for opiate-dependent patients: implications for buprenorphine treatment among correctional populations. J Drug Issues 2004; 34:451–480.

31. Dolan K, Hall W, Wodak A. Methadone maintenance reduces injecting in prison. Br Med J 1996; 312:1162.

32. Donny EC, Walsh SL, Bigelow GE, et al. High-dose methadone produces superior opioid blockade and comparable withdrawal suppression to lower doses in opioid-dependent humans. Psychopharmacology (Berl) 2002; 161:202–212.

33. Fudala PJ, Bridge TP, Herbert S, et al. Office-based treatment of opiate addiction with a sublingual-tablet formulation of buprenorphine and naloxone. N Engl J Med 2003; 349:949–958.

34. Murray JB. Effectiveness of methadone maintenance for heroin addiction. Psychol Rep 1998; 83:295–302.

35. Metzger DS, Woody GE, McLellan AT, et al. Human immunodeficiency virus seroconversion among intravenous drug users in- and out-of-treatment: an 18-month prospective follow-up. J Acquir Immune Defic Syndr 1998; 6:1049–1056.

36. Johnson RE, Chutuape MA, Strain EC, et al. A comparison of levomethadyl acetate, buprenorphine, and methadone for opioid dependence. N Engl J Med 2000; 343:1290–1297.

37. Fiellin DA, O'Connor PG. Clinical practice. Office-based treatment of opioid-dependent patients. N Engl J Med 2002; 347:817–823.

38. Liguori A, Morse WH, Bergman J. Respiratory effects of opioid full and partial agonists in rhesus monkeys. J Pharmacol Exp Ther 1996; 277:462–472.

39. Clark N, Lintzeris N, Gijsbers A, et al. LAAM maintenance vs methadone maintenance for heroin dependence. Cochrane Database Syst Rev (2), 2002:CD002210.

40. Johnson RE, Eissenberg T, Stitzer ML, et al. Buprenorphine treatment of opioid dependence: clinical trial of daily versus alternate-day dosing. Drug Alcohol Depend 1995; 40:27–35.

41. Bruce RD, Dvoryak S, Sylla L, Altice FL. HIV treatment access and scale-up for delivery of opiate substitution therapy with buprenorphine for IDUs in Ukraine – program description and policy implicaitons. Int J Drug Pol 2007: in press.

42. Greenstein RA, Evans BD, McLellan AT, et al. Predictors of favorable outcome following naltrexone treatment. Drug Alcohol Depend 1983; 12:173–180.

43. Roth A, Hogan I, Farren C. Naltrexone plus group therapy for the treatment of opiate-abusing health-care professionals. J Subst Abuse Treat 1997; 14:19–22.

44. Peck JA, Reback CJ, Yang X, et al. Sustained reductions in drug use and depression symptoms from treatment for drug abuse in methamphetamine-dependent gay and bisexual men. J Urban Health 2005; 82:i100–i108.

45. Kalichman SC, Rompa D. HIV treatment adherence and unprotected sex practices in people receiving antiretroviral therapy. Sex Trans Infect 2003; 79:59–61.

46. Bruce RD, Altice FL. Editorial comment: why treat three conditions when it is one patient? AIDS Read 2003; 13:378–379.

47. Basu S, Chwastiak LA, Bruce RD. Clinical management of depression and anxiety in HIV-infected adults. AIDS 2005; 19:2057–2067.

48. Anonymous. Treating 3 million by 2005: making it happen: the WHO Strategy: the WHO an UNAIDS global initiative to provide antiretroviral therapy to 3 million people with HIV/AIDS in developing countries by the end of 2005. Geneva: World Health Organization; 2003.

49. Bruce RD, Altice FL, Gourevitch MN, Friedland GH. Pharmacokinetic drug interactions between opioid agonist therapy and antiretroviral medications: implications and

management for clinical practice. J Acquir Immune Defic Syndr 2006; 41:563–572.

50. McCance Katz EF, Rainey PM, Friedland GH, et al. Effect of opioid dependence pharmacotherapies on zidovudine disposition. Am J Addict 2001; 10:296–307.

51. Sellers E, Lam R, McDowell J, et al. The pharmacokinetics (PK) of abacavir (ABC) and methadone (M) following co-administration: CNAA1012. Abstract No. 305. 39th Interscience Conference on Antimicrobial Agents and Chemotherapy, San Francisco, CA: 26–29 September 1999.

52. Smith P, Kearney B, Cloen D, et al. Tenofovir DF does not affect the pharmacokinetics or pharmacodynamics of methadone. Abstract no. 869. 2nd IAS Conference on HIV Pathogenesis and Treatment, Paris, France: July 2003.

53. Friedland G, Rainey P, Jatlow P, et al. Pharmacokinetics (pK) of didanosine (ddI) from encapsulated enteric coated bead formulation (EC) vs chewable tablet formulation in patients (pts) on chronic methadone therapy. 14th International AIDS Conference: 7–12 July 2002.

54. Altice FL, Friedland GH, Cooney EL. Nevirapine-induced opiate withdrawal among injection drug users with HIV infection receiving methadone. AIDS 1999; 13:957–962.

55. Clarke SM, Mulcahy FM, Tjia J, et al. The pharmacokinetics of methadone in HIV-positive patients receiving the non-nucleoside reverse transcriptase inhibitor efavirenz. Br J Clin Pharmacol 2001; 51:213–217.

56. McCance Katz E, Pade P, Friedland G, et al. Efavirenz is not associated with opiate withdrawal in buprenorphine-maintained individuals. 12th Conference on Retroviruses and Opportunistic Infections: February 2005.

57. McCance Katz EF. Antiretroviral therapy in injection drug users with HIV disease: using drug interactions to design more effective treatment. Presented at the 3rd International Workshop on Clinical Pharmacology of HIV Therapy, Washington, DC: April 2002.

58. McCance-Katz EF, Moody DE, Morse GD, et al. Interactions between buprenorphine and antiretrovirals. I. The nonnucleoside reverse-transcriptase inhibitors efavirenz and delavirdine. Clin Infect Dis 2006; 43(Suppl 4):S224–S234.

59. McCance Katz EF, Rainey PM, Friedland G, et al. The protease inhibitor lopinavir-ritonavir may produce opiate withdrawal in methadone-maintained patients. Clin Infect Dis 2003; 37:476–482.

60. Cantilena L, McCrea J, Blazes D, et al. Lack of pharmacokinetic interaction between indinavir and methadone (Abstract PI-74). Clin Pharmacol Ther 1999; 65:135.

61. Hsyu PH, Lillibridge JH, Maroldo L, et al. Pharmacokinetic(PK) and pharmacodynamic (PD) interactions between nelfinavir and methadone. Abstract No. 87 or 245. 7th Conference on Retroviruses and Opportunistic Infections, San Francisco, CA: 30 Jan–2 Feb 2000.

62. GlaxoSmithKline Product Information. Agenerase(r), amprenavir. GlaxoSmithKline, Research, Triangle Park, NC (revised September 2002).

63. Friedland GH, Andrews L, Argawala S, et al. Lack of an effect of Atazanavir on steady-state pharmacokinetics of methadone in chronically treated subjects. International Symposium on HIV and Emerging Infectious Disease, Toulon, France: June 2004.

64. Gerber JG, Rosenkranz S, Segal Y, et al. ACTG 401 Study Team. Effect of ritonavir/saquinavir on stereoselective pharmacokinetics of methadone: results of AIDS Clinical Trials Group (ACTG) 401. J Acquir Immune Defic Syndr 2001; 27:153–160.

65. Shelton MJ, Cloen D, DiFrancesco R, et al. The effects of once-daily saquinavir/minidose ritonavir on the pharmacokinetics of methadone. J Clin Pharmacol 2004; 44:293–304.

66. Clarke S, Mulcahy F, Bergin C, et al. Absence of opioid withdrawal symptoms in patients receiving methadone and the protease inhibitor lopinavir-ritonavir. Clin Infect Dis 2002; 34:1143–1145.

67. Boehringer Ingelheim Pharmaceuticals Inc. Product information: Aptivus(r), tipranavir. Boehringer Ingelheim Pharmaceuticals Inc. Rigdefield, CT (PI revised June 2005).

68. Bruce RD, Altice FL. Three case reports of a clinical pharmacokinetic interaction with buprenorphine and atazanavir plus ritonavir. AIDS 2006; 20:783–784.

69. McCance-Katz E, Pade P, Morse GD, et al. Interaction between buprenorphine and atazanavir (oral abstract). In: Program and Abstracts of the 68th Annual Meeting of the College on Problems of Drug Dependence (Phoenix). Philadelphia: College on Problems of Drug Dependence, 2006:44.

70. McCance-Katz EF, Moody DE, Smith PF, et al. Interactions between buprenorphine and antiretrovirals. II. The protease inhibitors nelfinavir, lopinavir/ritonavir, and ritonavir. Clin Infect Dis 2006; 43(Suppl 4):S235–S246.

71. Kreek MJ, Garfield JW, Gutjahr CL, et al. Rifampin induced methadone withdrawal. N Engl J Med 1976; 1976:1104–1106.

72. Cobb MN, Desai J, Brown LS, et al. The effect of fluconazole on the clinical pharmacokinetics of methadone. Clin Pharm Ther 1998; 63:655–662.

73. Broadhead RS, Altice FL. Safer Injection Facilities in North America: Their Place in Public Policy and Health Initiatives. J Drug Issues 2002; 32:329–356.

74. Broadhead RS, Borch C, van Hulst Y, et al. Safer injection sites in New York City: A utilization survey of injection drug users. J Drug Issues 2003; 33:533–538.

75. CDC. Compendium of HIV Prevention Interventions with Evidence of Effectiveness. Centers for Disease Control & Prevention. National Center or HIV, STD, and TB Prevention; 2001.

76. Pollack H, Khoshnood K, Blankenship K, et al. The impact of needle exchange-based health services on emergency department use. J Gen Int Med 2002; 17:341–348.

526

CHAPTER 45

Models of Care: HIV Care in the Urban USA

Richard D. Moore

Jeanne C. Keruly

Introduction

It is estimated that 1 million persons are infected with HIV in the USA, and approximately half of these are engaged in HIV care.[1] In the USA, most HIV care is concentrated in larger cities, reflecting the historical and current demography of the US HIV epidemic. The model of HIV care that developed in the USA was driven in large part by these demographics, and also by the strong influence of urban-based academic medical centers in the development of state-of-the-art treatment for HIV. The HIV care model has also been shaped by policies and guiding principles developed by the HIV/AIDS Bureau in the Health Resources and Services Administration (HRSA). This Bureau provides oversight of the largest governmental funds for HIV/AIDS care in the USA, the Ryan White Comprehensive AIDS Resources Emergency (CARE) Act, providing over US$2 billion dollars in 2004, and requires that an integrated and patient-centered approach be developed in centers that receive these funds.[2] In urban USA, HIV disproportionately affects vulnerable populations including the poor, minorities, underinsured, and injection drug users.[3] Ryan White CARE Act funds support medical and social services for this group. Bureau policies and principles are guided evidence indicating that integrated services and social service support improve access to care among vulnerable populations.[4-6]

The Johns Hopkins AIDS Service in Baltimore, Maryland is a large academic practice in an urban US medical center that incorporates the interests and expertise of specialists in HIV/AIDS and multiple other disciplines into an integrated framework. Importantly, it has also been shaped by external factors that include the regional epidemiology of HIV infection and the methods employed to finance HIV healthcare in Maryland and across the USA. This program will be used to describe the urban HIV care model in the USA. The Johns Hopkins AIDS Service also supports other models that are not typical of urban care centers, but support HIV care in communities of need.

The urban US model of HIV care is depicted in Figure 45.1. The USA has an economic and health infrastructure that supports the rapid introduction of novel medical therapies. This has provided those with HIV infection a wide-range of breakthrough treatments, and has simultaneously created the requirement that healthcare providers be experienced and expert in managing HIV infection, its complications, and the comorbidities associated with this disease. As the complexity of HIV treatment has grown, an increasing proportion of care in the USA has been done by specialists in HIV care.[1-8] These HIV specialists also serve as the primary care providers or HIV specialty providers for non-HIV providers in the community. As both morbidity and mortality have declined because of the effectiveness of current antiretroviral therapy,[9] HIV care must also now encompass the provision of more general medical preventive care and include treatment appropriate to the health of an aging population of women and men.

A clinical infrastructure which fosters easy access to diverse specialty care has developed in response

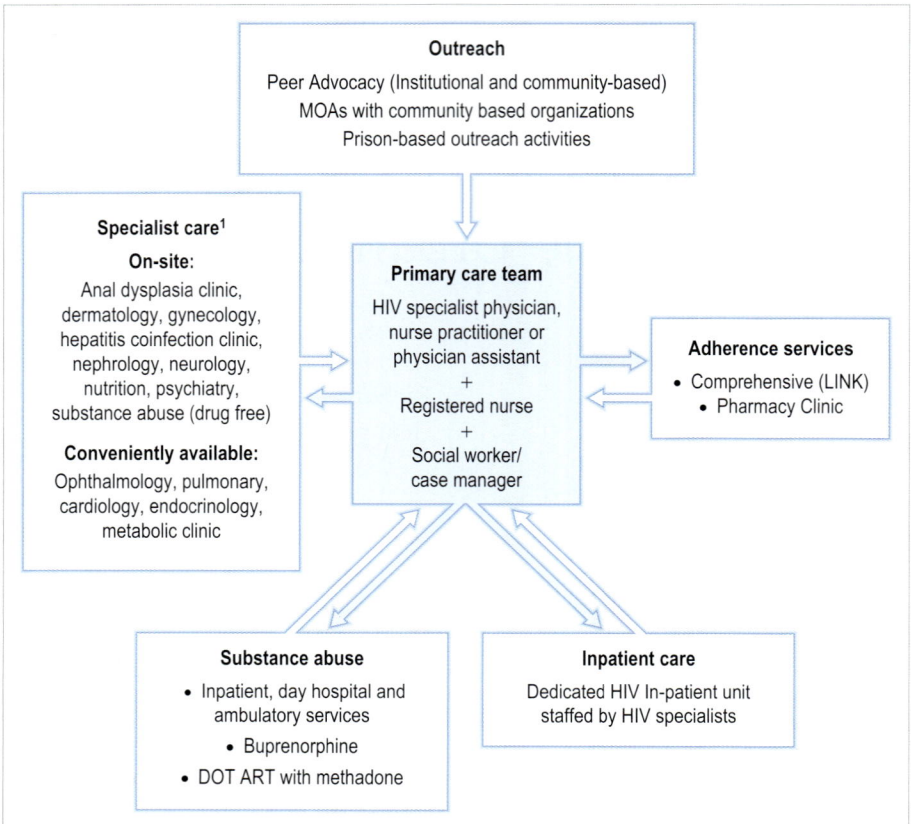

Figure 45.1 Johns Hopkins AIDS Service model of care. An example of urban US HIV care with comprehensive HIV, infectious diseases and general medical care for HIV-infected adult men and women provided in an integrated environment.

to the complex medical needs of HIV-infected persons. Under this model, comprehensive care is provided in a single location that affords prompt access to consultation with multiple disciplines, easy access to medical documentation on the patients, and the ability to modify the treatment plan based on emerging information. Specialists in endocrinology, cardiology, psychiatry, hepatology, neurology, etc. have become increasingly important for the comprehensive care of HIV-infected people. This model reflects the provision of diverse specialty care that is easily accessible to the patient and is congruent with one of the HRSA's principles to expand services to meet emerging need.[2] Highly utilized services are offered within the HIV outpatient clinic with other specialty services provided on the main medical campus. Other components of the model require accessibility after hours or extended hours to enhance access to a clinician with the goal of reducing emergency room utilization. In one study assessing emergency room use in NY Medicaid enrollees newly diagnosed with AIDS, clinics which offer on-call, evening or weekend hours, and had HIV expertise were found to have reduced use of emergency room utilization.[10]

Other disciplines and supportive services compliment the model and are critical to the long term success of treatment and access to medical services. Pharmacist evaluation and adherence support, medical coordination through registered nurse practice, and social support services through case management are major components of the HIV primary care model. Ancillary services frequently include an on site pharmacy, radiology, laboratory, and treatment room services. Patient group activities that offer counseling or general information on HIV and treatment, peer advocacy activity that encompasses outreach and adherence support provide additional depth to the program. Programmatic detail that is exemplary of this model of care is provided below.

The Johns Hopkins AIDS Service was founded in January 1984, as the first organized HIV clinical care service in Maryland, and it remains the largest care provider for HIV-infected persons in the region, having delivered care to over 10 000 patients since 1984. Urban HIV care in the USA reflects the demographics of poverty and minority race/ethnicity found in many inner-urban US cities. The Johns Hopkins Hospital is no different in that it is located in a census tract with a median household income that is only 1.5 times the poverty level for Maryland. In his bequest of US$7 million in 1873 to establish the University and Hospital that bears his name, Mr Johns Hopkins' will stated that the hospital was to 'compare favorably with any institution of like character in this country or in Europe' and, remarkably for its time, the hospital was to treat 'the poor of this city and state, of all races'.

The Johns Hopkins AIDS Service has approximately 27 000 patient visits/year for 3400 patients (Table 45.1). Most are from the Baltimore metropolitan area and their demographics reflect the regional HIV epidemic. The total number of HIV and AIDS cases reported in Maryland through to 31 December 2004 was 44 123.[11] In 2004, Maryland ranked ninth among the 50 states and DC in cumulative AIDS cases, and fourth in AIDS incidence (26.1 cases/100 000 population). Baltimore has the fifth highest AIDS case incidence rate of any major metropolitan area, 32.8/100 000 population. There are an estimated 40 000 injection drug users in Baltimore, and the city ranks third among US cities in drug-related emergency room visits. The predominant risk category for HIV transmission is injection drug use, accounting for 41% of all reported AIDS cases. African-Americans account for 83% of all cases, with women accounting for 37% of cases. With regard to third party payor, 60% are Medicaid recipients, 34% are 'no pay' and 6% have some form of commercial insurance. Approximately 5% of patients are homeless, but many more have no stable residence.

Although the clinic in the medical center is the largest practice site within the AIDS Service, satellite programs were implemented to address emerging and HIV medical care needs outside of the urban community (Fig. 45.2). This feature of the Johns Hopkins AIDS Service reflects the role that many US academic-affiliated HIV care centers have played in providing expanded clinical services to the surrounding communities and region. Although one model is for the HIV-infected person to travel to the urban-care center, the alternative model is for the provision of care in suburban and rural settings under the direct supervision of the central urban

Table 45.1 Characteristics of patients of the Johns Hopkins HIV clinical practice

	(%)
Age at enrollment	
Median	38 (years)
Range	18–97 (years)
Sex	
Male	69
Female	31
Race	
White	21
Black	76
Hispanic	1
Asian/other	1
HIV transmission route	
Injecting drug use (IDU) only	22
Homosexual only	25
Heterosexual contact only	25
IDU and heterosexual contact	21
IDU and homosexual contact	5
Other (including unknown routes)	2
Time from diagnosis of HIV to clinic enrollment	435 (median days)
History of AIDS-defining illness at enrollment	29
Antiretroviral naive at clinic enrollment	55
CD4 count at clinic enrollment (cells/mm^3)	
≤50	21
51–200	21
201–500	37
>500	22
Viral load at enrollment (copies/mL)	
<10 000	40
10 000–50 000	24
50 000–100 000	10
>100 000	26
Axis-1 mental disorder	26
Hepatitis C antibody positive	53

clinic. As an example, in 1994 a program was developed to provide HIV care in the surrounding counties. A team of HIV specialty providers, along with registered nursing and support staff, travel to 11 health department clinics in five suburban and three rural counties to deliver primary HIV care. The model used in the rural county program is also known as 'share-care' model, where the HIV specialist provides longitudinal follow-up that is HIV focused with a rural clinician providing the majority of care.[12,13] In both the surrounding county and rural

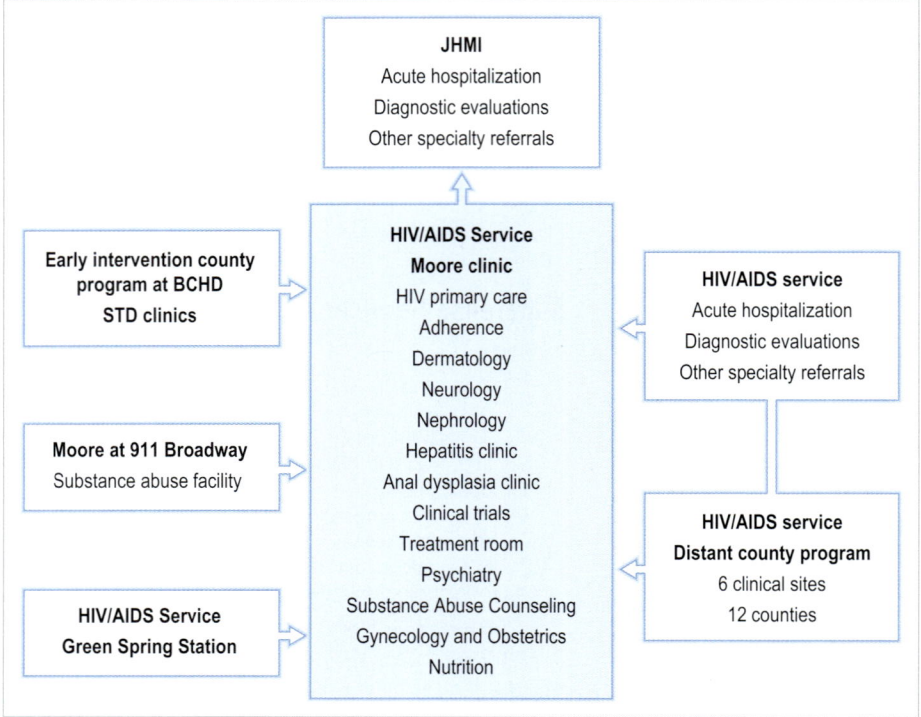

Figure 45.2 Organization of existing Johns Hopkins AIDS Service clinical programs.

program, the support services are provided by the health department staff, offering case management/advocacy on site in the respective health departments. In total, 650 patients access services through this satellite program. In 1997, HIV primary care services were extended to Baltimore County, which is contiguous to the city and has the second largest number of HIV cases in Maryland. This clinic is located in one of the Johns Hopkins larger ambulatory practice sites and has an access to extensive referral network. A small but critical satellite is located within a substance abuse facility, located two blocks from the main clinic and offers HIV care by HIV specialists.

In addition, there are linkages for specialty care with the Baltimore City Health Department's two STD clinics. Clinicians from the STD program provide early intervention HIV care in the STD clinic. Patients requiring more intensive and tertiary services transition to the Johns Hopkins HIV Clinic, while retaining the same primary care provider. This affords continuity of care while minimizing the anxiety of moving to a new facility for care. The uniqueness of this model is that all of these affiliated clinics have access to the totality of what is offered

on the main campus, providing for specialty care outside of HIV care that cannot easily be found in the community

Finally, this HIV care program makes use of collaborative relationships with community based organizations for referral of new patients. Full time peer advocates serve in an outreach capacity to counsel and support clients who are in need of services but are out of care. Peer activities extend to the acute inpatient facility and emergency room, supporting newly diagnosed patients who having difficulty adjusting to their diagnosis, and to patients in the ambulatory program who have fallen out of care. Outreach staff also liaison with the consumer advisory board and facilitate/organize a variety of patient education functions.

The remainder of this chapter will describe in more detail the specific components of an integrated HIV care model.

Primary HIV Care

This model of delivering primary HIV care is based on a team approach that combines a medical provider with a nurse and social worker. At Johns Hopkins, HIV primary care is provided by infectious diseases-trained physicians, generalists and mid-level practitioners (nurse practitioners and physician assistants) who specialize in HIV medicine. When trained and experienced in HIV medicine, each of these are effective providers of HIV care.[14,15]

Specialty Services

HIV infection and its associated co-morbidities affect multiple organ systems. The integration of sub-specialty care into HIV care is an efficient way to address these needs and provide the patient with the efficient delivery of comprehensive medical care. At Johns Hopkins, these sub-specialists include psychiatry/psychology, neurology, gynecology, dermatology, viral hepatitis, nephrology, endocrinology and gastroenterology. One study from an academic center provides evidence that the HIV multidisciplinary approach to on-site supportive care is effective in improving access to and retention in HIV primary care.[6] The effectiveness of a multidisciplinary specialty care on HIV clinical outcomes has not been assessed to date.

Because of the relatively high rate of axis-1 mental disorders, provision of on-site psychiatric service may be of particular importance. At Johns Hopkins, this service is staffed both by psychiatrists, psychologists and nurse therapists and is offered 5 days/week. A full-range of mental health and substance abuse care is provided, including inpatient and day-hospital care. Data from our clinical program demonstrates that patients with a mental disorder who are co-managed by psychiatry on-site have higher rates of HAART utilization and better clinical outcomes.[16]

Substance abuse accounts for a particularly prominent proportion of HIV transmission in urban USA. There is evidence of a relatively high prevalence of relapse and continuing use of illicit drugs which interferes with antiretroviral adherence, viral suppression and immunologic recovery.[17] Substance abuse care can be integrated with HIV care to potentially maximize the management of these co-morbidities. Johns Hopkins has done this by establishing an on-site HIV clinic within our hospital's substance abuse treatment clinic to provide HIV care at the same facility for which substance abuse care and methadone treatment is being delivered. This has been the location of a program to provide directly observed antiretroviral treatment (DOT-ART) to our patients in the setting of methadone maintenance.

This program has now provided DOT-ART to 60 patients. Compared with patients who are not in DOT-ART, this program has been successful in suppressing viral load and improving immune response. We have also implemented a HRSA-funded program of buprenorphine management of opiate abuse on-site in our main HIV clinic, further enhancing the ability to offer effective substance abuse care in conjunction with HIV treatment.[18]

Adherence Services

Adherence has emerged as one of the most important factors in the effectiveness of antiretroviral therapy.[19,20] This incorporation of adherence services into HIV practice is an important part of this care model. These services can be staffed by pharmacists, nurses, social workers and peer counselors. At Johns Hopkins, on-site adherence support is provided by clinical pharmacists who offer adherence evaluation, drug-drug interaction evaluation and dosing recommendations, medication tailoring and longitudinal support. An educational and training program for Fuzeon administration is managed by this service. A more intensive patient-tailored adherence support program is offered that includes a nurse educator, social support services and peer counseling. This readiness program that comprehensively assesses a patient's needs and develops a tailored plan for the introduction and maintenance of treatment. This more intensive program is targeted to patients who are identified with significant social, behavioral and economic needs.

Social Services

Poverty is a hallmark of HIV infection in inner-urban USA, and the need for comprehensive social services support has been integral in the delivery of effective HIV care. It is common that multiple social workers will support the operation of an urban HIV service. For example, at Johns Hopkins seven full-time social workers provide services. All patients are evaluated by social services at clinic enrollment, and approximately 70% of patients continue to access social work services longitudinally. As an outgrowth of this need, case management is based on a primary care model of care delivery which includes a comprehensive care plan for an enrollee who is a member of a special needs population (HIV/AIDS is legally defined as special needs in Maryland and several other states) and which uses a coordinated and continuous case management approach, involving the enrollee and, as appropriate, the enrollee's family, guardian, or caregiver, in all aspects of care, including primary, acute, tertiary, and home care. Case management services are mostly centered in the coordination of social support services while medical needs are coordinated through the primary care nurse. Case management activities typically include:

1. Providing an initial and on-going needs assessment to develop of a comprehensive, individualized care plan.
2. Linking the patient with the full range of available benefits.
3. Linking the patient with any additional needed services including: mental health, substance abuse, social, financial, counseling, educational, housing, and other required support services.
4. Ensuring timely and coordinated access to medically necessary and appropriate levels of care that support continuity of care across the continuum of service providers.
5. Initial and on-going assessment of the individual's needs with development of a comprehensive, individualized care plan that uses a multidisciplinary approach.
6. Linking to community substance abuse services when not available within the clinic or usual referral site.

Inpatient Care

Prior to HAART, AIDS-defining illness accounted for the admission diagnoses of over 80% of these patients. Almost 50% of the costs of care were accounted for by inpatient services.[21] Early in the US epidemic, Johns Hopkins established a dedicated AIDS inpatient unit which averaged 700–800 admissions/year and was staffed by an attending physician from the ID Division, an ID fellow who serves as chief resident, three Hopkins house staff and one or two sub-interns or students.

With the advent of HAART, the number of hospital days declined significantly as the outpatient visit rate simultaneously increased (Fig. 45.3). Since 1998, admissions have been maintained at a constant level, by both the large number of patients who are first diagnosed with advanced HIV and who present with an AIDS-defining illness, or other comorbidity such as viral hepatitis requiring hospital admission (Fig. 45.4).[22] The inpatient unit continues to serve an important role in HIV care at our facility by focusing specialized medical, nursing, social, nutritional and pharmacy services in a cost-effective manner. However, dedicated units such as this do not exist at all urban HIV care locations in the USA.

Other important components of a cost-effective comprehensive HIV service include an infusion/treatment room for discharged patients to receive specific treatments that cannot be arranged through

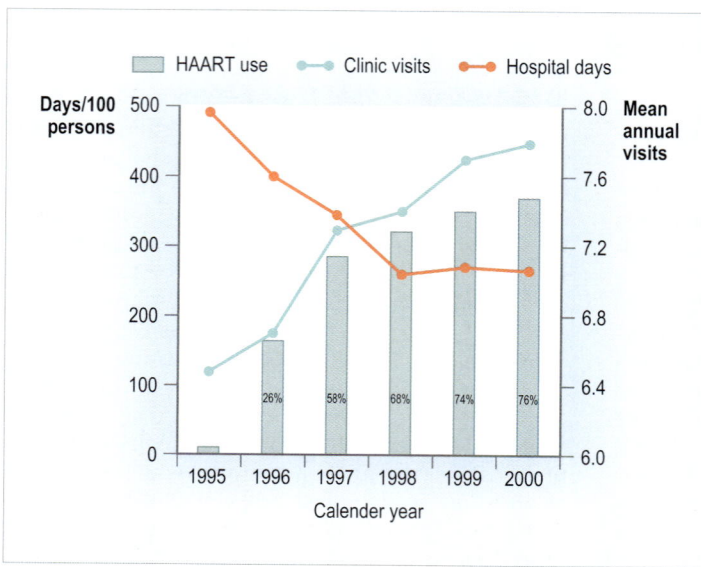

Figure 45.3 Healthcare resource use in HIV-infected persons from the Johns Hopkins AIDS Service.

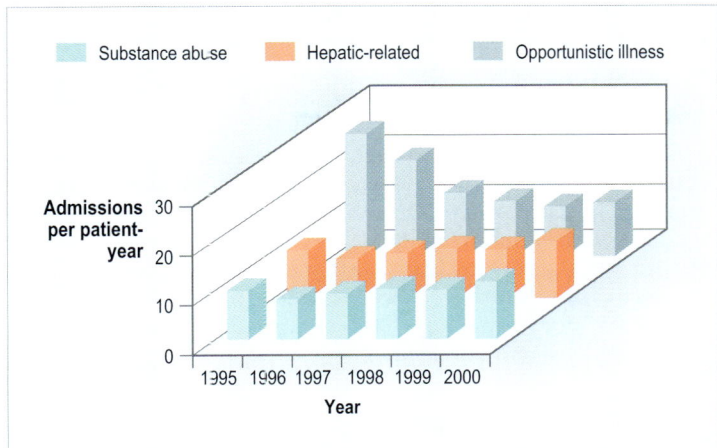

Figure 45.4 Principal diagnosis associated with hospitalization for patients of the Johns Hopkins AIDS Service.

home care. This site can also be used for ambulatory diagnostic procedures such as lumbar puncture and fine needle aspirations, and for hydration, blood transfusion and patient teaching for injection. Acute-care services can be offered, eliminating the need for many emergency room evaluations.

Clinical Research

Particularly in academic HIV care settings, research is an engine that has driven the remarkable growth in new and effective treatments for HIV. The National Institutes of Allergy and Infectious Diseases (NIAID)-sponsored AIDS Clinical Trials Units have been a part of the infrastructure of urban academic HIV care sites since 1987. In addition, multiple pharmaceutical industry-supported clinical trials have been conducted. The inner urban setting also provides the opportunity for participation in trials by minority race/ethnicity, women and injection drug users. For example, participation by these groups in clinical trials has been relatively high at Johns Hopkins, with 84% African-Americans, 19% women, and 22% with IDU as their risk group.

Observational AIDS research has also been an important component of our understanding of the natural history of HIV infection and disease since the founding of the Muticenter AIDS Cohort Study in 1986.[23] This is the model of an interval or classical cohort in which a population-specific characteristics is identified, enrolled, and then followed longitudinally over time with the interval collection of data relevant to the progression of the disease process. An alternative type of cohort study based within the clinical setting has emerged over the past decade to directly assess HIV care and the outcomes of care as it is practiced.[24] These so-called 'real-world' clinical cohorts are nested within a clinical care site and are designed to observe and record a wide variety of variables that allow the assessment of the utilization, benefits and toxicities of therapy, and the effect of therapy on the natural history of clinical HIV disease. These have been established in a number of care sites in North America, Europe, and around the world. Johns Hopkins established one of the first of these clinical cohorts in 1989 to collect HIV outcomes information. The Johns Hopkins data collection process was designed to capture a comprehensive array of sociodemographic, clinical, and therapeutic data as patients receive longitudinal care in the clinical setting. Included are laboratory, diagnostic, clinical, pharmaceutical, and demographic data collected in detail at the time of enrollment; these data are updated by full-time chart abstractors using outpatient and inpatient medical records, and by the Johns Hopkins Health System automated databases, vital records, insurance claims data and patient or provider interviews. The cohort has been the source of important information regarding resource utilization, cost of care, frequency of complications and comparative data across risk categories and other patient variables.[25]

Quality Assurance

Guidelines for the management of HIV infection have been an integral part of the care of HIV-infected persons for the past decade.[26] Standards of care are established for use of antiretroviral therapy and for prophylaxis and treatment of opportunistic illness, and a highly visible and aggressive program for adherence/compliance is in operation. These guidelines, and care guides such as *Medical Management of HIV Infection*[27] serve as 'clinical protocols' for HIV treatment. At Johns Hopkins, other quality assurance measures include regular reviews of the medical records of all providers to determine compliance with standards of care with emphasis on appropriate laboratory monitoring, preventative services and use of antiretroviral drugs. Feedback is provided to individual providers and patterns of poor performance become the subject of weekly conferences. There is a weekly provider conference to review the rapidly evolving medical information and case reviews. In addition, the annual Hopkins HIV Care Program conference is a 2-day review, which is mandatory for providers and strongly encouraged for support and ancillary staff. This conference is also attended by providers from throughout the region, which fosters a collaborative regional approach to HIV care.

Using the HIV Cohort data, both process and outcomes data can be collected. Assessments are done for survival, HIV-related complications, co-morbid conditions, resource utilization, quality of life, etc. Administrative decisions and practice guidelines have been fostered by critical examination and analyses using these observational data. At Johns Hopkins, overall program performance is monitored by a senior leadership committee with regular feedback to providers. Patient satisfaction surveys are conducted regularly by an independent agent; our program is compared with other clinics within the institution, regionally, and nationally. Surveys that are specific to address the concerns of the agencies responsible for distribution of clinical funds are conducted twice yearly with the support of the consumer advisory board.

A grievance process exists for patients to report complaints related to quality of care, expectations of services, and/or enrollment issues. The process requires a formal statement completed by the member and reviewed by the Program Administrator and Medical Director. All grievances and corresponding resolutions are documented and reported to the Medical Advisory Committee. Any grievance that cannot be resolved to the member's satisfaction will be referred to the Medical Advisory Committee for resolution.

Consumer and Community Advisory Boards

Community activism and participation has been a cornerstone of HIV care in the USA since early in the epidemic. Both clinical care and clinical research are commonly overseen by a Community or Patient Advisory Board (CAB) comprised of consumers of the HIV program and concerned members of the HIV community. Responsibilities include community linkage through local meetings, public relations, liaison with HIV service organizations and administration of the Community Advisory Board composed of patients and community leaders. Administrative staff may meet with the CAB to address concerns and to discuss strategies for making the clinical practice more consumer-friendly.

Financing HIV Care

In the USA, financing of healthcare is a composite system that can present barriers to care, particularly for high-cost illness, such as HIV. Unlike many Western countries, a universal healthcare delivery and financing system does not exist. Historically, employers have been responsible for much of the payment for healthcare; thus, the unemployed or underemployed are at risk for healthcare to be inaccessible or rationing of care when it is accessed. The spiraling costs of delivering healthcare in the USA present further financial barriers. Recent estimates indicate monthly costs ranging from US$512 for patients with a CD4 >500 cells to US$2344 for patients with a CD4 <50 cells.[1] As noted earlier, urban HIV care in the USA is predominantly the care of indigent patients, and therefore the major funder of HIV care is through state or federally supported programs. At the end of calendar year 2004, the insurance type of patients in The Johns Hopkins program was predominantly federal and state government, with <15% of the support from private and commercial sources.

Medicaid, a joint federal/state supported program to provide medical insurance to the poor, is the primary payer for approximately 53% of all adult patients with AIDS and approximately 90% of pediatric patients with HIV infection.[28] In the late 1990s, the growth of the Medicaid budget was ~10% per annum, attributed to both the increase in medical care costs and the number of low income persons who became eligible of Medicaid benefits. As a mechanism to reduce costs, Medicaid in a number of states has moved to a capitated managed-care model. Maryland was one the first states in the USA to move to a capitated Medicaid model in 1997.

Many states approached the issue of the high cost population with the assumption that managed care organizations would serve large patient populations in which the high cost users would be appropriately diluted by patients who have modest medical care requirements, thus providing an equalizing effect to achieve a reasonable economic balance. However, a single standard rate would be financially untenable if a high proportion of patients had exceptionally high costs, as was the situation with HIV/AIDS. The state of Maryland realized this and implemented a special AIDS capitation rate which was based on the historic experience with Medicaid payments for adult patients with AIDS. The rate for patients with AIDS was set at US$2161 per member per month (pmpm) for Baltimore City residents and US$1812 pmpm for Maryland residents outside of Baltimore. (The State used geographic residence as a proxy for socioeconomic adjustment.) Since its initial implementation, the rate has been adjusted to reflect actual expenditure data and to adjust for other co-morbidities, with a rate of US$3185 pmpm for City residents and US$2721 pmpm for other Maryland residents. Additionally, special capitation rate was approved for patients with HIV.

Even with this risk-adjusted rate, most clinical HIV programs could not maintain its existence and provide the depth of service without access to clinical care funds for the uninsured. Ryan White Comprehensive AIDS Resources Emergency (CARE) Act funding has been an integral component of financing of HIV care in the USA since 1991. For fiscal year 2006, it supported over US$2 billion of the HIV care delivered in the USA. Typical of most urban HIV care sites, 50% of new patients to the Johns Hopkins program lack any insurance and approximately 38% of patients who are on Medicaid will lapse in insurance necessitating some bridge funds to access care critical. The majority of funds (78%) is directed at supporting ambulatory clinical care, however other funding supports medication adherence (9%), the purchase of medications or co-payments for medicines (4%), outreach (3%), social work services (2%) and transportation (1%). Clinical care funding supports primary care providers, specialty providers and registered nurses who provide on-site care in the programs. Approximately 20% of the budget for ambulatory care is allocated for laboratory and radiology and 'vouchered' specialty services that are less commonly used.

Recipients of Ryan White clinical funds for the uninsured are contractually obligated to meet standards of care established by the Ryan White administrative agents of the respective Titles. Guiding principles established by HRSA for safe and accessible care for vulnerable populations are routinely monitored through site visits and an independent quality improvement program conducted by the Title I grantee.

Conclusion

As one of the oldest clinical services providing HIV care in the USA, the Johns Hopkins AIDS Service is an example of urban HIV care in the USA. The philosophy of providing both expert and comprehensive integrated care is the core of this HIV care model. Within this framework, quality care can be provided in an urban location with a high population rate of HIV-infection, as well as through an outreach network in suburban and rural areas where there is a relatively low population infection rate. Although many of these integrated services are important for the care of anyone with HIV, the demographics of HIV infection in an urban setting further define the expertise and ancillary services that we deliver. All of this is done within a national healthcare financing structure that leaves millions without healthcare payment and where a natural tension exists between cost and quality.

It should be noted that there is no consensus on the definition of an HIV/AIDS expert. This reflects the failure to define expertise on the basis of training criteria with a qualifying specialty board. Alternative criteria include >50 patients (lifetime of practice), adequate performance on a standardized test, adequate continuing education in HIV/AIDS.

References

1. Bozzette SA, Joyce G, McCaffrey DF, et al. Expenditures for the care of HIV-infected patients in the era of highly active antiretroviral therapy. N Engl J Med 2001; 344:817–823.
2. HRSA. Online. Available: http://hab.hrsa.gov/reports/funding.html (accessed 16 January, 2007).
3. Shapiro MF, Moron SC, McCaffrey DF, et al. Variations in the care of HIV-infected adults in the United States: results from the HIV Cost and Services Utilization Study. JAMA 1999; 281:2305–2315.
4. Soto TA, Bell J, Pillen MB. HIV/AIDS Treatment Adherence, Health Outcomes and Cost Study Group. Literature on integrated HIV care: a review. AIDS Care 2004; 16:43–55.
5. Messeri PA, Abramson DM, Aidala AA, et al. The impact of ancillary HIV services on engagement in medical care in New York City. AIDS Care 2002; 14:15–29.
6. Sherer R, Stieglitz K, Narra J, et al. HIV multidisciplinary teams work: support services improve access to and retention in HIV primary care. AIDS Care 2002; 14:S31–S44.
7. Kitahata MM, Koepsell TD, Dyo RA, et al. Physicians' experience with the acquired immunodeficiency syndrome as a factor in patient' survival. N Engl J Med 1996; 334:701–706.
8. Kitahata MM, Rompaey SE Van, Dillingham PW, et al. Primary care delivery is associated with greater physician

experience and improved survival among persons with AIDS. J Gen Intern Med 2003; 18:95–103.

9. Pallela F, Delaney KM, Moorman AC, et al. Declining morbidity and mortality among patients with advanced human immunodeficiency virus infection. HIV Outpatient Study Invest. N Engl J Med 1998; 338:853–860.

10. Markson LE, Houchens R, Fanning TR, et al. Repeated emergency department use by HIV-infected persons: effect of clinic accessibility and expertise in HIV care. J Acquir Immune Defic Syndr Hum Retrovirol 1998; 17:35–41.

11. AIDS Administration. The Maryland 2003 HIV/AIDS Annual Report. Maryland Department of Health and Mental Hygiene, 2003.

12. Graham RP, Forrester ML, Wysong JA, et al. HIV/AIDS in the rural United States: epidemiology and health services delivery. Med Care Res Rev 1995; 52:435–452.

13. Grace C, Soons K, Kutzko D, et al. Service Delivery for patients with HIV in a rural state: The Vermont Model. AIDS Patient Care STDs 1999; 13:659–666.

14. Wilson IB, Landon BE, Hirschhorn LR, et al. Quality of HIV care provided by nurse practitioners, physician assistants, and physicians. Ann Intern Med 2005; 143:729–736.

15. Landon BE, Wilson IB, McInnes K, et al. Physician specialization and the quality of care for human immunodeficiency virus infection. Arch Int Med 2005; 165:1133–1139.

16. Himelhoch S, Moore RD, Treisman G, et al. Does presence of an identified mental disorder in AIDS patients affect the initiation of antiretroviral treatment and duration of therapy? J Acquir Immune Defic Syndr 2004; 37:1457–1463.

17. Lucas G, Weidle PJ, Hader S, et al. Directly administered antiretroviral therapy in an urban methadone maintenance clinic: a nonrandomized comparative study. Clin Infect Dis 2004; 38:409–413.

18. Lucas GF. Buprenorphine in primary HIV care clinics: a big pill to swallow. Hopkins HIV Rep 2004; 16:5–7.

19. Paterson DL, Swindells S, Mohr J, et al. Adherence to protease inhibitor therapy and outcomes in patients with HIV infection. Ann Intern Med 2000; 133:21–30.

20. Bartlett JA. Addressing the challenges of adherence. J Acquir Immune Defic Syndr 2002; 29:2–10.

21. Hellinger F. The lifetime cost of treating a person with HIV. JAMA 1993; 270:474–478.

22. Gebo K, Diener-West M, Moore R. Hospitalization rates differ by hepatitis C status in an urban HIV cohort. J Acquir Immune Defic Syndr 2003; 34:165–173.

23. JHSPH. Online. Available: www.statepi.jhsph.edu/index. html (accessed 14 January, 2006).

24. Phillips AN, Grabar S, Tassie JM, et al. Use of observational databases to evaluate the effectiveness of antiretroviral therapy for HIV infection: comparison of cohort studies with randomized trials. EuroSIDA, the French Hospital Database on HIV and the Swiss HIV Cohort Study Groups. AIDS 1999; 13:2075–2082.

25. Moore RD. Understanding the clinical and economic outcomes of HIV therapy: the Johns Hopkins HIV clinical practice cohort. J Acquir Immune Defic Syndr Hum Retrovirol 1998; 17:38–41.

26. NIH. Online. Available: http://aidsinfo.nih.gov/Guidelines (accessed 13 January, 2006).

27. Bartlett J, Gallant J. Medical management of HIV infection. Baltimore, MD: Johns Hopkins Medicine Health Publishing Business Group; 2005.

28. Hellinger FJ. Cost and financing of care for persons with HIV disease: an overview. Healthcare Financ Rev 1998; 19:5–18.

CHAPTER 46

Antiretroviral Therapy of Drug-resistant HIV

Marianne Harris
P. Richard Harrigan
Julio S. G. Montaner

Introduction

Aims of HIV Treatment – Virologic Success and Failure

The goal of antiretroviral therapy is to achieve full suppression of HIV replication on a long-term basis. Full suppression of HIV replication is defined as an HIV-1-RNA level in plasma below the limit of quantification of the most sensitive commercial assays (typically <50 copies/mL). Fully adherent HAART-treated patients can be expected to maintain full suppression of HIV replication on a long-term basis, even if low-level plasma HIV-1-RNA (below 50 copies/mL) can be demonstrated when more sensitive experimental assays are used. Such low HIV-1-RNA levels are not associated with viral evolution and do not promote the emergence of resistant HIV variants in the short term. In fact, it has recently been suggested that this is the case even when isolated transient low-level 'blips' in plasma HIV-1-RNA levels (below 200 copies/mL) are detected.[1]

In contrast, HIV mutants with reduced susceptibility to antiretroviral drugs emerge promptly during partially suppressive therapy, as is usually the case when inadequate antiviral pressure is allowed to exist. Resistant HIV variants typically are persistent (even if they cannot be detected using standard drug resistance assays), and may re-emerge rapidly in the future when the selective conditions are favourable.[1,2]

Patient management depends on the extent of resistance mutations that have accumulated. If there is evidence of viral strains which are resistant to only one or two drugs (which is often the case after failure of first- or second-line therapy), current guidelines provide adequate recommendations based on replacing the failing drugs with three new active drugs, usually including at least one agent from a class to which that patient has not previously been exposed.[3,4] However, regimen standards are poorly-defined as patients move beyond first- and second-line regimens. After failure of several highly active antiretroviral therapy (HAART) regimens, a patient may harbor viral strains with reduced susceptibility to multiple drugs from several available drug classes, and the selection of an effective regimen becomes more challenging. Alternatively, there may be no evidence of resistance if the patient has been sufficiently non-adherent to therapy.

The management of patients with extensive HIV drug resistance is critically dependent on a thorough understanding of the determinants of prior treatment failure and resistance. It is critical to emphasize that chances for success with the next regimen are seriously hampered unless the prior determinants of treatment failure are dealt with adequately.

Assessing Determinants of Treatment Failure

Once HIV-1-RNA viral rebound has been confirmed by consecutive detectable plasma viral loads, the next step in patient assessment is to delineate the reasons why this has occurred, to avoid repeating the same mistakes and to help design an effective next regimen. Broadly, treatment failure and the consequent emergence of HIV resistant variants can be attributed to:

1. Patient factors (e.g. incomplete adherence).
2. Treatment factors (e.g. low potency regimens or drug interactions).
3. Viral factors (e.g. pre-existing decreased susceptibility as in primary infection with drug resistant virus or following exposure to partially suppressive therapy).

Patients may be unwilling or unable to take their antiretroviral drug regimens as prescribed. Irregular compliance and missed doses (even if infrequent) are a common cause of treatment failure and provide fertile ground for the development of drug-resistant HIV. Patients may be insufficiently motivated to take antiretrovirals correctly for a number of reasons, including inadequate preparation or psychological factors such as depression. Other psychosocial factors (including homelessness or active substance abuse), drug intolerances (e.g. nausea, fatigue, headache) or toxicities (e.g. peripheral neuropathy) may likewise render it difficult or impossible for patients to maintain the strict levels of adherence required for successful antiretroviral therapy. Complex regimens, such as those which entail a high pill burden and inconvenient schedules or food restrictions, may also conspire against consistent adherence. The situation is often further complicated by symptoms of co-morbid conditions (hepatitis C, addictions) and medications taken concomitantly to treat those conditions. While a complete medical and psychosocial history may delineate some of the contributing factors mentioned above, no standardized procedure exists for assessing a patient's motivation or adherence to antiretrovirals. Clearly a trusting physician–patient relationship is key in assessing the degree of adherence, determining the reasons why it may be suboptimal, and establishing a regimen best suited to the individual patient.[5] It is imperative to deal with these issues before moving on to the next regimen. Failure to do so will invariably compromise the chances for success with the next regimen, due to resistance mutations which accumulate during periods of suboptimal adherence, or (in patients with no evidence of drug-resistant virus) due to continued non-adherence.

For antiretroviral drugs to exert their maximum effect, they need to achieve adequate levels in the blood and target tissues. Aside from incomplete adherence, sub-therapeutic drug levels may be caused by malabsorption or drug-to-drug interactions. The absorption of some antiretroviral drugs is affected by whether they are taken with food or in a fasting state. Gastrointestinal symptoms such as diarrhea may cause chronic or intermittent poor drug absorption. Plasma drug levels can be significantly affected by pharmacokinetic interactions between antiretroviral drugs and concomitant medications, including other antiretroviral drugs, other prescription and over-the-counter medications, herbal products and supplements. For example, co-administration of the herbal products St John's wort or garlic supplements have been shown to significantly reduce plasma levels of some protease inhibitors.[6,7] A thorough medical and medication history can often identify some of these factors. A high degree of suspicion should be maintained in this area as antiretroviral drug interactions are often poorly understood and often not fully characterized, particularly when new drugs first become available for use in the clinic. This issue is further compounded by the plethora of non-medicinal and alternative therapies often used in the setting of HIV disease. Measurement of plasma levels of antiretroviral drugs is the most direct way of assessing the adequacy of drug levels and the effect of pharmacokinetic interactions; however, therapeutic drug monitoring in the context of antiretroviral therapy remains fraught with a number of issues.[8] These issues include: lack of access to the tests in some areas, uncertainty around the definition of target levels for individual agents in individual patients (particularly in the presence of varying degrees of HIV drug resistance), and technical difficulty in measuring intracellular levels of tri-phosphates, the active form of nucleoside reverse transcriptase inhibitors.

With the availability of a wide range of effective antiretroviral combinations, suboptimal regimen potency should not be a major issue, as long as therapy is prescribed in accordance with current guidelines.[3,4,9] However, therapeutic guidelines are subject to rapid evolution as new clinical trial data emerge. For example, initial treatment regimens consisting of triple nucleosides or those containing two nucleosides and an un-boosted protease inhibitor, while recommended in previous guidelines, have now been identified as being less potent than other treatment options currently available.[10–12] It is therefore not uncommon to encounter patients who have developed virological failure and eventually resistance, while being fully adherent to contemporary treatment guidelines. This is also the case for patients originally treated with single or double nucleosides, or for those treated with sequential addition of new drugs to a failing regimen, among others. Even if resistance testing was not done or unavailable at those times, these patients should be considered at high risk for harboring virus resistant to the components of the previously used partially suppressive regimens.

Emergence of Drug-resistant HIV during Treatment Failure

Whatever the underlying mechanism, insufficient drug pressure is associated with ongoing viral replication in the presence of drug. While this may be initially associated with wild-type virus circulating in plasma, selection of pre-existing mutants with decreased susceptibility to the specific drugs in the failing regimen eventually occurs. The time required to select for resistant mutants will depend on the genetic barrier posed by the regimen. Different drugs have different characteristics in this regard. The non-nucleoside reverse transcriptase inhibitors (NNRTIs) efavirenz and nevirapine have a low genetic barrier to the development of resistance. These agents can rapidly select for pre-existing single point mutations associated with decreased susceptibility to the NNRTI class, following which no residual antiviral activity on the part of these drugs can be expected. A similar phenomenon exists for enfuvirtide, with resistant mutants having no residual susceptibility to this agent.[13,14] Other agents, such as ritonavir-boosted protease inhibitors (PIs) provide a higher genetic barrier, requiring the accumulation of multiple mutations before a significant decrease in HIV-1 drug susceptibility to the specific PI can be demonstrated. Hence, *in vivo* antiviral potency decreases more gradually with the accumulation of resistance mutations for ritonavir-boosted protease inhibitors, as has been elegantly demonstrated for lopinavir/ritonavir.[15] In contrast, the nucleoside analog reverse transcriptase inhibitors lamivudine (3TC) and emtricitabine (FTC) offer a different pattern, with rapid development of *in vitro* resistance with the emergence of the 184V mutation and partial retention of antiviral potency *in vivo*.[16,17] The latter phenomenon has been at least partially attributed to the fact that some drug-resistant HIV mutants can be associated with decreased viral fitness.[18] From a practical standpoint, this is best illustrated by the fact that the plasma HIV-1 RNA levels tend to remain partially suppressed compared to pre-treatment levels following the emergence of resistance. Similarly, other nucleosides such as zidovudine and abacavir tend to have significant residual antiretroviral effect after the first emergence of *in vitro* resistance.

Over time, however, continued viral evolution allows for new mutations to emerge which will both compensate for the effect of earlier mutations on viral fitness and also increase the level of resistance and cross resistance within the drug class. This is typically associated with progressive increases in plasma HIV-1-RNA levels. Of note, circulating resistant HIV-1-RNA tends to drift back to wild type virus when treatment is discontinued. However, drug resistance is retained in the form of minority viral populations, and as integrated provirus, which can rapidly re-emerge when drug pressure is re-established. Failure to account for the phenomenon of archived drug-resistant mutants will lead to rapid virologic failure of a subsequent regimen and ultimately promote further resistance accumulation.

Evaluating the Extent of HIV-1 Drug Resistance

HIV drug resistance may be suspected clinically when plasma HIV-1-RNA levels are shown to be detectable while on antiretroviral drugs; however, the severity and extent of resistance cannot be determined using this approach. In fact, a significant number of patients presenting with detectable plasma HIV-1-RNA levels while on highly active antiretroviral therapy (HAART) will have completely wild-type virus circulating as a result of incomplete adherence. Unfortunately, this is not fully reassuring as the circulating wild-type HIV-1 is only a reflection of the predominating viral quasi-species and it cannot rule out the presence of minority resistant viruses. It has been clearly demonstrated that minority species with decreased susceptibility not detected by the standard resistance assays can negatively impact response to the next regimen.[19,20] More compelling yet is the experience in HIV-infected pregnant women who received single-dose nevirapine to prevent mother-to-child transmission (MTCT) of HIV. Although the intervention was able to reduce MTCT, exposure to a single dose of nevirapine was associated with decreased response rate to subsequent nevirapine-based triple-drug therapy. In fact, response rates were decreased in nevirapine-exposed mothers regardless of whether NNRTI mutations were present.[21,22] These results emphasize the importance of using resistance testing as a confirmatory tool when evaluating patients with detectable HIV-1-RNA levels while on treatment.

Genotypic and phenotypic methods are available to objectively characterize HIV-1 resistance. Geno-

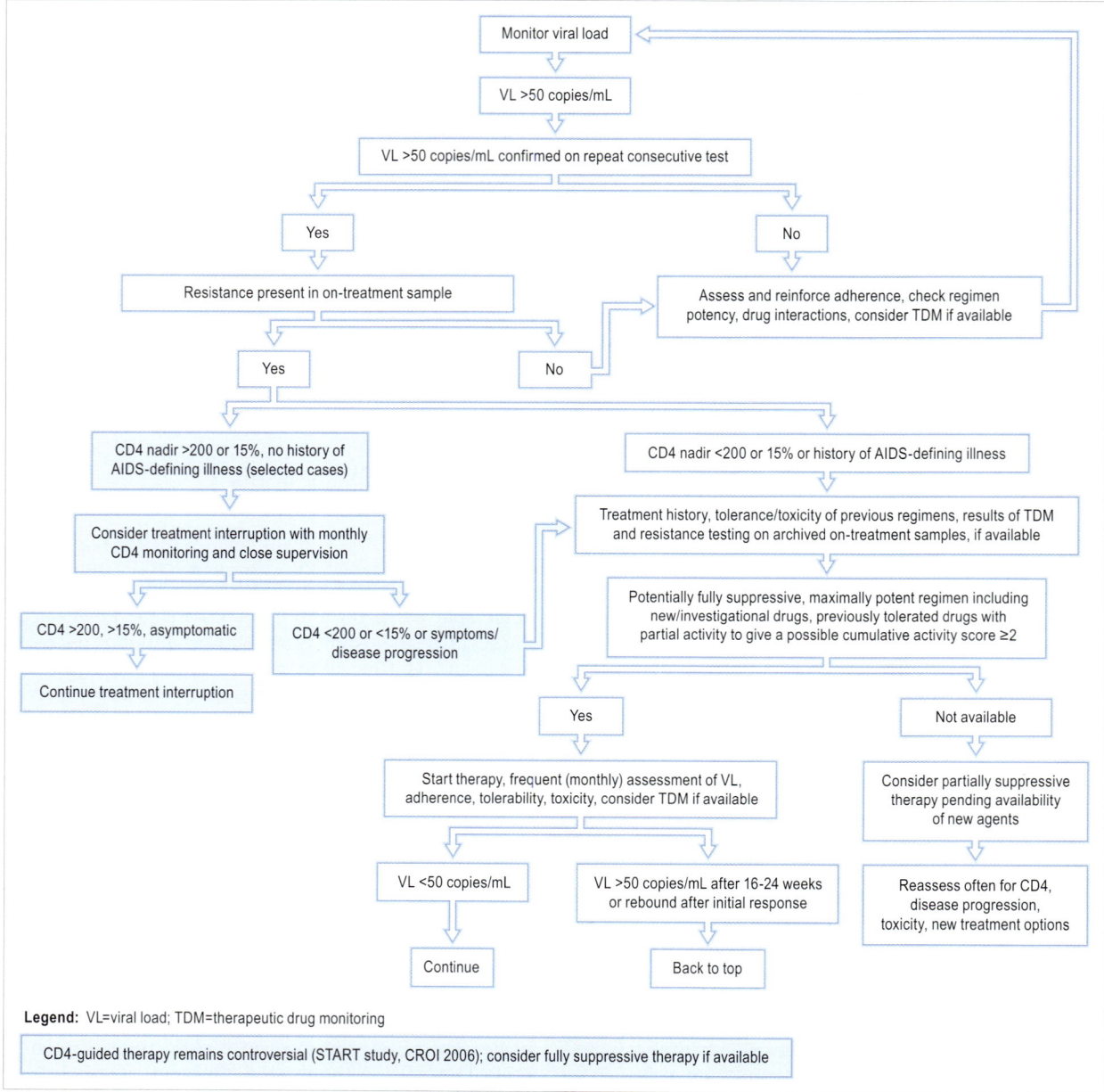

Figure 46.1 Monitoring viral load.

typing usually requires expert interpretation. This can be overcome to some extent using information from large relational databases, making it more practical for widespread clinical use.[23] Phenotypic testing provides a direct measurement of the level of resistance (or decreased susceptibility). However, this is more cumbersome, takes longer and is more expensive, making genotypic testing a more appealing tool for widespread clinical use. Both methods share several limitations: they often can only reflect resistance to the current regimen, they cannot reliably judge resistance to past regimens, they commonly underestimate resistance in patients off therapy, and they can only identify predominant viral quasi-species. In summary, both genotypic and phenotypic HIV drug resistance tests are valuable to confirm the existence of resistance but they cannot rule out resistance.

Interpretation of resistance tests has been predominantly based on the *in vitro* decreased susceptibility of a given clinical isolate when compared to a control wild-type virus (either measured in a phenotypic assay or inferred in a genotypic assay) or using a set of 'rules' (in a genotypic assay). More recently, a new approach to the interpretation of genotypic resistance testing results has been proposed and validated based on clinically derived breakpoints or clinical cutoffs (CCO) for HIV-1 resistance.[24] These analyses demonstrate that for some NRTIs and ritonavir-boosted protease inhibitors there is a broad range of resistance patterns against which the drugs retain partial antiviral efficacy. In contrast, for 3TC, FTC, NNRTIs, and enfuvirtide, resistance tends to be more of an 'all-or-nothing' phenomenon. Incorporation of these clinical cut-off values provides an attractive rational tool to objectively select the next optimal antiretroviral treatment regimen for treatment-experienced HIV-1+ subjects.

Management Options

MDRT

It is critical in the salvage setting that the patient's entire previous antiretroviral history be considered and whenever possible, resistance testing be performed on archived samples obtained while on previous failing regimens. The key objective at this stage is to develop a composite picture of the worst possible resistance profile, referred to as the 'Virtual Virus,' that needs to be targeted by the next treatment. It should be noted that while an individual patient may have developed resistance to multiple drugs over time, the patient's viral quasi-species will always retain a high degree of heterogeneity with respect to antiretroviral drug susceptibility. Also, it is important to emphasize that antiretroviral drugs may retain substantial residual antiretroviral potency after the development of *in vitro* resistance.

A salvage regimen should be constructed tailored to the specific needs of the patient, incorporating active drugs whenever possible to achieve a level of antiretroviral potency comparable with that of standard triple-drug regimens in treatment-naive patients. This may pose a significant challenge in patients harboring HIV with multiple drug resistance. In such instances, regimens consisting of mul-

tiple drugs (also known as multiple drug rescue therapy (MDRT), mega-HAART or giga-HAART) including a number of recycled drugs plus newly available and/or investigational drugs, have been used with substantial success.[25-30] Such regimens typically include five or more drugs, some of which may have retained varying degrees of antiviral activity. The selection of the specific drugs to be included in the multiple drug regimen should be based on a thorough understanding of the patient's prior history of antiretroviral drug exposure and treatment response, in terms of antiviral effect, tolerability and demonstrated resistance.

The use of multiple drug rescue regimens is often regarded as a very challenging proposition in terms of tolerability, toxicity, and cost. In this context, it is critically important to carefully optimize the salvage regimen taking into account the patient's cumulative level of drug resistance and current antiretroviral drug exposure using therapeutic drug monitoring and the inhibitory quotient as a guide. Clearly, this is an approach that should be reserved for situations where the risk of disease progression is considerable, as in patients presenting with at least three-class resistance/failure and a history of a previous AIDS-defining illness or a CD4 nadir below $200/mm^3$. While long-term use of a challenging multiple drug rescue regimen may be unsustainable, it is reasonable to use this approach as a temporary measure to prevent further viral evolution while awaiting the availability of newer second-generation drugs that may allow for simplification of the regimen.

New Drugs

New antiretroviral drugs, especially those active against resistant viruses within existing drug classes (e.g. tipranavir and TMC 114 within the protease inhibitors, and TMC 125 within the NNRTIs) and those active against new targets (the fusion inhibitor enfuvirtide) play a key role in the management of experienced patients. It is particularly important that the introduction of one or more new agents be done with adequate optimization of the backbone regimen using the same principles outlined above, to maximize the magnitude and durability of the therapeutic response. Patients on multiple drug rescue regimens including one or more new agents should be followed very closely with regard to efficacy, safety and tolerability issues. This represents a very rapidly evolving field and as such, it is critical that such patients be followed under the guidance of an experienced practitioner, who can rapidly translate the evolving state of the art in antiretroviral therapy into clinical practice.

Structured Treatment Interruptions

Structured treatment interruptions (STI) for the purpose of re-establishing HIV sensitivity or responsiveness to antiretroviral drugs are currently not recommended. In most clinical trials, this approach has failed to offer a virological benefit and perhaps more importantly, it has been associated with substantial loss of CD4 cell count and increased rate of disease progression events.[31-34]

Partially Suppressive Regimens

Patients with multiple-drug-resistant virus who cannot fully suppress HIV-1-RNA levels (e.g. due to extensive high-level resistance or patient's inability to tolerate a complex MDRT regimen) should be offered partially suppressive regimens, which can provide varying degrees of CD4 cell count preservation.[35,36] Frequent review of this treatment strategy is needed to avoid unnecessary toxicity and to take advantage of newer drugs to optimize the safety, tolerability and potency of the salvage regimen.

A Systematic Approach to the Patient with Multidrug Resistant Virus

First, the physician needs to identify where the patient is in the spectrum of HIV disease. This will include a full medical history and physical examination to identify past and present HIV-related symptoms and AIDS-defining conditions. A thorough review of all available laboratory results, particularly CD4 cell counts, since the time of HIV diagnosis is also needed to assess the rate of CD4 decline and the individual's CD4 nadir. This information is essential to assess the urgency of treatment. Immediate switch to a salvage regimen is warranted in patients with a prior AIDS defining illness, or CD4 nadir below 200/mm^3 for the absolute count or 15% for the CD4 fraction. Asymptomatic individuals without a history of AIDS-defining illness and with a CD4 nadir in excess of 200 cells/mm^3 do not have an immediate risk for disease progression or death and therefore they may be encouraged to defer salvage therapy as long as they tolerate a drug free interval with very close (monthly CD4 cell count) monitoring, even in the presence of a high viral

load.[37] Such patients should be offered treatment if symptoms develop, or the CD4 cell count decreases below 200/mm^3 or if the CD4 fraction decreases below 15%. However, CD4-guided treatment interruptions remain controversial pending results of further studies.

The next step is a thorough assessment of the extent of HIV drug resistance. Resistance testing results from assays performed on a recent blood sample have been shown to predict response to the subsequent regimen. It is now abundantly clear that virologic responses to salvage treatment improve with the number of active drugs in the salvage regimen. For example, in the TORO studies where heavily treatment-experienced patients received multiple-drug salvage regimens including enfuvirtide, which at the time was a new drug from a novel class (an HIV fusion inhibitor), therapeutic responses were better in patients whose background regimens included at least two other drugs to which their virus had been shown to be susceptible on baseline testing.[27,28,38] Maximal response rates were seen once patients had three active drugs in the regimen. Also of interest, in a post-hoc exploratory analysis, it was consistently found that for an equal number of 'active' drugs included in the regimen, the inclusion of enfuvirtide was associated with a slightly higher response rate. This lends support to the hypothesis that an active drug from a previously compromised drug class may have a lesser impact than an active drug from a previously unused drug class. Alternatively, this may relate to an intrinsic, yet to be characterized, attribute of enfuvirtide in this setting. Whatever the mechanism, these results argue strongly in favor of enfuvirtide as a cornerstone of most current salvage regimens.

Next, the limitations of treatment options need to be taken into account when considering potentially active drugs. As discussed above, the reasons for previous regimen failure must be identified and dealt with if possible, (e.g. psychosocial issues affecting adherence) or taken into account in designing future regimens (e.g. treatment-limiting toxicities which may recur on rechallenge with the same or similar agents). Drugs to which the patient has a clear history of a true intolerance must be avoided; examples would include abacavir or nevirapine in patients with a history of hypersensitivity reactions to those agents.[39,40] These should be differentiated from subjective tolerability problems such as gastrointestinal side effects, which may be amenable to symptomatic measures and do not necessarily rule out the use of the offending drug. In this context, subjective ritonavir intolerance has been a frequent problem. Given the very central role of ritonavir-boosting in modern HAART, this is an issue that needs to be aggressively pursued. Patients may feel the intolerance relates to ritonavir when it may have been due to the second protease inhibitor. Often, this can be resolved with a trial of ritonavir alone (100 mg once or twice daily) for a period of a few days. This should also provide an opportunity to establish symptomatic strategies or medications that may be needed to address this intolerance.

Co-morbidities and concomitant medications do not usually represent absolute contraindications to use of a certain agent. Notable exceptions include a history of recurrent pancreatitis for didanosine or stavudine; or use of ribavirin for hepatitis C for didanosine.[41,42] However, these factors need to be taken into account in terms of monitoring for the occurrence of toxicities and possible dosage adjustments.

Any previous pharmacokinetic data may be of use in identifying bioavailability issues that may necessitate pharmacologic boosting or dosage adjustments. The drug levels that can be achieved in the blood are a critical factor in achieving antiviral effect. As compared to the levels required to suppress wild-type drug-susceptible virus, higher drug levels are required to achieve a similar antiviral effect in treatment-experienced patients, to overcome intermediate degrees of HIV drug resistance. The relationship between drug levels and HIV drug resistance determines the activity of a drug in a given individual and has been described in terms of an inhibitory quotient (IQ), i.e. the ratio of minimum or trough drug concentration (C_{trough}) over the inhibitory concentration (IC) of the drug against that individual's virus (either IC50 or IC90).[43] IQ has been studied most extensively for protease inhibitors, and has been shown to correlate with antiviral response to regimens containing indinavir, nelfinavir, saquinavir, amprenavir, lopinavir, and atazanavir.[44-49] Pharmacologic boosting of most protease inhibitors (with the exception of nelfinavir) using small doses of ritonavir has enabled higher exposure to the co-administered protease inhibitor, particularly enhanced trough levels, and is recommended in the setting of drug-resistant virus.[50] One effect of ritonavir boosting is to increase C_{trough}, thereby increasing IQ, and in turn, enhancing the antiviral effect. However, in the setting of high-level resistance conferred by multiple accumulated HIV mutations, it may not be possible to achieve an effective IQ without reaching toxic drug levels.

Taking the above factors into account, the goal is to design a regimen with the maximum possible cumulative activity score, i.e. the sum of the expected activities (total or partial) of all the components of the regimen. The activity score for an individual drug can be viewed as fraction of potential activity or as the predicted contribution to the decrease in viral load. For example, a new drug from a class to which that patient has not previously been exposed, and thus would be expected to retain full susceptibility, would have an activity score of 1, equivalent to a predicted fraction of potential activity of 100%. A drug to which the patient's virus (past or present) is fully resistant would have an activity score of 0 and would not be expected to contribute to the virologic effect. However, a heavily treatment-experienced patient may have few (if any) remaining drugs with an activity score of 1. In this situation, the contribution of drugs that retain partial activity needs to be carefully considered. Objective data to validate this approach is limited; however, the recently developed clinical cut offs (CCO) for the interpretation of genotypic testing offers an objective tool to characterize antiviral activity of a drug as a function of the fold change in susceptibility of the virus against the specific drug.[14,24] Again, achievable plasma levels of drug are of key importance. For example, saquinavir, indinavir and lopinavir demonstrate a progressively wider range of intermediate susceptibility when pharmacologically boosted with ritonavir. For example, the upper CCO of unboosted saquinavir, associated with an 80% loss of antiviral activity, is 1.0, whereas ritonavir-boosted saquinavir retains antiviral activity against virus with a fold-change in susceptibility of up to 12.

Once an optimal salvage regimen has been designed and implemented taking all the above factors into account, frequent reassessment of the patient is critical. This should comprise assessment of tolerability and adherence, as well as regular analysis of laboratory tests for efficacy and toxicity. The frequency of reassessment will depend on a number of factors, including the clinical disease stage and complexity of the regimen, but generally should be at least once a month initially, until the patient's condition is stabilized and viral load is consistently undetectable. Failure of the regimen to achieve a virologic response promptly (within 16–24 weeks, depending on the baseline viral load) or viral load rebound after an initial response should be dealt with immediately and aggressively, to prevent further accumulation of further resistance mutations. Factors impacting adherence (e.g. subjective intolerance) and efficacy (e.g. resistance) should be re-evaluated and the patient counseled, symptomatic treatment initiated, and/or the regimen modified accordingly. Truly failing regimens should be discontinued, thus avoiding unnecessary toxicities and preserving future treatment options with new or investigational agents that may soon become available. In specific circumstances, partially suppressive regimens may be considered. These strategies should also be undertaken with regular clinical and laboratory monitoring, particularly with regard to clinical disease progression in patients with very low nadir CD4 cell counts (i.e. 100/mm^3 or below), to ensure that the current treatment strategy remains the most appropriate option for that patient at that time.

Conclusion

In summary, the ideal goal of antiretroviral therapy is to suppress viral replication as completely as possible, even in the face of drug-resistant HIV. Otherwise, accumulation of more drug-resistant HIV mutations is inevitable, which in turn will result in virologic failure, immunological decline and clinical disease progression. Reasons for previous therapy failure including patient-, regimen- and virus-related factors need to be thoroughly evaluated. This will include a comprehensive history of previous antiretroviral therapy and extensive resistance testing on archived samples taken during previous failing treatments, if possible. The next antiretroviral regimen must be carefully designed, taking into account the likelihood of cumulative resistance mutations and history of drug intolerance and toxicity. Regimen potency should be maximized by including as many agents as possible that are likely to be active against that patient's 'virtual virus,' either drugs from new classes or with unique resistance profiles from existing classes, and also considering drugs which may retain partial activity. Treatment adherence, tolerability, toxicity, and efficacy should be re-evaluated on a regular basis and the regimen or treatment strategy modified accordingly. The ultimate goal of antiretroviral therapy in patients with multidrug resistant HIV is to preserve immune function and quality of life, with the hope of sustaining the patient until the future availability of more compact, tolerable, and efficacious treatment options.

References

1. Siliciano RF. Scientific rationale for antiretroviral therapy in 2005. Abstract 179. 12th Conference on Retroviruses and Opportunistic Infections, Boston, MA: 22–25 February 2005.

2. Clavel F. HIV drug resistance: small changes, big differences. Abstract 180. 12th Conference on Retroviruses and Opportunistic Infections, Boston, MA: 22–25 February 2005.

3. Yeni PG, Hammer SM, Hirsch MS, et al. Treatment for adult HIV infection: 2004 Recommendations of the International AIDS Society – USA Panel. JAMA 2004; 92:251–265.

4. Department of Health and Human Services. Guidelines for the use of antiretroviral agents in HIV-1-infected adults and adolescents. Online. Available: http://AIDSinfo.nih.gov

5. Chesney M. Adherence to HAART regimens. AIDS Patient Care STDs 2003; 17:169–177.

6. Piscitelli SC, Burstein AH, Chaitt D, et al. Indinavir concentrations and St. John's wort. Lancet 2000; 355:547–548.

7. Piscitelli SC, Burstein AH, Welden N, et al. The effect of garlic supplements on the pharmacokinetics of saquinavir. Clin Infect Dis 2002; 34:234–238.

8. Back D, Gatti G, Fletcher C, et al. Therapeutic drug monitoring in HIV infection: current status and future directions. AIDS 2002; 16:S5–S37.

9. Gazzard B, BHIVA writing committee. British HIV Association (BHIVA) guidelines for the treatment of HIV-infected adults with antiretroviral therapy (2005). HIV Med 2005; 6:S1–S61.

10. Walmsley S, Bernstein B, King M, et al. Lopinavir-ritonavir versus nelfinavir for the initial treatment of HIV infection. N Engl J Med 2002; 346:2039–2046.

11. Gulick RM, Ribaudo HJ, Shikuma CM, et al. Triple-nucleoside regimens versus efavirenz-containing regimens for the initial treatment of HIV-1 infection. N Engl J Med 2004; 350:1850–1861.

12. Gerstoft J, Kirk O, Obel N, et al. Low efficacy and high frequency of adverse events in a randomized trial of the triple nucleoside regimen abacavir, stavudine and didanosine. AIDS 2003; 17:2045–2052.

13. Deeks S, Lu J, Hoh R, et al. Interruption of enfuvirtide in patients with enfuvirtide resistance. Abstract 680. 12th Conference on Retroviruses and Opportunistic Infections, Boston, MA: 22–25 February 2005.

14. Bacheler L, Winters B, Harrigan R, et al. Estimation of phenotypic clinical cut-offs for VircoType HIV-1 through meta analyses of clinical trial and cohort data. 44th ICAAC, Washington DC: October 2004.

15. Kempf DJ, Isaacson JD, King MS, et al. Analysis of the virological response with respect to baseline viral phenotype and genotype in protease-inhibitor-experienced HIV-1-infected patients receiving lopinavir/ritonavir therapy. Antiviral Ther 2002; 7:165–174.

16. Wainberg MA. Increased fidelity of drug-selected M184V mutated HIV-1 reverse transcriptase as the basis for the effectiveness of 3TC in HIV clinical trials. Leukemia 1997; 11(Suppl):85–88.

17. Anonymous. Randomised trial of addition of lamivudine or lamivudine plus loviride to zidovudine-containing regimens for patients with HIV-1 infection: the CAESAR trial. Lancet 1997; 349:1413–1421.

18. Wainberg MA. The impact of the M184V substitution on drug resistance and viral fitness. Expert Rev Antiinfective Ther 2004; 2:147–151.

19. Palmer S, Kearney M, Maldarelli F, et al. Multiple, linked human immunodeficiency virus type 1 drug resistance mutations in treatment-experienced patients are missed by standard genotype analysis. J Clin Microbiol 2005; 43:406–415.

20. Mellors J, Palmer S, Nissley D, et al. Low-frequency NNRTI-resistant variants contribute to failure of efavirenz-containing regimens. Abstract 39. 11th Conference on Retroviruses and Opportunistic Infections, San Francisco, CA: 8–11 February 2004.

21. Johnson J, Li JF, Morris L, et al. Resistance emerges in the majority of women provided intrapartum single-dose nevirapine. Abstract 100. 12th Conference on Retroviruses and Opportunistic Infections, Boston, MA: 22–25 February 2005.

22. Palmer S, Boltz V, Mortinson N, et al. Persistence of nevirapine-resistant HIV-1 in women after single-dose nevirapine therapy for prevention of maternal-to-fetal HIV-1 transmission. Proc Natl Acad Sci USA 2006; 103:7094–7099.

23. Larder B, Vroey V De, Dehertogh P, et al. Predicting HIV-1 phenotypic resistance from genotype using a large phenotype-genotype relational database. Antiviral Ther 1999; 4(Suppl):41.

24. Winters B, Rinehart A, Montaner J, et al. Validation of clinically relevant breakpoints for HIV-1 phenotypic resistance data. Abstract 705. 12th Conference on Retroviruses and Opportunistic Infections, Boston, MA: 22–25 February 2005.

25. Montaner JSG, Harrigan PR, Jahnke N, et al. Multiple drug rescue therapy for HIV-infected individuals with prior virologic failure to multiple regimens. AIDS 2001; 15:61–69.

26. Miller V, Cozzi-Lepri A, Hertogs K, et al. HIV drug susceptibility and treatment response to mega-HAART regimens in patients from the Frankfurt HIV cohort. Antiviral Ther 2000; 5:49–55.

27. Lalezari JP, Henry K, O'Hearn M, et al. Enfuvirtide, an HIV-1 fusion inhibitor, for drug-resistant HIV infection in North and South America. N Engl J Med 2003; 348:2175–2185.

28. Lazzarin A, Clotet B, Cooper D, et al. Efficacy of enfuvirtide in patients infected with drug-resistant HIV-1 in Europe and Australia. N Engl J Med 2003; 348:2186–2195.

29. Hicks C, et al. RESIST 1: A phase 3 randomized, multicenter trial comparing tipranavir/ritonavir to an optimized comparator protease inhibitor regimen in antiretroviral experienced patients: 24 week data. Abstract LBH-1137. 44th Interscience Conference on Antimicrobial Agents and Chemotherapy, Washington, DC: 30 October–2 November, 2004.

30. Hicks CB, Cahn P, Cooper PA, et al. Durable efficacy of tipranavir in combination with an optimized background regimen of antiretroviral drugs for treatment-experienced HIV-1-infected patients at 48 weeks in the Randomized Evaluation of Strategic Intervention in multi-drug resistant patients with Tipranavir (RESIST) studies: an analysis of combined data from two randomized open-label trials. Lancet 2006; 368:466–475.

31. Lawrence J, Mayers D, Huppler Hullsiek K, et al. Structured treatment interruption in patients with multidrug-resistant Human Immunodeficiency Virus. N Engl J Med 2003; 349:837–846.

32. Lawrence J, Hullsiek KH, Thackeray LM, et al. Disadvantages of structured treatment interruption persist in patients with multidrug-resistant HIV-1: final results of the CPCRA 064 study. JAIDS 2006; 43:169–178.

33. Ruiz L, Ribera E, Bonjoch A, et al. Role of structured treatment interruption before a 5-drug salvage antiretroviral regimen: the Retrogene study. J Infect Dis 2003; 188:977–985.

34. Walmsley S, LaPierre N, Loutfy M, et al. CTN 164: a prospective randomized trial of structured treatment interruption vs immediate switching in HIV-infected patients experiencing virologic failure on HAART. Abstract

580. 12th Conference on Retroviruses and Opportunistic Infections, Boston, MA: 22–25 February 2005.

35. Deeks SG, Wrin T, Liegler T, et al. Virologic and immunologic consequences of discontinuing combination antiretroviral-drug therapy in HIV-infected patients with detectable viremia. N Engl J Med 2001; 344:472–480.

36. Deeks SG, Barbour JD, Grant RM, Martin JM. Duration and predictors of CD4 T-cell gains in patients who continue combination therapy despite detectable plasma viremia. AIDS 2002; 16:201–207.

37. Toulson A, Harrigan R, Heath K, et al. Treatment interruption of antiretroviral therapy among patients with nadir CD4 cell counts >200 cells/mm^3. J Infect Dis 2005; 192:1787–1792.

38. Montaner J, DeMasi R, Delehanty J, et al. Analysis of virological response of enfuvirtide in TORO: Implications for patient management. Antiviral Ther 2003; 8(Suppl):S212.

39. GlaxoSmithKline. Ziagen Product Monograph. 21 December. Mississauga, Ontario: GlaxoSmithKline Inc; 2004.

40. Boehringer Ingelheim. Viramune Product Monograph. 30 August. Burlington, Ontario: Boehringer Ingelheim (Canada) Ltd; 2004.

41. Bristol-Myers Squibb. Zerit Product Monograph. 27 March. Montreal, Quebec: Bristol-Myers Squibb Canada Inc; 2001.

42. Bristol-Myers Squibb. Videx Product Monograph. Montreal, Quebec: Bristol-Myers Squibb Canada Inc; 2002.

43. Montaner J, Hill A, Acosta E. Practical implications for the interpretation of minimum plasma concentration/inhibitory concentration ratios. Lancet 2001; 357:1438–1440.

44. Kempf D, Hsu A, Jiang P, et al. Response to ritonavir (RTV) intensification in indinavir (IDV) recipients is highly correlated with virtual inhibitory quotient. Abstract 523. 8th Conference on Retroviruses and Opportunistic Infections, Boston MA.

45. Casado JL, Moreno A, Sabido R, et al. Individualizing salvage regimens: the inhibitory quotient (C_{trough}/IC50) as predictor of virological response. AIDS 2003; 17:262–264.

46. Marcelin AG, Lamotte C, Delaugerre C, et al. Genotypic inhibitory quotient as predictor of virological response to ritonavir-amprenavir in human immunodeficiency virus type 1 protease inhibitor-experienced patients. Antimicrob Agents Chemother 2003; 47:594–600.

47. Gonzalez de Requena D, Gallego O, Valer L, et al. Prediction of virological response to lopinavir/ritonavir using the genotypic inhibitory quotient. AIDS Res Hum Retroviruses 2004; 20:275–278.

48. Breilh D, Pellegrin I, Rouzes A, et al. Virological, intracellular and plasma pharmacological parameters predicting response to lopinavir/ritonavir (KALEPHAR study). AIDS 2004; 18:1305–1310.

49. Barrios A, Rendon AL, Gallego O, et al. Predictors of virological response to atazanavir in protease inhibitor-experienced patients. HIV Clin Trials 2004; 5:201–205.

50. King JR, Wynn H, Brundage R, Acosta EP. Pharmacokinetic enhancement of protease inhibitor therapy. Clin Pharm 2004; 43:291–310.

CHAPTER 47

Complementary and Alternative Medicine

Jason Tokumoto
Donald I. Abrams

Introduction

In developed countries, the availability and use of antiretroviral therapy has significantly decreased morbidity and mortality from human immunodeficiency virus-1 (HIV) infection. Unfortunately, most of the world's HIV-infected population does not have access to antiretroviral therapy and therefore must turn to locally available indigenous therapies or folk remedies. When these interventions are exported to the developed world, they may be used as complementary and alternative medicine (CAM). Even in countries where antiretroviral therapy is available, there is a high use of CAM.[1,2] Due to the use of CAM worldwide, it is important for anyone involved in HIV care to be aware of the various complementary/alternative modalities that patients may be using. For the purpose of this discussion, complementary and alternative medicine will be defined as any therapeutic modalities that are 'non-conventional' or any healthcare system that is not considered to be allopathic.

From a global perspective, studies looking at the use and types of CAM that are published in the English language are limited. The majority of studies assessing CAM use in HIV patients are from the USA. This chapter will focus on CAM use in the following four regions/sub-regions of the world:

1. Southern Africa
2. Asia/Thailand
3. North America/USA
4. Western Europe

Southern Africa

Southern Africa (South Africa, Botswana, Lesotho, Namibia, Rwanda, Mozambique, Central Africa Republic, Swaziland, Malawi, Zambia, Zimbabwe, Angola) is the most heavily affected region in the world with an estimated HIV prevalence >25%. This amounts to 11 500 000 HIV-infected individuals which represents about 30% of the global HIV positive population.[3]

Unfortunately, the majority of these HIV-infected individuals do not yet have access to adequate allopathic care and antiretroviral therapy. However, in this region, there is another system of care consisting of traditional healers who represent the first line of care for 70% of the population.[4] These traditional healers (n'angas in Zimbabwe) represent a broad range of practitioners, which includes herbalists (inyangas in South Africa), spiritualists, diviners (sangomas in South Africa), faith healers, and priests.[5-7] Historically, traditional healers have been providing treatment for sexually transmitted diseases although their explanation as to the causes of these diseases, modes of transmissions, and treatment vary among healers.[8] Traditional healers outnumber allopathic doctors by a hundred-fold or more and provide accessible and affordable care that is personal, culturally appropriate and trustworthy; therefore they are well-positioned to promote behavior change and to care for, support, and refer HIV-infected individuals.[4] Since 1990, the World Health Organization (WHO) has advocated for the inclusion of traditional healers in the National AIDS Programs and many

547

experts now agree that these healers bear much of the burden of HIV care and support in this area.[7,8]

Despite the WHO's recognition of traditional healers and the interest of these healers to learn about HIV and collaborate with formal healthcare workers, little progress has been made in actually working with these healers.[4,7,8] Furthermore, there is a lack of research on the impact these healers have on the HIV epidemic. A major focus has been on projects involving collaboration between traditional healers and formal healthcare workers in which traditional healers are educated in HIV/AIDS medicine. These healers then integrate this information into their practice. The main goal of these projects is HIV prevention rather than treatment.[8] In order for this to occur, it is vital that these healers have correct and adequate knowledge about HIV and do not disseminate misinformation as to the causes of AIDS or claim they have a cure for HIV. Although there are no follow-up studies assessing the impact these educated healers have on HIV prevention, compared with healers who are not educated about HIV, educated healers are more likely to conduct community education, counsel AIDS patients and their families, distribute condoms and refer the sick to appropriate care.[4]

Herbs are commonly used by these traditional healers but most of these herbs are ineffective against HIV. However, there are some herbs that have demonstrated *in vitro* activity against HIV. For example, 38 plants used for the treatment of infections in Rwandan traditional medicine were tested for *in vitro* activity against HIV.[9] Three plants, *Aspilia pluriseta* (Asteraceae), *Rumex bequaertii* (Polygonaceae), and *Tithonia diversifolia* (Asteraceae) showed *in vitro* anti-HIV activity. None of these herbs have yet been studied in the clinical setting.

In South Africa, the government has accredited 27 facilities to provide traditional and complementary medicine for HIV patients.[10] The South African Medical Research Council launched a study looking at the activity of the herb unwele (*Sutherlandia frutescens*) containing L-canavanine, which has known antiretroviral properties. There have been anecdotal reports of HIV patients taking L-canavanine and reporting improvement in their overall sense of well-being as well as appetite and weight.[11] However, *Sutherlandia* and another plant used for HIV, *Hypoxis hemerocallidea* (African potato), have both been shown to inhibit CYP3A4 activity which could result in potentially significant drug interactions if taken with licensed antiretroviral agents.[10]

In Harare City, Zimbabwe, a study conducted from 1996 to 1998 looked at the impact of traditional herbs on psychiatric illness and quality of life in HIV patients. There were 105 participants who received herbs or no herbs. These patients were followed-up on a 3-monthly basis. At the end of 6 months, based on multiple accepted standard neuropsychological measurement tools, the relative risk of psychiatric diagnosis was less in the group that took the herbs than those who did not ($P = 0.046$).[12] Furthermore, based on WHO quality of life measurement tools, the group that took herbs had better quality of life scores than those who did not ($P < 0.0001$).[13]

Asia/Thailand

Approximately 1.5% of the adults in Thailand are infected with HIV.[3] For these individuals, there are two health systems that they can turn to: conventional allopathic medicine and traditional Thai medicine. Traditional Thai medicine includes: Thai medicine: *phaet phaen thai* and folk medicine: *phaet pheun baan*. Thai medicine is formalized with practitioners who go through a testing process and receive a license. *Phaet phaen thai* was developed by Buddhist monks and generally includes the use of herbs and massage. *Phaet pheun baan* generally involves divinity and spiritual practices based on Buddhism.[14]

For Thai patients who have access to conventional care (antiretroviral therapy), a large number also incorporate CAM into their care as illustrated by a study[15] involving 160 HIV positive patients (107 males and 53 females) attending the outpatient clinic at the King Chulalongkorn Memorial Hospital in 2000. This study showed that 152 (95%) used complementary medicine and 124 (78%) saw a complementary provider. The most common complementary modalities used were: ritual remedies called 'Mor Pra', generally consisting of holy water used to prepare the remedy provided by the abbot of Buddhist temples (84.2%); biophysical approach ('Chee Wa Jit'), which is a regimen consisting of a vegetarian diet, several herbs, meditation, and coffee enema (67.1%); Thai traditional herb remedy known as 'Yar Mor' (55.3%); Chinese traditional herb remedies (52.6%); and vitamins (51.3%).

JinHuang, a Chinese herbal medicine that has *in vitro* activity against HIV, was demonstrated in another study, to be safe and to improve the quality of life of asymptomatic HIV-infected Thai patients.[16] This prospective study involved 21 patients who received *JinHuang* preparations consisting of six capsules and two bottles of liquid formula orally, three times a day for 6 months. It is unclear whether these patients were also receiving antiretroviral therapy.

No serious adverse events were reported, although increased bowel movements were common.

There is a dearth of information on the efficacy of Thai herbs on HIV. Two herbs used in traditional Thai medicine have been studied for their antiretroviral effect. One herb, *Coleus parvifolius* has potent *in vitro* activity against HIV[17] and another herb, *Clausena excavata* has immunomodulatory activity in the mouse immune system model.[18] None of these herbs have yet been studied in the clinical setting.

North America/USA

An estimated 850 000–950 000 individuals are infected with HIV in the USA[3] and despite the availability of antiretroviral therapy, studies have consistently shown a high use of CAM in these individuals.[1,19] In the Alternative Medicine Care Outcomes in AIDS (AMCOA) study,[19] which took place from 1995 to 1997, 63% of the 1675 HIV patients surveyed reported the use of 1600 different types of complementary therapy. The most commonly used complementary therapies in this study were prayer (58.3%), garlic (53%), massage therapy (48.8%), meditation (45.9%), and acupuncture (45.5%). Furthermore, in a telephone survey of 180 HIV positive patients who saw a complementary practitioner, these patients visited their complementary practitioner 12 times a year, while seeing their allopathic provider seven times a year.[20] The reasons for the high CAM use in HIV patients have been assessed and include: to (1) slow the progression of the disease; (2) relieve symptoms from HIV or side-effects from medications; (3) enhance the immune system, and (4) complement allopathic medicine.[20,21] Most patients do not generally use CAM in place of, but instead to supplement, allopathic medicine.[1]

A major problem regarding the use of CAM in the USA is that many providers do not know that their patients are using complementary medicine. In one study,[1] 33% of clinicians did not know that their HIV patients were using complementary medicine. This disconnection is due to either the patient not wanting to tell their provider for fear of losing the respect of the provider or the provider simply not asking. There are a number of reasons why it is important that the clinician is aware that their patient is using CAM. In one study,[1] 25% of patients were using a complementary modality with the potential for adverse effects. The patient may be using a complementary treatment that has no proven benefit, is costly, or is potentially harmful. A symptom may be due to the complementary treatment and not from HIV or conventional medications. Finally, there may be a potential for a pharmacokinetic interaction between prescribed antiretroviral agents and the CAM therapy, as described below.

There are hundreds of different CAM therapies that HIV patients might integrate into their care but the following are commonly used modalities: (1) Chinese medicine, (2) herbs, (3) acupuncture, (4) mind-body therapy, and (5) supplements (vitamins). For many of these interventions, there is little data on their safety profile and purported therapeutic value.

Chinese Medicine

Chinese medicine is a complex healing system in which the practitioner balances the 'energy' of the body by combining diet, exercise, acupuncture, and herbal remedies. Because Chinese medicine is a complex system involving multiple modalities, it may be difficult to study its effectiveness when using Western study methodologies. Two studies investigated the therapeutic value of Chinese herbal remedies in HIV positive individuals. The first study[22] was a double-blind, placebo-controlled study involving 30 patients who were randomized to either a mixture of Chinese herbs ('Enhance' and 'Clear Heat') or placebo. The group that took the mixture had a trend towards better quality of life scores and less HIV-related symptoms. In the other study,[23] which was also a double-blind, placebo-controlled study, 68 patients were randomized to either a mixture of 35 herbs that had either *in vitro* activity against HIV or was purported to help various symptoms such as nausea. At the end of 6 months of therapy, there was no difference in CD4 cell count, HIV viral load, disease progression, or quality of life scores.

Herbs

Many HIV patients use various herbs to treat HIV or its co-morbidities.[19,20] However, one of the major concerns about herbal preparations is that there are no strict regulated quality control standards. There are several plant derivatives that demonstrate *in vitro* activity against HIV but two of the more interesting compounds are calanolide A and prostratin. Calanolide A is derived from a Malaysian rainforest tree, *Calophyllum lanigerum* and functions like a non-nucleoside reverse transcriptase inhibitor. In a randomized, double-blind, placebo-controlled study,[24] 43 patients were randomized to receive various doses of calanolide A or placebo. The group that received the highest dose (600 mg twice a day) experienced a mean drop in HIV viral load of 0.81 $\log_{10}$ from baseline. This reduction was significantly greater than the placebo group ($P = 0.027$). Prostratin is a phorbol ester derived from the plant *Homalanthus nutans*. This herb is used by Samoan healers to treat various illnesses, including yellow fever. Prostratin has been shown to induce expression of HIV from latently HIV-infected cells *in vitro*.[25] Eradication of proviral HIV DNA from these latently infected cells has been a major obstacle in HIV treatment.

A common herb that HIV patients may use for depression is St John's wort. In standard pharmacokinetic investigations, St John's wort decreased indinavir trough blood levels by 81%.[26] St John's wort has also been shown to decrease nevirapine blood concentration levels by 20%.[27] This decrease in blood levels could result in drug resistance and virological failure. Thus, St John's wort should be avoided in patients who are taking either a protease inhibitor or non-nucleoside based regimen.

Two herbal agents that HIV patients may use for antiretroviral therapy associated hyperlipidemia are Cholestin and garlic. Cholestin is produced by red yeast fermented on rice. Cholestin has been shown to contain nine monacolins (statins) which inhibit HMG-CoA reductase. Two controlled trials (one in the USA and one in China) involving 390 non-HIV patients showed a drop in LDL cholesterol and triglycerides by about 20–30%.[28] A case of Cholestin-induced myopathy has been reported.[29] Garlic has purported anticholesterol activity but a potential problem with garlic is that it has been demonstrated to decrease saquinavir blood levels by about 50%.[30] Garlic should be used with caution in HIV individuals who are taking a protease inhibitor based regimen.

Elevated hepatic transaminases due to infections, alcohol, malignancies, and side-effects of medications are commonly seen in HIV positive individuals. An herb that HIV patients may use for its hepato-protective or hepato-restorative properties is milk thistle (active ingredient: silymarin).[31] Like St John's wort and garlic, milk thistle can decrease protease inhibitor blood levels. Milk thistle has been shown to decrease mean indivinar trough blood levels by 25%,[32] so it should be used with caution when using a protease inhibitor based regimen.

Diarrhea is common in the HIV population and is generally due to infection or side-effects of medications. A plant product that has demonstrated to be effective in controlling diarrhea is SP-303, which is an extract from the sap of the *Croton lechleri* tree. This sap is used by shamans in the Amazon rain forest to promote normal stool formation. In a randomized, double-blind, placebo-controlled study;[33] 51 AIDS patients who had >200 g of watery stool during a 24 h period and no anti-diarrheal agents 24 h prior to enrollment received either 500 g of SP-303 or placebo orally four times a day for 4 days. Some 48 of the 51 patients had no identified pathogen to account for the diarrhea. When both groups were compared over the 4-day study period, the treatment group had a significant decrease in stool weight ($P = 0.008$) and diarrhea frequency ($P = 0.04$). In an 8-week open label trial, a mixture of Chinese herbs called Source Qi showed no benefit in HIV patients with pathogen negative or nelfinavir-related diarrhea.[34]

One of the more controversial plants used for medicinal purposes is *Cannabis sativa* or marijuana. Estimated marijuana use by HIV-infected persons for medical or recreational purposes ranges from 14% to 43%.[35] There are several reasons for the use of marijuana in patients with HIV infection, including to decrease nausea, improve appetite, and relieve pain. Because medical marijuana is a politically sensitive issue, it has been difficult to assess the safety and benefits of marijuana as a therapeutic agent. In a randomized, placebo-controlled study,[36] the effect of marijuana on HIV viral load was assessed in 67 HIV individuals. Patients either received a 3.95%-tetrahydrocannabinol marijuana cigarette, a 2.5 mg dronabinol (Marinol) capsule, or a placebo capsule three times a day for 21 days. The results of the study showed that there was no increase in HIV viral loads, no decrease in CD4 cell counts and no clinically significant effect on protease inhibitor blood levels. At least over a 21-day period, marijuana appeared to be safe. In an open-label pilot study,[37] the benefit of smoking marijuana for painful HIV neuropathy was assessed. A total of 16 patients smoked 3.56%-tetrahydrocannibol marijuana cigarettes three times a day for 7 days. All patients experienced a decrease in pain scores and 10 patients had a >30% decrease in pain.

Acupuncture

Surveys have shown that up to 46% of HIV patients use acupuncture.[20] A common use for acupuncture is for pain relief due to peripheral neuropathy from HIV or side-effects of antiretroviral therapy. Despite the high use of acupuncture, there is a paucity of double-blind, placebo-controlled studies assessing the efficacy of acupuncture in this population. In a moderately sized trial,[38] 250 HIV patients with peripheral neuropathy were randomized to one of three options (all double-blinded) for 14 weeks: (1) a standardized acupuncture regimen (SAR) + amitriptyline or control points + amitriptyline or SAR + placebo amitriptyline or control points + placebo amitriptyline; (2) SAR or control points, and (3) amitriptyline or placebo amitriptyline. The SAR was created by acupuncturists. At the end of 14 weeks, there was essentially no difference in the level of pain reduction among all groups; neither acupuncture nor amitriptyline appeared better than placebo in reducing pain.

Mind-body Therapy

Mind-body interventions include prayer, meditation, hypnosis, and spiritual practice. In surveys inquiring about CAM, up to 60% of HIV positive individuals have reported using a mind-body therapy.[20]

Most of the studies on mind-body therapy have been either descriptive or exploratory. An intriguing mind-body intervention that has been studied in HIV positive individuals is distant healing, defined as 'a conscious dedicated act of mentation attempting to benefit another person's physical or emotional well-being at a distance.'[39] In a randomized double-blind study,[39] 40 AIDS patients were randomized to receive either 10 weeks of distant healing or no distant healing, while receiving 'standard medical care' from their provider. Patients in both groups were matched for age, CD4 cell count, and number of AIDS defining diagnosis. Distant healing was carried out by a self-identified healer (different healing and spiritual practices were used) and the healer and patient never met. At the end of 6 months, the distant healing group had less illness severity ($P = 0.03$), fewer new opportunistic infections ($P = 0.04$), fewer physician visits ($P = 0.01$), and fewer hospitalizations ($P = 0.04$). There was no change in CD4 cell count; viral loads were not assessed. Based on the results of this small study, the National Institute of Health has funded a larger randomized three arm trial to assess the effect of distant healing on HIV disease.

Vitamins

Studies have shown that serum levels of various vitamins and minerals are lower in HIV positive individuals compared with HIV negative individuals and that low levels of these vitamins and minerals are associated with a more rapid disease progression.[40] In longitudinal studies, higher intake of vitamins was associated with improved CD4 cell counts, delay in disease progression, and decreased mortality.[40]

Despite these observations, there are only a few randomized, double-blind, placebo-controlled studies assessing the benefits of vitamins in HIV positive individuals. In Africa, 1078 pregnant HIV-positive women were enrolled in a randomized, double-blind, placebo-controlled study[41] to assess the effects of daily vitamins on disease progression, CD4 cell count and HIV viral load. In addition to receiving antenatal iron and folic acid, the women were randomized to one of four groups: vitamin A only, multivitamins without vitamin A, multivitamins with vitamin A, or placebo. The CD4 cell count of these women ranged from 204 to 653 cells/mm^3 and HIV viral load from $\log_{10} 4.56 \pm 0.78$–4.66 ± 0.77. The median follow-up was 5.91 years. Results showed that the women who took multivitamins were significantly less likely to progress to AIDS or death (24.7% multivitamins only, 26.1% multivitamins + vitamin A, 29% vitamin A only, 31% placebo; $P = 0.04$). Furthermore, the women who took multivitamins had a mean CD4 cell count that was 48 cells/mm^3 higher than placebo ($P = 0.01$) and an HIV viral load that was $0.18 \log_{10}$ lower than placebo ($P = 0.02$). Vitamin A alone was no more beneficial than placebo.

Western Europe

There are approximately 520 000–680 000 HIV positive individuals in the 12 Western European countries.[3] Several surveys have indicated a high use of CAM by these individuals. In two European surveys[2] assessing CAM use in persons living with HIV conducted from 1996 to 1999, 58–63% used vitamins/minerals, 14–21% used homeopathy, and 20–25% used herbal products. Many of the participants in this survey were on antiretroviral therapy. Multiple regression analysis indicated that those individuals who used homeopathy were more likely to have HIV for a longer period of time, a higher educational level and a lower CD4 cell count.

In another survey[42] conducted in 1996 in Switzerland, involving approximately 129 HIV-infected persons, 80% used at least one complementary therapy. The most common CAM interventions were vitamins, special diets, supplements, meditation, phytotherapy, and homeopathy. About 50% of the participants took antiretroviral therapy. A survey[43] of 70 HIV-positive gay men in The Netherlands demonstrated that 71% used CAM alone or in combination with traditional medicine. Users of CAM were most likely to have symptomatic disease, little or no pain, and to be actively involved in their care.

Conclusion

Since there is a high use of CAM in people living with HIV, it is vital that any clinician caring for an HIV patient inquires about the use of CAM and counsel them as completely as possible regarding possible concerns. To do so effectively, clinicians must be supportive, non-judgmental, humble, and willing to learn more about CAM in order to have and maintain an open discussion with their patients. Armed with education, the clinicians can be a valuable source of accurate and unbiased information on complementary and alternative modalities. When alternative and complementary medicine is integrated into standard care, the following principles should be kept in mind:

1. Individualize care. Each patient and each healthcare provider brings a unique set of experiences, beliefs, and knowledge to the patient-provider relationship. This uniqueness must be respected.

2. Relationship. It is critical to establish a trusting and compassionate relationship. This will facilitate honest and open communication between the patient and provider.

3. Consumer awareness. Educate patients about the red flags of fraud. It is also important to educate patients that CAM does not automatically mean safe.

4. Non-exclusivity. Allopathic and CAM providers need to share their knowledge and work together rather than dismissing each other. The ultimate goal is to provide optimal care for our patients and this requires a comprehensive approach that integrates the better of these two modalities.

References

1. Hsiao AF, Wong MD, Kanouse DE, et al. Complementary and alternative medicine use and substitution for conventional therapy by HIV-infected patients. J Acquir Immune Defic Syndr 2003; 33:157–165.
2. Colebunders R, Dreezen C, Florence E, et al. The use of complementary and alternative medicine by persons with HIV infection in Europe. Int J STD AIDS 2004; 14:672–674.
3. UNAIDS/WHO. AIDS epidemic update: December 2004.
4. Homsy J, King R, Balaba D. Kabatesi. Traditional health practitioners are key to scaling up comprehensive care for HIV/AIDS in sub-Sahara Africa. AIDS 2004; 18:1723–1725.
5. Arkovitz MS, Manley M. Specialization and referral among the N'anga (traditional healers) of Zimbabwe. Trop Doct 1990; 20:109–110.
6. Green EC, Zokwe B, Dupree JD. The experience of an AIDS prevention program focused on South African traditional healers. Soc Sci Med 1995; 40:503–515.
7. Morris K. Treating HIV in South Africa-a tale of two systems. Lancet 2001; 357:1190.
8. Joint United Nations Programme on HIV/AIDS. Collaboration with traditional healers in HIV/AIDS prevention and care in sub-Sahara Africa. A literature review. Geneva, Switzerland: Joint United Nations Programme on HIV/AIDS; 2000.
9. Cos P, Hermans N, Bruyne T De, et al. Antiviral activity of Rwanda medicinal plants against human immunodeficiency virus type-1(HIV-1). Phytomedicine 2004; 9:62–68.
10. Mills E, Foster B, Heeswijk R, et al. Impact of African herbal medicines on antiretroviral metabolism. AIDS 2005; 19:95–97.
11. Morris K. South Africa tests traditional medicines. Lancet (Infectious Diseases) 2002; 2:319.
12. Sebit MB, Chandiwana SK, Latif AS, et al. Neuropsychiatric aspects of HIV disease progression: impact of traditional herbs on adult patients in Zimbabwe. Prog Neuropsychopharmacol Biol Psychiatry 2002; 3:451–456.
13. Sebit MB, Chandiwana SK, Latif AS, et al. Quality of life evaluation in patients with HIV-1 infection: the impact of traditional medicine in Zimbabwe. Cent Afr J Med 2000; 46:208–213.
14. Casino VJ Jr. (Re)placing health and healthcare: mapping the competing discourses and practices of 'traditional' and 'modern' Thai medicine. Health Place 2004; 10:59–73.
15. Wiwanitkit V. The use of CAM by HIV-positive patients in Thailand. Complementary Ther Med 2003; 11:39–41.
16. Maek-a-nantawat W. Pitisuttithum P, Bussaratid V, et al. 6-month evaluation of JinHuang Chinese herbal medicine study asymptomatic HIV-infected Thais. Southeast Asian J Trop Med Public Health 2003; 34:379–384.
17. Tewtrakul S, Miyashiro H, Nakamura N, et al. HIV-1 integrase inhibitory substances from Coleus parvifolius. Phytother Res 2003; 17:232–239.
18. Manosroi A, Saraphanchotiwitthaya A, Manosroi J. Immunomodulatory activities of fractions from hot aqueous extract of wood from Clausena excavata. Fitoterapia 2004; 75:302–308.
19. Greene KB, Berger J, Reeves C, et al. Most frequently used alternative and complementary therapies and activities by participants in the AMCOA study. J Assoc Nurses AIDS Care 1999; 10:60–73.
20. Fairfield KM, Eisenberg DM, Davis RB, et al. Patterns of use, expenditures and perceived efficacy of complementary and alternative therapies in HIV-infected patients. Arch Intern Med 1998; 158:2257–2264.
21. Langewitz W, Ruttimann S, Laifer G, et al. The integration of alternative treatment modalities in HIV infection: the patient's perspective. J Psychosom Res 1994; 38:687–693.
22. Burack J, Cohen M, Hahn J, et al. Pilot randomized controlled trial of Chinese herbal treatment for HIV-associated symptoms. J Acquir Immune Defic Syndr Hum Retrovirol 1996; 12:386–393.
23. Weber R, Christen L, Loy M, et al. Randomized, placebo-controlled trial of Chinese herb therapy for HIV-1 infected individuals. J Acquir Immune Defic Syndr 1999; 22:56–64.
24. Sherer R, Dutta B, Anderson R, et al. A phase IB study of (+)-calanolide A in HIV-1-infected, antiretroviral therapy in naïve patients. 7th Conference on Retroviruses and Opportunistic Infections, San Francisco, CA: 30 January–2 February 2000.
25. Korin YD, Brooks DG, Brown S, et al. Effects of prostratin on T-cell activation and human immunodeficiency virus latency. J Virol 2002; 76:8118–8123.

26. Markowitz JS, Donovan JL, DeVane CL, et al. Effect of St. John's wort on drug metabolism by induction of cytochrome P450 3A4 enzyme. JAMA 2003; 290:1500–1504.

27. De Maat MMR, Hoetelmans RMW, vanGorp ECM et al. A potential drug interaction between St. John's wort and nevirapine. First International Workshop on Clinical Pharmacology of HIV Therapy, Noordwijk, Netherlands: 30–31 March 2000.

28. Patrick L, Uzick M. Cardiovascular disease: C-reactive protein and the inflammatory disease paradigm: HMG-CoA reductive inhibitors, alpha-tocopherol, red yeast rice, and olive oil polyphenols. A review of the literature. Alternative Med Rev 2001; 6:248–271.

29. Smith DJ, Olive KE. Chinese red rice-induced myopathy. South Med J 2003; 96:1265–1267.

30. Piscitelli SC, Burstein AH, Welden N, et al. The effect of garlic supplements on the pharmacokinetics of saquinavir. Clin Infect Dis 2002; 34:234–238.

31. Saller R, Meier R, Brignoli R. The use of silymarin in the treatment of liver diseases. Drugs 2001; 61:2035–2063.

32. Piscitelli SC, Formentini E, Burstein AH, et al. Effect of milk thistle on the pharmacokinetics of indinavir in healthy volunteers. Pharmacotherapy 2002; 22:551–556.

33. Holodniy M, Koch J, Mistal M, et al. A double-blind, randomized, placebo-controlled phase II study to assess the safety and efficacy of orally administered SP-303 for the symptomatic treatment of diarrhea in patients with AIDS. Am J Gastroenterol 1999; 94:3267–3273.

34. Cohen MR, Mitchell TF, Bacchetti P, et al. Use of a Chinese herbal medicine for treatment of HIV-associated pathogen-negative diarrhea. Integrat Med 1999; 2:79–84.

35. Prentiss D, Power R, Balmas G, et al. Patterns of marijuana use among patients with HIV/AIDS followed in a public healthcare setting. J Acquir Immune Defic Syndr 2004; 35:38–45.

36. Abrams DI, Hilton JF, Leiser RJ, et al. Short-term effects of cannabinoids in patients with HIV-1 infection: a randomized, placebo-controlled clinical trial. Ann Intern Med 2003; 139:258–266.

37. Jay C, Shade S, Vizoso H, et al. The effect of smoked marijuana on chronic neuropathic and experimentally induced pain in HIV neuropathy: results of an open-label pilot study. 11th Conference on Retroviruses and Opportunistic Infections, San Francisco, CA: 8–11 February 2004.

38. Shlay JC, Chaloner K, Max MB, et al. Acupuncture and amitriptyline for pain due to HIV-related neuropathy: a randomized controlled trial. JAMA 1998; 280:1590–1595.

39. Sicher F, Targ E, Moore DII, et al. A randomized double-blind study of the effect of distant healing in a population with advanced AIDS. Report of a small scale study. West J Med 1998; 169:356–363.

40. Fawzi WW. Micronutrients and human immunodeficiency virus type-1 disease progression among adults and children. Clin Infect Dis 2003; 37:S112–S116.

41. Fawzi WW, Msamanga GI, Spiegelman D, et al. A randomized trial of multivitamin supplements and HIV disease progression and mortality. N Engl J Med 2004; 351:23–32.

42. Brauchli P, Reuteler I, Burki B, et al. Use of complimentary medical therapies in HIV/AIDS in Switzerland. Schweiz Med Wochenschr 1996; 126:1297–1305.

43. Knippels HMA, Weiss JJ. Use of alternative medicine in a sample of HIV-positive gay men: an exploratory study of prevalence and user characteristics. AIDS Care 2000; 12:435–446.

553

CHAPTER 48

The HIV-infected International Traveler

Malcolm John

Introduction

The advent of highly active antiretroviral therapy (HAART) has led to significant decreases in human immunodeficiency virus type 1 (HIV-1)-related morbidity and mortality with concomitant improved immunocompetence.[1-4] Despite this, the HIV-positive traveler is still at increased risk for opportunistic infections and other complications compared with HIV-negative travelers. This is especially true for HIV-infected travelers with low CD4 T-cell counts and those traveling to developing countries. Nonetheless, pre-travel health advice is often underutilized.[5,6]

One recent study of patients at an HIV clinic in a tertiary care hospital in North America, found that 46% of 290 surveyed individuals had traveled internationally within the previous 5 years. Only 44% of these individuals sought health advice before traveling.[6] Of those seeking pre-travel advice, only half told the provider that they were HIV-positive. International travel was associated with poor adherence to antiretrovirals and to risky sexual activity in these patients. A total of 93% of the 75 individuals not seeking pre-travel health advice believed such consultations were unnecessary. Such data are disturbing given that international travel increased steadily throughout the 1990s and early twenty-first century.[7]

Outbound overseas travel from the USA alone climbed to a high of almost 27 million by 2000 with travel to Asia, South America, and the Middle East growing by 93%, 130%, and 159%, respectively.[7] During this period, incident infections in returning international travelers continued to rise.[8] There has

also been increasing numbers of immigrants to developed countries who visit their countries of origin and return that are a population at high risk for tropical infections including tuberculosis (TB), malaria, food- and water-borne illnesses, hepatitis A, and sexually transmitted infections (STIs).[9] It is therefore important that persons living with HIV/AIDS and their pre-travel providers stay informed about preparations and precautions that should be taken by the HIV-infected person when traveling internationally today.

General Considerations

The quality of pre-travel health advice can vary greatly; thus, consultation with a travel medicine specialist is advisable. A study from the UK of 215 clinicians serving higher-education establishments in the UK showed that practitioners often gave good advice with respect to immunizations and malaria prophylaxis, but little on HIV and other risks.[10] Training in travel medicine was associated with more appropriate pre-travel health advice.

Pre-travel health advice for the HIV-infected international traveler should be sought as soon as possible. Consultation at least 6–8 weeks before travel is recommended to allow time for development of adequate responses to any necessary vaccinations. Use of resources such as travel clinics and travel related websites before traveling is appropriate. Detailed counseling and evaluation of the risks and benefits of preventive prophylaxis and vaccinations is essential.

Pre-travel advice should include a discussion of immunizations, malaria prophylaxis, traveler's diarrhea management, supplemental health insurance, accidents and injuries, motion sickness, jet lag, extremes of temperature and sun exposure, food and water safety, use of an emergency medical bracelet, list of medical services abroad, and possible arrangement of visits with physicians who speaks the traveler's language.[11] The last issue is especially important for extended visits so that adequate medical follow-up and medication supplies are maintained. A discussion of behavioral risk reduction while traveling is also essential. Boxes 48.1 and 48.2 summarize advice on items to take while traveling and what to do while traveling that should be part of a pre-travel consultation.

It is wise to reassess the stage of HIV prior to travel as low CD4 counts are the biggest predictor of risk of opportunistic infections (OIs) when traveling. However, changing medications just prior to travel is not encouraged in order to avoid complications from the medications occurring while traveling.

The Centers for Disease Control and Prevention (CDC) warns that some countries screen for HIV and deny entry to those who have AIDS or test positive for HIV (usually those entering for extended periods,

e.g. for work or study). Some countries also deny entry to those carrying antiretroviral medications; placing such medications in an empty vitamin or other medication container is one means of avoiding problems in such situations. More specific information is best obtained from the consular officials of

---

Box 48.1

What to take when traveling

- Adequate supply of medications (1–2 weeks' extra supply is advisable) and prophylactic agents (e.g. for malaria) for shorter trips, along with copies of prescriptions; attention should be given to any need for refrigeration of medications
- Documentation of vaccinations
- Medications for traveler's diarrhea, e.g. ciprofloxacin for 3 to 7 day courses of treatment or daily prophylaxis up to 3 weeks' duration; trimethoprim-sulfamethoxazole (TMP-SMX) recommended for children and pregnant women
- Mosquito netting (preferably treated with permethrin)
- Insect repellent that contains <30% Deet (N,N-diethylmetatoluamide)
- Medications for sinusitis and jet lag
- Condoms and other safe sex items
- First aid kit, including topical antibiotics
- Consider bringing own equipment for boiling water, purifying water by iodine treatment, and/or filtration of water using commercial filters using 1 micron or smaller filters
- Consider need for fluconazole, itraconazole, and isoniazid prophylaxis if CD4 T-cell count <100 cells/μL.

Box 48.2

What to do when traveling

Avoid behaviors that increase risk of new infections or complications.

- 'Boil it, peel it, cook it, or forget it', and WASH HANDS
- Avoid raw vegetables, fruit you have not peeled yourself, unpasteurized dairy products, cooked food not served steaming hot, and tap water, including ice; meat should be well-cooked, as undercooked beef, pork or fish can be a source of tapeworms
- Purify water in high-risk areas – boiling water is the best method of purification; tincture of iodine or tetraglycine hydroperiodide tablets is an alternative but the water must be used within a few weeks and the method cannot be relied on to kill Cryptosporidium unless the water is allowed to sit for 15 h before it is drunk; filtering water produces variable results especially for small bacteria or viruses and proper selection, operation, care, and maintenance of water filters are essential
- Avoid walking barefoot in areas with high risk of soil pathogens
- Avoid swimming in bodies of water that may be contaminated by other people and from sewage, animal wastes, and wastewater run-off; avoid swallowing water when swimming, even chlorinated water which may contain live organisms (e.g. Cryptosporidium, Giardia, hepatitis A, and Norwalk virus) which have moderate to very high resistance to chlorine; avoid swimming in areas of endemic schistosomiasis or water at risk of contamination from animals carrying Leptospira
- Use safe sex practices to avoid risks from acquiring sexually transmitted diseases. These risks include increased severity and complications (e.g. herpes outbreaks more prolonged and severe), risks related to acquiring new HIV strains (e.g. non-nucleoside reverse transcriptase inhibitors are not active against HIV-2)
- Avoid blood exposures (e.g. acupuncture, tattoos, injections with possibly unsterile needles, sharing razors, manicures and pedicures) that can lead to acquiring hepatitis C as hepatitis C-related cirrhosis is accelerated in those co-infected with HIV.

Table 48.1 Summary of vaccination recommendations

Routinely given	Given if travel indicates	Contraindicated
• Diphtheria-Tetanus • Hepatitis A • Hepatitis B • Influenza • Pneumococcal (*S. pneumonia*) (*H. influenza B* generally not recommended as HIV-positive adults generally infected with non-typable strains; children should be vaccinated)	• Japanese B encephalitis (many side-effects which are not unique to HIV-infected persons; use if at high risk e.g. >1 month in rural endemic area) • Measles (live vaccine should not be given if severe immunosuppression; use immunoglobulin if needed) • Meningococcal • Polio, inactivated (IPV) • Rabies (safe; pre-exposure prophylaxis generally not indicated) • Tick-borne encephalitis (only if high risk, e.g. forested endemic areas and drinking unpasteurized milk products) • Typhoid Vi (inactivated) • Yellow Fever (live vaccine should not be given if severe immunosuppression, instruct how to avoid mosquito bites and provide a vaccination waiver letter)	• BCG • Polio, live • Typhoid, live • Varicella-Zoster Virus, VZV (cholera vaccine no longer recommended or required)

Box 48.3

Useful travel resources

- CDC Traveler's Health site: www.cdc.gov/travel/index.htm
- CDC Malaria webpage: www.cdc.gov/malaria
- CDC Traveler's Help Hotline: 1-877-FYI-TRIP or 1-877-394-8747, toll free
- World Health Organization (WHO) homepage: www.who.int/en
- WHO International Travel & Health page: www.who.int/ith/en
- US Department of State HIV Testing Requirements List: www.travel.state.gov/travel/tips/brochures/brochures_1230.html
- US State Department Travel Warnings & Consular Information: http://travel.state.gov/travel/cis_pa_tw/tw/tw_1764.html

the individual nations; an unofficial list is kept by the US Department of State (which can be found online. See Box 48.3 for a list of travel resources.

Vaccinations

Concerns over vaccinating HIV-positive persons because of documented elevations in HIV viral loads have not borne out. Such viral load elevations are transient, resolving within 4–6 weeks and sooner if on HAART without any documented long-term deleterious effects.[12] All HIV-infected travelers should therefore be up-to-date on routinely recommended vaccines and those routinely recommended for HIV-positive individuals. Additional vaccines should be given based on the specific travel risk exposures to endemic infections. It should be noted that vaccine responses are generally inadequate if the patient's CD4 count is <100 cells/μL; best results are obtained if the CD4 count is >350 cells/μL.[13] The CDC's *Traveler's Health Yellow Book* states that antiretroviral drug-induced increased CD4 counts and not nadir counts should be used to categorize HIV-infected persons and that waiting 3 months post- immune reconstitution before immunization is advisable.

In general, inactivated vaccines are safe to administer and should be initiated 6–8 weeks before travel. Live vaccines, including BCG, should be avoided with two exceptions (Box 48.1):

- Live measles vaccine is recommended for non-immune travelers whose CD4 counts are >200 cells/μL as the clinical course of the disease is worse in those with HIV. Non-immune travelers with CD4 counts <200 cells/μL should receive the immune globulin if traveling to endemic areas (CDC, "Traveller's Health: Yellow Book").
- Yellow fever vaccine is of unknown risk and benefit to HIV-infected individuals; however, it should be offered to asymptomatic HIV-positive

individuals with minimal immune-suppression (avoid if CD4 counts <200 cells/µL) who cannot avoid potential exposure to the yellow fever virus. Those at risk who defer immunization should be instructed in methods to avoid mosquito bites and provided a vaccination waiver letter understanding that such a letter may not be accepted by some countries (CDC, www.cdc.gov/travel/hivtrav.htm).

Prophylaxis Considerations

Prophylaxis should be given for malaria to those at risk. Empiric treatment for traveler's diarrhea (TD) rather than primary prophylaxis is generally recommended. However, primary prophylaxis for TD can be considered for those who cannot afford to get ill, e.g. those with severely depressed CD4 counts (see sections below on Malaria and Enteric Infections for details).

Consider prophylaxis for those with severe immunosuppression (e.g. CD4 counts <100 cells/µL) at risk for TB or disseminated infections from endemic mycoses such as *Penicillium marneffei, Coccidioides immitis, Histoplasma capsulatum,* and *Paracoccidioides brasiliensis* as well as *Cryptococcus neoformans* (see below).

Selected Disease-specific Issues

HIV-infected travelers and their healthcare providers should review the risks of the following disorders and opportunistic infections to travelers to the developing world, especially to those with low CD4 counts:

- Enteric infections (e.g. salmonella) and wasting
- TB, bacterial respiratory infections (e.g. *S. pneumonia*)
- Malaria, leishmaniasis, Chagas disease, and other parasitic infections
- Penicilliosis and other disseminated endemic mycoses
- Other, e.g. new HIV infections, fevers.

Enteric Infections

Etiologies of traveler's diarrhea in HIV-infected travelers

The main enteric bacterial pathogen to which HIV-infected individuals are at increased risk of acquir-

ing is *Salmonella typhimurium* and other non-typhoidal *Salmonella* (NTS). HIV-positive patients have up to a 100-fold risk of infection compared with HIV-negative individuals in developing countries where NTS is the leading cause of diarrhea with fever.[14] Disease often relapses and can be difficult to treat effectively leading to significant morbidity and mortality. HIV-positive persons with *Salmonella* septicemia require chronic maintenance therapy to prevent recurrence.

Other common bacterial enteric infections in the HIV-positive traveler include enterotoxigenic *E. coli,* enteroaggregative *E. coli, Shigella,* and *Campylobacter,* especially among men who have sex with men. Other causes of TD include parasites, e.g. *Giardia, Isospora,* cryptosporidium, and *Cyclospora,* especially in Central America. Despite the fact that parasitic diarrheal diseases occur in the HIV-infected traveler, there appears to be little evidence that HIV infection increases the risk of intestinal helminth infections.[15,16] More rarely, one sees TD related to *Yersinia, Plesiomonas, Aeromonas* (more commonly in Southeast Asia), *Entamoeba,* and non-cholera *Vibrio* species. Rarely, cholera or polio is found. Viruses can cause TD in HIV-positive travelers as in HIV-negative persons although this may reflect infection prior to travel; rotavirus and Norwalk viruses are common agents in this group and have been implicated in outbreaks on cruise ships in the Caribbean. TD due to infection with hepatitis A can be avoided with proper immunization.

Prevention of TD in HIV-infected travelers

Some recommend empiric daily prophylaxis (e.g. ciprofloxacin 500 mg daily) for up to 3 weeks for those who must avoid TD.[13,15,17] This may include those with severely depressed CD4 counts and may be desired even if such travelers are already on tri-methoprim-sulfamethoxazole (TMP/SMX) for *Pneumocystis carinii* pneumonia (PCP) prophylaxis given the high rates of TMP/SMX resistance in enteric pathogens worldwide. Antibiotics recommended by the Infectious Disease Society of America include ciprofloxacin, norfloxacin, infaximin, and bismuth subsalicylate. Care should be taken to avoid contact with reptiles (e.g. snakes, lizards, iguanas, and turtles) as well as chicks and ducklings because of the risk for salmonellosis.[17]

As mentioned earlier, prevention of enteric infections in the HIV-positive traveler is best accomplished by ensuring safe water for drinking, brushing teeth, and making ice cubes. Bottled beverages, hot coffee and tea, beer, and wine, are considered safe for drinking. In addition, all fruits and vegetables must be washed and peeled, preferably by the travelers themselves; all meats and other foods should be cooked thoroughly to steaming hot. Boiling water is the best method of water purification and should be done until at least 1 min (3 min at >2000 m altitude) of vigorous boiling has been achieved. Tincture of iodine or tetraglycine hydroperiodide tablets is an alternative, but the water must be used within a few weeks and the method cannot be relied on to kill *Cryptosporidium* unless the water is allowed to sit for 15 h before it is drunk. Filtering water produces variable results especially for small bacteria or viruses and proper selection, operation, care, and maintenance of water filters is essential. Commercial filters should be labeled either 'Reverse osmosis,' 'Absolute pore size of 1 micron or smaller,' 'Tested and certified by NSF Standard 53 or NSF Standard 58 for cyst removal,' or 'Tested and certified by NSF Standard 53 or NSF Standard 58 for cyst reduction.' Reverse-osmosis filters provide broad protection but they are expensive, relatively large, and have small pores that are easily plugged by dirty water. Microstrainer filters with pore sizes in the 0.1–0.3 μm range do not remove viruses so disinfection with iodine or chlorine is still necessary.

The importance of preventing diarrheal disease in the HIV-infected traveler is underscored by the fact that wasting syndrome ('slim disease') has been associated with international travel in a study carried out among 4549 participants of the SWISS HIV Cohort Study.[18] Slim disease is a major health problem in developing nations consisting of chronic diarrhea associated with wasting in HIV-positive patients. There is also evidence that chronic parasitic infections of the intestines may negatively influence the natural history of HIV infection and chronically increase HIV viral loads.[19,20]

Treatment of TD in HIV-infected travelers

Empiric treatment for traveler's diarrhea (TD) should be given at the onset of diarrhea. This consists of antiperistaltic agents (e.g. loperamide) for mild diarrhea (<2 loose stools/day) which should not be used if there is high fever, blood in the stool, or symptoms persisting >48 h on antiperistaltic agents. Antibiotics should be combined with antiperistaltic agents for more severe diarrhea or diarrhea with fevers or constitutional symptoms. Medical attention should be sought if there any fevers with chills, bloody stools, or dehydration. Recommended antibiotics include ciprofloxacin 500 mg twice daily (or equivalent fluoroquinolone) for 3–7 days, or azithromycin 500 mg

once daily for 3 days for pregnant women, those in areas of increasing fluoroquinolone resistance (e.g. Thailand and Nepal), and children (5–10 mg/kg × 1). Single dose regimens such as azithromycin 1000 mg once can be attempted when taken early in the course of infection and with milder symptoms. TMP-SMX DS, 1–2 pills twice daily for 3–7 days is no longer the recommended first line treatment due to increased resistance worldwide (see suggested antibiotics under 'prevention of TD in HIV-infected travellers'). Since the FDA approved rifaximin in 2004 for diarrhea from non-invasive strains of *E. coli*, this drug is a reasonable alternative to ciprofloxacin especially in pregnant women and children, but there is little data to support this. Rifaximin is a poorly absorbed rifamycin derivative that has been shown to be as effective as ciprofloxacin in the management of TD in Mexico and Jamaica, perhaps attributable to its activity against a wide range of enteric bacteria.[21] It has also been shown to effectively prevent TD in travelers to Mexico.[22] Usual dose of rifaximin is 200 mg three times per day for 3 days. Its use should be limited to areas outside of Asia where the predominant cause of TD is Campylobacter rather than enterotoxigenic *E. coli* until further studies are done.

Respiratory Infections

Bacterial pneumonia

Bacterial infections are increased in HIV-infected individuals and bacterial pneumonias may be acquired during travel.[15] *Streptococcus pneumoniae* infections in particular may be problematic given the increased rates of penicillin/β lactam-resistant *S. pneumoniae* worldwide (often also resistant to TMP-SMX and macrolides). All travelers should be immunized with the 23-valent polysaccharide pneumococcal vaccine as part of their routine care. This may be repeated if not vaccinated within the previous 5 years.[17]

Tuberculosis

HIV-infected travelers are at increased risk for primary TB or reactivation upon return from developing countries or other areas with a high prevalence of TB. Care should be taken to avoid conditions that promote TB transmission such as crowded situations and contact with hospital, prison, or homeless shelter populations. TB skin testing should be assessed prior to travel as part of routine care and again 3 months after returning from developing countries.[23] Travelers with negative TB skin tests prior to travel to high-risk areas are at increased risk for primary infection but efficacy of treatment among this group has not been demonstrated. Decisions concerning using chemoprophylaxis in these situations must be considered individually and latent TB infections treated according to treatment guidelines.[17]

Other respiratory infections

PCP is not more common during travel and the incidence is lower in tropical areas than in North America. However, all at risk should be on appropriate chemoprophylaxis. HIV-positive travelers should note that the common cold and sinusitis are some of the more common health issues to affect all travelers and should bring along medications for symptomatic relief.

Emerging and Re-emerging Infections in HIV

Malaria

Despite mixed data in the past, it now appears that malaria interacts with HIV especially in advanced HIV disease and pregnancy, which has long been associated with more severe disease independent of HIV serostatus.[19] Malaria presentation changes with decreasing CD4 counts, with increased episodes of symptomatic parasitemia, increased density and duration of parasitemia, and prolonged fever and malaria can be more severe in areas of unstable disease transmission.[24-26] In addition, there is increased activation and replication of HIV during infection with malaria.[24] Changes in host-parasite interactions occur that may worsen malarial disease in HIV-positive persons on HAART.[19]

Prophylaxis for malaria should be given to those traveling to endemic areas. Some caution may be warranted as mefloquine has been shown to decrease ritonavir levels, a component of most protease-based HAART regimens, in healthy volunteers.[27] The clinical relevance of this is unclear. There is also concern that antiretrovirals with central nervous system effects such as efavirenz may worsen the neuropsychiatric effects of mefloquine. For this reason, doxycycline, chloroquine, atovaquones, and proguanil may be the preferred prophylaxis in travelers on HAART, but there is no contraindication to mefloquine. Those on TMP-SMX for PCP prophylaxis will have some protection against malaria. Malaria prophylaxis should be started prior to travel to monitor for any side effects and to achieve adequate drug levels in the body before being exposed

to infected mosquitoes. Use of the CDC's travel hotline (1-877-FYI-TRIP; 1-877-394-8747) or malaria website (www.cdc.gov/malaria) can help in assessing the risk of acquiring malaria and drug-resistant *P. falciparum* malaria.

Leishmaniasis

Visceral leishmaniasis (Kala-Azar) remains an emerging opportunistic infection among HIV-infected individuals. Co-infections with HIV and leishmania have occurred at significant rates in Eastern Africa, India, Brazil, and Europe and have been reported in 35 countries.[19] In Brazil and southwestern Europe, HIV-leishmania co-infection is promoted by the sharing of needles in intravenous drug use rather than the usual case of transmission by sandflies. When CD4 counts fall below 200–300 cells/μL, parasites spread to atypical sites, especially the gastrointestinal site. Only 50% of patients have fever and hepatosplenomegaly; cytopenias are very severe.[28] Diagnosis may be difficult as 50% of patients do not develop characteristic antibodies. Ultimately, diagnosis from visualization of parasites in peripheral blood monocytes may be possible given the high parasite burden in HIV-positive patients.[17,19] Polymerase chain reaction of the buffy coat of blood can yield the diagnosis in up to 100% of patients.[19] Treatment consists of stibogluconate or amphotericin B with 50–100% of patients responding. However, long-term suppressive treatment will be required, e.g. HAART with intermittent liposomal amphotericin B every 21 days until CD4 greater 350 cells/μL for 3–6 months.[29]

Chagas disease

Trypanosoma cruzi infection (Chagas disease) is accelerated and more severe in HIV infection.[19] The chronic phase of infection is characterized by persistent reactivation of Chagas disease with high levels of parasitemia in co-infected individuals in contrast with low-level parasitemia in HIV-negative persons.[30] Fever, cutaneous eruptions, and myocarditis similar to that seen in acute Chagas disease is often seen in contrast to the cardiac and GI involvement characteristic of disease in HIV-negative persons. CNS involvement such as meningoencephalitis that can be fatal, CNS abscesses, and granulomatous encephalitis is usually present in co-infected patients while it is rarely seen in HIV-negative patients.[19,31] Diagnosis in co-infected persons can be made by examination of the peripheral blood for spirochetes, PCR of the blood or tissue, or examination of tissue biopsies. Treatment for *T. cruzi* should be initiated earlier than usually done in HIV-negative persons, preferably in the asymptomatic phase of the disease. Life-long treatment with benznidazole or nifurtimox may be needed.[31]

Precautions should be taken to avoid infection if traveling in the Americas where the infection exists and spread by the bite of the reduviid bug. The risk of infection is significant for those with extended stays; infections of tourists are uncommon. To minimize risk of infection, avoid sleeping in substandard houses, use mosquito nets, and use insect repellents at night.

Other Parasitic Infections

Few major interactions exist between HIV and other emerging parasitic infections in travelers. The propensity for disseminated strongyloidiasis is associated with HTLV-1 not HIV-1 infection. The egg burden in schistosomiasis may be higher in HIV-infected persons and the time until re-infection may be shorter.[19] Onchocerciasis does not appear to be significantly affected by HIV infection, although cellular immune responses may be depressed in HIV-*Onchocerca volvulus* co-infected individuals.[19,32] There is little data on the impact of HIV on filariasis and loiasis.[19]

Penicilliosis

Penicilliosis, disseminated infection with the fungus *Penicillium marneffei*, has become an important opportunistic infection in AIDS patients in southeast Asia (especially northern Thailand) and southern China. The disease usually occurs when CD4 T-cell counts fall below 50 cells/μL.[33] Common presenting symptoms include fever, sweats, wasting, and skin lesions – often papules with central umbilication or nodules, but a wide range of skin eruptions are possible – in association with anemia, lymphadenopathy and hepatomegaly. Diagnosis is often made by bone marrow examination or skin biopsy, and less reliably from blood cultures. Treatment consists of amphotericin B followed by itraconazole. Chronic maintenance therapy with itraconazole is needed as post-treatment relapse is common.[34] Untreated, mortality is over 75%.[34] Penicilliosis can occur in AIDS patients with a remote history of only brief travel to endemic areas. Soil exposure is a known risk factor and should be avoided in endemic areas, especially during the rainy season. Prophylactic itraconazole at 200 mg/day for AIDS patients traveling in high-risk parts of endemic areas may be considered, especially for those with CD4 counts <100 cells/μL.

Other Endemic Mycoses

HIV-positive travelers with low CD4 counts are at risk for diseases from other endemic fungal infections. These include coccidioidomycosis in southwest USA, northern Mexico and South America, histoplasmosis with a worldwide distribution but primarily in the Americas and Africa, and paracoccidioidomycosis in Central America. These disseminated diseases are more common in the immunocompromised host with decreased cell-mediated immunity such as HIV-positive travelers with low CD4 counts. Disease can reflect new infection, reinfection, or reactivation of previous infections.

Prophylaxis with itraconazole at 100 mg/day can be considered for travelers with CD4+ T-lymphocyte counts <100 cells/μL who are at high risk for acquiring histoplasmosis because of occupational exposure or who travel to a community with a hyperendemic rate of histoplasmosis (>10 cases/100 patient-years) although there has not been demonstrated survival benefit in doing this.[17] Severely immunocompromised travelers should avoid activities known to be associated with increased risk such as creating dust when working with surface soil; cleaning chicken coops that are heavily contaminated with droppings; disturbing soil beneath bird roosting sites; cleaning, remodeling, or demolishing old buildings; and exploring caves.[17] Prophylaxis for the other endemic mycoses is generally not recommended. Avoiding the agents of coccidioidomycosis and paracoccidioidomycosis is not entirely possible, but at-risk travelers should avoid activities associated with increased risk including those involving extensive exposure to disturbed native soil, e.g. dust storms.[17]

Cryptococcus neoformans causes disseminated cryptococcosis, a common opportunistic infection worldwide in AIDS patients with CD4 cell counts <50 cells/μL. *C. neoformans* been found in soil samples from around the world in areas frequented by birds, especially pigeons and chickens but there has been no evidence linking exposure to pigeon droppings with an increased risk for acquiring cryptococcosis. Little can be done to avoid exposure to *C. neoformans*. Prophylaxis for those at risk is not commonly recommended but can be considered in the context of prophylaxis for other mycoses.

Travel-related Skin Disorders

Dermatologic lesions in the returning traveler are common in the HIV-infected and HIV-uninfected traveler alike. One prospective study of 269 returning travelers with skin disorder found that the most common skin lesions were cutaneous larva migrans (25%); pyodermas (18%); pruritic arthropod-reactive dermatitis (10%); myiasis (9%); tungiasis (6%); urticaria (5%); fever and rash (4%); and cutaneous leishmaniasis (3%).[35]

The appearance of skin lesions can give clues to their etiology[8]:

- Papules, usually pruritic: consider insect bites, scabies, seabather's eruption for rashes confined to skin covered by bathing suits, cercarial dermatitis for rashes involving exposed skin, onchocerciasis in long-term travelers, and drug eruptions
- Nodules: consider myiasis if painful boil-like lesions with central opening with intermittently visible fly larva, tungiasis (jiggers) especially if lesions mainly on soles of the feet and around toenails, loiasis if migratory areas of angioedema (Calabar swellings), acute East African trypanosomiasis and furuncles
- Ulcers: consider pyoderma if lesions painful (frequently bite-related with secondary infection from *S. aureus* or group A streptococci), leishmaniasis if lesions painless, and rickettsial diseases if an eschar is present
- Linear and migratory lesions: consider cutaneous larva migrans; larva currens due to strongyloidiasis if perianal cutaneous track present; and photodermatitis if painless, non-pruritic fixed linear streaks (from skin exposure to psoralen-containing products, e.g. limes).

Other Issues in the HIV-infected Traveler

New HIV Infections

In Western countries, where the B subtype is predominant, there is a steep increase in non B-subtypes and circulating recombinant forms, while new recombinants emerge worldwide. Travelers contribute to the spread of HIV-1 genetic diversity worldwide; in the developing world, migration of rural populations and civil war are additional contributing factors. The spreading of HIV-1 variants has implications for diagnostic, treatment (unknown clinical relevance at this time based on limited data), and vaccine development.[36]

Fever in the Returning HIV-positive Traveler

The evaluation of fever in the returning HIV-positive traveler should focus on the same etiologies as those in the HIV-negative traveler. Common causes are still most likely, such as sinusitis, pneumonia, urinary tract infection, drug fever. Important infectious causes of non-specific fevers include malaria, dengue, rickettsial diseases (e.g. RMSF, scrub typhus), leptospirosis, typhoid fever, tuberculosis, acute schistosomiasis, East African trypanosomiasis, viral hepatitis, and traveler's diarrhea.[8]

Conclusion

As individuals with HIV/AIDS continue to live longer in the era of HAART, we can expect increased rates of international travel in this population including those with depressed CD4 counts. Careful medical evaluation and appropriate pre-travel health advice will be increasingly important. Simple precautions and the use of a travel health expert can help minimize risks enabling all HIV-infected travelers to have safer and more enjoyable international travels.

References

1. Palella F, Delaney K, Moorman A, et al. Declining morbidity and mortality among patients with advanced human immunodeficiency virus infection. N Engl J Med 1998; 338:853–860.
2. van Sighem AI, van de Wiel MA, Ghani AC, et al. Mortality and progression to AIDS after starting highly active antiretroviral therapy. AIDS 2003; 17:2227–2236.
3. Autran B, Carcelain G, Debre P. Immune reconstitution after highly active anti-retroviral treatment of HIV infection. Adv Exp Med Biol 2001; 495:205–212.
4. Autran B, Carcelain G, Li TS, et al. Positive effects of combined antiretroviral therapy on CD4+ T cell homeostasis and function in advanced HIV disease. Science 1997; 277:112–116.
5. Kemper CA, Linett A, Kane C, et al. Travels with HIV: the compliance and health of HIV-infected adults who travel. Int J STD AIDS 1997; 8:44–49.
6. Salit IE, Sano M, Boggild AK, et al. Travel patterns and risk behaviour of HIV-positive people travelling internationally. Can Med Assoc J 2005; 172:884–888.
7. Bureau of Transportation Statistics. US International Travel and Transportation Trends, BTS02–03. Washington, DC: US Department of Transportation; 2002.
8. Ryan ET, Wilson ME, Kain KC. Illness after international travel. N Engl J Med 2002; 347:505–516.
9. Fulford M, Keystone JS. Health risks associated with visiting friends and relatives in developing countries. Curr Infect Dis Rep 2005; 7:48–53.
10. Porter JF, Knill-Jones RP. Quality of travel health advice in higher-education establishments in the United Kingdom and its relationship to the demographic background of the provider. J Travel Med 2004; 11:347–353.

11. Suh KN, Mileno MD. Challenging scenarios in a travel clinic: advising the complex traveler. Infect Dis Clin North Am 2005; 19:15–47.

12. Glesby M, Hoover D, Farzedegan H, et al. The effect of influenza vaccination on human immunodeficiency virus type 1 load: a randomized, double-blinded, placebo-controlled study. J Infect Dis 1996; 174:1332–1336.

13. Castelli F, Patroni A. The human immunodeficiency virus-infected traveler. Clin Infect Dis 2000; 31:1403–1408.

14. Gruenewald R, Blum S, Chan J. Relationship between human immunodeficiency virus infection and salmonellosis in 20- to 59-year-old residents of New York City. Clin Infect Dis 1994; 18:358–363.

15. Mileno MD, Bia FJ. The compromised traveler. Infect Dis Clin North Am 1998; 12:369–412.

16. McCombs SB, Dworkin MS, Wan PC. Helminth infections in HIV-infected persons in the United States, 1990-1999. Clin Infect Dis 2000; 30:241–242.

17. Kaplan JE, Masur H, Holmes KK. Guidelines for preventing opportunistic infections among HIV-infected persons–2002. Recommendations of the US Public Health Service and the Infectious Diseases Society of America. MMWR Recomm Rep 2002; 51:1–52.

18. Furrer H, Chan P, Weber R, et al. Increased risk of wasting syndrome in HIV-infected travellers: prospective multicentre study. Trans R Soc Trop Med Hyg 2001; 95:484–486.

19. Harms G, Feldmeier H. The impact of HIV infection on tropical diseases. Infect Dis Clin North Am 2005; 19:121–135.

20. Bentwich Z, Maartens G, Torten D, et al. Concurrent infections and HIV pathogenesis. AIDS 2000; 14:2071–2081.

21. DuPont HL, Jiang ZD, Ericsson CD, et al. Rifaximin versus ciprofloxacin for the treatment of traveler's diarrhea: a randomized, double-blind clinical trial. Clin Infect Dis 2001; 33:1807–1815.

22. DuPont HL, Jiang ZD, Okhuysen PC, et al. A randomized, double-blind, placebo-controlled trial of rifaximin to prevent travelers' diarrhea. Ann Intern Med 2005; 142:805–812.

23. Ericsson CD. Travellers with pre-existing medical conditions. Int J Antimicrob Agents 2003; 21:181–188.

24. Whitworth J, Morgan D, Quigley M, et al. Effect of HIV-1 and increasing immunosuppression on malaria parasitaemia and clinical episodes in adults in rural Uganda: a cohort study. Lancet 2000; 356:1051–1056.

25. French N, Nakiyingi J, Lugada E, et al. Increasing rates of malarial fever with deteriorating immune status in HIV-1-infected Ugandan adults. AIDS 2001; 15:899–906.

26. Grimwade K, French N, Mbatha DD, et al. HIV infection as a cofactor for severe falciparum malaria in adults living in a region of unstable malaria transmission in South Africa. AIDS 2004; 18:547–554.

27. Khaliq Y, Gallicano K, Tisdale C, et al. Pharmacokinetic interaction between mefloquine and ritonavir in healthy volunteers. Br J Clin Pharmacol 2001; 51:591–600.

28. Rosenthal E, Marty P, del Giudice P, et al. HIV and Leishmania coinfection: a review of 91 cases with focus on atypical locations of Leishmania. Clin Infect Dis 2000; 31:1093–1095.

29. Lopez-Velez R, Videla S, Marquez M, et al. Amphotericin B lipid complex versus no treatment in the secondary prophylaxis of visceral leishmaniasis in HIV-infected patients. J Antimicrob Chemother 2004; 53:540–543.

30. Sartori AM, Neto JE, Nunes EV, et al. Trypanosoma cruzi parasitemia in chronic Chagas disease: comparison between human immunodeficiency virus (HIV)-positive and HIV-negative patients. J Infect Dis 2002; 186:872–875.

31. Ferreira MS, Nishioka Sde A, Silvestre MT, et al. Reactivation of Chagas' disease in patients with AIDS: report of three new cases and review of the literature. Clin Infect Dis 1997; 25:1397–1400.

32. Sentongo E, Rubaale T, Buttner DW, et al. T cell responses in coinfection with Onchocerca volvulus and the human immunodeficiency virus type 1. Parasite Immunol 1998; 20:431–439.

33. Clezy K, Sirisanthana T, Sirisanthana V, et al. Late manifestations of HIV in Asia and the Pacific. AIDS 1994; 8:35–43.

34. Supparatpinyo K, Khamwan C, Baosoung V, et al. Disseminated *Penicillium marneffei* infection in southeast Asia. Lancet 1994; 344:110–113.

35. Caumes E, Carriere J, Guermonprez G, et al. Dermatoses associated with travel to tropical countries: a prospective study of the diagnosis and management of 269 patients presenting to a tropical disease unit. Clin Infect Dis 1995; 20:542–548.

36. Perrin L, Kaiser L, Yerly S. Travel and the spread of HIV-1 genetic variants. Lancet Infect Dis 2003; 3:22–27

CHAPTER 49

HIV Transmission and its Prevention in Africa

Catherine Hankins
Steffanie Strathdee
Salim Abdool Karim

Introduction

Sub-Saharan Africa has just over 10% of the world's population, but is home to more than 63% of all people living with HIV in the world: 24.5 million (21.6–27.4 million). HIV prevalence among adults aged 15–49 years is 6.1% (5.4–6.8%). In 2005, an estimated 2.7 million (2.3–3.1 million) people in the region became newly infected, while 2.0 million (1.7–2.3 million) adults and children died of AIDS.[1] Among young people aged 15–24 years, an estimated 4.6% (4.2–5.5%) of young women and 1.7% (1.3–2.2%) of young men were living with HIV in 2005.[2]

In this chapter, HIV transmission and prevention in the African context will be addressed, beginning with a look at the declines in HIV prevalence being observed in a few countries and the likely contributing factors for these prevention successes. Then essential prevention policy and programmatic actions will be discussed with reference to various countries. Finally the involvement of African researchers and communities in HIV prevention trials of promising new prevention tools will be reviewed.

HIV Prevalence Declines

The HIV epidemic appears to have reached a stable level in sub-Saharan countries such as Uganda, Tanzania, Sierra Leone, Senegal, Rwanda, Lesotho, Guinea, Ghana, and Botswana. This stability is occurring at prevalence proportions ranging from 0.9% in Senegal to 24.1% in Botswana.[1] Such stability is no cause for complacency because it represents active epidemic dynamics in a steady state with equal numbers of people dying as are being newly infected. Declines in adult national HIV prevalence appear to have begun in Uganda in the early 1990s, Zimbabwe in the mid-1990s and Kenya in the late 1990s. Peak HIV prevalence among adults aged 15–49 years was 13%, 29% and 10%, respectively. In urban areas of two eastern sub-Saharan African countries – Ethiopia and Rwanda – adult HIV prevalence has begun to decline while in Burundi's capital city it is now falling. West and Central African countries (where estimated national HIV prevalence is considerably lower than in the southern and eastern countries of the region) show no signs of changing HIV infection levels, except for urban parts of Burkina Faso where prevalence now appears to be declining.[1]

With close to one in three people infected with HIV globally living in southern Africa, this sub-region remains the epicenter of the pandemic. With the exception of Zimbabwe, countries of southern Africa show little evidence of declining epidemics. HIV prevalence levels remain exceptionally high, except for Angola, and might not yet have reached their peak in several countries, as the expanding epidemics in South Africa and Swaziland suggest.[1]

As these trends reveal, there is no single 'African' AIDS epidemic. Furthermore, national-level HIV prevalence data sometimes provide incomplete pictures of the real epidemic situation within a country.

HIV prevalence levels observed among pregnant women attending antenatal clinics differ by wide margins in most countries, depending on the location. Household surveys that include testing for HIV provide additional countrywide data on HIV prevalence since they include participants of both sexes from various age groups and include samples from remote rural areas which may not be included in antenatal surveys. However, if a significant share of respondents refuse to be tested it is difficult to interpret the results. Specific studies can also highlight localized variance within countries, emphasizing both the adaptability of HIV epidemics and their sensitivity to contextual factors. Prominent among these factors is the social and socioeconomic status of women, who are affected by HIV disproportionately in this region. Three-quarters of all women living with HIV worldwide are in sub-Saharan Africa. They make up a striking 59% of all adults living with HIV in the region today.

Prevention Successes in Africa: Cause of Declines in HIV Prevalence?

Three countries in East Africa, Uganda, Zimbabwe and Kenya, provide hopeful indications that serious AIDS epidemics can be reversed. Uganda was the first African country to show that prevention efforts can bring a widespread HIV epidemic under control. National HIV prevalence peaked at over 15% in the early 1990s before steadily declining during the mid- and late-1990s to reach an estimated adult HIV prevalence of 6.7% (5.7–7.6%) in 2005.[1] New HIV surveillance data indicate that HIV prevalence continues to decline among pregnant women in the capital, Kampala, and has remained stable elsewhere, including in most rural areas since 2001. There have been many attempts to determine after the fact what elements were the most critical in provoking and then maintaining the HIV prevalence declines observed in Uganda. Political leadership, open dialogue across all levels of society and combination prevention choices by individuals (Box 49.1) all are playing a role.

Uganda's prevention strategy focuses on a multipronged effort to provide information, education and communication through decentralized community orientated programs. Since 1996, Uganda has provided free, compulsory education for all young people from 6 to 13 years and is using its schools to deliver AIDS education. These collective efforts led to observed behavior changes: condom use by single women aged 15–24 years almost doubled between

---

Box 49.1

The ABCs of combination prevention[3]

Just as combination treatment attacks HIV at different phases of virus replication, combination prevention includes various safer sex behavior strategies that informed individuals who are in a position to decide for themselves can choose at different times in their lives to reduce their risk of exposing themselves or others to HIV.[4] These are often referred to as the ABCs of combination prevention.

A: Abstinence – not engaging in sexual intercourse or delaying sexual initiation. Whether abstinence occurs by delaying sexual debut or by adopting a period of abstinence at a later stage, access to information and education about alternative safer sexual practices is critical to avoid HIV infection when sexual activity begins or is resumed.

B: Being safer – by being faithful to one's partner or reducing the number of sexual partners. The lifetime number of sexual partners is a very important predictor of HIV infection. Thus, having fewer sexual partners reduces the risk of HIV exposure. However, strategies to promote faithfulness among couples do not necessarily lead to lower incidence of HIV unless neither partner has HIV infection and both are consistently faithful.

C: Correct and consistent condom use – condoms reduce the risk of HIV transmission for sexually active young people, couples in which one person is HIV-positive, sex workers and their clients, and anyone engaging in sexual activity with partners who may have been at risk of HIV exposure. Research has found that if people do not have access to condoms, other prevention strategies lose much of their potential effectiveness.

A, B, and C interventions can be adapted and combined in a balanced approach that will vary by cultural context, the population addressed and the stage of the epidemic.

1995 and 2001, and women in this age group are increasingly delaying sexual intercourse or abstaining entirely. In the capital, Kampala, almost 98% of sex workers surveyed in 2000 reported that they had used a condom the last time they had sex.[5] However, a 2004–2005 national household survey found condom use was erratic (only about half the men and women surveyed reported using a condom the last time they had sex with a casual partner), and almost one in three men (29%) compared with 4% of women said they had had more than one sexual partner in the previous year. Gender disparity is evident with HIV prevalence among women in urban areas twice that among men (13% compared with 7.3%). In rural areas, the prevalence of HIV in women was also higher (7.2% versus 5.6%). Finally, there is evidence of continued HIV-related stigma: roughly half the men and women surveyed said that if a family member contracted HIV they would prefer to keep that fact secret.[6]

Recent findings from a multi-year (1994–2003) study of 44 communities in Rakai in southern Uganda demonstrate that HIV prevalence declined sharply, from 20% in 1994–1995 to 13% in 2003 among women, and from 15–9% among men. Generally in Uganda, behavioral change has been considered to be responsible for such declines. For example, in Masaka district, which is next to Rakai, declining HIV incidence in the 1990s appeared to correlate strongly to behavior change.[7] However, in Rakai there were no significant increases in abstinence or fidelity. Furthermore, the proportion of young people who report multiple non-marital partners has increased considerably (from under 25% in 2000, to almost 35% in 2003), although condom use with casual partners is now more commonplace, particularly among men. While this probably helped in lowering HIV prevalence, most of the momentum appears to have been the result of higher mortality rates. Approximately 5% of the observed 6.2% decline in HIV prevalence in Rakai between 1994–2003 was likely due to increased mortality.[8] Tentative signs of a possible resurgence of HIV incidence among young men and women aged 15–24 years in Rakai, and elsewhere in Uganda, underline the need for revitalized HIV prevention strategies.

Recent reports from Zimbabwe suggest that changes in sexual behavior, including delaying sexual debut and reducing the number of casual partners, led to declining HIV prevalence. Between 2003 and 2005 in Zimbabwe, overall HIV prevalence declined from 22.1 to 20.1%, with the most significant declines seen in young men and women aged 15–24 years. The substantial increase in condom use since the early 1990s in Zimbabwe is likely associated with increasing AIDS awareness, relatively extensive health infrastructure and a growing fear of AIDS mortality. In the eastern province of Manicaland, where HIV prevalence in young women aged 15–24 years fell by half, from 16% in 1998 to 8% in 2003,[9] more women and men are delaying their sexual debut and avoiding casual sex liaisons. However, a significant part of the decline in HIV prevalence in Zimbabwe is attributable to high mortality rates. Zimbabwe cannot rest on its laurels: it needs to act

decisively to sustain the declining trend in HIV prevalence while reducing mortality through dramatic improvements in the provision of antiretroviral treatment for its citizens.

Kenya is the third country in which HIV prevalence among pregnant women has been declining, particularly in urban areas. As a result, national adult HIV prevalence is estimated to have fallen from 10% in the late 1990s to about 7% in 2003.[10] Various behavioral surveys show that the proportion of adults with more than one sexual partner is shrinking, more women are delaying their sexual debut, and condom use is rising. Increased mortality and the saturation of infection among people most at risk also appear to be factors contributing to the decline in HIV prevalence.[11] But there are troubling trends, with very high HIV prevalence in women attending some antenatal clinics, particularly on the coast where prevalence ranges from 14–30%.[12] Injecting drug use is now a factor in the epidemics in some cities and large towns including Nairobi, where 53% of injecting drug users, heroin users for the most part, have tested HIV positive.[13]

Essential Prevention Policy and Programmatic Actions

Implementing a strong national prevention program with sufficient coverage, scale and intensity to turn the epidemic around requires a strong national policy framework that reduces vulnerability, maximizes the accessibility and effectiveness of HIV prevention services, encourages safer behaviors, promotes gender equality and women's empowerment, and reduces stigma and discrimination. It also requires a clear understanding of the various dynamics of the country's epidemic and careful selection of an appropriate mix of HIV prevention programatic actions. Mounting such a comprehensive, evidence-informed response in a country requires political leadership and vision but also involvement of all levels and sectors of society.

The UNAIDS document *Intensifying HIV Prevention* articulates basic principles and strategies that form the basis of strong national HIV prevention plans.[14] National prevention programs should incorporate each essential programmatic and policy action; however, the relative emphasis of specific prevention measures will differ by setting, based on the nature and severity of national and sub-national epidemics. Boxes 49.2 and 49.3 contain the essential policy actions and the essential programmatic actions for effective HIV prevention, respectively.

Box 49.2

Essential policy actions for HIV prevention

1. Ensure that human rights are promoted, protected, and respected, and that measures are taken to eliminate discrimination and combat stigma.
2. Build and maintain leadership from all sections of society, including governments, affected communities, non-governmental organizations, faith-based organizations, the education sector, media, the private sector, and trade unions.
3. Involve people living with HIV, in the design, implementation, and evaluation of prevention strategies, addressing their distinct prevention needs.
4. Address cultural norms and beliefs, recognizing both the key role they play in supporting prevention efforts and the potential they have to fuel HIV transmission.
5. Promote gender equality and address gender norms and relations to reduce the vulnerability of women and girls, involving men and boys in this effort.
6. Promote widespread knowledge and awareness of how HIV is transmitted and how infection can be averted.
7. Promote the links between HIV prevention and sexual and reproductive health.
8. Support the mobilization of community-based responses throughout the continuum of prevention, care and treatment.
9. Promote programs targeted at HIV prevention needs of key affected groups and populations.
10. Mobilize and strengthen financial, human and institutional capacity across all sectors, particularly in health and education.
11. Review and reform legal frameworks to remove barriers to effective, evidence-based HIV prevention, combat stigma, and discrimination, and protect the rights of people living with HIV or vulnerable to or at risk of HIV.
12. Ensure that sufficient investments are made in the research and development of, and advocacy for, new prevention technologies.

Box 49.3

Essential programatic actions for HIV prevention

1. Prevent the sexual transmission of HIV.
2. Prevent mother-to-child transmission of HIV.
3. Prevent the transmission of HIV through injecting drug use, including harm reduction measures.
4. Ensure the safety of the blood supply.
5. Prevent HIV transmission in healthcare settings.
6. Promote greater access to voluntary HIV counselling and testing, while promoting principles of confidentiality and consent.
7. Integrate HIV prevention into AIDS treatment centers.
8. Focus on HIV prevention among young people.
9. Provide HIV-related information and education to enable individuals to protect themselves from infection.
10. Confront and mitigate HIV-related stigma and discrimination.
11. Prepare for access and use of vaccines and microbicides.

micro-credit interventions to increase their self-efficacy for risk reduction. For injecting drug users this may mean that needle exchange programs take place alongside access to substitution treatment and crucial ancillary services such as condoms, on-site HIV testing and counselling, screening for sexually transmitted infections and tuberculosis, provision of vaccines to prevent hepatitis A and B infections, abscess care, overdose prevention, and multivitamins. For women, because the legal, social, and economic disadvantages faced by women and girls in most societies greatly increase their vulnerability to HIV, gender-sensitive approaches are key when designing prevention programs as well as structural interventions to address underlying determinants of risk.

Below, we provide brief examples of different types of prevention programs addressing the general population in high prevalence African settings as well as populations at higher risk of HIV infection in Africa.

Mass Media Campaigns

Mass media can be used to disseminate accurate and culturally-appropriate HIV prevention information, foster behavior change and pro-social norms, and reduce HIV-related stigma by reaching a large and diverse audience through television, radio, print and/or commercial advertising, and the Internet.

HIV prevention programing can focus on individuals, couples, social networks or communities. Prevention programs have been developed for the general population, through mass-media or school-based education campaigns and through expanded access to HIV testing and counselling services. Particularly vulnerable populations require tailored prevention programs based on the route of exposure. For female sex workers this may mean that condom promotion and provision takes place alongside

Although some media campaigns have been based on 'scare tactics,' these approaches have been discouraged by most health professionals, activists and NGOs. In contrast, by highlighting prominent public figures with HIV infection, media campaigns can help put a 'face' on the epidemic. In 2002, the popular children's television program, 'Sesame Street,' introduced the first HIV-positive Muppet, 'Kami,' to promote education about AIDS in Africa and elsewhere. In Côte d'Ivoire, television soap operas on AIDS, such as 'SIDA dans la Cité' have promoted condom use and appear to have appealed to viewers who engage in risky behavior.[15] In Botswana, the radio drama called 'Makgabaneng' focuses on culturally specific HIV-related issues and encouraging changes in sexual behavior. Another program called 'Talk Back' provides primary and secondary schools with a television, video recorder, satellite dish, and decoder as part of an interactive AIDS education program that is broadcast by Botswana Television. The Internet has become a powerful media tool for disseminating AIDS education and HIV prevention messages. HIV information in a multitude of languages, which targets both broad and specific audiences serves to inform people who access websites, listservs, and chat rooms.

Workplace Programs

Increasingly, countries are focusing on the workplace as an essential venue for effective HIV prevention programs. In Zimbabwe, peer-education programs among factory workers led to a 34% reduction in the incidence of HIV infections compared with factories randomized to the arm with no such programs.[16] The government of Côte d'Ivoire called on all businesses with more than 50 employees to establish AIDS committees, while the government of Cameroon has worked toward concluding agreements requiring AIDS education for workers by 2005 with 50% of all businesses. In South Africa, periodic presumptive treatment of sexually transmitted infections (STIs) for mineworkers has reduced STIs among workers and among sex workers in the communities surrounding mines. Also in South Africa, an agreement between representatives of workers and employers has led to establishment of a network of roadside clinics that provide both health services and HIV prevention interventions.[17] In Malawi, the World Food Program is partnering with private companies, NGOs and the government to provide prevention information, condoms, treatment of sexually transmitted diseases, voluntary counselling and testing,

and referrals for HIV treatment to truck drivers and sex workers in two locations in Malawi. Fear of losing employment often discourages individuals from accessing available testing services. Workplaces with 'Know your status' campaigns administered jointly by managers and workers' representatives report improved uptake of testing, treatment, and prevention services. For example, trade unions in Rwanda that maintain solidarity funds to care for workers who test positive, report that nearly all their members have been tested for HIV.[18]

School-based Programs

Higher levels of education are, in and of themselves, associated with safer sexual behaviors and delayed sexual debut.[19,20] Furthermore, school attendance enables the delivery of school-based sexuality education and HIV prevention programming for students. A review of 11 studies of school-based HIV prevention programs in Africa, found that 10 of the studies demonstrated significant improvements in young people's HIV-related knowledge and that all studies assessing students' attitudes detected positive behavioral changes. The review found evidence that school-based programs can contribute to delayed sexual initiation, a reduction in the number of sexual partners, and increases in condom use, although producing sustained behavior change appears more difficult than increasing knowledge.[21]

Community-based Responses

In an effort to broaden and integrate governments' responses to the HIV epidemic, several countries in Africa have initiated community based programs. Examples of successful community initiatives now emanate from almost every country in Africa. In Burkina Faso, the International Building Workers Union supports a drama group called 'Yamwekre', which means 'Prick your conscience', that uses music, drama and poetry to educate communities about HIV, particularly young people and their parents. The AIDS Service Organisation, better known as TASO, in Uganda is a well known example providing both HIV prevention and AIDS treatment through a well established community outreach program. Some of its successful community initiatives include the training of traditional leaders to become involved in HIV prevention, AIDS awareness campaigns targeting the taxi industry, and the integration of HIV communicators into Community Health Worker programs as a platform for door-to-door education programs. Integration of HIV prevention counselling in a home-based antiretroviral treatment program, combined with voluntary counselling and testing for the partners of antiretroviral patients, resulted in a 70% drop in unprotected sex, including an 85% reduction in unprotected sex among married couples.[22]

Healthcare Settings: Safe Blood and Prevention of Transmission

Unsafe transfusions, although important in the past, now account for a relatively small fraction of HIV transmission in Africa. In order to ensure a safe blood supply in Africa, the Safe Blood for Africa™ Foundation was established as a multi-year, stepped implementation plan to establish the facilities and train the professionals needed to manage, track and test the millions of blood transfusions performed in sub-Saharan Africa. These programs are currently being implemented in 18 African countries, including Nigeria and Botswana, providing training for over 500 blood banking technicians a year, supplying test kits and supplies, and furnishing technical assistance. Despite this progress, ensuring the safety of the blood supply remains a particular challenge in times of emergency, when wars, civil strife, disasters or epidemics damage health infrastructure. It is important for public health systems to reduce and eventually stop paying for blood and to increase the use of voluntary donors, who are the least likely to transmit infections such as HIV and hepatitis. Only 40 countries in the world have achieved 100% voluntary blood donation.

Unsafe injections in healthcare settings account for an estimated 2.5% of new infections in sub-Saharan Africa.[23] Although unsafe injections account for substantially fewer new infections than sexual intercourse[24] adherence to sound infection control practices in healthcare settings, including prohibitions on the re-use of injection equipment, can eliminate these. Relatively inexpensive auto-disable syringes help prevent HIV transmission in healthcare settings by making re-use impossible and by eliminating the risk of inadvertent needlestick injuries. International guidelines recommend use of auto-disable syringes as the 'equipment of choice' for immunization initiatives however 38% of low- and middle-income countries were not using such syringes in their national vaccine programs in 2004.[25]

Risk of exposure to blood or other body fluids can be significantly lowered through workers' adherence to 'universal precautions,' which involves the routine use of gloves and other protective gear to prevent occupational exposures, safe disposal of sharps, and timely administration of a 4-week prophylactic course of antiretroviral prophylaxis if a worker does get exposed. Where workers have the potential to encounter blood or other body fluids in the course of their employment, employers have an obligation to train workers in infection control and to ensure ready access to protective gear and post-exposure prophylaxis. Even though it is existing policy in many African countries, universal precautions and post-exposure prophylaxis to prevent accidental needlestick injuries in healthcare settings are generally sub-optimally implemented.

Condom Promotion

Correct and consistent use of the male condom reduces the risk of sexual transmission by 80–90%,[26] Condom use should be actively promoted for all sexually active adults, particularly in countries with generalized epidemics in sub-Saharan Africa. Strong and sustained promotion of condoms is needed to overcome negative attitudes to condoms, particularly among men who may feel that condom use reduces sexual pleasure or impedes sexual intimacy with steady partners. In addition to condom social marketing, condoms should be also made available for free, as even extremely low prices for over-the-counter condoms can serve as a deterrent to use.[27] Observational studies, laboratory experiments and mathematical modelling indicate that female condoms also offer strong protection against infection[28] but lower public sector prices for female condoms are essential for their more widespread use. UNFPA, the largest public sector purchaser of male condoms, estimates the global supply of public sector condoms is <50% of that needed to ensure adequate condom coverage, with the gap estimated at 8.3 billion condoms. In 2005, the UNFPA launched a 5-year Global Program to Enhance Reproductive Health Commodity Security which seeks to catalyze national efforts to define, own and drive strategies to ensure access to all sexual and reproductive health technologies, including male and female condoms.[29]

Effective HIV Prevention for Women and Girls

In the long run, effective HIV prevention for women and girls requires policy reforms that empower women and promote gender equality. Men need to be a substantial part of the solution by taking responsibility for fidelity and safer sex; committing themselves to their daughters' education; alleviating women's burden of care; and embracing a zero-tolerance attitude towards violence against women.

Although effective HIV prevention for women involves easy access to HIV prevention services and commodities along with intensified research efforts to develop new prevention methods that women can control, these are insufficient without policy reforms to reduce women's vulnerability and longer-term efforts to develop new gender norms and influence the behavior and attitudes of men and boys. Central for effective HIV prevention is a strong commitment to universal education. Higher education levels for girls are associated with a higher age of marriage, reduced fertility, improved health-seeking behavior, lower vulnerability to genital cutting, and reduced risk of HIV and STIs.[30] Other policy actions that support HIV prevention for women and girls include legal reform to secure women's property and inheritance rights, implementation and enforcement of strong legal measures combating violence against women, enhanced global and regional collaboration to fight human trafficking, and mainstreaming of gender issues in programs and policies. Leaders in government, religion, business and the media have a major advocacy role to play through vocally leading efforts to promote equality and empowerment for women. Education sectors should prioritize initiatives to inculcate healthier gender norms among boys. The Global Coalition on Women and AIDS launched by UNAIDS in 2004 aims to increase global awareness of the epidemic's growing burden on women and girls and to catalyze effective action to address the many sources of women's vulnerability to HIV. The Coalition unites a broad array of stakeholders – including civil society groups, networks of women living with HIV, governments, and UN agencies – to advocate for policies that address fundamental gender inequities and that promote women's empowerment.

Preventing HIV among Female Sex Workers

HIV transmission between female sex workers and truck drivers is well known to occur along major highways in equatorial Africa.[31] A variety of prevention programs involving sex workers, some of which also engage their clients, can be found across the region. Beyond the provision of condoms, some interventions have been designed to empower sex workers as a way to expand their employment opportunities beyond sex work and increase their ability to negotiate safer sex. In Zambia, for example, where women fish-traders were often forced into sex in exchange for fish from fishermen, economic cooperatives were established to bargain collectively for fish and provide credit to women, which led to reductions in sexual exploitation.[32]

Diagnosis and Treatment of Sexually Transmitted Infections

Programs to control sexually transmitted infections (STIs) are widely implemented in Africa, with most utilizing the syndromic approach recommended by the World Health Organization. High HIV prevalence is seen in many STI programs in Africa; for example, more than half of patients attending STI clinics in 2000 in Swaziland were HIV positive, while seropositivity among STI clinic patients in Zimbabwe exceeded 70% in 1995/6. Untreated ulcerative sexually transmitted infections, such as syphilis, chancroid and genital herpes significantly increase the risk of sexual transmission of HIV. Prompt diagnosis and treatment of sexually transmitted infections represent an essential programmatic component of a strong and comprehensive response to AIDS.[33] However, more effective technologies are needed since syphilis control depends on therapies that have barely changed in 60 years[34] and herpes simplex type 2 appears to have been replacing chancroid as the major cause of genital sores in many countries. Efficacy in reducing HIV transmission of mass administration of acyclovir to treat genital herpes is being assessed in two large trials in Africa.

Marginalized Populations: Men who have Sex with Men and Injecting Drug Users

In the generalized epidemics experienced by many African countries the importance of addressing HIV prevention among marginalized communities such as injecting drug users and men who have sex with men (MSM) has not been well understood. With few exceptions, programs are limited to demonstration projects in selected countries in Africa. Part of the problem lies in the non-recognition of the existence of such communities, which precludes assessing and addressing their specific HIV prevention needs. In Kenya, homosexuality is considered illegal but sex between men is reportedly common in coastal regions of the country. A study of high school students in Zimbabwe reported that 4.6% of boys self-identified as homosexual,[35] a proportion which is similar to that in Western countries. Both primary prevention to prevent new infections and secondary prevention programs can be effective in reducing risky behaviors and interrupting the chain of HIV transmission if they actively involve men who have sex with men in culturally appropriate program design, implementation and evaluation. A meta-analysis of behavioral interventions designed to reduce high-risk sexual behavior among MSM concluded that interventions that promoted interpersonal skills, were delivered in community-level formats, or focused on younger or those at higher risk were most effective.[36] Few studies have been conducted to assess the efficacy of these interventions outside of Western countries. Cultural taboos against homosexuality may drive MSM underground, making this population more difficult to reach in the African context.

Although few HIV infections have been attributed to the use of contaminated injecting equipment among drug users in Africa, injecting drug use has been recognized in at least seven African countries, including Nigeria, Morocco, South Africa, Tanzania, and Kenya.[13,37] The major types of interventions aimed to reduce drug-related harms include drug substitution treatment, needle exchange programs (NEPs), outreach, and network-oriented interventions. Consistent associations have been documented between enrolment in substance treatment and reductions in HIV risk behaviors, with the most consistent reductions in HIV-related risk behaviors observed for medication-assisted therapies that block opiate receptors, particularly maintenance programs offering methadone[38] or buprenorphine. The public health impact of substitution treatment on HIV has been virtually non-existent in Africa because access to such programs is severely limited. In fact, in much of sub-Saharan Africa morphine supplies for pain relief in palliative care are in exceedingly short supply. In settings where drug substitution treatment is unavailable, prohibitively costly or illegal, harm reduction initiatives aim to expand IDUs' access to sterile syringes through needle exchange programs, physician prescription of syringes or allowing legal purchase of syringes over the counter at pharmacies. An important aim of such programs is to decrease the circulation of contaminated injecting equipment, thereby reducing the spread of blood-borne pathogens in the community. The overwhelming majority of studies provide strong evidence of the effectiveness of needle exchange programs in reducing high-risk injecting

behaviors among HIV-seronegative and HIV-seropositive IDUs. An international comparison showed that in 29 cities with established needle exchange programs, HIV prevalence decreased on average by 5.8% per year, but increased on average by 5.9% per year in 51 cities without NEP.[39] Studies assessing needle accessibility in the African context are lacking.

HIV Prevention Trials in Africa

Male Circumcision

More than 20 years of observational studies have revealed that circumcised males have lower HIV-infection rates than uncircumcised males. In 2005, researchers announced the results of a large scale efficacy trial recruiting over 3100 men aged 18–24 years in Orange Farm, South Africa, in an area where almost one in three adults are HIV-positive. The trial found that adult male circumcision reduced the men's risk of contracting HIV during sexual intercourse by over 60% during the 18-month study period.[40] Male circumcision likely helps to protect against HIV infection by removing Langerhans cells which are target cells in the inner foreskin for HIV entry and by reducing men's risk of acquiring some sexually transmitted infections that increase vulnerability to HIV.

Two other efficacy trials for adult male circumcision underway in Kenya and Uganda are designed to follow participants over a longer period to determine whether sexual risk behavior changes and whether benefits of the intervention are maintained. All three trials involve male circumcision under local anaesthesia using one of two techniques. A third study in Uganda is assessing the degree of protection that male circumcision may offer to female partners of HIV-positive men.

UNAIDS is coordinating implementation of a UN Work Plan on male circumcision which focuses on increasing the safety of current practices and on developing tools to assist countries in deciding on the place of male circumcision within comprehensive HIV programming should the other trials confirm the protective effect.[41]

Results of the efficacy trials are anticipated in 2007. If proven effective, male circumcision will increase available proven options for HIV prevention, but male circumcision does not eliminate the risk of HIV for men. It is critical that male circumcision does not cause the abandonment of existing effective strategies such as correct and consistent condom use, sex between two seronegative partners, delay in onset of sexual relations, reduction in sexual partners and abstinence from penetrative sex.

Pre-exposure Prophylaxis

Pre-exposure prophylaxis (PrEP) to prevent sexual- and possibly parenteral-transmission of HIV holds promise for serodiscordant couples, sex workers, men who have sex with men, and injecting drug users who may be exposed to HIV despite using precautions. Small-to-medium sized phase II trials are under way in Atlanta and San Francisco, with larger phase II/III studies underway or planned in Botswana, Ghana, and possibly Thailand. Some of these studies have been dogged by controversy. The main issues were the adequacy of pre-trial community consultation and informed consent, linkages to HIV treatment programs for those found to be infected at baseline or in the course of the study and, in the case of Thailand, the lack of access to sterile needles in a study designed to examine HIV transmission among injecting drug users. Two PrEP studies were cancelled (Cambodia, Nigeria) and another (Cameroon) postponed. A consultation in Seattle and a series of consultations led by UNAIDS in two African regions, Asia and Geneva involving community activists, researchers, sponsors and others helped identify the problems in trial design in this promising research area.[42] Trials have moved forward in six other sites.

Microbicides

A microbicide is a product, such as a gel or a cream that could be applied topically to genital mucosal surfaces to prevent or significantly reduce the transmission of HIV and other disease-causing organisms during sexual intercourse. Microbicides could also take other forms, including films, suppositories, and slow-releasing sponges or vaginal rings. Safe and effective microbicides will help women substantially reduce their vulnerability to HIV infection during sexual intercourse.

Several different mechanisms for microbicide action are being studied. An effective microbicide may be able to kill or otherwise immobilize HIV; it may form a barrier between the virus and the vaginal tissue; it could boost the natural defences of the vagina against HIV; or it could prevent the virus from multiplying once it enters cells.

A safe and effective microbicide has not yet been found, but many substances are being tested and nearly a dozen microbicides have entered human testing. As of June 2006, there are six large-scale efficacy trials, all of which involve African study sites, underway of five first and second generation microbicide products (surfactants and polymers). Various third and fourth generation options (formulations containing antiretroviral drugs or co-receptor specific blockers) are in the pipeline. They include fusion inhibitors – CCR5, gp120 and gp41 blockers and gels containing antiretroviral medications. Formulations being explored include non-coitally dependent products that could be applied daily or weekly, such as vaginal rings releasing preventive levels of antiretroviral drugs, other devices in which the microbicidal drug could be released on contact with semen and genetically modified lactobacilli, which would release anti-viral proteins. An effective microbicide is likely to be more than 5 years away.

HIV Vaccines

A vaccine to overcome HIV is our most compelling hope for bringing the global HIV epidemic under control. But developing a vaccine remains an enormous challenge for reasons related to inadequate resources, clinical trial and regulatory capacity concerns, intellectual property issues and scientific challenges. As of June 2006, there are more than 30 preventive AIDS vaccine candidates in early stages of human clinical trials in approximately two dozen countries around the world (including the promising Merck adenovirus vector vaccine, which may stimulate anti-HIV cell-mediated immunity). The Global HIV Vaccine Enterprise has rallied scientists, activists, funders and others worldwide around a Strategic Scientific Plan to rapidly advance progress towards effective HIV vaccines.[43] An effective HIV vaccine is likely to be 10 years or more away.

Synergistic interactions with the Global HIV Vaccine Enterprise and other global partners are helping ensure that the African perspective is fully taken into account. The African AIDS Vaccine Program (AAVP) was conceived in June 2000 as a network of African scientists and communities, working together to promote and facilitate HIV vaccine research and evaluation in Africa, through capacity building and regional and international collaboration. The AAVP secretariat is hosted by the WHO-UNAIDS HIV Vaccine Initiative (HVI) in Geneva, Switzerland, and the WHO Regional Office for Africa in Harare, Zimbabwe. The AAVP strives to build on local knowledge and resources and fosters collaboration and networking within Africa, as well as with major international partners such as the US National Institutes of Health, the Centers for Disease Control, the Department of Defence and the International AIDS Vaccine Initiative (IAVI) among others. AAVP maintains a high level of visibility and advocacy to promote the development of HIV vaccines that stimulate immune responses to the viral sub-types common in Africa. To ensure better preparedness in addressing various complex challenges related to HIV vaccine research and development in Africa, AAVP supports capacity strengthening, training activities and development and implementation of National HIV Vaccine Plans which define national policies and strategies relevant to HIV vaccine trials. AAVP supports the development and strengthening of national and regional regulatory, ethical, legal and community frameworks so that the highest standards for HIV vaccine-related research and clinical trials are attained in Africa. An external review of AAVP undertaken in June 2005 found that AAVP, serving as the 'Voice of Africa', had made significant contributions in advocating for HIV vaccine research and development addressing Africa's needs, and in supporting the establishment of appropriate policies and normative frameworks, thereby strengthening relevant clinical trial capacity in the African region.

The Future of HIV Prevention in Africa

Several important topics, such as HIV prevention in refugee camps and among internally displaced populations as well as HIV prevention in correctional settings and prisons, have not been covered in this brief review and others have been only summarily described. Nonetheless, it is clear that many highly effective prevention tools are not being used at the scale and intensity necessary to turn the epidemic around in much of sub-Saharan Africa. Promising developments of declining prevalence are being seen in several eastern African countries but excessive mortality is contributing to these declines and surely has played a role in bringing home the seriousness of the epidemic in hard hit communities. On the other hand, it is to be remembered that, in every country in sub-Saharan Africa, people who are not infected with HIV constitute the majority. In generalized epidemics, where much of transmission is occurring within discordant cohabiting partners, more attention needs to be given to increasing access to HIV testing either through free-standing voluntary counselling and testing (VCT) services where

testing is client-initiated, through home-based offers of testing or through provider-initiated HIV testing in healthcare settings. Regardless of who initiates the testing process it must always be conducted respecting the 3 Cs: confidentiality, informed consent and counselling.[44]

With an estimated 90% of people living with HIV in sub-Saharan Africa unaware of their HIV status and with fear of stigma and discrimination being major deterrents to HIV testing, decisive action from the top level of leadership down through every level of society is urgently required to address stigma and discrimination. It must address women's empowerment, homophobia, attitudes towards injecting drug users and sex workers and social norms that affect sexual behavior, including the low status and powerlessness of women and girls. Changes in laws and policies must be accompanied by social mobilization campaigns which engage all elements of civil society including networks and organizations of people living with HIV. Finally, a fully funded plan to achieve universal education is fundamental to reducing HIV-related stigma and HIV transmission.

References

1. UNAIDS. Report on the global AIDS epidemic. Geneva, Switzerland: UNAIDS; 2006.
2. UNAIDS. AIDS Epidemic Update. Geneva, Switzerland: UNAIDS; 2005.
3. UNAIDS. Report on the Global AIDS Epidemic. Geneva, Switzerland: UNAIDS; 2004.
4. Global HIV Prevention Working Group. Access to HIV prevention: closing the gap. 2003. Online. Available: www.kff.org/hivaids/200305-index.cfm
5. Ugandan Ministry of Health. HIV/AIDS Surveillance Report 13. Kampala: Ministry of Health; 2001.
6. Ministry of Health Uganda. Uganda HIV/AIDS Serobehavioral Survey 2004–05: Preliminary Report. Kampala: Ministry of Health; 2005.
7. Mbulaiteye SM, Mahe C, Whitworth JA, et al. Declining HIV-1 incidence and associated prevalence over 10 years in a rural population in south-west Uganda: a cohort study. Lancet 2002; 360:41–46.
8. Wawer M, et al. Declines in HIVI prevalence in Uganda: Not as simple as ABC. Abstract 27 LB. 12th Conference on Retroviruses and Opportunistic Infections, Boston, MA: 22–25 February 2005.
9. Gregson S, Garnett GP, Nyamukapa CA, et al. HIV decline associated with behavior change in eastern Zimbabwe. Science 2006; 311:664–666.
10. Ministry of Health Kenya. AIDS in Kenya. 7th edn. Nairobi: National AIDS and STI Control Program (NASCOP), Ministry of Health; 2005.
11. Cheluget B, Marum L, Stover J. Evidence of declining HIV prevalence and risk behavior in Kenya. Harare: Presentation to the UNAIDS Reference Group on Estimates, Modelling and Projections, 2004: 15–17 November.
12. Baltazar G. HIV sentinel surveillance 2004. Ministry of Health Kenya: Slide presentation. 2005: June.
13. Beckerleg S, Telfer M, Hundt GL. The rise of injecting drug use in east Africa: a case study from Kenya. Harm Reduct J 2005; 2:12.

14. UNAIDS. Intensifying HIV prevention. UNAIDS policy position paper: UNAIDS; 2005.

15. Shapiro D, Meekers D, Tambashe B. Exposure to the 'SIDA dans la Cite' AIDS prevention television series in Côte' d'Ivoire, sexual risk behavior and condom use. AIDS Care 2003; 15:303–314.

16. Katzenstein D, McFarland W, Mbizvo M, et al. Peer education among factory workers in Zimbabwe: providing a sustainable HIV prevention intervention. Abstract No. 33514. XII International Conference on AIDS, Geneva: 1998.

17. ILO. Guidelines for the transport sector. Geneva, Switzerland: ILO; 2005.

18. UNAIDS/ILO/ICFTU. Global reach: how trade unions are responding to HIV and AIDS, case studies of union actions. Geneva, Switzerland: UNAIDS/ILO/ICFTU; 2006.

19. UNICEF. Girls, HIV/AIDS and Education. Washington DC: UNICEF; 2005.

20. Prata P, Vahidnia F, Fraser A. Gender and relationship differences in condom use among 15-24-year-olds in Angola. Int Fam Plann Perspect 2005; 31:192–199.

21. Gallant M, Maticka-Tyndale E. School-based HIV prevention programs for African youth. Soc Sci Med 2004; 58:1337–1351.

22. Bunnell R. Changes in sexual behavior and risk of HIV transmission after antiretroviral therapy and prevention interventions in rural Uganda. AIDS 2006; 20:85–92.

23. Hauri AM, Armstrong GL, Hutin YJF. The global burden of disease attributable to contaminated injections given in healthcare settings. Int J STD AIDS 2004; 15:7–16.

24. Schmid GP, et al. Transmission of HIV-1 infection in sub-Saharan Africa and effect of elimination of unsafe injections. Lancet 2004; 363:482–488.

25. WHO. The safety of immunization practices improves over last five years, but challenges remain. News Release. Geneva: WHO; 2005.

26. Weller S, Davis K. Condom effectiveness in reducing heterosexual HIV transmission. Oxford: The Cochrane Library, 2002: Issue 2.

27. Cohen DA, Farley TA. Social marketing of condoms is great, but we need more free condoms. Lancet 2004; 364:13–14.

28. Hoffman S, et al. The future of the female condom. Int Fam Plann Perspect 2004; 30:139–145.

29. UNFPA. Sexual and reproductive health & HIV/AIDS: A framework for priority linkages. UNFPA; 2005. Online. Available: www.unfpa.org/upload/lib_pub_file/501_filename_framework_priority_linkages.pdf

30. Grown C, Gupta GR, Pande R. Taking action to improve women's health through gender equality and women's empowerment. Lancet 2005; 365:541–543.

31. Ntozi JP, Najjumba IM, Ahimbisibwe F, et al. Has the HIV/AIDS epidemic changed sexual behavior of high risk groups in Uganda? Afr Health Sci Dec 2003; 3:107–116.

32. Msiska R. An intervention study to develop and test the benefits of an enabling approach in reducing HIV transmission in a Fish Trading Community in Zambia. Lusaka: National AIDS Program; 1994.

33. Dallabetta G, Neilson G. Efforts to control sexually transmitted infections as a means to limit HIV transmission: what is the evidence? Curr HIV/AIDS Rep 2004; 1:166–171.

34. Hook EW, Peeling RW. Syphilis control – a continuing challenge. N Engl J Med 2004; 351:122–124.

35. Sibanda EN, Mlingo T, Chikomo N, et al. Awareness of the risks of HIV infection by Zimbabwean urban and rural high school attendees. Cent Afr J Med 2002; 48:112–116.

36. Johnson WD, Hedges LV, Ramirez G, et al. HIV prevention research for men who have sex with men: a systematic review and meta-analysis. J Acquir Immune Defic Syndr 2002; 30:S118–S129.

37. McCurdy SA, Williams ML, Kilonzo GP, et al. Heroin and HIV risk in Dar es Salaam, Tanzania: youth hangouts, mageto and injecting practices. AIDS Care 2005; 17:S65–S76.

38. Metzger DS, Navaline H. Human immunodeficiency virus prevention and the potential of drug abuse treatment. Clin Infect Dis Dec 2003; 37:S451–S456.

39. Hurley S, Jolley D, Kaldor J. Effectiveness of needle-exchange programs for prevention of HIV infection. Lancet 1997; 349:1797.

40. Auvert B, Taljaard D, Lagarde E, et al. Randomized, controlled intervention trial of male circumcision for reduction of HIV infection risk: the ANRS 1265 trial. PLoS Med 2005; 2:e298.

41. UNAIDS. Statement on South African trial findings regarding male circumcision and HIV. Geneva, Switzerland: Media release, 2005: July 26.

42. UNAIDS. Creating effective partnerships for HIV prevention trials: report of a UNAIDS Consultation, Geneva, 20–21 June 2005. AIDS 2006; 20:W1–W11.

43. Global HIV/AIDS Vaccine enterprise. The global HIV/AIDS vaccine enterprise: scientific strategic plan. PLoS Med 2005; 2:e25.

44. UNAIDS/WHO. Position statement on HIV testing. Geneva: UNAIDS/WHO; 2004: June.

CHAPTER 50

HIV Transmission and its Prevention in Asia

Stephen Kerr
Kiat Ruxrungtham

Introduction

The countries of east and southeast Asia are home to approximately 60% of the world's population and represent a diverse group of nations experiencing HIV epidemics of differing severity and stages. The country prevalence rates at the end of 2003 are shown in Table 50.1. Although these rates are low in comparison with those seen in African countries, the burden of HIV disease is comparatively high because of the large populations in this region: currently over 7.4 million people are living with HIV/AIDS,[1] and a significant proportion of infected people may not be aware of their HIV status. Moreover, without good prevention programs the risks of a worsening epidemic are considerable: the number of people infected with HIV in India and China alone is estimated to increase to 30–40 million by 2010.[2]

Rapid spread of HIV in Asia began during the second decade of the global epidemic, and the time course of the epidemics can be classified into three groups[3]: (1) Countries which experienced severe epidemics in the late 1980s and early 1990s, including Thailand, Cambodia and Myanmar where HIV prevalence is currently in excess of 1%; (2) Countries in which epidemics have been noticeably growing in the past 5 years, including China, India, Indonesia, Nepal and Vietnam; (3) Countries such as Bangladesh, Laos, the Philippines and South Korea, which continue to have low levels of HIV infection, even among high-risk individuals. Two main reasons for this wide variation in the speed of evolution and severity of the Asian epidemics are postulated to be differences in the size of the adult male population visiting commercial sex workers (CSW), and the

number of clients CSW have each night.[4] The diversity of Asian regional and national epidemics also relates to the sociological, cultural, ethnic and geographic diversity of Asian nations. Importantly, one should realize that HIV epidemiology is a dynamic process, so that low HIV prevalence in a particular country or region may change to a high prevalence in just a few years.

The lessons of AIDS-related devastation in Africa unfortunately went unheeded in much of Asia, and prevention success stories at the national level in the region remain comparatively few.[3] This chapter reviews the current status of HIV epidemics in Asia, and addresses the lessons and challenges which can be drawn from successful prevention and treatment campaigns in the region, to encourage more aggressive action for containing HIV epidemics in Asia.

High-Risk Groups, Patterns of Spread and Interventions that are known to be Successful in Reducing Risk

HIV is transmitted through blood and blood products, at mucosal surfaces through sexual contact and transmission from mother-to-child. Individual epidemics within Asian countries and regions have exhibited similar patterns, with HIV typically spreading first among injecting drug users (IDU), followed by CSW and men who have sex with men (MSM). These represent the three interrelated high-risk groups that serve as a reservoir of infection and fuel the HIV epidemics in Asia (Fig. 50.1).[3,5]

High-risk groups subsequently introduce HIV to the lower risk groups in the population by sexual

Table 50.1 HIV prevalence estimates in selected Asian countries

Country	Adults and children living with HIV, end 2003		HIV prevalence in adults aged 15–49, end 2003 (%)	
	Estimate	Low estimate – High estimate	Estimate	Low estimate – High estimate
Cambodia	170 000	100 000–290 000	2.6	1.5–4.4
Thailand	570 000	310 000–1 000 000	1.5	0.8–2.8
Myanmar	330 000	170 000–620 000	1.2	0.6–2.2
India		2 200 000–7 600 000		0.4–1.3
Nepal	61 000		0.5	
Malaysia	52 000	25 000–86 000	0.4	0.2–0.7
Vietnam	220 000	110 000–360 000	0.4	0.2–0.8
Singapore	4100	1300–8000	0.2	0.1–0.5
Indonesia	110 000	53 000–180 000	0.1	0.0–0.2
Laos PDR	1700	600–3600	0.1	<0.2
Pakistan	74 000	24 000–150 000	0.1	0.0–0.2
China	840 000	430 000–1 500 000	0.1	0.1–0.2
Philippines	9000	3000–18 000	<0.1	<0.2
Sri Lanka	3500	1200–6900	<0.1	<0.2
Japan	12 000	5700–19 000	<0.1	<0.2

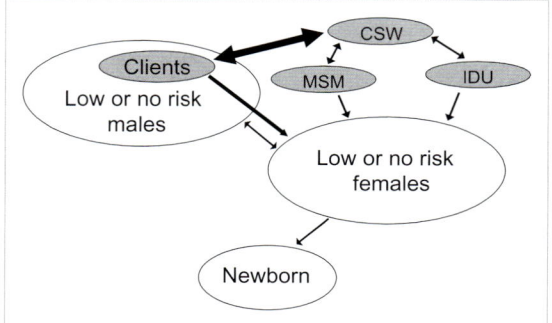

Figure 50.1 Diagrammatic representation of risk groups in Asian HIV epidemics, demonstrating multiple interlinked epidemics in higher risk populations (CSW, commercial sex worker, MSM, homosexual men, and IDU, injecting drug user) and their relationship with low risk groups (their immediate sexual partners). (Used by Permission, Tim Brown.)

transmission. CSW, IDU and MSM have regular partners with whom they are less likely to use condoms;[1,6] clients of CSW who have been infected transmit the virus to their female sexual partners. Indeed, most women who have been infected in Asia are the regular partners of high-risk males.[3,7] Women who have been infected can subsequently infect their children with HIV, driving the epidemic deeper into the population.

Injecting Drug Users

Unsafe injecting practices characterized by sharing needles leads to rapid increases in the prevalence of HIV among IDU because of the efficiency of transmission. Information about IDU and the prevalence within this high-risk group is scarce in some countries because sentinel surveillance systems are not in place. Prevalence changes in IDU over time in selected regions are shown in Figure 50.2A. Nine countries in the region have an estimated IDU population >100 000 (Bangladesh, China, India, Japan, Indonesia, Malaysia, Myanmar, Pakistan, and Vietnam); in Brunei, Indonesia, Malaysia, Myanmar, Pakistan, Singapore, Hong Kong, and Japan, IDU prevalence among adults is over 0.5%. In many regions within countries with established epidemics, it has been reported that >50% of IDU who have been tested are HIV positive.[5,8] Epidemics among IDUs seem to have an important role in supporting and escalating generalized epidemics,[9] possibly because a substantial proportion of IDU are clients of sex workers.[6] For this reason, harm reduction interventions are vital in averting infections. IDU in many parts of Asia have a good understanding of the risks of needle sharing, but this knowledge does not always translate into safe behavior.[5] IDU may be victimized by law enforcement agencies, and access to

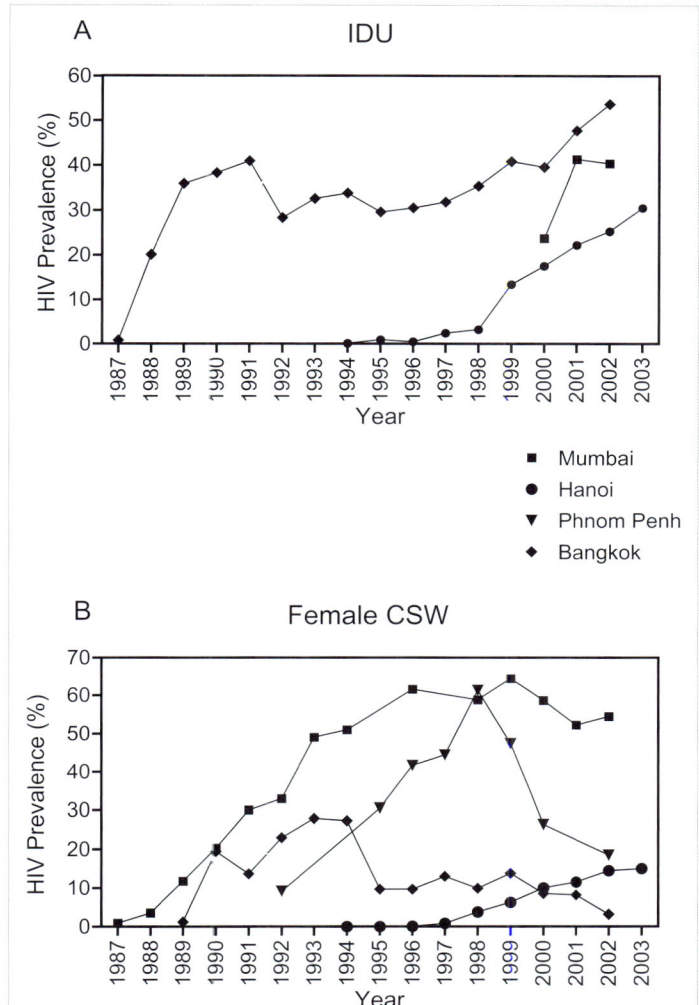

Figure 50.2A,B Graph showing changes in HIV prevalence in (A) IDU and (B) CSW in Asian surveillance populations.[46]

safe injecting equipment is often difficult. This is partly because authorities have difficulties in reconciling the provision of safe injecting equipment with other policies and international treaties that seek to control substance abuse by limiting supply and demand for illicit drugs, although this is not the case.[10]

There is strong evidence from many centers in both developed and less developed countries that participation in needle exchange programs decreases the prevalence of HIV among IDU.[11] Furthermore, there is good evidence from developed countries including Hong Kong that in addition to needle exchange programs, provision of oral substitution maintenance drugs such as methadone or buprenorphine will also assist in maintaining low seropreva-

lence rates.[1,11] Needle exchange programs have been successfully established in parts of northern Thailand, Hanoi, and Kathmandu,[11] and many other Asian countries are implementing educational outreach and needle exchange in an attempt to limit spread of HIV.[5,10] It is critical, particularly in countries with low seroprevalence rates among IDU, that such harm reduction strategies are implemented and expanded.

Heterosexual Transmission

Three factors seem to determine the dynamics of heterosexual HIV epidemics within Asian populations: the proportion of males who visit CSW, the number of clients that CSW have each night, and the rate of condom use within these sexual encounters.[4,12] The risk of sexual transmission of HIV increases with the number of sexual partners, since there is a greater chance of exposure to a partner who is already HIV-infected. Because of their high turnover of sexual partners, CSW who are predominantly female, (but also CSW who are transsexual and male), are at particularly high risk of acquiring HIV infection when condoms are not used during sex. HIV prevalence changes in female CSW in selected regions over time are shown in Figure 50.2B.

Brown and Peerapatanapokin[12] have developed a sophisticated computer simulated model exploring the interplay between behavioral, biological, and epidemiological inputs which shape the epidemic. Developed using comprehensive information derived from the Thai and Cambodian epidemics, the model accurately replicates the pattern of spread within these countries, and is a useful tool for assessing how changes in the factors described above will impact on the epidemic evolution in other Asian regions. This model recognizes that several determinants will impact on the efficiency and rate of epidemic spread from high-risk groups to the general population, and to a large extent, these determinants account for the diversity in rate of epidemic evolution in Asian countries. Behavioral modifiers include the proportion of men visiting CSW, the proportion of times a condom is used during sex or that safe injecting practices are followed, the rate at which preventive measure are adopted by high-risk groups in response to educational interventions, and the duration of time spent in a high-risk group.[12] Biological modifiers include presence of other sexually transmitted infections or genital inflammation which can facilitate HIV transmission,[13] proportion of circumcised males, the relative efficiency of HIV transmission depending on the risk behavior, and the timing of introduction of the virus into high-risk populations.[3] Another modifier is the degree of overlap between people in high-risk groups, since some individuals may exhibit more than one high-risk behavior (Fig. 50.1).[12]

The modifiers that are most amenable to intervention are those in the behavioral category, and among those, the proportion of men in a country who visit sex workers and the percentage of clients and sex workers who use condoms are important targets to slow the rate of epidemic development.[3,5,12,14] Across Asia there are wide variations in both. In Thailand in the early 1990s, approximately 20% of adult males were visiting sex workers, but this later reduced to 10% in response to the HIV epidemic.[3] Surveys in a number of countries suggest that between 2% and 15% of men have visited a CSW in the preceding year, making this the most frequent risk factor for HIV transmission in Asia.[1,5] Within countries there is also variation between the proportion of men in the general population who visit CSW compared with those who have a higher disposable income and occupations which allow them to travel. Among this latter group, the percentage of men buying sex in the previous year was approximately 3 times higher in China, and approximately 10 times higher in Vietnam and Indonesia.[3,5,15,16]

The proportion of direct and indirect sex workers using condoms is similarly variable within and between countries. For example, direct sex workers in Vietnam reported consistent condom use in 67% of encounters with clients, but indirect sex workers reported consistent condom use 81% of the time.[17] Behavioral surveillance data from 2002 found that among brothel-based sex workers, consistent use of condoms with recent clients ranged from 2% in Bangladesh, 10% in Indonesia, 30% in the Philippines and 54% in Nepal.[5] These data are supported by studies which demonstrate variable patterns of consistent condom use among the male clients of female CSW.[15,16,18]

Regional variations in consistent use of condoms may relate to differences in knowledge about HIV transmission and safe sexual practices. In some countries, particularly those with a low HIV prevalence, knowledge about HIV is poor. For example, in East Timor, some CSW had never heard of AIDS.[5] In countries where HIV is growing rapidly, misconceptions about HIV transmission routes exist among CSW.[19,20] However, increasing knowledge about HIV is not the only important factor: even when condoms are freely available and sex workers are well educated about their use in HIV prevention, CSW often choose not to use them if the client refuses.[1,14,19]

Programs in Thailand and Cambodia have provided good evidence that large-scale interventions addressing sexual transmission of HIV in a less-developed country setting lead to significant reductions in risk behavior with subsequent reductions in new HIV infections and STIs.[21-24] A nationwide epidemic among CSW and their clients was first noted in Thailand in 1989. In 1990–2001, the Royal Thai Government launched the 100% condom campaign targeting not only CSW, but all groups within the general population. The campaign focused on education about HIV and its prevention in an attempt to reduce the number of men visiting sex workers, and to promote condom use in all commercial and casual

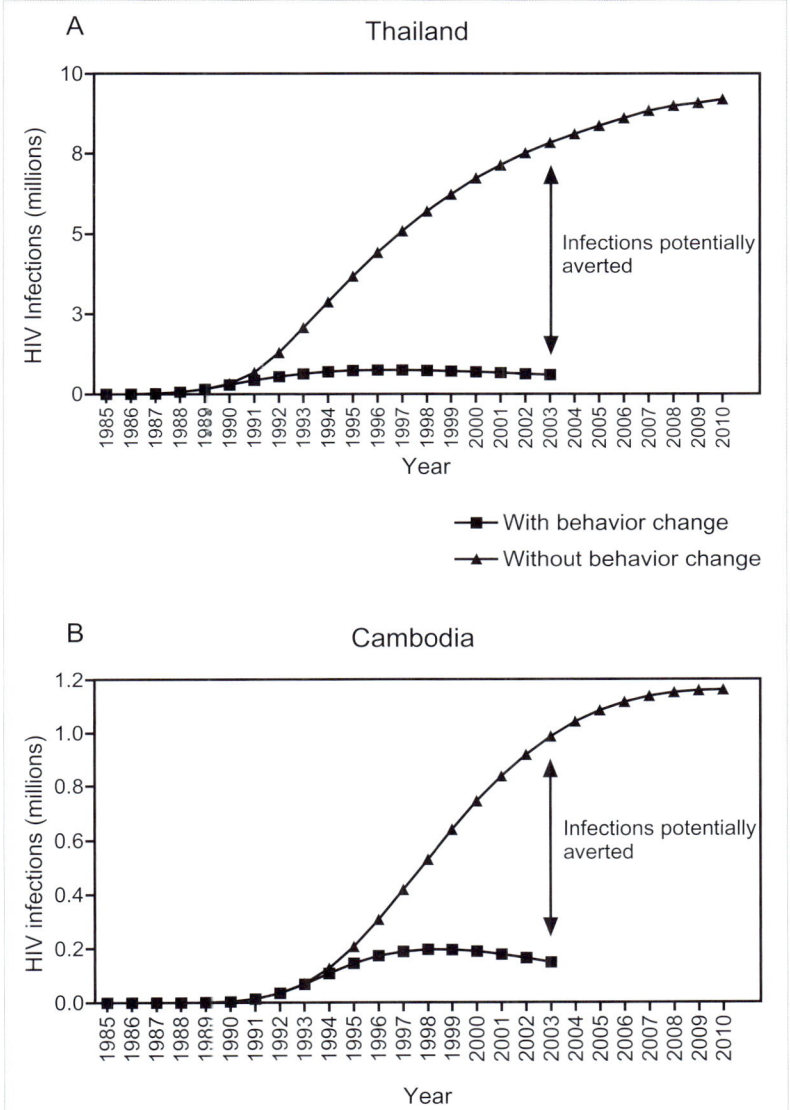

Figure 50.3A,B Graph showing observed HIV prevalence compared with expected HIV prevalence in the absence of behavior change in (A) Thailand and (B) Cambodia. The behavior changes were a reduction by 50% in the number of men visiting CSW, and an increase to 90% or higher of condom use in sex work.[24,25]

sexual interactions. The Royal Thai Government mobilized funds to support such programs in every government ministry, in addition to non-government organisations (NGOs), communities and the private sector. As a result, fewer men visited sex workers and condom use in brothels rose to >90%. Moreover, consultations at STI clinics were reduced by 90% and the prevalence rates among army conscripts halved within a few years.[22,23] It is estimated that these behavior changes have prevented millions of infections in Thailand in the past 15 years (Fig. 50.3A).[25] Cambodia displayed a similar degree of

political commitment in dealing with its own epidemic: the 100% condom use program coupled with behavior change communication strategies and STI services for high-risk populations have led to a reduction in the incidence of STIs and decreasing prevalence of HIV among high-risk groups. Behavior changes in Cambodia have similarly averted many HIV infections (Fig. 50.3B).[21,24]

Evidence from India supports the efficacy of community level HIV prevention programs to increase condom use among CSW.[20] However, to significantly impact on the epidemic, focused interventions are necessary with all high-risk groups in addition to low-risk groups in the population.

Voluntary counselling and testing (VCT) programs are also an important strategy for reducing risk behaviors. VCT combines confidential discussion on HIV status with counselling for positive individuals with education on reducing the risk of HIV transmission. Studies generally show that such interventions reduce risk behaviors in individuals who test positive for HIV, although the extent of risk reduction may depend on levels of program uptake and access to effective treatment modalities.[26,27] Before such programs are implemented, it is important to educate the community and health professionals to address negative attitudes towards people who have HIV.[28]

Men who have Sex with Men

MSM continue to be an important risk group in regional epidemics in Asia. Little data have been collected on this topic, probably because of cultural taboos discussing male-male sex. Indeed, most Asian countries do not include MSM in their ongoing HIV surveillance. Nevertheless, recent seroprevalence studies in many countries have described serious epidemics in this high-risk group.[29-32] In a study in Beijing in 2001 and 2002, the prevalence of HIV-1 among MSM was 3.1%, with 49% of the participants reporting unprotected anal intercourse with men and 22% reporting unprotected anal or vaginal intercourse with women during the 6 months preceding the study.[30] In 2003, a study in MSM from Bangkok reported an HIV prevalence rate of 17.3%; the proportion of participants reporting consistent condom use with casual partners and regular partners was 80% and 54.4%, respectively. In Jakarta, a study conducted in 2002 reported HIV prevalence of 22% among transgender sex workers, 3.6% among male sex workers, and 2.5% among MSM identifying as homosexual. Between 53.1% and 64.8% of subjects in these groups reported recent unprotected sex.[32] In Vietnam, India, and Cambodia, MSM have frequently reported recent unprotected anal sex with men or anal/vaginal sex with women.[33-35] These findings of inconsistent condom use with both male and female sexual partners, and the efficiency of HIV transmission by anal sex highlights that in the Asian region, MSM are an important link between high-risk and low-risk populations.

Because data defining the magnitude of the HIV epidemic in MSM have been scarce, countries have frequently ignored this risk group when designing their prevention and intervention strategies. To date, no Asian countries have developed comprehensive prevention programs for MSM, and for this reason evidence for effective interventions in an Asian context is limited. A recent meta-analysis of studies primarily conducted in the West demonstrated that behavioral interventions including peer group discussion significantly reduced rates of unprotected anal intercourse,[36] however the usefulness of interventions in effecting sustained behavior change in MSM has waned over time. In Asia, MSM is a diverse category that encompasses homosexual relationships between men who identify as gay, sex between heterosexual men and transgender sex workers, culturally sanctioned transgender groups (such as *waria* in Indonesia and *katoey* in Thailand), and men whose self-reported sexual orientation is inconsistent with their self-reported sexual behavior. Such diversity necessitates a good understanding of the attitudes to and knowledge about HIV and risk behavior so that prevention and intervention strategies will adequately target specific areas where knowledge is lacking or where behavior needs to be modified. The high prevalence rates among MSM in many regions, together with the behavioral data describing the magnitude of unsafe sexual practices suggest that urgent action is required to prevent a worsening epidemic.

New Approaches for Prevention of HIV Transmission: Scaling-up Antiretroviral Therapy (ART)

Prevention strategies based on the use of therapeutic agents have had mixed success. To date, an effective HIV vaccine has not been developed, and candidate HIV vaccines have been disappointing in clinical trials.[37] Another approach is the use of topical microbicides to prevent the sexual spread of HIV. Recently, a number of agents have been developed that target mechanisms of HIV infection without interfering with the body's natural defences, but definitive evidence of efficacy in human clinical trials is lacking.[38]

Expanded access to antiretroviral therapy (ART) offers new opportunities to strengthen prevention efforts in Asia. Infectiousness of HIV is directly related to the inoculum dose, and viral load seems to be an important predictor of sexual spread of HIV. In support of this, in a study of monogamous HIV-1 discordant couples in Uganda, compared with those with plasma viral loads <3500 copies/mL the risk of transmission or acquisition of HIV was approximately 12 times higher for those with plasma viral loads >50 000 copies/mL, and no transmission occurred in couples where the HIV-infected partner had a viral load <1500 copies/mL.[39] It therefore follows that programs which increase access to ART and reduce the concentration of virus in the blood and genital tract will reduce the transmissibility of HIV. There is some evidence to support this conjecture. A cohort study in San Francisco demonstrated a decrease in HIV infectivity following widespread use of HAART.[40] Additional evidence comes from the experience of Taiwan, which implemented a policy to provide HAART without cost to all HIV-infected citizens in 1997. In subsequent years the HIV transmission rate decreased by 53%, but the incidence of syphilis in the same period was unchanged.[41] In addition to decreased infectivity, this decreased rate of HIV transmission supports the hypothesis that increased access to treatment will provide incentives for HIV testing, which bring people into the health system before they become symptomatic. This will in turn increase opportunities for delivering and reinforcing messages on prevention. This aspect is particularly important since prevention gains may be offset should resistance develop or risk behaviors increase.

Within resource limited settings in Asia, Thailand has the most experience with bringing ART programs to scale. Thailand's ART program began in 1992 as a program of AZT monotherapy. This evolved over time to include dual and triple therapy, but mainly in a clinical research setting. In 2000, the Thai Ministry of Public Health established a pilot Access to Care initiative, as a first step towards national access to ART. At the same time, the Royal Thai Government decided to strengthen national capacity to manufacture antiretrovirals through the Government Pharmaceutical Office (GPO). In 2002, the GPO started to produce a fixed dose combination of stavudine, lamivudine and nevirapine (GPO-VIR) at the price of 1200 Baht (US$30) per month. In 2002–2003 access to care was further expanded with the National Access to Antiretroviral Program for People with HIV/AIDS (NAPHA program) with a commitment to provide triple ART as the standard of care to all HIV/AIDS persons for whom ART is medically indicated. Under this program, the number of people living with HIV/AIDS accessing treatment was approximately 40 900 in August 2004 and was projected to increase to 50 000 by December 2004.[3]

Thailand's experience offers some insights to other Asian nations seeking to expand access to ART. First, committed leadership is necessary at the policy level, with commitment and continued effort from all sectors of society, including people living with HIV and AIDS to mount a successful national response.[22,23] Second, ART and monitoring modalities need to be available at a price that will permit treating large numbers of individuals. Third, infrastructure needs to be developed so that healthcare workers can initiate and have appropriate laboratory facilities to monitor treatment with highly active antiretroviral therapy (HAART). Fourth, patients need to be educated about HAART and the importance of adherence. Fifth, locally relevant behavioral and clinical research is important to inform policy options.[42] Finally, adequate international supplemental support should be sought to cover the costs of these programs. Despite the achievements to date, in Thailand as in other Asian countries, there are some important challenges ahead in expanding access to ART. For example, sustaining access to care will require continued effort as people begin to fail first line regimens in a situation where resources are limited.

New HIV Testing Strategy to Identify New Incident Cases of HIV and Help Track HIV in Asia

To trace highly contagious, newly infected persons creates new opportunities for HIV surveillance and prevention. Recent studies have reported promising results with new HIV testing methodologies including de-tuned anti-HIV antibody testing and nucleic acid amplification, for their utility in finding newly or recently infected individuals.[43-46] Thailand and India are among the Asian countries currently implementing and evaluating this approach, which if effective will enhance national HIV prevention and control programs, which are currently in use.

Lessons Learnt and Challenges for Asia

The prevention success stories in Thailand and Cambodia are largely attributable to the commitment shown when their leaders made HIV/AIDS a national health priority. Beside the committed leadership issue, two other key determinants were required for sustained success in HIV prevention: committed HIV prevention programs at various levels within the country, and committed action by the community. With current infrastructures, recent economic crises, and burdens from other urgent epidemics such as SARS and avian influenza, there are serious concerns whether these two countries can sustain their capacity to keep the HIV epidemic under control.

Unfortunately the prevention successes of these two countries are not being well replicated in other Asian countries. What is likely to happen in the countries in transition such as China, Indonesia, and in countries with very low HIV prevalence? In the absence of extensive prevention programs to reduce HIV transmission in at-risk populations comprising clients and sex workers, IDUs and MSM, one might expect that they will see steadily climbing HIV prevalence. The first step as well as the real challenge, is to convince Country leaders to make the HIV pandemic one of their National priorities. International HIV/AIDS organizations such as WHO, UNAIDS, and the International AIDS society together with local experts and the community need to take this challenge seriously, and establishing effective and evidence-based programs in highly populated countries such as China, India and Indonesia should be an urgent priority.

Conclusion

HIV epidemics in Asia show considerable diversity in their rate and extent of spread, but share common elements in terms of the risk behaviors and transmission patterns. IDU, CSW, and MSM represent the three high-risk and interlinked groups that server as a reservoir for spreading HIV to the general population. Regionally relevant, effective prevention programs now provide good evidence for changing the course of HIV epidemics: Thailand and Cambodia have demonstrated that even in the face of a severe epidemic, targeted interventions are successful if implemented both with high coverage and intensity. Some countries in the region have seemingly been protected to date, but risk serious epidemics if prevention services are denied to those who need them. When designing intervention strategies, it is important to consider the social, political and cultural contexts which shape risk behaviors in any particular country, so that appropriate and effective prevention strategies can be implemented. The provision of effective antiretroviral treatment must be seen as a complimentary strategy to other behavioral and risk reduction interventions. Commitment and integrated action by country leaders, healthcare providers and all sectors of the community is essential so that effective prevention and treatment programs can become a reality for all Asian Countries.

References

1. UNAIDS/WHO. AIDS epidemic update. Geneva: UNAIDS/WHO, 2004: December.
2. National Intelligence Council. The next wave of HIV/AIDS: Nigeria, Ethiopia, Russia, India and China. 2002. Online. Available: www.cia.gov/nic/special_nextwaveHIV.html (accessed 29 March 2005).
3. Ruxrungtham K, Brown T, Phanuphak P. HIV/AIDS in Asia. Lancet 2004; 364:69–82.
4. Chin J, Bennett A, Mills S. Primary determinants of HIV prevalence in Asian-Pacific countries. AIDS 1998; 12: S87–S91.
5. Monitoring the AIDS Pandemic Network, AIDS in ASIA. Face the facts. A comprehensive analysis of the AIDS epidemics in Asia. 2004. Online. Available: www.fhi.org/en/HIVAIDS/pub/survreports/aids_in_asia.htm
6. Pisani E, Dadun PK, Sucahya O, et al. Sexual behavior among injection drug users in 3 Indonesian cities carries a high potential for HIV spread to noninjectors. J Acquir Immune Defic Syndr 2003; 34:403–406.
7. Solomon S, Buck J, Chaguturu SK, et al. Stopping HIV before it begins: issues faced by women in India. Nat Immunol 2003; 4:719–721.
8. Aceijas C, Stimson GV, Hickman M, et al. Global overview of injecting drug use and HIV infection among injecting drug users. AIDS 2004; 18:2295–2303.
9. Saidel TJ, Des Jarlais D, Peerapatanapokin W, et al. Potential impact of HIV among IDUs on heterosexual transmission in Asian settings: scenarios from the Asian Epidemic Model. Int J Drug Policy 2003; 14:63–74.
10. Wodak A, Ali R, Farrell M. HIV in injecting drug users in Asian countries. Br Med J 2004; 329:697–698.
11. Wodak A, Cooney A. Effectiveness of sterile needle and syringe programming in reducing HIV/AIDS among injecting drug users. Geneva: WHO; 2004.
12. Brown T, Peerapatanapokin W. The Asian epidemic model: a process model for exploring HIV policy and program alternatives in Asia. Sex Transm Infect 2004; 80:i19–i24.
13. Celum CL, Robinson NJ, Cohen MS. Potential effect of HIV type 1 antiretroviral and herpes simplex virus type 2 antiviral therapy on transmission and acquisition of HIV type 1 infection. J Infect Dis 2005; 191:S107–S114.
14. Tucker JD, Henderson GE, Wang TF, et al. Surplus men, sex work, and the spread of HIV in China. AIDS 2005; 19:539–547.
15. Lau JT, Tsui HY. Behavioral surveillance surveys of the male clients of female sex workers in Hong Kong: results of three population-based surveys. Sex Transm Dis 2003; 30:620–628.
16. Parish WL, Laumann EO, Cohen MS, et al. Population-based study of chlamydial infection in China: a hidden epidemic. JAMA 2003; 289:1265–1273.
17. Minh TT, Nhan T do, West GR, et al. Sex workers in Vietnam: how many, how risky? AIDS Educ Prev 2004; 16:389–404.
18. Wee S, Barrett ME, Lian WM, et al. Determinants of inconsistent condom use with female sex workers among men attending the STD clinic in Singapore. Sex Transm Infect 2004; 80:310–314.
19. Lau JT, Tsui HY, Siah PC, et al. A study on female sex workers in southern China (Shenzhen): HIV-related knowledge, condom use and STD history. AIDS Care 2002; 14:219–233.
20. Basu I, Jana S, Rotheram-Borus MJ, et al. HIV prevention among sex workers in India. J Acquir Immune Defic Syndr 2004; 36:845–852.
21. Saphonn V, Sopheab H, Sun LP, et al. Current HIV/AIDS/STI epidemic: intervention programs in Cambodia, 1993-2003. AIDS Educ Prev 2004; 16:S64–S77.
22. Ainsworth M, Beyrer C, Soucat A. AIDS and public policy: the lessons and challenges of 'success' in Thailand. Health Policy 2003; 64:13–37.

23. UNDP. Thailand's response to HIV/AIDS: Progress and challenges. Bangkok: United Nations Development Program; 2004.

24. Cambodian Working Group on HIV/AIDS Projections. Projections for HIV/AIDS in Cambodia: 2000-2010. Phnom Penh: National Center for HIV/AIDS Dermatology and STD; 2002.

25. Brown T. Tackling the HIV/AIDS epidemic in Asia. In: Asia-Pacific population and policy. Honolulu: East West Center; 2004.

26. Hogan DR, Salomon JA. Prevention and treatment of human immunodeficiency virus/acquired immunodeficiency syndrome in resource-limited settings. Bull World Health Organ 2005; 83:135–143.

27. The Voluntary HIV-2 Counselling and Testing Efficacy Study Group. Efficacy of voluntary HIV-1 counselling and testing in individuals and couples in Kenya, Tanzania, and Trinidad: a randomised trial. Lancet 2000; 356:103–112.

28. Hesketh T, Duo L, Li H, et al. Attitudes to HIV and HIV testing in high prevalence areas of China: informing the introduction of voluntary counselling and testing programs. Sex Transm Infect 2005; 81:108–112.

29. Go VF, Srikrishnan AK, Sivaram S, et al. High HIV prevalence and risk behaviors in men who have sex with men in Chennai, India. J Acquir Immune Defic Syndr 2004; 35:314–319.

30. Choi KH, Liu H, Guo Y, et al. Emerging HIV-1 epidemic in China in men who have sex with men. Lancet 2003; 361:2125–2126.

31. van Griensven F, Thanprasertsuk S, Jommaroeng R, et al. Evidence of a previously undocumented epidemic of HIV infection among men who have sex with men in Bangkok, Thailand. AIDS 2005; 19:521–526.

32. Pisani E, Girault P, Gultom M, et al. HIV, syphilis infection, and sexual practices among transgenders, male sex workers, and other men who have sex with men in Jakarta, Indonesia. Sex Transm Infect 2004; 80:536–540.

33. Dandona L, Dandona R, Gutierrez JP, et al. Sex behavior of men who have sex with men and risk of HIV in Andhra Pradesh, India. AIDS 2005; 19:611–619.

34. Colby DJ. HIV knowledge and risk factors among men who have sex with men in Ho Chi Minh City, Vietnam. J Acquir Immune Defic Syndr 2003; 32:80–85.

35. Girault P, Saidel T, Song N, et al. HIV, STIs, and sexual behaviors among men who have sex with men in Phnom Penh, Cambodia. AIDS Educ Prev 2004; 16:31–44.

36. Herbst JH, Sherba RT, Crepaz N, et al. A meta-analytic review of HIV behavioral interventions for reducing sexual risk behavior of men who have sex with men. J Acquir Immune Defic Syndr 2005; 39:228–241.

37. Pope M, Haase AT. Transmission, acute HIV-1 infection and the quest for strategies to prevent infection. Nat Med 2003; 9:847–852.

38. Shattock R, Solomon S. Microbicides–aids to safer sex. Lancet 2004; 363:1002–1003.

39. Quinn TC, Wawer MJ, Sewankambo N, et al. Viral load and heterosexual transmission of human immunodeficiency virus type 1. Rakai Proj Study Group N Engl J Med 2000; 342:921–929.

40. Porco TC, Martin JN, Page-Shafer KA, et al. Decline in HIV infectivity following the introduction of highly active antiretroviral therapy. AIDS 2004; 18:81–88.

41. Fang CT, Hsu HM, Twu SJ, et al. Decreased HIV transmission after a policy of providing free access to highly active antiretroviral therapy in Taiwan. J Infect Dis 2004; 190:879–885.

42. Duncombe C, Kerr SJ, Ruxrungtham K, et al. HIV disease progression in a patient cohort treated via a clinical research network in a resource limited setting. AIDS 2005; 19:169–178.

43. Pilcher CD, Fiscus SA, Nguyen TQ, et al. Detection of acute infections during HIV testing in North Carolina. N Engl J Med 2005; 352:1873–1883.

44. Guy RJ, Breschkin AM, Keenan CM, et al. Improving HIV surveillance in Victoria: the role of the 'detuned' enzyme immunoassay. J Acquir Immune Defic Syndr 2005; 38:495–499.

45. Janssen RS, Satten GA, Stramer SL, et al. New testing strategy to detect early HIV-1 infection for use in incidence estimates and for clinical and prevention purposes. JAMA 1998; 280:42–48.

46. United States Bureau of the Census. HIV/AIDS Surveillance database. Washington, DC: US Census Bureau; 2004. Online. Available: www.census.gov/ipc/www/hivaidsd.html

CHAPTER 51

HIV Transmission and its Prevention in Eastern Europe

Kasia Malinowska-Sempruch

Introduction

It is hard to keep hopeful about the global HIV epidemic. The past 25 years have witnessed a constant and continuous rise in the number of people living with HIV around the world. With five million new infections in 2005, the total number of people living with HIV globally has reached an estimated 40.3 million people, up from 37.5 million in 2003. Despite recent, much heralded efforts to expand access to lifesaving antiretroviral medications, more than three million people died of AIDS-related illnesses in 2005, including over 500 000 children.[1] Yet these shocking figures would be even higher if strides had not been made over the past 25 years to identify and implement effective HIV care and prevention strategies. Successful interventions in certain parts of the world, such as Uganda and Senegal, have focused broadly on general populations. Others have been designed primarily to reach high-risk communities, such as effective activities targeting gay men in USA and sex workers in Thailand.

It is not always easy, or even appropriate, to integrate these specific strategies elsewhere for various cultural, economic, social, and political reasons. Even so, these cases offer powerful, relevant lessons for policymakers and public health officials around the world who hope to help their countries join the small, but increasing number of HIV prevention success stories.

Unfortunately, seemingly obvious HIV prevention lessons from targeting other populations are often ignored when it comes to offering services for drug users. For example, Thailand, which successfully curbed HIV infection rates among its vulnerable sex worker populations with a pragmatic national program that set out to ensure condom use in every sex work establishment, ignored international experience and lessons learned within its own borders when it came to addressing the problem among drug users. Instead of striving for 100% needle coverage for injection drug users (IDUs), a logical corollary to its stated goal of 100% condoms and care coverage for sex workers, the national government chose instead the route of stigmatization, persecution and even extrajudicial killings in response to the country's drug problem.[2] While declining among every other sub-population in Thailand, the HIV infection rate among drug users hovers near 50%, a similar rate to that seen in the early 1990s.[3]

The Thai government is not alone in making short-sighted decisions that harm drug users and, ultimately, contribute to the continuing spread of HIV. Other countries, including a number of Thailand's middle-income neighbors in Asia, have repressive policies regarding drug use, with governments routinely harassing users while neglecting to take measures to protect the health of this vulnerable population. Repressive attitudes concerning addiction, treatment, and social integration remain popular in many corners of the world, despite the negative local public health consequences and increased scientific evidence supporting progressive policies coming from many Western European countries.

The regressive policies currently in place in many parts of the world are especially troubling when one considers the explosiveness with which HIV can move through drug-using communities if effective prevention efforts are not in place. Shared needles are especially efficient transmitters of HIV. When HIV is introduced into a drug-using community, the rates of infection can surge from 0 to 50% in a matter of weeks. In Svetlagorsk, Russia, for example, 67% of IDUs were infected within 1 year of the first HIV case.[4] Similarly, in the Yili prefecture of Xianjiang, China, the percentage of IDUs with HIV rose from 9% to 76% between January and August of 1996.[5] Such data shows that transmission among IDUs can become self-perpetuating, with even modest levels of risk behavior leading to substantial rates of infection once HIV prevalence reaches 20% among this group.[6] Globally, 10% of all infections are among IDUs, although that percentage is rising and already tops 30% outside of sub-Saharan Africa.[7]

Emerging Dual Epidemics in the Former Soviet Union and Central and Eastern Europe

Countries in Eastern Europe (CEE) and the Former Soviet Union (FSU) are experiencing some of the fastest growth rates of HIV around the globe.[3] Unique among the world's HIV epidemics, the majority of infections in the region to date (an estimated 87%[9]) are attributable to injection drug use. The region's epidemic is greatly shaped by ongoing transitions in the wake of the Soviet Union's collapse in the early 1990s. Over the past decade, large segments of the population, particularly young people, have been greatly impacted by faltering economies, social dislocation and crumbling public health and education services. Even in countries that have witnessed a growth of a middle class in recent years, much of the population has yet to recover from the loss of communist-era safety nets. Increased economic and social vulnerability combined with the ready availability of heroin and other opiates – widely available due to the region's position on a main drug-trafficking route from opium producing Afghanistan to Western Europe – have resulted in an explosion of drug use from Kyrgyzstan to Estonia. Conservative estimates indicate that 3.2 million people in CEE/FSU currently inject illicit drugs,[10] making up nearly one-quarter of the world's total of 13.2 million IDUs.[11]

Not surprisingly, HIV has thrived in this climate of weak economies and heavy drug use. According to the Joint United Nations Programme on HIV/AIDS (UNAIDS), perhaps 150 000 individuals in CEE/FSU were HIV positive in 1995. Just 8 years later, however, the estimate had risen to 1.6 million people.[10] Infections rates climb across the region, with Estonia, Russia and Ukraine faring the worst. In each of these countries, HIV prevalence rates among the adult population exceed 1%.[1] In terms of sheer numbers, the situation is most severe in Russia, by far the most populous country in the region. In March 2005, there were nearly 333 332 individuals in Russia officially registered as having HIV.[12] This figure reflects only reported cases and many put the actual number of individuals living with HIV as estimated to be up to four times higher – at least one million, nearly all of whom contracted the virus in the past 5 years.[7] The surge in HIV infections can only mean that the number of annual deaths, currently relatively low at just under 7000, will rise inexorably for the foreseeable future. Hopes are already diminishing for a nation where 80% of those infected are younger than 30.[7]

In February 2005, an official from one of Russia's main HIV/AIDS monitoring agencies declared that a growing number of infections are attributable to sexual contact.* With hundreds of thousands of drug users, many of whom are sexually active, infected, transmission to partners and other segments of the population is increasingly common. Thus, it is quite likely that the failure to curb the epidemic among drug users and concomitant disregard for their health needs affect an ever-growing segment of the general population. Although these numbers pale in comparison to similar data from sub-Saharan Africa – home to about 65% of the nearly 40.1 million people living with HIV at the end of 2005[1] – the speed with which this relatively new epidemic is spreading and the vulnerability of many people in the region not yet infected are cause for great concern.

Nearly all observers believe the dual crises of HIV and drug abuse will only deepen. A highly publicized report from the World Bank in 2003 estimated that even under the most optimistic scenario, the cumulative number of people infected with HIV in the region would rise to 2.3 million in 2010 and 5.4 million in 2020.[13] Several UN agencies and international non-governmental organizations (NGOs) also released reports detailing the region's growing epidemic.[14-18] If projections from these groups are realized, the epidemic will have reached levels seen

---

*The official, Larisa Dementyeva, represents the Russian Consumer Control's HIV/AIDS monitoring department.

nowhere else but sub-Saharan Africa – and will undoubtedly have catastrophic effects on public health, economies, social stability, and national security of regions already struggling with many challenges.

Regrettably, it is precisely the countries where the needs of drug users are the most urgent that often harbor the most repressive policies towards drug users. Across the former Soviet Union in particular, drug users' risk of contracting HIV is heightened by social marginalization and punitive responses to their behavior by authorities – both of which help keep most users underground and isolated. This greatly limits their ability and willingness to obtain information and services that can help safeguard their health and the health of those around them. For a variety of reasons, epidemiological research and advocacy from concerned groups have yet to promote a sense of urgency among the region's policymakers. The scenario is distressingly similar to the situation in Africa two decades ago, when clear signs of a burgeoning (in that region primarily sexually transmitted) epidemic were largely ignored. Whatever lessons there might be from the consequences of that inaction have not been learned by those with relevant oversight and responsibility in the former Soviet Union and many neighboring countries.

Harm Reduction: The Effective Yet Neglected Intervention

In the HIV arena, the goal of harm reduction is to diminish the individual and social harms associated with drug use – especially the risk of HIV infection – through an approach emphasizing human rights, public health, and pragmatism. In practice, harm reduction encompasses a wide range of drug user services including needle and syringe exchange, substitution therapy (such as methadone maintenance), health education, medical referrals, and support services. In many parts of the world where injection drug use has been a main driver of the HIV epidemic, including Canada, The Netherlands and Switzerland, harm reduction strategies are the cornerstone of HIV prevention approaches that have largely been effective.[19] The results of one of the most comprehensive studies, a review of data from 81 cities across Europe, Asia, and North America with and without needle-exchange programs (NEPs), found that, on average, HIV seroprevalence increased by 5.9% per year in the 52 cities without NEPs and decreased by 5.8% per year in the 29 cities with NEPs.[20] Based on this and other studies, most leading

public health agencies and organizations, including the World Health Organization, UNAIDS, the US National Institutes of Health and the American Medical Association, have concluded that needle exchange is safe, cost-effective and, most importantly, helps prevent new infections.

In Russia and neighboring countries of the former Soviet Union, more than 200 harm reduction programs have been implemented since the late 1990s. In Russia, for example, an estimated 75 needle/syringe exchange programs were operating at the beginning of 2004.[21] Most of them offer drug users a variety of services including sterile syringes and needles, condoms, counselling and information, and referrals to other health and social services. Unlike in Croatia, however, the number of programs currently operating in these regions does not come close to meeting the needs of drug users, especially as drug use rates continue to climb and HIV-related illnesses become more common. Authorities' staunch opposition has kept methadone illegal in Russia for any purpose, even as the drug has been used successfully for more than three decades, not just in nearby Croatia, but also in populous countries such as Germany[22] and Spain.[23] It is important to note that even the US government supports the use of methadone in treating addiction to heroin and other opiates.[24] The estimated coverage rate – how many IDUs have consistent access to harm reduction services – is just 2% in the region, far too small to have a significant impact on HIV incidence among drug users.[9]

A lack of political support for harm reduction is the primary limiting factor in the expansion of such services. Like many of their US counterparts, government officials in most countries in the former Soviet Union have not been swayed by the growing body of evidence supporting the efficacy of harm reduction interventions. Drug users are often considered social misfits who deserve whatever health problems they might acquire. Most people do not believe that drug addiction is a medical condition that is best addressed through interventions that avoid shaming or punishing the user. Law enforcement authorities and other policymakers throughout the region generally remain opposed to harm reduction.

Echoing arguments made in the US and other countries endorsing more punitive approaches to drug users, these officials claim that the harm reduction approach increases drug use and represents the first step toward drug legalization. A look at international drug policy in the last 20 years undermines the fallacious assumptions held by opponents of harm reduction. In the USA, for example, the federal government in 1982 launched a high-profile 'war on drugs' that focused on punitive responses to illegal drug use, such as mandatory minimum sentences for drug use and possession. Government officials have cited this 'war' as justification for imposing and maintaining a ban on federal funding for domestic needle-exchange programs. Despite these aggressive policies and the billions of dollars spent to enforce them, illegal drug use in the USA has remained stable or even increased since then.[25] Meanwhile, studies conducted around the world over the past two decades indicate that access to comprehensive harm reduction services often *decreases* illegal drug use because programs prompt users to emerge from their marginalized and stigmatized positions in society to access health and social services that can help them to change behavior.[26-28]

Beyond the well-rehearsed arguments that harm reduction encourages drug use, officials in the region often defend their policies by noting obligations to comply with international drug-control guidelines mandated by three United Nations conventions: the 1961 Single Convention on Narcotic Drugs, the 1971 Convention on Psychotropic Substance, and the 1988 Convention against Illicit Traffic in Narcotic Drugs and Psychotropic Substances. These conventions attempt to lay out a framework for controlling illegal substances and include extensive measures against illegal trafficking that require states to work towards the elimination of drug use. While the reduction of drug trafficking and control of illicit narcotics may be worthy goals, the agreements do not require participating nations to safeguard the health and rights of vulnerable populations, including those whose actions may harm no-one but themselves, such as most individuals addicted to drugs. The conventions can thus be interpreted to justify severe drug control policies, including mandatory minimum incarcerations and pave the way for physical abuse and other harsh treatment of drug users. International pressure, especially from the USA, to adhere to these treaties and the lack of awareness and understanding of harm reduction principles exacerbate leaders' tendencies to develop strict drug control policies that primarily punish, rather than effectively treat, drug users.

Most international public health organizations agree that rigidly interpreting these conventions, two of which came into existence prior to HIV becoming a global epidemic, is a short-sighted and poorly conceived strategy. Recent policies towards drug users in the former Soviet Union bear out their

belief that the public health and human rights consequences are clearly and profoundly negative. In Central Asia, for example, authorities continue to emphasize confinement over treatment, therefore condemning drug users to overcrowded prisons where needles are shared and HIV rates are surging at an even faster rate than among the population at large. A large percentage of these prisoners are or will be infected with tuberculosis (TB), which itself has reached epidemic levels in the former Soviet Union.[29] TB is now the most common killer of HIV-infected people in the region, and in prisons alone, >30% of those with TB have a multi-drug-resistant strain of the disease. Prison sentences, even for minor offenses, now often become death sentences.

There are reasons to hope that these harsh policies may be changing in some parts of the region, a development that would help remove significant barriers to effective HIV prevention and treatment. In May 2004, Russia decriminalized personal possession of illicit substances.[30] Moreover, the decision was applied retroactively, leading to the release of over 30 000 drug offenders from prison. Though conservative leaders have since attempted to overturn the decision to decriminalize, the victory of harm reduction advocates shows that key legislative reform in the region can be achieved. An effective, comprehensive response to the growing HIV epidemic in the region necessitates the conversion of more key leaders and policymakers and the introduction of supportive policies and enforcement that can allow scale up of harm reduction services for drug users.

Human Rights and HIV

Experience over the last 20 years has shown that there is a direct relationship between respect for people's human rights and their vulnerability to HIV: the more discrimination individuals face, the greater their chances of transmitting HIV. When drug users are subjected to mass arrest or harassment from authorities, they are driven further underground and are less likely to access HIV prevention information or effective treatment. The unfolding tragedy in the former Soviet Union is just the latest example of this development.

The interconnection between realizing people's human rights and HIV prevention has gained increased attention over the past decade. Accordingly, there are several international documents and treaties that address human rights and HIV. For example, the Declaration of Commitment adopted during the UN General Assembly Special Session on

HIV/AIDS (UNGASS), held in 2001, stated that the 'realization of human rights and fundamental freedoms for all is essential to reduce vulnerability to HIV/AIDS'.[31] The declaration also included language recognizing that harm reduction measures, including the provision of sterile injection equipment, were indeed effective at reducing HIV transmission and that it is necessary to offer a wide range of non-discriminatory HIV prevention programs. Other treaties that speak to human rights and disease include the Universal Declaration of Human Rights, the International Covenant on Civil and Political Rights, the International Covenant on Economic, Social and Cultural Rights, and the International Guidelines on HIV/AIDS Prevention.[32] The attention paid to these treaties, along with the establishment of the Global Fund, the first truly international and transparent mechanism for distributing funding for HIV prevention and care activities, are indications of growing recognition that HIV must be considered a global problem that does not respect national borders and can only be confronted with international engagement and collaboration.

Moving from recognition to action is a slow process, however. Several countries that have signed some or all of these treaties have failed to implement key provisions, as evidenced by continued obstruction of viable and widespread harm reduction programs in much of the former Soviet Union. The lack of enforcement mechanisms associated with these documents means that nations failing to meet their commitments face less consistent or targeted pressure to change policies. And even within the texts and subsequent conversations about the treaties, there has been very little focus on the rights of drug users and the impact of drug policy on the spread of HIV.

Meanwhile, reports from the region disclose that drug users are the victims of a litany of human rights violations perpetrated by law enforcement and other authorities, including beatings, financial and sexual extortion, impromptu detainment without charge and corruption. In Kazakhstan, for example, a 37-year-old woman described an encounter with police after purchasing drugs from a dealer:

[T]here were two policemen, it was daytime, they led me into a nearby building in ruins and started to beat me . . . I was beaten in the head, and on my body, with their fists, I didn't fall down, but then they let me go.[33]

In Russia, a director of an NGO that provides support to drug users and HIV-positive people told a researcher, 'Planting drugs is common. If the police stop a drug user and see needle marks on his arm, they plant drugs and then beat him or do what they want'.[34]

It is perhaps not surprising that such abuse persists given the apparent contradiction between current drug control policies, as defined by the UN conventions, and the major international human rights declarations. In fact, police abuse of drug users and other vulnerable people, including youth, sex workers and Roma, seem inevitable under a law enforcement approach, which is usually the preferred option for authorities who want to appear tough on crime. When police infringe on the rights of vulnerable populations, it is not only the international treaties that are violated, but national constitutions as well. For example, Article 19 of Russia's Constitution guarantees citizens broad protection from discrimination when seeking to exercise the rights granted them under the Constitution, including the right to health.[35] Yet harassment and punitive policies based primarily on discrimination prevent most drug users from accessing services and taking appropriate measures to protect themselves from HIV and potential health problems associated with drug use.

HIV Treatment Concerns

As the HIV infection rates in the region have surged in recent years, whatever little attention is paid to HIV tends to be focused on prevention. In wealthier countries in North America and Western Europe, the introduction of life-prolonging HIV therapies in the late 1990s dramatically reduced AIDS death rates, while aiding prevention efforts. Offering life-extending hope to individuals who just a decade before would have been offered only palliative care, this development played a major role in influencing many individuals, particularly those most at risk, to get tested for HIV. It is no longer possible, if it was ever, to distinguish between prevention and treatment.

Despite the proven effectiveness of the medications, there is still work to be done in encouraging people to be tested and seek treatment, even in wealthy countries where medications are provided free of charge or through individuals' insurance. Perhaps one-quarter of the 900 000 estimated HIV-positive individuals in the USA, for example, are not aware that they have been infected and thus are not receiving the treatment they might need. Among the reasons cited for this gap in the USA are lingering stigma, the epidemic's increasing concentration in poorer or marginalized communities such as African-Americans, substandard outreach efforts and powerful opposition to realistic education about sex and other potentially risky behaviors from certain parts of the country.[36]

Though these lingering barriers to treatment are important to recognize and understand, the element of hope that treatment brings to vulnerable populations cannot be dismissed. Without the belief that they may access treatment for HIV, drug users and other individuals vulnerable for contracting HIV have little inclination to get tested. Yet if they know their HIV status, they are better prepared to protect their own health and the health of those around them. Whether encouraged from abroad or generated domestically, efforts to prevent the spread of HIV in CEE/FSU can only be successful if implemented in tandem with strategies to increase access to treatment.

Despite the efficacy of the medications and proven models for distributing across a variety of patients and contexts, treatment availability remains severely limited across the region. According to a recent report from the World Health Organization and UNAIDS, just 5.4% of the estimated 94 000 HIV-positive Russians who need ARV therapy were receiving it by the end of 2004.[37] The corresponding percentages were equally dismal in neighboring countries such as the Ukraine (5.4% of the 17 300 patients currently in need), Kazakhstan (3% of 1050) and Uzbekistan (0% of 1250).[38]

In most of these countries, the primary obstacles to increasing access to treatment have been the high cost of medicines and insufficient allocation of resources for this purpose. The ever-growing availability of lower-priced drugs and, in most of the region, financial assistance from the Global Fund and other outside sources, will likely help reduce the first problem. Perhaps even more important than funding is the political commitment of leaders in countries confronting the epidemic. Several countries in recent years delayed submitting applications to the Global Fund, for instance, or mismanaged the application process as key decision makers failed to step in and push the process forward.* Most EEC and FSU governments' own spending on HIV/AIDS treatment fails to match the urgency or scale of the problem.

---

*In the Ukraine, the Global Fund took the unprecedented step, in April 2004, of replacing the original entities, including the Ukrainian Ministry of Health, that had been chosen to oversee the disbursal of Round 1 funds. The ministry and its partners were accused of mismanagement and incompetence.

In the current climate, it is unclear whether HIV-positive IDUs would benefit even if ARV therapies were more widely available in these contexts. They are often placed last on the list of those eligible for treatment or denied access altogether, based on the assumption that they would be unable or unwilling to adhere to complicated drug regimens. The lack of trust between people who inject drugs and government service providers can also serve as a barrier to treatment. These fears are borne out in recent data that shows only 5% of HIV-positive Russians receiving antiretroviral therapy are former or current drug users,[7] even though this group represents a significant majority of all infected.

Some policymakers justify withholding or obstructing effective services for IDUs on the grounds that drug users' behavior indicates that they have no interest in protecting their health and cannot be trusted to adhere to treatment and other kinds of programs. The first assumption can be readily disproved by the steady stream of clients seeking out and obtaining clean needles and other harm reduction services at existing projects in the region, not to mention the waiting lists at some sites. The assumption that IDUs cannot be trusted to comply with HIV and other treatment regimens is equally specious. Successful efforts to offer HIV treatment to IDUs have been documented in Brazil, Argentina, and a number of urban settings in the USA and in Europe.[39]

Making abstinence a condition for support – a common requirement of many health providers – is also a flawed policy, because it imposes restrictions that many users are not emotionally or physically prepared to meet. If they are not offered the support that they need in their current state, they have less incentive or desire to change behaviors, such as sharing needles, that can spread HIV, hepatitis and other blood-borne diseases.

Given that the majority of the more than one million people infected with HIV in the region are drug users, it also seems unconscionable to even wonder whether it is appropriate to offer HIV treatment to this group. Failing to provide treatment reduces the effectiveness of all other prevention strategies. The only question that the international and national public health communities should be asking now is *how* to provide care. Some of the answers are already available in various parts of the world, including France (Paris), the USA (New York City and New Haven, Connecticut) and Poland (Chorzów), where AIDS physicians and other caregivers offer a range of services that support drug users' adherence.[39] These services may include social, legal and economic assistance as well as access to methadone maintenance. A comprehensive and non-judgmental provision of a range of services successfully attracts and retains drug users needing support and treatment.

Substitution treatment programs provide drug users with access to methadone, buprenorphine or other drugs that can help reduce and control the use of more dangerous street-based drugs and improve drug users' adherence to other forms of treatment. These programs have been shown to be highly effective for many users and have been an integral part of certain individuals' ability to maintain in HIV treatment. Despite the importance and proven efficacy of substitution treatment, many drug treatment specialists in the FSU and CCE consider abstinence treatment as the only worthy option, even though the suitability and effectiveness of this type of treatment for many patients has been called into question. Drug users are faced with a lack of realistic options to help treat their addiction. This situation, combined with the threat of punitive responses if their continuing drug use is discovered, convinces many drug users to avoid seeking assistance altogether.

While small pilot substitution treatment programs exist in most of the Eastern European counties, this is not the case throughout much of the former Soviet Union. Limited pilots of methadone substitution currently are functioning in only a few tiny countries, including Moldova, Lithuania, Estonia, and Kyrgyzstan. Similar programs are on the brink of being established in two others, Georgia and Uzbekistan. Countries in the region where the need is greatest lag far behind, however. Even though methadone is registered in the Ukraine, national drug control authorities prevent doctors from offering it to patients. In Russia, methadone is illegal for any purpose and discussion of substitution treatment is quickly stifled. By some measures, an estimated 800 000 people in just three countries – Russia, Ukraine and Kazakhstan – could benefit from substitution therapy if available now. None have access to it at the present moment.

Although a growing number of people across Central and Eastern Europe and the former Soviet Union recognize that aggressive and immediate action must be taken to address the HIV epidemic among drug users, including expanded access to harm reduction services, their ability to change attitudes and policies is limited. What is needed is top-down political engagement, accompanied by appropriate resources and monitoring. Discriminated against and in many cases harassed, incarcer-

ated, or otherwise abused, drug users in the region have, perhaps predictably, in many cases not been able to protect themselves from HIV. As with all vulnerable individuals who have faced discrimination, they are much more inclined to successfully change their behavior when policies and programs are in place that are designed to improve their health and assist in integrating them into society, where they can play useful roles in devising appropriate strategies to reach their peers. Leading by example is the only way governments can help to remove social and economic discrimination and, by extension, curb the growing regional HIV epidemic. If individuals with power continue to refuse to engage a rights-based approach to providing services for drug users, the price to pay, in terms of spoiled opportunities and lost lives, will be very high indeed.

References

1. UNAIDS/WHO. AIDS epidemic update: December 2005. Online. Available: www.unaids.org/epi/2005/ doc/ EPIupdate2005_pdf_en/epi-update2005_en.pdf
2. Human Rights Watch Report. The war on drugs, HIV/AIDS, and violations of human rights in Thailand. Online. Available: www.hrw.org/campaigns/aids/2004/thai.htm
3. Avert. HIV AIDS and Thailand. Online. Available: www. avert.org/aidsthai.htm
4. Dehne K, Kobyscha Y. The HIV epidemic in Central and Eastern Europe: Update 2000. A report to a second strategy meeting to better coordinate regional support to national responses to HIV/AIDS in Central and Eastern Europe. Copenhagen: World Health Organization.
5. UNAIDS/UNODCCP. Drug use and HIV vulnerability. Geneva/Vienna, Joint United Nations Programme on HIV/ AIDS/United Nations Office for Drug Control and Crime Prevention; 2000.
6. Des Jarlais DC, Marmor M, Friedmann P, et al. HIV incidence among injection drug users in New York City, 1992–1997: Evidence for a declining epidemic. Am J Public Health 2000; 90:352–359.
7. UNAIDS. AIDS epidemic update, December 2004. Online. Available: www.unaids.org
8. United Nations Development Program. Meeting the challenge: Addressing HIV/AIDS in Easter Europe and the CIS region. Online. Available: www.undp.org/hiv/docs/ regional_reps/europe_cis_regional_report.pdf
9. Open Society Institute. Harm Reduction Developments 2005: Countries with injection-driven HIV epidemics. Online Available: www.soros org/initiatives/health/focus/ ihrd/articles_publications/publications/ihrdreport_ 20060417
10. UNODC. Estimated IDU and HIV prevalence among general populations and in prison settings, September 2005.
11. Aceijas C, Stimson GV, Hickman M, et al. United Nations Reference Group on HIV/AIDS prevention and care among IDU in developing and transitional countries, global overview of injecting drug use and HIV infection among injecting drug users. AIDS 2004; 18:2295–2303.
12. Russian Federal AIDS Centre. AIDS Foundation East West. Online. Available: www.afew.org
13. World Bank report. Reversing the tide: Priorities for HIV/ AIDS prevention in Central Asia, released September 2003. Online. Available: www.worldbank.org/eca/aids

14. UNAIDS. Online. Available: www.unaids.org
15. UNDP. Online. Available: www.undp.org
16. SOROS. International Harm Reduction Development Program of the Open Society Institute. Online. Available: www.soros.org/initiatives/ihrd
17. Human Rights Watch. Online. Available: www.hrw.org
18. Transatlantic Partners Against AIDS. Online. Available: www.tpaa.net
19. Gibson DR, Flynn NM, Perales D. Effectiveness of syringe exchange programs in reducing HIV risk behavior and HIV seroconversion among injecting drug users. AIDS 2001; 15:1329–1341.
20. Hurley S, Jolly DJ, Kaldor JM. Effectiveness of needle-exchange programmes for prevention of HIV infection. Lancet 1997; 349:1797–1800.
21. Csete J, Cohen J. Lessons not learned: Human rights abuses and HIV/AIDS in the Russian Federation. Human Rights Watch 2004; 16:5.
22. Gerlach R. Drug-substitution treatment in Germany: A critical overview of its history, legislation and current practice. J Drug Issues 2002; 32:503–521.
23. Agència de Salut Pública in Barcelona. Information about methadone maintenance programs. Online. Available: www.aspb.es
24. US Office of National Drug Control Policy: Additional information about methadone's effectiveness. Online. Available: www.whitehousedrugpolicy.gov/publications/factsht/methadone
25. Cato Institute. Online. Available: www.cato.org/dailys/12-02-04.html
26. Watters JK, Estilo MJ, Clark GL, et al. Syringe and needle exchange as HIV/AIDS prevention for injection drug users. JAMA 1994; 271:115–120.
27. Normand J, Vlahov D, Moses LE, editors. Preventing HIV transmission: The role of sterile needles and bleach.

Washington DC: National Academy Press; 1995:224–226, 248–250.
28. Paone D, Des Jarlais DC, Gangloff R, et al. Syringe exchange: HIV prevention, key findings, and future directions. Int J Addict 1995; 30:1647–1683.
29. World Health Organization. Online website. Available: www.who.org
30. Moscow Times. No more jail terms for drug possession, 14 May, 2004.
31. UN General Assembly Special Session on HIV/AIDS. Online. Available: www.un.org/ga/aids/coverage
32. Alexandrova A. AIDS, drugs, and society. International Debate Association, 2002.
33. Human Rights Watch. Fanning the flames: How human rights abuses are fueling the AIDS epidemic in Kazakhstan. June 2003. Online. Available: www.hrw.org/reports/2003/kazak0603
34. Human Rights Watch. Lessons not learned: Human rights abuses and HIV/AIDS in the Russian Federation. May 2004. Online. Available: http://hrw.org/reports/2004/russia0404
35. Constitution of the Russian Federation. Adopted 12 December 12, 1993, as amended in 1996, 2001 and 2003, Art. 19.
36. National Institute of Allergy and Infectious Diseases. July 2004. Online. Available: www.niaid.nih.gov/factsheets/aidsstat.htm
37. WHO. Progress on global access to HIV antiretroviral therapy report. Online. Available: www.who.int/3by5/fullreportJune2005.pdf
38. WHO Country Reports. June 2005. Online. Available: www.who.int/countries/en
39. SOROS. Breaking down barriers: Lessons on providing HIV treatment to injection drug users, Open Society Institute, 2004. Online. Available: www.soros.org/initiatives/ihrd/articles_publications/publications/arv_idus_20040715

CHAPTER 52

Vaginal Microbicides Against HIV

Zeda F. Rosenberg

Mark Mitchnick

Paul Coplan

Introduction

As the HIV pandemic enters its third decade, women are becoming infected at an increasing rate. Since 2002, the number of women living with HIV has increased in every region. East Asia experienced the sharpest increase with 56% in 2 years, followed by Eastern Europe and Central Asia, with 48%. In sub-Saharan Africa, 76% of young people aged 15–24 living with HIV are female. In Russia, 38% of people living with HIV were women, compared with 24% in 2001.[1]

Biological differences between men and women result in women's exposure to higher levels of virus for longer periods of time during sexual intercourse. Additionally, in young women, immature cervico-vaginal tissue is likely to be damaged during sex, thus more easily allowing HIV entry. Confounding this biological predisposition are widespread cultural, economic, and political disparities that make it difficult for women to insist that condoms are used during sex or to leave a risky partnership.

As a result, new HIV prevention technologies that can be initiated by women, may not necessarily be contraceptive, and are culturally acceptable, are urgently needed. Microbicides, products that women can use vaginally to kill or inactivate HIV introduced during sex, are being developed to address this need.

Mechanisms of Action of Microbicides

During sexual intercourse, HIV enters the vagina in the seminal fluid as either free virus or within infected lymphocytes. While the precise mechanisms of transmission across vaginal mucosal surfaces are not known, it is possible that either free virus or virally-infected cells can migrate across the mucosal surface through intracellular junctions. Additionally, virus and cells may gain direct access to the sub-mucosal tissues through breaks in the epithelium, resulting from disease or sexual trauma.[2]

Once virus or virally-infected cells gain entry to the submucosal tissues, infection of CD4$^+$ T cells and macrophages can occur.[3] The predominant co-receptors used by HIV in these cell types are CCR5 and CXCR4. However, the virus can also be carried from the vaginal lumen by dendritic cells (DC) that normally circulate through mucosal tissue to identify invading pathogens. HIV can enter immature DC in mucosal tissues via a family of mannose-specific C-type lectin receptors, including DC-SIGN.[4] After a period of time (hours to days), locally infected T cells and macrophages migrate away from the vagina to the lymph nodes spreading the infection systemically. Similarly, HIV that is captured by DC is also rapidly transported through the submucosa to local lymph nodes where presentation to and infection of

CD4[+] T cells occurs. Thus, microbicides must be designed to act before virus, virus-infected cells, or virus-transporting cells leave the cervicovaginal tissue.

In many ways, microbicides are analogous to treatment strategies because both microbicides and therapeutic antiretrovirals are intended to prevent HIV infection of uninfected cells. In fact, many of the drugs currently used in therapy are appropriate microbicide candidates. Microbicides do, however, differ from therapeutics in one major way: they can attack the virus in the vagina, before it spreads throughout the body. This affords microbicide developers the opportunity to use drugs that may not be successful when taken orally but are useful when applied topically. It also means that some existing drugs, while not effective enough to cure HIV infection once it has a stronghold, may be effective enough to block it from entering the body. Thus, microbicide researchers have a wide variety of established available drugs and approaches that can and are being pursued.

Classes of microbicide drugs now under development are generally divided into four categories: membrane disruptive agents, attachment/fusion/entry (AFE) inhibitors, reverse transcriptase inhibitors and dendritic cell uptake inhibitors.

Membrane Disruptive Agents

The membrane disruptive agents were among the first candidate microbicides to be developed. Many of these products were originally marketed as vaginal spermicides that contained nonoxynol-9 (N-9), octoxynol-9, or benzalkonium chloride. These chemicals destroy the outer coating of cells (such as sperm) and pathogens (such as enveloped viruses), which renders the latter non-infectious. While very effective at killing HIV and other sexually-transmitted pathogens in vitro, the selectivity index (i.e. the ratio of HIV inhibition to host cell toxicity) of this category of agents is very low, such that cell death in vitro occurs at or near the same concentrations that kill HIV.[5]

Since N-9-containing spermicides were readily available in most countries, safety and efficacy trials were conducted to determine their effect on HIV acquisition. Although the potential for toxicity was acknowledged, the potential benefits were large given the relentless growth of the HIV epidemic, particularly among women. Several randomized controlled clinical trials failed to demonstrate a protective effect of N-9-containing products on HIV and STD (gonorrhea and chlamydia) transmission.[6,7] Indeed, one study of a 52.5 mg N-9-containing gel showed a trend towards increased HIV transmission and higher incidence of lesions with epithelial disruption, particularly among women with frequent daily use.[8]

The results from this study as well as more recent preclinical research on N-9 have highlighted the need to carefully examine the potential for mucosal irritation. Current approaches include determination of cumulative damage to cells in vitro; measurement of proinflammatory cytokines and anti-inflammatory factors in cell culture as well as in vaginal fluids in women following single and multiple applications of candidate microbicides.[5]

Two products with membrane disruptive activity, C31G and SLS are currently in clinical testing for efficacy and expanded safety, respectively (Table 52.1). Published studies suggest that these products have lower in vitro cytotoxicity than N-9.[9,10]

AFE Inhibitors

AFE inhibitors hinder the binding of HIV to its target cells, and the initial interactions that take place immediately after binding, thus interfering with the earliest steps of infection. These drugs are comprised of several distinct subclasses depending on whether they act at the viral level prior to target cell attachment or at the cell surface.[11] The majority of microbicides that are currently in large-scale efficacy trials (carrageenan, cellulose sulfate, naphthalene sulfonate polymer, Carbopol 974P) attack the virus in a similar way: a negatively charged polymer (the drug) attracts a positively charged group on HIV's surface (gp120), binding it and rendering the virus non-infectious.[2] Carbopol 974P also may have an inhibitory effect on HIV by virtue of its pH buffering capacity in the presence of seminal plasma.[12] SPL7013, a dendrimer with a polyanionic outer surface, is currently being tested in safety trials. It has been shown to prevent infection in female pigtailed macaques in a dose-dependent manner.[13]

Other AFE inhibitors interact in a very specific manner, with gp120 molecules on the surface of HIV. Cyanovirin, a protein isolated from blue-green algae, irreversibly binds to HIV gp120 and has been shown to prevent sexual transmission of simian-human immunodeficiency (SHIV) to macaques.[14] A vaginal gel containing high doses of monoclonal antibodies to gp120 has similarly been shown to inhibit infection by vaginal exposure to SHIV in macaques.[15]

Table 52.1 Products currently in development

	Pre-clinical	Safety	Efficacy
Entry/fusion inhibitors	Cyanovirin BMS 806 Plant lectins New polyanions		PRO2000 Carraguard™ Cellulose sulfate Buffer gel
NRTI		PMPA	
NNRTI	DABO	UC781 TMC120 MIV 150	
Membrane-disruptive agents		SLS	
Unclassified	Drug-expressing lactobacilli	Praneem	
Combinations	NRTI/NNRTI NRTI/Polyanion NNRTI/Polyanion NRTI/NNRTI/Polyanion AFE combinations		

Another potential pathway to interrupt HIV transmission involves targeting cellular co-receptors such as CD4 and CCR5 that are required for HIV attachment and fusion. Vaginal application of high doses of a CCR5 receptor ligand, PSC-RANTES, protected rhesus macaques against SHIV vaginal challenge.[16] Vaginal administration of gel-formulated CMPD 167, a CCR5-specific small molecule, resulted in complete protection of SHIV infection in only 2 of 11 animals. However, early viral loads in the remaining animals were statistically lower than in controls.[17] More recent studies have resulted in considerably higher numbers of protected animals with CCR5 blocking compounds both alone and in combination.[18]

Reverse Transcriptase Inhibitors (RTIs)

The concept of applying HIV therapeutic strategies to vaginal microbicide development was first described in 1996.[19] Since that time, several RTIs have been developed preclinically and have entered safety studies in women. The first such product was vaginal tenofovir gel, a nucleotide RTI, which was shown to be safe and well tolerated in both HIV-uninfected and infected women.[20] More recently, non-nucleoside RTIs have been developed preclinically as microbicides and are currently being tested for safety in human trials.[21,22]

Dendritic Cell Uptake Inhibitors

Since vaginal mucosal dendritic cells may play an important role in the dissemination of HIV to T cells, drugs that block the dendritic cell receptor for HIV (DC-SIGN) will be important in prevention of sexual transmission.[23] Although DC-SIGN may not be involved in the local spread of HIV within cervical tissue, it facilitates the uptake of virus by migratory cells. Current approaches to the inhibition of dendritic cell uptake of HIV include monoclonal antibodies to DC-SIGN, soluble DC-SIGN and mannin.[24] The polyanions also appear to have some activity against DC-SIGN.

Microbicide Product Development

In Vitro Studies

The drug development pathway for microbicides follows a well-defined pathway to determine safety and efficacy.[25,26] Products should initially be shown to have good activity against circulating strains of HIV and low *in vitro* cytotoxicity. This is particularly important to ensure that the vaginal and cervical surfaces are not disrupted even if the virus is. Studies progress from the simplest rapid assays in cell lines with laboratory adapted HIV and progress to tests for safety and efficacy using clinically relevant strains in explanted tissue models. It is important that these products do not disturb normal vaginal defenses such as an intact vaginal epithelium or hydrogen-peroxide producing lactobacilli that maintain a protective low pH environment intravaginally. In addition, microbicides should not cause significant inflammation because inflammatory chemicals, cytokines, recruit additional immune target cells into the area and may enhance HIV replication.[27]

The selection algorithm for lead candidates commonly involves an initial determination of the compound's mechanism of action using rapid virus infectivity assays based on *in vitro* cell lines. Its selectivity index (ratio of activity to toxicity) is also calculated. Given the risks of toxicity induced enhancement of HIV transmission, selectivity indices of 100 or higher are generally preferred. The product's activity is then further analyzed under physiological conditions that mimic the circumstances under which HIV is transmitted in humans. These conditions include testing for activity in the presence of semen, cervical mucous, and blood, and over a range of pH values.

Additional assays are subsequently performed with different HIV clades and primary isolates using primary cell cultures of peripheral blood mononuclear cells, macrophages, and dendritic cells, both alone and in co-culture with T cells. A subsequent step in the algorithm involves blocking HIV infection in cervical explants. Studies have shown that cervical explants contain the cell populations below the genital epithelial surface that are either directly infected by HIV or transmit HIV to susceptible cells.[28] Some unique considerations for microbicides include their impact on natural vaginal defense mechanisms such as the presence of hydrogen-peroxide producing lactobacilli.[29] Formulated products are also tested for their effect on vaginal pH as well as condom compatibility.

Other important factors in selection of lead candidates, particularly those intended for wide access in resource-poor settings, include cost of the active pharmaceutical ingredient, chemical/thermal stability, intellectual property, ease of manufacture, and ease of formulation. Regulatory requirements are also taken into consideration.

Animal Models

While *in vitro* toxicity and efficacy are important factors in determining the viability of a candidate microbicide, preclinical *in vivo* animal studies may provide data that is more relevant to the human experience. However, these models cannot be validated until a microbicide has been shown to be safe and efficacious in women. Until that time, several different animal models of safety and efficacy are performed. The 10-day rabbit vaginal irritation model is traditionally used to determine preclinical safety prior to the first phase I trial in women. If the candidate agent is absorbed, systemic toxicology studies in rats and dogs are generally conducted. For longer term vaginal exposure in women, 6- and 9-month vaginal studies are performed in rats and rabbits.[26]

For biological plausibility of efficacy, murine models of herpes simplex virus transmission can be employed for products with non-specific viral activty.[31] Immunocompromised mice injected with human lymphocytes are also used for microbicide-induced inhibition of HIV transmission.[32] While used infrequently for microbicide development, infection of cats via feline immunodeficiency virus infected cells has been shown to be inhibited by a N-9 containing gel.[33]

The most commonly used model for microbicide efficacy involves vaginal exposure of macaques to SIV/SHIV. In general, macaques more closely resemble humans than do rodent species, particularly in vaginal ecology and virus transmission. Two models of vaginal transmission are currently utilized in microbicide studies. The first is based on a single, high-dose intravaginal challenge within 15 min of microbicide application.[34] Animals are often pretreated with hormones to thin the vaginal epithelium and increase virus transmission. A second model that is thought to more closely approximate to HIV transmission in humans, involves multiple exposures to low doses of virus at weekly intervals.[35] Both of these models have been used to study protection from infection by a number of microbicide candidates.[36]

Microbicide Delivery Approaches

A critical step in microbicide development is the design of the delivery vehicle for the drug – its formulation. It can be a gel, lotion, film or solid such as a foaming tablet. It may also be a vaginal ring or other device designed to deliver the drug over an extended period of time. Formulation will help determine a drug's efficacy and, as importantly, its acceptability to the user. Depending upon the mechanism of action of the microbicide, specific formulations can keep the active ingredient in the vaginal lumen, on the epithelial surface, or within the tissue. Formulations can also be designed to fit with a desired application schedule. For example, some gels or creams can deliver a drug over a 24-h period.

In a separate but complementary approach, antiretrovirals can be loaded into a long-term delivery device such as a vaginal ring, designed to stay in place for 30 days or more. For certain types of drugs, this approach allows for prolonged, persistent drug delivery while minimizing many compliance issues.

Formulations can also be designed to have anti-inflammatory properties, be lubricating or drying, act as spermicides, and possibly have activity against other sexually transmitted infections.[37] Selection of the appropriate formulation to maximize the activity of each active is also made with cost, stability, and manufacturing ease in mind. And, as important, how the product looks, feels, smells, tastes are all critical since a highly effective microbicide that no one likes to use will not prevent infection.

Clinical Development

As is generally the case in traditional therapeutic drug development, vaginal microbicides are tested in successive phases for safety and efficacy. The initial safety studies are carried out in small numbers of healthy women at low risk of HIV or STD infection. The endpoints for these studies are local vaginal toxicity (as measured by colposcopic evidence of damage to the vaginal and cervical epithelium including ulceration, other lesions, erythema, and edema), systemic safety, and tolerability. In traditional drug development, Phase II trials are expanded safety and preliminary efficacy studies which often employ surrogate endpoints that help determine 'proof of concept.' However, because microbicides are designed to prevent rather than treat HIV infection and are tested in healthy women, there are no surrogate markers for predicting acquisition of HIV infection. Whereas a Phase II microbicide trial would generate expanded safety data, it would produce limited or no insights with respect to the plausibility of product effectiveness.[38] As a result, the traditional Phase I, II, and III nomenclature does not apply. For microbicides, the successive phases end up being early safety, expanded safety, and efficacy, with the latter being designed as either proof of concept or pivotal trials.

The conduct of one or two pivotal efficacy trials to evaluate an investigational microbicide requires substantial human and financial resources. The statistical power of the trials is driven by the number of new HIV infections that occur among women who were HIV-negative at the start of the trial; proof of concept trials accrue 70–100 new HIV infections and pivotal efficacy trials accrue 200–400 new HIV infections during the course of the trial. The efficacy of the microbicide determines the ratio of HIV cases in randomized treatment arms. The incidence of HIV infection in the study population determines the sample size that needs to be enrolled to reach the number of new HIV infections in a period of time. While the prevalence of HIV infection in a population can be relatively easily determined from cross-sectional surveys or sentinel surveillance at ante-natal clinics, the incidence of HIV infection is more difficult to determine and is likely to change rapidly. The clinical evaluation of microbicide efficacy is therefore constrained by the large, resource-intensive trials that require several thousand study participants, yet are essential to demonstrating efficacy to the standards required by drug regulatory agencies.

A key ethical principal of the conduct of HIV prevention efficacy trials is that participants receive appropriate risk-reduction counseling, condoms, and treatment for sexually-transmitted infections. Although participants are counseled that the efficacy of the preventative is not known and that half of the participants receive a placebo, there is a concern that efficacy will be assumed and risk behavior will increase during the trials. However, lower or equal risks of HIV infection among study participants enrolled in microbicide and vaccine efficacy trials have been found compared with the risk of HIV infection prior to enrollment in the study.[39] This is likely due to the higher level of medical care, counseling and provision of condoms that participants receive.

Regulatory Issues

Since microbicides represent a new indication without proven efficacy to date, regulatory authorities in both developed and developing countries lack experience in microbicide approval. With few exceptions, the regulatory agencies in developing countries lack the resources necessary to conduct multifaceted reviews of applications for licensure. These agencies often rely on approval and use experience in the USA or Europe, where new products must demonstrate a favorable risk-benefit profile for US and European populations. Although requirements for safety and efficacy are essential in all countries, risk-benefit profiles of microbicides differ enormously between developed countries and regions where HIV infection is higher by two orders of magnitude.

The US Food and Drug Administration (FDA) has raised concerns that use of microbicides could decrease condom use, resulting in a net increase in HIV infection rates. To address this issue, the FDA would like to see data from an efficacy trial that is designed with a no-gel arm in addition to the standard two-arm active versus placebo trial. Such a three-arm study for a single microbicide would require many more participants, clinical sites, and resources. More importantly, the addition of a no-gel arm would violate the principle that randomized, controlled, double-blinded trials are the standard for determining efficacy. The third arm was also recommended to address concerns that placebo gels may either reduce or enhance HIV infection. However, since this arm is clearly unblinded, behavioral differences in risk behavior in the comparator arm cannot be excluded. The placebo gel issue could be addressed more easily by *in vitro* or preclinical studies than in efficacy trials.[40]

Conclusion

The first generation of microbicides has now entered large clinical trials to determine efficacy (Table 52.2). These compounds work by either binding to the virus or its target cells (entry inhibitors) or by disrupting the viral envelope (membrane disruptive agents), the virus' outermost layer. Whereas first generation microbicides currently in large-scale efficacy trials are relatively non-specific in their mechanism of action, newer products are being developed that target specific molecules on HIV or the cells they infect (Table 52.3). The products currently being

Table 52.3 HIV microbicides in clinical safety trials

Candidate microbicide	Mechanism of action
Dapivirine	NNRTI
SPL7013	Entry inhibitor
SLS	Membrane disruptive agent
Tenofovir/PMPA	NRTI
Thiocarboxanilide	NNRTI

tested are also single agents. Future product development efforts are focusing on antiretroviral drugs that specifically target steps in mucosal HIV infection. These efforts also seek to combine more than one active ingredient in the same formulation, analogous to the therapeutic HIV drug 'cocktails', since HIV therapy has proven over and over again that single agent approaches are not effective over the long term in controlling HIV replication. There is good reason to believe the same will hold true for microbicides. The plan is to disable the virus before it reaches any vulnerable tissue but, failing complete success, combination microbicides will also deliver powerful antiretrovirals to the vaginal cells allowing them to ward off any virus that does invade.

References

1. Joint United Nations Programme on HIV/AIDS (UNAIDS). 2004 Report on the Global AIDS Epidemic, Executive Summary, June 2004, and Women and AIDS Fact Sheet. Geneva: UNAIDS; 2004: NAIDS Epidemic Update.
2. Shattock R, Moore J. Inhibiting sexual transmission of HIV infection. Nat Rev Microbiol 2003; 1:25–34.
3. Hu J, Gardner MB, Miller CJ. Simian immunodeficiency virus rapidly penetrates the cervicovaginal mucosa after intravaginal inoculation and infects intraepithelial dendritic cells. J Virol 2000; 74:6087–6095.
4. Geijtenbeek TB, van Kooyk Y. DC-SIGN: a novel HIV receptor on DCs that mediates HIV-1 transmission. Curr Top Microbiol Immunol 2003; 276:31–54.
5. Hillier SL, Moench T, Shattock R, et al. In vitro and in vivo: the story of Nonoxynol 9. J Acquir Immune Defic Syndr 2005; 39:1–8.
6. Roddy RE, Zekeng L, Ryan KA, et al. A controlled trial of nonoxynol 9 film to reduce male-to-female transmission of sexually transmitted diseases. N Engl J Med 1998; 339:504–510.
7. Roddy RE, Zekeng L, Ryan KA, et al. Effect of nonoxynol-9 gel on urogenital gonorrhea and chlamydial infection: a randomized controlled trial. JAMA 2002; 287:1117–1122.
8. Van Damme L, Ramjee G, Alary M, et al. COL-1492 Study Group. Effectiveness of COL-1492, a nonoxynol-9 vaginal gel, on HIV-1 transmission in female sex workers: a randomised controlled trial. Lancet 2002; 360:971–977.
9. Gagne N, Cormier H, Omar RF, et al. Protective effect of a thermoreversible gel against the toxicity of nonoxynol-9. Sex Transm Dis 1999; 26:177–183.
10. Krebs FC, Miller SR, Catalone BJ, et al. Comparative in vitro sensitivities of human immune cell lines, vaginal and

Table 52.2 HIV microbicides in clinical efficacy trials

Candidate microbicide	Mechanism of action
C31G	Membrane disruptive agent (surfactant)
Carbopol 974P	Vaginal defense enhancer
Carrageenan	Entry inhibitor
Cellulose sulfate	Entry inhibitor
Naphthalene sulfonate polymer	Entry inhibitor

cervical epithelial cell lines, and primary cells to candidate microbicides nonoxynol 9, C31G, and sodium dodecyl sulfate. Antimicrob Agents Chemother 2002; 46:2292–2298.

11. Moore JP, Doms RW. The entry of entry inhibitors: A fusion of science and medicine. Proc Natl Acad Sci USA 2003; 100:10598–10602.

12. Zeitlin L, Hoen TE, Achilles SL, et al. Tests of buffer gel for contraception and prevention of sexually transmitted diseases in animal models. Sex Trans Dis 2001; 28:417–423.

13. Jiang YH, Emau P, Cairns JS, et al. SPL7013 gel as a topical microbicide for prevention of vaginal transmission of SHIV89.6P in macaques. AIDS Res Hum Retroviruses 2005; 21:207–213.

14. Tsai CC, Emau P, Jiang Y, et al. Cyanovirin-N inhibits AIDS virus infections in vaginal transmission models. AIDS Res Hum Retroviruses 2004; 20:11–18.

15. Veazey RS, Shattock RJ, Pope M, et al. Prevention of virus transmission to macaque monkeys by a vaginally applied monoclonal antibody to HIV-1 gp120. Nat Med 2003; 9:343–346.

16. Lederman MM, Veazey RS, Offord R, et al. Prevention of vaginal SHIV transmission in rhesus macaques through inhibition of CCR5. Science 2004; 306:485–487.

17. Veazey RS, Klasse PJ, Ketas TJ, et al. Use of a small molecule CCR5 inhibitor in macaques to treat simian immunodeficiency virus infection or prevent simian-human immunodeficiency virus infection. J Exp Med 2003; 198:1551–1562.

18. Moore JP. Topical microbicides become topical. N Engl J Med 2005; 352:298–300.

19. Pauwels R, De Clercq E. Development of vaginal microbicides for the prevention of heterosexual transmission of HIV. J Acquir Immune Defic Syndr Hum Retrovirol 1996; 11:211–221.

20. Mayer KH, Maslankowski L, El-Sadr W, et al. Safety and tolerability of vaginal tenofovir gel (TFV) in HIV-uninfected and HIV-infected women (HPTN 050). Abstract No. ThOrB1373. XV International AIDS Conference; 2004.

21. Balzarini J, Naesens L, Verbeken E, et al. Preclinical studies on thiocarboxanilide UC-781 as a virucidal agent. AIDS 1998; 12:1129–1133.

22. Van Herrewege Y, Michiels J, Van Roey J, et al. In vitro evaluation of nonnucleoside reverse transcriptase inhibitors UC-781 and TMC120-R147681 as human immunodeficiency virus microbicides. Antimicrob Agents Chemother 2004; 48:337–339.

23. Geijtenbeek TB, Torensma R, van Vliet SJ, et al. Identification of DC-SIGN, a novel dendritic cell-specific ICAM-3 receptor that supports primary immune responses. Cell 2000; 100:575–585.

24. Hu Q, Frank I, Williams V, et al. Blockade of attachment and fusion receptors inhibits HIV-1 infection of human cervical tissue. J Exp Med 2004; 199:1065–1075.

25. Mauck C, Rosenberg Z, Van Damme L. Recommendations for the clinical development of topical microbicides: an update. AIDS 2001; 15:857–868.

26. International Working Group on Microbicides (IWGM). Recommendations for the nonclinical development of topical microbicides for prevention of HIV transmission: An update. J Acquir Immune Defic Syndr 2004; 36:541–552.

27. Fichorova RN, Bajpai M, Chandra N, et al. Interleukin (IL)-1, IL-6, and IL-8 predict mucosal toxicity of vaginal microbicidal contraceptives. Biol Reprod 2004; 71:761–769.

28. Greenhead P, Hayes P, Watts PS, et al. Parameters of human immunodeficiency virus infection of human cervical tissue and inhibition by vaginal virucides. J Virol 2000; 12:5577–5586.

29. Watts DH, Rabe L, Krohn MA, et al. The effects of three nonoxynol-9 preparations on vaginal flora and epithelium. J Infect Dis 1998; 180:426–437.

30. Zeitlin L, Whaley KJ, Hegarty TA, et al. Tests of vaginal microbicides in the mouse genital herpes model. Contraception 1997; 56:329–335.

31. Maguire RA, Bergman N, Phillips DM. Comparison of microbicides for efficacy in protecting mice against vaginal challenge with herpes simplex virus type 2, cytotoxicity, antibacterial properties, and sperm immobilization. Sex Transm Dis 2001; 28:259–265.

32. Di Fabio S, Roey J Van, Giannini G, et al. Inhibition of vaginal transmission of HIV-1 in Hu-SCID mice by the non-nucleoside reverse transcriptase inhibitor TMC120 in a gel formulation. AIDS 2003; 17:1597–1604.

33. Moench TR, Whaley KJ, Mandrell TD, et al. The cat/feline immunodeficiency virus model for transmucosal transmission of AIDS: nonoxynol-9 contraceptive jelly blocks transmission by an infected cell inoculum. AIDS 1993; 7:797–802.

34. Sodora DL, Gettie A, Miller CJ, et al. Vaginal transmission of SIV: assessing infectivity and hormonal influences in macaques inoculated with cell-free and cell-associated viral stocks. AIDS Res Hum Retroviruses 1998; 14:S119–S123.

35. Otten RA, Adams DR, Kim CN, et al. Multiple vaginal exposures to low doses of R5 simian-human immunodeficiency virus: strategy to study HIV preclinical interventions in nonhuman primates. J Infect Dis 2005; 191:164–173.

36. Weber J, Nunn A, O'Connor T, et al. 'Chemical condoms' for the prevention of HIV infection: evaluation of novel agents against SHIV(89.6PD) in vitro and in vivo. AIDS 2001; 15:1563–1568.

37. Garg S, Tambwekar KR, Vermani K, et al. Development pharmaceutics of microbicide formulations. Part II: formulation, evaluation, and challenges. AIDS Patient Care STDS 2003; 17:377–399.

38. Harrison PF, Rosenberg Z, Bowcut J. Topical microbicides for disease prevention: status and challenges. Clin Infect Dis 2003; 36:1290–1294.

39. Bartholow BN, Buchbinder S, Celum C, et al. for the VISION/VAX004 Study Team. HIV sexual risk behavior over 36 months of follow-up in the world's first HIV vaccine efficacy trial. J Acquir Immune Defic Syndr 2005; 39:90–101.

40. Coplan PM, Mitchnick M, Rosenberg ZF. Public health. Regulatory challenges in microbicide development. Science 2004; 304:1911–1912.

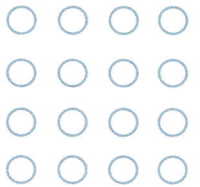

CHAPTER 53

Implications and Management of Malnutrition

Heather Southwell

Introduction

> If we could give every individual the right amount of nourishment and exercise, not too little and not too much, we would have found the safest way to health.
>
> Hippocrates c. 460–377 BC

Tens of millions around the world lack appropriate nourishment, with the largest number of malnourished individuals in third world countries located in Africa, Asia, and South America; the same regions that are most affected by human immunodeficiency virus (HIV).[1] Malnutrition may develop as a result of starvation, general undernutrition, one or more specific nutrient deficiencies, or nutrient imbalances. An unhealthy deficit or excess of any nutrient will impact how the body performs. Subsequently, body systems lacking or experiencing a significant imbalance in the essential building blocks or necessary substrates malfunction. Malnutrition in people living with HIV/AIDS (PLWHA) adds another dimension by worsening an otherwise weakened immune system. Dietary interventions can be planned to improve nutritional status, abate malnutrition, boost immune function and enhance response to therapies for many diseases.

The objectives of this chapter will be to understand malnutrition; to appreciate the relationship of nutrition and immune function; to provide nutrition information on treating malnutrition so immune function improves; and to present information on nutrition care for malnourished individuals.

Malnutrition

In order to comprehend malnutrition, it is important to understand how to determine a person's basic nutritional needs. The fundamental nutrition requirements of a human body include the energy necessary for essential tasks such as maintaining core body temperature and vital organ processes. This is measured as Resting Energy Expenditure (REE). Equations have been determined from studies based on healthy populations that estimate the REE. Once the REE is calculated, it is multiplied by a stress factor and an activity factor to determine energy requirements beyond basic needs such as movement and wound healing. A few of these equations include the Harris-Benedict[2] and Mifflin-St Jeor,[3] both of which use weight, height and age as predictors in sex-specific equations and Cunningham which uses fat free mass (FFM) as the predictor (Table 53.1).[4] Fat free mass is a more accurate basis of metabolic rate than weight, height and age but requires equipment that may not be available in many situations for its proper measurement. A simple estimate of energy needs when only weight is available multiplies weight in kg by a factor of 30 for weight maintenance, a factor of 35–50 to promote weight gain, and a factor of 25 to promote weight loss.

Malnutrition manifests itself in many different forms. Marasmus, or cachexia, results from inadequate energy intake, or starvation, over a long period of months or years. Regardless of an inadequate energy intake, the body still requires energy for basic needs. This basic energy requirement has

Table 53.1 Predictive equations for resting metabolic rate (RMR) in kcal/day

Harris and Benedict (1919)[2]	
Men	RMR = 66.47 + (13.75 × weight) + (5.0 × height) − (6.75 × age)
Women	RMR = 665.09 + (9.56 × weight) + (1.84 × height) − (4.67 × age)
Mifflin et al. (1990)[3]	
Men	RMR = (9.99 × weight) + (6.25 × height) − (4.92 × age) + 5
Women	RMR = (9.99 × weight) + (6.25 × height) − (4.92 × age) − 161
Cunningham (1991)[4]	
Men and women	RMR = 370 + (21.6 × FFM)

All equations use weight in kg, height in cm and age in years. FFM, fat free mass.

already been introduced as the REE. The nervous system, muscle, liver, red blood cells, bone marrow, phagocytes and fibroblasts all require glucose as their energy source. Under normal, well-fed situations, the diet provides this glucose or the body accesses the liver's short-term glycogen reserves. Once these limited reserves are depleted, the body begins breaking down skeletal muscle protein to use the amino acids as sources of glucose, also known as gluconeogenesis. The body also creates energy from the breakdown of adipose tissue into fatty acids. The fatty acids are metabolized resulting in ketones, which can be utilized as a partial substitute for the glucose. As the starvation process is prolonged, muscle protein is catabolized at a decreased rate and fat metabolism increases to continue to meet the body's energy needs. These modified body processes lead to weight loss, including wasting of lean body mass and fat stores. As a result, the proteins that would usually be earmarked for immune cell function are not available and immune function is reduced. Serum proteins often remain within normal ranges or are moderately reduced.

Kwashiorkor develops due to inadequate dietary protein intake. This type of malnutrition occurs more rapidly than marasmus, in a matter of weeks. Given sufficient energy intake, the lean body mass and fat stores are generally unaffected. Serum proteins are severely impacted, resulting in significant reduction in serum albumin, prealbumin and transferrin. These patients often exhibit edema and anemia. Immune function is depressed and wound healing is prolonged.

Diagnosis of marasmic kwashiorkor occurs when there is a deficit in both protein and energy intake. This protein energy malnutrition (PEM) results in an extreme loss of body weight, body fat, and lean body mass. Nutrient restriction severely limits protein synthesis and cell division, which severely depresses serum proteins and immune function.[5] As a result of the depressed immune system, the mortality rate increases with increased infections and poor wound healing.

Malnutrition in PLWHA can also manifest itself as wasting syndrome. The US Centers for Disease Control and Prevention (CDC) defines AIDS wasting syndrome as 'the involuntary loss of 10% of baseline body weight plus either chronic diarrhea (two loose stools per day for more than 30 days) or chronic weakness and documented fever (for 30 days or more, intermittent or constant) in the absence of a concurrent illness or condition other than HIV infection that would explain the findings'.[6] The CDC developed this definition initially to define AIDS in the absence of an opportunistic infection or malignancy prior to the use of CD4 count <200. This definition has now been adopted for other research and clinical purposes.

Wasting characterized the early years of the HIV/AIDS epidemic, prior to widespread use of combination antiretroviral therapy (ART). It is still prevalent in areas where ART is not readily available, such as the developing countries most impacted by malnutrition. In Africa, HIV/AIDS is often referred to as the 'slim' disease for this reason. This wasting is distinguished by loss of lean body mass and is unrelated to fat wasting, also known as lipoatrophy, lipodystrophy or fat redistribution syndrome.

Nutritional Requirements for HIV/AIDS

The existing equations for estimating energy expenditure are typically not appropriate for use in the HIV-positive population. PLWHA experience higher REE than HIV-negative controls.[7-9] The use of highly active antiretroviral therapy (HAART)[8,9] and higher HIV viral loads[9] may also increase their REE. Therefore, an increased energy requirement to maintain body weight and physical activity levels is recommended in asymptomatic HIV-infected adults and to achieve normal growth in asymptomatic HIV-infected children. Asymptomatic adults and children should increase their energy intakes by 10% above the estimated energy requirements of otherwise healthy individuals. For symptomatic HIV-infected adults and those struggling with opportunistic infections, energy requirements increase by 20–30% to maintain body weight. Children experiencing weight loss may need to increase their energy intakes by 50–100% over the normal intake of healthy uninfected children.[10]

Beyond the increased need for energy intake in PLWHA, other macronutrients may be necessary in higher amounts based on the presence of opportunistic infections and nutritional status. The body requires proteins and their building blocks, amino acids, to make and maintain cells, create hormones and enzymes, maintain muscles and organs and as part of the immune response. During infections, amino acids are diverted from normal functions for synthesis of immunoglobulins, lymphokines, C-reactive proteins, and production of other necessary proteins.[11] Apart from periods of infection, protein intake should at least meet the normal requirements of the general population of 10–35% of total energy intake, or 0.8 g protein per kg body weight.[12] During times of infection and PEM, 1.2–1.5 g protein per kg body weight may be required.

Fat needs of the general healthy population are 30–35% of total energy needs.[12] Individual alterations in protein and fat intake are recommended based on other symptoms experienced which will be covered later in this chapter.

Malnutrition and the Immune System

Infections can impair nutritional status and conversely, a malnourished state allows infections to invade, leading to a vicious cycle of continued malnutrition and infection. Malnutrition both impacts and is impacted by infections, leading to changes in metabolism and food intake. Depressed appetite, or anorexia, is a common side-effect of infections.[13] Even if the individual is able to consume sufficient energy and nutrients from their food intake, infections can change the gastrointestinal tract integrity leading to impaired nutrient and drug absorption. This malabsorption prevents the body from efficiently using the available nutrients in the food consumed. Without adequate nutrients absorbed or consumed, the body's supplies of energy, protein, vitamins and minerals are depleted. The metabolic

rate may vary as the body uses fat and lean body mass as energy sources. Infections and associated fevers also increase the REE.

Along with this synergism, malnutrition and infection influence one another, depending on the infection. The clinical courses of some infections (i.e. pneumonia, diarrhea, and tuberculosis) are without doubt adversely affected by undernutrition. Nutritional status hardly impacts other diseases, for instance viral encephalitis or tetanus. Nutrition moderately influences some viral infections such as HIV and influenza virus.[14,15] Studies by the Institute of Nutrition of Central America and Panama (INCAP) in the 1950s demonstrated that with any infection, nutritional status declined in some manner. The specific defense mechanisms influenced by nutritional status include humoral antibody production, phagocyte activity, cell-mediated immunity, complement formation, and T-lymphocyte formation.[16]

Decreased oral intake is another reason for altered metabolism and malnutrition. Reduced food consumption occurs as a result of a decreased desire for food or an inadequate food supply. The desire for food declines with anorexia, which can be triggered by infections, diarrhea, or medications. The effect of medication on appetite can be a direct side-effect of the medication itself, be due to consuming a large pill burden, or result from a medication schedule that may require avoiding food around the time of taking the pills. Even if the individual has an appetite, oral infections such as *Candida*, can cause oral pain and decrease food intake. Lastly, fatigue, as a result of the disease state, impedes food preparation and appetite with a consequent diminished oral intake.

Many times, despite a good appetite, other elements cause an unintentional decline in nutrient consumption. Food insecurity results from poverty, famine or war. Power imbalances by gender and household hierarchies impact how food is allocated and distributed. HIV/AIDS further aggravates this food insecurity by reducing the labor capacity, agricultural production and thus income. Illness reduces the entire household's labor as healthy members shift their attentions and earnings to assisting sick members of the family.[17]

The severity and impact of malnutrition depends on the rate of cell proliferation, protein synthesis and the availability of nutrients for various metabolic pathways. During times of stress and infection, when substrates are necessary to mount an immune response, malnutrition puts an extra burden on the body by not providing all the necessary building blocks. Protein energy malnutrition leads to limited protein synthesis and cell division, which along with negatively affecting other body systems, eventually weakens the immune system's ability to mount a defense.[5]

Micronutrients and the Immune System

Although clinical malnutrition rarely occurs with a deficit of just one nutrient, there are a few micronutrients that impact the immune system more than others. Important micronutrients for the immune system, and specifically HIV, are zinc, iron, selenium, vitamin A, vitamin C, vitamin E and the B vitamins (Table 53.2). Nutrition deficiencies can negatively impact the immune system by decreasing the host's line of defense through a variety of means.

These include decreased antibody production, decreased phagocyte activity, altered tissue and mucosal integrity, poor wound healing and collagen formation, and changes in endocrine activity.[14]

Trace Minerals

Zinc is often the first trace mineral referred to when covering nutrition and immunity. Zinc is essential during times of growth[18] and immune function.[19,20] Zinc is required in the activity of more than 100 enzymes involved in carbohydrate and fat metabolism, protein degradation and synthesis, nucleic acid synthesis and heme synthesis.[21] Zinc deficiency has been shown to decrease cell-mediated immunity and is required for CD4 regeneration.[19,20] Often

Table 53.2 The role and source of selected micronutrients

Micronutrient	Role	Food Source
Minerals		
Iron	Oxygen transport; cell growth and differentiation; immune function	Heme: red meats, fish, poultry. Non-heme: legumes, dried fruit, fortified cereals, grains
Selenium	Antioxidant; regulation of thyroid hormones	Seafood, liver, meat, nuts, whole grains, wheat germ, dairy, eggs
Zinc	Component in enzymes and proteins; carbohydrate and fat metabolism; immune function; sense of taste; wound healing; DNA synthesis; growth and development during pregnancy, childhood and adolescence	Oysters, red meat, poultry, beans, nuts, whole grains, fortified cereals
Vitamins		
Vitamin A (beta-carotene)	Vision; reproduction; embryonic development and growth; maintenance of skin, gastrointestinal, and pulmonary linings	Liver, dairy products, egg yolks, yams, pumpkin, palm oil, leafy green, yellow, and orange fruits, vegetables
Vitamin B_1 (thiamin)	Energy metabolism; supports appetite and nervous system function	Whole grains, cereals, chicken, fish, meat, pork
Vitamin B_2 (riboflavin)	Energy metabolism; supports normal vision and skin integrity	Dairy, bread, organ meats, whole grains, leafy green vegetables
Vitamin B_3 (niacin)	Energy metabolism; supports skin integrity; nervous and digestive systems	Dairy, eggs, meat, poultry, nuts, whole grains
Vitamin B_6 (pyridoxine)	Coenzyme in amino-acid metabolism; nucleic acid and protein synthesis	Legumes, nuts, eggs, meats, fish, whole grains, fortified cereal
Vitamin B_{12} (cobalamin)	Coenzyme in nucleic acid metabolism; nerve cell maintenance	Red meat, poultry, fish, dairy
Vitamin C (ascorbic acid)	Antioxidant; immune function; wound healing; co-factor in collagen formation; increases non-heme iron absorption	Citrus, tomatoes, berries, kiwi, mango, potatoes, winter squashes
Vitamin E	Antioxidant; protects cell structures	Vegetable oils, nuts, leafy green vegetables, fortified cereals, fish
Folate	Coenzyme in nucleic and amino-acid metabolism; immune function	Legumes, citrus fruit, whole wheat, leafy green vegetables, poultry, pork, shellfish

children in developing nations experience inadequate nutrient intake as well as infections that deplete any nutritional stores they may have been able to generate during the breast-feeding period. Zinc supplementation in the face of inadequate intake and deficiency can significantly improve growth,[18] increase resistance to infections, and reduce the duration and severity of persistent diarrhea.[22-25] Indicators of serum concentrations of some micronutrients, including zinc, acutely decrease during infection because of the acute-phase response (APR).[26] Therefore, it is important to consider the extent of APR activation when assessing indicators of zinc status and the necessity for supplementation.

The National Academies' Institute of Medicine determined the Dietary Reference Intake (DRI) of zinc for healthy individuals to be 11 mg/day for adult men, 8 mg/day for adult women, 11–12 mg/day for pregnant and lactating adult women, and 3–5 mg/day for children. Vegetarians may need up to 50% more dietary zinc given the presence of phytates in most vegetable sources which hinder zinc absorption.[27] Phytates will be discussed later in the chapter. Excess zinc supplementation is harmful and potentially toxic, above the tolerable upper intake levels determined by the Institute of Medicine. The upper level for adults is 40 mg/day, 34 mg for 14–18 year olds, 23 mg for children aged 9–13 years, 12 mg for children aged 4–8 years and 4–7 mg for infants under the age of 3 years.[27] Red meat, poultry, and oysters are excellent sources of dietary zinc. Plant sources are beans, nuts, whole grains, and fortified cereals.

Iron is an integral component of various aspects in the human body. This mineral is an essential part of many proteins and enzymes; regulates T-lymphocyte function; is involved in oxygen transport; and is crucial for cell growth and differentiation. Iron is the most prevalent micronutrient deficiency affecting the world. The United Nations Children's Fund (UNICEF) estimates 45% of children under the age of 5 years and 40% of women of childbearing age are iron deficient.[28] Iron deficiency is associated with impairments of cell-mediated immunity and innate immunity.[29] These immune impairments include a decline in lymphocyte proliferation, maturation and differentiation, decreased cytokine production, and decreased macrophage and neutrophil function.[21] Beyond the effect iron has on the immune system, its deficiency causes anemia that leads to fatigue and reduced productivity. People experiencing this are less likely to be able to work, prepare meals, or perform family responsibilities. The negative effects

on children are especially significant as growth and brain development are retarded leading to a lifetime of problems.[21] Zidovudine (AZT), an antiretroviral medication, and chronic infection can both lead to anemia. Iron deficiency compounds this anemia that HIV patients may be experiencing.[30]

Food sources of iron include both animal and plant forms. In animals, iron is derived from hemoglobin in red blood cells of red meats, fish and poultry. Plant sources provide non-heme iron, which is structurally different from heme iron with a lower bioavailability.[27] Iron-rich plant foods include legumes, broccoli, dried fruit, and fortified cereals and grains. The bioavailability of non-heme iron will improve with the consumption of vitamin C rich foods in the same meal as iron-rich plant foods as well as food processing practices which will be discussed later in the chapter. The DRI for iron is 18 mg/day for women of childbearing age (19–50 years), 27 mg/day for pregnancy and 9 mg/day for lactation, 8 mg/day for adult men, 7 mg/day for toddlers (1–3 years), and 10 mg/day for children aged 4–8 years.[27]

The role of selenium in the body is primarily as a component in selenoproteins, which are involved in defending against oxidative stress, regulating thyroid hormone metabolism and the regulation of redox reactions of vitamin C. The DRI for selenium is 15–20 µg/day for infants, 20 µg for toddlers (1–3 years old), 30 µg for children 4–8 years, 40 µg for children ages 9–13, 55 µg for men and women 14–70 years. Pregnancy increases requirements to 60 µg and lactation increases them further to 70 µg/day. Good dietary sources include seafood, liver, meat, nuts, whole grains, wheat germ, dairy and eggs. Selenium intake varies geographically depending on the selenium content of the soil in which plant products are grown.[31]

Water-soluble Vitamins

The water-soluble vitamin folate is required for DNA and RNA synthesis in cells. Deficiency of folate leads to reduced host resistance and impaired lymphocytic functions. Examples include decreased T-lymphocytes and decreased CD8 cells proliferation in response to activation.[32,33] Other signs and symptoms of folate deficiency include slow growth in children, megaloblastic anemia, behavioral disorders, loss of appetite, sore tongue, weight loss, and digestive disorders such as diarrhea.[34] Dietary sources of folate include beans, legumes, citrus fruits, whole wheat, leafy green vegetables, poultry, pork, liver, and shellfish. The recommended folate intake for individuals, based on the US National Academies' Institute of Medicine DRI, is 400 µg/day for adult men and women. Pregnant and lactating women are encouraged to take 600 µg and 500 µg/day, respectively.[34] Food consumption often does not meet the increased requirements thus supplementation is encouraged in pregnancy and lactation.

Water-soluble vitamin C, or ascorbic acid, aids in recovery from infections and wound healing. It also works as an antioxidant, protecting against the cellular damage caused by free radicals. Collagen is reliant on vitamin C to act as a cofactor in its formation. Collagen is an essential protein in connective tissue, bones and teeth. Inadequate ascorbic acid leads to impaired wound healing, as insufficient collagen is available to bind the connective tissues together. Inadequate collagen causes capillary breakdown, which leads to symptoms of scurvy. Deficiency symptoms include internal hemorrhage, bruising, raised red spots around hair follicles, and bleeding gums. The DRI for vitamin C is 75 mg/day for adult women, 85 mg and 120 mg/day for pregnant and lactating adult women, respectively, 90 mg/day for adult men, 15 mg/day for toddlers and 25 mg/day for children aged 4–8 years.[31]

Dietary sources are essential to provide ascorbic acid for the function of body cells but also work to improve the bioavailability of other nutrients such as non-heme iron. Vitamin C rich foods include citrus foods, tomatoes, berries, melons, kiwi, mango, potatoes, winter squashes, cranberries, and pineapple.

Vitamin B_6 is important to the maintenance of the immune system. This nutrient is required for normal nucleic acid and protein synthesis. A deficiency of vitamin B_6 depresses both cellular-mediated immune function and humoral responses to antigens. A vitamin B_6 deficiency produces dermatitis and oral lesions, which decreases tissue integrity thus allowing the entrance of secondary infections.[33] Good food sources of vitamin B_6 include beans, nuts, legumes, eggs, meats, fish, whole grains and fortified bread, and cereals. The DRI for vitamin B_6 is 1.3 mg for adult women and men (aged <50 years), 1.7 mg for older men (aged >51 years), 1.5 mg for older women (aged > 51 years), 1.9 mg and 2.0 mg for pregnant and lactating women.[34]

Fat-soluble Vitamins

Fat-soluble vitamin A, or its precursor beta-carotene, is integral to vision and for maintaining the integrity of skin as well as gastrointestinal and pulmonary linings. Adequate vitamin A helps to ensure these mucosal tissues are healthy and able to prevent infectious agent entry. Vitamin A deficiency increases host susceptibility to infections via humoral and cell-mediated immune mechanisms.[33] DRI for vitamin A (retinol) is 4000 IU/day for adult women, 5000 IU for adult men, 2000 IU for toddlers (1–3 years), 2500 IU for children aged 4–6 years and 4000 IU for teenagers.[27] Dietary sources of vitamin A include eggs, meat, dairy, liver, and fish oils. The precursor form, beta-carotene, is found in orange and green fruits, and vegetables such as carrots, pumpkin, sweet potatoes, winter squashes, cantaloupe, apricots, broccoli, and spinach.

Toxic intakes of vitamin A are easily achieved via supplementation. Upper limits of tolerance for vitamin A have been set at 10 000 IU/day for adults, 2000 IU for toddlers ages 1–3 years, 3000 IU for children aged 4–8 years, 5665 IU for children aged 9–13 years, and 9335 IU for teenagers aged 14–18 years. Hypervitaminosis A can lead to toxic symptoms such as birth defects, liver abnormalities and reduced bone mineral density that may result in osteoporosis.[27]

Studies in African pregnant women provided them with either a multivitamin alone or with a vitamin A supplement versus a placebo. Women who received vitamin A, either paired with a multivitamin or vitamin A alone, resulted in an increased risk of vertical transmission. Adding vitamin A to the multivitamin regimen also reduced the benefit of adding a multivitamin to the regimen of Africans.[35,36] Both low and high levels of vitamin A intake are potentially harmful, so supplements should be suggested with caution in this population unless a clinical deficiency is apparent.[37]

Good Nutritional Practices

A large number of people living in the developing world subsist on a monotonous diet of starchy staples without availability or financial resources to expand their diet to include all essential nutrients. Good nutrition involves eating a variety of foods given no one food provides all essential nutrients. Staples, or grains, should make up the largest part of every meal. They offer a relatively concentrated source of energy, some protein, and many important immune-boosting micronutrients (i.e. selenium, zinc, iron, vitamins B_6, and E). Whole grains provide a filling, inexpensive, nutritious basis of a meal.

Protein-rich foods provide amino acids, vitamins and minerals essential for maintaining lean body mass and the immune system. Depending on the cultural beliefs (i.e. religious restrictions) or economic status, animal-based proteins, and dairy products should be included as often as possible, whereas, plant-based protein (i.e. legumes, soy products, nuts, and seeds) should be consumed daily.

Fruits and vegetables are important parts of the daily diet. Table 53.2 lists important nutrients that impact the immune system and provide essential vitamins and minerals to all systems of the body. Dark green, yellow, orange, and red fruits and vegetables are especially good sources of vitamins A, C and folate.

Concentrated sources of energy such as fats and oils as well as sugars and sweet foods offer an easy means of increasing energy intake without the need to consume large quantities of foods. By adding fats or oils to other foods such as grains and vegetables or utilizing the natural fats in foods while cooking, extra energy will be supplied in the foods consumed. This provides the body with more energy in a smaller portion of food. Concentrated sources of energy are especially important during times of depressed appetite and intake when the body is not able to consume large quantities. On the other hand, concentrating energy in a food without many other nutrients present should be avoided when an individual is able to consume sufficient food.

Clean and safe water and fluids are the last aspect of a healthy diet. The human body is made largely of water. To maintain appropriate hydration status, a minimum of 64 fluid ounces (1.5 L) should be consumed each day. During times of high temperatures, sweating, diarrhea, and vomiting extra fluids are required to make up for fluid losses. Water, juices, soups, and sauces are all good sources of fluids. Caffeinated beverages, such as coffee, tea, and colas, should be limited during times of dehydration as they increase fluid excretion and further exacerbate the dehydrated state.

Dietary Treatment of Side-effects that Lead to Malnutrition

During illness, many traditional treatments exclude solid foods and rely on liquid nutrition such as gruels and other low energy, low protein liquids. These meal replacements can exacerbate the malnutrition people experience from infections by cutting back on available energy, protein, and micronutrients. It is important to focus on maximizing both energy and protein while treating malnutrition rather than just focusing on high-energy intake.[38]

Vitamin and/or mineral supplementation has been studied to determine any improvement in health results from this relatively inexpensive treatment. African studies of HIV-positive individuals found a multivitamin led to a decrease in oral and gastrointestinal complications associated with HIV.[35] These studies also demonstrated a positive relationship between multivitamin supplementation and improved HIV status, prolonged progression to AIDS and delay initiation of antiretroviral therapy (ART).[35,39]

Another means of improving nutrient intake besides supplementation is to improve the bioavailability of nutrients from food itself. The absorption of divalent cations, including zinc, iron and calcium will be decreased in the presence of phytates. This is due to negatively charged phytates chelating divalent cations, thus making them unavailable for the body to absorb and use. Phytic acid or phytates are present in many vitamin-rich plant foods that make the basis of diets for many people, such as cereals and unfermented soy products. Many cultures do not have wide access to animal protein or religious doctrines prohibit certain animal proteins to be included in the diet. To combat this, low bioavailability food-based interventions may be appropriate.

Interventions that increase nutrient bioavailability include education on dietary diversification and food processing modifications. Dietary interventions may include increasing production and consumption of nutrient-dense foods, especially animal proteins. Animal protein offers a good source of vitamin B_{12}, protein, zinc, and heme-iron. Heme-iron is more bioavailable than non-heme iron that is found in plants. Other dietary diversification education should focus on eating a variety of foods from all the food groups. As availability dictates, selecting from all of the food groups including grains, fruits, vegetables, dairy, protein-rich foods, and fats provides a variety of essential nutrients (Table 53.2).

Food processing interventions include incorporating absorption enhancers of the low bioavailable nutrients or improving food processing or cooking procedures. Absorption enhancers include adding ascorbic acid or vitamin C rich foods (Table 53.2) to enhance the non-heme iron found in plant foods. Food processing interventions to improve zinc's absorption includes germinating, fermenting or soaking the maize and/or legumes to lower the phytates thus less zinc is chelated and unavailable. The ultimate goal to improve nutritional status is to improve availability and access to food, the nutrient balance of the overall diet and improve utilization of food.

Studies[40] in African villages incorporated principles of diet education and food processing changes. Intervention villages received education on including fish and a wider variety of foods as well as how to process their highly maize-based diet to improve nutrient bioavailability. Their diets resulted in improved intake of vitamin B_{12}, calcium, heme-iron and vitamin A compared with control villages. Food preparation that included soaking the maize before cooking with it decreased the phytate content and thus resulted in significantly more bioavailable zinc. In the long term, the intervention group displayed improved lean body mass and decreased incidence of infections.

Diarrhea and Malabsorption

Diarrhea is a common occurrence worldwide. The World Health Organization (WHO) estimates 3.2% of worldwide deaths are caused by diarrheal disease.[1] HIV/AIDS has been known in Africa as 'slim disease' or a disease of wasting, often due to the fact that PLWHA often experience diarrhea. As part of the vicious cycle of malnutrition (Fig. 53.1), diarrhea leads to a decreased appetite and the associated malabsorption disallows the body to absorb necessary nutrients; leading to weight loss and further problems.

Foods to focus on consuming during times of diarrhea include refined starches and soluble fiber foods (i.e. white rice, maize meals, white bread, noodles, potatoes). Other easily digested foods should be included, such as soft fruits and cooked vegetables (i.e. bananas, applesauce, mangoes, papaya, watermelon, pumpkins, carrots). Boiled or steamed soft proteins such as eggs, skinless chicken and fish provide the important amino acids essential to continue nourishing the body during diarrheal episodes. Foods should be consumed warm rather than very hot or very cold to improve digestion. Small, frequent snacking every 2–3 hours is less likely to worsen diarrhea than large bulky meals. As a result of the dehydrated state caused by diarrhea, adequate fluid intake is essential. Individuals should drink sufficient fluids such as boiled or bottled water, diluted fruit juices, broth-based soups, and herbal teas.

Avoid foods that may worsen diarrhea such as whole grains, insoluble fiber, and gas producing foods (Table 53.3). Lactose intolerance may exacerbate the malabsorption so avoiding dairy products may improve symptoms in patients with suspected or known lactose intolerance. Spicy and fatty foods may also worsen symptoms. Given the fluid loss that occurs during diarrhea foods that naturally cause dehydration such as foods and drinks containing caffeine (i.e. coffee, tea, chocolate, and colas) and alcohol should be avoided. Avoid concentrated beverages such as strong fruit juices, nutrition supplements, and sodas as they exacerbate both diarrhea and fluid loss.

Combating Weight Loss

Making the most of each bite of food can be achieved by choosing concentrated sources of energy. These sources include staple grains and certain starchy fruits and vegetables such as cereals, rice, maize, sorghum, millet, potatoes, yams, and bananas. Other sources of energy-packed foods include legumes, soy products, nuts, seeds, meats, eggs, fish, oils, and fats. Beyond choosing naturally concentrated foods, adding calories to other foods improves energy and

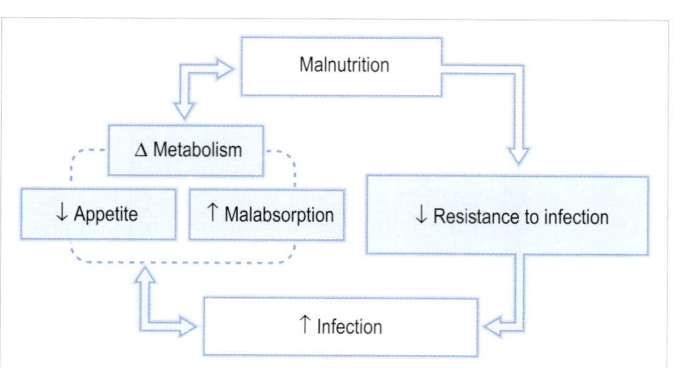

Figure 53.1 The cycle of malnutrition and infection.

Table 53.3 Nutrition management of symptoms

Symptom	Nutrition actions
Anorexia	Small, frequent meals every 2–3 h Limit liquids during the meal drink liquids between meals or snacks Light exercise Multivitamin and mineral supplement *Avoid*: strong smelling foods
Diarrhea	Drink plenty of fluids Small, frequent meals every 2–3 h Soluble fiber rich foods (i.e. porridge, sorghum, cassava, banana, mango, potatoes, yams, rice, lentils, barley, oats, millet, peas) Prepare foods by low-fat cooking methods (i.e. boiling, steaming, baking) *Avoid*: 　Frying foods 　Caffeine-rich foods and drinks (i.e. coffee, colas, chocolate) 　Gas-producing foods (i.e. legumes, cabbage, onions, peppers, sodas) 　Lactose containing foods (i.e. dairy, milk, cheese) 　Spicy and fatty foods 　Whole grains
Nausea and vomiting	Small, frequent meals every 2–3 h Drink plenty of fluids (small amounts throughout the day) Eat first, then drink liquids after the meal Dry or salty foods (i.e. crackers, dry toast) Ginger (candied ginger, ginger tea, fresh ginger) *Avoid*: spicy, fatty, or strong smelling foods and caffeine
Thrush and oral/ esophageal pain	Soft, bland foods (i.e. porridge, banana, eggs, soups, puddings) Cold or room temperature foods and drinks *Avoid*: spicy, salty, sugary or sticky foods and citrus fruits
Loss or altered sense of taste	Add flavor enhancers (salt, spices, herbs, fats) Use non-metal utensils (wood or plastic) Check for zinc deficiency
Constipation	Insoluble fiber (i.e. whole grains, seeds, nuts, berries, greens, fruits with peels, brown rice) Drink plenty of fluids Exercise as tolerated
Weight loss	Small, frequent meals every 2–3 h Drink fluids with calories Calorie-dense foods (i.e. grains, starchy fruits and vegetables, nuts, seeds, fats and oils, beans, animal proteins)

nutrient intake. Food additions can include powdered milk, oils, butter, sugar, or syrups into mixed ingredient dishes (i.e. porridges, cereals, sauces, and mashed potatoes.)

Lack of appetite is one of the most common side-effects of HIV/AIDS. It can be caused by infections, pain, depression, medication, and fatigue. Eating smaller meals or snacks every 2–3 h improves appetite and food intake. Exercise can also improve appetite, lean body mass and a sense of well-being. It is often easier to drink liquids than it is to eat solid foods, so people should be encouraged to eat first then drink fluids after and between meals to maximize energy intake.

Nausea

Small, frequent meals and snacks help to control nausea. Consuming small amounts of food every 2–3 hours can help tame nausea. Sitting up while eating and for 1 hour after a meal is helpful. Separating solid and liquid foods, with only a few sips of water during the meal may allay nausea. Foods to eat and drink during bouts of nausea and vomiting include soft, refined foods, as described in the section on diarrhea, as well as dry salty foods (i.e. toast, crackers, or dry cereal). Drinking sips of water, lemon juice, or ginger tea may also help to calm the stomach. Fatty, greasy, strong smelling, and sweet foods often worsen nausea and vomiting and should be avoided.

Thrush and Oral Pain

To avoid a decline in nutrient consumption during times of oral and esophageal pain and thrush soft, bland foods should be selected. Cold or room temperature foods are less likely to irritate. These include mashed foods, scrambled eggs, bananas, soups, and porridge. Foods that will irritate mouth and esophageal sores are acidic, spicy, salty, or sticky foods. Liquids such as citrus juices, sugary beverages, alcohol, and hot drinks should be avoided as well.

Loss or Altered Sense of Taste

During times of taste loss or alteration, adding salt, spices, herbs, lemon juice, and fats can enhance food's flavors. An individual should be encouraged to chew food thoroughly and to move it around the mouth to stimulate taste receptors. Utilizing non-metal (i.e. plastic or wood) utensils may also improve an altered sense of taste. Zinc deficiency may alter taste sensations and determination of zinc status should be pursued in the face of prolonged taste loss.

Conclusion

Good nutrition is key to achieving and maintaining good health and protect against infections. In the event of an infection, adequate nourishment improves the course of the infection and allows for the increased energy and nutrient requirements in the disease state. Many side-effects of infection and malnutrition such as diarrhea, fatigue, nausea, and altered taste may be improved with dietary interventions. There is a synergistic relationship between malnutrition and HIV/AIDS that lasts from the early, asymptomatic time of infection, and throughout the disease span.

A trained dietitian or nutritionist is an excellent resource to be consulted for assessment of nutritional status. A nutritionist is able to offer advice

during the asymptomatic stage of HIV on positive nutrition practices and awareness of early signs of malnutrition. Individualized nutrition education can cover symptom control and provide appropriate means of nutritionally treating significant weight changes, decreased food intake, signs of nutrient deficiency, and other metabolic complications of HIV including lipid abnormalities and glucose intolerance. A trained nutrition professional can provide appropriate nutrition advice to help stave off malnutrition and to treat it when necessary.

References

1. WHO. World Health Report 2004: Changing history. Geneva: World Health Organization; 2004.
2. Harris JA, Benedict FG. A biometric study of basal metabolism in man. Publication No. 279. Washington DC: Carnegie Institution of Washington; 1919.
3. Mifflin MD, St. Jeor ST, Hill LA, et al. A new predictive equation for resting energy expenditure in healthy individuals. Am J Clin Nutr 1990; 51:241–247.
4. Cunningham JJ. Body composition as a determinant of energy expenditure: a synthetic review and a proposed general prediction equation. Am J Clin Nutr 1991; 54:963–969.
5. Chandra RK. Rosette-forming T-lymphocytes and cell-mediated immunity in malnutrition. Br Med J 1974; 3:608–609.
6. Centers for Disease Control and Prevention. 1993 revised classification system for HIV infection and expanded surveillance case definition for AIDS among adolescents and adults. MMWR 1992; 41:16–17.
7. Grunfeld C, Pang M, Shimuzu L, et al. Resting energy expenditure, caloric intake, and short-term weight change in human immunodeficiency virus infection and the acquired immunodeficiency syndrome. Am J Clin Nutr 1992; 55:455–460.
8. Batterham MJ, Morgan-Jones J, Greenop P, et al. Calculating energy requirements for men with HIV/AIDS in the era of highly active antiretroviral therapy. Eur J Clin Nutr 2003; 57:209–217.
9. Shevitz AH, Knox TA, Spiegelman D, et al. Elevated resting energy expenditure among HIV-seropositive persons receiving highly active antiretroviral therapy. AIDS 1999; 13:1351–1357.
10. WHO. Nutrient requirements for people living with HIV/AIDS: report of a technical consultation. Geneva, Switzerland: World Health Organization; 2003.
11. Scrimshaw NS, SanGiovanni JP. Synergism of nutrition, infection, and immunity: an overview. Am J Clin Nutr 1997; 66:464s–477s.
12. Institute of Medicine, Food and Nutrition Board. Dietary reference intakes: energy, carbohydrate, fiber, fat, fatty acids, cholesterol, protein, and amino acids. Washington, DC: National Academy Press; 2002.
13. Martorell R, Yarbrough C, Yarbrough S, et al. The impact of ordinary illnesses on the dietary intakes of malnourished children. Am J Clin Nutr 1980; 33:345–350.
14. Scrimshaw NS, Taylor CE, Gordon JE. Interactions of nutrition and infection. Geneva: World Health Organization; 1968.
15. Chandra RK. Nutrition, immunity and infection: From basic knowledge of dietary manipulation of immune responses to practical application of ameliorating suffering and improving survival. Proc Natl Acad Sci 1996; 93:14304–14307.

16. Scrimshaw NS. Historical concepts of interactions, synergism and antagonism between nutrition and infection. J Nutr 2003; 133:316s–321s.

17. Uganda Ministry of Health STD/AIDS Control Programme and the Uganda Action for Nutrition. Nutritional Care and Support for People Living with HIV/AIDS in Uganda: Guidelines for Service Providers, 2004. Online. Available: www.fantaproject.org

18. Brown KH, Peerson JM, Rivera J, et al. Effect of supplemental zinc on growth and serum zinc concentrations of prepubertal children: a meta-analysis of randomized controlled trials. Am J Clin Nutr 2002; 75:1062–1071.

19. Bhaskaram P. Immunology of mild micronutrient deficiencies. Br J Nutr 2001; 85:75s–80s.

20. Fraker PJ, King LE, Laakko T, et al. The dynamic link between the integrity of the immune system and zinc status. J Nutr 2000; 130:1399s–1406s.

21. Field CJ, Johnson IR, Schley PD. Nutrients and their role in host resistance to infection. J Leukoc Biol 2002; 71:16–32.

22. Penny ME, Peerson JM, Marin RM, et al. Randomized, community-based trial of the effect of zinc supplementation, with and without other micronutrients, on the duration of persistent childhood diarrhea in Lima, Peru. J Pediatr 1999; 135:208–217.

23. Sandstead HH, Penland JG, Alcock NW, et al. Effects of repletion with zinc and other micronutrients on neuropsychologic performance and growth of Chinese children. Am J Clin Nutr 1998; 68:470s–475s.

24. Sazawal S, Black RE, Bhan MK, et al. Efficacy of zinc supplementation in reducing the incidence and prevalence of acute diarrhea - a community-based, double-blind, controlled trial. Am J Clin Nutr 1997; 66:413–418.

25. Black RE. Zinc deficiency, infectious disease and mortality in the developing world. J Nutr 2003; 133:1485s–1489s.

26. Wieringa FT, Dijkhuizen MA, West CE, et al. Estimation of the effect of the acute phase response on indicators of micronutrient status in Indonesian infants. J Nutr 2002; 132:3061–3066.

27. Institute of Medicine, Food and Nutrition Board. Dietary reference intakes: Vitamin A, vitamin K, arsenic, boron, chromium, copper, iodine, iron, manganese, molybdenum, nickel, silicon, vanadium, and zinc. Washington, DC: National Academy Press; 2001.

28. UNICEF. Vitamin and mineral deficiency: a global progress report. UNICEF, 2004: The micronutrient initiative. Online. Available: www.micronutrient.org

29. Ahluwalia N, Sun J, Krause D, et al. Immune function is impaired in iron-deficient, homebound, older women. Am J Clin Nutr 2004; 79:516–521.

30. Richman DD, Fischl MA, Grieco MH, et al. The toxicity of azidothymidine (AZT) in the treatment of patients with AIDS and AIDS-related complex. A double-blind, placebo-controlled trial. N Engl J Med 1987; 317:192–197.

31. Institute of Medicine, Food and Nutrition Board. Dietary reference intakes for vitamin C, vitamin E, selenium, and carotenoids. Washington, DC: National Academy Press; 2000.

32. Courtemanche C, Elson-Schwab I, Mashiyama ST, et al. Folate deficiency inhibits the proliferation of primary human $CD8^+$ T lymphocytes in vitro. J Immunol 2004; 173:3186–3192.

33. Beisel WR. Single nutrients and immunity. Am J Clin Nutr 1982; 35:S417–S468.

34. Institute of Medicine. Food and Nutrition Board. Dietary reference intakes: thiamin, riboflavin, niacin, vitamin B6, folate, vitamin B12, pantothenic acid, biotin, and choline. Washington, DC: National Academy Press; 1998.

35. Fawzi WW, Msamanga GI, Spiegelman D, et al. A randomized trial of multivitamin supplements and HIV disease progression and mortality. N Engl J Med 2004; 351:23–32.

36. Fawzi WW, Msamanga GI, Antelman G, et al. Effect of prenatal vitamin supplementation on lower-genital levels of HIV type 1 and interleukin type 1 at 36 weeks of gestation. Clin Infect Dis 2004; 38:716–722.

37. Tang AM, Graham NM, Saah AJ. Effects of micronutrient intake on survival in human immunodeficiency virus type 1 infection. Am J Epidemiol 1996; 143:1244–1256.

38. Sirisinha S, Suskind R, Edelman R, et al. Complement and C3-proactivator levels in children with protein-calorie malnutrition and effect of dietary treatment. Lancet 1973; 1:1016–1020.

39. Kanter AS, Spencer DC, Steinberg MH, et al. Supplemental vitamin B and progression to AIDS and death in black South African patients infected with HIV. J Acquir Immune Defic Syndr 1999; 21:252–253.

40. Gibson RS, Yeudall F, Drost N, et al. Experiences of a community-based dietary intervention to enhance micronutrient adequacy of diets low in animal source foods and high in phytate: A case study in rural Malawian children. J Nutr 2003; 133:3992s–3999s.

CHAPTER 54

Antiretroviral Therapy in Resource-poor Settings: Challenges, Research Priorities, Opportunities

Joep M. A. Lange
Elly Katabira
Papa Salif Sow

Introduction

For a long time after the introduction of antiretroviral therapy in the developed world, this treatment did not even begin to reach the masses of HIV-infected people in resource-poor settings. In the days of mono- and dual-drug therapy, global and national policymakers widely felt that the limited clinical benefit of these expensive and complex drugs did not warrant their widespread use in the poorest regions of the world. Even when the introduction of HAART in 1996 in the developed world immediately led to striking reductions of HIV-related morbidity and mortality, there was still very little push to extend the use of these life-saving drugs to resource-poor settings. Although it was now hard to argue the clinical benefits of HAART, this therapy was still considered to be far too expensive and complex for anything but sophisticated medical environments.

It is our personal belief that the fact the International AIDS Conference in 2000 was held for the first time in sub-Saharan Africa (Durban, South Africa), the region hardest hit by the HIV epidemic, accelerated a breakthrough in scaling up access to HAART in resource-poor settings. UN bodies, pharmaceutical companies, and the global HIV/AIDS community simply could not face going to Durban, without having something to offer. Shortly before the Durban conference, UNAIDS and five major pharmaceutical companies announced an agreement on significant price reductions of antiretrovirals for least-developed nations, especially in sub-Saharan Africa (the Accelerating Access Initiative).

This was followed by a United Nations General Assembly Special Session (UNGASS) on HIV/AIDS in 2001, clearly stating that antiretroviral treatment, next to HIV prevention, is an essential component of the fight against HIV/AIDS. The World Health Organization (WHO) subsequently included antiretrovirals in the Essential Medicines list and formulated guidelines for the development of a public health approach to treatment of HIV infections in resource-poor settings.[1] New and substantial funding mechanisms, such as the World Bank's Multicountry AIDS Program (MAP), the Global Fund to Fight AIDS, TB and Malaria (GFATM), and President Bush's Emergency Plan for AIDS Relief (PEPFAR) were established. Through its '3 by 5' initiative, the WHO set the target to have three million people in resource-poor settings on antiretroviral therapy by the end of 2005.[2] In the meantime, prices of a number of antiretrovirals continued to fall; partially as the result of generic competition.

Although the '3 by 5' target was not met, these developments – increased political commitment, both globally and nationally; vastly increased funding opportunities; sound treatment guidelines; and, decreasing drug prices – have led to impressive rises in the numbers of people receiving HAART. It is estimated that globally, over 1.3 million people were receiving HAART at the end of 2005. The scale-up in Africa has been the most dramatic: rising from just 100 000 people receiving HAART at the end of 2003 to 810 000 at the end of 2005.[3]

However, 1.3 million people still only represent 20% of the estimated 6.5 million people in immediate need of HAART and formidable obstacles remain a realization of the 2010 'universal access' target set by the G8 Summit. Moreover, the delivery of antiretroviral therapy in resource-poor settings usually takes place in environments that are very different from those in the developed world, posing specific challenges. This chapter attempts to identify some of those challenges and, where appropriate, also tries to identify priorities for research that can advance antiretroviral treatment under these difficult circumstances. It concludes by taking a long-term view. The focus is on sub-Saharan Africa.

Challenges to Providing Antiretroviral Therapy in Sub-Saharan Africa

Lack of Healthcare Workers and Medical Infrastructure

Even before the HIV/AIDS epidemic, the public health sector in sub-Saharan Africa was very much under-resourced, with limited possibilities to diagnose, prevent, and treat many of the diseases that abound, including those of non-infectious origin, such as hypertension, diabetes mellitus, and stroke. Because of poor working conditions and low salaries, retainment rates of doctors and nurses in the public sector in many sub-Saharan countries are appallingly low.[4] The HIV/AIDS epidemic has not only greatly increased demands on an already malfunctioning health sector, but also further attenuated the workforce by its lethal effect on infected healthcare workers. Among the low numbers of healthcare workers available, few have expert knowledge about the treatment of HIV infection. This does not only apply to sub-Saharan Africa, but also to a number of Asian countries.[5] Many training programs are closing this knowledge gap, but if it proves to be impossible to retain sufficient numbers of healthcare workers, much of this will be in vain. The shortages of doctors and nurses prompt the involvement of less qualified healthcare workers or even community members in the delivery of care. This means that treatment algorithms have to be very clear and simple.

Community-based care has been successfully introduced in rural Haiti,[6] and deserves to be further explored in sub-Saharan Africa.

In a number of countries, poor management of drug supplies and drug distribution has led to interruptions in antiretroviral drug supply to patients. This is highly unfortunate in a disease where adherence to therapy is essential to prevent development of viral drug resistance, especially with drug regimens that include drugs with greatly different elimination half lives, such as the NNRTI-containing first-line regimens that are nearly universally used in resource-poor settings.

Limited Monitoring Facilities

This is a consequence of the limited medical infrastructure and limited resources. In most sub-Saharan African settings, $CD4^+$ lymphocyte enumeration is not available, making the decision to initiate antiretroviral therapy based purely on clinical criteria.

This implies that antiretroviral treatment is usually initiated very late in the course of infection, leading to many cases of immune reconstitution inflammatory syndrome (IRIS) and high mortality rates following the initiation of therapy.[3] Because of the large numbers of co-morbidities and the high risk for IRIS, HAART should be initiated sooner rather than later in sub-Saharan Africa than in the developed world.[7]

The ability to measure plasma HIV-1 RNA load (pVL) is even more limited than that of $CD4^+$ lymphocyte enumeration. Treatment failure is thus usually diagnosed based on declining numbers of $CD4^+$ cells or clinical disease progression. Since these are usually preceded by virological failure, extensive viral drug resistance may have developed by the time that treatment failure is diagnosed. There is a great need for the development of affordable and simple pVL assays that can be used at the point of care.[3]

Cost of Care, Dictating Treatment Choices

Healthcare budgets in sub-Saharan African countries are generally extremely low, with annual *per capita* spending often being <US$20. The annual cost of even the cheapest available HAART regimen for the poorest countries currently is around US$150, and in many settings, this low price is theory rather than reality. This implies that for a long time, the HAART scale-up will be dependent on substantial

contributions from the international donor community. Middle-income countries form a specific problem, because they do not qualify for similar drug price reductions as the least developed countries, making some governments reluctant to initiate large antiretroviral treatment programs. However, we should also recognize the fact that governments make choices, and can only applaud the shining example of Brazil, where the government, after succumbing to pressure from civil society, has managed to provide effective universal free access to HAART to its HIV-infected population. In Brazil, domestic generic medicine production and the resulting increased bargaining power *vis a vis* research-based pharma companies (through being able to credibly use the mechanism of compulsory licensing) have led to significant price reductions of antiretrovirals.[8] Similar engagement and pressure from civil society is lacking in many African countries.

Cost-considerations have favored widespread use of a generic fixed dose HAART combination (FDC) of d4T/3TC/NVP in sub-Saharan Africa. In the light of the emergency situation and the drive to put as many people as quickly as possible on treatment, this is understandable, but the long-term costs of this 'cheap' choice should not be ignored. In the developed world, nobody today would initiate HAART with this specific drug combination. Although the short-term tolerance of the FDC in question is generally good, after a few years of treatment, the majority of people, due to the d4T component of the regimen, will develop the disfiguring syndrome of body fat redistribution, with complete loss of facial fat.[9,10] Apart from the human suffering this will cause, it will certainly have a negative impact on antiretroviral uptake and it would be wiser to spend a bit more money on better HAART regimens. Fortunately, the new WHO treatment guidelines recommend to move away from d4T-containing regimens.[3]

Another consequence of resource constraints is limited availability of adequate second line antiretroviral drug regimens. Those are generally PI-based and considerably more expensive than the NNRTI-based first line regimens. In quite a few countries, second line regimens contain recycled NRTIs and a suboptimal (unboosted) PI. An additional, unrelated problem with boosted PIs is the need for RTV refrigeration. The new Kaletra® formulation does away with that, but it is uncertain when that will be available in sub-Saharan Africa (see below). Moreover, this does not solve the RTV issue for other PIs than lopinavir.

Third-line or salvage therapy is simply out of reach in most resource-poor settings and also does not figure in the public health approach that WHO is advocating.[2,3]

Regulatory Environment

The regulatory environment in sub-Saharan Africa and many other resource-poor countries is not conducive to the rapid approval of new antiretrovirals. For drugs that have become part of mainstay regimens in the developed world, it may take years before they are available to patients in resource-poor settings. Part of the reason may be that the regulatory filing in developing countries occurs at a later stage than in the USA and Europe. But then, pharmaceutical companies, even when they offer a product considered to be an essential drug at not-for-profit prices, have to go through cumbersome and different procedures country by country that consume unnecessary resources and cost human lives. Surely, innovative mechanisms should be put in place to improve the regulatory situation. Proposals to accept licensing by the FDA or EMEA for essential drug availability in resource-poor settings are floating.[11]

Pediatric Treatment

Antiretroviral drug choices for adult treatment may be more limited in resource-poor settings than in the developed world but the situation is even more dire for pediatric treatment options. Relatively few antiretrovirals are available in pediatric formulations.

In settings where adult FDCs are the only available first-line drugs, children, if treated at all, usually receive arbitrary dosages of (broken) adult tablets.[12]

HIV/TB Co-infections

Dual HIV/TB infections form an exceptional challenge. Worldwide, 14 million people are co-infected with these pathogens and TB is a leading cause of death among people living with HIV.[13] HIV infection increases the risk of reactivating latent *M. tuberculosis* infection, placing HIV-positive persons at increased risk for developing TB.[14] HIV infection also increases the risk of rapid TB progression after primary *M. tuberculosis* acquisition or reinfection.[15] TB may accelerate the progression of HIV disease via immune activation and is associated with a higher mortality and shorter survival in HIV-positive persons.[16] The risk of TB increases as the HIV-related immune deficiency progresses; similarly, the highest mortality rates associated with TB occur in persons with the greatest immune deficiency.[17] However, there already is a rapid increase in TB incidence soon after infection with HIV.[18] The presentation of TB in those with advanced HIV disease is often atypical, and a documented bacteriological diagnosis may be more difficult to make.[19] Concomitant treatment of HIV and TB poses difficulties. In those with dual infections who initiate anti-HIV therapy (antiretroviral treatment) in advanced stages of HIV infection, there is a high rate of immune reconstitution disease, leading to considerable early morbidity and mortality.[20] There are overlapping drug toxicities[21] and pharmacological interactions between anti-TB drugs and antiretroviral agents considerably narrow antiretroviral treatment choices in those who need concomitant treatment.[22] The optimal timing of treatment of tuberculosis and HIV in co-infected patients clearly presents a research priority. Lastly, it is no exaggeration to state that successful global control of TB very much depends on our ability to prevent and treat HIV infections.

Linking Prevention to Treatment

The number of new HIV infections taking place in 2005 approached five million, 3.2 million of those occurring in sub-Saharan Africa. From these figures, it is clear that current efforts to rapidly expand and sustain antiretroviral therapy will be severely undermined without a more effective concomitant prevention effort.[23] Despite successes in curbing the HIV/AIDS epidemic in individual countries, global figures continue to grow. More people became infected with HIV in 2005 than in any year before.[23]

We cannot afford to continue to debate the relative merits of prevention versus treatment. This is a false dichotomy. Mathematical modeling, comparing a range of scenarios through 2020, shows that our best option is to scale-up treatment and prevention jointly. This strategy, as compared with more treatment-centered or prevention-centered strategies, will lead to the lowest number of new infections, the highest numbers of deaths averted and, in the long-term could also lead to dramatic reductions in resource needs for antiretroviral treatment.[24]

A specific problem regarding prevention versus treatment is the use of single-dose NVP to prevent mother-to-child transmission (PMTCT) of HIV, whereas NNRTI-based regimens are also the dominant first line therapy in resource-poor settings. One of the characteristics which make single-dose NVP

regimen effective in PMTCT – the long terminal half-life of the drug – also leads to development of viral NVP resistance in significant proportions of mothers and infants exposed in this manner.[25,26] A recent study confirmed the expectation of those with an understanding of HIV virology that intrapartum NVP has a negative impact on success rates of subsequent maternal treatment with NVP-containing HAART.[27] Strategies to maximize benefits of both antiretroviral prophylaxis against mother-to-child transmission of HIV-1 and chronic antiretroviral therapy for mothers and HIV-infected children are urgently needed.[28]

Conclusion

The Antiretroviral Scale-up as a Catalyst to Build Sustainable Healthcare Systems

After years of lost opportunity, we are currently still in the phase of an emergency response to scale-up antiretroviral therapy. HIV is a lifelong infection, however, and HIV treatment, once started should be taken lifelong. Despite all the recent progress that has been made, sustainable treatment of all those in need of antiretroviral therapy asks for more than an emergency response. It asks for HIV treatment embedded in the delivery of general healthcare, in the context of viable healthcare systems, with viable financing mechanisms and retainment of healthcare workers. To accomplish this, sub-Saharan Africa for a long time will need a considerable influx of donor money. Yet, that donor money should be used more creatively, and be targeting long-term solutions beside the emergency response, be targeting private sector initiatives next to the overburdened public sector. Sustainable financing of healthcare is only possible through the 'solidarity principle' of health insurance schemes. These are rare in sub-Saharan Africa and usually limited to people employed by large or medium sized companies. Uninsured people when confronted with a health problem usually have to make out-of-pocket expenses, which may push them into the poverty trap.[29] A substantial proportion of donor money should be used to extend insurance schemes to broader groups of the population. This will prevent aggravating poverty of those who get sick, generate predictable income for healthcare providers, help prevent healthcare worker attrition and make it attractive to invest in healthcare.

If we fail to recognize this, all the billions spent now eventually will not leave anything that lasts. If we do take a long-term view, the current momentum for the antiretroviral scale-up provides a unique opportunity to empower the poor and build sustainable healthcare systems in Africa and other resource-poor settings.

References

1. WHO. Scaling up antiretroviral therapy in resource-limited settings: guidelines for a public health approach. Geneva: World Health Organization; 2002.
2. WHO. Treating 3 million by 2005: making it happen. Geneva: World Health Organization; 2003.
3. WHO. Antiretroviral therapy for HIV infection in adults and adolescents in resource-limited settings: towards universal access: recommendations for a public health approach. Geneva: World Health Organization; 2006.
4. UNDP. Human Development Report 2004. UNDP.
5. Treat Asia. Treat Asia Special Report: expanded availability of HIV/AIDS drugs in Asia creates urgent need for trained doctors. Bangkok, Thailand: Treat Asia; 2004.
6. Farmer PE, Leandre F, Mukherjee JS, et al. Community-based approaches to HIV treatment in resource-poor settings. Lancet 2001; 358:404–409.
7. Braitstein P, Brinkhof MW, Dabis F, et al. Mortality of HIV-1-infected patients in the first year of antiretroviral therapy: comparison between low-income and high-income countries. Lancet 2006; 367:817–824.
8. Teixeira PR, Vitoria MA, Barcarolo J. Antiretroviral treatment in resource-poor settings: the Brazilian experience. AIDS 2004; 18:S5–S7.
9. Brinkman K, Smeitink JA, Romijn JA, Reiss P. Mitochondrial toxicity induced by nucleoside-analogue reverse-transcriptase inhibitors is a key factor in the pathogenesis of antiretroviral therapy-related lipodystrophy. Lancet 1999; 354:1112–1115.
10. Van der Valk M, Casula M, Weverling GJ, et al. Prevalence of lipoatrophy and mitochondrial DNA content of blood and subcutaneous fat in HIV-1-infected patients randomly allocated to zidovudine- or stavudine-based therapy. Antivir Ther 2004; 9:385–393.
11. UNGASS. United Nations General Assembly Special Session on HIV/AIDS. 2006.
12. Puthanakit T, Oberdorfer A, Akarathum N, et al. Efficacy of highly active antiretroviral therapy in HIV-infected children participating in Thailand's national access to antiretroviral program. Clin Infect Dis 2005; 41:100–107.
13. International AIDS Conference. Stop TB partnership. TB/HIV: facts at a glance. Online. Available: www.stoptb.org/events/internationalaidsconference/xv/assets/ InfoPack/ 1GB.pdf
14. Bucher HC, Griffith LE, Guyatt GH, et al. Isoniazid prophylaxis for tuberculosis in HIV infection: a meta-analysis of randomized controlled trials. AIDS 1999; 13:501–507.
15. Daley CL, Small PM, Schecter GF, et al. An outbreak of tuberculosis with accelerated progression among persons infected with the human immunodeficiency virus: an analysis using restriction-fragment length polymorphisms. N Engl J Med 1992; 326:231–235.
16. Whalen CC, Nsubuga P, Okwera A, et al. Impact of pulmonary tuberculosis on survival of HIV-infected adults: a prospective epidemiologic study in Uganda. AIDS 2000; 14:1219–1228.
17. Shafer RW, Bloch AB, Larkin C, et al. Predictors of survival in HIV-infected tuberculosis. AIDS 1996; 10:269–272.
18. Sonnenberg P, Glynn JR, Fielding K, et al. How soon after infection with HIV does the risk of tuberculosis start to increase? A retrospective cohort study in South African gold miners. J Infect Dis 2005; 191:150–158.
19. Jones BE, Young SM, Antoniskis D, et al. Relationship of the manifestations of tuberculosis to CD4 cell counts in patients with human immunodeficiency virus infection. Am Rev Respir Dis 1993; 148:1292–1297.
20. French MA, Price P, Stone SF. Immune restoration disease after antiretroviral therapy. AIDS 2004; 18:1615–1627.
21. Lee WM. Drug-induced hepatotoxicity. N Engl J Med 2003; 349:474–485.
22. De Maat MM, Ekhart GC, Huitema AD, et al. Drug interactions between antiretroviral drugs and co-medicated agents. Clin Pharm 2003; 42:223–282.
23. UNAIDS and WHO. AIDS epidemic update. December 2005: UNAIDS and World Health Organization; 2005.
24. Salomon JA, Hogan DR, Stover J, et al. Integrating HIV prevention and treatment: from slogans to impact. PLoS Med 2005; 2:50–56.
25. Jackson JB, Becker-Pergola G, Guay LA, et al. Identification of K103N resistance mutation in Ugandan women receiving nevirapine to prevent HIV-1 vertical transmission (HIVNET 012). AIDS 2001; 14:111–115.
26. Eshleman SH, Mracna M, Guay LA, et al. Selection and fading of resistance mutations in women and infants receiving nevirapine to prevent HIV-1 vertical transmission (HIVNET 012). AIDS 2001; 15:1951–1957.
27. Jourdain G, Ngo-Giang-Huong N, Le Coeur S, et al. Intrapartum exposure to nevirapine and subsequent maternal responses to nevirapine-based antiretroviral therapy. N Engl J Med 2004; 351:229–240.
28. McIntyre J. Controversies in the use of nevirapine for the prevention of mother-to-child transmission. 12th Conference on Retroviruses and Opportunistic Infections, Boston, MA: 22–25 February 2005; Abstract 8.
29. Preker AS, Langenbrunner JC, editors. Spending wisely, buying health services for the poor. Washington DC: World Bank; 2005.

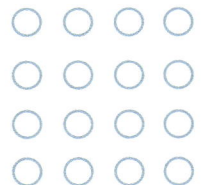

CHAPTER 55

Antiretroviral Treatment and Follow-up of HIV-infected Children in Resource-limited Settings

Sibyl Geelen

Philippa Musoke

Introduction

The majority of all HIV-infected children under the age of 15 years live in sub-Saharan Africa. The high burden of pediatric HIV infection in Africa is a direct result of the high prevalence of HIV infection among women of child-bearing age, very few of whom have access to HIV mother-to-child transmission intervention programs. HIV/AIDS is a major cause of infant and childhood mortality. Recent data from HIV mother-to-child transmission studies in sub-Saharan countries indicate that 7.6% of non-HIV-infected children, but 52% of HIV-infected children, die before 2 years of age.[1] These figures emphasize the urgent need for programs on the care and treatment of HIV-infected children in these parts of the world. Whereas antiretroviral therapy is part of standard care and has markedly improved the prognosis of HIV-infected children in resource-rich countries, very few children from resource-limited countries have access to these drugs.

Clinical Aspects

The clinical manifestations of HIV in children are described in Chapter 41. Selected clinical data on HIV-infected children in resource-limited areas are presented briefly below.

Common childhood infections and other diseases, such as acute pneumonia, otitis media, diarrhea, septicemia, and failure to thrive, occur frequently in both HIV-infected and uninfected children in resource-limited settings. However, these infections tend to occur more frequently and their course is often more severe in HIV-infected children, leading to a higher case fatality rate. For example, HIV infection was a strong predictor of death in Tanzanian children hospitalized with pneumonia,[2] and respiratory disease accounted for the majority of deaths in HIV-positive children in autopsy studies performed in Botswana and Kenya.[3,4] *Streptococcus pneumoniae* is the most common bacterial pathogen in respiratory disease, but *Pneumocystis jiroveci* (formerly called *Pneumocystis carinii*) is a common pathogen in African HIV-infected children with severe pneumonia, and especially in infants. Graham and co-workers[5] detected *P. carinii* in ≈10% of 150 Malawian infants younger than 6 months of age admitted with severe pneumonia. Bakeera-Kitata and co-workers[6] from Uganda, diagnosed *P. carinii* pneumonia (PCP) in 16.5% of 121 children <5 years of age, admitted with severe pneumonia. A total of 60% of these children were <6 months of age. Chintu and co-workers[7] diagnosed PCP at autopsy in 29% of Zambian children who died from respiratory illness, and Ruffini and Mahdi[8] found evidence of PCP in 48.6% of South African children between 2 and 24 months hospitalized for severe pneumonia.[3,5–9]

Tuberculosis (TB) is an important clinical problem in HIV-infected children in both African and Asian countries. HIV seroprevalence rates of 42% and 37% have been reported in South African and Zambian children with TB, but rates up to 67% have been reported in children in India. Common manifestations of tuberculosis in HIV-infected children are persistent cough, fever, and failure to thrive, but signs and symptoms may be non-specific and mimic those of other infections, such as acute bacterial pneumonia, bronchiectasis, lymphocytic interstitial pneumonitis (LIP), or *Pneumocystis jiroveci* pneumonia. Manifestations of TB also tend to be more severe and progress more rapidly in HIV-infected children, and children with advanced HIV disease often suffer from extrapulmonary and disseminated TB. Tuberculosis in children is a primary infection, in contrast with adults in whom TB usually results from reactivation of latent tuberculosis. With limited laboratory support, establishing a definite diagnosis may be difficult. Early during the course of HIV infection, the tuberculin skin reaction may be positive in exposed children; however, in children with profound immunosuppression due to malnutrition or to advanced HIV infection, tuberculin skin testing is often negative. The optimal treatment strategies for co-infection with HIV and TB still need to be determined.[10-12] Preliminary data from a recent placebo-controlled randomized trial conducted in Cape Town, South Africa in children between 8 weeks and 12 years showed that long-term isoniazid prophylaxis significantly reduced mortality.[13]

Malaria is a cause of significant morbidity and mortality in many areas where HIV is prevalent. While the frequency of malaria in HIV-infected children and uninfected children appears to be similar, there are reports that the course of malaria in HIV-infected children is different. Some investigators found a more complicated course in HIV-infected children, with increased hospitalization and severe anemia, whereas others did not.[14-17] The clinical response to antimalarial therapy does not differ between the two groups. Recently, Kublin and co-workers[18] reported a significant increase in the HIV viral load during malarial attacks in adult patients from a rural area in Malawi,[18] but it is not known whether this phenomenon also occurs in children.

While measles is infrequently encountered in children living in settings where preventive immunization is standard care, it is a serious disease and a major cause of morbidity in many sub-Saharan African regions. Studies of measles in HIV-infected and other immunocompromised children in the USA and Europe have shown that measles may present without the typical rash and cause higher rates of complications, such as pneumonitis and encephalitis. Children also show prolonged shedding of the measles virus. Data on the interaction between measles and HIV infection in African children are less clear. Mortality has not been found to be consistently higher in HIV-infected children versus uninfected children, although it may be increased in subsets of children. As in non-HIV-infected children, vaccination lowers mortality in HIV-infected African children.[19-21]

The risk of developing malignancies is increased in children with HIV disease. Non-Hodgkin lymphoma, predominantly Burkitt's lymphoma, is the most frequently diagnosed malignancy in reports from centers in the USA and Thailand.[22-24] While Kaposi's sarcoma rarely occurs in HIV-infected children living in Europe and North America, it does occur in children living in Africa. The prevalence of this condition is highest in East and Central Africa and is associated with the epidemiology of human herpes virus 8 (HHV8).[25-27] In contrast to African adults and adolescents with severe immunosuppression, young HIV-infected children are not frequently infected with cryptococcal meningitis and toxoplasmic encephalitis. A likely explanation for this phenomenon is that exposure to these pathogens has not yet occurred; disease in adults usually results from reactivation of these pathogens.[9] However, in older children and adolescents, cryptococcal meningitis may occur and may have an insidious onset with headache as the only presenting sign. And, when presenting with focal seizures, CNS toxoplasmosis or tuberculous meningitis should be considered. Where available, imaging of the brain (CT scan) may be helpful in making the diagnosis but presumptive treatment may have to be started if investigative facilities are limited.

Failure to thrive and growth retardation is an important sign of HIV infection and a sensitive indicator of disease progression in HIV-infected children, regardless of where they live. While stunting (appropriate weight for height z-scores) is associated with early stages of HIV infection, chronic malnutrition and wasting are associated with more advanced stages of the disease. In resource-limited areas, HIV-infected children are at a significantly higher risk of malnutrition during the course of HIV infection. Low birth weight, recurrent infections, and inadequate nutrition all add to the risk of developing severe wasting.[9,28-30]

There is no clear understanding of the causes of death among children in resource-limited settings in general, and among HIV-infected children in particular. Most studies have focused on single clinical conditions or on post-mortem findings,[3,7] but in practice, several conditions occur concurrently, such as HIV infection, tuberculosis, and malaria, and the outcome of these diseases is influenced by living conditions, such as inadequate nutrition, lack of clean water, and access to care.[4,31]

Diagnostic Issues

Because the clinical manifestations of HIV infection in children overlap with those of other pediatric infections and diseases, it may be difficult to distinguish between HIV-associated conditions and other diseases without specific diagnostic testing.

Rapid tests or alternative tests based on antibodies can be used to diagnose HIV infection in children older than 18 months. However, establishing a definite diagnosis of HIV infection in infants younger than 18 months requires virologic tests that directly detect virus such as HIV-DNA- PCR or HIV-RNA-PCR. The availability of these expensive diagnostic facilities in resource-constrained areas is limited, but the value of simpler and cheaper alternatives (e. g. ultra-sensitive p24 antigen determination[32]) to diagnose HIV infection in infants has yet to be determined.

Assays to determine CD4 counts or percentages are more widely available and can assist in the decision whether to start or defer antiretroviral therapy in children. In children under 6 years, the use of the CD4 percentage is preferred to the absolute CD4 cell count because the CD4 percentage does not change with age whereas the absolute cell count does.

As in adults, in HIV-infected children the total lymphocyte count is also significantly correlated with the risk of mortality. A recent meta-analysis confirmed that total lymphocyte count in children was a strong predictor of short-term disease progression. In children older than 2 years, the prognostic value was higher than in younger ones.[33,34]

It should be noted, however, that immunologic indices differ in populations, and the optimal cut-off value for the total lymphocyte count to use in pediatric populations from various areas of the world has not yet been determined.[35,36] Moreover, a recent study by Lau and co-workers[37] conducted with adults, has indicated that not only the absolute total lymphocyte count but also a rapid decline in the count is indicative of an increased likelihood of progression of the HIV infection.[37]

Disease Staging

Two international pediatric clinical classification systems are available for HIV disease: the Centers for Diseases Control and Prevention (CCD) pediatric clinical staging system (see Ch. 41) and the WHO pediatric clinical staging system (Box 55.1). Both systems can be used to assess the need for antiretroviral therapy.

The WHO pediatric staging system, revised in 2005, is based on clinical conditions for which a presumptive diagnosis is possible on the basis of clinical signs or simple investigations. Therefore, the WHO staging system is more suitable for use in settings with limited diagnostic facilities. Part of the clinical staging conditions, however, require more advanced diagnostic tools.

The WHO criteria for a presumed HIV clinical stage 4 diagnosis for infants and children under the age of 18 months in situations where virologic testing is not possible, are presented in Box 55.2.

If CD4 testing is available, clinical staging should be combined with immunologic staging using the WHO (Table 55.1)[38] or CDC (see Ch. 41) pediatric

Table 55.1 WHO pediatric immunologic staging: CD4+ T-cell levels in relation to the severity of immunosuppression

Level of immunosuppression	Age			
	≤11 months	12–35 months	36–59 months	≥5 years
Not significant immunosuppression	>35%	>30%	>25%	>500/mm³
Mild immunosuppression	30–35%	25–30%	20–25%	350–499/mm³
Advanced immunosuppression	25–29%	20–24%	15–19%	200–349/mm³
Severe immunosuppression	<25% (<1500/mm³)	<20% (<750/mm³)	<15% (<350/mm³)	<200/mm³ or <15%

Source: WHO 2006: WHO case definitions of HIV for surveillance and revised clinical staging and immunological classification of HIV-related diseases in adults and children (www.who.int/hiv).

Box 55.1

WHO pediatric clinical staging of HIV disease

Clinical Stage 1

- Asymptomatic
- Persistent generalized lymphadenopathy (PGL) (pain less enlarged lymph nodes >1 cm at two or more non-contagious sites lexclusive inguinal, without known cause and persisting for 3 months or more).

Clinical Stage 2

- Unexplained persistent hepatosplenomegaly
- Papular pruritic eruptions
- Seborrheic dermatitis
- Extensive wart infection (extensive facial, >5% of body area or disfiguring)
- Extensive molluscum contagiosum
- Fungal nail infections
- Recurrent oral ulcerations (two or more in 6 months)
- Linear gingival erythema
- Angular cheilitis
- Unexplained persistent parotid enlargement
- Herpes zoster (>1 episode/12 months)
- Recurrent or chronic upper respiratory tract infections: otitis media, otorrhea, sinusitis (twice or more episodes in any 6-month period).

Clinical Stage 3

- Moderate unexplained malnutrition or wasting not adequately responding to standard therapy
- Unexplained persistent diarrhea (14 days or more)
- Unexplained persistent fever (above 37.5°C intermittent or constant and for >1 month)
- Persistent oral candidiasis (after the first 6 weeks of life)
- Oral hairy leukoplakia
- Acute necrotizing ulcerative gingivitis or periodontitis
- Lymph node tuberculosis
- Pulmonary tuberculosis
- Severe recurrent presumed bacterial pneumonia.
- Chronic HIV-associated lung disease including bronchiectasis
- Symptomatic lymphoid interstitial pneumonitis (LIP)
- Unexplained anemia (<8 g/dL), and/or neutropenia (<500/mm^3) and/or thrombocytopenia (<50 000/mm^3).

Clinical Stage 4

- Unexplained severe wasting, stunting, or severe malnutrition, not responding to standard therapy
- Pneumocystis pneumonia
- Recurrent severe bacterial infections (e.g. empyema, pyomyositis, bone or joint infection, or meningitis, but excluding pneumonia) (current episode plus one or more in previous six months)
- Chronic herpes simplex infection (orolabial or cutaneous of >1 month's duration or visceral at any site)
- Extrapulmonary TB
- Kaposi sarcoma
- Esophageal candidiasis
- CNS toxoplasmosis (outside the neonatal period)
- HIV encephalopathy.

Box 55.1

WHO pediatric clinical staging of HIV disease—cont'd

- CMV infection (CMV retinitis or infection affecting another organ other with onset at age older than one month of life)
- Extrapulmonary cryptococcosis, including meningitis
- Disseminated endemic mycosis (e.g. extrapulmonary histoplasmosis, coccidiomycosis, penicilliosis)
- Chronic cryptosporidiosis (with diarrhea lasting >1 month)
- Chronic isosporiasis
- Disseminated non-tuberculous mycobacteria infection
- Acquired HIV associated rectovaginal fistula
- Cerebral or B-cell non-Hodgkin's lymphoma
- Progressive multifocal leukoencephalopathy (PML)
- Symptomatic HIV-associated cardiomyopathy or HIV-associated nephropathy.

Sources: WHO case definitions of HIV for surveillance and revised clinical staging and immunological classification of HIV-related disease in adults and children (www.who.int/hiv).

Box 55.2

Clinical criteria for presumptive diagnosis of severe HIV disease among infants and children aged under 18 months in situations where virological confirmation of HIV infection is not available

A presumptive diagnosis of severe HIV disease should be made if the infant is:

- confirmed HIV-antibody positive
- Diagnosis of anyother AIDS-indicator condition(s)* can be made or;
- symptomatic with two or more of the following clinical signs
  - oral candidiasis/thrush
  - severe pneumonia
  - severe wasting/malnutrition
  - severe sepsis.

Other factors that support the diagnosis of severe HIV disease in an HIV seropositive infant include:

- recent HIV-related maternal death or advanced HIV disease in the mother
- CD4 <20%.

Confirmation of the diagnosis of HIV infection should be sought as soon as possible.

*AIDS-indicator conditions include some but not all HIV Stage 4 conditions seen in children such as *Pneumocystis* pneumonia, esophageal candiasis, cyptococcal meningitis, cerebral toxoplasmosis, unexplained wasting or malnutrition.
Source: WHO case definitions of HIV for surveillance and revised clinical staging and immunological classification of HIV-related disease in adults and children (www.who.int/hiv).

immunologic classification system to determine whether antiretroviral therapy is required.

Laboratories often provide absolute CD4 counts without CD4 percentages, however, these percentages can be calculated if leucocyte count and differential are also determined.

If neither CD4 percentages nor counts can be determined, the total lymphocyte count may be helpful as a substitute. Recent WHO guidelines on antiretroviral treatment of infants and children in resource limited settings, provide cut-off values for age-related total lymphocyte counts that can be used for the initiation of antiretroviral therapy in settings where CD4 determination is not available (Table 55.2).[38]

Antiretroviral Therapy in Children in Resource-limited Settings

The health and survival of HIV-infected children can be improved by means of co-trimoxazole prophylaxis, routine immunizations, appropriate infant feeding practices, and nutritional supplementation.[9,40,41] A randomized controlled study from Zambia demonstrated a significant protective effect of co-trimoxazole against morbidity and mortality in HIV-infected children,[40] but only antiretroviral therapy improves the long-term prognosis. The ability to provide comprehensive care to HIV-infected children, including antiretroviral agents,

Table 55.2 **When to initiate antiretroviral therapy in children in resource-limited settings (clinical and immunological criteria for initiating antiretroviral therapy in infants and children)**

WHO pediatric clinical stage	Antiretroviral therapy
Clinical stage 4	Treat all
Presumptive clinical stage 4 (infants <18 months, no virologic diagnosis possible)	Treat all Confirmation of the diagnosis of HIV infection should be sought as soon as possible

Clinical stage 3	If <11 months: treat all.
	If ≥12 months: majority of children should be treated.
	Specific considerations:
	    in children with pulmonary TB, the clinical status and CD4 level should be used to determine the need for and timing of ART in relation to TB treatment.
	    in children with lymphocytic interstitial pneumonitis, oral hairy leukoplakia or thrombocytopenia CD4 levels may be taken into account.

Clinical stage 2 or 1	Use CD4 levels to guide decisions on antiretroviral therapy
	  ≤11 months CD4 <25% (<1500/mm³)
	  12–35 months CD4 <20% (<750/mm³)
	  36–59 months CD4 <15% (<350/mm³)
	  ≥5 years CD4 <200/mm³ or <15%
	If CD4 levels are not available, decisions may be guided by total lymphocyte counts
	  ≤11 months TLC <4000 mm³
	  12–35 months TLC <3000 mm³
	  36–59 months TLC <2500 mm³
	  ≥5 years TLC <2000 mm³

Source: WHO: Antiretroviral therapy for HIV infection in infants and children: towards universal access. Recommendations for a publoic health approach. WHO 2006 (www.who.int/hiv).

depends on the availability of local resources and infrastructure, and qualified professionals able to deliver HIV care and treatment. Very few children currently have access to antiretroviral therapy but numbers are likely to increase in the future as access to antiretroviral treatment programs improves.

Guidelines for the initiation and choice of ART regimens for children in resource-limited settings have been developed by WHO and ANECCA,[9,39,42] and most countries have national guidelines. Recommendations for children are based on age, clinical staging, the presence of tuberculosis, pre-exposure to single-dose nevirapine during PMTCT, and the availability of immunologic and virologic tests.[9,39,42]

Taking diagnostic limitations into account, recommendations for the initiation of ART usually distinguish between children older and younger than 18 months, and accommodate settings with and without available CD4 testing.

Because the number of total lymphocytes and CD4 cells tends to fluctuate during intercurrent illnesses, abnormal results should be confirmed before therapeutic decisions are made. Table 55.2[38] summarizes the criteria for initiating antiretroviral therapy recommended by WHO.[39]

Several factors should be considered when choosing an antiretroviral treatment regimen for children. The availability of particular antiretroviral drugs and suitable pediatric formulations, as well as the costs of the drugs, will often be the primary factors determining the choice of the regimen. As in adults, the combination of two NRTIs (zidovudine or stavudine or abacavir plus lamivudine) and 1 NNRTI (nevirapine or efavirenz) is most commonly recommended as the first-line regimen in antiretroviral treatment-naive children by most national guidelines, by WHO and ANECCA (Table 55.3).[9,38,43]

Preliminary reports suggest that antiretroviral treatment of children is resource-constrained settings is feasible and improves the clinical condition of most children, with increases of CD4 counts and HIV-suppression.[44-47] Kline and co-workers[46] reported on the results obtained with a comprehensive care program for children, including the use of antiretroviral therapy, in Constanta, Romania. Most of the 452 children received a lopinavir-based HAART regimen. To limit costs, CD4 and HIV-RNA were measured at about 6-month intervals in only a subset of children. After a median 67 weeks of follow-up, about 90% of

Table 55.3 First-line regimens as recommended by WHO and ANECCA

	Recommended first-line regimens	Comments

Treatment naive child	2 NRTI plus 1 NNRTI
	Preferred
	  ZDV *or* d4T *or* ABC
	  Plus 3TC
	  Plus NVP or EFV (>3 years)
	Alternatives
	  ZDV *or* d4T *or* ABC
	  Plus 3TC
	  Plus PI
		Stavudine is an effective antiretroviral drug. However, prolonged use is more frequently associated with metabolic complications such as lipo-atrophy/dystrophy than ZDV and ABC
		When serious anemia is present stavudine or abacavir is a good alternative.
		Future switching of stavudine to zidovudine may be considered.
		Do not combine: ZDV/d4T and D4T/ddI.
		Efavirenz cannot yet be used in children <3 years because of lack of an appropriate formulation and dosing information in this age group.
		Girls who may become pregnant should not be treated with efavirenz (possible teratogenic effects of EFV).

Child with HIV and TB co-infection, present prior to the initiation of antiretroviral therapy	If condition of child allows: first complete TB treatment, defer antiretrovirals
	or defer antiretrovirals for 2 weeks to 2 months (depending on the child's condition).
	In case of co-treatment of TB and HIV with use of rifampicin the preferred ART regimen is:
	  ZDV *or* d4T *or* ABC
	  Plus 3TC
	  Plus EFV in child >3 years and/or >10 kg.
	If EFV cannot be used, the alternatives are limited:
	Neither NVP nor a PI-based regimen are optimal choices.
	WHO advises to use a triple NNRTI regimen in this case (ZDV, 3TC, ABC *or* d4T, 3TC, ABC).
	However, a 3-NRTI HAART based regimen has been shown less efficacious in adult studies (lower virologic potency).
		Rifampicin interacts with many antiretrovirals, decreasing antiretroviral drug levels and increasing rifampicin levels.
		The choice of ART regimen is usually extra complicated by the limited options for pediatric drug formulations.
		
		Co-administration of NVP with rifampicin is not advised. The concentration of NVP has been shown to be decreased by 20–58%; Virologic consequences are uncertain.
		When no other options are available, a dosage increase of 30% may be considered, but carefully monitor for hepatotoxicity.

TB occurring while child is already on antiretroviral therapy. Child requiring antiretroviral treatment after failure of single-dose nevirapine prophylaxis in PMTCT regimen	Switch of regimen is advised if nevirapine is used. For options: see above. 2 NRTIs plus protease inhibitor	

Sources: WHO 2005,[38] ANECCA 2004,[9] CDC 2005.[43]

the children continued taking their HAART. The treatment was well tolerated, CD4 counts improved, growth velocity normalized, and rates of hospitalization and annual mortality declined markedly from 8–19% in the previous 4 years to 3%.[46] Eley and co-workers[45] described their short-term experience in treating 80 children and their parents in Cape Town, South Africa. Most children had advanced disease with severe immunosuppression, but responded well to HAART.[45] Fassinou and co-workers[47] reported their experience with the treatment of 159 children in Cote d'Ivoire between 2000 and 2002. Branded as well as generic drugs were prescribed. The majority of children responded well and the authors conclude that antiretroviral treatment appeared as effective as in developed countries.[47] Puthanakit and co-workers[44] treated 107 Thai children between 2 and 14 years, most of them with severely advanced disease (median CD4 percentage of 3% and plasma HIV-RNA level of 5.4 $\log_{10}$). The children received a combination of stavudine, lamivudine, and either nevirapine or efavirenz, all generic and/or adult formulations. After 72 weeks of HAART, the median CD4 percentage was 21%, and 76% of the patients had an HIV-RNA level <50 copies/mL.

Finally, Medicin Sans Frontières recently reported the short-term follow-up (mean 6.9 months) of 1840 children <13 years on antiretroviral treatment in 11 countries in Africa and Asia. In this group, the majority of children also had advanced HIV disease when started on ART. Some 65% were treated with a combination of stavudine, lamivudine plus nevirapine, often using breakable adult tablets. The probability of survival after 6 months in this group was 91%, and for the group treated for >1 year, the probability of survival was 88%.[48]

These preliminary results are encouraging and demonstrate that antiretroviral treatment of children is feasible and can be effective in settings with limited facilities. One should realize, however, that these reports all represent a relatively short-term follow-up of <2 years. Further follow-up should give insight of the long-term efficacy and sustainability of these programs.

Moreover, several other important issues remain to be resolved. Appropriate and child-friendly drug formulations are not widely available, and, as a consequence, children are often treated with adult formulations (e.g. fixed dose tablets). While this approach may be effective in older children, as Puthanakit and co-workers[44] have shown, it may lead to suboptimal treatment in infants and small children as a result of underdosing or overdosing of antiretroviral drug components. New pediatric formulations (e.g. fixed dose combinations) are being developed and tested in the field. Solid formulations, such as fixed dose and crushable tablets, would be useful, because they are more easy to administer and less expensive than syrups, and have no specific storage requirements.[42] Many HIV-infected children are shifting between caregivers or staying with a very sick mother. Others are staying with an elderly grandmother who is responsible for many children and syrups tend to be harder to administer (P.M. pers comm). Moreover, syrups come in larger bulk and therefore are harder to hide, especially where the mother has not disclosed her status to family members.

Extensive use of stavudine, currently recommended as a first-line drug in many national guidelines and a standard component of various less expensive generic drug preparations, should be avoided because of its association with lipoatrophy and dystrophy. This complication occurred in up to 40% of children after prolonged use of antiretroviral regimens consisting of protease inhibitors and NRTIs, especially stavudine.[49,50] Zidovudine is therefore preferred in the first-line regimen but stavudine remains a good alternative if the child has severe anemia or if zidovudine is not available.

The optimal strategy for starting antiretroviral therapy, and indeed the optimal regimen, for HIV and tuberculosis co-infection is not known. Rifampicin interacts with many antiretrovirals, which may reduce levels of antiretroviral drugs and cause suboptimal therapy (see Ch. 31). Furthermore, clinical symptoms of tuberculosis may temporarily worsen as a result of an immune reconstitution inflammatory syndrome if antiretroviral therapy is started together with tuberculosis drugs. When tuberculosis is present prior to the initiation of antiretroviral treatment, the approach used by most experts is to treat the tuberculosis first and defer antiretroviral therapy for at least 2 months if the clinical condition of the child allows this. If the child develops tuberculosis while being treated with antiretrovirals, the drug regimen may need to be modified. If modification is not possible or combined treatment is not tolerated by the child, temporary interruption of antiretroviral treatment may sometimes be necessary (Table 55.3).[9,38,43]

Another important issue that should be taken into consideration when deciding whether to start antiretroviral treatment is the possibility of HIV resistance. Because of its simple design, nevirapine single-dose monoprophylaxis is currently one of the most frequently used HIV-mother-to-child intervention strategies in resource-limited settings. Although effective in lowering transmission rates by about 42%, a major drawback of this method is the selection of HIV-1 variants that are resistant to antiretroviral drugs. Resistant mutants have been detected in up to 69% of mothers and in up to 87% of infants after a single dose of nevirapine.[51-53] These mutations appear to fade with time, but a recent study indicated that they may persist for a year or longer.[54] Moreover, previous use of nevirapine as monotherapy, to prevent mother-to-child transmission, has been shown to compromise the efficacy of this drug in the future. A nevirapine-containing regimen was less efficacious in achieving virologic suppression in women who had received intrapartum nevirapine and who had developed detectable nevirapine resistance mutations than it was in women who did not develop such mutations.[55] However, the long-term clinical and virologic outcome of these women, and especially in women who were exposed to single-dose NVP more than 6 months prior to starting HAART, is not clear yet.

Preliminary data from infants in Botswana, perinatally exposed to single-dose NVP plus AZT, also show a less favorable virologic response with subsequent antiretroviral therapy.[56]

Therefore, a first-line regimen of two NRTIs plus a protease inhibitor is recommended if antiretroviral treatment is needed in these children.[9] However, because of cost, many sites in sub-Saharan Africa continue to use nevirapine based regimens in infants and children, exposed to single-dose nevirapine. The debate on the clinical impact of nevirapine exposure at birth on later HAART efficacy continues and studies in children are ongoing.

Therapy Failure and Second-line Regimens

As in adults, treatment failure in children is often caused by poor adherence. Other factors such as insufficient drug levels or an inadequate potency of the first-line regimen may also be responsible.[39] Treatment failure can be defined as clinical, immunologic of virologic. Because viral load testing is currently unavailable for routine monitoring in most resource-limited settings, the diagnosis of treatment failure will depend on clinical and/or immunologic grounds.

Clinical treatment failure and switching to a second-line regimen should be considered in case of disease progression to a new or recurrent WHO pediatric stage 3 or 4 condition in a child receiving antiretroviral therapy for at least 6 months (Table 55.4).[38,39,43]

WHO pediatric stage 3 and 4 clinical signs considered particularly important as clinical indicators of treatment failure are:

- Lack of or decline in growth rate in children who show an initial response to treatment (moderate or severe unexplained malnutrition not adequately responding to standard therapy despite adequate nutritional support and without other explanation), or
- loss of neurodevelopmental milestones or development of encephalopathy, or
- occurrence of new opportunistic infections or malignancies, or recurrence of infections, such as oral candidiasis that is refractory to treatment or oesophageal candidiasis.

Although defined as a stage 3 condition, the development of pulmonary tuberculosis alone is regarded as an exception and switching may not be necessary if the child responds well to tuberculostatic therapy.[39]

It may also be extremely difficult to discriminate between progression of clinical symptoms due to treatment failure or to the immune reconstitution inflammatory syndrome (IRIS). IRIS is caused by an inflammatory response to infectious pathogens present in the child as a result of immune recovery (see Ch. 18). This condition is common in adults, but has also been described in children.[57,58]

Before switching to a second line on the basis of presumed clinical failure, adherence should be ensured, and the child should have received adequate nutrition and treatment for opportunistic infections (Table 55.4).[38,39,43]

Antiretroviral therapy usually increases CD4 values. If this is not the case in a child on ART, the antiretroviral regimen should be reviewed and an alternative treatment option should be considered. Table 55.4[38,43] summarizes the criteria for treatment failure in children based on the pediatric CD4 values. Total lymphocyte counts may be used to guide initiation of ART where CD4 assays are unavailable (Table 55.2),[38] but should not be used to judge treatment response, because TLCs poorly predict treatment success.[39]

It is difficult to advise on second-line regimens in case of therapy failure in resource limited settings. Because cross-resistance often occurs within a drug

Table 55.4 When to consider treatment failure and switching to second-line therapy

Indication of clinical failure: occurrence of a new or recurrent WHO pediatric clinical stage symptom	
	Advice on switching to second-line
WHO stage 1 symptom	Do not switch to other regimen
WHO stage 2 symptom	Check for adherence to treatment Closely monitor clinical events Check CD4
WHO stage 3 symptom	Check for adherence to treatment Treat and manage co-infections and/or opportunistic infections[a] Consider nutritional issues in case of signs of growth failure Consider regimen switch
WHO stage 4 symptom	Check for adherence to treatment Treat and manage co-infections and/or opportunistic infections[a] Consider nutritional issues in case of signs of growth failure Switch regimen
Indication of immunologic failure: guided by CD4 cell count or percentage	
	Consider switch to second-line if:
Prior to considering switching to second line, check if the child has had at least 24 weeks of treatment and check adherence to therapy. Preferably at least two CD4 measurements should be available	Development of age-related severe immunodificiency after initial immune recovery New progressive age-related severe immunodeficiency, confirmed with at least one subsequent CD4 measurement Rapid rate of decline to below threshold of age-related severe immunodeficiency (especially if <15% in child 12–35 months of age, <10% in child 36–59 months of age, <100/mm^3 if ≥5 years of age).
Indication of virologic failure	
	Consider switch to second-line if:
At least two measurements (taken 1 week apart) should be performed before considering a change in therapy.	HIV-RNA not suppressed to undetectable levels after 4–6 months of antiretroviral therapy Repeated detection of HIV-RNA in children who initially had an undetectable level in response to antiretroviral therapy (If the HIV RNA increase is limited (i.e. <5000 c/mL) continued observation with more frequent evaluation of HIV RNA levels should be considered. Development of resistance mutations is likely to occur.

[a]Differentiation from the immune reconstitution inflammatory syndrome (IRIS) is important; also see text for specific remarks on the occurrence of pulmonary TB in a child receiving ART.
Source: WHO case definitions of HIV for surveillance and revised clinical staging and immunological classification of HIV-related disease in adults and children (www.who.int/hiv).

class, choosing drugs that the patient has not taken previously, may not be sufficient.

Common cross-resistance patterns occur, e.g. between zidovudine and stavudine and may include other NRTIs (depending on the mutations that have emerged), between lamivudine and emtricitabine, and between nevirapine and efavirenz (single mutations). For protease inhibitors, class resistance occurs only after at least 2–3 mutations.[43]

Ideally, a new regimen is based on the treatment history of the patient combined with resistance testing; however, resistance testing is currently not a feasible option in the majority of resource limited settings and second-line drug options are limited, especially for children. As a consequence, the choice of a reasonable second-line regimen will mainly depend on the local availability and affordability of alternative antiretroviral drugs.

If available, a child failing a first-line regimen with 2 NRTIs and a NNRTI should receive a potent, PI-based second-line regimen consisting of two new NRTI agents plus one ritonavir boosted PI.

Preparing for Antiretroviral Therapy, Follow-up, Monitoring, and Support for the Child and Family

In general, antiretroviral therapy is rarely considered an emergency, but for children under 1 year of age, antiretroviral therapy should be initiated in a timely manner because of the high mortality rate in this age group. In Table 55.5[9] the steps to successful therapy in children are summarized and advice about monitoring and follow-up is provided. Several important medical and social conditions should be assessed prior to starting ART. The child's baseline physical condition and laboratory values should be determined and his or her medical eligibility for ART should be assessed according to national or local guidelines. In most settings, depending on the facilities, laboratory evaluation includes a full blood count, including leukocyte and differential, ALT, chest X-ray, CD4 percentage or count or total lymphocyte count, and, if available, determination of the HIV-RNA concentration.

But it is at least as important to assess the mother's/caregiver's readiness to take 'responsibility' for antiretroviral therapy. Experience from both adults and children in Western countries shows that incomplete adherence is the most common reason for therapy failure and the emergence of HIV resistance.[59-61] Since young children rely on adults for the administration of their medications, it is of crucial importance to optimize the ability of the caregiver to guarantee administration of the antiretroviral drugs. Before antiretroviral treatment is started, the caregiver should understand the ins and outs of the regimen (which drugs, frequency, potential side-effects), the expected outcome of treatment, the need for life-long therapy, and the consequences of poor adherence. The caregiver should know that children, depending on their age, can control adherence by spitting out, vomiting, or refusing medication, and healthcare providers should help families to find ways to give medication to young children. It has been shown that the readiness of the parent to accept the necessary care for the child and comply with the advice is related to the acceptance of the HIV status of the child. Also, the caregiver's perception of medication efficacy is a significant predictor of child adherence.[62,63] It is important to take time to prepare the caregiver adequately, to identify potential barriers that may interfere with adherence, and to discuss and resolve these barriers as far as possible before antiretroviral therapy is started. Involvement of another caregiver to support the mother or guardian at time on initiation of therapy in case of sickness or death is critical to the success of the therapy.

In the initial months and first year after the start of antiretroviral therapy, follow-up visits should be planned regularly, to check on the medical condition of the child and possible side-effects, to determine whether the medication is administered correctly and to support and encourage the mother/caregiver, particularly when drug administration is difficult. If therapy goes well and the child recovers, then follow-up visits can be planned for once every 3–6 months (Table 55.4).[38,43] The intensity of laboratory and clinical monitoring of the efficacy of antiretroviral therapy will depend on local resources and manpower. In settings with limited resources and laboratory support, improved growth is an important indicator of successful therapy.[46,64] At every visit, both the caregiver and the child should be reminded about the importance of adherence because barriers to adherence may change over time.

For adolescents, young people between 10 and 19 years, specific issues have to be taken into account. This period in life is associated with major biological and social changes and adolescents are not a homogeneous group. Healthcare workers taking care of adolescents should tailor their guidance to the developmental stage and social context of the adolescent and to their specific needs. A major goal will be to help the adolescent to take responsibility for his/her own treatment.[9]

Psychosocial support of the child or adolescent, the caregivers and siblings is an essential component of comprehensive care for HIV-infected children and families. All members of HIV-infected families face many dark clouds related to the nature of the disease. They often have to cope with serious illness and bereavement of family members and experience feelings of fear, anger, sadness, depression, and despair. Parents feel guilty towards their child and fear rejection because of stigma associated with HIV/AIDS. Denial of their own diagnosis is not unusual, and trying to hide the HIV diagnosis from even close relatives may result in isolation and complicates adherence to ART. When parents are very ill or die, children may not only have to cope with severe emotional stress but also with grave socioeconomic consequences. They may have to take over the care for younger siblings, or shift between caregivers themselves; sometimes they lose their home and possibilities for education.

Counselling and psychosocial interventions aim to support the child and family to cope with these issues and to help find ways to solve problems.[9] Child peer support groups, and support groups for

Table 55.5 Steps to successful antiretroviral therapy in children

Preparation of the child and mother/caregiver
  Child
    Has HIV diagnosis been confirmed?
    Has a comprehensive clinical and laboratory assessment been conducted, including FBC, ALT and chest X-ray?
    Has the child's illness been categorized using the WHO or CDC classification scheme?
    Have the results of CD4 testing or TLC been reviewed?
    Has the HIV-RNA level been determined? (if available)
    Is the child eligible for antiretroviral therapy according to the WHO or CDC criteria?
  Mother/caregiver
    Has the mother/caregiver received information on antiretroviral drugs expected outcomes, potential side-effects?
    Did the mother/caregiver receive information on the expected visit schedule?
    Has the importance of adherence been discussed?
    Have barriers to adherence been discussed and resolved as far as possible? (if needed with support of community support groups)

Assessing the mother/caregiver's readiness
    Has the mother/caregiver disclosed the HIV status to anyone?
      Do the other people in the household know about the child's diagnosis?
    Does the mother/caregiver understand antiretroviral treatments, expected outcomes, potential side-effects?
    Who will give the medications to the child?
      Does this person know when and how much to give?
      Does this person know how to store the medication?
    Does the mother/caregiver have an understanding of the importance of strict adherence and the consequences of inadequate adherence?
    Does the mother/caregiver recognize the need for the child to take ARV for life, even if symptoms improve and the child feels better?
    Does the mother/ caregiver have a plan for when to give ARV and how not to miss doses?
    Does the mother/caregiver appreciate the need for intensive monitoring and follow-up?
    Is there support in the household/family?
    Is the living situation stable?
    Has the child tasted the medications?
    How does the child's developmental level influence the ability to take medications?
    Have the healthcare providers observed medication administration?

Monitoring and counselling during antiretroviral therapy
  Frequency of visits: check for local guidelines
    Common scheme:
      Year 1: week 2, 4, 8, 12, 24, 36, 48: check for correct administration of antiretrovirals and improvement of the child's clinical condition.
      Year 2 and on: If therapy goes well, visits can be spaced to once per 3–6 months.
  Clinical monitoring (every visit)
    Determine the child's growth (weight, height)
      Monitor head circumference in children <2 years
    Assess physical condition of the child, treat intercurrent illnesses
      Assess neurodevelopment once or twice a year
    Calculate drug doses based on weight, size and/or age
      Adjust dosage when necessary
      Dosage is weight dependent and must be adjusted for significant weight gain/loss
      A practical advice is to adjust the dose after every 5 kg weight gain
      Failure to adjust for weight gain can lead to underdosage and development of resistance
      Failure to adjust for weight loss can lead to overdosing and toxicity
    Review dose changes and reasons for changes with the family.
    Consider concomitant medications. Can they be given with the prescribed ARV treatment?
    Assess for side-effects and toxicities, both immediate and long term
      Each medication creates a particular set of worries.

Table 55.5 Steps to successful antiretroviral therapy in children—cont'd

Laboratory monitoring
Full blood count and ALT: week 4 after start antiretroviral treatment:
    If normal, then twice yearly.
CD4 percentage/count (if available): twice yearly
If CD4 assay is not available: use total lymphocyte counts
HIV-RNA concentration (if available): twice yearly.

Counseling
Reassess knowledge
Assess adherence: missed doses in previous weeks, reason?
Anticipate non-adherence during crisis periods for the patients
Support and encourage family adherence efforts
Celebrate treatment success.

Source: Adapted from ANECCA 2004.[9]

caregivers and other family members can play a vital role in this process.

Access to ART programs gives hope and a future to the child and its caregivers but it may take time before the family actually believe this to be true.

For the long-term success of antiretroviral therapy in children, it is important to ensure the well-being of not only the child but also of the other family members. In particular, the mother's health is of crucial importance to the child's future and chance of survival.[1] Care and treatment programs should therefore preferably be family focused.

Conclusion

Antiretroviral therapy is standard care and has dramatically improved the prognosis of HIV-infected children in affluent countries. Unfortunately, in those areas where the burden of HIV-infected children is highest, only a few children currently have access to adequate care and antiretroviral treatment. The prognosis of the vast majority of infected children remains extremely poor and there is an urgent need to start antiretroviral treatment in as many children as possible. Recent clinical care programs have shown that improved care and effective antiretroviral treatment of HIV-infected children in resource-limited settings is feasible and effective. These results are encouraging and should stimulate initiatives to extend pediatric treatment programs. Efforts should be undertaken to address specific pediatric needs, such as the development of appropriate and child-friendly drug formulations. An integrated approach that incorporates treatment of infected parents/caregivers and siblings probably offers the best chance to ensure long-term sustain-

ability of pediatric antiretroviral treatment programs. It will be a challenge to expand family programs into areas with a high need while at the same time ensuring a good quality of care.

References

1. Newell ML, Coovadia H, Cortina-Borja M, et al. Mortality of infected and uninfected infants born to HIV-infected mothers in Africa: a pooled analysis. Lancet 2004; 364:1236–1243.
2. Villamor E, Misegades L, Fataki MR, et al. Child mortality in relation to HIV infection, nutritional status, and socioeconomic background. Int J Epidemiol 2005; 34:61–68.
3. Ansari NA, Kombe AH, Kenyon TA, et al. Pathology and causes of death in a series of human immunodeficiency virus-positive and negative pediatric referral hospital admissions in Botswana. Pediatr Infect Dis J 2003; 22:43–47.
4. Chakraborty R. Infections and other causes of death in HIV-infected children in Africa. Paediatr Resp Rev 2004; 5:132–139.
5. Graham SM, Mtitimila EI, Kamamga HS, et al. Clinical presentation and outcome of *Pneumocystis carinii* pneumonia in Malawian children. Lancet 2000; 355:369–373.
6. Bakeera-Kitata S, Musoke P, Dowing R, et al. *Pneumocystis carinii* in children with severe pneumonia at Mulago Hospital, Uganda. Ann Trop Paediatr: Int Child Health 2004; 3:227–235.
7. Chintu C, Mudenda V, Lucas S, et al. Lung diseases at necropsy in African children dying from respiratory illnesses: a descriptive necropsy study. Lancet 2002; 360:985–990.
8. Ruffini DD, Mahdi SS. The high burden of *Pneumocystis carinii* pneumonia in African HIV-1-infected children hospitalized for severe pneumonia. AIDS 2002; 16:105–112.
9. Tindyebwa D, Kayita J, Musoke P, et al. ANECCA (African Network for the Care of Children affected by AIDS). Handbook on Paediatric AIDS in Africa. 2004. Online. Available: www.fhi.org/en/HIVAIDS/guide/mans1/htm.
10. Mahdi SA, Huebner RE, Deodens L, et al. HIV-1 co-infection in children hospitalized with tuberculosis in South Africa. Int J Tuberc Lung Dis 2000; 4:448–454.
11. Luo C, Chintu C. Bhat, et al. HIV infection in Zambian children with tuberculosis changing seroprevalence and evaluation of a TCZ free region. Tuberc Lung Dis 1994; 75:110–115.

12. Swaminathan S. Tuberculosis in HIV- infected children. Paediatr Resp Rev 2004; 5:225–230.

13. Zar H, Cotton M, Lombard C, et al. Early and unexpected benefit of isoniazid in reducing mortality in HIV-infected children in an area of high tuberculosis prevalence. Abstract No. LbOrB12. International AIDS Conference, Bangkok, Thailand: 11–16 July 2004.

14. Kalyesubula I, Musoke-Mudido P, Marum L, et al. Effects of malaria infection in human immunodeficiency virus type 1-infected Ugandan children. Pediatr Infect Dis J 1997; 16:876–881.

15. Grimwade K, French N, Mbatha DD, et al. Childhood malaria in a region of unstable transmission and high human immunodeficiency virus prevalence. Pediatr Infect Dis J 2003; 22:1057–1063.

16. Van Eijk AM, Ayisi JG, Ter Kuile FO, et al. Malaria and human immunodeficiency virus infection as risk factors for anemia in infants in Kisumu, Western Kenya. Am J Trop Hyg 2002; 67:44–53.

17. Greenberg AE, Nsa W, Ryder RW, et al. Plasmodium falciparum malaria and perinatally acquired human immunodeficiency virus type 1 infection in Kinshasa, Zaire. A prospective, longitudinal cohort study of 587 children. N Engl J Med 1991; 325:105–109.

18. Kublin JG, Patnaik P, Jere CS, et al. Effect of plasmodium falciparum malaria on concentration of HIV-1-RNA in the blood of adults in rural Malawi: a prospective cohort study. Lancet 2005; 365:233–240.

19. Kaplan LJ, Daum RS. Smaron, et al. Severe measles in immunocompromised patients. JAMA 1992; 267:1237–1241.

20. Kernahan J, McQuillin J, Craft AW. Measles in children who have malignant disease. Br Med J 1987; 295:15–18.

21. Perry RT, Mmiro F, Ndugwa C. Measles Infection in HIV-infected children. Ann N Y Acad Sci 2000; 918:377–380.

22. Mueller BU, Pizzo PA. Malignancies in pediatric AIDS. Curr Opin Pediatr 1996; 8:45–49.

23. Biggar RJ, Frisch M, Goedert JJ. Risk of cancer in children with AIDS. AIDS-Cancer Match Registry Study Group. JAMA 2000; 284:205–209.

24. Sanpakit K, Veerakul G, Kriengsuntornkij W, et al. Malignancies in HIV-infected children at Siraj Hospital. J Med Assoc (Thai) 2002; 85:S542–S548.

25. Newton R, Ziegler J, Beral V, et al. A case control study of human immunodeficiency virus infection and cancer in adults and children residing in Kampala, Uganda. Int J Cancer 2001; 92:622–627.

26. Athale UH, Patil PS, Chintu C, et al. Influence of HIV epidemic on the incidence of Kaposi's sarcoma in Zambian children. J Acquir Immune Defic Syndr Hum Retrovirol 1995; 8:96–100.

27. Amir H, Kaaya EE, Manji KP, et al. Kaposi's sarcoma before and during a human immunodeficiency virus epidemic in Tanzanian children. Pediatr Infect Dis J 2001; 20:518–521.

28. McKinney RE. Growth delay, failure to thrive, and wasting in the HIV-infected child. Pediatr Infect Dis J 1995; 6:32–39.

29. Lepage P, Msellati P, Hitimana DG, et al. Growth of human immunodeficiency virus type 1-infected and uninfected children: a prospective cohort study in Kigali, Rwanda, l998-l993. Pediatr Infect Dis J 1996; 15:479–485.

30. Villamor E, Fataki MR, Bosch RJ, et al. Human immunodeficiency virus infection, diarrheal disease and sociodemographic predictors of child growth. Acta Paediatr 2004; 93:372–379.

31. Mulholland EK, Adegbola RA. Bacterial infections-a major cause of death among children in Africa. N Engl J Med 2005; 1:75–77.

32. Sherman GG, Stevens G, Stevens WS. Affordable diagnosis of human immunodeficiency virus infection in infants by p24 antigen detection. Pediatr Infect Dis J 2004; 23:173–176.

33. Mofenson LM, Harris DR, Moyle J, et al. Alternatives to HIV-RNA concentration and CD4 counts to predict mortality in HIV-infected children in resource-poor settings. Lancet 2003; 362:1625–1627.

34. HIV Paediatric Prognostic Markers Collaborative Study. Use of total lymphocyte count for informing when to start antiretroviral therapy in HIV-infected children: a meta-analysis of longitudinal data. Lancet 2005; 366: 1868–1874.

35. Enbree J, Bwayo J, Nagelkerke N, et al. Lymphocyte subsets in human immunodeficiency virus type 1-infected and uninfected children in Nairobi. Pediatr Infect Dis J 2001; 20:397–403.

36. Lugada ES, Mermin J, Kaharuza F, et al. Population-based hematologic and immunologic reference values for a healthy Ugandan population. Clin Diagn Lab Immunol 2004; 11:29–34.

37. Lau B, Gange SJ, Phair JP, et al. Use of total lymphocyte count and hemoglobulin concentration for monitoring progression of HIV infection. J Acquir Immune Def Syndr 2005; 39:620–624.

38. WHO. Antiretroviral treatment of HIV infection in infants and children in resource limited settings, towards universal access: recommendations for a public health approach. WHO 2005 revision, draft October 2005. Geneva: World Health Organization; 2005. Online. Available: www.who. int/hiv/pub/guidelines/paedARTguideDRAFT_ webreviewNOV05%20_2_.pdf

39. WHO. Interim WHO clinical staging of HIV/AIDS and HIV/ AIDS case definitions for surveillance. Geneva: World Health Organization; 2005. Online. Available: www.who. int/3by5/publications/documents/arv_guidelines/en

40. Chintu C, Bhat GJ, Walker AS, et al. CHAP trial team. Co-trimoxazole as prophylaxis against opportunistic infections in HIV-infected Zambian children (CHAP): a double-bind randomised placebo-controlled trial. Lancet 2004; 364:1865–1871.

41. Van Kooten Niekerk NK, Knies MM, Howard J, et al. The first five years of the family clinic for HIV at the Tygerberg Hospital: Family demographics, survival of children and early impact of antiretroviral therapy. J Trop Pediatr 2005; 52:3–11.

42. WHO. Scaling up antiretroviral therapy: revision. Geneva: World Health Organization; 2003. Online. Available: www. who.int/3by5/publications/documents/arv_guidelines/en

43. CDC. Guidelines for the use of antiretroviral agents in HIV-1-infected adults and adolescents. CDC, 2005: Online. Available: http://AIDSinfo.nih.gov

44. Puthanakit T, Oberdorfer A, Akarathum N, et al. Efficacy of highly active antiretroviral therapy in HIV-infected children in Thailand's national access to antiretroviral program. CID 2005; 41:100–107.

45. Eley B, Nutall J, Davies MA, et al. Initial experience of a public sector antiretroviral treatment programme for HIV infected children and their infected parents, S. Afric Med J 2004; 94:643–646.

46. Kline MW, Matusa RF, Copalu L, et al. Comprehensive pediatric human immunodeficiency virus care and treatment in Constantia, Romania: implementation of a program of highly active antiretroviral therapy in a resource-poor setting. Pediatr Infect Dis J 2004; 23:696–700.

47. Fassinou P, Elenga N, Rouet F, et al. Highly active antiretroviral therapies among HIV-1-infected children in Abidjan, Cote d'Ivoire. AIDS 2004; 18:1905–1913.

48. AIDS working group. Epicentre, Medicins sans Frontieres. Very satisfactory outcomes can be achieved in children treated with highly active antiretroviral treatment under programme conditions in resource limited settings: the experience of Medicins Sans Frontieres. Abstract WE OaBo201. 3rd IAS Conference on HIV Pathogenesis and Treatment, Rio de Janeiro: 2005.

49. McComsey GA, Leonard E. Metabolic complications of HIV therapy in children. AIDS 2004; 18:1753–1768.

50. European Paediatric Lipodystrophy Group. Antiretroviral therapy, fat redistribution and hyperlipidaemia in HIV-infected children in Europe. AIDS 2004; 18:1443–1451.

51. Eshelman SH, Mracna M, Guay LA, et al. Selection and fading of resistance mutations in women and infants

receiving nevirapine to prevent HIV-1 transmission (HIV-NET 012). AIDS 2001; 15:1951–1957.

52. Eshelman SH, Hoover DR, Chen S, et al. Nevirapine (NVP) resistance in women with HIV-1 subtype C, compared with subtypes A and D, after the administration of single-dose NVP. J Infect Dis 2005; 192:30–36.

53. Eshelman SH, Hoover DR, Hudelson SE, et al. Development of nevirapine resistance in infants is reduced by the use of infant-only single dose nevirapine plus zidovudine postexposure prophylaxis for the prevention of mother-to-child transmission of HIV-1. J Infect Dis 2006; 193:479–481.

54. Flys T, Nissley DV, Claasen CW, et al. Sensitive drug-resistance assays reveal long term persistence of HIV-1 variants with the K103N nevirapine (NVP) resistance mutation in some women and infants after the administration of single-dose NVP : HIVNET 012. J Infect Dis 2005; 192:1–3.

55. Jourdain G, Ngo-Giang N, Le Coeur S, et al. Intrapartum exposure to nevirapine and subsequent maternal responses to nevirapine-based antiretroviral therapy. N Engl J Med 2004; 351:229–240.

56. Lockman S, Shapiro RL, Smeaton LM, et al. Response to antiretroviral therapy after a single, peripartum dose of nevirapine. New Engl J Med 2007; 356:135–147.

57. Puthanakit T, Oberdorfer P, Punjaisee S, et al. Immune reconstitution syndrome due to bacillus Calmette-Guerin after initiation of antiretroviral therapy in children with HIV infection. Clin Infect Dis 2005; 41:1049–1052.

58. Puthanakit T, Oberdorfer P, Akarathum N, et al. Immune reconstitution syndrome after highly active antiretroviral therapy in human immunodeficiency virus-infected Thai children. Pediatr Infect Dis J 2006; 25:53–58.

59. Paterson DL, Swindells S. Mohr, et al. Adherence to protease inhibitor therapy and outcomes in patients with HIV infection. Ann intern Med 2000; 133:21–30.

60. Reddington C, Cohen J, Baldillo A, et al. Adherence to medication regimens among children with human immunodeficiency virus infection. Pediatr Infect Dis J 2000; 19:1148–1153.

61. Gibb DM, Goodall RL, Giacometti V, et al. Adherence to prescribed antiretroviral therapy in human immunodeficiency virus-infected children in the PENTA 5 trial. Pediatr Infect Dis J 2003; 22:56–62.

62. Brouwer CNM, Lok CL, Wolffers L, et al. Psychosocial and economic aspects of HIV/AIDS and counselling of caretakers of HIV infected children in Uganda. AIDS care 2000; 12:535–540.

63. Steele RG, Grauer D. Adherence to antiretroviral therapy for pediatric HIV infection: review of the literature and recommendations for research. Clin Child Fam Psychol Rev 2003; 6:17–30.

64. Benjamin DK, Miller WC, Ryder RW, et al. Growth patterns reflect response to antiretroviral therapy in HIV-positive infants: potential utility in resource-poor settings. AIDS Patient Care 2004; 18:35–43.

CHAPTER 56

Epidemiology, Natural History and Treatment of HIV-2 Infections

Maarten F. Schim van der Loeff

Introduction

In 1986, 3 years after the discovery of HIV-1, another retrovirus was identified, and named HIV-2.[1,2] It was isolated from West African patients with AIDS and its discovery caused concern that another devastating epidemic was at hand. Quite soon, it was shown that HIV-2 is less transmissible, is characterized by slower disease progression, and is geographically limited to West Africa and countries with direct ties to that region. The probable explanation of the epidemiological differences is that the plasma viral load in HIV-2 infected persons tends to be much lower than in HIV-1 infected persons.[3–6] In this chapter, the epidemiology, natural history, interactions with HIV-1, and treatment of HIV-2 are discussed. The comparison with HIV-1 is central to this chapter (see Table 56.1).[3–32]

Epidemiology

The transmission routes of HIV-2 are the same as for HIV-1: vaginal intercourse, anal intercourse, mother-to-child transmission, blood transfusion, parenteral (e.g. needle-stick incidents, needle sharing among intravenous drug users).[7] The efficiency of heterosexual transmission of HIV-2 is about $^1/_3$–$^1/_4$ that of HIV-1.[33,8] This can be explained by the generally lower plasma viral load, but no data have been published to prove this. Heterosexual intercourse is thought to account for the large majority of HIV-2 infections worldwide.

Prevalence and Incidence

The prevalence of HIV-2 exceeds 5% in the adult general population in only one country, Guinea-Bissau.[34] In other West African countries the prevalence in the general population is usually around 1 or 2%. Among high-risk groups higher prevalences have been observed (e.g. among female commercial sex workers: 38% in Southern Senegal,[35] 27.5% in The Gambia,[36] 41% in Abidjan, Cote d'Ivoire).[37] Outside West Africa, the infection is found in Portugal (the former colonial power in Guinea-Bissau), where 4% of AIDS cases are caused by HIV-2, and sporadically elsewhere in Europe.[38–41] In the USA, only one case of HIV-2 infection was detected among 7 000 000 blood donors over a 4-year period (1997–2000).[42] Sporadic cases of HIV-2 have also been detected in Asia (e.g. India, Korea) and South America (e.g. Brazil).

All repeated cross-sectional studies from West African countries have shown stable or declining prevalences of HIV-2; this was the case in diverse populations like female commercial sex workers,[33,36,37,43–46] an occupational cohort,[34] pregnant women,[34,37,47–49] STD patients,[50,51,51A] and the general population.[52]

There are very few studies reporting incidence rates of HIV-2. In a peri-urban community in Guinea-Bissau the incidence was 0.5 per 100 person-years of observation (pyo);[53] among female commercial sex workers in Dakar the incidence rate was 1.1 per 100 pyo.[33] Three cohort studies reported incidence rates over different time periods; among commercial sex workers in Dakar the incidence was stable[33] and in an occupational cohort and in a peri-urban

Table 56.1 Comparing HIV-1 and HIV-2

Characteristic	HIV-1	HIV-2
Epidemiological		
Geographic spread[7]	Worldwide	West Africa; rare elsewhere
Risk factors[7]	History of STDs, laboratory evidence of STIs, multiple partners, history of commercial sex	Same
Age with highest prevalence	20–34 years	40–55 years
Epidemic trend	Variable	Stable or declining in most countries
Global number of cases[7]	40 000 000	2 000 000[a]
Transmission routes[7]	Heterosexual, homosexual, mother-to-child, blood transfusions, needle sharing/incidents	Same
Mother-to-child-transmission[4]	20–40%	1–4%
Sexual transmission[8]		$1/3$–$1/4$ of that of HIV-1
Clinical		
Median time to progression to AIDS[5,6,22]	10 years	>10 years
Kaposi's Sarcoma[17]	Common	Less common
Proportion of infected subjects that develop AIDS if not treated	>99%	Unknown, but much lower
Independent predictors of AIDS and mortality[5,6,15]	High PVL and low CD4	High PVL and low CD4
Excess mortality (compared with uninfected adults)[18]	10-fold	2–3 fold
Virological		
Closest simian virus	SIV_{cpz}	SIV_{sm}
Homology to closest simian virus	Distant	75–85%
Presumed timing of zoonotic event[12]	1930	1940
Presumed number of zoonotic events	1 (causing worldwide HIV-1 group M epidemic) several (causing sporadic N and M infections)	8 (equal to number of subtypes)
Subtypes[9,10,11,23]	Within group M: A,B,C,D,F, G,H, I,J,K, and several circulating recombinant forms	A,B,C,D,E,F,G,H
Genes	*pol, gag, env, nef, tat, rev, vif, vpr* *vpu*	Same *vpx*
Plasma viral load[3,5,14,19]	Usually high: 10 000–100 000 copies/ml	Usually low: undetectable to 1000 copies/ml; $1/3$–$1/5$ of subjects have undetectable PVL
Proviral load (in asymptomatic subjects)[13,14,16,24,25]	Similar	Similar
Use of co-receptors[21]	CCR5 and CXCR4	Broader: CCR5 and CXCR4 and several others
Sensitive to NNRTI[20]	Yes	No
Immunological		
CD4 decline[14,26]	Fast	Slow
Immune activation[27,28]	High	Low
Neutralizing antibodies	Efficient, broad specificity	Less efficient, narrow specificity
CTL[29,30,31]	Common, mostly against *gag*	Same
Apoptosis of T cells[27,32]	High	Low
Cross-reactive responses to other HIV[29]	46% of patients have CTL responses to HIV-2 peptides	27% of patients have CTL responses to HIV-1 peptides

STD, sexually transmitted disease; STI, sexually transmitted infection; PVL, plasma viral load; SIV, simian immunodeficiency virus; cpz, chimpanzee; sm, sooty mangabey; CTL, cytotoxic T lymphocyte; NNRTI, non-nucleoside reverse transcriptase inhibitor; PBMC, peripheral blood mononuclear cell. [a]Author's estimate.

community in Bissau the rates were falling over time in men and stable in women.[34,52] Because all studies report stable or declining incidences and prevalences in West Africa, and no new HIV-2 epidemics have been observed outside West Africa, HIV-2 should not be considered an emergent epidemic, but an epidemic in decline.

In striking contrast to HIV-1, the highest prevalence of HIV-2 is not observed in young adults (15 to 34 years) but in older adults. This is the case in all study populations, whether female commercial sex workers, clinic patients, pregnant women or the general population. HIV-2 infection is very rare in children, even in Guinea-Bissau. The higher prevalence among older people could be the result of a cohort effect (lifelong infection with low mortality), or of an increased susceptibility of older persons, especially women.[54,55] The low prevalence among children is due to the very low mother-to-child transmission rate of 4%, which again can be attributed to the lower plasma viral load in HIV-2-infected pregnant women.[4]

Origin of HIV-2 and of the Epidemic

The trend of a declining epidemic raises one of the fundamental, still unanswered questions about HIV-2: which events created the epidemic, and what has changed so that the epidemic is no longer sustained? HIV-2 is genetically indistinguishable from the simian immunodeficiency virus of the sooty mangabey (SIV$_{sm}$)[56] monkey. The natural habitat of the sooty mangabey (Cercocebus torquatus atys) is West Africa. Based on the large degree of genetic homology, the geographic overlap, and the fact that human–monkey contacts are common in West Africa, most researchers maintain that SIV$_{sm}$ is the source of HIV-2.[57] In a phylogenetic tree, most subtypes of HIV-2 cluster closer to specific strains of SIV$_{sm}$ than to each other.[58,59] Therefore it is assumed that the eight different clades of HIV-2[9-11] represent at least eight different zoonotic events.

HIV-1 is thought to originate from chimpanzee SIV (SIV$_{cpz}$); the exact details of this zoonotic event are unknown and are controversial.[60,61] Back-calculations using mutation rates of the viral genome as a molecular clock have estimated the timing of the original transmission from chimpanzee to human at about 1930.[62,63] In analogy to HIV-1, these back-calculations have recently been done for HIV-2. Based on partial sequences of 33 samples, the most likely date of the zoonotic event giving rise to the HIV-2 subtype A epidemic was estimated to be 1940 (± 16 years).[12]

Assuming that one person or a few persons became infected with HIV-2 clade A through contact with a sooty mangabey, it is still unclear how this led to an epidemic. It is theoretically possible that the virus used to be more virulent than it is now, but this is unlikely: there is no record of an epidemic of an AIDS-like syndrome in West Africa prior to 1985. So, if we assume that the virulence of the virus has not substantially changed over time, there must have been an increase in transmission that amplified a small outbreak into a large epidemic. This could have been due to an increase in unscreened blood transfusions on a large scale, high rates of sexual partner change, many concurrent sexual partnerships or presence of co-factors enhancing sexual transmission like sexually transmitted infections (STIs), or non-sterile injections. Several of these factors may have been present at the same time in Guinea-Bissau, especially in the period from 1963 to 1974, when a war of independence was fought against Portugal. The transmission of the virus may not be efficient enough to maintain ongoing epidemic spread in the absence of important amplifiers such as frequent commercial sex, high levels of STIs, and unscreened blood transfusions.

Marx hypothesized that re-use of unsterilized needles may have been responsible for both the HIV-1 and HIV-2 epidemics.[57] In West Africa, various mass vaccination and treatment campaigns against yaws, yellow fever, and small pox were conducted in the final decades of the colonial era,[64] and these may have been responsible for mass inoculations with HIV-2. There is no proof for this and it does not explain why HIV-2 became epidemic in Guinea-Bissau and nowhere else.

Natural History

HIV-2 infection can lead to disease manifestations, including AIDS, that are similar to those seen in HIV-1 infection. Not all infected persons progress to clinical disease, and the extent of non-progressors is not known. In Senegal 85% of HIV-2 infected women in a sero-incident cohort remained free of disease 8 years later.[65,66] In Guinea-Bissau, several persons aged over 80 years were HIV-2 infected and symptom-free; the date of infection in these octogenarians is uncertain but is presumed to be some decades ago. There are case reports of persons who have been infected 20 years or more without clinical signs and symptoms.

Although the average progression to symptomatic disease and premature death is much slower in

HIV-compared with HIV-1, fast disease progression does occur.[40] Once patients have a CD4 count below 200 cells/μL[67] or they have AIDS[67A], the mortality rate is similar to that in HIV-1. In The Gambia, the median time to death after AIDS was 12.6 months. This was significantly longer than that of HIV-1 infected patients, and the difference was attributed to the higher CD4 count at time of AIDS in HIV-2 compared with HIV-1 infected patients.[67A]

As in HIV-1 infection, lower CD4 counts are associated with symptomatic HIV-2 infection and mortality. The CD4 count is an independent predictor of mortality.[67] In a clinic-based study in The Gambia the mortality rate among HIV-2 infected women with CD4 count ≥500 cells/μL was 8.1 per 100 pyo; in those with CD4 counts between 200 and 500 cells/μL it was 18.4 per 100 pyo; and among those with CD4 count <200 cells/μL it was 83.6 per 100 pyo.[67] Also in community-based studies from The Gambia and Guinea-Bissau[5,6,13] mortality rates were significantly higher in the groups with lower CD4 counts. In the clinic-based study from The Gambia the mortality rates were similar between HIV-1 and HIV-2 infected patients with CD4 counts below 200 cells/μL, but were significantly lower for HIV-2 infected patients compared to HIV-1 infected patients in the group with CD4 cell counts ≥500 cells/μL.[67]

Plasma and Proviral Load

The plasma viral load (PVL) in HIV-2 infected persons tends to be much lower than in HIV-1 infection.[3,4,14] In a community-based sample of 130 HIV-2 infected persons in rural Guinea-Bissau, the median PVL was only 347 copies/mL.[5] In a cross-sectional clinic-based study in The Gambia, 17 of 23 asymptomatic patients (74%) had undetectable PVL.[3] In the latter study it was also shown that the PVL varied with disease stage. Among patients with CD4% >28%, the median PVL was 460 copies/mL; among those with CD4% between 14% and 28%, the median PVL was 28 000 copies/mL; and among those with CD4% <14% the median PVL was 65 000 copies/mL.[3] In a clinic-based study in Senegal, plasma viral load predicted CD4 decline in HIV-2, like in HIV-1 infection. The annual rate of decline of the CD4 count among asymptomatic HIV-2 patients was $1/4$ that of asymptomatic HIV-1 patients (4.1% versus 15.9%).[14] The difference in loss of CD4 cells could be attributed to the lower plasma viral load in HIV-2 infected patients, and was not determined by the HIV type per se.[14]

HIV-2 plasma viral load is an independent and strong predictor of mortality.[5,6,15] In a community-based study in Guinea-Bissau, the mortality rate among HIV-2 infected persons rose 1.7 times (95% Confidence Interval 1.2–2.3, $P = 0.002$) for each $\log_{10}$ increase of virus copies/mL.[5] In a study among women recruited during pregnancy in The Gambia, the mortality rate among infected persons with undetectable PVL and normal CD4% was not significantly different from that of women without HIV infection.[6] In a multivariate analysis, PVL and CD4 count were independent predictors of mortality, but HIV type (HIV-1 or HIV-2) was not.[6] Thus in HIV-2 infection, like in HIV-1 infection, plasma viral load is a crucial predictor of disease progression.

Integrated viral DNA (provirus) is the source of all plasma virions. HIV-2-infected patients have DNA viral loads similar to those in HIV-1 patients,[13,14,16,68] but the plasma concentration of virions is lower in HIV-2 infection.[3] This could be explained in several ways. Perhaps a larger proportion of HIV-1 proviruses is actively replicating. Another possibility is that in HIV-1 infection, more DNA is integrated and replication-competent compared with HIV-2. It is also possible that in HIV-1 infection, high proviral DNA levels exist in other compartments than blood. Finally, it may be that HIV-2 virions are cleared more efficiently.[14] In six long-term non-progressing HIV-2 infected patients with undetectable plasma viral load and normal CD4 counts, it could be demonstrated that replication-competent virus was present in peripheral blood mononuclear cells (PBMCs), albeit at extremely low concentrations.[69]

Clinical Features

Although clinical AIDS in HIV-2 is similar to that in HIV-1, a few differences have been observed. Despite a similar prevalence of HHV8 infection, HIV-2 infected subjects had a much lower incidence of Kaposi's sarcoma in a study from The Gambia.[17] An autopsy study from Cote d'Ivoire found that HIV-2 infected patients were more likely to have severe multi-organ cytomegalovirus (CMV) infection, HIV encephalitis, and cholangitis than HIV-1 infected patients, suggesting a more prolonged terminal disease course.[70] Tuberculosis (TB) is a major opportunistic infection for HIV-2 infected patients, and its incidence increases strongly with decreasing CD4 counts.[71] In a clinic-based study from The Gambia, no difference in TB incidence was observed between HIV-1- and HIV-2-infected persons with similar CD4 counts. A study among hospital patients in Dakar found that chronic diarrhea and diarrhea caused by bacterial infections were more frequent in HIV-2 compared with HIV-1-infected patients with AIDS; oral candidiasis and chronic fever were more frequent in HIV-1 patients with AIDS.[72]

The median CD4 count among HIV-2 patients with AIDS varied between 73 and 358 cells/μL in several studies from West Africa and Paris.[39, 67A,72-75] In a clinic-based study in The Gambia, the median CD4 count at the time of AIDS diagnosis was 176 cells/μL in HIV-2 patients ($n = 87$), which was significantly higher than the 109 cells/μL in HIV-1 patients ($n = 341$).[67A]

The median CD4 count near the time of death was found to be between 61 and 146 cells/μL in HIV-2 infected patients.[67A,70,76] This is higher than the usual CD4 count at time of death reported from HIV-1 infection, but most studies on HIV-1 were done in developed countries with better end-of-life care than in most of Africa.

One of the first epidemiological studies on HIV-2, conducted in Bissau in 1987–1988,[77] showed that the mortality associated with HIV-2 infection was much lower than that usually found in HIV-1 infection. All subsequent studies have confirmed this.[5,6,53,67,73,78] In a seroprevalent clinical cohort in The Gambia, HIV-2 patients had a lower mortality than HIV-1 patients, but this lower mortality was limited to those with a normal CD4 count (>500/μL). Among those with a CD4 count <200/μL, the mortality rate was similar between HIV-1- and HIV-2-infected subjects.[67] This could be explained in two ways. The first possibility is that all HIV-2-infected subjects experience a deterioration of their immune system, but this decline is slower than in HIV-1 infection. Once the CD4 count has declined to below 200/μL, patients are at high risk of fatal opportunistic infections and there is no difference in mortality. The other possibility is that those with HIV-2 infection fall in either of two categories: those whose immune system is not affected at all by the infection, and those whose immune system is damaged by the infection, at a rate similar to HIV-1. This question is unresolved and long-term follow-up of an incident cohort would be required to answer it.

HIV-2 infection in children is rare, even in endemic areas, due to the low mother-to-child transmission risk of 4%.[4] There are few data on the clinical course of HIV-2 in children. In the only prospective long-term observational study of children with perinatally acquired HIV infection (median follow-up time 6.6 years), conducted in The Gambia, three out of eight HIV-2 infected children died (38%) compared

with 12 out of 17 HIV-1 infected children (71%) and 40 out of 448 children of HIV-uninfected mothers (9%). The mortality rate of HIV-2-infected children was significantly higher than that of uninfected children ($P = 0.02$), but the difference with HIV-1-infected children did not reach statistical significance ($P = 0.08$).[79]

HIV-1 and HIV-2 Interactions

Dual Infection

Using type-specific antibody tests, it became evident that both HIV-1 and HIV-2 circulated in West Africa. Samples of some people in West Africa showed dual serological reactivity, and it was not clear whether this was mainly due to antibody cross-reactivity, dual infection, or an infection with a third, unknown virus.[80] Quite early on, it was demonstrated by PCR that dual infection with both HIV-1 and HIV-2 did occur.[81,82] Later improvements in PCR techniques showed that a large proportion of people with dually reactive samples (up to 86%) is truly dually infected.[83,84]

HIV-2 does not Protect against HIV-1 Infection

In 1995, Travers and co-workers[85] reported that HIV-2 seemed to offer protection against subsequent HIV-1 infection in a cohort of commercial sex workers in Dakar; this caused excitement and hope as it could lead to the development of a vaccine against HIV-1.[18] Several research groups in Guinea-Bissau,[34,86] Cote d'Ivoire,[87,88] and The Gambia[89,90] examined this putative effect in other cohorts. None of the seven analyses so far have been able to reproduce this finding, so currently available epidemiological data do not support a protective effect of HIV-2 infection against incident HIV-1 infection.[91] The investigators of the cohort in which the original finding was made, have provided no updates of the effect in that cohort since 1999,[66,92,93] so it is unknown whether the effect in that cohort persisted, or declined over time, or even reversed. Two studies compared the distribution of HIV-1 subtypes among singly infected and HIV-1 and HIV-2 dually infected subjects, and found no differences in frequencies.[94,95] This argues against a possible protective effect of HIV-2 that is limited to certain HIV-1 subtypes.

HIV-2 does not Protect against Progression of HIV-1 Disease

Two cross-sectional studies from West Africa have examined the pattern of PVL and CD4 count in dually infected patients. In these studies it was found that in patients with low CD4 counts, the PVL of HIV-1 is very high and that of HIV-2 very low.[96,97] This contrasts with singly infected HIV-2 patients with low CD4 counts, in whom the PVL tends to be high.[3,96] In dually infected patients with normal CD4 counts, the PVL of HIV-2 tended to be comparable with that in singly HIV-2 infected subjects. In all CD4 strata, the PVL of HIV-1 appeared similar to that in HIV-1-singly infected subjects.[96] This suggests that in patients with progressing immunodeficiency, HIV-1 is out-competing HIV-2, and that the disease progression is dictated by HIV-1 rather than HIV-2.

There is only one long-term study analyzing the survival and mortality of subjects with dual HIV infection.[67] Among patients of the genito-urinary (GU) clinic in Fajara, The Gambia, the mortality rate of 107 dually infected patients was similar to that of HIV-1-infected patients, and worse than that of HIV-2-infected patients. This was true overall, and after adjusting for baseline CD4 count. These data do not support suggestions that HIV-2 infection could mitigate the course of HIV-1 infection.

HIV-1/HIV-2 Recombination

If a person is infected with two or more subtypes of HIV-1, these can re-combine their genomes to form new strains of HIV-1, and these can be transmitted. Some of the recombinant strains are successful in spreading, e.g. CRF01_AE in Thailand and CRF02_AG in West Africa.[98] Recombinations of the genetically rather distant groups O and M have been described,[99–101] but so far no recombinations of HIV-1 and HIV-2 have been reported. Construction of chimeric HIV-1/SIV viruses indicate that this is biologically possible.[102,103] Curlin and co-workers[104] searched for recombinations in the *env* gene of 46 dually infected patients in Senegal, but found none. It is possible that these recombinations are very rare or that their productive existence is constrained by biological factors.[104]

Treatment of HIV-2 Infection

As PVL and CD4 count are key predictors of disease progression in both HIV-1 and HIV-2,[5,6,14,15] it appears logical to use the same principles in their treatment. The mortality rate of HIV-2 infected subjects with undetectable PVL and normal CD4 count is not increased compared with uninfected people,[6] and these people may never need treatment. Randomized controlled clinical trials for treatment of HIV-2 infection have not been done, and at the time of writing, there are no agreed international treatment guidelines specific to HIV-2. Available clinical data are case reports,[105,106] case series,[41,39,107] and cohorts.[108,109] The suggestions for treatment given here are based on the few available clinical data, on *in vitro* studies, and on extrapolation of what is known from treatment of HIV-1 infection.

Initiating Treatment

ART should be started when the patient has AIDS. Symptomatic, non-AIDS, disease should not be an indication for treatment, as the symptoms or conditions may be unrelated to HIV-2. This is especially important in sub-Saharan Africa, where the background incidence of HIV-associated conditions is relatively high.[110] Patients with a CD4 count <200 cells/μL should be started on ART. For those with a CD4 count between 200 and 350 cells/μL, ART should be considered, and those with CD4 counts above 350 cells/μL should be monitored but treatment could be deferred (Table 56.2).

Objective of Treatment

The objective of treatment should be to reduce the PVL to undetectable levels. As there is no commercially available plasma viral load assay, it will be difficult in practice to monitor PVL outside specialized research centers where in-house assays have been developed.[3,14,19,111–113] Therefore monitoring of

Table 56.2 Suggested guidelines for initiating antiviral therapy of patients with HIV-2 infection

Disease stage		Recommendation
Clinical	CD4 count	
AIDS	Any CD4 count	Start ART
Symptomatic or asymptomatic	≤200 CD4 cells/μL	Start ART
	>200 and ≤350 CD4 cells/μL	Consider ART[a]
	>350 CD4 cells/μL	Defer ART

[a]When plasma viral load is high (e.g. >10 000 copies/mL), there is more reason to start ART than when plasma viral load is low. ART, antiviral therapy.

CD4 count may be the only option, but this will be showing treatment failure at a later stage than monitoring plasma viral load.

Resistance and Adherence

HIV-2 is inherently resistant to the non-nucleoside analog reverse transcriptase inhibitor (NNRTI) class of drugs.[20,114-116] The virus can become resistant to nucleoside-analog reverse transcriptase inhibitors (NRTIs) and to protease inhibitors (PIs).[41,117] Although no data are available, it is assumed that adherence is as crucial in HIV-2 as in HIV-1 to prevent resistance formation and maintain suppression of plasma viral load. In recent years, resistance mutations in HIV-2 have been identified, but the interpretation of genotypic resistance data in HIV-2 is difficult and no agreed guidelines exist.[118-120] Some mutations appear to have the same significance as in HIV-1 infection (e.g. M184V conferring resistance against lamivudine and Q151M conferring resistance against NRTIs),[108,109,121] but other mutations may have an impact different to that in HIV-1.[118,119]

Choice of Drugs

Although *overall,* HIV-2 is a less virulent virus than HIV-1, patients that have progressing infection, with HIV-associated symptoms, high PVL, and decreasing CD4 count, have a poor prognosis, similar to HIV-1 infected patients.[6,67] Therefore they should be treated as vigorously as HIV-1-infected patients, with at least three drugs. NNRTIs are not active against HIV-2.[20,114-116] NRTIs and PIs are effective, although clinical studies suggested that nelfinavir is less effective against HIV-2 than against HIV-1.[41,108,109] Amprenavir and atazanavir are not active against HIV-2 *in vitro.*[20,116] In *in vitro* studies, HIV-2 strains appeared to be naturally resistant against the fusion inhibitor enfuvirtide.[116] This means that there are far fewer therapeutic options for HIV-2 patients. A first option could be a combination of two NRTIs and a boosted PI, e.g. indinavir or lopinavir.[109] The choice of a salvage regimen will be even more restricted than in HIV-1.[109,119]

Long-term Benefits

There are no data showing the long-term benefits of ART in HIV-2. A study of 18 ARV treated patients in Cote d'Ivoire showed a doubling of the CD4 count after 12 months of treatment, from 82 to 163 cells/µL, but this was not statistically significant.[108] In The Netherlands, 11 out of 13 HIV-2-infected patients treated with ZDV-3TC-IND/RTV had successful suppression of plasma viral load during the entire course of treatment (median duration 91 weeks, range 52–234 weeks). The CD4 count increased from a median 90 cells/µL to a median 270 cells/µL.[109]

Treatment of HIV-1 and HIV-2 Dual Infection

Some patients are infected with both HIV-1 and HIV-2 and in West Africa this is not uncommon.[67] In these patients HIV-1 is the virus that dictates disease progression, with low HIV-2 PVL and high HIV-1 PVL.[96,97] This has led some researchers to advocate that treatment should be directed against HIV-1 only.[97] This may be dangerous as exemplified by a patient whose HIV-1 PVL was successfully suppressed, but who nevertheless progressed due to unsuppressed HIV-2 PVL.[122] Therefore, drugs should be chosen that cover both infections, so NNRTIs, some PIs (e.g. nelfinavir and amprenavir), and enfuvirtide should be avoided.[20,116]

Treatment of HIV-2-Infected Children

Mortality among children with HIV-2 is higher than in seronegative children and this suggests that children with HIV-2 infection need the same care as HIV-1-infected children. There are no published data from clinical trials or even cohort studies or patient series that could guide the treatment of HIV-2-infected children. The same principles as in treatment of HIV-1-infected children should guide the management of pediatric HIV-2 infection, with the caveat about the choice of antiretroviral drugs mentioned above.

Conclusion

HIV-2 is an infection of public health interest in West Africa, where up to 2 million people may be infected; an unknown proportion of these will suffer from HIV-2 induced immunodeficiency and premature mortality. Antiretroviral treatment is effective against HIV-2, but no evidence-based guidelines for treatment exist. It is suggested that principles and guidelines for treatment of HIV-1 are used, while avoiding the use of NNRTIs, which are not effective against HIV-2, some protease inhibitors (amprenavir, nelfinavir), and enfuvirtide. HIV-2 is a human model for HIV-1 infection and elucidation of its lower pathogenicity may provide clues for an effective vaccine against HIV-1.[21]

There are four crucial questions regarding HIV-2 that are unanswered. The first question is: Why did a zoonotic event lead to a localized HIV-2 epidemic in Guinea-Bissau and why is this epidemic now in decline? In recent decades, several animal pathogens jumped the species barrier and caused epidemics in humans (among others: HIV-1, HIV-2, the corona virus causing SARS, Ebola virus, prions causing variant Creutzfeldt–Jakob disease). In the case of HIV-1 and HIV-2, some widely discussed hypotheses have held medical interventions responsible for the epidemics. It seems important to trace the origin of these epidemics, whether that means confirming or rejecting these hypotheses. Phylogenetic analyses on a larger scale than have been done so far, and epidemic modeling studies that try to fit the existing data, can contribute to answering this question.

The second question is: What proportion of people that are HIV-2-infected develop immunodeficiency or AIDS, and die prematurely? This proportion needs to be known to better understand the pathogenesis of HIV-2 infection, to inform patients about their prognosis, and to help identify factors that may determine non-progression. Estimates based on prevalent cohorts are biased; long-term follow-up of seroconverters is needed to answer this question. There are few such cohorts and all are small; collaboration between research groups in West Africa could help to answer this question.

The third question is: Why does HIV-2 infection usually not lead to high plasma viral loads, in spite of proviral loads similar to HIV-1? This could be due to characteristics inherent to the virus, or to a more efficient immune response, or to generally lower levels of immune activation. This question could be examined by detailed comparative virological and immunological studies.

The final unanswered question: Is the virological, immunological, and clinical response of HIV-2 infected people to highly active antiretroviral therapy similar to that in HIV-1-infected people? The first observational data are suggesting this is the case. In order to establish effective, evidence-based treatment regimens for HIV-2 disease, clinical trials and cohort studies of antiretroviral therapy should be conducted in HIV-2-infected patients.

Acknowledgments

I would like to thank Hilton Whittle, Koya Ariyoshi and Andreas Hansmann for their comments on a draft of this chapter.

References

1. Clavel F, Guyader M, Guetard D, et al. Molecular cloning and polymorphism of the human immune deficiency virus type 2. Nature 1986; 324:691–695.
2. Brun-Vezinet F, Rey MA, Katlama C, et al. Lymphadenopathy-associated virus type 2 in AIDS and AIDS-related complex. Clinical and virological features in four patients. Lancet 1987; 1:128–132.
3. Berry N, Ariyoshi K, Jaffar S, et al. Low peripheral blood viral HIV-2 RNA in individuals with high CD4 percentage differentiates HIV-2 from HIV-1 infection. J Hum Virol 1998; 1:457–468.
4. O'Donovan D, Ariyoshi K, Milligan P, et al. Maternal plasma viral RNA levels determine marked differences in mother-to-child transmission rates of HIV-1 and HIV-2 in The Gambia. MRC/Gambia Government/University College London Medical School working group on mother-child transmission of HIV. AIDS 2000; 14:441–448.
5. Berry N, Jaffar S, Schim van der Loeff M, et al. Low level viremia and high CD4% predict normal survival in a cohort of HIV type-2-infected villagers. AIDS Res Hum Retroviruses 2002; 18:1167–1173.
6. Hansmann A, Schim van der Loeff M, Kaye S, et al. Contrasts in plasma viral load, CD4% and survival in a community-based cohort of HIV-1 and HIV-2 infected women in The Gambia. J Acquir Immun Defic Syndr 2005; 38:335–341.
7. Schim van der Loeff MF, Aaby P. Towards a better understanding of the epidemiology of HIV-2 (review). AIDS 1999; 13:S69–S84.
8. Gilbert PB, McKeague IW, Eisen G, et al. Comparison of HIV-1 and HIV-2 infectivity from a prospective cohort study in Senegal. Stat Med 2003; 22:573–593.
9. Chen Z, Luckay A, Sodora DL, et al. Human immunodeficiency virus type 2 (HIV-2) seroprevalence and characterization of a distinct HIV-2 genetic subtype from the natural range of simian immunodeficiency virus-infected sooty mangabeys. J Virol 1997; 71:3953–3960.
10. Yamaguchi J, Devare SSG, Brennan CA. Identification of a new HIV-2 subtype based on phylogenetic analysis of full-length genomic sequence. AIDS Res Hum Retroviruses 2000; 16:925–930.
11. Damond F, Worobey M, Campa P, et al. Identification of a highly divergent HIV type 2 and proposal for a change in HIV type 2 classification. AIDS Res Hum Retroviruses 2004; 20:666–672.
12. Lemey P, Pybus OG, Wang B, et al. Tracing the origin and history of the HIV-2 epidemic. Proc Natl Acad Sci U S A 2003; 100:6588–6592.
13. Ariyoshi K, Berry N, Wilkins A, et al. A community-based study of human immunodeficiency virus type 2 provirus load in a rural village in West Africa. J Infect Dis 1996; 173:245–248.
14. Gottlieb GS, Salif Sow P, Hawes SE, et al. Equal plasma viral loads predict a similar rate of CD4+ T cell decline in human immunodeficiency virus (HIV) type 1- and type 2-infected individuals from Senegal, West Africa. J Infect Dis 2002; 185:905–914.
15. Ariyoshi K, Jaffar S, Alabi A, et al. Plasma RNA viral load predicts the rate of CD4 T cell decline and death in HIV-2 infected patients in West Africa. AIDS 2000; 14:339–344.
16. Berry N, Ariyoshi K, Jobe O, et al. HIV type 2 proviral load measured by quantitative polymerase chain reaction correlates with CD4+ lymphopenia in HIV type 2-infected individuals. AIDS Res Hum Retroviruses 1994; 10:1031–1037.
17. Ariyoshi K, Schim van der Loeff M, Cook P, et al. Kaposi's Sarcoma in the Gambia, West Africa is less frequent in Human Immunodeficiency Virus type 2 than in Human Immunodeficiency Virus type 1 infection despite a high prevalence of Human Herpes virus 8. J Hum Virol 1998; 1:193–199.

18. Cohen J. Can one type of HIV protect against another type? (News; Comment). Science 1995; 268:1566–1566.

19. Andersson S, Norrgren H, da Silva Z, et al. Plasma viral load in HIV-1 and HIV-2 singly and dually infected individuals in Guinea-Bissau, West Africa. Arch Intern Med 2000; 160:3286–3293.

20. Parkin NT, Schapiro JM. Antiretroviral drug resistance in non-subtype B HIV-1, HIV-2 and SIV. Antivir Ther 2004; 9:3–12.

21. Guillon C, Blaak H, Van der Ende ME, et al. Human immunodeficiency virus type-2, an AIDS virus with two faces. Curr Top Virol 2004; 4:75–87.

22. Morgan D, Mahe C, Mayanja B, et al. HIV-1 infection in rural Africa: is there a difference in median time to AIDS and survival compared with that in industrialized countries? AIDS 2002; 16:597–603.

23. Gao F, Yue L, Robertson DL, et al. Genetic diversity of human immunodeficiency virus type 2: evidence for distinct sequence subtypes with differences in virus biology. J Virol 1994; 68:7433–7447.

24. Gomes P, Taveira NC, Pereira JM, et al. Quantitation of human immunodeficiency virus type 2 DNA in peripheral blood mononuclear cells by using a quantitative-competitive PCR assay. J Clin Microbiol 1999; 37:453–456.

25. Damond F, Gueudin M, Pueyo S, et al. Plasma RNA viral load in human immunodeficiency virus type 2 subtype A and subtype B infections. J Clin Microbiol 2002; 40:3654–3659.

26. Jaffar S, Wilkins A, Ngom PT, et al. Rate of decline of percentage CD4+ cells is faster in HIV-1 than in HIV-2 infection. J Acquir Immune Defic Syndr Hum Retrovirol 1997; 16:327–332.

27. Michel P, Balde AT, Roussilhon C, et al. Reduced immune activation and T cell apoptosis in human immunodeficiency virus type 2 compared with type 1: correlation of T cell apoptosis with beta2 microglobulin concentration and disease evolution. J Infect Dis 2000; 181:64–75.

28. Sousa AE, Carneiro J, Meier-Schellersheim M, et al. CD4 T cell depletion is linked directly to immune activation in the pathogenesis of HIV-1 and HIV-2 but only indirectly to the viral load. J Immunol 2002; 169:3400–3406.

29. Zheng NN, Kiviat NB, Sow PS, et al. Comparison of human immunodeficiency virus (HIV)-specific T-cell responses in HIV-1- and HIV-2-infected individuals in Senegal. J Virol 2004; 78:13934–13942.

30. Whittle HC, Ariyoshi K, Rowland-Jones S. HIV-2 and T cell recognition. Curr Opin Immunol 1998; 10:382–387.

31. Jaye A, Sarge-Njie R, Schim van der Loeff M, et al. No differences in cellular immune responses between asymptomatic human immunodeficiency virus type 1 and type 2- infected Gambian patients. J Infect Dis 2004; 189:498–505.

32. Machuca A, Ding L, Taffs R, et al. HIV type 2 primary isolates induce a lower degree of apoptosis 'in vitro' compared with HIV type 1 primary isolates. AIDS Res Hum Retroviruses 2004; 20:507–512.

33. Kanki PJ, Travers KU, Mboup S, et al. Slower heterosexual spread of HIV-2 than HIV-1. Lancet 1994; 343:943–946.

34. Norrgren H, Andersson S, Biague AJ, et al. Trends and interaction of HIV-1 and HIV-2 in Guinea-Bissau, west Africa: no protection of HIV-2 against HIV-1 infection. AIDS 1999; 13:701–707.

35. Kanki P, M'Boup S, Marlink R, et al. Prevalence and risk determinants of human immunodeficiency virus type 2 (HIV-2) and human immunodeficiency virus type 1 (HIV-1) in west African female prostitutes. Am J Epidemiol 1992; 136:895–907.

36. Hawkes S, West B, Wilson S, et al. Asymptomatic carriage of Haemophilus ducreyi confirmed by the polymerase chain reaction. Genitourin Med 1995; 71:224–227.

37. Greenberg A, Coulibaly IM, Kadio A, et al. Trends in the HIV-1 and HIV-2 epidemics in Abidjan, Cote d'Ivoire: 11 years of HIV serosurveillance at Project Retro-CI. Abstract B041. Xth International Conference on AIDS and STD in Africa; December 1997.

38. Machuca A, Soriano V, Gutirrez M, et al. Human immunodeficiency virus type 2 infection in Spain. The HIV-2 Spanish Study Group. Intervirology 1999; 42:37–42.

39. Matheron S, Pueyo S, Damond F, et al. Factors associated with clinical progression in HIV-2 infected-patients: The French ANRS cohort. AIDS 2003; 17:2593–2601.

40. van der Ende ME, Schutten M, Ly TD, et al. HIV-2 infection in 12 European residents: virus characteristics and disease progression. AIDS 1996; 10:1649–1655.

41. Smith NA, Shaw T, Berry N, et al. Antiretroviral therapy for HIV-2 infected patients. J Infect 2001; 42:126–133.

42. Delwart EL, Orton S, Parekh B, et al. Two percent of HIV-positive U. S. blood donors are infected with non-subtype B strains. AIDS Res Hum Retroviruses 2003; 19:1065–1070.

43. Pepin J, Dunn D, Gaye I, et al. HIV-2 infection among prostitutes working in The Gambia: association with serological evidence of genital ulcer diseases and with generalized lymphadenopathy. AIDS 1991; 5:69–75.

44. Pepin J, Morgan G, Dunn D, et al. HIV-2-induced immunosuppression among asymptomatic West African prostitutes: evidence that HIV-2 is pathogenic, but less so than HIV-1. AIDS 1991; 5:1165–1172.

45. Wilkins A, Oelman B, Pepin J, et al. Trends in HIV-1 and HIV-2 infection in The Gambia. AIDS 1991; 5:1529–1530.

46. Peeters M, Koumare B, Mulanga C, et al. Genetic subtypes of HIV type 1 and HIV type 2 strains in commercial sex workers from Bamako, Mali. AIDS Res Hum Retroviruses 1998; 14:51–58.

47. De Cock KM, Adjorlolo G, Ekpini E, et al. Epidemiology and transmission of HIV-2. Why there is no HIV-2 pandemic. JAMA 1993; 270:2083–2086.

48. Djomand G, Greenberg AE, Sassan-Morokro M, et al. The epidemic of HIV/AIDS in Abidjan, Cote d'Ivoire: a review of data collected by Projet RETRO-CI from 1987 to 1993. J Acquir Immune Defic Syndr Hum Retrovirol 1995; 10:358–365.

49. Schim van der Loeff MF, Sarge-Njie R, Ceesay S, et al. Regional differences in HIV trends in The Gambia: results from sentinel surveillance among pregnant women. AIDS 2003; 17:1841–1846.

50. Mabey DC, Tedder RS, Hughes AS, et al. Human retroviral infections in The Gambia: prevalence and clinical features. Br Med J 1988; 296:83–86.

51. Pepin J, Quigley M, Todd J, et al. Association between HIV-2 infection and genital ulcer diseases among male sexually transmitted disease patients in The Gambia. AIDS 1992; 6:489–493.

51A. Schim van der Loef MF, Awasana AA, Sarge-Njie R, et al. Sixteen years of HIV surveillance in a West African research clinic reveals divergent epidemic trends of HIV-1 and HIV-2. Int J Epidemiol 2006; 35:1322–1328.

52. Larsen O, da Silva Z, Sandstrom A, et al. Declining HIV prevalence and incidence among men in a community study from Guinea-Bissau. AIDS 1998; 12:1707–1714.

53. Poulsen AG, Aaby P, Larsen O, et al. 9-year HIV-2-associated mortality in an urban community in Bissau, west Africa. Lancet 1997; 349:911–914.

54. Aaby P, Ariyoshi K, Buckner M, et al. Age of wife as a major determinant of male-to-female transmission of HIV-2 infection: a community study from rural West Africa. AIDS 1996; 10:1585–1590.

55. Holmgren B, Aaby P, Jensen H, et al. Increased prevalence of retrovirus infections among older women in Africa. Scand J Infect Dis 1999; 31:459–466.

56. Hirsch VM, Olmsted RA, Murphy-Corb M, et al. An African primate lentivirus (SIVsm) closely related to HIV-2. Nature 1989; 339:389–392.

57. Marx PA, Alcabes PG, Drucker E. Serial human passage of simian immunodeficiency virus by unsterile injections and the mergence of epidemic human immunodeficiency virus in Africa. Phil Trans R Soc Lond B 2001; 356:911–920.

58. Gao F, Yue L, White AT, et al. Human infection by genetically diverse SIVsm-related HIV-2 in West Africa. Nature 1992; 358:495–499.

59. Chen Z, Telfer P, Gettie A, et al. Genetic characterization of new West African simian immunodeficiency virus SIVsm: geographic clustering of household-derived SIV strains with human immunodeficiency virus type 2 subtypes and genetically diverse viruses from a single feral sooty mangabey troop. J Virol 1996; 70:3617–3627.

60. Hooper E. The river: a journey back to the source of HIV and AIDS. London: Allen Lane and Penguin Press; 1999.

61. Weiss RA. Natural and iatrogenic factors in human immunodeficiency virus transmission. Phil Trans R Soc Lond B 2001; 356:947–953.

62. Korber B, Muldoon M, Theiler J, et al. Timing the ancestor of the HIV-1 pandemic strains. Science 2000; 288:1789–1796.

63. Yusim K, Peeters M, Pybus O, et al. Using human immunodeficiency virus type 1 sequences to infer historical features of the acquired immunodeficiency syndrome epidemic and human immunodeficiency virus evolution. Phil Trans R Soc Lond B 2001; 356:855–866.

64. Antal GM, Causee G. The control of endemic treponematoses. Rev Infect Dis 1985; 7:220–226.

65. Marlink R, Kanki P, Thior I, et al. Reduced rate of disease development after HIV-2 infection as compared to HIV-1. Science 1994; 265:1587–1590.

66. Kanki PJ. Human Immunodeficiency Virus Type 2 (HIV-2). AIDS Rev 1999; 1:101–108.

67. Schim van der Loeff MF, Jaffar S, Aveika AA, et al. Mortality of HIV-1, HIV-2 and HIV-1/HIV-2 dually infected patients in a clinic-based cohort in The Gambia. AIDS 2002; 16:1775–1783.

67A. Martinez-Steele E, Avieka Awasana A, Corrah T, et al. Is HIV-2 induced AIDS different from HIV-1 associated AIDS? Data from a West African clinic. AIDS 2007; 21:317–324.

68. Popper SJ, Sarr AD, Gueye-Ndiaye A, et al. Low plasma human immunodeficiency virus type 2 viral load is independent of proviral load: low virus production in vivo. J Virol 2000; 74:1554–1557.

69. Blaak H, Boers PH, Schutten M, et al. HIV-2-infected individuals with undetectable plasma viremia carry replication-competent virus in peripheral blood lymphocytes. J Acquir Immune Defic Syndr 2004; 36:777–782.

70. Lucas SB, Hounnou A, Peacock C, et al. The mortality and pathology of HIV infection in a West African city. AIDS 1993; 7:1569–1579.

71. Van der Sande MAB, Schim van der Loeff MF, Cashdollar R, et al. Incidence of tuberculosis and survival after its diagnosis in patients infected with HIV-1 and HIV-2. AIDS 2004; 18:1933–1941.

72. Ndour M, Sow PS, Coll-Seck AM, et al. AIDS caused by HIV1 and HIV2 infection: are there clinical differences? Results of AIDS surveillance 1986-97 at Fann Hospital in Dakar. Senegal Trop Med Int Health 2000; 5:687–691.

73. Norrgren H, Da Silva ZJ, Andersson S, et al. Clinical features, immunological changes and mortality in a cohort of HIV-2-infected individuals in Bissau, Guinea-Bissau. Scand J Infect Dis 1998; 30:323–329.

74. Whittle H, Egboga A, Todd J, et al. Clinical and laboratory predictors of survival in Gambian patients with symptomatic HIV-1 or HIV-2 infection. AIDS 1992; 6:685–689.

75. Le Guenno BM, Barabe P, Griffet PA, et al. HIV-2 and HIV-1 AIDS cases in Senegal: clinical patterns and immunological perturbations. J Acquir Immune Defic Syndr 1991; 4:421–427.

76. Matheron S, Mendoza-Sassi G, Simon F, et al. HIV-1 and HIV-2 AIDS in African patients living in Paris (letter). AIDS 1997; 11:934–936.

77. Poulsen AG, Kvinesdal B, Aaby P, et al. Prevalence of and mortality from human immunodeficiency virus type 2 in Bissau, West Africa. Lancet 1989; 1:827–831.

78. Ricard D, Wilkins A, N'Gum PT, et al. The effects of HIV-2 infection in a rural area of Guinea-Bissau. AIDS 1994; 8:977–982.

79. Schim van der Loeff MF, Hansmann A, Aveika AA, et al. Survival of HIV-1 and HIV-2 perinatally infected children in The Gambia. AIDS 2003; 17:2389–2394.

80. De Cock KM, Brun-Vezinet F, Soro B. HIV-1 and HIV-2 infections and AIDS in West Africa. AIDS 1991; 5:21–28.

81. Evans LA, Moreau J, Odehouri K, et al. Simultaneous isolation of HIV-1 and HIV-2 from an AIDS patient. Lancet 1988; 2:1389–1391.

82. Rayfield M, De Cock K, Heyward W, et al. Mixed human immunodeficiency virus (HIV) infection in an individual: demonstration of both HIV type 1 and type 2 proviral sequences by using polymerase chain reaction. J Infect Dis 1988; 158:1170–1176.

83. Ishikawa K, Fransen K, Ariyoshi K, et al. Improved detection of HIV-2 proviral DNA in dually seroreactive individuals by PCR. AIDS 1998; 12:1419–1425.

84. Walther-Jallow L, Andersson S, Da Silva Z, et al. High concordance between polymerase chain reaction and antibody testing of specimens from individuals dually infected with HIV types 1 and 2 in Guinea-Bissau. AIDS Res Hum Retroviruses 1999; 15:957–962.

85. Travers K, Mboup S, Marlink R, et al. Natural protection against HIV-1 infection provided by HIV-2. Science 1995; 268:1612–1615.

86. Aaby P, Poulsen AG, Larsen O, et al. Does HIV-2 protect against HIV-1 infection? (letter). AIDS 1997; 11:939–940.

87. Wiktor SZ, Nkengasong JN, Ekpini ER, et al. Lack of protection against HIV-1 infection among women with HIV-2 infection. AIDS 1999; 13:695–699.

88. Ghys PD, Diallo MO, Ettiegne-Traore V, et al. Effect of interventions to control sexually transmitted disease on the incidence of HIV infection in female sex workers. AIDS 2001; 15:1421–1431.

89. Ariyoshi K, Schim van der Loeff M, Sabally S, et al. Does HIV-2 infection provide cross-protection against HIV-1 infection? (letter). AIDS 1997; 11:1053–1054.

90. Schim van der Loeff MF, Aaby P, Ariyoshi K, et al. HIV-2 does not protect against HIV-1 infection in a rural community in Guinea-Bissau. AIDS 2001; 15:2303–2310.

91. Greenberg AE. Possible protective effect of HIV-2 against incident HIV-1 infection: review of available epidemiological and in vitro data. AIDS 2001; 15:2319–2321.

92. Kanki PJ, Eisen G, Travers KU, et al. HIV-2 and natural protection against HIV-1 infection. Science 1996; 272:1959–1960.

93. Travers K, Eisen G, Hsieh C, et al. HIV-2 provides natural protection against HIV-1 infection. Abstract A072. Xth International Conference on AIDS and STDs in Africa; December 1997; Abidjan.

94. Andersson S, Norrgren H, Dias F, et al. Molecular characterization of human immunodeficiency virus (HIV)-1 and -2 in individuals from Guinea-Bissau with single or dual infections: predominance of a distinct HIV-1 subtype A/G recombinant in West Africa. Virology 1999; 262:312–320.

95. Gottlieb GS, Sow PS, Hawes SE, et al. Molecular epidemiology of dual HIV-1/HIV-2 seropositive adults from Senegal, West Africa. AIDS Res Hum Retroviruses 2003; 19:575–584.

96. Alabi AS, Jaffar S, Ariyoshi K, et al. Plasma viral load, CD4% and survival of HIV-1, HIV-2, and dually infected Gambian patients. AIDS 2003; 17:1513–1520.

97. Koblavi-Deme S, Kestens L, Hanson D, et al. Differences in HIV-2 plasma viral load and immune activation in HIV-1 and HIV-2 dually infected persons and those infected with HIV-2 only in Abidjan, Cote D'Ivoire. AIDS 2004; 18:413–419.

98. McCutchan FE. Understanding the genetic diversity of HIV-1. AIDS 2000; 14:31–44.

99. Takehisa J, Zekeng L, Miura T, et al. Triple HIV-1 infection with group O and group M of different clades in a single Cameroon patient. J AIDS Hum Retrovirol 1997; 14:81–82.

100. Takehisa J, Zekeng L, Ido E, et al. Human immunodeficiency virus type 1 intergroup (M/O) recombination in Cameroon. J Virol 1999; 73:6810–6820.

101. Peeters M, Liegecis F, Torimori N, et al. Characterisation of a highly replicative intergroup M/O human immunodeficiency virus type I recombinant isolated from a Cameroonian patient. J Virol 1999; 73:7368–7375.

102. Shibata R, Sakai H, Kiyomasu T, et al. Generation and characterization of infectious chimeric clones between human immunodeficiency virus type 1 and simian immunodeficiency virus from an African green monkey. J Virol 1990; 64:5861–5868.

103. Kuwata T, Igarashi T, Ido E, et al. Construction of human immunodeficiency virus 1/simian immunodeficiency virus strain mac chimeric viruses having *vpr* and/or *nef* of different parental origins and their in vitro and in vivo replication. J Gen Virol 1995; 76:2181–2191.

104. Curlin ME, Gottlieb GS, Hawes SE, et al. No evidence for recombination between HIV type 1 and HIV type 2 within the envelope region in dually seropositive individuals from Senegal. AIDS Res Hum Retroviruses 2004; 20:958–963.

105. Clark NM, Dieng-Sarr A, Sankale JL, et al. Immunologic and virologic response of HIV-2 infection to antiretroviral therapy. AIDS 1998; 12:2506–2507.

106. Houston SC, Mieczinski LJ, Mashinter LD. Rapid progression of CD4 cell decline and subsequent response to salvage therapy in HIV-2 infection. AIDS 2002; 16:1189–1191.

107. Mullins C, Eisen G, Popper S, et al. Highly active antiretroviral therapy and viral response in HIV type 2 infection. Clin Infect Dis 2004; 38:1771–1779.

108. Adje-Toure CA, Cheingsong R, Garcia-Lerma JG, et al. Antiretroviral therapy in HIV-2-infected patients: changes in plasma viral load, CD4+ cell counts, and drug resistance profiles of patients treated in Abidjan, Cote d'Ivoire. AIDS 2003; 17:49–54.

109. van der Ende ME, Prins JM, Brinkman K, et al. Clinical, immunological and virological response to different antiretroviral regimens in a cohort of HIV-2-infected patients. AIDS 2003; 17:55–61.

110. Morgan D, Mahe C, Mayanja B, et al. Progression to symptomatic disease in people infected with HIV-1 in rural Uganda: prospective cohort study. Br Med J 2002; 324:193–196.

111. Schutten M, van den Hoogen B, van der Ende ME, et al. Development of a real-time quantitative RT-PCR for the detection of HIV-2 RNA in plasma. J Virol Methods 2000; 88:81–87.

112. Soriano V, Gomes P, Heneine W, et al. Human immunodeficiency virus type 2 (HIV-2) in Portugal: clinical spectrum, circulating subtypes, virus isolation, and plasma viral load. J Med Virol 2000; 61:111–116.

113. Popper SJ, Sarr AD, Travers KU, et al. Lower human immunodeficiency virus (HIV) type 2 viral load reflects the difference in pathogenicity of HIV-1 and HIV-2. J Infect Dis 1999; 180:1116–1121.

114. Cox S, Aperia K, Albert J, et al. Comparison of the sensitivities of primary isolates of HIV type 2 and HIV type 1 to antiretroviral drugs and drug combinations. AIDS Res Hum Retrovir 1994; 12:1725–1728.

115. Witvrouw M, Pannecouque C, Laethem KV, et al. Activity of non-nucleoside reverse transcriptase inhibitors against HIV-2 and SIV. AIDS 1999; 13:1477–1483.

116. Witvrouw M, Pannecouque C, Switzer WM, et al. Susceptibility of HIV-2, SIV and SHIV to various anti-HIV-1 compounds: implications for treatment and postexposure prophylaxis. Antivir Ther 2004; 9:57–65.

117. van der Ende ME, Guillon C, Boers PH, et al. Antiviral resistance of biologic HIV-2 clones obtained from individuals on nucleoside reverse transcriptase inhibitor therapy. J Acquir Immune Defic Syndr 2000; 25:11–18.

118. Descamps D, Damond F, Matheron S, et al. French ANRS HIV-2 Cohort Study Group. High frequency of selection of K65R and Q151M mutations in HIV-2 infected patients receiving nucleoside reverse transcriptase inhibitors containing regimen. J Med Virol 2004; 74:197–201.

119. Nkengasong JN, Adje-Toure C, Weidle PJ. HIV antiretroviral drug resistance in Africa. AIDS Rev 2004; 6:4–12.

120. Damond F, Brun-Vezinet F, Matheron S, et al. Polymorphism of the Human Immunodeficiency Virus Type 2 (HIV-2) Protease Gene and Selection of Drug Resistance Mutations in HIV-2-Infected Patients Treated with Protease Inhibitors. J Clin Microbiol 2005; 43:484–487.

121. Rodes B, Holguin A, Soriano V, et al. Emergence of drug resistance mutations in human immunodeficiency virus type 2-infected subjects undergoing antiretroviral therapy. J Clin Microbiol 2000; 38:1370–1374.

122. Schutten M, van der Ende ME, Osterhaus AD. Antiretroviral therapy in patients with dual infection with human immunodeficiency virus types 1 and 2. N Engl J Med 2000; 342:1758–1760.

647

CHAPTER 57

Affordable CD4 T-cell Enumeration and HIV/AIDS Viral Load Monitoring in Resource-poor Settings

Tobias F. Rinke de Wit

Introduction

Recent developments in the field of HIV/AIDS therapy in resource-poor settings are spectacular and raise hope that highly active antiretroviral therapy (HAART) will become a reality for substantially more HIV-infected people. For a considerable period of time, the most important drawback of HAART was its cost. This impediment is now gradually disappearing: prices of drugs have decreased considerably. The accelerated access initiative (AAI), a collaborative effort of five UN organizations and the major pharmaceutical industries, has achieved important price reductions of branded HAART drugs (down to 5–10%). Manufacturers of generic antiretroviral (ARV) drugs are continuously offering further price reductions. The Clinton Foundation has negotiated prices of so-called fixed dose combinations (FDC) of generic ARVs down to US$140 per patient per year. In support of these efforts, the World Health Organization (WHO) is regularly updating a list of manufacturers of safe HAART drugs approved for UN purchase. In addition, the WHO has launched its '3 by 5' initiative (HAART for 3 million people by the year 2005). Although this effort will most likely prove to be too ambitious, it will contribute to further strengthening the option of (generic) ARVs for resource-poor countries. Meanwhile, various large international institutions are releasing substantial amounts of money to support the implementation of nationwide HAART programs. The most important players in this field are the US President's Emergency Plan for HIV/AIDS Relief (PEPFAR; US$15 billion), the Global Fund to Fight AIDS, Tuberculosis and Malaria (GFATM; US$6.1 billion) and the World Bank Multi-country AIDS Program (MAP; US$1.1 billion).

Although these developments are promising, there is no room for complacency since a substantial gap remains between 'solving the money issue' and actual large-scale implementation of HAART in the developing world. Moreover, as long as there are countries where the public-sector spending on prescription drugs each year is <US$2 *per capita*, it remains questionable whether HAART is a realistic option, even if the drugs are for free.

It goes beyond the scope of this chapter to discuss in detail the multitude of issues that still hamper access to HAART for the developing world. Instead, this chapter concentrates on one of the next hurdles to be taken: simplifying and reducing the costs of laboratory monitoring of HAART. Unfortunately, the most important laboratory markers for HAART monitoring (CD4 T-cell enumeration and viral load (VL) determination) are quite expensive, are technically challenging, and suffer from lack of external quality control. On the other hand, the Clinton Foundation has negotiated price reductions for CD4 and VL equipment and reagents with most of the major manufacturers. In addition, there are various research groups and industries working on more affordable technologies for CD4 T-cell enumeration and VL determination in resource-poor settings. This chapter provides an overview of the state-of-the art in this field.

Laboratory Monitoring Remains Expensive

In general, it could be stated that the absence of laboratory facilities should not be a reason to refrain from implementing HAART in a resource-poor setting. In principle, good clinical follow-up is sufficient, provided it is combined with a serious effort in guaranteeing adherence, for example through direct observed therapy (DOT), as applied in tuberculosis (TB) control programs.[1] It should be emphasized that HAART does not cure the patient and constant alertness is required from both the patient (adherence) and the counsellor-clinician (monitoring) to avoid sub-optimal use of the medication, which may result in potentially catastrophic, massive drug resistance in the developing world.

However, if a laboratory is at hand, HAART monitoring should ideally consist of performing hematology (full blood count), some basic blood chemistry (minimally three markers, e.g. ALAT, creatinine, and glucose), enumeration of CD4 T cells and measurement of VL at regular intervals. In addition, some extra lab tests have to be performed at intake and during follow-up if indicated (e.g. hepatitis B and hepatitis C serology, syphilis, and pregnancy test). Table 57.1 gives an example of a laboratory and medical costs for a patient during the first year of HAART. In this example, a rather ideal situation is depicted, where both CD4 T-cell enumeration and VL determination are available.

Prices of the various tests and activities depicted in Table 57.1 are averages from private clinics and laboratories in more than 20 countries in Africa that have been assessed by PharmAccess Foundation.[2] Since the Clinton Foundation, US$140/year ARV prices are subject to a list of conditions, a more realistic annual bottom-price of US$240 has been taken. Under these assumptions, it can be concluded from Table 57.1, that there is little difference between the medical expenses (US$405) and the laboratory-related expenses (US$468) of a patient on HAART. In fact, the laboratory monitoring costs will be higher in many circumstances. In general, it should be stated that the laboratory prices mentioned in this manuscript are based on inquiries made in the years 2004 and 2005 and are subject to future changes.

Hematology and Blood Chemistry

Hematology (full blood count) is often possible in resource-poor settings, since this minimally requires a microscope and a small hematocrit centrifuge. Quality control and proficiency testing can be organized through central laboratories, which quite often are equipped with automatic hematological counters. Blood chemistry is a bit more expensive, since it needs a spectrophotometer, which involves maintenance and expensive reagents (e.g. Reflotron) that sometimes need a cold chain for transport. However, some internal quality control of blood chemistry can be provided by the laboratory reagent kits and in general, these tests do not impose major challenges to resource-poor laboratories.

CD4 T-cell Enumeration

CD4 T cells are important markers, not only for making the correct decisions when to start HAART, but also to measure the success or failure of a given ARV combination or to make informed decisions on initiating prophylactic treatment of opportunistic infections (Table 57.2).

Although there is no consensus for application in the developing world, the start of HAART is usually recommended when CD4 T-cell counts are between 200–350/μL whole blood.[3] The cut-off point for starting HAART is an important issue, not only because it has implications for the incidence of opportunistic infections, but also regarding costs. Cohort study data indicate that as a rule of thumb, 50% of all HIV-infected patients in a country with a mature HIV epidemic qualify for HAART when 350 cells/μL is taken as a cut-off, but only 25% qualifies with the lower cut-off (200 cells/μL).[4] Taking a higher cut-off value will thus make access to a HAART program more expensive. On the other hand, earlier start of treatment will avoid occurrence of opportunistic infections that are often expensive to treat.

Choice of Technology for CD4 T-cell Enumeration

The choice of technology to be used for CD4 T-cell enumeration is dependent on a variety of issues. One could make a choice based on the setting and throughput (number of lab tests required per time unit) of the laboratory:

Table 57.1 Comparison of medical and laboratory monitoring costs of a patient on HAART, year 1

	Pre-intake	Intake	Week 2	Week 4	Week 8	Week 12	Week 24	Week 36	Weeks 48–52	Total
Physician consult	10	10		10		10	10	10	10	70
Counselor consult	5	5	5	5	5	5	5	5	5	45
ARVs[a]		10	10	20	20	60	60	60		240
Co-medication					50	Average				50
Total medical										405
HIV serology	10									10
Full blood count		5	5	5	5	5	5	5	5	40
Chemistry 3 markers		9	9	9	9	9	9	9	9	72
CD4 T cells	20	20			On indication		20		20	80
Pregnancy		5			On indication					5
HIV VL		75			On indication		75		75	225
Hepatitis B		5			On indication					5
Hepatitis C		10			On indication					10
Syphilis TPPA/RPR		5			On indication					5
Urine glucose	2	2	2	2	2	2	2	2	2	16
Total laboratory										468

ARVs, antiretrovirals.

Table 57.2 HAART initiation, success and failure criteria as defined by CD4 and VL

HAART initiation
   Adults: <200/μL → immediate; 200–350/μL → consider
   Children: <15% → immediate; 15–20% → consider

HAART success
   Median CD4 increase 100–200/μL in the first year
   Median CD4 increase 100/μL in next years
   VL decline of 1.0–2.0 log in first 2–8 weeks
   VL decline to <LDL in 24 weeks

HAART failure
   <25–50 CD4/μL increase per year, measured by at
      least 3 CD4 tests
   VL decline <0.5–0.75 log by week 4
   VL decline <1.0 log by week 8
   VL remains >LDL after 24 weeks
   VL increase above nadir with >0.5 log
   Repeated VL blips → increase VL monitoring frequency

HAART, highly active antiretroviral therapy; VL, viral load.

- **Point of care laboratory**: low throughput – either referral to regional laboratory or manual technologies (Dynabeads, Cytospheres) or, eventually a battery operated PointCARE technology
- **Regional laboratory**: medium throughput – single platform flow cytometry (FACScount, EasyCD4, CyFlow)
- **Central reference laboratory**: high throughput – double platform flow cytometry (FACScan, FACScalibur, Coulter XL), or pan-leukogating (PLG) technology.

Point of Care Laboratory

The simplest way of quantifying CD4 T cells is by manual technologies, using synthetic beads and simple microscopy for read-out. Currently, the most efficient methods for low volume applications are Dynabeads[5] and Cytospheres.[6] Dynabeads cost US$3–4 per test and need an investment of US$750 for a magnet and rotating wheel. Cytospheres are easier to use but more expensive (up to US$8 per test). Equipment investments for Cytospheres are low: only a light microscope with a 40× objective, a 0.1 mm hemacytometer and a manual counter are required.

Both Dynabeads and Cytospheres are widely used in laboratories in the developing world.[7] However, there are important disadvantages when using these techniques. First, microscope reading of the results is difficult, it needs trained technicians, and it is prone to subjective interpretation. As a result of this, only limited numbers of blood samples can be tested on a daily basis (10–15 tests per technician), as there is a serious 'fatigue factor' associated with such manual technology. In the higher ranges of CD4 T-cell counts, Dynabeads tend to underestimate results, since samples are not diluted and high numbers of cell nuclei have to be counted, which is difficult for the human eye.[8] Conversely, the use of Cytospheres involves the risk that CD4 positive monocytes are mistaken for CD4 T cells and therefore CD4 counts are overestimated.[9] Another problem is the fact that both Dynabeads and Cytospheres need fresh blood (<6 h) for proper performance, which significantly limits the action radius of a laboratory, since no blood preservatives can be used with those technologies. The incompatibility of both Dynabeads and Cytospheres with blood preservatives precludes the laboratory to participate in external proficiency testing schemes, like QASI and NEQAS. Finally, both Dynabeads and Cytospheres need cold storage and transport of essential reagents and are not designed for determination of the percentage of CD4 T cells, which is an essential marker for pediatric applications.

An alternative for manual technologies could be the PointCARE machine, a new CD4 T-cell testing system based on side-angle light scatter detection of immuno-conjugated CD4 gold particles on CD4 positive lymphocytes. The PointCARE system is simple to operate, can be performed on blood tubes without opening them (reducing biohazards) and has internal quality control systems. The equipment is compact, can be run on batteries and the test is FDA approved. However, the test needs a large blood sample (5 mL) and cannot be used for batch-wise analyses (throughput time of 1 sample is in the order of 30 min). PointCARE currently provides an absolute CD4 T-cell count, a CD4 T-cell percentage, a total white blood cell count (WBC) and a percentage WBC. The equipment is relatively expensive compared with manual technologies (US$17 500); reagents are in the same price range (Table 57.3). In the near future the option of measuring hemoglobin will be added, which (in combination with battery-power) could make the PointCARE machine ideal for field-settings.

Although other manual CD4 T-cell enumeration technologies have long been declared obsolete (TRAx, Capcellia, Zymmune, Immunoalkaline phosphatase essay), the current pressure to deliver laboratory services to rapidly evolving national HAART programs occasionally revitalizes them. Recently,

Table 57.3 Comparison of CD4 T-cell enumeration technologies[a]

Technique	Features	Throughput/ day	Price of equipment (US$)[b]	Price (US$/ test)[b]	CD4%	Time to result (min)	Sample volume (µL)	External QA/QC	Age of blood sample	Cold chain	Remarks	Maintenance service	Company
Cytospheres	Latex beads Light microscopy Manual count rosettes	15	1500	5–8	No	30–45	100	No	<6 h	Yes	Subjective interpretation (eye fatigue), overestimations. >10 tests/week for reproducibility. FDA approved.	No	Beckman Coulter
Dynabeads	Magnetic beads Light or fluorescent microscopy	15	2500 (light) 6000 (fluorescent)	3–5	No	30–45	125	No	<6 h	Yes	Subjective interpretation Underestimations at high CD4 levels. >10 tests week for reproducibility.	No	Dynal Biotech
FACScount	Dedicated single platform, fully automated no RBC lysis	30–40	25 000	8–10	No	15	50	Yes	<3 days	Yes	Obliged to use kit, requires accurate reverse pipetting. FDA approved.	5000/year	Becton & Dickinson
PointCARE	Single platform flow cytometer, fully automated, closed system	20	17 500	5–7	Yes	30	5000	No	<3 days	No	Fully automatic, slow (3 tests/h), no blood handling, lots of waste tubes. FDA approved.	1400/year	Beckman Coulter
CyFlow	Dedicated single platform, no lyse no wash	50–100	21 000	3–5	Yes	15	50	No	<3 days	Yes	No independent validation, unstable volumetric counting software not user friendly	Limited	Partec
EasyCD4	Single platform flow cytometer Minimal sheath fluid, small test volume, RBC lysis	30–50	40 000	2–3	No	30	10	?	<3 days	Yes	Can be done on finger-pricks (pediatric use); 10 µL of whole blood is sufficient. Minimal waste, no external QA possible. Undergoing evaluation.	Limited	Guava Technologies Inc.
FACSscan FACScalibur Coulter XL Cytoron	Can be used with pan leukogating	300	>50 000	6	Yes	20–30	100	Yes	<5 days	Yes	Gold standard equipment, in principle designed for research, technically complex. FDA approved.	5000/year	Becton & Dickinson Beckman Coulter

[a]Up-to-date reporting of options for CD4 T-cell enumeration is provided through the 'Afford CD4 website', available at: www.affordcd4.com [b]Considerably lower prices can be negotiated at bulk-procurement level, through National AIDS Control Programs or initiatives like the Clinton Foundation.

TRAx in combination with dried blood spot (DBS) sampling technology was recommended.[10] However, DBS cannot discriminate between CD4 molecules derived from CD4 T-cells versus those from monocytes. Especially in AIDS patients, who have downregulated CD4 expression, decreased CD4 T-cells and increased monocytes because of bacterial infections (including tuberculosis), the monocyte-derived CD4 will skew the TRAx enzyme-linked immunosorbent assay (ELISA)-based T-cell enumeration to an unknown extent, making DBS-TRAx CD4 counts highly unreliable.[11]

Regional Laboratory

The gold standard for CD4 enumeration remains flow cytometry. The easiest instruments to use are the single-platform (volumetric) flow cytometers, like the FACScount, the CyFlow or the EasyCD4 machines. Table 57.3 provides a comparison of these technologies and puts them in the context of other CD4 T-cell counting strategies. The common finding is that cytometers remain expensive (ranging from US$17 500–35 000) and their maintenance contracts (up to US$5000/year) are not affordable or not existing for most resource-poor settings. Reagent prices vary between US$3 (CyFlow) and US$8–10 (FACScount) per test. Most machines are fine for medium throughput situations ($\approx$50 tests/day), with the exception of the slow PointCARE apparatus, which can handle a maximum of only 20 samples per day.[12] Although most machines can measure the percentage CD4 T cells (the important pediatric marker), the FACScount is not fit for this parameter and the CyFlow can only do this after adding lysing solution. On the other hand, the FACScount is compatible with external proficiency testing, which is not (yet) the case for the PointCARE or CyFlow machines. All machines need cold transport and cold storage of reagents and kits, a significant disadvantage in tropical settings. For those machines that are not volumetric (FACScount and EasyCD4), beads have to be used for absolute CD4 T-cell enumeration. Beads are expensive and need very accurate and precise (reverse) pipetting. The CyFlow CD4 machine has been used in Africa,[13] but there are reports of CD4 underestimations,[14] vulnerability to air bubbles,[15] and the machine has not been independently validated and as such is not recommended by WHO standards.

The FACScount is the only stand-alone flow cytometer that has proven its robustness in resource-poor settings for a period of more than 10 years, and is supported by a well-functioning (preventive) maintenance system.

Central Reference Laboratory

For high throughput settings (national reference laboratories in capital cities), there are other research-type flow cytometers, like the B&D FACScan and FACScalibur, and the Coulter XL. These flow cytometers are even more expensive and either need an additional blood cell counter (dual platform technology) or expensive beads for CD4 T-cell quantification. Table 57.3 summarizes some characteristics of these high throughput machines.

Recent developments allow for a more affordable use of these heavyweight research type flow cytometers. Clever gating strategies avoid the prescribed batteries of expensive monoclonal antibodies and enable the laboratory to use fewer and often generic reagents. The bare minimum is the primary CD4-gating technology,[16] which only uses a generic CD4 monoclonal antibody. An alternative is the pan-leukogating (PLG) technology, which requires CD45 and CD4 antibodies (www.plgCD4.net).[17] PLG measures both absolute and percentage of CD4 T cells and can do this on blood samples of up to 5 days for approximately US$6/test. The methodology is quickly gaining popularity and excellent results have been obtained in >25 settings in South Africa.[17A]

Centralized high throughput CD4 T-cell enumeration can be greatly improved in efficiency when good blood preservatives are available that allow for substantial travelling times of blood samples at ambient temperatures. Transfix is a standardized fixative developed by UK NEQAS and supplied by the UK Public Health Laboratory Service. Transfix is added 1/10 to fresh whole blood and allows accurate CD4 T-cell enumeration[18] even after 10 days at 25°C. Cytochex is a non cross-linking fixative designed to preserve white blood cells in whole blood (1:1). This reagent can keep blood samples stable for a full week at 4°C.[8] In general, it should be kept in mind that the adding of preservatives automatically adds costs, increases contamination risk and introduces a level of inaccuracy (pipetting errors). It is recommended that blood-drawing tubes are prepared with fixed quantities of blood anticoagulants and preservatives to avoid these issues.

Finally, CD4 T-cell enumeration should always be supported by an independent external quality control program. A program with over 8 years of international experience of proficiency testing in both Francophone and Anglophone countries all over the world is the one offered by Health Canada: the Quality Assessment and Standardization for Immunological Measures Relevant to HIV/AIDS (QASI) program.[19] QASI provides an external quality assessment program (EQAP) for CD4 T-cell counts where none is available. The EQAP shipments include challenge survey material that contains simulated specimens. The program collects, processes and analyzes EQAP data and provides rapid return of survey results to assure maximum time for remedial action. The QASI program is backing a recently developed African program named WHO/South African NHLS/QASI collaborative REQAS (Regional External Quality Assessment Scheme). REQAS supports five fixed date shipments per year, of which one or two are also supported by QASI.

Pipeline CD4 Technologies

As mentioned earlier, spectacular technological improvements and/or price reductions of the existing CD4 T-cell enumeration technologies are not expected. A breakthrough could come from alternative technologies with entirely different approaches, however. An interesting variation on the manual microscope-based CD4 T-cell enumeration for point of care applications involves the use of microchips to miniaturize an antibody-based cell-capture system. This microchip could subsequently be read using digital camera technology and analyzed through an associated computer algorithm. An attractive feature is the fact that very minute blood samples are required (<16.5 µL), which makes the technology fit for pediatric applications (and possibly for finger pricks). The reader is estimated to cost US$3000 and the test would be in the US$1–2 range. The assay is simple to perform, has short analysis time (<15 min), needs no sample preparation, produces little waste, and could reduce reagent cost up to 90%, since the miniaturized systems requires only small volumes of monoclonal antibodies. In addition, the assay could be developed into a multiplex system that can measure other relevant markers such as viral load, hemoglobulin, and liver enzymes, which are relevant to HAART monitoring. LabNow is developing a CD4 test along these lines and a prototype has recently been favorably field-tested.[20]

The University of Twente, in the Netherlands is developing a non-flow cytometry-based device (the Easy Count), which is based on magnetic sorting and optical image analysis of CD4 T cells. This machine could eventually be marketed for US$1000–2000.

However, the first prototypes had difficulty with separating monocytes from CD4 T cells and to date, little progress has been made in solving this issue.

A newer system is the SemiBio Ligand Catcher. This uses a treated microscope slide to which CD4 T cells adhere and which can be made visible using digital camera technology. The attractive feature of this system is the fact that samples can be fixed and transported for a long time before analysis. Disadvantages are the expected costs per test: US$15–20, despite the low capital costs for the machine.[21]

Choice of Technology for VL Determination

As for CD4 T-cell enumeration, the choice for HIV viral load (VL) determination technologies is dependent on the setting of the laboratory:

- **Point of care laboratory**: low throughput – referral to regional laboratory (DBS)
- **Regional laboratory**: medium throughput – either P24 determination, Cavidi assay or referral to central reference laboratory
- **Central reference laboratory**: high throughput – 'classical' VL determination (PCR, bDNA, NASBA, real time PCR, LCR).

Point of Care Laboratory

VL determination in small, low throughput laboratories is not a realistic option with the current methodologies. Rather, patients should be referred to regional or central laboratories. Alternatively, finger-prick blood samples could be sent to the central reference laboratories by using special anticoagulated blood sampling PPT-tubes or by dried blood spot/dried plasma spot (DBS/DPS) technology.[22] The advantage of this method is that samples can be stored for prolonged time periods (up to 1 year; storage at 4°C for short periods or at −20°C for periods longer than 1 month is recommended). Shipment can be done at ambient temperatures by normal mail (as long as a desiccant is used), RNA can be isolated and tested in batches, which reduces costs. Several VL technologies can accommodate DBS/DPS, including the Rainbow real time Primagen Rainbow NASBA, the Roche Amplicor HIV-1 Monitor and the bioMerieux NucliSens HIV-1 QT assays, although the protocols have not been formalized yet. DBS/DPS sampling thus increases the action radius and efficiency of central reference labs. There are some reports that DBS/DPS works very well for pediatric applications, but the small sample size might collect too few events for reliable measurement of adult VL (W. Stevens, pers comm). This problem might be overcome by the 'Sample Tanker' that can accommodate 1 mL of plasma sample and allows for shipment at ambient temperatures.[23]

Regional Laboratory

Regional laboratories can be advised to either collect blood samples through DBS or to perform small-scale, low-throughput determinations of markers that are a proxy for the 'classical' VL. These alternative markers are measured through a modified p24 ELISA[24] or an ultra-sensitive reverse transcriptase assay (Cavidi).[25] Table 57.4 summarizes some assay characteristics.

The classical HIV-1 p24 assay has been improved by heat-denaturation and signal-amplification techniques. The assay needs less equipment than any RNA-based VL assay. Apart from a dry heat block, the most important device required is an ELISA reader, which historically is present in many laboratories, since ELISA was the standard for HIV serology prior to the rapid HIV tests. However, it should be kept in mind that ELISA-based technology requires continuous maintenance and well-trained lab technicians. Heat-denatured p24 ELISA is quite sensitive, has a good linearity and correlates well with plasma RNA levels. The test is marketed for a list price of US$6–8 (PerkinElmer Life Sciences, Boston, MA), which is far more affordable than RNA-based VL tests. Recent evaluations have indicated that the heat denatured p24 ELISA can be applied to any group M HIV-1 subtype and (in contrast to the VL assays) also to HIV-1 group O viruses.[26] The assay is far less prone to contamination risks than RNA-based VL tests, is less technologically complex, and could allow for a high throughput (96-wells plates). On the other hand, the p24 assay is vulnerable to the existence of p24/ap24 complexes, which need to be completely denatured in order to get the correct measurement of pg of p24 in plasma. Since (non-specific) immune activation is common in resource-poor settings,[27] this could compromise complete heat-denaturation of p24/ap24 complexes, leading to underestimations of VL. Since p24/ap24 complexes are less prevalent in (newborn) children and sero-converters, the new p24 assay can be recommended as an early diagnostic tool for HIV-1 infection in these subjects.[28] The assay is not very robust leading to variable results between technicians and laboratories and depends on the composition of the denaturation buffer.[29] The sensitivity of the p24 assay is less than that of the RNA-based VL assays and clinical cut-off is at the equivalent level of RNA-based VL >30 000 copies/mL.[30]

The ExaVir assay measures the *in vitro* activity of HIV-1 reverse transcriptase recovered from HIV-1 virions in plasma. Since an enzyme activity is measured, there are no primers or monoclonal antibodies required. Therefore, the ExaVir assay is less prone to contamination and independent of HIV-1 subtype, extending its use to the rare HIV-O and HIV-N groups. The assay is very specific and fairly sensitive and compares well with the RT-PCR based gold standard. A conversion factor has been calculated, multiplying the fg/mL result with 210 to get the classic HIV RNA copies/mL; lower limit of detection is in the order of the equivalent of 2000 RNA copies/mL.[31] The ExaVir RT test is moderately expensive (US$10–20), but requires considerable laboratory equipment, including: rocking table, vacuum pump, incubator, plate washer, plate reader, and magnetic spinner (approx. US$20 000). The test is also fit for measuring viral resistance against non-nucleoside reverse transcriptase inhibitors, as well as some nucleoside reverse transcriptase inhibitors (Table 57.4). The ExaVir kit does not contain a positive control, since this should be a live attenuated HIV-1 strain, which as a bio-hazardous agent, imposes challenges on the shipment of the kit. If the kit arrives thawed, it should be used within 1 week. Plasma samples to be tested should be <6 h old, otherwise storage is required in an (expensive) −80°C freezer. The required volume of plasma (1 mL) poses challenges to drawing sufficient blood samples from infants. Finally, the ExaVir RT extraction process is tedious and it takes 2–3 days for the assay to be completed, since there is a prolonged 33°C incubation step (an uninterrupted power supply is needed).

For both heat-denatured p24 and ExaVir RT assays, the literature demonstrates a wide degree of variability when compared with the VL gold standards. This can be expected, since different biological parameters are measured: the p24 assay for example does not measure virion-associated molecules, like the RNA-based VL assays do. In addition, the sensitivity of p24 and ExaVir assays remains sub-optimal,[32] and to date there are too few clinical evaluations to interpret the results of these assays in light of HAART.

Central Reference Laboratory

The gold standard for VL determination remains the number of RNA copies/mL of plasma, as measured

Table 57.4 Comparison of VL determination technologies

Technique	Features	Target	Price of equipment (US$)[b]	Price (US$/test)[b]	Unit	Sample volume	HIV-1 variants	Dynamic range	Remarks	Contamination risk	Company
P24 ELISA	Heat denaturation + signal amplification to improve sensitivity	P24 protein		6–8	pg/mL		(subtype D?) M+O	500–6 250 000	Diagnosis acute infections + pediatric. Technically challenging, mixed evaluation results, dependent on buffer used.	Low	Perkin Elmer
ExaVir Load Quantitative HIV-RT	Reverse transcriptase enzyme activity	RT enzyme		10–20	fg/mL[a]		M+O+N	>400	Also fit for resistance monitoring NNRTI, AZT, d4T, long performance time. Less prone to contamination.	Low	Cavidi Tech AB
Cobas Amplicor HIV-1 Monitor v1.5	RT-PCR based	gag	30 000	50 / 17 (Amplicare)	copies/mL	0.5 mL	M	50–75 000 (ultra) 400–750 000	FDA approved, PCR technology is patented (US$10/test), colorimetric.	High	Roche
NucliSens EasyQ	Isothermal NASBA	gag	21 000	30	copies/mL	0.2–1 mL	(subtype G?) M	40–10 000 000 (ultra)	FDA approved, electro-chemilumin-escence. FDA approved, chemiluminescence detection method.	High	bioMerieux
Versant Quantiplex HIV-1 RNA 3.0 (bDNA)	Branched DNA >80 probes TMA signal amplification	pol	58 000	60	copies/mL	0.5–1 mL	M (+O)	400–10 000 000 50–500 000		Low	Bayer
LCx	RT-PCR + ligase chain reaction	pol	?	?	copies/mL	<1 mL	M+O	50–1 000 000 (ultra) 178–5 000 000	VL values are generally a bit higher	High	Abbott Laboratories
Retina HIV-1 Rainbow	Molecular beacon	LTR	18 500	25	copies/mL	0.2–1 mL	(subtype G) M+O+N	50–1 000 000		Medium	Primagen

[a]Conversion factor: 1 fg RT = 220 copies RNA. [b]Considerably lower prices can be negotiated at bulk-procurement level, through National AIDS Control Programs or initiatives like the Clinton Foundation.

by the various RNA-based amplification technologies (summarized in Table 57.4). All of the RNA-based technologies are high-throughput assays, fit for central reference laboratories. All assays have been extensively validated and three of them are FDA-approved (Cobas Amplicor HIV-1 Monitor 1.5, Nuclisens QT and Quantiplex HIV-1 RNA 3.0). Clinicians are familiar with the interpretation of RNA-based VL results, as expressed in numbers or logs of numbers of RNA copies/mL plasma. Most of the assays work with DBS/DPS, but protocols need formalization. However, drawbacks remain the price of equipment and tests (Table 57.4), the complexity of their technology requiring highly skilled laboratory technicians, the maintenance of the equipment, the risk of contamination (not for the bDNA assay), and unknown performance with (newly emerging) HIV-1 subtypes and recombinants. All RNA-based VL assays can be performed in an ultra-sensitive variation, lowering the lower detection limit (LDL) to <50 copies/mL. However, this adaptation often requires an expensive ultracentrifuge. In general, RNA-based VL assays assume the presence of a fairly sophisticated laboratory, including additional expensive equipment, such as biological safety cabinets, 12-channel pipettes, dry heat block incubators, refrigerated centrifuges, vacuum systems, separate laboratory rooms and −80°C freezers. All of these items, including maintenance costs, labour costs of well-trained laboratory technicians, and shipment costs of kits, contribute to the real price of a VL test and should be kept in mind when comparing options.

An alternative assay is the Real Time PCR (e.g. TaqMan) for viral RNA or proviral DNA.[33] Most real time PCR methods are 'home made' and thus the reagents for this assay are relatively cheap. However, the equipment is expensive, the assay is not yet standardized (variability in reagents and no QA from manufacturer, leading to lack of reproducibility), it is prone to contamination and clinically not yet sufficiently validated. There are two vendors (bioMerieux and Roche) that offer commercial Real Time assays and this technology is certainly promising.

Conclusion

It is still questionable whether true quantitative CD4 T-cell enumeration and VL determination is really required. This is not only an issue for resource-poor settings, but eventually also for the industrialized world. Which difference between two consecutive measurements of CD4 will actually lead to the important clinical decision that HAART failed and

that second-line therapy is indicated? To date, a rule of thumb is that CD4 differences of >2-fold are considered different from each other (as are VL measurements of >0.5 log difference). However, studies that quantify the underlying natural diurnal and seasonal CD4 T-cell variations of people living in resource-poor settings, are lacking. In addition, there are inadequate data on CD4 normal values in non-Caucasoid subjects. Both of these parameters could play crucial roles in the interpretation of CD4 T-cell enumeration data in resource-poor settings. Possibly a CD4 T-cell slope, instead of a single absolute estimate, would be more informative. Similar arguments could be held for the measurement of HIV-1 VL.

A more practical approach could be to invest in the development of less sensitive, semi-quantitative technologies for both CD4 T-cell enumeration and VL determination. Carefully designed semi-quantitative bins should be defined that are crucial for clinical decision making. For example, for CD4 T-cell enumeration, a 3-bin test could be recommended that determines CD4 counts of <200, between 200 and 350, and >350. This test would be sufficient to produce all information that is required by a clinician to make informed decisions about when to start HAART, when to start prophylactic treatment of opportunistic infections, and whether the HAART is successful. The application of such a test for children, where percentage CD4 T cells are more important, would however be limited. For VL, similar 3-tier bins could be defined, for example: <10 000, between 10 000 and 100 000, and >100 000 RNA copies/mL.

Thus, the ideal CD4 T-cell or VL test to be developed should be: sensitive, specific, simple, need minimal laboratory equipment, maintenance independent, cheap, have long expiry reagents, should not suffer from contamination, should be independent of HIV subtype, should not need cooled shipping and storage, and should produce meaningful semi-quantitative results. A US$1 semi-quantitative dipstick for both CD4 and VL would be ideal and efforts are underway to develop such a test.

Until new breakthrough CD4 and VL tests are available, the 'old' technologies will have to be used and optimized, and efforts should continue to reduce their costs. In light of this, the negotiations of the Clinton Foundation can be commended. These have resulted in an 80% price reduction by five medical technologies companies of their HIV/AIDS-related equipment and reagents for an increasing number of counties in the world. Even though this is a remarkable achievement, it is not realistic to expect further substantial price reductions of HAART monitoring laboratory technology in the near future. Rather, a completely new generation of (fluorophore) technologies should make the difference, bringing down the hardware costs to only several thousands of dollars and the reagents to <US$1/test.

In conclusion, the decision of which technology to use for CD4 T-cell enumeration and VL determination depends on a multitude of factors, including performance (dynamic range, specificity, sensitivity, reproducibility) and throughput, sophistication of the lab, training of laboratory technicians, availability of technical and maintenance support, cost of equipment and test kits, availability of (external) QA/QC possibilities, independent evaluation status and clinical validation, expected HIV-1 subtypes, specimen shipment flexibility, required storage temperatures, contamination issues and possibly even turn-around time, possibility of performing the test in batches, etc. The choices are manifold and complex and therefore, it is recommended that the WHO issue guidelines that help laboratory managers in various resource-poor settings to make informed decisions which would enable them to monitor HAART in the most effective and meaningful way.

Acknowledgments

The author wishes to acknowledge the critical comments and suggestions of D. Glencross and W. Stevens (University of Witwatersrand), T. Peter (Clinton Foundation), F. Mandy (Health Canada) and A. Kliphuis (PharmAccess).

References

1. Farmer P, Leandre F, Mukherjee JS, et al. Community-based approaches to HIV treatment in resource-poor settings. Lancet 2001; 358:404–409.
2. PharmAccess Foundation. [Prices are based on 2005 analyses and are subject to changes]. Internal database: PharmAccess Foundation; 2005.
3. WHO. Scaling up antiretroviral therapy in resource-limited settings: Treatment guidelines for a public health approach. Geneva: WHO; 2003. Online. Available: www.who.int/hiv/pub/prev_care/en/arvrevision2003en.pdf
4. Ethio-Netherlands AIDS Research Project. Analysis of CD4 T-cell counts of HIV+ factory workers at enrolment in cohort study. (Unpublished data.) Ethio-Netherlands AIDS Research Project; 2000.
5. Lyamuya EF, Kagoma C, Mbena EC, et al. Evaluation of the FACScount, TRAx CD4 and Dynabeads methods for CD4 lymphocyte determination. J Immunol Meth 1996; 195:103–112.
6. Carella AV, Moss MM, Provost V, et al. A manual bead assay for the determination of absolute CD4+ and CD8+ lymphocyte counts in human immunodeficiency virus-infected individuals. Clin Diagn Lab Immunol 1995; 2:623–625.
7. Diagbouga S, Chazallon C, Kazatchkine MD, et al. Successful implementation of a low-cost method for enumerating CD4+ T lymphocytes in resource-limited settings: the ANRS 12–26 study. AIDS 2003; 15:2201–2208.
8. Crowe S. Data presented at the Forum for Collaborative AIDS Research, Boston: March 2005. Online. Available: www.hivforum.org/uploads/Crowe1.pdf
9. Mandy F, Bergeron M, Fernandez-Repollet E, et al. How to select, evaluate and maintain correct CD4 T-cell counting methods for HIV/AIDS treatment. XIV International AIDS conference. Skills Building Workshop SB68, July 11 2002, Barcelona, Spain.
10. Mwaba P, Cassol S, Pilon R, et al. Use of dried whole blood spots to measure CD4+ lymphocyte counts in HIV-1 infected patients. Lancet 2003; 362:1459–1460.
11. Shapiro HM, Many FF, Rinke Wit TF de, et al. Dried blood spot technology for CD4+ T-cell counting. Lancet 2004; 363:164–165.
12. Scott L, Kirkpatrick D, Hansen P, et al. PointCARE CD4 testing: the new kid on the block, session 126, poster 742. 12th Conference on Retroviruses and Opportunistic Infections (CROI): 2005.
13. Imade GE, Badung B, Pam S, et al. Comparison of a new, affordable flow cytometric method and the manual magnetic bead technique for CD4 T-lymphocytes counting in a northern Nigerian setting. Clin Diagn Lab Immunol 2005; 12:224–227.
14. Spira T. Forum for Collaborative AIDS Research Meeting, Warsaw, Poland: 2003.
15. Dieye TN, Vereecken C, Diaw PA, et al. Evaluation of an affordable instrument for absolute CD4 counting in resource-poor settings against two reference clinical flow cytometers. IAS. Online. Available: www.ias.se/abstract/show.asp?abstract_id=10762
16. Janossy G, Jani I, Gohde W. Affordable CD4(+) T-cell counts on 'single-platform' flow cytometers I. Primary CD4 gating. Br J Haematol 2000; 111:1198–1208.
17. Glencross D, Scott LE, Jani IV, et al. CD45-assisted PanLeucogating for accurate, cost-effective dual-platform CD4+ T-cell enumeration. Cytometry 2002; 50:69–77.
17A. Glencross DK, Mendelow BV, Stevens WS. Laboratory monitoring of HIV/AIDS in a resource-poor setting. S Afr Med J 2003; 93:262–263.
18. Jani V, Janossy G, Iqbal A, et al. Affordable CD4+ T-cell counts by flow cytometry. II. The use of fixed whole blood in resource-poor settings. J Immunol Meth 2001; 257:145–154.
19. Mandy F, Bergeron M, Houle G, et al. Impact of the international program for Quality Assessment and Standardization for immunological measures relevant to HIV/AIDS: QASI. Cytometry 2002; 50:111–116.
20. Rodriguez WR, Christodoulides N, Floriano PN, et al. A microchip CD4 counting method for HIV monitoring in resource-poor settings. PLoS Med 2005; 2:e182. Online. Available: www.plosmedicine.org
21. AIDSMAP. Online. Available: www.aidsmap.com/en/docs/A1527BEC-D49E-456D-B402-6EDEA4A1B7F0.asp
22. Brambilla D, Jennings C, Aldrovandi G, et al. Multicenter evaluation of use of dried blood and plasma spot specimens in quantitative assays for human immunodeficiency virus RNA: measurement, precision, and RNA stability. J Clin Microbiol 2003; 41:1888–1893.
23. Research Think Tank. Online. Available: www.researchthinktank.com/OTHER/publications/posters-2004.06.10-IHDRW01.pdf
24. Schupbach J, Boni J, Flepp M, et al. Antiretroviral treatment monitoring with an improved HIV-1 p24 antigen test: an inexpensive alternative to tests for viral RNA. J Med Virol 2001; 65:225–232.
25. Malmsten A, Shao XW, Aperia K, et al. HIV-1 viral load determination based on reverse transcriptase activity recovered from human plasma. J Med Virol 2003; 71:347–359.
26. Ribas SG, Ondoa P, Schupbach J, et al. Performance of a quantitative human immunodeficiency virus type 1 p24 antigen assay on various HIV-1 subtypes for the follow-up

of human immunodeficiency type 1 seropositive individuals. J Virol Meth 2003; 113:29–34.

27. Kassu A, Tsegaye A, Petros B, et al. Distribution of lymphocyte subsets in healthy human immunodeficiency virus-negative adult Ethiopians from two geographic locales. Clin Diagn Lab Immunol 2001; 8:1171–1176.

28. Sherman GG, Stevens G, Stevens WS. Affordable diagnosis of human immunodeficiency virus infection in infants by p24 antigen detection. Pediatr Infect Dis J 2004; 23:173–176.

29. Stevens G, Rekhviashvili N, Scott LE, et al. Evaluation of two commercially available, inexpensive alternative assays used for assessing viral load in a cohort of human immunodeficiency virus type 1 subtype C-infected patients from South Africa. J Clin Microbiol 2005; 43:857–861.

30. Sterling TR, Hoover DR, Astemborski J, et al. Heat-denatured human immunodeficiency virus type 1 protein 24 antigen: prognostic value in adults with early-stage disease. J Infect Dis 2002; 186:1181–1185.

31. Greengrass V, Dunne A, Hocking J, et al. Evaluation of Cavidi ExaVir quantitative HIV RT load kit for monitoring HIV viral load, session 133, poster 958. 11th Conference on Retroviruses and Opportunistic Infections (CROI): 2004.

32. Antunes R, Figueiredo S, Bartolo I, et al. Evaluation of the clinical sensitivities of three viral load assays with plasma samples from a paediatric population predominantly infected with human immunodeficiency virus type 1 subtype G and BG recombinant forms. J Clin Microbiol 2003; 41:3361–3367.

33. Lewin SR, Vesanen M, Kostrikis L, et al. Use of real-time PCR and molecular beacons to detect virus replication in human immunodeficiency virus type 1-infected individuals on prolonged effective antiretroviral therapy. J Virol 1999; 73:6099–6103.

CHAPTER 58

Essential Medicines for HIV/AIDS

Hans V. Hogerzeil

The Concept of Essential Medicines

Essential medicines are those that satisfy the priority healthcare needs of the population. They are selected on the basis of disease prevalence, evidence on efficacy, safety and comparative cost-effectiveness. The selection of essential medicines is one of the core principles of a national drug policy because it helps to set priorities for all aspects of the pharmaceutical system. This is a global concept which can be applied in any country, in private and public sectors and at different levels of the healthcare system.

There is good evidence that clinical guidelines and essential medicines lists, when properly developed, introduced and supported, improve prescribing quality and lead to better health outcomes (Fig. 58.1).[1-4] But there is also an economic argument. First, in developing countries pharmaceuticals are the second biggest budget line in the health system, after salaries. Second, new essential medicines are expensive. For example, even with good differential pricing lumefantrine-artemisinine is 25 times more expensive than chloroquine, the first-line antimalarial it is supposed to replace; atovaquone-proguanil is about 400 times as expensive. Life-saving antiretroviral combinations cost US$150–250 per year while 38 countries have <US$2 per person per year available for all medicines.[5] The selection of new essential medicines for public supply, subsidy or reimbursement has enormous financial implications for developing countries.

The advantages of limited lists are therefore both medical and economical. From a medical point of view, they lead to better quality of care and better health outcomes and help focus quality control, drug information, prescriber training and medical audit. Economically they lead to better value for money, to lower costs through economies of scale and to simplified systems of procurement, supply, distribution, and reimbursement. All of this is even more important in resource-poor situations where the availability of drugs in the public sector is often erratic. Under such circumstances, measures to ensure a regular supply of essential drugs will result in real health gains and in increased confidence in the health services.

The concept of essential medicines was launched in 1977 with the publication of the first WHO Model List of Essential Medicines (Box 58.1). Since then, the List was revised every 2 years. Both its content and the process by which it is updated are intended as a model for developing countries.

In 2002, WHO completed a rigorous overhaul of the process to update the list. An important change was that affordability changed from a precondition into a consequence of the selection. For example, before 2002, effective but expensive medicines, such as single-dose azithromycin for trachoma, were not listed because of their high price. Under the new definition (Box 58.2), 12 antiretroviral medicines for HIV/AIDS were listed, irrespective of their high cost at that time. Their listing now implied that these medicines should become affordable to all patients who need them.

Within a country, market approval of a pharmaceutical product is usually granted on the basis of efficacy, safety and quality, and rarely on the basis of a comparison with other products already on the market, or cost. This regulatory decision defines the

---

Box 58.1

Useful resources available from WHO

The WHO Model List of Essential Drugs

The WHO Model List of Essential Drugs is a model for national programs and reimbursement decisions. It has been updated every 2 years since 1977. The Model List of 2005[6] contains about 300 active ingredients and is divided into a main list and a complementary list. Drugs are specified by international non-proprietary name (INN) or generic name without reference to brand names or specific manufacturers. As a model product, the Model List aims to identify cost-effective medicines for priority conditions, linked to evidence-based clinical guidelines and with special emphasis on public health aspects and considerations of value of money.

The WHO Essential Medicines Library

In addition to the information on whether a medicine is in the Model List or not, it is important for national or institutional selection committees to have access to information that supports the selection of essential medicines, such as summaries of relevant WHO clinical guidelines, the most important systematic reviews, important references and indicative cost information. Other information is linked to the WHO Model Formulary, international nomenclature, ATC/DDD classifications and quality-assurance standards.

The WHO Model Formulary

The WHO Model Formulary[7] presents model formulary information on all medicines on the Model List. Besides being a useful reference to individual prescribers, it is mainly intended as a starting point for developing national or institutional formularies. For this reason, the text of the formulary is also available in electronic format for national adaptation in Arabic, English, Russian, and Spanish, with a practical manual for national committees.

The WHO Medicines website: www.who.int/medicines

All WHO publications on essential medicines, including the Model List, Model Formulary, Essential Medicines Library, guidelines for national drug policies, information on prices, quality, patent status, regulatory status are freely available on this website.

Box 58.2

Definition of essential medicines (WHO 2002)

Essential medicines are those that satisfy the priority healthcare needs of the population. They are selected with due regard to disease prevalence, evidence on efficacy and safety, and comparative cost-effectiveness. Essential medicines are intended to be available within the context of functioning health systems at all times, in adequate amounts, in the appropriate dosage forms, with assured quality, and at a price the individual and the community can afford. The implementation of the concept of essential medicines is intended to be flexible and adaptable to many different situations; exactly which medicines are regarded as essential remains a national responsibility.[8]

---

siderations of value for money. This second step leads to a national list of essential drugs. A list of essential drugs is best developed for different levels of care, and on the basis of standard treatment guidelines for common diseases and complaints that can and should be diagnosed and treated at that level. National lists of essential medicines are used to guide the procurement and supply of medicines in the public sector, reimbursement schemes, medicine donations and local medicine production; they also help define the training of health workers. In short, essential medicines lists provide the scientific and public health basis for focus and expenditure in the pharmaceutical sector.

In many countries, it has taken several years and several editions of treatment guidelines and lists of essential medicines before a more or less stable product was developed which was accepted by most prescribers and actually used for training, procurement and supply. Although time-consuming, the wide involvement of a large number of prescribers, academic departments, health facilities and professional organizations is crucial. It is also important to stress the point that essential medicines are not second-rate medicines for poor people, but that they represent the most cost-effective treatments for a given condition. Over time, prescribers increasingly recognize and trust the value of the clinical guidelines.

By the end of the century, 156 countries had official essential medicines lists, of which 127 had been updated in the previous 5 years (Fig. 58.2). Most countries have national lists and some have provincial or state lists as well. Many international organi-

availability of a medicine in the country. In addition, most public drug procurement and insurance schemes have mechanisms to limit procurement or reimbursements of drug costs. For these decisions, an evaluation process is necessary, based on a comparison between various drug products, and on con-

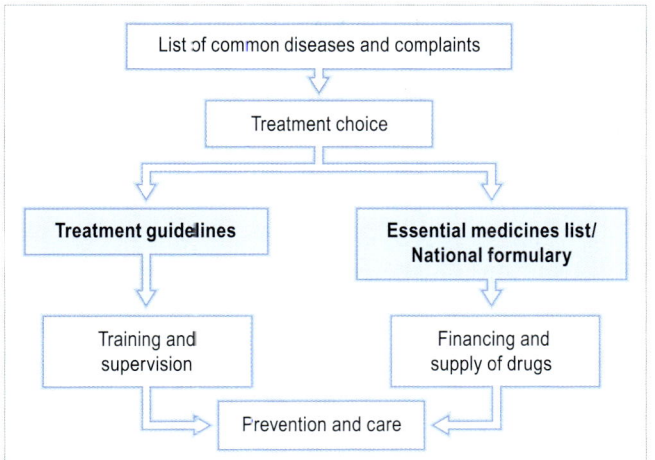

Figure 58.1 Link between selection of essential medicines, clinical guidelines and the supply system. (From the WHO Department of Medicines Policy and Standards.)

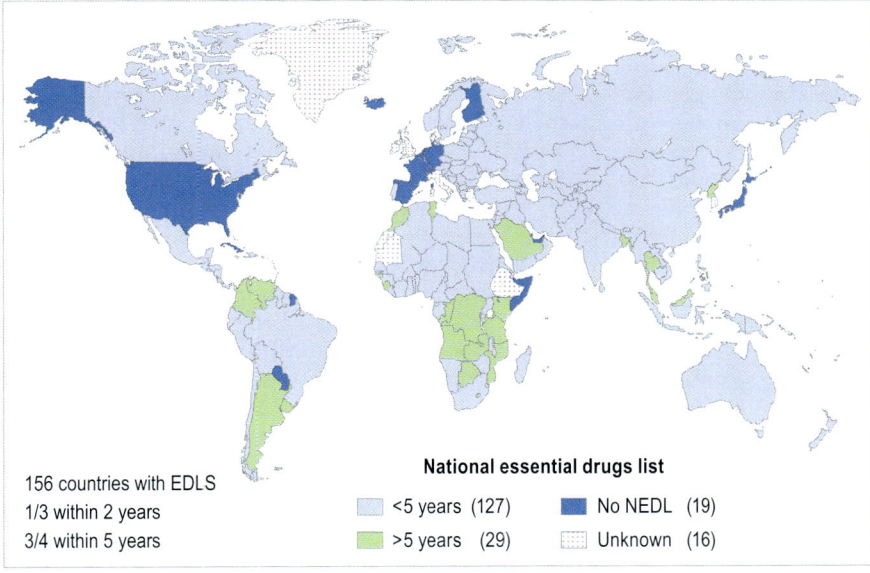

Figure 58.2 Countries with a national list of essential medicines (January 2000). (From the WHO Department of Medicines Policy and Standards.)

zations, including UNICEF and UNHCR, as well as non-governmental organizations and international non-profit supply agencies, have adopted the essential medicines concept for their supply systems. Several developed countries, such as Australia, also use the same approach.

Access to Essential Medicines for HIV/AIDS

Access to essential medicines, including those for HIV/AIDS, depends on four factors: rational selection, affordable prices, sustainable financing, and reliable health systems. Each of these four aspects is essential, and all four are needed. Any discussion on access to medicines for AIDS therefore has to start with the question: access to which medicines?

Much media and patient attention is focused on highly active antiretroviral treatment (HAART). For example, in October 2003, the Director-General of the World Health Organization, Dr Lee Yong-wook, declared the lack of such treatment a global emergency. Yet much more is needed. When opportunistic infections, tuberculosis, palliative and terminal care are added, a total of around 120 essential medicines are necessary for comprehensive care of patients with AIDS.

In practice, this implies that every national or institutional AIDS program must first agree on the clinical guidelines for HIV/AIDS, and draw up a list of essential medicines accordingly. The most sustainable solution is that the clinical guidelines be included in the national clinical guidelines used for training and supervision, and that the list of essential medicines for HIV/AIDS be included in the national list of essential medicines for supply and reimbursement. When the national list of essential medicines for HIV/AIDS has been agreed upon and published, focused efforts can start to increase funding for these medicines through government supply, bilateral support, donations, Global Fund grants, World Bank loans, etc.

There are many ways to improve affordability of essential medicines, including those for HIV/AIDS. In general, the best mechanism is competition. Competition is best guaranteed by the availability of several similar products of assured quality, and price transparency. Globally, wholesale prices for generic medicines from not-for-profit suppliers are published by WHO and Management Sciences for Health.[9] A special website presents sources and prices of essential medicines for HIV/AIDS.[10] Prices of raw materials are also published, in support of national production. In addition, national price surveys can be performed, price negotiations can be started and pricing policies can be developed, including generic policies. In case of high prices linked to patent protection and failure of price negotiations, voluntary or compulsory licenses can be issued for local production or importation of generic products. Parallel import (import of a registered branded product from another country in which its market price is lower) is not generally recommended as it undermines differential pricing agreements and leads, in the long run, to higher prices for the poorer countries.

With regard to quality, there is always a tendency to buy the cheapest medicines irrespective of quality. This is a dangerous approach which needs to be resisted. The product with the lowest price can only be chosen when minimum quality standards are guaranteed. Within the UN system (but also used by the Global Fund and the World Bank), WHO operates a programme of prequalification of suppliers and products for the treatment of HIV/AIDS, tuberculosis, and malaria, based on a rigorous system of international assessments of the product dossiers and manufacturing site inspections.[11] By early 2005, over 100 products had been listed for use by the UN system; this service is of great practical relevance for national procurement agencies.

Access to Essential Medicines as a Human Right

Human rights concern the relationship between the state and the individual; they generate state obligations and individual entitlements. The WHO Constitution of 1946 set out the first articulation of health as a human right in an international legal instrument. It states that 'The enjoyment of the highest attainable standard of health is one of the fundamental rights of every human being without distinction of race, religion, political belief, economic or social condition.' Article 25.1 of the Universal Declaration of Human Rights (1948) states that 'Everyone has the right to a standard of living adequate for the health of himself and of his family, including food, clothing, housing and medical care and necessary social services.' The 'right to health' (short for the right to the enjoyment of the highest attainable standard of health) is also recognized in many other international and regional treaties.

The International Covenant on Economic, Social and Cultural Rights (ICESCR) of 1966, ratified by 151 countries,[12] provides an authoritative interpretation of the right to health. The implementation of the ICESCR is monitored by the Committee on Economic, Social and Cultural Rights, which regularly issues general comments, one of which is particularly relevant to essential medicines.[13,14] While the Covenant provides for progressive realization and acknowledges the limits of available resources, State parties have an immediate obligation to take deliberate and concrete steps towards the full realization of Article 12 and to guarantee that the right to health will always be exercised without discrimination of any kind.

By ratifying a treaty, the government becomes legally bound by its provisions. This means that government legislation, policies, and practices need to be in conformity with the right to health and other health-related human rights. In recent years, there is an increasing trend towards litigation in this regard. A total of 59 cases are known, in which access to essential medicines was successfully claimed, partially on the basis of the human rights treaties ratified or acceded to by the government. Most cases refer to life-saving medicines for HIV/AIDS and show that international human rights principles, if enshrined in constitutional provisions, can promote the realization of individual rights at the national level; and that skilful litigation can promote government accountability in fulfilling constitutional and international treaty obligations.[15]

Rational Use

About half of the medicines used are not prescribed in the most cost-effective manner: overprescription, unnecessary prescription, wrong doses, overuse of antibiotics, overuse of injections and prescriptions not in line with clinical guidelines are very common. After that, about half the patients do not adhere to the treatment: many never collect the medicines of the prescription, do not follow the instructions or interrupt the treatment before it is completed. All this leads to enormous medical and economic waste. The situation is not any better in the treatment of HIV/AIDS and tuberculosis. The need for long-term adherence to chronic treatment and the risk of emerging resistance add to the problem.

There are many proven effective ways to promote rational and cost-effective prescribing,[16] such as the use of clinical guidelines and essential medicines lists, drugs and therapeutic committees, and problem-based undergraduate training in pharmacotherapy. In general, a combination of interventions is more effective than isolated measures. In the case of treatment of HIV/AIDS, the use of clinical guidelines and standard protocols for use by doctors and other health workers is the best option; especially for treatment and follow-up in rural clinics. The most cost-effective use of expensive laboratory tests and promoting long-term adherence to treatment need further study.

National Medicine Policies: Integration and Sustainability

Different aims and objectives of a national pharmaceutical program are often contradictory. For example, reimbursement restrictions may lead to irrational alternative prescribing, and support to the national pharmaceutical industry usually results in higher domestic medicine prices. A national medicines policy, when developed in a consultative way, helps to bring out and resolve such diverging interests.[17] The policy then becomes the expression of government commitment to a common goal and a framework for action. For example, the 1996 national medicine policy of South Africa[18] strongly focuses on equity. By the turn of the century, 109 developing countries had developed a national medicines policy.

With regard to HIV/AIDS, in many developing countries the needs are so overwhelming that drastic nationwide measures are needed. In addition, several aspects of the problem touch upon other departments, such as the medicine regulatory agency (for speedy registration of medicines, quality assurance, licensing of national production), supply and distribution (for inclusion of HIV/AIDS medicines in the regular medicine supply system), and human resources (for clinical guidelines and prescriber training programs); or other ministries, such as the Ministry of Finance (for additional funding for essential medicines, tax reductions, inclusion of HIV/AIDS medicines in health insurance and reimbursement schemes), the Ministry of Trade (for international trade agreements, patent legislation, compulsory licenses), and the Ministry of Education (for undergraduate and in-service training). Sustainability of access and rational use of medicines for HIV/AIDS is therefore best guaranteed by full integration into the national pharmaceutical system and the national medicines policy. Creating a vertical system of supply and training may seem tempting for quick results, but does not create or guarantee sustainability in the long run.

Are AIDS Medicines Different from other Essential Medicines?

Technically, the 120 essential medicines needed for the prevention and treatment of AIDS are no different from other essential medicines. First, many of these 120 medicines are used for other conditions as well. Second, most antiretroviral medicines are not specifically expensive anymore (anti-cancer medicines are much more costly). Third, if HAART has to be given on a named-patient basis, the existing procedure for opioid narcotics can be used. From a managerial or technical point of view, there is no reason to create separate systems for AIDS medicines, and many good reasons not to do it.

Politically, medicines for AIDS are indeed different – but then, especially the antiretroviral medicines. The international community has clearly exposed the shameful lack of access to life-saving HAART and politicians, international organizations and the pharmaceutical industries have responded. As better access to HAART is only slowing picking up, and as many large countries such as the Russian

Federation, India and China are only starting with their epidemics, this political momentum needs to be maintained. However, the political attention for HAART does not have to be translated into managerial exceptions and unnecessary cumbersome parallel supply systems. The more the selection, procurement, quality assurance, and distribution of essential medicines for AIDS is integrated into the regular pharmaceutical system, and the more international technical and financial support is directed towards supporting these systems rather than creating parallel systems, the better the limited number of health workers in developing countries can focus on what really matters: treating the patients.

References

1. Grimshaw J, Russell IT. Effect of clinical guidelines on medical practice: a systematic review of rigorous evaluations. Lancet 1993; 342:1317–1322.
2. Woolf SH, Grol R, Hutchinson A, et al. Clinical guidelines: potential benefits, limitations and harms of clinical guidelines. Br Med J 1999; 318:527–530.
3. Kafuko J, Bagenda D. Impact of national standard treatment guidelines on rational drug use in Uganda health facilities. Kampala: UNICEF/Uganda; 1994.
4. Laing RO, Hogerzeil HV, Ross-Degnan D. Ten recommendations to improve use of medicines in developing countries. Health Pol Plan 2001; 16:13–20.
5. WHO. WHO Medicines Strategy 2004–2007. Geneva: World Health Organization; 2004.
6. WHO. The Use of Essential Drugs, including the 14th WHO Model List of Essential Drugs, revised March 2005. Geneva: World Health Organization; 2005. Technical Report Series (in press).
7. WHO. The WHO Model Formulary. Geneva: World Health Organization; 2004.
8. WHO. The selection and use of essential medicines. Report of the WHO Expert Committee, 2002 (including the 12th Model List of Essential Medicines). Technical Report Series 914. Geneva: World Health Organization; 2003:15.
9. Management Sciences for Health. Online. Available: www.msh.org
10. WHO. Online. Available: www.who.int/medicines ['sources and prices for medicines for HIV/AIDS'].
11. WHO. Online. Available: www.who.int/medicines ['prequalification'].
12. United Nations High Commissioner for Human Rights. Database of signed/ratified treaties. New York: United Nations. Online. Available: www.unhchr.ch
13. Committee on Economic, Social and Cultural Rights. The right to the highest attainable standard of health. 11/08/2000: CESCR, 2000: General Comment 14, para 12(a). E/.12/2000/4.
14. WHO. Model List of Essential Drugs. WHO Drug Inf 1999; 13:4.
15. Hogerzeil HV, Samson M, Casanovas JV, Ratimani-Ocora L. Is access to essential medicines a part of the fulfilment of the right to health enforceable through the courts? Lancet 2006; 368:305–311.
16. WHO. Policy perspectives on medicines, No. 5. Promoting rational use of medicines: core components. Geneva: World Health Organization; 2002.
17. WHO. How to establish and implement a national drug policy. Geneva: World Health Organization; 2001.
18. Ministry of Health. National drug policy of South Africa. Pretoria: Ministry of Health; 1996.

CHAPTER 59

Pharmacoeconomics of HIV/AIDS Treatment

Máirín Ryan

Introduction

Treatment of HIV/AIDS imposes a significant financial burden, and therefore expenditure on drug therapy has been the subject of detailed analysis. Cost of care information is required to assess the economic impact of treatment, to compare the cost-effectiveness of alternative treatment strategies, to determine the affordability of interventions and to facilitate healthcare resource planning.

Differences in terms of prevalence and models of care are evident between high and lower income countries. Antiretroviral therapy constitutes a large part of cost of care in high income countries, whereas in low income countries, smaller proportions of HIV-infected patients receive antiretroviral therapy and inpatient care constitutes a greater proportion of expenditure. Comparison of cost of care between healthcare systems is compromised by differences in relative costs of constituents of care as well as differences in the methods used to calculate overall costs. Costs of treatment are lower in less-developed countries but the impact on the healthcare system may account for a greater proportion of healthcare resources and represent a far greater burden due to higher prevalence of disease.[1]

Pharmacoeconomics

The fundamental economic problem is scarcity. Economic scarcity means that choices have to be made in allocating healthcare resources. The basic task of an economic evaluation is to identify, measure, value, and compare the costs and consequences of alterna-

tive uses for the healthcare budget, thereby facilitating priority setting and hence resource allocation.[2] Economic evaluation of pharmaceutical products (pharmacoeconomics) is increasingly used, reflecting the recognition that healthcare decision makers are placing increased emphasis on value for money from healthcare interventions.

Methods of Economic Evaluation

All methods of pharmacoeconomic evaluation share the common feature of comparing inputs (cost) with outcomes (benefits) resulting from drug intervention. The cost of drug therapy relates not only to the price of the drug but also includes direct and indirect costs. Direct costs include costs of staff and capital. Indirect costs might include loss of earnings, loss of productivity and cost of travel to hospital. Many of these costs are difficult to measure, as are intangible costs for pain or other distress a patient might suffer. As costs are expressed in monetary terms, the difference between economic evaluations resides in the measurement of benefits. Such benefits may be measured in natural units such as years of life saved following antiretroviral therapy. Benefits may also be measured in terms of utility units such as quality of life. This combines assessment of physical activity such as degree of mobility and psychosocial outcomes such as anxiety and ability to cope. The Quality Adjusted Life Year (QALY) is a measure of health outcome, which includes quality and quantity of life. An alternative measure of health outcome frequently used in economic evaluations in developing world settings is the Disability Adjusted Life Year (DALY), which also attempts to reflect quality and quantity of life. Types of pharmacoeconomic evaluations frequently used include cost minimization analysis (CMA), cost-effectiveness analysis (CEA) and cost utility analysis (CUA).

Cost Minimization Analysis

This method of analysis can be used when the treatments being evaluated have similar health outcomes. The comparison is limited to analyzing the costs. Generic substitution may be considered an example of cost-minimization strategy. In the developing world setting, the WHO pre-qualification procedure attempts to provide reassurance about the quality of generic ARVs produced and marketed under exemptions in the Doha Declaration. Although the cost minimization approach is easily understood, it cannot be used to assess drug therapies with different outcomes.

Cost-effectiveness Analysis (CEA)

If two or more drug therapies have the same treatment objective but different degrees of efficacy, then cost-effectiveness analysis may be performed. When comparing therapies, the important question for resource allocation is how much additional benefit is achieved for the additional cost incurred. It is essential therefore to calculate the incremental cost-

effectiveness of one therapy (A) over the other (B); this is expressed as the incremental cost-effectiveness ratio (Fig. 59.1). Frequently, the results of such an evaluation, i.e. incremental cost-effectiveness ratios are demonstrated on the cost-effectiveness plane (Fig. 59.2). Interventions with higher effectiveness and lower cost (quadrant 2) are said to dominate and can easily be accepted, whereas those with lower effectiveness and higher cost (quadrant 4) are rejected. In developing nations, decision makers may occasionally be forced to consider interventions in quadrant 3, i.e. lower cost and lower effectiveness. In wealthy industrialized countries, new interventions frequently fall into quadrant 1, i.e. higher effectiveness but at greater cost.

Cost Utility Analysis (CUA)

This form of analysis enables the effects of treatment on patient quality of life and survival to be considered together by converting both into a common unit of measure. The outcome measure most commonly used is the quality adjusted life year (QALY). The cost-effectiveness of HAART in high income countries has been estimated in a number of studies revealing ICERs of the order of US$10 000–30 000 per QALY.[3,4,5] In such healthcare settings, ICERs less than the widely accepted cost-effectiveness threshold of US$50 000/QALY are considered cost-effective,

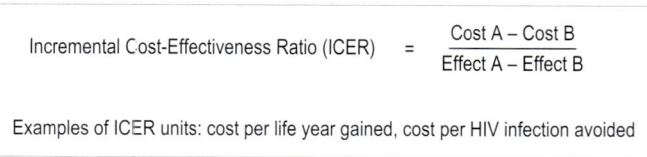

Incremental Cost-Effectiveness Ratio (ICER) $= \dfrac{\text{Cost A} - \text{Cost B}}{\text{Effect A} - \text{Effect B}}$

Examples of ICER units: cost per life year gained, cost per HIV infection avoided

Figure 59.1 The incremental cost-effectiveness ratio.

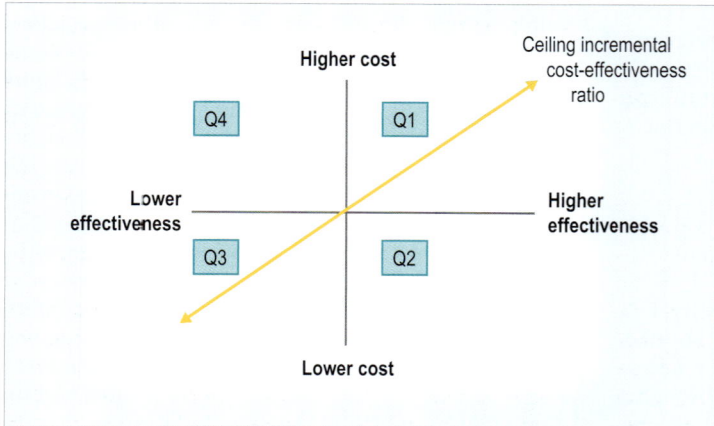

Figure 59.2 The cost-effectiveness plane.

thereby suggesting that HAART is an efficient use of healthcare dollars.

Cost of Illness Studies

The main constituents of healthcare costs for HIV-infected patients include expenditure on drug therapy, outpatient clinical and diagnostic monitoring, and inpatient care. Per-patient costing may be achieved according to a top-down or bottom-up approach. *Top-down costing* involves calculating the total cost of providing all services and dividing by the number of patients accessing the service to estimate cost per patient. *Bottom-up costing* involves measuring resource utilization, e.g. numbers of outpatient visits, monitoring tests, inpatient days and quantity of drugs dispensed to individual patients and multiplying by unit costs to provide mean estimates of cost per patient. Top-down costing is easier and less time consuming to perform but relationships between patient characteristics and resource utilization and costs are weakly defined. The bottom-up approach can be more time-consuming, complex and difficult to perform but provides more useful data in relating use of services and costs to patient characteristics. Standardized guidelines on costing approaches are available and when adhered to, greatly enhance the comparability and generalizability of data from individual costing analysis.[2,6,7]

An alternative approach to the analysis of patient level data is to model the cost of care based on population characteristics and expected patterns of care dictated by treatment guidelines and/or expert opinion. This approach, also known as macro-planning, has been more commonly adopted in the developing world setting, where accurate observational data is scarce and budgeting the cost of care prior to availability of these interventions is the objective.

Impact of HAART on Resource Utilization and Cost of Care in Developed Countries

In developed countries, the adoption of triple combination therapy as standard of care antiretroviral therapy in 1995 replacing mono and dual therapy, as well as the paradigm shift to initiating treatment earlier in disease progression before CD4 counts had decreased to $<200 \times 10^6$/L, resulted in major changes in the pattern of resource utilization for HIV care. Triple combination or highly active antiretroviral therapy (HAART) is associated with high drug

acquisition costs of approximately US$12 000–18 000 per patient per year, resulting in greater expenditure on antiretroviral therapy.

Frequently, cost of illness data before and after the adoption of HAART is presented as part of a cost consequence analysis, i.e. accompanied by information on the association of HAART with unprecedented improvements in clinical outcomes. In a pivotal US observational cohort study, Palella and co-workers[8] demonstrated a marked decrease in morbidity and mortality associated with HAART in severely immunosuppressed patients (CD4 $<100 \times 10^6$/L).[8] Mortality decreased from 29.4 per 100 person years in 1995 to 8.8 per 100 person years in the second-quarter of 1997. Increased intensity of antiretroviral therapy was associated with a stepwise reduction in morbidity and mortality. Moore and Bartlett[9] postulated in 1996 that the enhanced clinical outcomes associated with HAART would result in the higher cost of antiretroviral therapy being offset by decreased expenditure on the management of opportunistic infection as well as decreased hospitalization costs. In the pre-HAART era, hospitalization accounted for the largest category of expenditure on HIV healthcare. After the introduction of HAART, hospital costs declined rapidly and antiretroviral therapy now accounts for the largest proportion of the cost of care.[4,10] Mouton and co-workers[11] reported dramatic reductions in healthcare resource use among patients at 10 French centers receiving HAART. An increase in the proportion of patients receiving ARVs from 36% to 53% coincided with a 35% reduction in hospitalizations over a year, as well as reductions of 35% and 46% in new AIDS cases and mortality, respectively.[11] A greater impact in terms of reduced mortality and decreased hospitalization was observed for centers who initiated HAART earlier in disease progression. Dramatic reductions in inpatient healthcare resource utilization have been reported across the developed world.[12] In Ireland, the introduction of HAART coincided with a 44% reduction in hospitalization, and a 68% reduction in the incidence of AIDS defining illnesses.[10]

In the USA, the introduction of HAART was initially associated with an overall reduction in the total cost of care as the high acquisition cost of antiretrovirals was offset by savings on management of complications of HIV disease.[13,14,15] The direct cost of care across all HIV-infected adults in the USA declined from about US$1800 to <US$1400 per patient per month during the first 36 months of care after the introduction of HAART.[4] Subsequently, other analyses in the USA demonstrated an increase in

per patient costs and increased cost of managing cohorts.[16] Increase in the total cost of managing cohorts was largely attributable to increased numbers of patients in care as a result of increased survival. Some other developed world countries have reported total cost savings,[12,17] whereas others have reported modest increases in per patient expenditure coincident with substantial improvements in morbidity and mortality.[10,18]

The extent to which the cost of intensification of antiretroviral strategies is offset by decreased expenditure on inpatient care and the management of opportunistic disease is dependant on the specific characteristics of the cohort and of the healthcare system, in which the impact of the new strategies is evaluated. The relative cost of constituents of HIV healthcare vary widely between countries. The cost of antiretroviral therapy is of the order of 1.5 times more expensive in the USA compared with European countries but the cost of hospitalization is more than twice as expensive.[14,19,20] As the majority of savings associated with HAART are derived from decreased hospitalization costs, these strategies will prove most cost-effective in centers with more expensive inpatient care.

The degree of immunosuppression of the cohort is also important. In a less immunosuppressed cohort, the incremental increase in the total cost of care will be greater because the addition of HAART will have little impact on inpatient resource use and will result in an overall increase in resource utilization. Indeed, it has been suggested that overall savings in the total cost of providing care for a Californian Veterans Affairs HIV-infected cohort as a consequence of HAART compared with a slight increase in expenditure for a Denver Veterans Affairs cohort might be due to a greater degree of immunosuppression in the pre-HAART era among the Californian group, i.e. 81% and 55%, respectively.[15]

Patient characteristics that have been shown to impact on the total cost of care include: gender, ethnicity, socioeconomic status, duration of illness, and level of disease progression. Several studies have demonstrated higher costs of care among patients with lower CD4 counts in the pre- and post-HAART era.[13,20,21,22] Lower CD4 counts are associated with increased HIV progression and therefore increased risk of opportunistic infection and hospitalization. Anis and co-workers[23] showed that drivers of increased drug expenditure among HIV patients in British Columbia in the pre-HAART era included increased patient age, poorer socioeconomic status, greater levels of disease progression by CD4 counts, hospitalization, and duration of illness.[23] Bozette

and co-workers[4] showed that among a nationally representative cohort in the USA, the introduction of HAART did not result in cost savings on hospitalization among persons of color, injection drug users and the underinsured who had limited access to HAART and consequently reduced clinical and economic benefits.[4]

Cost of Illness in Developing Countries

There is a relative paucity of observational costing analyses of the components of HIV/AIDS care in developing countries despite the fact that >50–70% of inpatients in some low and middle income countries are HIV-infected.[24,25] One study in Zimbabwe reported inpatient costs for HIV-infected patients to be of the order of twice that for non-HIV infected patients, which could be explained by higher direct costs per patient (drugs, diagnostic tests), and longer average duration of stay.[25] Comparing the results of this study to the cost of home-based care in Zimbabwe indicated that the cost of a home visit in a rural area (Z$1317 = US$2000) equalled the cost of 2.7 inpatient days in the rural district hospital.[26] However, a large proportion of the cost of home-based care was not of direct benefit to the patient (56–75% spent getting to the patient), therefore suggesting that home-based care may not represent the most efficient use of resources. In contrast to the Zimbabwe study of inpatient care, a detailed bottom-up costing analysis in a Kenya teaching hospital found no difference in the cost or mean length of stay between HIV-infected and non-infected patients (mean cost per admission $163 (US$2000), mean length of stay 9.3 days).[27] The authors suggest that similar costs between the two groups probably reflects the limited provision of care available beyond basic clinical services.

Few studies to date have reported on the costs of treating HIV-infected children in developing countries. One study of a small cohort of children (n = 54) enrolled in the Drug Access Initiative in Cote d'Ivoire measured the cost of care for HIV-infected children before and after access to HAART.[28] Follow-up periods before and after HAART were 310 and 638 children months, respectively. Mean costs per year for direct medical costs including drug therapy, clinical, and diagnostic monitoring, outpatient visits and transport costs were €666.13 pre-HAART and €3037.81 post-HAART. Morbidity decreased 2- to 3-fold with treatment. Drugs and monitoring tests accounted for 84% and 8% of the costs post-HAART. However, there have been substantial decreases in the acquisition cost of antiretroviral therapy since this study was carried out.

Decline in Cost of Antiretroviral Therapy Acquisition Cost in the Developing World

Antiretroviral therapy consisting of three of more drugs from branded originator companies is associated with high acquisition costs, considered expensive even in high income countries and puts such treatments beyond the reach of the majority of patients living in middle to low income countries. A number of initiatives in recent years such as drastic reductions in the price of ARVs, simplification of treatment and monitoring strategies and increased donor funds have made it possible for people in poor countries to begin accessing life saving therapy. In 2000, five UN organizations joined in partnership with five (later six) ARV originator companies in the Accelerated Access Initiative (AAI) with the aim of 'making HIV/AIDS drugs more affordable and accessible in developing countries' through a 'preferential pricing' mechanism.[29] Using the AAI as a framework, the price of branded ARVs has fallen >10-fold in 11 developing countries. Further price reductions were achieved with the introduction of generic ARVs locally produced in countries such as Brazil, Thailand, and India. The decision of the Joint Clinical Research Center in Uganda in 2001 to use imported generic drugs led to a 20–45% decrease in the cost of the most frequently used ARV combinations in Uganda.[30] Finally, the Doha Declaration in 2001 recognized that HIV/AIDS qualifies as a national emergency in developing countries and therefore authorizes the use of compulsory licensing allowing a third party to use a patent without the owner's consent under the current rules of the World Trade Organization.[31] Current least expensive prices offered by generic countries to some national ARV programs are of the order of US$1/day. Further work is necessary to reduce the cost of and complexity of laboratory and clinical monitoring to ensure that these low prices combined with increased donor funding leads to further expansion in access for large numbers of infected individuals.

Macroplanning Analyses of the Cost of HIV Treatment and Care

The substantial decrease in the acquisition cost of antiretroviral therapy as well as the advent of simpli-fied regimens and monitoring protocols have coincided with an increased urgency to make HIV treatment available in developing countries. The availability of increased funding through national funding initiatives and international donors, e.g. Global Fund has required budget analysis of the implementation of national ARV programs. A number of macroplanning approaches have been developed, e.g. AIDS Treat Cost (ATC) modelling software developed by Partners for Health Reform Plus.[32] The ATC model estimates the costs and resources required to implement an ARV program under various assumptions and scenarios that can be tailored to country-specific situations. ATC modelling has been applied to planning of ARV programs in Zambia, Uganda, Cambodia, Nigeria, etc. Applying the ATC model in Zambia has estimated the average annual incremental cost per patient for a first-line HAART regimen to be US$488 (US$2003), with drugs and monitoring tests accounting for 57% and 36%, respectively.[33] The model estimates of providing HAART to all who are clinically eligible are US$50 million in the first year rising to US$160 million in the second year, due to increasing prevalence associated with improved survival and increased use of more expensive second line regimens. The model highlights that human resource constraints may be even more important than financial constraints as providing universal access to HAART over 5 years, would require twice the total number of laboratory technicians and half the number of doctors currently available in the public health system. Building human capacity is therefore a high priority.

South Africa has the most resources of the high prevalence sub-Saharan countries but also suffers with the greatest burden of disease with approximately 5 million HIV-infected individuals representing approximately 25% of the population. Prior to the announcement of the national ARV program, a number of costing studies were conducted to inform policy. The studies include:

- demographic models to estimate the number of patients on treatment each year under different scenarios
- estimates of ARV costs per patient per year
- estimates of the number and cost of consultations per patient per year
- estimates of laboratory testing costs per patient per year.

Using different coverage levels of those requiring therapy by 2007, the direct cost of ARV based care in 2007 was estimated at R409 million (10%) to R11 billion (90%) with ARV costs of the order of R5000 per patient per year.[34,35] An older study had costed 80% coverage in 2007 at R13–70 billion using much higher ARV costs of R44 000 per patient per year.[36] In a review of these costing studies, the key determinant of anticipated costs was identified to be the level of universal coverage. The main barrier to achieving universal coverage at levels estimated in the costing studies even if financial resources are available is the current deficient infrastructure of the public healthcare system, not least gaps in healthcare personnel capacity.[37] Other key determinants include ARV and laboratory monitoring costs as well as the costs of clinical consultations.

Impact of HAART on Resource Utilization and Cost of Care in the Developing World

Brazil, a middle income country with an HIV prevalence of 0.6%, was the first developing country to provide universal access to antiretroviral therapy as a component of its comprehensive prevention and care package. Approximately 125 000 patients received antiretroviral therapy in 2002. From 1996, when HAART became standard of care until 2002, it is estimated that 60 000 AIDS cases, 90 000 deaths and 358 000 AIDS-related hospital admissions have been averted. AIDS defining illnesses have declined by 60–80%. HAART has achieved net savings of US$200 million with the cost of antiretroviral therapy offset by savings in outpatient and hospitalization costs. Large reductions in the cost of antiretroviral therapy achieved through local production and strong negotiation with pharmaceutical companies underpin the cost savings achieved by the Brazil national program.[38]

Introducing HAART as a constituent of the healthcare package provided by an electricity company in Cote d'Ivoire to its employees in December 1999 resulted in dramatic health benefits for workers and proved cost-saving for the company. Prior to the introduction of HAART, HIV was the leading cause of death for employees. Comparing the 12-month period before and 24-month period after introduction of antiretroviral therapy, there was a 5-fold increase in voluntary counselling and testing; a 94% decrease in HIV-related absenteeism; an 81% decrease in HIV-related hospitalizations; a 78% decrease in new AIDS cases, and a 58% decrease in HIV-related mortality. The company achieved a net saving over the 2-year period of US$294 000 on healthcare costs. In addition, the program made

savings of US$287 000 due to reduced absenteeism and of US$194 000 on funeral costs. This case study demonstrated substantial cost-savings for industry, social, economic, and health benefits for workers and increased uptake of VCT and other prevention services. It has provided a best practice model for other Ivorian businesses.[39]

Pharmacoeconomic Modelling

Pharmacoeconomic evaluation frequently requires the construction of models, which effectively provide a framework to synthesize data from different sources, e.g. efficacy trials, observational cohort and epidemiology data, local cost and pattern of care data to reflect local circumstances. Decision analytic models include decision-tree analysis that incorporates strategic choices, probabilities of subsequent events and final outcomes. Examples of this approach include economic evaluations of alternative strategies to prevent mother-to-child transmission (PMTCT) of HIV (Fig. 59.3). The expected cost per patient outcome for each strategy is calculated as the sum of costs weighted by their probability of occurrence for each treatment strategy. The different strategies can then be compared in terms of their different expected costs.

Much of the economic work in developing countries has focussed on the cost-effectiveness of strategies to prevent transmission and in particular mother-to-child transmission of HIV. Earlier regimens, such as short course AZT and AZT/3TC, were shown to have ICERs ranging from cost saving to US$3000 per infection averted. Marseille and coworkers[40] conducted a cost-effectiveness analysis of the HIVNET 012 short course nevirapine regimen compared with the AZT regimen and demonstrated a highly favorable cost-effectiveness ratio of US$298/infection averted and US$11.29/DALY for targeted treatment at 30% seroprevalence.[40] This evidence has underpinned the roll out of nevirapine based PMTCT programs across the developing countries.

Alternative techniques, such as Markov modeling, which represents stochastic processes, i.e. random processes which evolve over time, are particularly suited to chronic disease such as HIV disease. In such a model, HIV disease may be divided into distinct states, e.g. HIV, AIDS, death (Fig. 59.4). Transition probabilities are assigned for movement between these states and estimates of resource use are attached to each state and transitions within the model. Running the model over a large number of cycles enables the estimation of long-term costs and

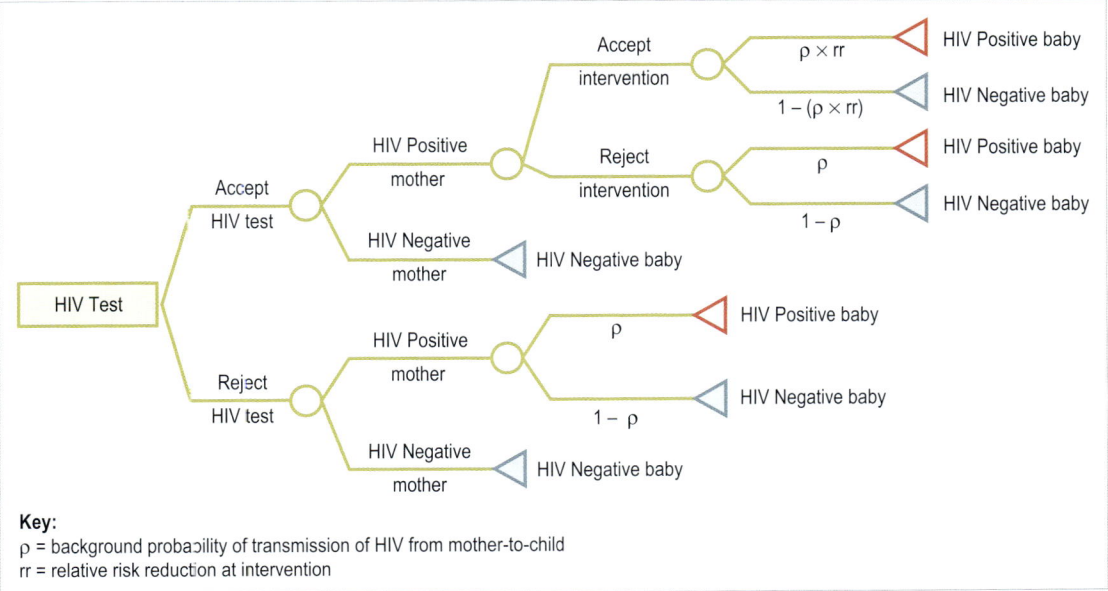

Figure 59.3 Decision-tree to determine cost-effectiveness of antiretroviral intervention to reduce mother-to-child transmission if HIV infection. ρ, background probability of transmission of HIV from mother-to-child; rr, relative risk reduction at intervention.

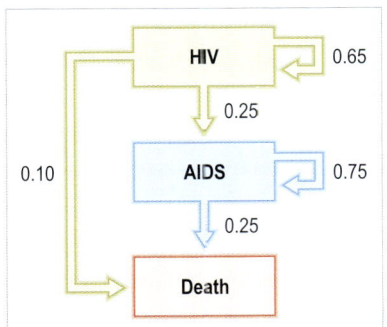

Figure 59.4 Markov model to determine the cost-effectiveness of HAART to treat HIV disease.

outcomes associated with the disease and a particular healthcare intervention.

In a review of published economic studies of HIV interventions in developing countries, Creese and co-workers[41] recalculated the results of a South African study using more recent drug costs of US$350/year to give a cost-effectiveness ratio of US$1800 per life year gained for HAART treatment of 25% of those infected in South Africa.[41] The authors concluded that this relatively high ICER compared with those for a range of prevention interventions (US$1–731 per DALY gained) rendered HAART not

cost-effective. A more recent South African study using data from the donor funded (Médecins sans Frontières) ART program in Khayelitsha, Cape Town, resulted in ICERs of US$984 per life year gained.[42] Another South African study produced ICERs ranging from cost-saving to US$1772 per life year gained for patients initiating HAART at different WHO stages of HIV disease.[43] Some commentators have suggested that a suitable cut off for cost-effectiveness in developing countries is the *per capita* GDP, i.e. US$4627 per capita for 2004 in South Africa. Using this criteria, HAART is cost-effective in the South African context, in contrast to the analysis by Creese and co-workers.[41]

Specific Considerations in Interpreting Developing World Cost Data

There are a number of factors which must be taken into consideration when interpreting cost of care studies from different developing countries. Costs are frequently quoted in US dollars (US$), but these figures may be based on current direct currency conversions or alternatively, on purchasing power parities. Costs will have been measured at a particular point in time but given the erratic nature of inflation in many developing countries, may no longer represent present-day costs. A number of reviews of economic analyses of HIV/AIDS interventions in developing countries have highlighted deficiencies in transparency and quality of the methodologies employed.[41,44] There have been ongoing drastic reductions in the price of some of the key determinants of the cost of care, including the cost of ARVs and of monitoring tests. In addition, much work is underway to examine the effectiveness of alternative models for delivery of care, e.g. use of public private partnerships in Botswana and South Africa in which private healthcare infrastructure including personnel is employed to treat public patients or, alternatively, using community-based models employing large numbers of non-healthcare personnel to deliver care rather than the traditional hospital-based approach used in high income countries. All of these issues may have considerable impact on the comparability, transferability, and interpretation of cost of care studies from different healthcare settings and different time periods.

Conclusion

Much work has been undertaken to demonstrate the cost-effectiveness of expensive antiretroviral strategies in high income countries. While these analyses have demonstrated that ART is cost-effective, the high acquisition cost appropriately limits use to the most efficient strategies as outlined in various standardized guidelines. Additional work has focussed on other aspects of care, such as the economic impact of initiating therapy at different stages of disease and the cost-effectiveness of the use of resistance testing to guide antiretroviral selection.[45,46]

Much work is needed to further clarify how limited resources for HIV/AIDS interventions in developing countries can be best utilized to maximize health outcomes. This work requires high quality local cost data as well as data on the efficacy of HAART regimens in these settings. Collecting this data alongside the expansion of ARV treatment programs is of paramount importance to identify the most cost-effective approaches and thereby save the greatest number of lives for the fixed budget available.

References

1. Beck E, Miners A, Tolley K. The cost of HIV treatment and care; a global review. Pharmacoeconomics 2001; 19:13–39.

2. Drummond M, O'Brien B, Stoddart G, et al. Methods for the economic evaluation of health care programmes. 2nd edn. Oxford: Oxford Medical Publications; 1997.

3. Freedberg K, Losina E, Weinstein M, et al. The cost-effectiveness of combination antiretroviral therapy for HIV disease. N Engl J Med 2001; 344:824–831.

4. Bozette S, Joyce G, McCaffrey D, et al. Expenditures for the care of HIV-infected patients in the era of highly active antiretroviral therapy. N Engl J Med 2001; 344:817–823.

5. Sendi P, Bucher H, Harr T, et al. Cost-effectiveness of highly active antiretroviral therapy in HIV-1 infected patients. Swiss HIV Cohort Study AIDS 1999; 13:1115–1122.

6. Gold M, Siegel J, Russell L, et al. Cost-effectiveness in health and medicine. Oxford: Oxford University Press; 1996.

7. Kumaranayake L, Pepperall J, Goodman H, et al. Costing guidelines for HIV prevention strategies 2000. London: Health Economics and Financing Program, Health Policy Unit, London School of Hygiene and Tropical Medicine. 2000. Online. Available: www.hivtools.lshtm.ac.uk/downloads/costings/costgui.pdf

8. Palella F, Delaney K, Moorman A, et al. Declining morbidity and mortality among patients with advanced human immunodeficiency virus infection. N Engl J Med 1998; 338:853–860.

9. Moore R, Bartlett J. Combination antiretroviral therapy in HIV infection: an economic perspective. Pharmacoeconomics 1996; 10:109–113.

10. Ryan M. A study of the impact of highly active antiretroviral therapy on the pharmacoepidemiology and pharmacoeconomics of HIV infection. PhD thesis, Trinity College Dublin; 2001.

11. Mouton Y, Alfandari S, Valette M, et al. Impact of protease inhibitors on AIDS-defining events and hospitalisations in 10 French AIDS reference centers. Federation National des Centers de Lutte contre le SIDA. AIDS 1997; 11:101–105.

12. Tramarin A, Campostrini S, Postma M, et al. A multicenter study of patient survival, disability, quality of life and cost of care. Pharmacoeconomics 2004; 22:43–53.

13. Gebo K, Chaisson R. Folkemer, et al. Costs of HIV medical care in the era of highly active antiretroviral therapy. AIDS 1999; 13:963–969.

14. Keiser P, Nassar N, Kvanli M, et al. Protease inhibitor-based therapy is associated with decreased HIV-related health care costs in men treated at a Veterans Administration hospital. J Acquir Immune Defic Syndr Hum Retrovirol 1999; 20:28–33.

15. Mole L, Ockrim K, Holodniy M. Decreased medical expenditures for care of seropositive patients: the impact of highly active antiretroviral therapy at a US veterans medical center. Pharmacoeconomics 1999; 16:307–315.

16. Bozette S. The economics of HIV in the HAART era. Clinical Care Options. 2004. Online. Available: www.clinicaloptions.com/hiv/treatment/pe (accessed May 2003).

17. Flori Y, le Vaillant M. Use and cost of antiretrovirals in France 1995–2000. Pharmacoeconomics 2004; 22:1061–1070.

18. Krentz H, Auld M, Gill M. The changing direct costs of medical care for patients with HIV/AIDS, 1995-2001. CMAJ 2003; 169:106–110.

19. Bozette S, Berry S, Duan N, et al. The care of HIV-infected adults in the United States. HIV Cost and Services Utilization Study Consortium [see comments]. N Engl J Med 1998; 339:1897–1904.

20. Ryan M, Merry C, Ryan C, et al. population based study of the cost of inpatient care for HIV-infected individuals in an Irish teaching hospital. Ir Med J 2004; 97:200–202.

21. Krentz H, Auld M, Gill M. The high cost of medical care for patients who present late (CD4 <200 cells/μL) with HIV infection. HIV Med 2004; 5:93–98.

22. Kennelly J, Tolley K, Ghani A, et al. Hospital costs of treating haemophiliac patients infected with HIV. AIDS 1995; 9:787–794.

23. Anis A, Hogg R, Yip B, et al. Modelling the potential economic impact of viral load-driven triple drug

combination antiretroviral therapy. Pharmacoeconomics 1998; 13:697–705.

24. Hassig S, Perriers J, Baende E, et al. Ana analysis of the economic impact of HIV infection among patients at Mama Yemo Hospital, Kinshasa, Zaire. AIDS 1990; 4:883–887.

25. Hansen K, Chapman G, Chitsike I, et al. The costs of HIV/AIDS care at government hospitals in Zimbabwe. Health Policy Plan 2000; 15:432–440.

26. Hansen K, Woelk G. Jackson, et al. the cost of home-based care for HIV/AIDS patients in Zimbabwe. AIDS Care 1998; 10:751–759.

27. Guinness L, Arthur G, Bhatt S, et al. costs of hospital care for HIV-positive and HIV-negative patients at Kenyatta National Hospital, Nairobi, Kenya. AIDS 2002; 16:901–908.

28. Laguide R, Elenga N, Fassinou P, et al. Direct costs of medical care for HIV-infected children before and during HAART in Abidjan, Côte d'Ivoire, 2000-2002. In: Moatti JP, Coriat B, Souteyrand Y, et al., eds. Economics of AIDS and access to HIV/AIDS care in developing countries. Issues and Challenges. Paris: ANRS; 2003.

29. WHO/UNAIDS. Accelerating Access Initiative. Widening access to care and support for people living with HIV/AIDS. Progress report. 14th International AIDS Conference, Barcelona: July 2002.

30. Ferriman A. Doctors demand immediate access to antiretroviral drugs in Africa. Br Med J 2001; 322:1012.

31. World Trade Organisation. The Doha Declaration on the TRIPS Agreement and Public Health. Adopted by the ministerial conference, 4th session, Doha: 14 November 2001.

32. Bautista S, Dmytraczenko T, Kombe G, et al. Costing of HIV/AIDS treatment in Mexico. Bethesda, MD: The Partners for Health Reformplus Project; 2003: Technical report No. 020. Online. Available: www.phrplus.org (accessed March 2005).

33. Kombe G, Smith O. The costs of antiretroviral treatment in Zambia. Bethesda, MD: The Partners for Health Reformplus Project; 2003: Technical report No. 029. Online. Available: www.phrplus.org (accessed March 2005).

34. Boulle A, Kenyon C, Skordis J, et al. Exploring the costs of a limited public sector antiretroviral treatment program in South Africa. S Afr Med J 2002; 92:811–817.

35. Geffen N, Nattrass N, Raubenheimer C. The cost of HIV prevention and treatment interventions in South Africa. Cape Town: Center for social science research, University of Cape Town; 2003.

36. Abt Associates Inc. Impending catastrophe revisited. Lovelife 2001.

37. Ryan M, Tchum I, Coakley P, et al. Healthcare worker crisis in Africa threatens the fight against HIV/AIDS. Ir Med J 2005; 98:61.

38. Teixeira P, Vitoria MA, Barcarolo J. The Brazilian experience in providing universal access to antiretroviral therapy. In: Moatti JP, Coriat B, Souteyrand Y, et al. eds. Economics of AIDS and access to HIV/AIDS care in developing countries. Issues and challenges. Paris: ANRS; 2003.

39. Eholie S, Nolan M, Gaumon AP, et al. Antiretroviral treatment can be cost-saving for industry and life-saving for workers: a case study from Cote d'Ivoire's private sector. In: Moatti JP, Coriat B, Souteyrand Y, et al., eds. Economics of AIDS and access to HIV/AIDS care in developing countries. Issues and challenges. Paris: ANRS; 2003.

40. Marseille E, Kahn J. Mmiro et al. Cost-effectiveness of single dose nevirapine regimen for mothers and babies to decrease vertical HIV-1 transmission in sub-Saharan Africa. Lancet 1999; 354:803–809.

41. Creese A, Floyd K, Alban A, et al. Cost-effectiveness of HIV/AIDS interventions in Africa : a systematic review of the evidence. Lancet 2002; 359:1635–1642.

42. Cleary S, McIntyre D, Boulle A. The cost-effectiveness of antiretroviral treatment in Khayelitsha, South Africa – a primary data analysis. Cost Effec Resour Alloc 2006; 4:20 (Epub).

43. Badri M, Maartens G, Mandalia S, et al. Cost-effectiveness of highly active antiretroviral therapy in South Africa. PLoS Med 2006; 3:e4.

44. Kumaranayake L. Cost-effectiveness and economic evaluation of HIV/AIDS related interventions: the state of the art. State of the Art: AIDS and Economics 2002. Online. Available: www.policyproject.com/pubs/other/SOTAecon.pdf (accessed March 2005).

45. Schackman B, Freedberg K, Weinstein M, et al. Cost-effectiveness implications of the timing of antiretroviral therapy in HIV-infected adults. Arch Intern Med 2002; 162:2478–2486.

46. Chaix C, Grenier-Sennelier C, Clenbergh P, et al. economic evaluation of drug resistance genotyping for the adaptation of treatment in HIV-infected patients in the VIRADAPT study. J Acquir Immunes Defic Syndr 2000; 24:227–231.

CHAPTER 60

Logistics and Models of Implementing HAART in Resource-constrained Settings

Ernest Darkoh-Ampem

Introduction

The special considerations and concerns associated with the provision of HAART in the developing world largely relate to: (1) the requirement of long-term sustained perfect to near-perfect adherence; (2) the potential of developing epidemics of resistant strains of virus in the event of non-adherence; (3) the advanced epidemic and unprecedented large scale at which these relatively expensive medications would have to be provided in settings where the capacity and systems have traditionally been weak, and (4) the lack of time necessary to build the systemic capacity to reach and treat such large numbers especially considering the high proportion with already advanced disease and who unfortunately, are largely are still unaware of their HIV status. According to the UNAIDS it was estimated 39.4 million (range 35.9–44.3 million) people living with HIV as of December 2004.[1] An estimated 25.4 million of this number are in sub-Saharan Africa. As of the end of 2003, UNAIDS also estimated that only 400 000 patients were on HAART in the developing world. The challenge of ensuring timely, equitable, appropriate, and clinically sound access of HAART for such large numbers of people in the economically underdeveloped world is daunting. Most developing countries have experienced long and intense legacies of underdevelopment and had severe problems in providing even basic healthcare services for their populations long before the emergence of HIV/AIDS. The political, economic, social, cultural, technological, legal, and environmental problems are deep, and in most countries have been the norm rather than the exception. It is precisely these systemic weaknesses that need to be addressed if HAART is to be successfully, appropriately, and timeously made available to the millions who are in need in the developing world and other resource constrained settings. This chapter will:

- Define the basic generic supply chain framework for implementing antiretroviral treatment programs
- Describe the challenges of implementation in economically underdeveloped countries
- Discuss lessons learned and insights gained from programs that have been implementing HAART in economically underdeveloped settings
- Based on the challenges and lessons learned, and propose a program modeling framework for providing rapid large scale HAART in resource-constrained settings
- Propose a framework for linking prevention and treatment
- Discuss outstanding challenges going forwards
- Summarize conclusions for the way forward for countries, program implementers, and key decision makers.

677

The Supply Chain for HAART

The system interventions (health and other) necessary to motivate and support an individual through the process of discovering their HIV status, all the way to the point where they receive the necessary interventions (follow-up, management of opportunistic infections and/or HAART) is referred to as the direct supply chain for HAART. There are also numerous cross-cutting supportive functions that feed into the direct supply chain and make it function. There are about 12 direct supply chain components and 10 cross-cutting supportive functions (Fig. 60.1). Each of these direct and cross-cutting functions in turn has numerous sub-components that must all function together in a well coordinated and concerted manner.

Combined, these functions therefore represent the work elements or 'work streams' associated with implementing a successful HAART program, against which a large array of staff of widely varying technical expertise are deployed. Table 60.1 gives a description of each component and the activities entailed therein. It is important to emphasize that these steps can be implemented through a wide range of models with different cost structures, ranging from grass-roots community-based models to high-end tertiary care settings.

Each of the direct supply chain components/ workstreams listed above is supported by some or all of the cross-cutting/supportive functions listed below. It is critical to note that some of the cross-cutting functions also support other cross-cutting functions (e.g. staff recruitment and retention and training cuts across all components). These activities are explained in detail in Table 60.2.

Challenges of Implementation in Economically Underdeveloped Countries

The fundamental challenge economically underdeveloped countries face is one where health systems coping capacity ('supply') is often grossly inadequate to meet the 'demand' for services. Programmatically, the main challenge is that of how to systematically and cost effectively identify and appropriately treat the numbingly large and widely dispersed target population (most of whom do not currently know their status and will present as critically ill, if not identified early), whilst maintaining high levels of adherence and compliance over the long term.

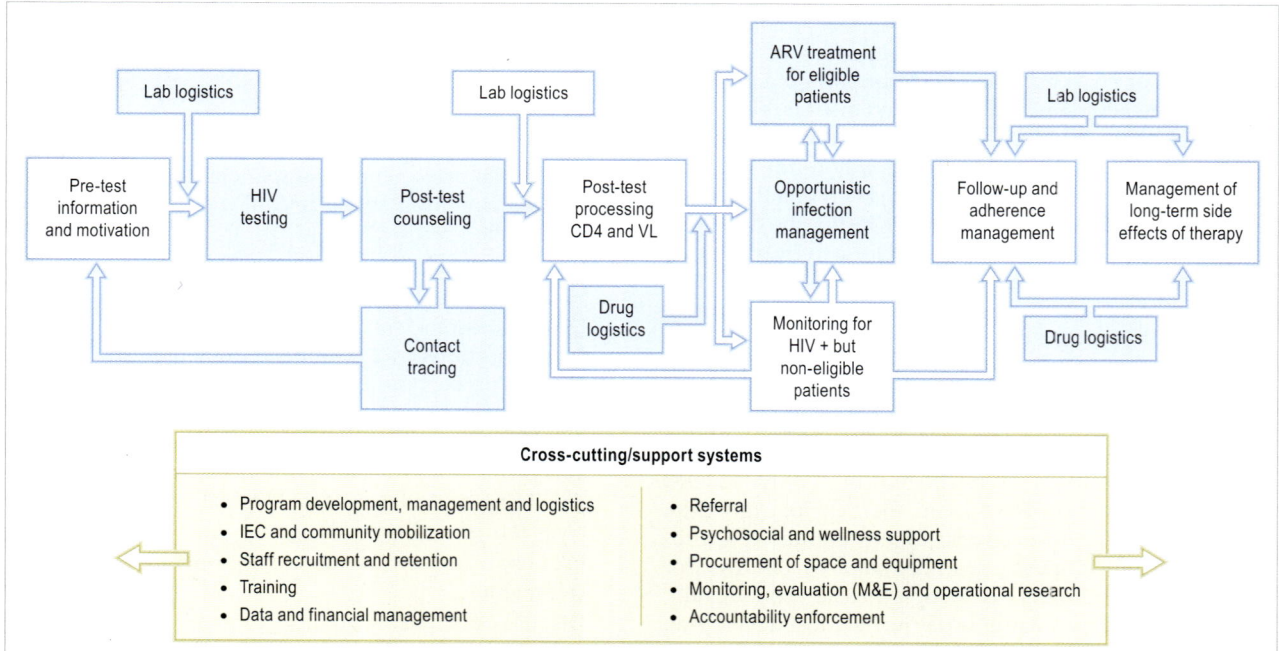

Figure 60.1 Key workstreams for implementing a national ARV program. (From BroadReach Healthcare Implementation and Assessment Strategy. ©BroadReach Healthcare, LLC.)

Table 60.1 Direct supply chain workstreams and their key activities

Direct supply chain workstreams	Description of key activities
Pre-test information and motivation	This includes all activities aimed at motivating populations and individuals to seek and make themselves available for HIV testing. Activities include: Large-scale public mass media campaigns Establishment and enforcement of national testing policies, non-discrimination and equity assurance laws and statutes Community mobilization treatment literacy campaigns including facilitated group discussions in communities and providing group information, education and/or counseling in health facilities or other relevant forums with 'captive' audiences Targeted intensive one-to-one counseling for individuals who require it as a motivation to complete an HIV test.
Laboratory logistics (for HIV and other diagnostic tests)	Includes all activities that ensure: Availability of laboratories as well as relevant laboratory equipment, reagents, kits and other consumables necessary for a HIV testing to be done Specimens and samples are handled, transported and processed in a timely and appropriate manner Once testing is completed, timely results are accurately reported back to the appropriate source.
HIV testing	Includes all activities associated with the actual testing of individuals through a variety of: Outlets: e.g. public, private, NGO, or faith-based health facilities (hospitals, clinics, laboratories); stand-alone voluntary testing centers, mobile testing services Processes: Individual voluntary testing, routine diagnostic testing, general routine testing (e.g. as part of clinic visit differential diagnosis, annual physical examinations or associated with other key life events such as marriage, pregnancy, etc.) Modalities: ELISA, rapid test, Western blot, infant PCR Staff: Doctors, nurses, laboratory technicians, counselors, community health workers, etc. associated with the outlets listed above (and per formal national regulatory and licensure requirements).
Post-test counseling	Includes activities and processes associated with: Informing individuals of their HIV test results (positive or negative) Advising/educating them appropriately Providing necessary immediate psychosocial support and referral to additional services as necessary.
Contact tracing	Activities and processes associated with systematically identifying and ultimately testing current and past sexual partners and young children of HIV-infected individuals.
Post-test processing	Includes all clinical and laboratory diagnostic activities associated with determining eligibility for HAART and subsequently monitoring those who are HIV-positive but not yet eligible for therapy (as determined by specific national guidelines). Laboratory and clinical diagnostic parameters monitored typically processed include: CD4, viral load, total lymphocyte count, hematology, blood chemistry (in particular liver function), TB, pregnancy, weight, chest X-ray and review of systems.
Drug logistics	Includes all activities spanning the manufacture of the drugs, formulation of national guidelines and regimen selection, in-country registration of medications and necessary formulations, forecasting demand, procurement, storage, distribution and ultimate dispensing of HAART and other necessary medications (e.g. for management of opportunistic infections) to patients.
Provision of HAART for eligible patients	Includes all day-to-day activities associated with establishing and maintaining adequate health systems capacity and processes through which individuals receive and are appropriately maintained on HAART over the long term through a variety of outlets, processes, modalities and staff.

Table 60.1 Direct supply chain workstreams and their key activities—cont'd

Direct supply chain workstreams	Description of key activities
Monitoring HIV-positive but not yet eligible patients	Includes all day-to-day activities associated with establishing and maintaining adequate health systems and community-based capacity through which individuals receive supportive care and monitoring services such that they are initiated on HAART at a time which maximizes therapeutic benefits and maintains their livelihood (i.e. before they are too sick to support themselves).
Management of opportunistic infections	Includes all day-to-day activities associated with establishing and maintaining adequate health systems' capacity and processes through which individuals' opportunistic infections are effectively diagnosed, managed and morbidity is minimized (for both those on HAART and those HIV positive but not yet eligible).
Patient/client follow-up and adherence management	Includes all day-to-day activities associated with establishing and maintaining adequate health systems' capacity and processes through which high levels of adherence and compliance are maintained in the HIV positive population being managed under care and treatment. Specific initiatives may include the establishment and maintenance of adequate: Paper and electronic-based data management systems Patient tracking, referral and follow-up protocols and systems Communication systems through which timely information can be disseminated and shared between relevant stakeholders (especially patients, providers and managers).
Management of long-term side-effects of HAART	Includes activities associated with establishing and maintaining adequate health systems and community-based capacity through which long-term side-effects of HAART (e.g. cardiovascular disease) will be addressed for what are likely to become very large proportions of national populations on HAART.

Table 60.2 Cross-cutting supportive functions and their key activities

Cross-cutting supportive functions	Description and key activities
Program development, management and logistical support	This includes all activities that ensure the program (or relevant program components) are appropriate and functioning to specification. Elements include: Program conceptualization Conducting assessments and investigations Developing strategies, operational plans, budgets, guidelines, and protocols Ensuring workstreams, daily activities, managerial and supervisory (performance monitoring) aspects are functioning in a well coordinated manner.
Information, education, communication (IEC) and community mobilization	This includes all internal and external stakeholder communications necessary for the well coordinated accomplishment of individual supply chain component objectives and the overall program goals. Internally IEC and mobilization efforts are aimed at achieving common understanding and operational alignment among implementers and suppliers of different services. Externally, efforts are aimed at informing, educating and ultimately influencing the behavior of both the general public as well as potential and actual patients. IEC and mobilization efforts also serve a critical demand management function by offloading some of the patient education burden from health facility staff and ensuring that patients are adequately informed so as to access services in a manner that maximizes benefits and minimizes stress on the health system.

Table 60.2 Cross-cutting supportive functions and their key activities—cont'd

Cross-cutting supportive functions	Description and key activities
Staff recruitment and retention	Although doctors and nurses are critical for providing healthcare, the mapping out of the supply chain and cross-cutting functions makes it clear that staffing considerations go well beyond theses two cadres. If, for example, the workers at the loading dock at the harbor do not perform their job of offloading imported medications in a timely and efficient manner, it may mean that the drugs are not there to dispense to a patient who may have traveled many hundreds of km to a clinic. All the direct supply chain components and cross-cutting/supportive functions therefore require maintenance of adequate numbers of staff with the appropriate sets of skills. Staff deficits mean that recruitment efforts must be launched and this in turn requires that correct expertise for recruitment be in place with adequate capacity. Furthermore, existing staff must be retained to the extent possible to avoid an ever-expanding and accelerating deficit.
Training	Each supply chain component requires an element of training and/or sensitization of staff. Due to its novelty in the developing world, most health professionals did not receive relevant training in how to administer and manage patients on HAART. Training therefore must span basic and advanced clinical aspects of HAART for those who will prescribe and dispense it. It must also encompass all elements associated with the running of and managing the relevant supply chain and patient service logistics, e.g. training staff how to use computers, manage patient records, operate new lab equipment, perform new tests, fill out forms, process and transport samples, refer patients, use reporting forms, communicate with patients, etc. The large need and multiple areas requiring training and critical staff shortages necessitate the identification of novel training models and modalities that can be implemented rapidly while minimizing disruption to ongoing health services. Furthermore, training programs must be able to continuously update training of existing staff while accommodating any new staff joining the system.
Data and financial management	*Timely information* is the cornerstone of all decision making. All of the supply chain elements listed have a strong data and information management component. This includes the capture, analysis, and dissemination of data and information for internal and external needs of all policy/decision makers and participants in the direct supply chain activities and their supportive cross-cutting functions. Everything from an individual's CD4 or viral load, to the number of staff planning to take vacation next month matters. Financial management is also critical as the basic foundation which fuels project activities. This includes budgeting, fundraising, securing, and distributing funds as well as the efficient and appropriate spending of money with appropriate accounting mechanisms in place. Numerous systems and modalities must either be established or adapted to accomplish the data and financial management information needs. More importantly, these systems must communicate and work in a well coordinated and consistent manner or the entire program will experience severe setbacks and possibly outright failure.
Referral	Referral is a critical element in ensuring appropriateness and continuity of services. This is the process through which individuals and information are channeled through the appropriate set of interventions and services in a manner that assures the desired results and outcomes. The supply chain gives a good picture of the numerous actors who come into play and a well functioning referral system with clearly understood operational protocols ensures the streamlined delivery of a coherent setoff services. Referral is complex and involves coordinated data management and communication across a wide array of cadres, departments, institutions, sectors, and governance bodies. Although the movement of a patient from a clinic, to a hospital, to their home, seems simple, the background communication necessary for health providers to ensure the patient is appropriately managed can be dauntingly complex, especially in environments of chronic understaffing.

Table 60.2 Cross-cutting supportive functions and their key activities—cont'd

Cross-cutting supportive functions	Description and key activities
Psychosocial and wellness support	As individual make their way through the steps detailed in the supply chain, they have numerous interaction points with various personnel in the health system. Collectively, this array of providers constitutes the 'health team' and it is the teams' duty to ensure the physical, social, and mental wellness of the patient/client. An individual interacting with the health system typically has numerous psychosocial needs, ranging from simple reassurance to deep professional psychological input. In poor countries, the public sector health facilities offer the only venue through which the poor can receive care, and therefore provision social welfare (nutrition, legal recourse, housing etc) support becomes a critical component of providing meaningful and contextually appropriate services. Although a health facility may not provide all these services, it is at least necessary to be able to refer clients to them and at each interaction point (including at managerial level), the roles and responsibilities of staff to provide the necessary support must be well defined and operationalized.
Procurement of space and equipment	All of the supply chain elements and cross-cutting support functions require an element of space and/or equipment in order to be performed. Space is necessary for treating patients, providing waiting areas, providing testing and other diagnostics. Management and program staff also require working/office space. Staff also require housing for themselves and their families. The technological needs to support service provision are also quite significant, ranging from the basic (office supplies, telephones, fax machines, computers, printers, photocopiers, weighing scales, stethoscopes, pressure cuffs) to the more complex (IT-based patient/hospital management systems, CD4 and viral load analysers, special refrigerators, resistance testing equipment). Transportation is also a critical function for staff to support program logistics and demands the procurement and use of a variety of transportation modalities (motorcycles, automobiles, special trucks, airplanes, etc.).
Monitoring, evaluation (M&E) and operational research	As mentioned earlier, the supply chain elements also denote the workstreams that must be performed. Each workstream must in turn deliver a desired outcome in line with the overall goals of the program. Therefore for each workstream, input, output, and outcome measures and indicators need to be developed and monitored to ensure optimum functionality of the system and ultimately achieve the desired impact. This involves defining what is going to be monitored, how it will be monitored, the modalities to be used to monitor, the information flows necessary, and how the information will be fed back in a process of continuous improvement. Individual patient, facility, program, and system level data and information has to be monitored, evaluated and used to make appropriate decisions. The monitoring and evaluation framework is therefore inseparably linked to the data management system and utilizes many of the same modalities, ranging from paper and voice-based systems to computerized electronic modalities. In developing countries, it is critical that the data management and M&E modalities employed be contextually appropriate and not detract from the workflow. Operational research enables the program to identify ways of improving processes and outcomes (or achieving the same outcomes more cost-efficiently). All processes associated with the supply chain require operational research in order to continuously improve service provision and cost-efficiency.
Accountability enforcement	This is the process through which any bottlenecks and deficits in the above mapped supply chain are addressed in a timely and appropriate manner. At the core of accountability enforcement is the issue of governance and executive sponsorship. The project management framework must therefore incorporate this aspect to ensure smooth functioning. Strategies for enforcing accountability include: – Ensuring a well designed project management framework with highest level of executive sponsorship and clear roles and responsibilities and appropriate governance, reporting forums and technical guidance committees. – Structuring incentive systems for staff in a manner that encourages achievement of the desired results (e.g. outcome-relevant performance based reward systems). – Ensuring that the program objectives and goals appear in the performance plans of key senior management officials.

Supply-side Challenges

In economically underdeveloped countries, there usually exist severe capacity and capability challenges associated with all elements of the supply chain and cross-cutting supportive functions. In these countries, the supply chain therefore represents both the work that needs to be done and the supply-side challenges. However, even prior to getting to the supply chain, there are a series of national and health systems capacity deficits that must be addressed. They include everything from availability of political will, political instability, management capability and adequate finances, to human resources, infrastructure, technology and appropriate care models necessary for actual service provision. These challenges are referred to as the 'sliding-bottlenecks' (Fig. 60.2) because as a particular bottleneck is addressed, another then becomes the critical rate limiting step.

A whole separate text could be written for each of the supply-side challenges so this chapter cannot explore them in detail. However, a few key issues do deserve special consideration.

Weakness of fundamental health delivery models

The first is whether the models of healthcare delivery in the developing world are appropriate to address the problem at hand. Most developing countries have built health systems along the lines of Western medical models which require highly specialized staff (doctor, nurses, pharmacists, laboratory technicians, etc.) and 'brick and mortar' health facilities. Such models tend to be suitable for low prevalence conditions which do not require long-term follow-up. Health systems were overstretched even before HIV made an appearance, so the fact that adult prevalence in some African countries exceeds 40%, puts the problem well out of the bounds that most current health systems can manage.

Irreconcilable human resource, skills, infrastructure, and technology barriers

These specialized and resource-intensive models greatly compound (and are compounded by) staff shortages that are particularly severe and essentially insurmountable in the foreseeable to future. Doctor and nurse to patient ratios on the continent of Africa (the most severely affected continent) are shockingly low and with the continuing 'brain drain,' are likely to get even worse. The grave shortage of health workers is best framed according to WHO Director Dr Lee Jong Wook in a Canadian Press communiqué of November 2005, by Helen Branswell: 'with a population of 682 million, sub-Saharan Africa has just 600 000 healthcare workers; Canada with a population totaling less than 5% of sub-Saharan Africa has 500 000 healthcare workers'.[2]

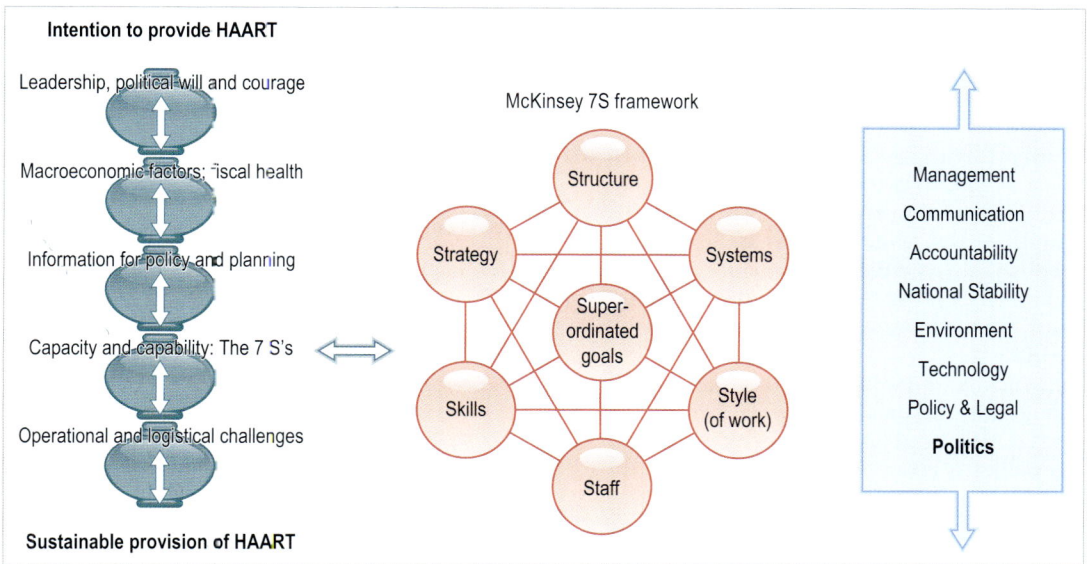

Figure 60.2 Supply-side challenges: The sliding bottlenecks. (From BroadReach Healthcare Implementation and Assessment Strategy. ©BroadReach Healthcare, LLC.)

In addition to formal hospital and clinic staff, other cadres necessary to support the comprehensive supply chain and its cross-cutting functions (Fig. 60.1) are often lacking, most notably staff with good management, planning, and logistics skills. This is compounded by the lack of basic physical infrastructure and equipment for patient care, laboratory, and pharmacy services. Many countries still cannot ensure availability of basic enablers, such as clean water, roads, and electricity for the majority of their populations. This makes technology rollout difficult even in the best of circumstances. Furthermore, the current technologies available for key diagnostic tests such as CD4, viral load and resistance testing are large, non-portable, expensive, electricity dependent, and require specialized staff to operate. The area of resistance monitoring and management of long-term side-effects of HAART will pose increasing challenges as the size population on treatment increases and treatment failure begins to set in. Currently, there are severe skills deficits in the areas of resistance testing and interpretation. There is also a critical lack of simplified failure management guidelines that can be operationalized on a public health level and be implemented in district level facilities and community clinics.

Systems deficits

Systems (management, logistics, financial, monitoring) tend to be weak, making it difficult to run efficient and cost-effective programs at large enough scale to meet the needs of the broader population. The core essence of a HAART program is the provision of monitoring and follow-up services. Few countries had good patient or program level monitoring and evaluation systems prior to the advent of HIV (were not providing good follow-up for lifetime chronic disease conditions like hypertension and diabetes). The high burden of HIV severely raises the bar and amplifies the acute systems deficits with respect to being able to effectively monitor chronic 'well' patients as they move between health facilities, other service providers and the communities in which they live.

Few economically underdeveloped countries have effective budgeting, financial claims and management systems for their public health sectors. Authority to spend money is often restricted to senior-most management who are typically far removed from the implementation interface. Budgets are inflexible and funding is slow to be disbursed, hampered by numerous bureaucratic obstacles and often, absence of clear mechanisms for spending. Even if disbursed, procurement and financial management systems tend to be procedurally dense, slow, and bureaucratic.

Often, line managers responsible for programs have no budgetary or hiring and firing authority and therefore cannot drive performance. Ability to conduct basic financial functions, such as expenditure tracking, cost accounting and cost sharing (e.g. instituting user fees and co-pays) becomes virtually impossible. As such, even if large sums of money were to materialize, there exist severe capacity constraints to being able to spend it speedily, effectively and appropriately. This is not to mention the serious and often egregious levels of corruption that concurrently need to be addressed to ensure funds go where intended.

Structured healthcare financing obstacles

Finally, there are often constraints associated with what funds can be used for. This is particularly so in the case of donor funds. Funding agencies rightfully attempt to institute accountability by strictly delineating fund use and earmarking funds for specific use. However, these criteria do not necessarily align well with the recipient in-country systems, capacity and priorities. As such, strictly focused funding often results in growth of vertical non-integrated programs that further fragments capacity and strain the already weak systems.

Demand-side Challenges

Demand-side challenges are those associated with accessing and serving the population being targeted for HAART. The primary demand-side challenge is the unprecedented large burden of disease that HIV represents in many economically underdeveloped countries. The burden of disease issue is further greatly complicated by the following additional challenges:

1. Most individuals in economically underdeveloped countries do not know their HIV status and as such are not 'identifiable' for service provision. This situation has arisen from a combination of factors including fear, lack of availability of testing infrastructure, and equipment, and a long legacy of acclimating to the previous paradigm that HAART would not be an option for developing countries (little incentive to test).

2. The relatively small initial 'identifiable' HIV positive population tends to be that of those

who are already very sick with low CD4 counts. These patients are very resource intense and take up a disproportionately large amount of resources, effort, and time. Even with relatively small numbers, they overwhelm the existing 'novice trained' health staff (usually understaffed), leading to long queues.

3. Triage at health facilities exacerbates the situations above by further moving only the sickest of the sick to the front of the line each day. This creates a *de facto* eligibility criteria of 'clinically unstable' as opposed to one based on CD4. Creating a 'first come first served' model at all HAART locations can therefore potentially result in model of perpetually insatiable demand as only the sickest of the sick become eligible on any given day. To make matters worse, such individuals, even if successfully initiated on therapy, would have lost their livelihoods and ability to support themselves or their families by that point; a fact which nullifies many of the national productivity preservation justification arguments for providing HAART in the first place.

4. The bulk of populations in need are in hard to reach rural areas and spread over large varied geographic terrains where poverty is high and lack of service capacity is usually much more pronounced.

5. Highly rural areas are not appealing and enabling environments for health workers (even if available) to live and work due to lack of basic amenities (housing, electricity, and running water), social/recreational outlets and availability of good caliber educational facilities for children. As such, rural areas cannot draw the required service providers into their communities.

6. Sociocultural norms and a policy/legal environment make it difficult to identify and systematically reach highly-infected 'taboo' or disenfranchised groups, such as commercial sex workers, immigrants, and marginalized ethnic groups. For example, in many countries, commercial sex work is illegal, making it difficult to even identify the practice within populations.

7. The presence of groups who are dependent on proxy-care givers such as children, people with psychological or physical disabilities. With children for example, most countries do not yet have policies supporting HIV screening for all

pregnant women and newborns. This means that the first interaction with an HIV positive child is often at the point where they are critically ill and seeking care, which often is too late.

8. There are a large number of different languages and dialects across the target populations which makes it difficult to provide adequate and appropriate programming and communication support for individuals who require HAART.

9. Numerous sociocultural beliefs and practices that either affect the ability to identify individuals in need of services, or that negatively impact the efficacy of services provided, for example, the interaction between allopathic medicine and traditional/spiritual medicine may result in dangerous conflicting messages. This is of concern, given that large numbers of people depend on traditional/spiritual healers as their primary first-line healthcare providers in developing countries.

Lessons learned and insights gained from programs implementing HAART in economically underdeveloped and resource-constrained settings

1. Although money is a critical enabler, the main challenge is that of building systems capacity (health and other) to address all aspects of the epidemic. As such, HIV/AIDS remediation must be viewed in the context of the overall national development agenda.

2. Capacity buildup is a sigmoid as opposed to a linear function. Initial capacity that is brought on line saturates quickly and patient enrollment can only increase if additional capacity is provided; a difficult and slow process. This is due to learning curve effects and initial cohorts of highly resource intensive patients being imposed on a small established base of trained (i.e. functional) staff at program commencement. With existing hospital and specialized-staff-based models (meant for low prevalence conditions), capacity is particularly difficult to scale up.

3. Private sector, NGOs and civil society present a large untapped well of human resources, unique enabling skill sets, implementation frameworks and flexible resources not typically found in the public sector. Examples of expertise include program management,

685

financial administration and claims management, risk management, 'capitated' disease management models, social marketing, information technology (e.g. networking and data management), advocacy, policy, planning, actuarial, and risk modeling, etc. As such, public-private partnerships can greatly 'catalyze' implementation and scale-up of HAART if implemented under an appropriate well coordinated framework, which effectively networks all the elements together.

4. Incidence of serious side-effects (warranting regimen change) is relatively low (according to data from Haiti and Botswana). With defined (and enforced) treatment guidelines, HAART lends itself well to simple treatment algorithms, parts of which can be administered by a wide range of non-specialist health staff under supervision (general practitioners, nurses, medical students, and community health workers) with outcomes comparable or better than those in the more economically developed countries.[3]

5. Private sector models in Africa (South Africa in particular) that utilize remote decision support to leverage the expertise of HIV specialists over a larger number of field-based general practitioners (in some cases across borders) can achieve equivalent or better treatment outcomes than those achieved in highly resourced developed countries. One of the companies that offers such services, 'Aid for AIDS', provides treatment for over 25 000 people living with HIV (of whom over 17 000 are on HAART) and have achieved outcomes equivalent or better than US CDC and British Columbia Study data.[4]

6. Large scale lack of knowledge of HIV status in the population creates a 'crisis management' operating paradigm, which disables programs from being able to plan and allocate resources rationally, equitably, and cost effectively.

7. Availability of treatment and relevant supportive services empowers the health system to 'normalize' and mainstream HIV care into primary care activities, and to be more aggressive and proactive in normalizing routine, ethical and systematic testing, screening, and follow-up of populations.

8. Slow, phased launches lead to severe incapacitating overcrowding and therefore program rollout must be very rapid so that the true dispersed demand distribution can be assessed and resources allocated rationally. Furthermore, each new site launched tends to experience the same 'teething' problems, so there is little benefit in delaying between launches as the same issues/problems arise each time and it is easier to address the issues *en mass* for large numbers of sites (effectively batch and condense the learning curve period).

9. The HAART supply chain and cross-cutting supportive functions provide many opportunities for concretely linking treatment and prevention. As such, the established treatment capacity can be used to improve the targeting and measurability of prevention initiatives by providing numerous interaction points through which prevention can be driven with a now, highly identifiable and traceable target population.

10. Due to the wide spectrum of opportunistic conditions and infections through which HIV/AIDS presents, building capacity to address HIV/AIDS can strengthen the overall health system and improve care and management for other disease conditions, if done in a well integrated manner.

11. The large majority of pre-HAART and on-HAART patients are essentially well. Prior to needing HAART, most people are functionally well and ambulatory. Likewise, after initiation of HAART, most patients again become or remain functionally well. The main workload is therefore associated with monitoring large populations of 'well' patients in the community, something hospitals and clinics are not designed for. Setting up robust effective M&E systems (that can track patients between health facilities and communities) as an early critical priority greatly increases a program's ability to experiment with different provision models (as any negative outcome can be quickly identified and remedied).

12. The core of a successful HAART program is not physical infrastructure, rather it is systems and processes, which allow patients to take drugs on a prescribed and consistent basis.

Program Frameworks for Providing Rapid Large-scale HAART in Resource-constrained Settings

The two previous sections have articulated the challenges and lessons learned. Unfortunately, most programs attempting to roll out HAART on a large scale are relatively new, so there are as yet no proven solutions. That said, by looking at the on-the-ground realities (system capacity constraints) and applying lessons learned, and a set of reasonable logic tested assumptions, a framework can be developed to guide programmatic efforts, in terms of achieving rapid large scale, with acceptable quality of care afforded by appropriate levels of monitoring.

Extrapolating from the challenges and lessons learned, the following conclusions can be reached, that define the attributes of 'winning' models and inform the design of new large rapidly scaleable HAART programs. Therefore, a 'winning' model is one that:

- is built around a feasible intrinsically scaleable model with appropriate goals, objectives, deliverables, timeframes and responsibilities spelled out
- has accountability and performance enforced from the highest levels of authority in each participating institution
- is large in scale from the outset and establishes simultaneous access in as many locations as possible with minimum scale-up time an/or requirements
- is community-based (because that is where the people are) and can responsively manage millions of 'well' individuals
- is built on a robust, functional and responsive Monitoring and Evaluation (M&E) system
- aggressively addresses the demand-side issues (see Demand-side Challenges above) in order to identify the bulk of the eligible population and reach them before they are critically ill
- identifies, monitors and links non-eligible individuals to HAART at the optimum time (while still maintaining livelihood and averting severe morbidity)
- harnesses and utilizes *all* formal and informal healthcare capacity (public, private, NGO, FBO, community, individual)
- creates 'docking stations' and enforces guidelines for all providers to 'plug in' and work together in a concerted, well coordinated manner
- leverages rare expertise over larger numbers of less skilled providers in the field by providing rapid training and continuous supervision (e.g. through high or low 'tech' 'telemedicine') allowing extension of rare skills sets (e.g. management of resistance related treatment

failure) to remote areas and to challenging populations (e.g. children)
- is as minimally dependent as possible on highly skilled professional staff and 'brick and mortar' health facilities
- optimizes and maximizes use of existing resources by continuously applying principle that 'no health professional should do work that someone less qualified can do'
- has strong referral and communication channels between all participating stakeholders
- identifies and uses simplified point-of-care technologies and tools to enable key diagnostics (like CD4, hematology and chemistries) to be done in the community, with minimal need for highly specialized staff
- utilizes simplest possible, yet effective regimens (lowest pill burden), diagnostic protocols and treatment algorithms, which confer the best public health clinical benefit, maximize future options and minimize side-effects and the risk of resistance
- has efficient financial flow and management systems which allow rapid deployment, utilization and tracking of funds.

Based on the attributes above, a picture of a viable, rapidly scaleable, far-reaching HAART model of service provision begins to emerge. Essentially, it is a model that organizes a wide array of existing providers into a provider network composed of participants who collectively provide all the necessary supply-side elements. Concurrently, the demand-side is also organized by identifying, defining and mobilizing 'organized units of demand' through which most of the supportive and care functions can be channeled. The supply-side network is then matched to the organized demand-side population under a unifying centralized expert support and coordinating structure (public -private partnership) which centralizes rare expertise and provides support to both sides (Fig. 60.3). The expert support center centralizes rare expertise as well as any backroom functions (e.g. financial claims, bulk procurement) that are critical but not necessary to replicate at every point-of-care. Figure 60.4 details the services such a coordinating unit can provide on a national or regional basis. It could be envisioned that numerous public-private decision support and coordination centers being distributed across a continent and leveraging rare resources and expertise over a large and widely distributed base of providers and people under treatment and care. Figure 60.5 is a high-level

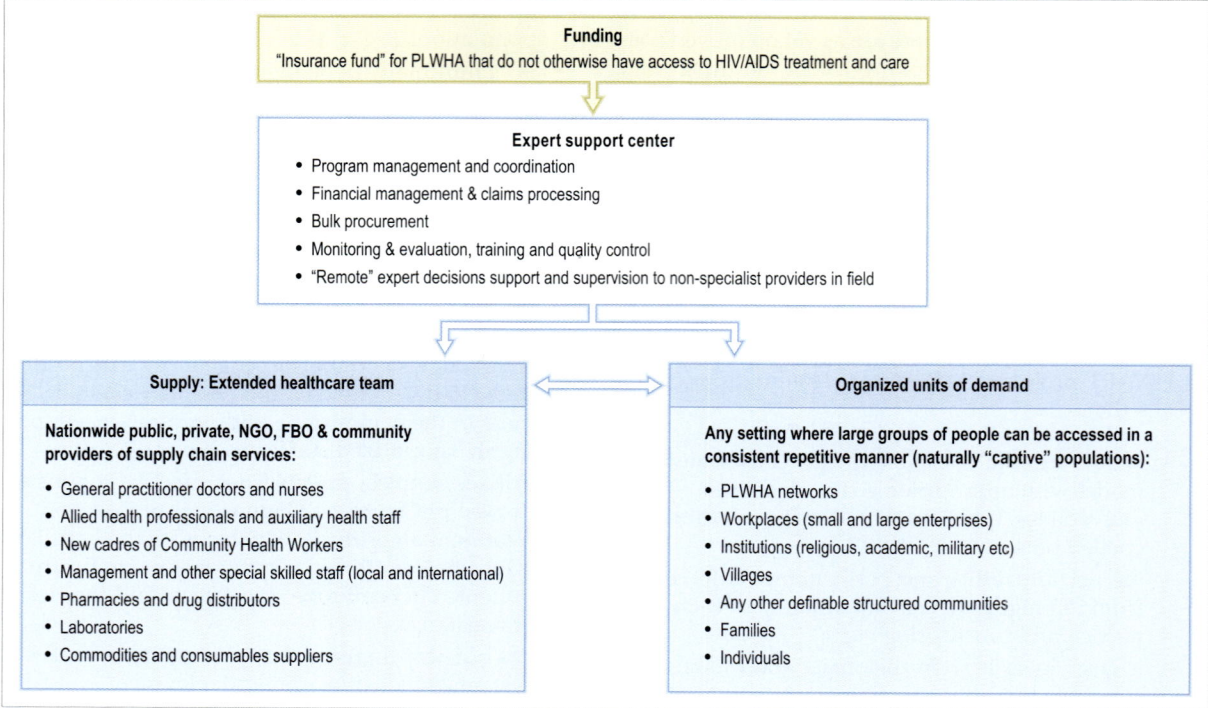

Figure 60.3 Networked model of matching supply and demand-side needs at scale. (From BroadReach Healthcare Implementation and Assessment Strategy. ©BroadReach Healthcare, LLC.)

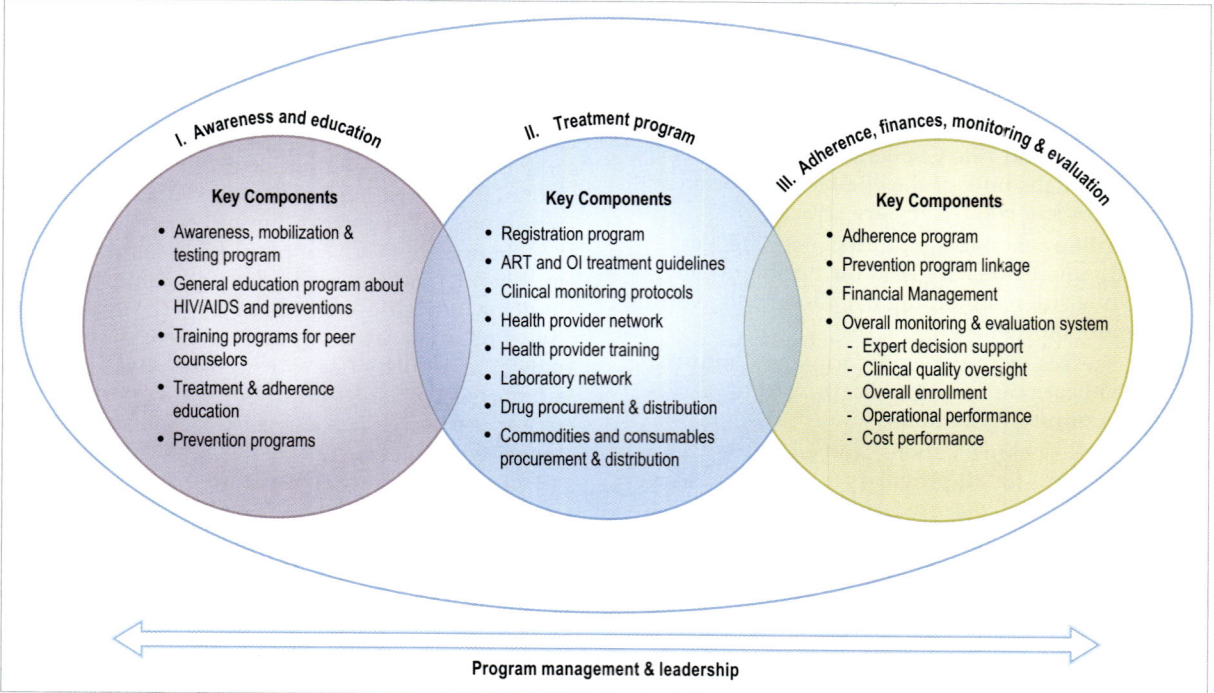

Figure 60.4 Regional decision support center service components. (From BroadReach Healthcare Implementation and Assessment Strategy. ©BroadReach Healthcare, LLC.)

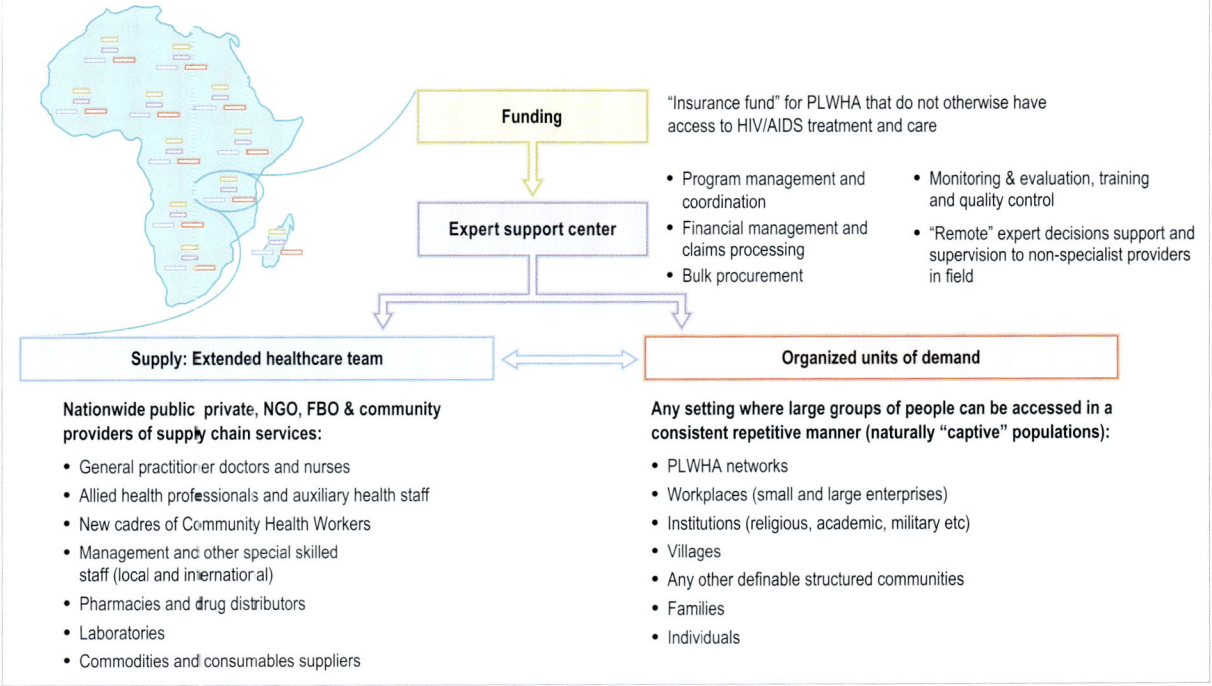

"Insurance fund" for PLWHA that do not otherwise have access to HIV/AIDS treatment and care

Funding

Expert support center

- Program management and coordination
- Financial management and claims processing
- Bulk procurement

- Monitoring & evaluation, training and quality control
- "Remote" expert decisions support and supervision to non-specialist providers in field

Supply: Extended healthcare team

Organized units of demand

Nationwide public private, NGO, FBO & community providers of supply chain services:

- General practitioner doctors and nurses
- Allied health professionals and auxiliary health staff
- New cadres of Community Health Workers
- Management and other special skilled staff (local and international)
- Pharmacies and drug distributors
- Laboratories
- Commodities and consumables suppliers

Any setting where large groups of people can be accessed in a consistent repetitive manner (naturally "captive" populations):

- PLWHA networks
- Workplaces (small and large enterprises)
- Institutions (religious, academic, military etc)
- Villages
- Any other definable structured communities
- Families
- Individuals

Figure 60.5 Expanded vision of public capacity maximization. (From BroadReach Healthcare Implementation and Assessment Strategy. ©BroadReach Healthcare, LLC.)

schematic depiction of how such a network could be replicated across a continent (Africa in this case).

In addition to addressing most of the supply and demand side-deficits and offering unprecedented scalability, such a model offers the following additional potential benefits:

- Ability to implement a wide array of other primary care activities (e.g. other chronic disease care and monitoring, management of complex side-effects, and resistance-related treatment failure) through such a wide distributed network with reach into rural areas and special hard-to-reach populations with a vast improvement in ability to monitor and follow-up patients in the community
- Reversal of dependency on government and empowers communities and individuals to take responsibility for their health and play a much more proactive role in preventing further morbidity and mitigating the effects of the epidemic in their lives
- Emphasizes maintenance of wellness and prevention in the community, as opposed to largely managing critical illness (like pure

hospital and clinic model) and as such, is likely to achieve substantial cost savings
- Obviates the need for impossibly large numbers of specialized staff while promoting cost and effort sharing across a much wider array of participants (including individuals) resulting in a health system that is more likely to be sustainable in the long term
- Has the potential to reach into highly rural areas as long as individuals with the right aptitude can be identified in the community, trained and linked to a functional decision support framework (helps address difficulties associated with getting skilled staff to live in rural areas and for extending reach of rare skills like pediatric HIV management).

Framework for Linking Prevention, Treatment, and Care Activities

As treatment initiatives in the developing world are launched, the million dollar question is whether treatment will promote or detract from prevention efforts. Popular belief is that treatment with HAART may indeed serve to promote and support prevention by:

- providing an incentive for individuals to get tested and as such empower them to make conscious choices related to how they will manage their risk going forward
- affording access to large numbers of identifiable HIV positive and negative individuals to whom targeted individualized interventions can be given and *monitored* longitudinally
- potentially decreasing infectivity of individuals by decreasing viral load.

If one believes that knowledge of individual status is a key element of prevention, then it stands to reason that availability of HAART provides the engine to drive a key outcome (knowledge of status) that is critical to the fulfillment of prevention objectives. Experience with implementing large-scale HAART in countries like Botswana provides compelling evidence that availability of HAART activates a virtuous loop resulting in decreased transmission of the virus over time. Figure 60.6 schematically depicts this loop. If this proves to be true, provision of HAART may indeed be one of the best prevention strategies. Naturally, there is potential risk associated with large-scale availability of HAART (e.g. decrease in risk perception) and this is why strong monitoring and evaluation systems are critical, so that negative trends can be identified early and remedied.[5]

Beyond the theoretical constructs however, there are some clear and tangible operational ways of linking prevention and treatment. As mentioned before, the supply chain and cross-cutting functions detailed in Figure 60.1 can be implemented through a variety of models ranging from advanced tertiary care facilities to community health workers providing door-to-door services. The fundamental elements remain the same, regardless. It is just a matter of *how* they are accomplished. Therefore, if truly large-scale models can be developed to fulfill all elements of the supply chain (and cross-cutting functions), then opportunities afforded to concretely link prevention activities, if exploited well, could result in an equally large-scale ability to drive much better targeted prevention programs based on the fact that the treatment supply chain affords health workers and managers access to ever increasing numbers of *identifiable* HIV positive and negative individuals. The testing interface provides the first interaction and from that point, everyone (positive or negative) should be enrolled into a wellness program. Subsequent points in the supply chain provide opportunities for targeted interactions including:

- Providing behavior change advice, education and supplies such as condoms
- Monitoring of desirable prevention behavior change at subsequent interactions
- Providing referral to psychosocial support, social welfare services and prevention programs (e.g. safe blood).

Furthermore, each point along the supply chain allows for improved management coordination and program integration (joint planning, budgeting,

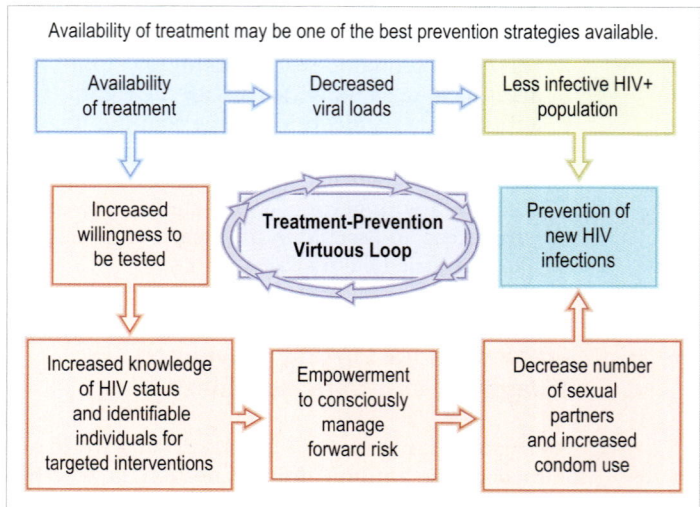

Figure 60.6 Operationalizing links between prevention, testing, and treatment. (From BroadReach Healthcare Implementation and Assessment Strategy. ©BroadReach Healthcare, LLC.)

training etc). A system can be envisioned where after an HIV test, a positive individual who is eligible for therapy, receives intensive counseling and education about protecting their sexual partners, is encouraged to be faithful, is dispensed condoms with their HAART, and the effectiveness of these interventions supported and monitored during subsequent visits.

Likewise a person who tests negative can be recruited into a safe blood donation program (an area where most countries have critical life-threatening shortages) at the VCT center and provided with a set of programmatic interventions to keep them negative as part of a blood donor pool. Tables 60.3 and 60.4 look at each element of the supply chain and cross-

Table 60.3 Direct-supply chain activities and their potential linkage to prevention

Direct-supply chain activities	Potential linkage to prevention
Pre-test information and motivation	Ensure prevention messages are reinforced (abstinence, be faithful, use condoms) Incorporate demonstration of condom usage and distribute condoms and information on protection options as part of counseling sessions Ensure a clear link between VCT, PMTCT, STI, TB, and HAART programs as well as other social welfare services
Lab and testing logistics	Utilize HAART phlebotomy activities and staff for safe blood program Use phlebotomy interaction as an opportunity to distribute condoms and information on protection options.
HIV testing	Reinforce prevention messages Capture contact details for future targeted messaging and education Distribute information on protection options.
Post-test counseling	Reinforce prevention messages Demonstrate condom usage and distribute condoms Recruit HIV-negative clients into safe blood program Directly link VCT and PMTCT clients to HAART program Recruit individuals into a longitudinal routine testing program Distribute condoms and information on protection options, STI prevention and reproductive health.
Contact tracing	Contact partners and children and do all the above.
Post-HIV test processing (CD4, VL, chemistry and hematology etc.)	Reinforce prevention messages Distribute condoms and information on protection options Ensure linkage into ARV program.
Drug logistics	Merge OI prophylaxis with ARV logistics and dispensing Merge OI prophylaxis with testing activities mentioned above.
ARV treatment/ provision	Provide targeted prevention interventions to population on HAART Prescribe condoms and monitor use in subsequent appointments Perform condom demonstrations and distribute Provide information on protection options Provide safe sex, STI prevention and reproductive health education.
Clinical management of opportunistic infections	Ensure all presenting with OIs are tested for HIV Aggressive prevention education on protecting partners and avoiding re-infection Provide OI treatment and prophylaxis Perform condom demonstrations and distribute Provide information on protection options, STI prevention, and reproductive health.
Monitoring of HIV+ non-eligible	Provide aggressive targeted prevention initiatives Provide OI prophylaxis Distribute condoms and information on protection options, STI prevention, and reproductive health.
Follow-up, adherence management and management of long-term side-effects	Provide all of the above where applicable.

Table 60.4 Cross-cutting supportive functions and their potential linkage to prevention

Cross-cutting supportive functions	Potential linkage to prevention
Assessment, planning and project management	Joint assessment and planning for ARV, PMTCT, safe blood, routine testing, prophylaxis, behavior change and other primary care programs (holistic approach).
Follow-up and adherence management	Build on HAART follow-up system and infrastructure to provide other prevention oriented services.
IEC and community mobilization	Joint and integrated IEC campaigns encompassing treatment and prevention Piggy-back other initiatives on HAART community mobilization models Link to workplace programs, private sector initiatives and school programs.
Training	Integrate HAART program training with prevention training (e.g. condom demonstrations, role plays etc.) Extend hard hitting joint prevention and treatment training into schools Integrate HAART training into pre-service training for all health professionals (supports 'de-verticalization' of staff capacity).
Data management	Use HAART data management systems to track key treatment and prevention indicators, e.g. STI incidence, episodes of unprotected sex, and routine testing data, etc. Use HAART data management system as foundation to monitoring of other chronic healthcare conditions.
Referral	Strengthen linkages between clinical activities and social support/welfare services in the communities Refer negative testers to safe blood program and provide incentives Refer positives into supportive and HAART-related services.
Psychosocial and wellness support	Incorporate prevention messages and disseminate information on protection options.
Procurement of space and equipment	Done with holistic integrated services model in mind serving all health needs (in manner that strengthens overall health capacity).
Monitoring, evaluation, and research	Done holistically across integrated prevention, treatment and general healthcare programs (supports 'de-verticalization').
Accountability enforcement	Done holistically across integrated prevention, treatment and general healthcare programs (supports 'de-verticalization').

cutting functions, respectively and suggest concrete ideas for linking prevention and treatment as well as integrating other related programmatic activities so as to reduce 'verticalization' and redundancy.

Outstanding Challenges Going Forward

Despite there being existing large-scale solutions and modalities that can be leveraged to create and enhance capacity at large scale as articulated in this chapter, there are two key areas that will be difficult to surmount in the short term and require a combination of new scientific thought and technological innovation. These are the areas of laboratory monitoring and the management of long term side-effects

and treatment failure due to viral resistance. Current technologies for monitoring critical parameters such as CD4 and viral load are large, expensive, electricity loading, and specialist-operator dependent. These tests are fundamental to monitoring treatment progress but unfortunately cost and expertise considerations mean that developing countries are limited in their ability to deploy more than one or two machines countrywide. This results in crippling logistical problems associated with laboratory testing and timely result reporting. There is an urgent need for technological innovation in this area to enable easy decentralized deployment of these technologies in a manner that does not require specialists (for drawing blood or for operating machine) and where results are available within minutes of

Need point of care technologies which provide instant results.

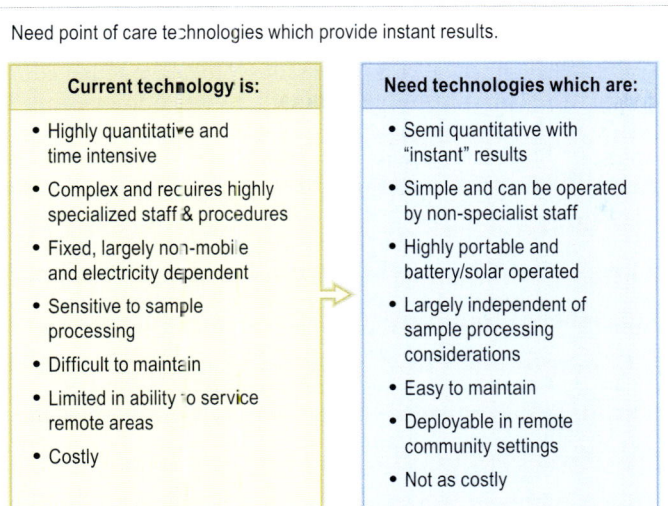

Current technology is:	Need technologies which are:
• Highly quantitative and time intensive	• Semi quantitative with "instant" results
• Complex and requires highly specialized staff & procedures	• Simple and can be operated by non-specialist staff
• Fixed, largely non-mobile and electricity dependent	• Highly portable and battery/solar operated
• Sensitive to sample processing	• Largely independent of sample processing considerations
• Difficult to maintain	• Easy to maintain
• Limited in ability to service remote areas	• Deployable in remote community settings
• Costly	• Not as costly

Figure 60.7 New laboratory technologies needed. (©BroadReach Healthcare, LLC.)

Need point of care technologies which provide instant results.

Current protocols:	Need protocols which are:
• Are dependent on complex centralized technology	• Simple and practical
• Require VERY highly specialized staff	• Operable on a population level basis and decentralized
• Lack consensus even among experts	• Minimally dependent on expensive technology
• Not easy to operationalize at large scale	• Adaptable across a wide range of cadres of staff
• Are VERY costly	

Figure 60.8 Failure management and long-term side-effect protocols needed. (©BroadReach Healthcare, LLC.

the test. The necessary attributes are summarized in Figure 60.7.

The issue of dealing with viral resistance and associated treatment failure, as well as the management of long-term side-effects of antiretrovirals also poses a critical challenge to the scientific and public health communities. Currently, there are no widely agreed large-scale public health protocols on how to manage treatment failure in a community-based setting. Capacity to manage long-term side-effects for, e.g. cardiovascular disease is also severely lacking. Figure 60.8 summarizes the key scientific inputs required.

Conclusions

The Way Forward

Large-scale provision of HAART is a new area and most programs are trying to find their way. In this chapter, an attempt has been made to highlight certain key programmatic 'must haves' in order to achieve rapid large-scale distribution. HIV/AIDS poses unprecedented challenges which have merely unearthed the innate weaknesses and capacity constraints of existing health provision models in the developing world. These deficits existed long before the advent of HIV/AIDS and are the result of many decades of underdevelopment, instability, and poor management. If a system cannot distribute aspirin or clean water effectively, then it is almost certain it will struggle to distribute antiretroviral drugs. Therefore, as decision makers and program managers approach this issue, they should take a systems approach to establish foundational elements that will improve the overall provision of health services and thus, HIV-related service provision will improve. That said, the time critical nature of the HIV epidemic and staggering number of lives at stake forces all involved to conceptualize new models that can achieve and deliver good quality large scale services without the luxury of the time required to build a large capacity of highly specialized staff and associated infrastructure. It is clear that individuals spend a small fraction of their life within the confines of health facilities and the majority of it in the community. However, the community is precisely where the resources and modalities for care, monitoring, and effective follow-up are severely lacking.

Drawing from implementation experience on the ground and lessons learned, this chapter has attempted to propose a program modeling and development framework that addresses most of the existing challenges, while delivering scalability commensurate with the burden of disease. The key message is that all involved must have the courage to explore new models and cross operational boundaries in a manner never attempted before. The shackles of familiarity must be broken if the full magnitude of the HIV/AID pandemic is to be contained. It is critical that decision makers and program managers orient efforts around the actual numbers of individuals and design programs that realistically have a chance at reaching those numbers while they are still alive (which in most cases means less than a 5-year timeframe). This will require pulling together expertise and resources from all sectors and opening up the solution space beyond the traditional notions of how and where healthcare can be delivered. For example, breakthroughs are necessary in the areas of simplified portable laboratory technologies and there is a need to create new protocols for managing complex issues like viral resistance related treatment failure and complex long term side-effect of HAART. This demands openness and evidence-based (as opposed to ideologically driven), nimble responsiveness to new lessons. Finally, financial and environmental realities in economically underdeveloped countries demand models that maximize the use of existing resources and focus on maintaining wellness (as opposed to only addressing catastrophic disease). This fundamental 'maintenance of wellness' tenet should form the foundational bedrock on which health systems in developing countries are built in order to turn the dream of achieving sustainable health systems into a reality.

References

1. UNAIDS. AIDS Epidemic Update. December 2004:77.
2. Canadian Press. Global: urgent need for health-care workers in poor AIDS afflicted countries: WHO press article by Helen Branswell. Friday 5 November 2004.
3. Behforouz HL, Farmer PE, Mukherjee JS. From directly observed therapy to accompagnateurs: enhancing AIDS treatment outcomes in Haiti and in Boston. Clin Infect Dis 2004; 38:S429–S436.
4. Aid for AIDS (AfA). Comparison data to US CDC and British Columbia Study cohorts. Capetown, South Africa: AfA database.
5. Darkoh R, Mazonde H. Antiretroviral therapy in Botswana. Merck and Gates Foundations Partnership (ACHAP). Gaborone, Botswana: Ministry of Health; July 2004.

CHAPTER 61

Universal Access to Antiretroviral Therapy: The Brazilian Experience

Mauro Schechter

Marie Charles

Introduction

The first AIDS case in Brazil was diagnosed in 1982. By 1990, the number of cases had risen to 10 000, leading the World Bank to predict that Brazil would face an estimated 1 200 000 cases of HIV/AIDS within one decade. At the time, the situation looked bleak and many feared that the HIV epidemic was out of control. Government agencies were not responding adequately and seemed in denial of the severity of the situation. However, by 2000, the actual number of HIV infections was half the World Bank had anticipated.

What changed and how did Brazil manage to turn what seemed to be a looming disaster into a success story that might provide valuable lessons for developing countries facing their own HIV/AIDS crisis? How did Brazil, a developing country, manage to curb the infection rate and save hundreds of thousands of lives?

Brazil's success at curbing the HIV/AIDS epidemic is the result of a multi-sector approach to HIV/AIDS prevention and treatment at an early stage of the epidemic. The forces that came together to prevent the World Bank's predictions from coming true include a strong governmental response, civil society mobilization, consistent prevention messages, comprehensive treatment, and a national scale-up of the public health system.

Background

In 1985, after 21 years of military government in Brazil, power was peacefully turned over to civilian leaders. Brazil is currently a Federal Republic with an estimated population of 184 million, of which over 75% are Catholics. It is the fifth most populous country in the world, with an average life expectancy of 68 years. However, Brazil is still ranked 72nd on the Human Development Index; a ranking that reflects the large income disparities between the rich and the poor in the country.[1] The gross national *per capita* income is similar to that of South Africa, at approximately $2800/year.[2]

The AIDS epidemic in Brazil shares many epidemiological characteristics with the epidemic in many other developing countries. In the early 1980s, the majority of infected individuals were well-educated men, 20–44 years of age. At that time, the leading modes of transmission were male homosexual sex and needle-sharing between intravenous drug users. Over time, however, the epidemic shifted into the general population and the number of heterosexually acquired infections has risen sharply.[3,4] At present, new infections and AIDS cases are increasingly more frequent in women and in individuals with fewer years of formal education; a marker for lower socioeconomic status.[5,6]

Faced with dire predictions and the beginning of a generalized epidemic, a strong response was set in motion, through a multi-sector strategy, which involved national and provincial governments, civil society, comprehensive prevention measures, and health system enhancement. In concert, these measures had a substantial impact on the course of the HIV epidemic, saved numerous lives, and had a largely undocumented positive effect on the social and economic fabric of the country.

The Brazilian Government

The 1985 re-democratization of Brazil's political system allowed for substantial reforms to be made to the public healthcare system. Three core principles underlined the new system: universal access, free treatment, and decentralized administration. These reforms were further solidified in 1988, when Health was declared a constitutional right, and set the stage for a successful national AIDS program by creating the necessary legal and regulatory environment.[6] Since then, despite economic, civil, and religious challenges, successive governments demonstrated that they understood the threat the epidemic represented, as well as the risks associated with paralysis and denial.

Brazil's efforts to combat the epidemic began in earnest in 1985 when guidelines for the National AIDS Program (NAP) were established. The plan involved the multi-sector strategy previously mentioned, and its potential effectiveness was greatly strengthened by the simultaneous implementation of all of these activities. Specifically, the national plan included active involvement of civil society; balanced prevention and treatment efforts; frank, direct and consistent messages; and a practical, locally developed, public health approach.

Civil Society

A combination of forces, including re-democratization, reduction of stigma and discrimination against HIV-infected individuals, as well as a strong sense of social responsibility within the homosexual community, the group first to be affected by the epidemic, paved the way for non-governmental organizations to play major roles as activists and as passionate disseminators of HIV prevention messages. As in many countries, AIDS in Brazil was highly stigmatized in 1985. Not uncommonly, HIV-infected patients were fired by their employers, denied access to healthcare by hospitals, and dropped by health insurance companies. The stigmatization of HIV-infected individuals, in turn, attracted considerable attention from several civil-rights organizations and led to a decisive response from a variety of sectors from civil society.[6] Initially, these grass roots movements were active mainly in Sao Paulo and in Rio de Janeiro, but they quickly spread to other regions of the country.

The Brazilian Interdisciplinary AIDS Association (ABIA), one of the first national non-governmental organizations (NGO) that focused on HIV/AIDS, was established in Rio de Janeiro in 1986. A well-known Brazilian dissident Herbert de Souza, better known as Betinho, founded ABIA. Betinho was also one of the first public figures to announce that he was HIV-infected as a result of blood transfusions received for hemophilia in Canada several years before, while living in that country as a political refugee. ABIA became a clearinghouse for information on HIV-infection and AIDS, focusing on policy analysis, advocacy, public education, and research, as well as providing legal assistance to HIV-infected persons, in an effort to combat discrimination.[6] Rapidly, similar organizations sprouted in other cities, ultimately leading to an extensive and engaged network of non-governmental organizations, who have conducted numerous prevention projects nationwide. Many of these NGOs work closely with and/or are sponsored by the National AIDS Program, which, in turn, draws project funding from designated loans by the World Bank.

Although the NAP had the capacity and political power to implement potentially successful prevention and treatment policies, only NGOs had the necessary legitimacy and on-the-ground expertise to respond to the particular needs of specific communities, to link up with high-risk groups, such as injection drug users and prostitutes, and to deliver targeted messages that could resonate within each community. Thus, collaboration of governmental and non-governmental organizations has been key to the development of more effective prevention campaigns.[6] Many consider the close collaboration between NGOs and NAP one of the main strengths of the Brazilian response. Conversely, others strongly criticize the financial dependency of many NGOs on governmental funds that was almost inevitably created, potentially limiting their ability to criticize government decisions.

Prevention

A comprehensive and effective prevention strategy should consist of the simultaneous implementation of several components. These include:

- Promoting of behavioral change and delayed initiation of sexual activity
- Promoting of condom use at all times
- Strengthening prevention and treatment of sexually transmitted diseases
- Setting-up testing programs and encouraging voluntary counseling and testing
- Maintaining a safe blood supply
- Ensuring infection control procedures in healthcare settings
- Providing harm reduction programs for injection drug users
- Preventing mother-to-child transmission of HIV
- Providing support and education programs for people living with HIV/AIDS
- Enacting policy reforms focusing on needle exchange and condom use.

All these components were integral parts of the Brazilian response to HIV/AIDS.

Many contend that cultural norms in Brazil, which include sexual openness, have fueled the HIV/AIDS epidemic, while others argue that willingness to openly discuss sex and sexuality has greatly enabled and enhanced the implementation of effective prevention programs. These include general messages, aiming to reach the entire population, as well as specifically targeted messages aimed at certain groups considered more vulnerable, such as men who have sex with men, prostitutes, and injection drug users. Additionally, nationwide there are several programs that provide easy access to condoms and to the exchange of needles and syringes.

Brazil is largely a Catholic country, with 75% of the population identifying themselves as Catholics. Not surprisingly, the Catholic Church is a very powerful and influential player in all aspects of Brazilian life. The Vatican religious doctrine opposes the use of condoms. Accordingly, several prominent church members in Brazil strongly and publicly condemn the use of condoms. Nonetheless, every time the Church authorities in Brazil release a message indicating that the Church does not condone condom use, the government issues an immediate, respectful, and strong rebuttal, stressing that abstinence is a matter of personal choice, while condom promotion is of public health importance.

The results of the campaigns to promote the use of condoms demonstrate the power of an integrated effort, even when having to contend with such an influential opponent as the Catholic Church. In the beginning of the epidemic, fewer than 5% of Brazilians reported using condoms at their first sexual relationship. By 2001, condom use at the first sexual relationship had grown exponentially to approximately 80%, a level similar to that reported in Western Europe and in the USA. In parallel with the increase in condom use, there has been an increase in purchases of male condoms by the Ministry of Health. In 1993, the government purchased and distributed 18 million units; by 2001, 250 million condoms were purchased by the Ministry of Health and were made available at a subsidized rate or were distributed for free. Besides being made available in brothels, condoms are being distributed to all segments of the population, including senior citizens and high school students, as well as distributed at public gatherings, such as carnivals.[7-9]

Overall, changes in HIV prevalence rates in sentinel populations confirm the effectiveness of Brazil's prevention messages[10,11]:

- HIV prevalence among IDUs decreased from 49% in 1997 to 9.7% in 2001
- HIV prevalence rate among prostitutes fell from 17.8% in 1996 to 6.1% in 2000
- HIV prevalence rate among MSM decreased from 10.8% in 1999 to 4.7% in 2001
- HIV prevalence rate among pregnant women fell from 1.2% in 1997 to 0.6% in 2001.

HIV Care and Treatment

The Brazilian response to the epidemic relied on a balanced approach that included AIDS care and HIV prevention. Brazil was the first developing country to provide free and universal access to antiretroviral therapy to all who need it. In 1991, AZT was made available on a very limited scale. In 1996, a law was passed guaranteeing free and universal access to treatment through the public healthcare system, including antiretroviral drugs. It is worth mentioning that in the 1990s many, including the World Bank, were against providing treatment to developing countries. They believed that, with limited resources, funds should be preferentially directed to prevention.[12] Brazil was, thus, the first country to realize that prevention and treatment are inextricably intertwined, an approach presently endorsed by the World Bank.[13]

One of the most notable aspects of the Brazilian response is the delivery of prevention messages and programs through public healthcare centers and clinics, thus integrating treatment and prevention. This is an effective way to reinforce and broaden the reach of prevention messages, yet one so often overlooked in many developing countries.

The 1996 law ensured the provision of drugs to all HIV-infected individuals who qualify for treatment according to locally developed guidelines. In order to provide this unprecedented access to treatment, the healthcare system needed to be scaled up at various levels.[14]

Treatment guidelines needed to be developed and periodically updated. Thus, an external and independent advisory expert committee was created in late 1996 and was given the responsibility to establish HIV treatment criteria.[14] It was (and still is) composed of local experts who meet periodically to review the latest scientific developments in order to develop and adjust treatment guidelines accordingly. Given its independence from the NAP, the advisory committee ensures that treatment guidelines are established strictly based upon scientific evidence and good clinical judgment. During the first few years, Brazilian guidelines were somewhat more conservative vis-à-vis indications for starting treatment than their contemporary US and European guidelines. Over the ensuing years, guidelines in the USA, Europe, and Brazil converged. Presently, they are very similar.[15]

To guarantee the continuous success of any program of free and universal access to treatment, it is essential to ensure the permanent availability of safe and affordable antiretroviral drugs. AZT first became available in Brazil in 1991 and soon thereafter began to be produced locally.[5,6,14] With the arrival of protease inhibitors in 1996 and the subsequent approval of various other antiretrovirals, the Ministry of Health predictably faced a significant increase in medication costs, in the complexity of drug procurement and distribution, and in training needs for healthcare workers. The spiraling costs of the program called into question the viability and long-term sustainability of the program of free and universal access to antiretroviral drugs. Thus, in 1997, the government declared the AIDS epidemic a matter of national emergency.[5,6] International laws concerning intellectual property rights only came into effect in Brazil in 1999. This allowed the government and local drug manufacturers to make generic copies of

antiretroviral medications that were already available at that time, without infringing international intellectual property laws. Considering that international trade agreements allow for compulsory licensing of drugs in cases of national emergency, Brazil has successfully used this prerogative as an instrument to bargain for better prices for drugs registered after 1999 and thus protected by intellectual property laws. While the decision to discuss compulsory licensing has created a heated international debate on intellectual property and public health needs, it should be noted that Brazil has yet to break the patent of any antiretroviral drug.

As a direct result of these policies, the annual cost for antiretroviral medications per patient on treatment was reduced by 67% between 1997 and 2002. Since then, it has decreased even further to the current level of approximately $1000 per patient per year.[5] In 1999, 43% of all antiretrovirals used in the country were locally produced generics and 57% were brand-name drugs. By 2001, 63% of antiretrovirals used in the program were locally produced generics. In 2002, the costs of antiretroviral drugs amounted to only 1.5% of the budget of the Ministry of Health.

A balanced prevention and treatment approach requires a reliable healthcare infrastructure, which not only must be able to cope with the increased patient load without compromising care for other conditions and diseases, but must also be able to successfully deliver prevention messages. Thus, beyond the availability of treatment guidelines and medications, Brazil needed to expand its specialized healthcare system in order to meet these new challenges. Early in the epidemic, Brazil's healthcare infrastructure was largely inadequate. The government recognized that it was necessary to take major steps to adequately address the HIV/AIDS epidemic, including:

- Integration of AIDS care with overall medical care
- Creation of more treatment facilities, priority being given to areas with the highest HIV prevalence
- Regionalization of the healthcare system, giving the necessary autonomy for each region to address its own specific needs
- Establishment of a hierarchical healthcare system, with well defined referral systems
- Creation of a national network of voluntary testing and counseling (VCT) sites, as well as dissemination of guidelines for counseling and testing

- Establishment of a national system for procurement and distribution of drugs and laboratory reagents and supplies
- Development of programs of continuous education and training on HIV-related issues to physicians and healthcare workers, including wide dissemination of the national treatment guidelines.

In order to ensure patient confidentiality and adherence to the national treatment guidelines, as well as to allow for adequate planning of the necessary drug supplies, a computerized system was locally developed, linking patients, clinics, laboratories, and pharmacies into one central database. Under this system, which is yet to be fully implemented on a national scale, each patient carries a card with a unique identifier number. This number is entered into the database at every point of contact with the healthcare system, allowing for optimal monitoring of the effectiveness of the program and fine-tuning when necessary.

The Brazilian program also realized early on that even in settings where antiretrovirals are univer-

sally available, the importance of treatment and prophylaxis for opportunistic infections could not be underestimated. In Brazil, the steep decline in AIDS-related deaths has paralleled reports from the USA and Western Europe. Moreover, similar to the USA and Europe, improvements in survival and the beginning of the decline in AIDS deaths preceded the widespread availability of potent drugs (Figs. 61.1 and 61.2).[16] This, in turn, suggests that other factors, besides the availability of antiretroviral drugs, were contributing to the declining mortality. This hypothesis is reinforced by studies, such as the one performed in Europe that showed that even for patients who were not on antiretroviral drugs, AIDS-related mortality rates declined from 92.7 per thousand to 50.3 per thousand between 1995 and 1997.[17] In the USA, the incidence of most opportunistic infections started to decline in the early 1990s, long before effective antiretroviral drugs became available.[18] A similar phenomenon occurred in Brazil. With the exception of tuberculosis (TB), the incidence of which started to decline only after effective antiretroviral drugs became widely available; the decline in the incidence of the major opportunistic

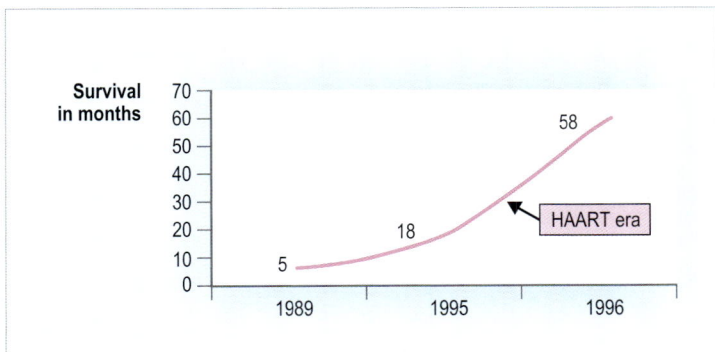

Figure 61.1 Median survival after AIDS diagnosis in Brazil.[16]

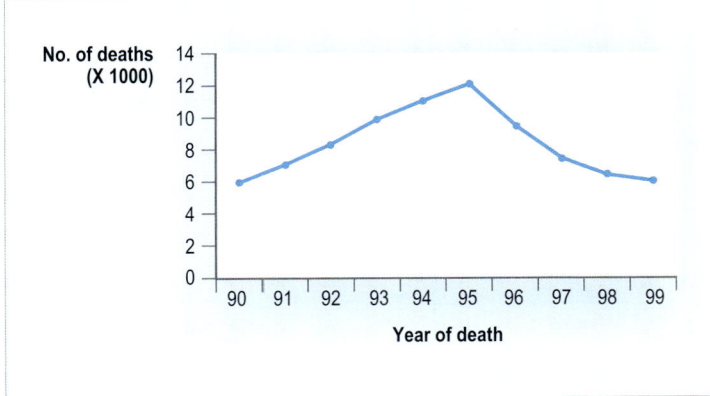

Figure 61.2 AIDS-related deaths, Brazil 1990–1999 (Online. Available: www.aids.gov.br).

infections preceded the widespread availability of highly active antiretroviral therapy (Fig. 61.3). One of the possible reasons for differences in observed changes in the incidence of TB in comparison with other opportunistic infections is that, in Brazil, primary prophylaxis with cotrimoxazole was always frequently prescribed, whereas chemoprophylaxis for TB was not. It is also noteworthy that the use of antiretrovirals has been shown to effectively prevent the development of active TB.[19] There are also data from Brazil and elsewhere to show that primary TB chemoprophylaxis can have a substantial impact on the survival of HIV-infected individuals (Fig. 61.4).[20] As a whole, these data strongly argue for the continuous importance of prevention of opportunistic infections, even in settings where antiretrovirals are widely available, a lesson learned very early on by the Brazil NAP.

The Net Effect of Brazil's Efforts to Stem the HIV Epidemic

As treatment and care became widely available throughout the public health system, there was a considerable decline in the estimated under-reporting of cases. Concomitantly, attendance to free VCT sites vastly exceeded initial projections and has remained reasonably stable ever since. In turn, the greater than expected attendance to VCT sites allowed prevention messages to reach a larger audience.

The estimated national prevalence of HIV infection in the adult population declined from 1.2 in the mid-1990s to 0.6% in 2001. Between 1996 and 2004, the number of individuals receiving free antiretroviral drugs increased from <20 000 to >150 000.

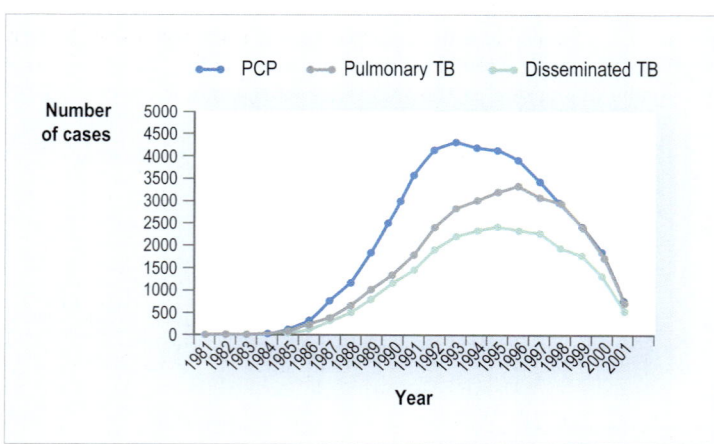

Figure 61.3 PCP and tuberculosis in patients with AIDS, Brazil 1991–2001 (Online. Available: www.aids.gov.br).

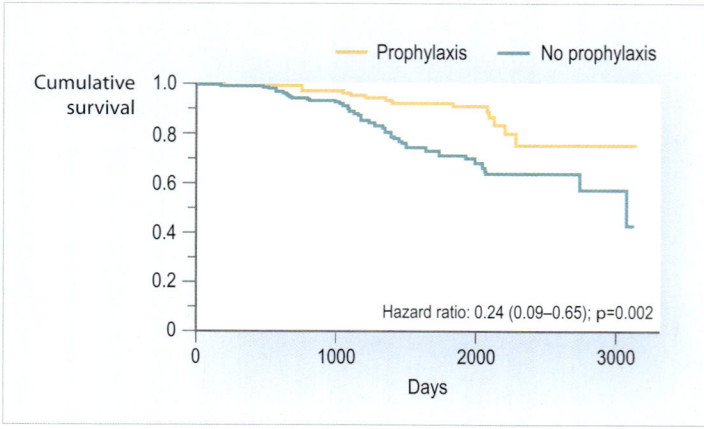

Figure 61.4 TB prophylaxis and survival among PPD+, HIV-infected patients.[20]

During approximately the same period, the overall incidence of opportunistic infections decreased by 80%, the incidence of TB decreased by 72%, and there was a 7-fold reduction (or 358 000) in hospital admissions. During the same period, deaths due to AIDS have plummeted by 60–80% and the decline in life expectancy has leveled off, thereby greatly mitigating the societal impact of the HIV epidemic.[3,14]

While the government spent approximately $250 million, or 1.5% of the total health budget, on antiretroviral drugs in 2002, the decrease in hospital admissions and incidence of opportunistic infections resulted in estimated net savings of $1 billion between 1996 and 2001.[14] As previously mentioned, as the government negotiated lower prices with brand-name manufacturers and more drugs were locally manufactured, the costs of therapy per patient gradually decreased, allowing more patients to receive free treatment. In 1999, the Brazilian government spent $336 million to treat 75 000 patients, whereas in 2000, 110 000 patients were being treated for approximately $250 million, a figure that remained stable while the number of patients on treatment increased to over 150 000.

As the Brazilian response to the AIDS epidemic gained increasing international recognition, Brazil signed several bilateral and multilateral agreements with other developing countries to assist them in scaling-up their treatment programs and, in some cases, with the local manufacturing of antiretroviral medications.

Conclusion

Arguably, South Africa, a country with economic characteristics similar to Brazil, represents the most poignant example of what can happen when there is no or limited government support or when action is not taken at a time when the epidemic is still in its early stages. In 1990, the prevalence rate in the general population was <1%. By 2001, the estimated prevalence of HIV in the general adult population in South Africa had risen to 20.1 %; by 2002, 26.5 % of pregnant women were HIV positive. Voluntary testing and counseling services only became available in 2000, and prevention of mother-to-child transmission was started in late 2001. The government took no action on treatment until mid-2003. As a result, it has been estimated that, due to the AIDS epidemic, an excess of 10 million deaths will have occurred by 2015, as well as a decrease in total labor force by 21%. It is also forecasted that by 2015 there will be 4.7 million orphans and the population will

be 44% smaller than it would have been were it not for the AIDS epidemic.[21-23]

Some of the most populous nations in the world, including China and India, have rapidly emerging epidemics still with low HIV prevalence rates, a situation not dissimilar to that which Brazil faced in the mid-1990s. Many of these countries share other characteristics with Brazil: sharp disparities between rich and poor, rapid economic growth with high mobility from rural to urban areas, displaced workers, and insufficient healthcare systems.

The pillars to Brazil's success can be summarized in a few words: early response; strong government support; active civil society involvement; balanced prevention and treatment efforts; direct prevention messages; comprehensive medical care; and decentralized action under strong, yet democratic, centralized leadership.

Brazil's success conclusively demonstrates that it is possible to curb the epidemic, provided all pieces of the puzzle are simultaneously put in place. There is no reason to believe that other countries cannot follow in Brazil's shoes.

References

1. UNDP. Human Development Reports. UNDP 2003. Online. Available: www.hdr.undp.org
2. World Bank. World Development Indicators. World Bank 2005. Online. Available: www.worldbank.org
3. Teixeira P, Vitoria MA, Barcarolo J. The Brazilian experience in providing universal access to antiretroviral therapy. Economics of AIDS and access to HIV/AIDS care in developing countries. Issues and challenges. ANRS.
4. Reardon C. AIDS: How Brazil turned the tide. Ford Foundation; 2002: Summer. Online. Available: www. fordfound.org/publications
5. Galvão J. Access to antiretroviral drugs in Brazil. Lancet 2002; 360:1862–1865.
6. Galvão J. Brazil and access to HIV/AIDS drugs: a question of human rights and public health. Am J Public Health 2005; 95:1110–1116.
7. Kaiser Network. Brazil to distribute more than 3 million condoms to high school students for HIV, pregnancy prevention. Kaiser Daily HIV/AIDS Report; 2003: 18 August. Online. Available: www.kaisernetwork.org
8. Kaiser Network. Brazil to distribute condoms to people over 60. Kaiser Daily HIV/AIDS Report; 2001: 10 September. Online. Available: www.kaisernetwork.org
9. Kaiser Network. Brazil to distribute 11M condoms during carnival festivities to prevent spread of HIV, other STDs. Kaiser Daily HIV/AIDS Report; 2005: 21 January. Online. Available: www.kaisernetwork.org
10. National STD/AIDS Program. Positive response: The experience of Brazilian AIDS program. Brasilia: Ministry of Health of Brazil, 2002. Online. Available: www.aids.gov.br/ final/biblioteca/resposta/resp_ingles.pdf
11. Telles DPR, et al. Factors associated with declining HIV infection rates among IDUs in Rio de Janeiro in Brazil. Abstract MoPeC3399. IAC, Barcelona: 7–12 July 2002.
12. World Bank. Confronting AIDS: public priorities in a global epidemic. New York: Oxford University Press; 1997.

13. Piot P, Feachem RG, Lee JW, et al. Public health. A global response to AIDS: lessons learned, next steps. Science 2004; 304:1909–1910.
14. Levi GC, Vitoria MA. Fighting against AIDS: the Brazilian experience. AIDS 2002; 16:2373–2383.
15. Yeni PG, Hammer SM, Hirsch MS, et al. Treatment for adult HIV infection: 2004 recommendations of the International AIDS Society-USA Panel. JAMA 2004; 292:251–265.
16. Marins JRP, Leda FJ, Sanny YC, et al. Dramatic improvement in survival among adult Brazilian AIDS patients. AIDS 2003; 17:1675–1682.
17. Mocroft A, Vella S, Benfield T, et al. Changing patterns of mortality across Europe in patients infected with HIV-1. Lancet 1998; 9142:1725–1730.
18. Kovacs JA, Masur H. Prophylaxis against opportunistic infections in patients with human immunodeficiency virus infection. N Engl J Med 2000; 342:1416–1429.
19. Santoro-Lopes G, Pinho AMF, Harrison LH, et al. Reduced risk of tuberculosis among patients with advanced HIV infection treated with HAART in a Brazilian cohort. Clin Infect Dis 2002; 34:543–546.
20. Pinho AMF, Santoro-Lopes G, Harrison LH, et al. Chemoprophylaxis for tuberculosis and survival of HIV-infected patients in Brazil. AIDS 2001; 15:2129–2135.
21. World Bank. The long-run economic costs of AIDS: Theory and an application to South Africa. World Bank; 2003. Online. Available: www1.worldbank.org/hiv_aids/docs/BeDeGe_BP_total2.pdf
22. Garbus L. HIV/AIDS in South Africa. Country AIDS Policy Analysis Project, 2003: October. Online. Available: www.hivinsite.org
23. Bureau for Economic Research. The macroeconomic impact of HIV/AIDS in South Africa. Bureau for Economic Research, Economic Research Note. 2001: January.

CHAPTER 62

Surveillance of Antiretroviral Drug Resistance in Resource-poor Settings

Inge Derdelinckx
Charles Boucher

Scaling-up of Antiretroviral Treatment Programs in Resource-poor Settings

The use of highly active antiretroviral therapy (HAART) in developed countries has led to a dramatic and sustained drop in the mortality rate of AIDS patients in these countries. However, until recently, few people from countries with limited resources had access to life preserving but expensive antiretroviral drugs. The Declaration of Commitment on HIV/AIDS, unanimously adopted in 2001 by 189 member states at the first-ever Special Session of the United Nations Assembly on HIV/AIDS, called for the delivery of the 'highest attainable standard treatment for HIV/AIDS' in all countries.[1] It was decided to scale-up the antiretroviral (ARV) treatment programs to meet the needs of people living with HIV/AIDS in resource-limited settings by using standardized and simplified ARV regimens based on the best scientific evidence. Several initiatives worldwide are providing resources for this effort, including individual country drug-access initiatives, the Global Fund against AIDS, TB and Malaria, the World Health Organization, the US Government's Emergency Plan for AIDS Relief and many others.

The goal of therapy is to durably inhibit viral replication so that the patient can attain and maintain an effective immune response to most microbial pathogens. Even though the scale-up of ARV treatment in resource-limited settings is expected to reduce the rate of AIDS complications, and greatly reduce mortality, major concerns exist about the potential generation of an epidemic of drug resistant strains of HIV. The high error rate of HIV-1 RT and the rapid turnover of the virus population contribute to the generation of the extensive genetic variation in the HIV-1 quasi-species. Under drug selective pressure, drug resistant variants can be selected. The clinical significance of antiretroviral drug resistance has been shown to negatively affect treatment outcomes in patients failing treatment, however, the impact of baseline drug resistance on treatment response of the first regimen is less well studied.

Given the complexity and open-ended nature of HIV treatment and the need to begin programs quickly, fears have been raised that drug resistance could emerge quickly in resource limited countries, spreading rapidly and quickly rendering anti-HIV drugs useless.

HIV Drug Resistance in the Scale-up of Antiretroviral Treatment Programs: What to Expect

The widespread use of ARV treatment in developed countries has led to the development of HIV drug resistance (Box 62.1). Some surveys show that 75% of treated patients with detectable viral load harbor a drug resistant virus.[2] Also, drug resistant variants

Box 62.1

Factors influencing the occurrence of HIV drug resistance in resource-poor settings

Factors reducing the risk

- Triple therapy can be prescribed as first-line treatment
- The prescribed regimens are simple and well tolerated
- Knowledge on importance of adherence and its management can be implemented
- Currently ART coverage is limited

Factors increasing the risk

- Lack of trained healthcare workers
- Poorly supervised ART programs
- Failure of drug delivery due to budgetary or logistical problems
- Bad quality of drugs due to insufficient control mechanisms
- Inadequate storage of treatment at particular (low) temperature
- Mono- or bi-therapy due to illegal prescription of therapy or financial problems
- Absence of viral load monitoring
- Absence of second-line regimen
- Mother-to-child transmission programs, especially those using single-dose nevirapine
- Increased stigma, negatively affecting adherence

can be transmitted to newly infected patients, potentially jeopardizing ARV treatment programs. In Europe, a large retrospective study found 10% of patients infected with a resistant virus.[3] The high prevalence of drug resistance in industrialized countries stems partly from the administration of suboptimal regimens in the pre-HAART era. The delayed roll-out of ARV treatment programs in resource-limited countries, by contrast, can rely on the experience gathered in countries where treatment has been in place for a longer time. Especially, the use of mono- and bi-therapy could be avoided with the implementation of standardized treatment regimens. Also, a simple and well-tolerated regimen, with as few pills and as few daily doses as possible, can be prescribed. Adherence, a major issue in the prevention of HIV drug resistance, could potentially be better addressed in these settings based on the lessons learnt in industrialized countries. Although comparisons between studies must be made with caution, because of varying definitions and modes of ascertaining adherence, reports of adherence levels above 90% in China,[4] Senegal,[5] and South-Africa

were encouraging and compare favorably with those reported from Europe and North America where adherence is around 70%.

However, serious concerns have been raised regarding the emergence of HIV drug resistance due to the rapid scale-up of treatment in resource-limited settings. Poorly supervised, poorly managed ART programs could lead to the rapid increase of resistance. Especially, the lack of trained healthcare workers could lead to suboptimal use of ARV treatment and suboptimal follow-up of patients on treatment. Failure in drug delivery, due to budgetary or logistical reasons, could lead to (involuntary) treatment interruptions and could attribute to the emergence of drug resistance. Other logistical issues, such as the storage of treatment at a particular temperature could be hard to establish in settings with electricity failures, which are not infrequent in resource-limited settings. Also, concerns have been raised about illegal prescription of ARV. Failure to control the quality of drugs could also lead to suboptimal drug levels in the patient, and thus potentially lead to the development of drug resistance.

The laboratory monitoring of patients on treatment in these settings is generally limited. In most countries, no information on viral load is available. Treatment failure is therefore defined on clinical or immunological grounds, leading to a late switch to a second-line regimen compared with Western countries. This way, the virus could accumulate several HIV drug resistance mutations giving rise to broad cross-resistance and therefore not only lower the efficacy of second-line regimens, but also increase the possibility of transmitting a resistant strain. Issues related to adherence are also of concern. Less adherence have been linked to stigmatization[6] and limited resources when having to pay for treatment themselves.[7]

In an attempt to predict the emergence of an HIV drug-resistant epidemic in Africa, Blower and colleagues used mathematical modeling.[8] They predicted that, at currently planned levels of treatment coverage over the next decade in Africa – i.e. only 5–10% of infected individuals will receive treatment – the transmission rates of drug-resistant HIV would remain below 5%.

HIV Drug Resistance in Untreated Populations in Resource-limited Countries

Where a number of studies have documented the increasing transmission of HIV drug resistance in the developed world, data on this topic in resource-limited settings are limited. Data are increasingly being gathered and generally show very low prevalence rates of HIV drug resistance among untreated patients, not exceeding rates of 5%.[9–12]

HIV Drug Resistance in Treated Populations in Resource-limited Countries

Unregulated Use of ART

Unregulated use of ART may lead to the rapid emergence of resistant viral strains limiting future therapeutic options and increase the risk of transmission of resistant virus. Various studies have demonstrated this in countries where ART has been administered without proper infrastructure to monitor patients. Vergne and colleagues showed that, in Gabon, 58% of patients who had received unsupervised ART without an adequate health infrastructure developed major ART resistance mutations.[13]

Use of Non-suppressive ART

The use of non-suppressive ART has also shown to contribute to the occurrence of drug-resistant HIV. In the context of the UNAIDS-WHO Drug Access Initiative, started in 1998, ART was frequently prescribed as bi-therapy given the high cost of the treatment. This not only gave rise to high levels of virologic failure, but also resulted in high levels of HIV drug resistance.[14] In Uganda, in the context of the same initiative, where patients and their families were responsible for paying all of their medical care, drugs and laboratory tests, approximately one-third of patients on HAART and just over one-half of those prescribed two NRTIs, had resistance to at least one drug.[9]

HIV Drug Resistance in Programs to Reduce the Transmission from Mother-to-Child

Mother-to-child transmission (MTCT) is a great cause of new HIV infections, with >800 000 newly-infected infants each year, of them 90% in Africa. In the ACTG 076 trial, it was first demonstrated that with a short course of antiretroviral treatment, this transmission risk could be reduced.[15] In this study in

which zidovudine was given to the mother pre- and intrapartum as well as to the infant for the first 6 weeks of life, MTCT of HIV-1 was reduced by 70%. In industrialized countries, the programs for the prevention of MTCT (PMTCT) were further optimized and the use of triple combination therapy in pregnant women along with an optimal package of interventions, including cesarean section and formula feeding, has further reduced the rate of MTCT to 1–2%.[16] However, this strategy was not feasible in resource-constrained settings and a number of alternative strategies were tested. In the HIV Network on Prevention Trials (HIVNET) 012, performed in Uganda, it was reported that a single 200 mg dose of nevirapine (NVP) given to the mother at the time of delivery followed by a single 2 mg/kg dose given to the infant within 72 h of birth resulted in a reduction in MTCT of 50% at 14–16 weeks after treatment, compared with a short course of ZDV and its persistent benefit extended to 18 months after treatment.[17,18] This was an easy regimen to administer, was inexpensive, required no additional health-care infrastructure and could potentially be deployed widely and rapidly in even the most rural settings, thus making it the intervention of choice in resource-restricted countries for PMTCT programs. However, a great disadvantage of the regimen was the emergence of HIV drug resistance after the administration of single dose (SD)-NVP. In HIVNET 012, NVP resistance was detected in 25% of women and in 46% of infants.[19] Moreover, with more sensitive techniques, NNRTI-associated resistance mutations can be detected in the majority of women (65%) exposed to NVP at 6–36 weeks postpartum.[20,21] It is not surprising that mutations associated with NNRTI resistance would emerge with the administration of a drug for which the occurrence of rapid, single-step, high-level resistance have been described for years, especially since SD NVP regimen has a median half-life of 61 h resulting in prolonged low blood levels. Several factors have been associated with the development of NVP resistance: viral subtype (subtype C > subtype D > subtype A), a high baseline viral load[22] and the number of maternal doses of NVP.[23] The development of resistance could have serious implications for the prevention of MTCT of subsequent pregnancies. It could also jeopardize the treatment of the mothers and their HIV-positive offspring since most resource-constrained countries use an NNRTI-based first-line regimen. The findings of a study among Thai women suggested that women who received intrapartum NVP in combination with zidovudine prophylaxis were less likely to have virologic suppression after 6 months of postpartum treatment with a NVP-containing regimen.[24] Larger clinical trials are underway and others are planned, in order to provide more definitive data on the clinical implications of these findings. Several studies are evaluating methods avoiding the occurrence of resistance with these regimens. In one trial, 1413 pregnant women were randomized to receive single-dose NVP alone or in combination with either 4 or 7 days of Combivir treatment. Compared with the high proportion of resistant strains in the group of women treated with SD NVP (57%), this proportion was substantially lower in the group treated with the additional Combivir (13% and 9%, respectively for the 4 and 7 days CBV arm). Infant resistance was reduced from 78% to 13% and 0%, respectively.[25]

Given all these short comings, bringing single-dose NVP to the mothers who need it is an enormous challenge that few public health services in the developing world are managing to meet. At time of writing, only 10% of the mothers in Africa who need the drug are currently receiving it. Therefore, the current World Health Organization (WHO) guidelines still recommend the use of the SD NVP as a minimal recommendation, but suggest the use of zidovudine in combination with NVP as the regimen of choice.

Evaluation of HIV Drug Resistance for Public Health Purposes

As more people receive ART in Africa, concerted international efforts are being put in place to monitor HIV drug resistance. In this respect, WHO has established a Strategy for HIV Drug Resistance Prevention, Surveillance, and Monitoring. Together with its advisory body, HIVResNet, consisting of the world's experts on HIV drug resistance and several implementing partners, like the European UNITE MORE project, programs were drafted aimed at using standardized methods for the evaluation of drug resistance in both treated and untreated populations in countries where treatment is being scaled-up. Information gained in these programs should help countries make appropriate decisions in selecting first- and second-line regimens and may provide important data for program management and policy. Currently, WHO does not recommend the use of resistance testing for the monitoring of the individual patient until other, more basic monitoring tools are in place and generalized. WHO proposes two

different protocols for the monitoring of HIV drug resistance.

HIV Drug Resistance Transmission Surveillance

Studies assessing the prevalence of HIV drug resistance among untreated patients show large discrepancies. Geographical differences, differences in study population, duration of HIV infection, transmission mode, gender or race make comparison between these studies often very difficult. Also, the use of different resistance assays and different interpretation methods give variable results. In addition, most performed studies are retrospective in design and study small numbers. Worldwide, several efforts have been made to standardize these studies. Within the SPREAD project, for instance, clinicians, virologists, and epidemiologists from European countries work together to implement a structured and quality controlled European surveillance program. The aim of the program is to determine the prevalence of resistance transmission within the different risk groups and to identify risk factors enhancing the risk of transmission in a prospective and representative way.

The WHO has developed a minimum-resource method called the HIV drug resistance threshold survey for use in resource-limited countries, specifically targeting geographic areas where antiretroviral therapy is already in use or is being rapidly scaled-up. The purpose of this protocol is to study the extent of transmitted resistance and focuses on recently infected populations. The protocol is designed for use as a supplement to unlinked anonymous HIV sentinel serosurveys, conducted routinely in many resource-limited countries with generalized epidemics. It is proposed to study the specimens of women who are under the age of 25 and in their first pregnancy, attending antenatal care clinics. In other epidemics, the protocol will need to be adapted and other entry points defined (e.g. voluntary counseling and testing sites). Using a method based on binomial sequential sampling, up to 47 consecutively collected eligible specimens will be genotyped to detect mutations known to be associated with resistance to antiretroviral drugs. Prevalence of resistance will not be estimated precisely, but will be classified (for each drug or drug-class) as <5%, 5–15% and >15%. Depending on the classification, different public health actions will be recommended. In case a high prevalence is found, more extended steps might be adopted to enable more insight in the characteristics of the spread of resistant strains. Surveys using more extensive data collection forms, like the ones used in the Spread network, could be organized.

Monitoring of HIV Drug Resistance Emerging in Treated Populations

In a second protocol, WHO proposes the Monitoring of HIV viral suppression and HIV drug resistance in populations receiving ART in resource-limited settings. Populations achieving viral suppression while on therapy are less likely to develop HIVDR. Therefore, the single most important measure in determining programatic success is the proportion of the population taking ART who achieve sustained viral suppression at 1 year. Programmatic achievement of >70% viral suppression in populations at 1 year after commencement of ART is the HIVResNet suggested standard to minimize the emergence of HIVDR. In patients not achieving a suppressed viral load, resistance testing will be performed, thus evaluating resistance profiles in patients failing therapy after 1 year. Together with results from HIVDR Surveillance studies, the HIVDR Monitoring study results can contribute to an overall analysis and interpretation to assist decision makers to adjust treatment programs at local and national levels. Action may be proposed to improve adherence, assure an uninterrupted supply of good quality drugs. Results from studies can also assist in making informed care and treatment policy decisions at national and global levels, regarding the durability of first-line regimens and the potential composition of second-line regimens.

HIV Drug Resistance Testing in Resource-poor Settings

Sequencing is most commonly used for the determination of HIV drug resistance and provides information on an entire viral nucleotide sequence. A well organized molecular diagnostic laboratory with highly specialized personnel for the processing of the samples, the use of dedicated equipment and the interpretation of the results is needed. At this moment, most resource-limited countries lack the capacity for HIV drug resistance testing. Many countries are in the process of purchasing equipment and setting up genotyping facilities in inexperienced

laboratories. Also, the set-up of WHO/HIVResNet global Surveillance program requires accurate and comparable laboratory data. For this purpose, WHO has designed the WHO/HIVResNet Global Laboratory Network. In this network, guidelines and recommendations will be developed on specimen type, specimen storage and testing procedures for HIV drug resistance testing. Also, materials will be developed for the assistance of the capacity building of laboratories for the performance of molecular diagnostic work and sequencing in particular. Since a lot of existing laboratories lack the capacity, the network will provide the opportunity for extensive twinning between experienced and less experienced laboratories, with possibility for back-up procedures, extensive training in the sequencing technique and support for the laboratory capacity building. A global HIV drug resistance program will also be developed and proficiency panels will be provided. For a laboratory to enter the network, specific criteria will be developed and assessment visits organized. Supranational laboratories will be identified for the organization of the training and twinning in one region.

Dried Blood Spots for HIV Drug Resistance Testing

Presently, the standard specimen for HIV drug resistance genotyping is plasma or serum. Their necessity to be stored and shipped in frozen conditions provides extra challenges in resource-limited settings, where freezers are not always available and electricity not always reliable. In these settings, the collection of dried blood spots (DBS) would provide an attractive alternative. Since no laboratory manipulations are needed, the collection of dried blood spots is relatively easy. Short-term storage can be done at ambient temperature, allowing centers without freezers to collect samples and send the samples to facilities where freezers (−20°C) can provide long-term storage. Another advantage is the ease of transportation: dry ice is not needed and the filters can be shipped as non-infectious material, thus substantially reducing the cost of the specimen collection. Dried blood and dried plasma spots have been shown to be used as an easy and inexpensive means for the collection and storage of specimens under field conditions for the diagnosis of HIV infection and the monitoring of antiretroviral therapy.[26,27] At the present time, data suggest that DBS are a suitable method to collect blood for HIVDR testing, although genotyping procedures on DBS have still to be standardized and validated by laboratories performing the analysis.[28]

Subtype Variability in Resource-limited Settings

Two types of HIV exist, HIV-1 and HIV-2. HIV-1 can further be divided into three distinct groups, group M (main), O (outlier), and N (non-M, non-O). Group M, the predominant HIV-1 group, comprises 11 subtypes (A–K). Antiretroviral drugs were designed, tested, and validated primarily in North America and Europe, where HIV-1 group M subtype B strains predominate. However, non-B subtypes predominate in the rest of the world. CRF02_AG predominate in West-Africa, multiple subtypes exist in Central Africa, subtypes A and D predominate in East Africa and subtype C in Southern Africa.[29]

Until recently, due to lack of data on ART use in Africa, there was speculation whether persons infected with subtype B virus had similar patterns of drug resistance mutations as those infected with subtype B strains. Some limited studies in non-B subtypes have shown a strong correlation between the presence of major mutations and phenotypic resistance, similar to mutations seen in subtype B infections under similar treatment regimens. However, differences occur. Some mutations occur as natural polymorphisms in non-B subtypes and were described as minor genotypic resistance mutations in B subtypes (L10I/V, K20I, M36I in protease). Also, tissue culture experiments with efavirenz have shown that subtype C isolates developed the V106M mutation, conferring high level cross resistance to all NNRTIs.[30] A study of single-dose NVP to prevent mother-to-child-transmission of HIV showed that selection of genotypic mutations associated with resistance to NVP occurred more frequently in women infected with subtype D than in women infected with subtype A viruses.[31]

Genotypic assays are currently commercially available to detect HIV-1 genotypic resistant mutations. These assays were developed and validated mostly on clinical specimens obtained from persons infected with HIV-1 subtype B viruses. Thus, limited information is available on the performance of these assays on HIV-1 non-B subtypes. The high degree of sequence heterogeneity that characterizes HIV-1 subtypes may limit their performance in geographic areas where HIV-1 non-B subtypes predominate. However, limited available data point towards

an adequate detection of mutations in different subtypes.[32]

Strategies to Limit the Occurrence of Drug Resistance in Resource-limited Countries

Pivotal in the reduction of the occurrence of HIV drug resistance is the implementation of a good ARV program. Several issues are important: initiated treatment should be as potent and simple as possible in order to maximize the suppression of viral replication, maximize adherence and reduce infectiousness of the population. Health infrastructure should be optimized and uninterrupted drug supplies and quality assurance of the drugs guaranteed. Good programs allowing for the monitoring and evaluation of the ARV programs should be put in place to provide information to policy makers to take actions

---

Box 62.2

Actions to minimize the occurrence of HIV drug resistance

To implement a well managed ART program

- State-of-the-art guidelines for prevention, treatment and care of HIV infection
- Well trained health care workers
- Adequate adherence measures
- Adequate health care facilities
- Timely supply of drugs
- Controlled quality of drugs
- Program to monitor and evaluate the treatment outcomes of the ART program

To form a committee on HIV drug resistance to develop a plan on HIV drug resistance for the country, including:

- Ministry of Health
- Laboratory experts
- Clinicians
- Epidemiologists
- NGO
- Patient organizations
- WHO, UNAIDS

To organize studies on HIV drug resistance

- In untreated recently infected populations in specific geographic settings where HIV drug resistance is expected to occur first
- In treated populations

accordingly. Treatment should continue to be provided free of charge in order to limit treatment interruption. For the accomplishment of these tasks, the commitment of the national government is necessary (Box 62.2).

Conclusion

Antiretroviral drug resistance is an inevitable consequence when providing long-term treatment and should not be seen as a limitation for providing antiretrovirals to patients in resource-poor settings. The rapid expansion of HIV/AIDS treatment access is an urgent public health necessity. However, efforts should be undertaken to reduce the development of drug resistance as much as possible by providing healthcare infrastructures that will maximize the effectiveness of treatment and minimize the risk for drug resistance. Programs to monitor the prevalence of drug resistance will help in evaluating the situation and providing a basis for appropriate public health action.

Acknowledgments

Inge Derdelinckx is supported by the Unite More project, funded by the European Commission (LSHP-CT-2004-516030).

References

1. United Nations General Assembly on HIV/AIDS. Declaration of Commitment HIV/AIDS. No. 55. New York: United Nations; 2001.
2. Richman DD, Morton SC, Wrin T, et al. The prevalence of antiretroviral drug resistance in the United States. AIDS 2004; 18:1393–1401.
3. Wensing AMJ, van de Vijver DAMC, Angarano G, et al. on behalf of the SPREAD Program. Prevalence of drug-resistant HIV-1 variants in untreated individuals in Europe: implications for clinical management. J Infect Dis 2005; 192:958–966.
4. Fong OW, Ho CF, Fung LY, et al. Determinants of adherence to highly active antiretroviral therapy (HAART) in Chinese HIV/AIDS patients. HIV Med 2003; 4:133–138.
5. Laniece I, Ciss M, Desclaux A, et al. Adherence to HAART and its principal determinants in a cohort of Senegalese adults. AIDS 2003; 17:S103–S108.
6. Nachega JB, Stein DM, Lehman DA, et al. Adherence to antiretroviral therapy in HIV-infected adults in Soweto, South Africa. AIDS Res Hum Retroviruses 2004; 20:1053–1056.
7. Oyugi JH, Byakika-Tusiime J, Charlebois ED, et al. Multiple validated measures of adherence indicate high levels of adherence to generic HIV antiretroviral therapy in a resource-limited setting. J Acquir Immune Defic Syndr 2004; 36:1100–1102.
8. Blower S, Bodine E, Kahn J, McFarland W. The antiretroviral rollout and drug-resistant HIV in Africa: insights from empirical data and theoretical models. AIDS 2005; 19:1–14.
9. Weidle PJ, Kityo CM, Mugyenyi P, et al. Resistance to antiretroviral therapy among patients in Uganda. J Acquir Immune Defic Syndr 2001; 26:495–500.
10. Toni T, Masquelier B, Bonard D, et al. Primary HIV-1 drug resistance in Abidjan (Cote d'Ivoire): a genotypic and phenotypic study. AIDS 2002; 16:488–491.
11. Vergne L, Kane CT, Laurent C, et al. Low rate of genotypic HIV-1 drug-resistant strains in the Senegalese government initiative of access to antiretroviral therapy. AIDS 2003; 17(Suppl):31–38.
12. Toni TD, Recordon-Pinson P, Minga A, et al. Presence of key drug resistance mutations in isolates from untreated patients of Abidjan, Cote d'Ivoire: ANRS 1257 study. AIDS Res Hum Retroviruses 2003; 19:713–717.
13. Vergne L, Malonga-Mouellet G, Mistoul I, et al. Resistance to antiretroviral treatment in Gabon: need for implementation of guidelines on antiretroviral therapy use and HIV-1 drug resistance monitoring in developing countries. J Acquir Immune Defic Syndr 2002; 29:165–168.
14. Adje C, Cheingsong R, Roels TH, et al. High prevalence of genotypic and phenotypic HIV-1 drug-resistant strains among patients receiving antiretroviral therapy in Abidjan, Cote d'Ivoire. J Acquir Immune Defic Syndr 2001; 26:501–506.
15. Connor EM, Sperling RS, Gelber R, et al. Reduction of maternal-infant transmission of human immunodeficiency virus type 1 with zidovudine treatment. Pediatric AIDS Clinical Trials Group Protocol 076 Study Group. N Engl J Med 1994; 331:1173–1180.
16. European Collaborative Study. Mother-to-child transmission of HIV infection in the era of highly active antiretroviral therapy. Clin Infect Dis 2005; 40:458–465.
17. Guay LA, Musoke P, Fleming T, et al. Intrapartum and neonatal single-dose nevirapine compared with zidovudine for prevention of mother-to-child transmission of HIV-1 in Kampala, Uganda: HIVNET 012 randomised trial. Lancet 1999; 354:795–802.
18. Jackson JB, Musoke P, Fleming T, et al. Intrapartum and neonatal single-dose nevirapine compared with zidovudine for prevention of mother-to-child transmission of HIV-1 in Kampala, Uganda: 18-month follow-up of the HIVNET 012 randomised trial. Lancet 2003; 362:859–868.
19. Eshleman SH, Mracna M, Guay LA, et al. Selection and fading of resistance mutations in women and infants receiving nevirapine to prevent HIV-1 vertical transmission (HIVNET 012). AIDS 2001; 15:1951–1957.
20. Flys T, Nissley DV, Claasen CW, et al. Sensitive drug-resistance assays reveal long-term persistence of HIV-1 variants with the K103N nevirapine (NVP) resistance mutation in some women and infants after the administration of single-dose NVP: HIVNET 012. J Infect Dis 2005; 192:24–29.
21. Johnson JA, Li JF, Morris L, et al. Emergence of drug-resistant HIV-1 after intrapartum administration of single-dose nevirapine is substantially underestimated. J Infect Dis 2005; 192:16–23.
22. Eshleman SH, Hoover DR, Chen S, et al. Nevirapine (NVP) resistance in women with HIV-1 subtype C, compared with subtypes A and D, after the administration of single-dose NVP. J Infect Dis 2005; 192:30–36.
23. Moodley D, Moodley J, Coovadia H, et al. A multicenter randomized controlled trial of nevirapine versus a combination of zidovudine and lamivudine to reduce intrapartum and early postpartum mother-to-child transmission of human immunodeficiency virus type 1. J Infect Dis 2003; 187:725–735.
24. Jourdain G, Ngo-Giang-Huong N, Le CS, Intrapartum exposure to nevirapine and subsequent maternal responses to nevirapine-based antiretroviral therapy. N Engl J Med 2004; 351:229–240.
25. McIntyre J, Martinson N, Gray G, et al. for the Trial 1413 Investigator Team. Single dose nevirapine combined with a

short course of Combivir for prevention of mother to child transmission of HIV-1 can significantly decrease the subsequent development of maternal and infant resistant virus. Antivir Ther 2005; 10:S4.

26. Brambilla D, Jennings C, Aldrovandi G, et al. Multicenter evaluation of use of dried blood and plasma spot specimens in quantitative assays for human immunodeficiency virus RNA: measurement, precision, and RNA stability. J Clin Microbiol 2003; 41:1888–1893.

27. Mwaba P, Cassol S, Pilon R, et al. Use of dried whole blood spots to measure CD4+ lymphocyte counts in HIV-1-infected patients. Lancet 2003; 362:1459–1460.

28. Garcia-Lerma JG, McNulty A, Jennings C, et al. Evaluation of dried blood spots for HIV-1 drug resistance testing. Antivir Ther 2005; 10:S49.

29. Peeters M, Toure-Kane C, Nkengasong J. HIV-1 genetic subtypes in Africa: implication for diagnosis, antiretroviral therapy, pathogenesis and vaccine development. AIDS 2003; 17:2547–2560.

30. Brenner B, Turner D, Oliveira M, et al. A V106M mutation in HIV-1 clade C viruses exposed to efavirenz confers cross-resistance to non-nucleoside reverse transcriptase inhibitors. AIDS 2003; 17:1–5.

31. Eshleman SH, Becker-Pergola G, Deseyve M, et al. Impact of human immunodeficiency virus type 1 (HIV-1) subtype on women receiving single-dose nevirapine prophylaxis to prevent hiv-1 vertical transmission (HIV Network for Prevention Trials 012 study). J Infect Dis 2001; 184:914–917.

32. Bile EC, dje-Toure C, Borget MY, et al. Performance of drug-resistance genotypic assays among HIV-1 infected patients with predominantly CRF02_AG strains of HIV-1 in Abidjan, Cote d'Ivoire. J Clin Virol 2005; 32:60–66.

CHAPTER 63

Post-exposure Prevention

Adelisa L. Panlilio
Denise M. Cardo

Introduction

HIV infection is a concern in the healthcare setting because there is a risk of occupational transmission from infected patients to susceptable healthcare personnel (HCR). Despite improved methods of preventing exposures, occupational exposures continue to occur. Although preventing blood exposures is the primary means of preventing occupationally acquired HIV infection, appropriate post-exposure management, including post-exposure prophylaxis (PEP)* is an important element of workplace safety. PEP for occupational exposures was first recommended by the US Public Health Service (PHS) in 1996, with subsequent updates to HIV PEP regimens recommended in 1998, 2001, and 2005.[1–4] What follows is a summary of the most recent guidelines. Recommendations for HIV PEP after non-occupational exposure are described elsewhere.[5]

Post-exposure Prophylaxis

Rationale for post-exposure prophylaxis

Factors that influence the decision to recommend the use of PEP for occupational exposures include the pathogenesis of HIV infection, particularly events occurring during the course of early infection; the

---

*The findings, views, and recommendations contained herein are those of the authors and should not be construed as official Centers for Disease Control and Prevention or US Department of Health and Human Services positions. The use of trade names and commercial sources is for identification only and does not imply endorsement by the US PHS or the US Department of Health and Human Services.

biologic plausibility that infection can be prevented or ameliorated by using antiretroviral drugs; direct or indirect evidence of the efficacy of specific agents used for prophylaxis; and the risk/benefit of PEP to exposed HCP. The following discussion considers each of these issues.

Role of pathogenesis in considering antiretroviral prophylaxis

Information about primary HIV infection indicates that there is a brief 'window of opportunity' before systemic infection occurs, during which post-exposure intervention with antiretroviral agents may modify viral replication. Data from studies in animal models and *in vitro* tissue studies suggest that dendritic cells in the mucosa and skin may be the initial target for HIV infection or capture and have an important role in initiating HIV infection of CD4+ T cells in regional lymph nodes.[6] In a primate model of simian immunodeficiency virus (SIV) infection, infection of dendritic-like cells occurred at the site of inoculation during the first 24 h following mucosal exposure to cell-free virus.[7] Over the subsequent 24–48 h, migration of these cells to regional lymph nodes occurred, and virus was detectable in the peripheral blood within 5 days. Theoretically, initiation of antiretroviral PEP soon after exposure may prevent or inhibit systemic infection by limiting the proliferation of virus in the initial target cells or lymph nodes.

Animal studies

Interpretation of data from animal studies has been difficult, partly because of problems identifying an animal model comparable with humans.[8] Differences in controlled variables (e.g. choice of viral strain (based on the animal model used), inoculum size, route of inoculation, time of prophylaxis initiation, and drug regimen) have made it difficult to extrapolate the results of early studies to humans. Most animal studies have used SIV or other non-human retroviruses that have different pathogenetic mechanisms from HIV-1 in humans. Furthermore, most studies used a higher inoculum and different route for exposure than would be seen in needlestick injuries. In the animal studies in which PEP appeared effective, efficacy was greatest when prophylaxis was begun before or within a few hours after exposure; there was no apparent effect when drugs were begun later than 24–36 h post-exposure.[8,9]

More recently, refinements in methodology have resulted in more relevant studies; in particular, the mucosal exposure routes have been used and viral inocula have been reduced to levels more analogous to human exposures but sufficient to cause infection in control animals.[10,11] These studies provide encouraging evidence of postexposure chemoprophylactic efficacy in the experimental setting.

Human studies

There are limited indirect data that can be used to assess the efficacy of PEP after occupational exposures in humans. Because of the relative infrequency of seroconversion after an occupational exposure to HIV-infected blood, a prospective trial would require enrollment of thousands of exposed HCP to achieve the statistical power necessary to directly demonstrate PEP efficacy. During 1987–1989, the Burroughs-Wellcome Company sponsored a prospective placebo-controlled clinical trial among HCP to evaluate 6 weeks of zidovudine (ZDV) prophylaxis; however, this trial was terminated prematurely because of low enrolment.[12] In view of current indirect evidence of PEP efficacy, it is unlikely that a placebo-controlled trial in HCP would ever be considered ethical.

A retrospective case-control study of HCP that assessed potential risk factors for HIV transmission after percutaneous exposure found that use of ZDV as PEP was associated with a reduction in the risk of HIV infection by approximately 81% (95% CI = 43–94%).[13] Limitations of this study include its retrospective nature, the small number of cases, and having cases and controls from different cohorts.

Additional supportive data on the efficacy of PEP come from studies of perinatal HIV transmission. In a randomized, controlled, prospective trial (AIDS Clinical Trial Group protocol ACTG 076), in which

ZDV was administered to HIV-infected pregnant women and their infants, the administration of ZDV during pregnancy, labor, and delivery and to the infant reduced transmission by 67%.[14] Only 9–17% (depending on the assay used) of the protective effect of ZDV was explained by reduction of the HIV viral load in the maternal blood, suggesting that ZDV prophylaxis in part involves a mechanism other than the reduction of maternal viral burden.[15] Subsequent studies of various PEP regimens to prevent perinatal transmission lend further support to the role of antiretroviral agents as prophylaxis against HIV-infection transmission.[16,17]

The limitations of all of these studies in animals and humans must be considered when reviewing evidence of PEP efficacy. The extent to which data from animal studies can be extrapolated to humans is largely unknown, and the exposure route for mother-to-infant HIV transmission is not similar to occupational exposures; therefore these findings may not be directly applicable to PEP in HCP.

Reports of failure of PEP

The protection against HIV infection provided by PEP is not absolute, as demonstrated by 22 reported instances of failure of PEP to prevent HIV infection in HCP.[3,18,19] In 16 of the cases, ZDV was used as a single agent; in two cases, ZDV and didanosine (ddI) were used in combination; and in four cases, three or more drugs were used for PEP. Some 14 of the source patients were known to have been treated with antiretroviral therapy before the exposure. Antiretroviral resistance testing of the virus from the source patient was performed in eight instances, and in five, the HIV transmitted was found to have decreased sensitivity to ZDV and/or other drugs used for PEP. In addition to possible exposure to an antiretroviral-resistant strain of HIV, other factors that may have contributed to these apparent failures may include a high titer and/or large inoculum exposure, delayed initiation and/or short duration of PEP, and possible factors related to the host (e.g. cellular immune system responsiveness) and/or to the source patient's virus (e.g. presence of syncytia-forming strains). Summary information about the cases of PEP failure involving combinations of antiretroviral agents is shown in Table 63.1.

Antiretroviral Agents for PEP

Antiretroviral agents from four classes of drugs are currently available for the treatment of HIV disease.[20,21] These include the nucleoside or nucleo-

Table 63.1 Reported instances of failure of combination drug post-exposure prophylaxis (PEP) to prevent HIV-infection among health-care personnel exposed to HIV-infected blood through percutaneous injury

Year of incident	Device	PEP regimen[a]	Time to first dose (hrs)	No. days to onset of retroviral illness	No. days to document seroconversion[b]	Source-patient HIV-infection status	On antiretrovirals	Virus resistant to antiretrovirals?[c]
1992[d]	Biopsy needle	ZDV, ddl	0.5	23	23	AIDS, terminally ill	Yes	Unknown
1996[e]	Hollow-bore needle	ZDV, ddl[f]	1.5	45	97	Asymptomatic HIV infection	No	Not tested
1997[e]	Large-bore, hollow-bore needle	3 drugs[g]	1.5	40	55	AIDS	Yes	No
1998[h]	Hollow-bore needle	ZDV, 3TC, ddl, IDV	0.67	70	83	AIDS	Yes	Yes
1999[i]	Unknown sharp	ddl, d4T, NVP[j]	2	42	100	AIDS	Yes	Yes
2001[k]	Phlebotomy needle	ZDV, 3TC, IDV[l]	1.6	24	<100	AIDS	Yes	Yes

[a]ZDV = zidovudine; ddl = didanosine; 3TC = lamivudine; IDV = indinavir; d4T = stavudine; and NVP = nevirapine.

[b]By enzyme immunoassay for HIV-1 antibody and Western blot.

[c]By genotypic or phenotypic resistance testing.

[d]*Source:* Jochimsen EM. Failures of zidovudine postexposure prophylaxis. Am J Med 1997; 102(Suppl 5B):52–55.

[e]*Source:* Lot F, Abiteboul D. Infections professionnelles par le VIH en France chez le personnel de santé. Bull Epi Hebdom 1999; 18:69–70.

[f]ZDV and ddl taken for 48 hours and then changed to ZDV alone.

[g]ZDV, 3TC, and IDV taken for 48 hours and then changed to d4T, 3TC, and IDV.

[h]*Source:* Perdue B, Wolde Rufael D, Mellors J, Quinn T, Margolick J. HIV-1 transmission by a needlestick injury despite rapid initiation of four-drug postexposure prophylaxis [Abstract no 210]. In: Program and abstracts of the 6th Conference on Retroviruses and Opportunistic Infections. Chicago, IL: Foundation for Retrovirology and Human Health; 1999.

[i]*Source:* Beltrami EM, Luo C-C, de la Torre N, Cardo DM. Transmission of drug-resistant HIV after an occupational exposure despite combination postexposure prophylaxis with a combination drug regimen. Infect Control Hosp Epidemiol 2002; 23:345–348 and CDC, unpublished data.

[j]ZDV and 3TC taken for one dose and then changed to ddl, d4T, and NVP; ddl was discontinued after 3 days as a result of severe vomiting.

[k]*Source:* Hawkins DA, Asboe D, Barlow K, Evans B. Seroconversion to HIV-1 following a needlestick injury despite combination post-exposure prophylaxis. J Infect 2001; 43:12–15.

[l]ZDV, 3TC, and IDV initially and then changed after 1st dose to d4T, ddl, NVP; then ddl discontinued after 8 days; and d4T, NVP taken for 4 weeks.

tide reverse transcriptase inhibitors (NRTIs), non-nucleoside reverse transcriptase inhibitors (NNRTIs), protease inhibitors (PIs), and a single fusion inhibitor. Only antiretroviral agents that have been approved by the Food and Drug Administration (FDA) for treatment of HIV infection are recommended as PEP by the US PHS. This document summarises the PHS recommendations on use of PEP regimens that are based on the level of risk for HIV transmission represented by the exposure (Tables 63.2, 63.3, Box 63.1).

Toxicity and drug interactions of antiretroviral agents

An important goal when administering PEP is completion of a 4-week PEP regimen when PEP is indicated. Toxicity and side-effects among HCP have been cited as reasons why many HCP were unable to complete a full 4-week course of HIV PEP. Because all of the antiretroviral agents have been associated with side-effects (Table 63.4), the toxicity profile of these agents, including the frequency, severity, duration, and reversibility of side-effects, is an important consideration in selection of HIV PEP regimens. Most data on adverse events have been reported primarily for persons with established HIV infection receiving prolonged antiretroviral therapy and therefore may not reflect the experience in uninfected persons who take PEP for a limited time. At least anecdotally, antiretroviral agents appear to be less well tolerated by HCP taking them as PEP than by HIV-infected patients taking these agents as long-term treatment.

Side-effects are frequently reported by persons taking antiretroviral agents as PEP.[22-27] Several series reported that a large proportion of HCP did not complete a full 4 weeks of therapy because of an inability to tolerate the drugs.[23,25,26] Data from the National Surveillance System for Health Care Workers (NaSH),

Table 63.2 Recommended HIV post-exposure prophylaxis (PEP) for percutaneous injuries

Exposure type	Infection status of source				
	HIV-positive, class 1[a]	HIV-positive, class 2[a]	Source of unknown HIV status[b]	Unknown source[c]	HIV-negative
Less severe[d]	Recommend basic 2-drug PEP	Recommend expanded 3-drug PEP	Generally, no PEP warranted; however, consider basic 2-drug PEP[e] for source with HIV-risk factors[f]	Generally, no PEP warranted; however, consider basic 2-drug PEP[e] in settings in which exposure to HIV-infected persons is likely	No PEP warranted
More severe[g]	Recommend expanded 3-drug PEP	Recommend expanded 3-drug PEP	Generally, no PEP warranted; however, consider basic 2-drug PEP[b] for source with HIV-risk factors[f]	Generally, no PEP warranted; however, consider basic 2-drug PEP[b] in settings where exposure to HIV-infected persons is likely	No PEP warranted

[a]HIV-positive, class 1 – asymptomatic HIV infection or known low viral load (e.g., <1,500 ribonucleic acid copies/mL). HIV-positive, class 2 – symptomatic HIV infection, acquired immunodeficiency syndrome, acute seroconversion, or known high viral load. If drug resistance is a concern, obtain expert consultation. Initiation of PEP should not be delayed pending expert consultation, and, because expert consultation alone cannot substitute for face-to-face counselling, resources should be available to provide immediate evaluation and follow-up care for all exposures.
[b]For example, deceased source person with no samples available for HIV testing.
[c]For example, a needle from a sharps disposal container.
[d]For example, solid needle or superficial injury.
[e]The designation 'consider PEP' indicates that PEP is optional; a decision to initiate PEP should be based on a discussion between the exposed person and the treating clinician of the risks versus benefits of PEP.
[f]If PEP is offered and taken and the source is later determined to be HIV-negative, PEP should be discontinued.
[g]For example, large-bore hollow needle, deep puncture, visible blood on device, or needle used in patient's artery or vein.

Table 63.3 Recommended HIV post-exposure prophylaxis (PEP) for mucous membrane exposures and nonintact skin[a] exposures

Exposure type	Infection status of source				
	HIV-positive, class 1[b]	HIV-positive, class 2[b]	Source of unknown HIV status[c]	Unknown source[d]	HIV-negative
Small volume[e]	Consider basic 2-drug PEP[f]	Recommend basic 2-drug PEP	Generally, no PEP warranted[g] (2001 guidelines also state consider basic 2-day PEP for some risk factors)	Generally, no PEP warranted (2001 guidelines also state consider basic 2-day PEP in settings where exposure to HIV-infected persons is likely)	No PEP warranted
Large volume[h]	Recommend basic 2-drug PEP	Recommend expanded 3-drug PEP	Generally, no PEP warranted; however, consider basic 2-drug PEP[f] for source with HIV-risk factors[g]	Generally, no PEP warranted; however, consider basic 2-drug PEP[f] in settings in which exposure to HIV-infected persons is likely	No PEP warranted

[a]For skin exposures, follow-up is indicated only if evidence exists of compromised skin integrity (e.g., dermatitis, abrasion, or open wound).
[b]HIV-positive, class 1 – asymptomatic HIV infection or known low viral load (e.g., <1,500 ribonucleic acid copies/mL). HIV-positive, class 2 – symptomatic HIV infection, AIDS, acute seroconversion, or known high viral load. If drug resistance is a concern, obtain expert consultation. Initiation of PEP should not be delayed pending expert consultation, and, because expert consultation alone cannot substitute for face-to-face counseling, resources should be available to provide immediate evaluation and follow-up care for all exposures.
[c]For example, deceased source person with no samples available for HIV testing.
[d]For example, splash from inappropriately disposed blood.
[e]For example, a few drops.
[f]The designation 'consider PEP' indicates that PEP is optional; a decision to initiate PEP should be based on a discussion between the exposed person and the treating clinician of the risks versus benefits of PEP.
[g]If PEP is offered and taken and the source is later determined to be HIV-negative, PEP should be discontinued.
[h]For example, a major blood splash.

CDC's occupational surveillance system for occupational exposures and infections in hospitals for the period June 1995 through December 2004 indicate that almost half (46.9%) of 921 HCP with at least one follow-up visit after starting PEP experienced one or more symptoms. The symptom reported most frequently was nausea (26.5%) followed by malaise and fatigue (22.8%) (CDC, unpublished data). Similar data have been reported from the Italian Registry of Antiretroviral Postexposure Prophylaxis (IRAPEP) that includes data primarily on HCP taking PEP, but also collects data on persons taking PEP after non-occupational exposures.[24,27] In multivariate analysis, those taking protease-inhibitor-including regimens were more likely to experience PEP-associated side-effect and to discontinue PEP prematurely (<28 days).[27] Because side-effects are frequent and particularly because they are cited as a major reason for not completing PEP regimens as pre-

scribed, the selection of regimens should be heavily influenced towards those that are tolerable for short-term use.

In addition, all of the approved antiretroviral agents may have potentially serious drug interactions when used with certain other drugs. For this reason, careful evaluation is required of concomitant medications including over-the-counter medications and supplements (e.g. herbals) being used by an exposed person before prescribing PEP. Anyone receiving these drugs should be monitored closely for toxicity (Table 63.4).[28–30] Protease inhibitors and NNRTIs, in general, have the most potential for significant interactions with other drugs. Information about potential drug interactions can be found in Tables 63.5 and 63.6, as well as in the adult and adolescent HIV treatment guidelines,[20] and more detailed information is in the manufacturers' package inserts. Tables 63.5 and 63.6 list drugs that

Box 63.1

Recommended HIV PEP Regimens for Occupational HIV Exposure

- Two-drug regimens
  - Zidovudine (ZDV) + (lamivudine (3TC) or emtricitabine (FTC))
  - or
  - Stavudine (d4T) + (3TC or FTC)
  - or
  - Tenofovir (TDF) + (3TC or FTC)
  - or
  - Didanosine (ddI) + (3TC or FTC)

Avoid d4T + ddI or should it be Avoid ddi + d4T

Expanded Regimen

Basic regimen plus one of the following:
Lopinavir/ritonavir (Kaletra)
Nelfinavir (NFV)
or
Saquinavir + ritonavir (RTV)
Atazanavir (ATV)
ATV + RTV
Indinavir
Indinavir + RTV
Efavirenz
Fosamprenavir (FOSAPV)
(FOSAPV) + RTV

Antiretroviral Agents Generally not Recommended for Use as PEP

Nevirapine
Delavirdine
Abacavir
Zalcitabine

Antiretroviral Agent for use as PEP Only with Expert Consultation

Enfuvirtide

should not be administered concomitantly with PIs and efavirenz, respectively, because of interactions.

Selection of HIV PEP regimens

Determining which agents and how many to use as well as when to alter a PEP regimen is largely empiric.[31] In HIV-infected patients, combination regimens with three or more antiretroviral agents have proved superior to monotherapy and dual-therapy regimens in reducing HIV viral load, reducing the incidence of opportunistic infections and death, and delaying onset of drug resistance.[20,21] Guidelines for the treatment of HIV infection, a condition usually involving a high total body burden of HIV, recommend the use of three or more drugs;[20,21]

however, the applicability of these recommendations to PEP remains unknown.

A combination of drugs with activity at different stages in the viral replication cycle (e.g. nucleoside analogues with a PI) theoretically could offer an additive preventive effect in PEP, particularly for occupational exposures that pose an increased risk of transmission or transmission of a resistant virus. Although the use of a three (or more)-drug regimen may be justified for exposures that pose an increased risk of transmission, it is uncertain whether the potential added toxicity of a third (or even fourth) drug is justified for lower-risk exposures, especially in the absence of data supporting increased efficacy of more drugs in the context of occupational PEP. A recent modeling study has concluded that offering two-drug regimens remains a viable option, primarily because the benefit of completing a full course of the two-drug regimen exceeds the benefit of adding the third agent (and risking non-completion).[32] In addition, the total body burden of HIV is substantially lower among exposed HCP compared with persons with established HIV infection. For these reasons, the recommendations provide guidance for two- and three (or four)-drug PEP regimens that are based on the level of risk for HIV transmission represented by the exposure (Tables 63.2, 63.3, Box 63.1). Guidelines from elsewhere (e.g. New York State, European Union) recommend different HIV PEP regimens.[33,34]

Resistance to antiretroviral agents

Known or suspected resistance of the source virus to antiretroviral agents, particularly to those that might be included in a PEP regimen, is a concern for those who make decisions about PEP.[35,36] Drug resistance occurs to all of the currently available antiretroviral agents, and cross-resistance within drug classes is frequent.[37] Although occupational transmission of drug-resistant HIV strains, despite PEP with combination drug regimens, has been reported,[3,18,19] the relevance of exposure to a resistant virus to transmission and transmissibility is still not well understood.

Determining the presence of antiretroviral drug resistance is often difficult because patients generally take more than one antiretroviral agent. Resistance testing of the source virus at the time of exposure is impractical as the results will not be available in time to influence the choice of the initial PEP regimen. There are no data that suggest that modification of a PEP regimen after resistance testing results become available (usually 1–2 weeks) improves

Table 63.4 Primary side effects and toxicities associated with antiretroviral agents used for HIV postexposure prophylaxis, by class and agent

Class and agent	Side effects and toxicities
Nucleoside reverse transcriptase inhibitors (NRTIs)	Class warnings: All drugs in this class have the potential to cause lactic acidosis with hepatic steatosis
Zidovudine (Retrovir™; ZDV; AZT)	Anemia, neutropenia, nausea, headache, insomnia, muscle pain, and weakness
Lamivudine (Epivir™; 3TC)	Abdominal pain, nausea, diarrhea, rash, and pancreatitis
Stavudine (Zerit™; d4T)	Peripheral neuropathy, headache, diarrhea, nausea, insomnia, anorexia, pancreatitis, elevated liver function tests (LFTs), anemia, and neutropenia
Didanosine enteric coated (Videx EC™; ddl)	Pancreatitis, neuropathy, diarrhea, abdominal pain, and nausea
Abacavir (Ziagen™; ABC)	Nausea, diarrhea, anorexia, abdominal pain, fatigue, headache, insomnia, and hypersensitivity reactions
Emtricitabine (Emtriva™; FTC)	Headache, nausea, vomiting, diarrhea, and rash. Skin discoloration (mild hyperpigmentation on palms and soles) primarily among nonwhites
Nucleotide analogue reverse transcriptase inhibitor (N₁RTI)	Class warnings: All drugs in this class have the potential to cause lactic acidosis with hepatic steatosis
Tenofovir (Viread™; TDF)	Nausea, diarrhea, vomiting, flatulence, and headache
Class and agent	Side effect and toxicity
Nonnucleoside reverse transcriptase inhibitors (NNRTIs)	
Nevirapine (Viramune™; NVP)	Rash (including cases of Stevens-Johnson syndrome), fever, nausea, headache, hepatitis, fatal hepatic necrosis, and elevated LFTs
Delavirdine (Rescriptor™; DLV)	Rash (including cases of Stevens-Johnson syndrome), nausea, diarrhea, headache, fatigue, and elevated liver fuction test
Efavirenz (Sustiva™, EFV)	Rash (including cases of Stevens-Johnson syndrome), insomnia, somnolence, dizziness, trouble concentrating, abnormal dreaming, and teratogenicity
Protease inhibitors	
Indinavir (Crixivan™; IDV)	Nausea, abdominal pain, nephrolithiasis, and indirect hyperbilirubinemia
Nelfinavir (Viracept™; NFV)	Diarrhea, nausea, abdominal pain, weakness, and rash
Ritonavir (Norvir™; RTV)	Weakness, diarrhea, nausea, circumoral paresthesia, taste alteration, and increased cholesterol and triglycerides
Saquinavir (Fortovase™; SQV)	Diarrhea, abdominal pain, nausea, hyperglycemia, and elevated LFTs
Fosamprenavir (Lexiva®; FOSAPV)	Nausea, diarrhea, rash, circumoral paresthesia, taste alteration, and depression
Atazanavir (Reyataz™; ATV)	Nausea, headache, rash, abdominal pain, diarrhea, vomiting
Class and agent	Side effect and toxicity
Lopinavir/Ritonavir (Kaletra™; LPV/RTV)	Diarrhea, fatigue, headache, nausea, and increased cholesterol and triglycerides
Fusion inhibitor	
Enfuvirtide (Fuzeon®; T-20)	Local injection site reactions, bacterial pneumonia, insomnia; depression, peripheral neuropathy, and cough

Sources: Package inserts; Panel on Clinical Practices for Treatment of HIV Infection. Guidelines for the use of antiretroviral agents in HIV-infected adults and adolescents – April 7, 2005. Washington, DC: National Institutes of Health; 2005. Available at http://aidsinfo.nih.gov/guidelines/default_db2.asp?id=50.

Table 63.5 Prescription and over-the-counter drugs that should not be administered with protease inhibitors because of drug interactions[a]

Drug	Comment
Antimycobacterials: rifampin	Decreases plasma concentrations and area under plasma concentration curve of the majority of protease inhibitors by approximately 90%, which might result in loss of therapeutic effect and development of resistance
Benzodiazepines: midazolam, triazolam	Contraindicated because of potential for serious or life-threatening events (e.g., prolonged or increased sedation or respiratory depression)
Ergot derivatives: dihydroergotamine, ergotamine, ergonovine, methylergonovine	Contraindicated because of potential for serious or life-threatening events (e.g., acute ergot toxicity characterized by peripheral vasospasm and ischemia of the extremities and other tissues)
Gastrointestinal motility agent: cisapride	Contraindicated because of potential for serious or life-threatening events (e.g., cardiac arrhythmias)
HMG-CoA reductase inhibitors ("statins"): lovastatin, simvastatin.	Potential for serious reactions (e.g., myopathy, including rhabdomyolysis) Use atorvastatin cautiously and start with the lowest possible starting dose and monitor for atorvastatin-associated adverse events
Neuroleptic: pimozide	Contraindicated because of potential for serious or life-threatening events (e.g., cardiac arrhythmias)
Inhaled steroids: fluticasone	Coadministration of fluticasone and ritonavir-boosted protease inhibitors are not recommended unless the potential benefit to the patient outweighs the risk of systemic corticosteroid side effect
Herbal products: St. John's wort (hypericum perforatum), garlic (might lower saquinavir levels)	Coadministration might reduce plasma concentrations of protease inhibitors, which might result in loss of therapeutic effect and development of resistance

[a]This table does not list all products that should not be administered with protease inhibitors (atazanavir, lopinavir/ritonavir, fosamprenavir, indinavir, nelfinavir, saquinavir). Product labels should be consulted for additional information regarding drug interactions.
Sources: US Department of Health and Human Services. Guidelines for the use of antiretroviral agents in HIV-1-infected adults and adolescents. Washington, DC: US Department of Health and Human Services; 2005. Available at http://www.aidsinfo.nih.gov/guidelines/adult/AA_040705.pdf; University of California at San Francisco Center for HIV Information. Database of antiretroviral drug interactions. Available at http://hivinsite.ucsf.edu/InSite?page=ar-00-02.

efficacy of PEP.[38] Resistance should be suspected in source patients when there is clinical progression of disease or a persistently increasing viral load and/or decline in CD4 T-cell count despite therapy, or a lack of virologic response to therapy.

PEP regimens may need to be tailored depending on the drugs to which the source virus is known or suspected to be resistant.

Recommendations for the Management of HCP Potentially Exposed to HIV

Exposure prevention remains the primary strategy for reducing occupational blood-borne pathogen infections. Nevertheless, because occupational exposures continue to occur, appropriate post-exposure management is an essential element of workplace safety.

Definition of Healthcare Personnel and Exposure

The term healthcare personnel refers broadly to all paid and unpaid persons working in healthcare settings who have the potential for exposure to infectious materials, including blood, tissue, and specific body fluids, and medical supplies, equipment, or environmental surfaces contaminated with these

Table 63.6 Prescription and over-the-counter drugs that should not be administered with efavirenz because of drug interactions[a]

Drug	Comment
Antifungal: voriconazole	Contraindicated because efavirenz substantially decreases voriconazole plasma concentrations
Benzodiazepines: midazolam, triazolam	Contraindicated because of potential for serious or life-threatening events (e.g., prolonged or increased sedation or respiratory depression)
Ergot derivatives: dihydroergotamine, ergotamine, ergonovine, methylergonovine	Contraindicated because of potential for serious or life-threatening events (e.g., acute ergot toxicity characterized by peripheral vasospasm and ischemia of the extremities and other tissues)
Gastrointestinal motility agent: cisapride	Contraindicated because of potential for serious or life-threatening events (e.g., cardiac arrhythmias)
Herbal products: St. John's wort (hypericum perforatum), garlic (might lower saquinavir levels)	Coadministration might reduce plasma concentrations of protease inhibitors, which might result in loss of therapeutic effect and development of resistance

[a]This table does not list all products that should not be coadministered with efavirenz. Efavirenz product labeling should be consulted for additional information regarding drug interactions.
Source: Sustiva package insert, April 2005; US Department of Health and Human Services. Guidelines for the use of antiretroviral agents in HIV-1-infected adults and adolescents. Washington, DC: US Department of Health and Human Services; 2005. Available at http://www.aidsinfo.nih.gov/guidelines/adult/AA_040705.pdf; University of California at San Francisco Center for HIV Information. Database of antiretroviral drug interactions. Available at http://hivinsite.ucsf.edu/InSite?page=ar-00-02.

body substances. These personnel may include but are not limited to emergency medical service personnel, dental personnel, laboratory personnel, autopsy personnel, nurses, nursing assistants, physicians, technicians, therapists, pharmacists, students and trainees, contractual staff not employed by the healthcare facility, and persons not directly involved in patient care but potentially exposed to blood and body fluids (e.g. clerical, dietary, housekeeping, maintenance, and volunteer personnel). The same principles of exposure management could be applied to other workers who have potential for occupational exposure to blood and body fluids in other settings.

An exposure that might place HCP at risk for HIV infection is defined as a percutaneous injury (e.g. a needlestick or cut with a sharp object) or contact of mucous membrane or non-intact skin (e.g. exposed skin that is chapped, abraded, or afflicted with dermatitis) with blood, tissue, or other body fluids that are potentially infectious. In addition to blood and visibly bloody body fluids, semen and vaginal secretions also are considered potentially infectious. Although semen and vaginal secretions have been implicated in the sexual transmission of HIV, they have not been implicated in occupational transmission from patients to HCP. The following fluids are also considered potentially infectious: cerebrospinal fluid, synovial fluid, pleural fluid, peritoneal fluid,

pericardial fluid, and amniotic fluid. The risk for transmission of HIV infection from these fluids is unknown; the potential risk to HCP from occupational exposures has not been assessed by epidemiologic studies in healthcare settings. Feces, nasal secretions, saliva, sputum, sweat, tears, urine, and vomitus are not considered potentially infectious unless they are visibly bloody. The risk for transmission of HIV infection from these fluids and materials is extremely low.[39]

Any direct contact (i.e. contact without barrier protection) to concentrated virus in a research laboratory or production facility is considered an exposure that requires clinical evaluation. For human bites, the clinical evaluation must include the possibility that both the person bitten and the person who inflicted the bite were exposed to blood-borne pathogens. Transmission of HIV infection only rarely has been reported by this route, but not following an occupational exposure.[40,41]

HIV PEP

The US PHS recommendations (Tables 63.2, 63.3, Box 63.1) apply to situations in which a worker has had an exposure to a source person who has HIV infection or is likely to be HIV infected. These recommendations are based on the risk for HIV infection after different types of exposure and limited data regarding the efficacy and toxicity of PEP. If PEP is offered and taken, and the source is later determined to be HIV-negative, PEP should be discontinued. Although HIV-negative sources could be in the window period for seroconversion, there have been no documented transmissions reported in the USA involving exposure sources in the window period.[42] Rapid HIV testing of source patients can facilitate timely decisions about use of HIV PEP after occupational exposures to sources of unknown HIV status. Because most occupational HIV exposures do not result in the transmission of HIV, potential toxicity must be carefully considered when prescribing PEP. When possible, because of the complexity of selecting HIV PEP regimens, these recommendations should be implemented in consultation with persons having expertise in antiretroviral therapy and HIV transmission. Re-evaluation of exposed HCP should be strongly encouraged within 72 h post-exposure, especially as additional information about the exposure or source person becomes available.

Timing and duration of PEP

PEP should be initiated as soon as possible, preferably within hours of exposure, rather than days. If there is a question about which antiretroviral drugs to use, or whether to use a basic or expanded regimen, it is better to start the basic regimen immediately than to delay PEP administration. The optimal duration of PEP is unknown. Because 4 weeks of ZDV appeared protective in occupational and animal studies, PEP probably should be administered for 4 weeks, if tolerated. Although animal studies suggest that PEP is unlikely to be effective when started later than 24–36 h post-exposure, early treatment of HIV infection may be beneficial.[43]

Recommendations for the Selection of Drugs for HIV PEP

Determining which agents and how many to use or when to alter a PEP regimen is primarily empiric.[34] Those selecting a drug regimen for HIV PEP must strive to balance the risk for infection against the potential toxicities of the agent(s) used. Because PEP is potentially toxic, its use is not justified for exposures that pose a negligible risk for transmission (Tables 63.2, 63.3). In general, the regimens recommended here should be viewed as suggestions for initial HIV PEP regimens that could be changed should additional information about the source of

the occupational exposure, such as possible treatment history, and antiretroviral drug resistance be obtained and/or expert consultation be provided. Given the complexity of choosing and administering HIV PEP, consultation with an infectious diseases consultant or other physician with experience in the use of antiretroviral agents is recommended whenever possible, if doing so will not delay the timely initiation of PEP.

When selecting a PEP regimen, the comparative risk represented by the exposure and information about the exposure source, including history of and response to antiretroviral therapy based on clinical response, CD4+ T-cell counts, viral load measurements, and current disease stage should be considered. When the source person's virus is known or suspected to be resistant to one or more of the drugs considered for the PEP regimen, the selection of drugs to which the source person's virus is unlikely to be resistant is recommended; expert consultation is advised. If this information is not immediately available, initiation of PEP, if indicated, should not be delayed; changes in the PEP regimen can be made after PEP has been started, as appropriate. For HCP who initiate PEP, re-evaluation of the exposed person should occur within 72 h post-exposure, especially as additional information about the exposure or source person becomes available.

The US PHS recommends stratifying HIV PEP regimens based on the severity of exposure and other considerations, such as concern for antiretroviral drug resistance in the exposure source (Tables 63.2, 63.3, Box 63.1). Most HIV exposures will warrant a two-drug regimen, using two NRTIs (Tables 63.2, 63.3, Box 63.1). NRTI combinations that can be considered for PEP include ZDV and lamivudine (3TC) or emtricitabine (FTC); stavudine (d4T) and 3TC or FTC; and tenofovir (TDF) and 3TC or FTC; and didanosine (ddI) and 3TC or FTC. In the previous PHS guideline, a combination of d4T and ddI was considered one of the first choice PEP regimens; but this regimen is no longer recommended because of concerns about toxicity (especially neuropathy and pancreatitis) and the availability of alternative regimens that are more tolerable.[3]

The addition of a third (or even a fourth) drug should be considered for exposures that pose an increased risk for transmission or which involve a source in whom antiretroviral drug resistance is likely. The addition of a third drug for PEP following high-risk exposures is based on demonstrated effectiveness in reducing viral burden in HIV-infected persons. However, no definitive data exist that demonstrate increased efficacy of three- versus two-drug regimens as HIV PEP. Previously, indinavir (IDV), nelfinavir (NFV), efavirenz (EFV), or abacavir (ABC) were recommended as first-choice agents for inclusion in an expanded PEP regimen.[3] PHS is now recommending that expanded PEP regimens be primarily protease inhibitor-based, with lopinavir/ritonavir (Kaletra) being the preferred PI for use in expanded PEP regimens. Other protease inhibitors acceptable for use in expanded PEP regimens include atazanavir, fosamprenavir, ritonavir-boosted indinavir, ritonavir-boosted saquinavir, or nelfinavir (Box 63.1). Although side-effects may be common with the NNRTIs, EFV may be considered for expanded PEP regimens, especially when resistance to protease inhibitors in the source person's virus is known or suspected. Caution is advised when EFV is used in women of child-bearing age because of the risk of teratogenicity.

Drugs that may be considered as alternatives to the above regimens, with warnings about side-effects and other adverse event are efavirenz and ddI with either 3TC or FTC. The fusion inhibitor enfuvirtide (T20), has theoretical benefits for the use in PEP since its activity occurs prior to viral-host cell integration; however, it is not recommended for routine HIV PEP because of the mode of administration (subcutaneous, twice daily). Furthermore, use of enfuvirtide has the potential for production of anti-enfuvirtide antibodies that cross react with HIV gp41. This could result in a false positive enzyme-linked immunoassay (EIA) diagnostic HIV antibody test in HIV uninfected patients. A confirmatory western blot test would be expected to be negative in such cases. Enfuvirtide should only be used with expert consultation.

Antiviral drugs NOT recommended for use as PEP, due mostly to higher risk of adverse events (some serious or life-threatening), include abacavir, delavirdine, and zalcitabine, and as noted previously, the combination of ddI and d4T. Nevirapine should not be included in PEP regimens, except with expert consultation because of serious side-effects including hepatotoxicity (with one instance of fulminant liver failure requiring liver transplantation); rhabdomyolysis; and a hypersensitivity syndrome reported among persons taking nevirapine as PEP.[44]

Because of the complexity of selection of HIV PEP regimens, consultation with persons having expertise in antiretroviral therapy and HIV transmission is strongly recommended. Some institutions have assured appropriate consultation by requiring consultation with the hospital epidemiologist and/or infectious diseases consultant in situations where HIV PEP use is being considered or indicated. There are several situations in which this is especially important, such as management of a pregnant or breast-feeding worker, management of a worker exposed to a treatment-experienced source, etc (Box 63.2).

Box 63.2

Situations for which expert[a] consultation is advised

- Delayed (i.e. later than 24–36 h) exposure report:
  - the interval after which there is no benefit from PEP is undefined
- Unknown source (e.g. needle in sharps disposal container or laundry):
  - decide use of PEP on a case-by-case basis
  - consider the severity of the exposure and the epidemiologic likelihood of HIV exposure
  - do not test needles or other sharp instruments for HIV
- Known or suspected pregnancy in the exposed person:
  - does not preclude the use of optimal PEP regimens
  - do not deny PEP solely on the basis of pregnancy
- Breast-feeding in the exposed person:
  - does not preclude the use of optimal PEP regimens
  - do not deny PEP solely on the basis of breast-feeding
- Resistance of the source virus to antiretroviral agents:
  - influence of drug resistance on transmission risk is unknown
  - if the source person's virus is known or suspected to be resistant to one or more of the drugs considered for the PEP regimen, a selection of drugs to which the source person's virus is unlikely to be resistant is recommended
  - resistance testing of the source person's virus at the time of the exposure is not recommended
  - initiation of PEP should not be delayed while awaiting results of resistance testing, if obtained
- Toxicity of the initial PEP regimen:
  - adverse symptoms, such as nausea and diarrhea are common with PEP
  - symptoms often can be managed without changing the PEP regimen by prescribing antimotility and/or antiemetic agents
  - in other situations, modifying the dose interval (i.e. taking drugs after meals, administering a lower dose of drug more frequently throughout the day, as recommended by the manufacturer), may help alleviate symptoms when they occur

[a]Local experts and/or the National Clinicians' Post-Exposure Prophylaxis Hotline (PEPline; 1-888-448-4911)

Follow-up of Exposed HCPs

Post-exposure testing

HCP with occupational exposure to HIV should receive follow-up counseling, post-exposure testing, and medical evaluation regardless of whether they receive PEP. HIV-antibody testing should be performed for at least 6 months post-exposure (e.g. at 6 weeks, 12 weeks, and 6 months). Extended HIV follow-up (e.g. for 12 months) is recommended for HCP who become infected with HCV following exposure to a source co-infected with HIV and HCV. It is unclear whether extended follow-up is indicated in other circumstances (e.g. exposure to a source co-infected with HIV and HCV in the absence of HCV seroconversion or for exposed persons with a medical history suggesting an impaired ability to amount an antibody response to acute infection). Although rare instances of delayed HIV seroconversion have been reported,[45] the infrequency of this occurrence does not warrant adding to exposed persons' anxiety by routinely extending the duration of post-exposure follow-up. However, this should not preclude a decision to extend follow-up in an individual situation based on the clinical judgment of the exposed person's healthcare provider. HIV testing should be performed on any exposed person who has an illness consistent with an acute retroviral syndrome, regardless of the interval since exposure. When HIV infection is identified, the individual should be referred for medical management to a specialist knowledgeable in the area of HIV treatment and counseling.

HIV-antibody testing using EIA should be used to monitor for seroconversion. Direct virus assays (e.g. HIV p24 antigen EIA or tests for HIV RNA) to detect infection in exposed HCP generally are not recommended.[46] The relatively high rate of false-positive results of these tests in this setting could lead to unnecessary anxiety and/or treatment.[47,48] Despite the ability of direct virus assays to detect HIV infection a few days earlier than EIA, the infrequency of occupational seroconversion and increased costs of these tests do not warrant their routine use in this setting.

- HIV-antibody testing should be performed for at least 6 months post-exposure
- Direct virus assays for routine follow-up of HCP are *not* recommended
- HIV testing should be performed on any exposed person who has an illness compatible with an acute retroviral syndrome.

Monitoring and management of PEP toxicity

If PEP is used, HCP should be monitored for drug toxicity by testing at baseline and again 2 weeks after starting PEP. The scope of testing should be based on medical conditions in the exposed person and the toxicity of drugs included in the PEP regimen. Minimally, laboratory monitoring for toxicity should include a complete blood count and renal and hepatic function tests. Monitoring for evidence of hyperglycemia should be included for HCP whose regimens include any PI; if the exposed person is receiving IDV, monitoring for crystalluria, hematuria, hemolytic anemia, and hepatitis also should be included. If toxicity is noted, modification of the regimen should be considered after expert consultation; further diagnostic studies may be indicated.

Exposed HCP who choose to take PEP should be advised of the importance of completing the prescribed regimen. Information should be provided about potential drug interactions and the drugs that should not be taken with PEP, the side-effects of the drugs that have been prescribed, measures to minimize these effects, and the methods of clinical monitoring for toxicity during the follow-up period. They should be advised that the evaluation of certain symptoms (e.g. rash, fever, back or abdominal pain, pain on urination or blood in the urine, or symptoms of hyperglycemia – increased thirst and/or frequent urination) should not be delayed.

HCP who fail to complete the recommended regimen often do so because of the side-effects they experience (e.g. nausea, diarrhea). These symptoms can often be managed with antimotility and antiemetic agents or other medications that target the specific symptoms, without changing the regimen. In other situations, modifying the dose interval (i.e. administering a lower dose of drug more frequently throughout the day, as recommended by the manufacturer), may facilitate adherence to the regimen. Serious adverse events should be reported to FDA's MedWatch program.

Although recommendations for follow-up testing, monitoring, and counseling of exposed HCP are unchanged from previous guidelines,[3] greater emphasis is needed on improving follow-up care provided to exposed HCP. This may result in increased adherence to HIV PEP regimens, better management of associated symptoms with ancillary medications or regimen changes, improved detection of serious adverse effects, and serologic testing in a larger proportion of exposed personnel to determine if infection is transmitted after occupational exposures. Closer follow-up should in turn provide some reassurance to healthcare personnel who understandably become very anxious after these events.[49,50] The psychological impact on HCP of needle-sticks or blood and body fluid exposure should not be underestimated. Psychological counseling of HCP should be an essential component of the management and care of exposed HCP.

References

1. Centers for Disease Control and Prevention Update: provisional Public Health Service recommendations for chemoprophylaxis after occupational exposure to HIV. MMWR 1996; 45:468–472.
2. Conters for Disease Control and Prevention. Public Health Service guidelines for the management of health-care worker exposures to HIV and recommendations for postexposure prophylaxis. MMWR Recomm Rep 1998; 47:1–33.
3. Centers for Disease Control and Prevention. US Public Health Service. Updated US Public Health Service guidelines for the management of occupational exposures to HBV, HCV, and HIV and recommendations for postexposure prophylaxis. MMWR Recomm Rep 2001; 50:1–52.
4. Centers for Disease Control and Prevention. Updated US Public Health Service guidelines for the management of occupational exposures to HIV and recommendations for postexposure prophylaxis. MMWR Recomm Rep 2005; 54:1–17.
5. Centers for Disease Control and Prevention. Antiretroviral postexposure prophylaxis after sexual, injection-drug use, or other nonoccupational exposure to HIV in the United States: recommendations from the US Department of Health and Human Services. MMWR Recomm Rep 2005; 54:1–20.
6. Piguet V, Blauvelt A. Essential roles for dendritic cells in the pathogenesis and potential treatment of HIV disease. J Invest Derm 2002; 119:365–369.
7. Spira AI, Marx PA, Patterson BK, et al. Cellular targets of infection and route of viral dissemination after an intravaginal inoculation of simian immunodeficiency virus into rhesus macaques. J Exp Med 1996; 183:215–225.
8. Black RJ. Animal studies of prophylaxis. Am J Med 1997; 102:S39–S44.
9. Tsai C-C, Emau P, Follis KE, et al. Effectiveness of postinoculation (R)-9-(2-phosphonylmethoxypropyl) adenine treatment for prevention of persistent simian immunodeficiency virus SIVmne infection depends critically on timing of initiation and duration of treatment. J Virol 1998; 72:4265–4273.
10. McClure HM, Anderson DC, Ansari AA, et al. Nonhuman primate models for evaluation of AIDS therapy. In: AIDS: anti-HIV agents, therapies and vaccines. Ann NY Acad Sci 1990; 616:287–298.
11. Otten RA, Smith DK, Adams DR, et al. Efficacy of postexposure prophylaxis after intravaginal exposure of pig-tailed macaques to a human-derived retrovirus (human immunodeficiency virus type 2). J Virol 2000; 74:9771–9775.
12. LaFon SW, Mooney BD, McMullen JP, et al. A double-blind, placebo-controlled study of the safety and efficacy of Retrovir (zidovudine, ZDV) as a chemoprophylactic agent in health care workers exposed to HIV. Abstract 489. 30th Interscience Conference on Antimicrobial Agents and Chemotherapy; 1990; Washington, DC: American Society for Microbiology.
13. Cardo D, Culver DM, Ciesielski C, et al. A case-control study of HIV seroconversion in health care workers after percutaneous exposure. N Engl J Med 1997; 337:1485–1490.
14. Connor EM, Sperling RS, Gelber R, et al. Reduction of maternal-infant transmission of human immunodeficiency virus type 1 with zidovudine treatment. N Engl J Med 1994; 331:1173–1180.
15. Sperling RS, Shapiro DE, Coombs RW, et al. Maternal viral load, zidovudine treatment, and the risk of transmission of human immunodeficiency virus type 1 from mother to infant. N Engl J Med 1996; 335:1621–1629.
16. Wade NA, Birkhead GS, Warren BL, et al. Abbreviated regimens of zidovudine prophylaxis and perinatal transmission of the human immunodeficiency virus. N Engl J Med 1998; 339:1409–1414.
17. De Cock K, Fowler MG, Mercier E, et al. Prevention of mother-to-child HIV transmission in resource-poor countries: translating research into policy and practice. JAMA 2000; 283:1175–1182.
18. Jochimsen EM. Failures of zidovudine postexposure prophylaxis. Am J Med 1997; 102:S52–S55.
19. Hawkins DA, Asboe D, Barlow K, et al. Seroconversion to HIV-1 following a needlestick injury despite combination post-exposure prophylaxis. J Infect 2001; 43:12–18.
20. Panel on Clinical Practices for Treatment of HIV Infection. Guidelines for the use of antiretroviral agents in HIV-infected adults and adolescents. 10 October 2006. Online. Available: http://aidsinfo.nih.gov/guidelines/GuidelineDetail.aspx?MenuItem=Guidelines&Search=Off&/GuidelineID=7&ClassID=1 (accessed 2 February 2007).
21. Yeni PG, Hammer SM, Hirsch MS, et al. Treatment for adult HIV infection: 2004 recommendations of the International AIDS Society-USA Panel. JAMA 2004; 292:251–265.
22. Wang SA, Panlilio AL, Doi PA, et al. Experience of healthcare workers taking postexposure prophylaxis after occupational HIV exposures: findings of the HIV Postexposure Prophylaxis Registry. Infect Control Hosp Epidemiol 2000; 21:780–785.
23. Swotinsky RB, Steger KA, Sulis C, et al. Occupational exposure to HIV: experience at a tertiary care center. J Occup Environ Med 1998; 40:1102–1109.
24. Puro V, De Carli G, Orchi N, et al. Short-term adverse effects from and discontinuation of antiretroviral post-exposure prophylaxis. J Biol Regul Homeost Agents 2001; 15:238–242.
25. Russi M, Buitrago M, Goulet J, et al. Antiretroviral prophylaxis of health care workers at two urban medical centers. J Occup Environ Med 2000; 42:1092–1100.
26. Garb JR. One-year study of occupational human immunodeficiency virus postexposure prophylaxis. J Occup Environ Med 2002; 44:265–270.
27. Puro V, DeCarli G, Soldani F, et al. Adverse drug reactions associated with PEP. Poster #711. 10th Conference on Retroviruses and Opportunistic Infections, Boston, MA: February 2003.
28. University of California San Francisco Center for HIV Information. Database of antiretroviral drug interactions. Online. Available: http://hivinsite.ucsf.edu/InSite?page=ar-00-02.
29. Andrade A, Flexner C. Genes, ethnicity, and efavirenz response: clinical pharmacology update from the 11th CROI. Hopkins HIV Rep 2004; 16:1–7.
30. de Maat MM, Ekhart GC, Huitema AD, et al. Drug interactions between antiretroviral drugs and comedicated agents. Clin Pharm 2003; 42:223–282.
31. Gerberding JL. Clinical practice. Occupational exposure to HIV in health care settings. N Engl J Med 2003; 348:826–833.
32. Bassett IV, Freedberg KA, Walensky RP. Two drugs or three? Balancing efficacy, toxicity, and resistance in postexposure prophylaxis for occupational exposure to HIV. Clin Infect Dis 2004; 39:395–401.
33. New York State Department of Health AIDS Institute. HIV prophylaxis following occupational exposure. 2005. Online. Available: www.hivguidelines.org/public_html/oe/oe.pdf (accessed 14 June 2005).
34. Puro V, Cicalini S, De Carli G, et al. on behalf of the European Occupational Post-Exposure Prophylaxis

Study Group. Towards a standard HIV post exposure prophylaxis for healthcare workers in Europe. Eurosurveillance Mon 2004; 9:40–43. Online. Available: www.eurosurveillance.org/em/v09n06/0906-222.asp (accessed 14 June 2005).

35. Beltrami EM, Cheingsong R, Heneine WM, et al. Antiretroviral drug resistance in human immunodeficiency virus-infected source patients for occupational exposures to healthcare workers. Infect Control Hosp Epidemiol 2003; 24:724–730.

36. Hirsch MS, Brun-Vézinet F, D'Aquila RT, et al. Antiretroviral drug resistance testing in adult HIV-1 infection: recommendations of an international AIDS Society-USA panel. JAMA 2000; 283:2417–2426.

37. Tack PC, Bremer JW, Harris AA, et al. Genotypic analysis of HIV-1 isolates to identify antiretroviral resistance mutations from source patients involved in health care worker occupational exposures (letter). JAMA 1999; 281:1085–1086.

38. Puro V. Genotypic resistance tests for the management of postexposure prophylaxis. Scand J Infect Dis Suppl 2003; 35: S93–S98.

39. Bell DM. Occupational risk of human immunodeficiency virus infection in healthcare workers: an overview. Am J Med 1997; 102:9–15.

40. Richman KM, Rickman LS. The potential for transmission of human immunodeficiency virus through human bites. J Acquir Immune Defic Syndr 1993; 6:402–406.

41. Pretty IA, Anderson GS, Sweet DJ. Human bites and the risk of human immunodeficiency virus transmission. Am J Forensic Med Pathol 1999; 20:232–239.

42. Do AN, Ciesielski CA, Metler RP, et al. Occupationally acquired human immunodeficiency virus (HIV) infection: national case surveillance data during 20 years of the HIV epidemic in the United States. Infect Control Hosp Epidemiol 2003; 24:86–96.

43. Kinloch-de Loës S, Hirschel BJ, Hoen B, et al. A controlled trial of zidovudine in primary human immunodeficiency virus infection. N Engl J Med 1995; 333:408–413.

44. CDC. Serious adverse events attributed to nevirapine regimens for postexposure prophylaxis after HIV exposures. MMWR 2001; 49:1153–1156.

45. Ciesielski CA, Metler RP. Duration of time between exposure and seroconversion in healthcare workers with occupationally acquired infection with human immunodeficiency virus. Am J Med 1997; 102:S115–S116.

46. Busch MP, Satten GA. Time course of viremia and antibody seroconversion following human immunodeficiency virus exposure. Am J Med 1997; 102:S117–S124.

47. Rich JD, Merriman NA, Mylonakis E, et al. Misdiagnosis of HIV infection by HIV-1 plasma viral load testing: a case series. Ann Intern Med 1999; 130:37–39.

48. Roland ME, Elbeik TA, Kahn JO, et al. HIV RNA testing in the context of nonoccupational postexposure prophylaxis. J Infect Dis 2004; 190:598–604.

49. Armstrong K, Gorden R, Santorella G. Occupational exposure of health care workers (HCWs) to human immunodeficiency virus (HIV): stress reactions and counseling interventions. Soc Work Health Care 1995; 21:61–80.

50. Meienberg F, Bucher HC, Sponagel L, et al. Anxiety in health care workers after exposure to potentially HIV-contaminated blood or body fluids. Swiss Med Wkly 2002; 132:321–324.

CHAPTER 64

Selected NGOs Active in HIV and Web Links

Sahai Burrowes

Laurence Peiperl

Introduction

Non-governmental organizations (NGOs) have been pioneers in providing antiretroviral treatment (ART) to people living with HIV in resource-poor countries. In the late 1990s, NGOs began small pilot treatment projects for men and women in urban slums and poor rural areas. These projects were crucial in demonstrating that ART is feasible in these settings and that resource-poor countries can provide affordable HIV treatment if they have access to low-cost antiretroviral (ARV) drugs. By adapting treatment protocols to local conditions, simplifying monitoring regimens, decentralizing service delivery, and transferring some treatment monitoring and implementation duties from doctors to nurses, other clinical staff, or community health workers, these projects were able to achieve clinical results that were comparable with those in developed countries.[1,2]

NGOs used these early successes to pressure governments and international institutions to develop cheaper, simpler ARV regimens, relax trade laws to allow the production and importation of generic drugs, and to increase funding for HIV treatment in resource-poor countries. This advocacy has had impressive results; although as of June 2005, only 1 million of the 6 million people in resource-poor countries who need ART have access to it, great strides have been made in expanding access since the call of 'treatment for all' was raised at the XIII International AIDS conference in Durban, South Africa in 2000.[3] For example, the prices of ARV drugs have dropped significantly and the financial resources available for treatment programs have increased dramatically through the creation of funding mechanisms such as the Global Fund to Fight AIDS, Tuberculosis and Malaria (GFATM) and the President's Emergency Plan for AIDS Relief (PEPFAR).* At the writing of this chapter, several large ARV treatment programs in the countries most heavily affected by HIV were in their start-up stages.

Although most of these new treatment programs will be implemented by government-run health facilities, national and international NGOs will remain central to the effort to scale-up treatment rapidly. Their ongoing pilot projects will be crucial to the development of innovative treatment delivery systems. Moreover, international NGOs are largely responsible for providing technical assistance, training, and logistical support for government programs. National NGOs, particularly religious organizations, also play an important role in providing treatment, particularly in remote rural areas.

---

*PEPFAR is an initiative announced by President Bush of the USA that commits US$15 billion over 5 years to fight HIV. Originally, 14 countries were designated as targets for the program: Botswana, Cote d'Ivoire, Ethiopia, Guyana, Haiti, Kenya, Mozambique, Namibia, Nigeria, Rwanda, South Africa, Tanzania, Uganda, and Zambia. Vietnam was added to the list in June 2004 and the PEPFAR legislation allows the president to designate other countries as focus countries as long as they had existing HIV programs in 2003. Of the funds promised in the initiative, 55% is earmarked for HIV treatment; 15% for palliative care; 20% for HIV prevention; and 10% for support to orphans and vulnerable children.

This chapter will provide an overview of NGOs that have been at the forefront of providing HIV treatment in resource-poor countries and guidance on how to access information about their work (see also Table 64.1). The chapter focuses on organizations providing clinical care: ART, prophylaxis and treatment of opportunistic infections, and interventions to prevent mother-to-child transmission of HIV. It does not discuss the many organizations that are involved in primarily HIV-education and HIV-prevention work or those that mainly provide other important services in the HIV-care continuum such as counseling and testing, psychosocial support, or homecare. We also attempt to focus on organizations that provide intensive technical support and direct care rather than those that provide funding exclusively. Finally, although research projects sometimes provide a large portion of the treatment in resource-poor countries, particularly to vulnerable groups like children, for the sake of brevity we have chosen not to include the many organizations that are involved primarily in conducting research rather than providing long-term care.

International NGOs

Médecins Sans Frontières

Médecins Sans Frontières (MSF), one of the NGOs most experienced in providing HIV treatment in resource-poor settings, has been at the forefront of advocacy efforts to make cheaper and simpler treatment regimens available to populations in need.

MSF began pilot HIV programs in Cameroon, South Africa and Thailand in 2000. As of December 2005, the organization was providing ART to more than 57 000 patients including 3500 children in 29 countries: Angola, Benin, Burkina Faso, Cambodia, Cameroon, China, Congo-Brazzaville, Democratic Republic of Congo, Ecuador, Ethiopia, Guatemala, Guinea, Honduras, Indonesia, Kenya, Laos, Malawi, Mozambique, Myanmar, Nigeria, Peru, Rwanda, South Africa, Tanzania, Thailand, Uganda, Ukraine, Zambia, and Zimbabwe.[4] The programs are based in a variety of settings ranging from hospitals in capital cities to small clinics in rural areas and slums.

MSF's treatment programs provide a comprehensive package of care including health education, condom distribution, voluntary counseling and testing (VCT), interventions for the prevention of mother-to-child transmission of HIV (PMTCT),

nutritional and psychosocial support, treatment and prophylaxis of opportunistic infections, and ART.[5] Usually, treatment is provided free of charge.

One of MSF's first ART programs was the Khayelitsha project in Cape Town, South Africa. In April 2000, MSF and the Western Cape provincial government set up three clinics dedicated to HIV within Khayelitsha's primary healthcare centers. These clinics began offering ART in May 2001. After 2 years of operations, the three clinics were serving over 1800 HIV-infected clients per month.[5] MSF is now in the process of handing over this program to the provincial government.

Another large MSF project is the comprehensive HIV care program at Chiradzulu District hospital in Malawi, which has been providing ART to a poor rural population for several years. The program, initiated in 1997, at first focused on HIV prevention. In 1999, HIV care was added and in 2001, management of opportunistic infections, PMTCT, and ART. By March 2004, the program had provided ART to 2194 patients.[7]

Where to get more information

The MSF International's website has general information on MSF's work (www.msf.org). Information on specific projects can be found at the various national MSF program sites, which are linked from the MSF home page. Information on the group's experiences delivering ART and its various press releases, advocacy briefs, and pricing documents can be found on its 'Campaign for Access to Essential Medicines' website (www.accessmed-msf.org).

Partners in Health

Partners in Health (PIH), a small non-governmental organization affiliated with Harvard Medical School, has also been a strong proponent of access to ART in resource-poor settings. PIH initiated one of the early pilot programs providing ART to HIV-infected people living in very poor rural areas in Haiti. Like MSF's pilots, this project was crucial in demonstrating that successful ART was possible in these settings.

In 1988, PIH and its sister organization Zanmi Lasante began providing HIV testing and counseling free of charge to the residents of the Central Plateau in Haiti at the Clinique Bon Sauveur. PMTCT activities began there in 1995, and in 1997, the clinic began offering post-exposure prophylaxis to exposed health workers and rape victims.[8] The clinic now serves approximately 7000 HIV-infected patients, 700 of whom were receiving ART in 2003 through the 'HIV Equity Initiative' pilot project.[9]

PIH's HIV Equity Initiative pilot used a directly observed therapy (DOT) community-based care model to deliver ARVs. PIH developed this model in its efforts to treat multidrug-resistant tuberculosis in Haiti and Peru. In the model, community health workers called *accompagnateurs* visit patients daily. During these visits, they deliver the day's dose of ARV drugs and other care and support services, while supervising the patients to ensure treatment compliance. The *accompagnateurs* are trained to recognize common ARV side-effects and signs of HIV-related illness. All medical consultations, drugs, social service, and social support are provided free of charge.

According to an interim analysis conducted in 2001, the majority of the HIV patients under treatment in this program achieved undetectable viral loads.[2] The group is one of the implementing organizations in GFATM's US$67 million grant to Haiti, which was awarded in 2002. With these funds PIH will be expanding its HIV and tuberculosis treatment program to four new sites in Lascahobas, Belladère, Boucan Carré, and Thomonde. The Zanmi Lasante clinic has also been designated as a teaching site for US Centers for Disease Control and Prevention's HIV training programs in the Caribbean.[9]

Where to get more information

The PIH website contains background information on the organization and its work, links to articles and papers written about the project, publication ordering information, patient stories, and links to PIH's clinical manuals for tuberculosis and HIV care (www.pih.org). Of note is the PIH Guide to the Community-Based Treatment of HIV in Resource-Poor Settings (www.pih.org/inforesouces/pihguide-hiv.html), which describes the treatment protocols used in the HIV Equity Initiative.

French Red Cross

The French Red Cross has been providing ART in sub-Saharan Africa since 1994, when it set up its first 'day care center' (DCC) in Congo-Brazzaville. These centers, which are small clinics usually located in larger health facilities, provide HIV testing, ART and monitoring, treatment for opportunistic infections, prevention counseling, and clinical care. In addition, the DCCs serve as training centers for local health

staff.[10] Patients pay a nominal fee for services. The French Red Cross has since opened 10 more clinics in sub-Saharan Africa and two in Cambodia.* According to the organization, 10 000 patients had received care through the centers as of 2003, 2000 of whom were receiving ART.

To compliment its ART provision, the French Red Cross has set up a PMTCT clinic in Congo-Brazzaville that provides ARV prophylaxis and distributes infant formula. The PMTCT center has screened 4000 women, of whom 200 received PMTCT interventions.[10] The organization has also started nutritional rehabilitation centers linked to the DCCs in Senegal and Burkina Faso, which provide food, nutritional counseling, and cooking lessons to those on therapy. In Cambodia, the group has started a pediatric caring center in Phnom Penh.

Where to get more information

The French Red Cross's website has basic background information on the organization's activities (www.croix-rouge.fr/goto/actions/sida/index.asp). Information is only available in French.

MTCT-Plus

MTCT-Plus is an initiative led by Columbia University's Mailman School of Public Health that provides clinical protocols, funding, training, drug procurement, data management, program evaluation, and technical support to health facilities in resource-poor countries. The initiative, started in February 2003, currently supports PMTCT interventions and HIV treatment through 13 programs, in nine countries[†,11].

The MTCT-Plus initiative has pioneered a family-centered approach to HIV care in antenatal care settings. PMTCT interventions are the entry point to care in the program; pregnant women who participate in the program receive PMTCT interventions, HIV clinical care, prevention counseling, nutrition counseling, family planning services, and other supportive care, as well as ART when indicated. Their children, spouses, and direct family members are also eligible to receive HIV care and treatment services. As of March 2005, approximately 7095

---

*The African care centers are in Morocco (1), Senegal (1), Burkina Faso (2), Gabon (3), Republic of Congo (2), and Niger (1).
†MTCT-Plus programs are located in Cameroon, Cote d'Ivoire, Kenya, Mozambique, South Africa, Rwanda, Uganda, Zambia, and Thailand.

patients were enrolled in the program. Approximately 35% of patients (2472) are children.[12]

In February 2004, The Mailman School of Public Health received a grant from the PEPFAR initiative for the 'Multicountry Columbia Antiretroviral Program' (MCAP), which will provide family-centered ART at health facilities in Kenya, Mozambique, Rwanda, South Africa, and Tanzania.[13] Columbia University has also partnered with the Clinton Foundation to create the Dominican HIV/AIDS Treatment Initiative, which supports the national roll-out of HIV treatment in the Dominican Republic. The Initiative provides technical assistance to the Ministry of Health and clinical training at both governmental and NGO sites. At the end of 2004, the program had 17 functioning treatment sites, enrolling patients. A total of 28 sites are planned by the end of 2006. The MTCT-Plus Initiative, MCAP, and the Dominican HIV/AIDS Treatment Initiative all operate under Columbia University's International Center for AIDS Care and Treatment Programs (ICAP).

Where to get more information

The MTCT-Plus website provides a thorough overview of the program, summaries of project site activities, and news stories about the program (http://www.mtctplus.org/). It also contains links to the pediatric dosing tables, conference presentations, and the organization's *Pediatric Clinical Manual,* and the *Columbia Clinical Manual*, which is available in English, French, Portuguese, Spanish, and Thai. Information on the new MCAP program can be found at www.columbia-mcap.org

Baylor College of Medicine

The Baylor College of Medicine has been a leader in offering treatment to HIV-infected children in resource-poor countries. The Baylor International Pediatric AIDS Initiative (BIPAI) is a research-focused treatment project that currently provides treatment in Romania, Ukraine, Mexico, and 10 countries in Africa. In Romania, 452 children have begun ART through the program since November 2001.[14] In Botswana, Baylor has worked with the government to set up a center of excellence at the Princess Marina Hospital, where more than 1000 children and 200 families are in care.[14]

Where to get more information

The Baylor International Pediatric AIDS Initiative website (http://bayloraids.org) provides an over-view of Baylor's international work as well as an image library on pediatric HIV care, an archive of pediatric HIV-infection case studies, a training on pill swallowing for children, and the *Baylor HIV Curriculum for the Health Professional.*

Médecins du Monde/Medicos del Mundo/Doctors of the World

Médecins du Monde (MDM) is an international non-governmental organization founded in 1980 that has been active in HIV prevention and harm reduction work in marginalized groups such as commercial sex workers and injecting drug users. MDM currently runs ART programs in Cambodia and South Africa, and PMTCT programs in Tanzania, Ethiopia, and Haiti.[15]

Where to get more information

MDM's website contains information on the history of the organization, links to national affiliates, and an overview of its programs (www.mdm-international.org). The site's HIV information page has links to MDM's HIV strategy paper and summaries of the organization's HIV projects. Information is provided in English and French. (www.mdm-international.org/international/pages/sidapremierdecembre.htm).

Family Health International

Family Health International (FHI) has been active in STI prevention since the early 1970s. In 2002, a grant from USAID enabled FHI's ongoing IMPACT project to set up ARV 'learning sites' in Ghana, Rwanda, and Kenya to explore the challenges around introducing ART in resource-poor settings.[16] In 2003, the program started VCT, PMTCT services, clinical care and ART delivery at 17 sites.[17] As of April 2005, 5800 new patients were receiving ART through the programs.[18]

FHI has recently received US$34 million from PEPFAR to lead a 5-year project to help the government of Guyana expand its HIV prevention care and treatment programs.[19] The project, the Guyana HIV Reduction and Prevention Pro-ject (GHARP), provides VCT and other PMTCT services.[20]

Where to get more information

The FHI website (www.fhi.org/en/index.htm) has a wealth of information on the organization's HIV work. It contains:

- policy briefs on the major issues in HIV care, treatment, and prevention (www.fhi.org/en/HIVAIDS/pub/fact/index.htm)
- overviews of FHI's country programs (www.fhi.org/en/HIVAIDS/country/index.htm)
- a large library of FHI publications, curricula, manuals and program tools for free download (www.fhi.org/en/HIVAIDS/pub/index.htm).

Country-specific resources can be found by scrolling through the site's country pages (www.fhi.org/en/HIVAIDS/country/index.htm).

PharmAccess International

PharmAccess International is a non-profit organization based in the Netherlands that provides support services to help in the scale-up of HIV care and treatment in resource-poor countries. Examples of the services they provide include the following:

- Clinical expertise and assistance with clinical guideline development
- Site assessments and the creation of site accreditation criteria and standards
- Training of healthcare providers
- Creation of data management systems
- Project management assistance and help-desk support
- Procurement and distribution of ARV medications and reagents.

Currently, PharmAccess International is involved in treatment projects in 30 sub-Saharan African countries as well as projects in Russia, Suriname, Honduras, and Vietnam.

Where to get more information

The PharmAccess website contains information on the program's services, projects and partners (www.pharmaccess.org).

Harvard University

Harvard University (Cambridge, MA, USA) is involved in a variety of HIV treatment research and intervention projects around the world. Of note is: The Harvard School of Public Health's 'Botswana-HAI Partnership for HIV Research and Education' program (www.aids.harvard.edu), which has created a treatment research laboratory and training center in Botswana and has supported the KITSO AIDS Training Program (www.aids.harvard.edu/kitso/

index.html). Information on Harvard's programs can be found on the Harvard School of Public Health's AIDS Initiative website (www.aids.harvard.edu).

The Harvard School of Public Health recently received a 5-year US$107 million grant from PEPFAR for its 'AIDS Treatment Care and Prevention Initiative', which will be used for the rapid expansion of ART programs in Nigeria, Botswana, and Tanzania. The project plans to treat 8000 people in Nigeria, 4000 in Botswana, and 3000 in Tanzania in its first year. Over the course of the 5-year grant, 75 000 will be treated.[21]

Religious Non-governmental Organizations

According to the Catholic Medical Missions Board, religious healthcare organizations provide up to half of the health services available in most resource-poor countries.[22] For example, in Kenya, mission hospitals provide 40% of hospital beds and have been at the forefront of HIV treatment provision. By the end of 2002, 34 of the 57 mission hospitals in the country were providing ART.[23] Religious organizations are some of the world's largest NGOs and have extensive networks of health facilities that reach areas that are often unserved or underserved by government facilities and other NGOs. Religious organizations have the additional strength of trusting, longstanding relationships with their communities. Through hundreds of hospices, mission hospitals, and home-based care programs, these organizations have been heavily involved in providing palliative care and psychosocial support for people living with HIV in remote rural areas. They also run many of the programs that care for children orphaned by HIV. Their involvement in HIV treatment is more recent but is expected to expand dramatically as donors seek to build upon these organizations' healthcare networks, in order to scale-up treatment services.

Catholic Relief Services

Catholic Relief Services (CRS) has been supporting palliative care and home-based care projects in resource-poor countries for several years. In 2004, the organization received US$335 million over 5 years from PEPFAR to lead the 'AIDSRelief Consortium', which will provide ART in nine countries: South Africa, Zambia, Nigeria, Kenya, Rwanda, Uganda, Tanzania, Haiti, and Guyana.[24] The other members of the consortium are the University of Maryland Institute of Human Virology, the Catholic

Medical Mission Board, New York Interchurch Medical Assistance, and the Maryland Futures Group. The consortium plans to care for 14 900 patients in the first year and 137 600 by year 5 of the project.[24]

Where to get more information

The CRS website has background information on CRS's HIV work and press releases on the AIDSRelief project (www.catholicrelief.org).

Catholic Medical Missions Board

The Catholic Medical Missions Board (CMMB) supports the work of religious healthcare organizations by donating medicines, providing training and supplying program volunteers.

The main HIV activity of CMMB is the 'Born to Live' program, which provides PMTCT services at 42 religious health facilities in South Africa, Kenya, Zambia, Swaziland, Nigeria, Haiti, and Papua New Guinea. In 2004, CMMB started a national scale-up of PMTCT programs at 60 religious health facilities in Kenya with the Kenyan Catholic Bishops Conference and the Christian Health Association of Kenya.[25]

Where to get more information

The CMMB website has background information on CMMB's projects, including its HIV work (www.cmmb.org).

Mildmay

Mildmay is a non-denominational Christian organization based in London. In 1998, it created a center of excellence for HIV care in Kampala, Uganda that has treated approximately 6000 patients since its inception. The center provides comprehensive care and support for HIV-infected patients, including ART. It also serves as a regional training center on HIV care and treatment. The clinic is one of the few in the country that provides treatment for children. The organization has opened a second pediatric clinic in Zimbabwe and has recently received a US$1.7 million grant from PEPFAR to expand ARV treatment in Uganda.[19]

Where to get more information

The Mildmay website has general information about the organization's work in Uganda and the UK and detailed information on the training courses offered by the program (www.mildmay.org.uk).

Local Non-governmental Organizations

In addition to the international organizations discussed above, many local organizations provide HIV care and treatment. HIV care and treatment projects often involve partnerships between the local and international organizations.

Sub-Saharan Africa

- **The Lighthouse** is a Malawian organization that started as a home-based care program in 1997 and added VCT and clinical services in 2000. It now provides ART to about 750 patients[26]
- **Reach Out Mbuya** is a community-based organization that provides ART testing and counseling, and food assistance to needy families in the slums of Kampala, Uganda. As of October 2005, the project was providing ART to about 800 clients (www.reachoutmbuya.org)[27]
- **The AIDS Support Organization (TASO)** has clinics throughout Uganda that provide testing and basic medical care. The organization has recently received a US$3.7 million grant for care, treatment, and prevention activities from PEPFAR[28] (www.tasouganda.org)
- **The Southern African Catholic Bishops Conference (SACBC) AIDS Office** supports HIV care projects throughout South Africa. It recently received funding from Catholic Relief Services through PEPFAR for a community-based ARV treatment program. In this project, health facilities with affiliated home-care projects are staffed with a medical doctor, a professional nurse, and a project coordinator, all of whom are trained in government-accredited ARV management courses. These staff in turn train home-based care workers to be adherence monitors and treatment supporters. After intensive adherence training, patients are started on treatment. Home-based caregivers visit the patients regularly and monitor them for adherence, side-effects and nutrition with further monitoring done at the health facility during the patient's monthly consultation. As of January 2005, the project was operational at seven of the 22 proposed sites, with approximately 300 patients on treatment.[29]

India

- **Aids Research and Control Center (ACORN)** is a technical resource center that works closely with the Government of Maharashtra State, India and the University of Texas, Houston USA. It is one of the three NGOs chosen to administer the ART component of India's 2004 GFATM grant.[30]
- **YRG-CARE:** YRG-CARE is a non-profit organization based in Chennai, India that provides training, education, HIV care and treatment, and research. The organization currently provides care to 5000 HIV-infected people. It is one of implementing organizations in India's 2004 GFATM grant[30] (www.yrgcare.org).

Cambodia

- **The Center of Hope:** The Center of Hope is a treatment clinic at the Sihanouk Hospital in Phnom Penh, Cambodia. It is staffed and managed by HOPE worldwide and also receives major support from Japan Relief for Cambodia. It currently provides HIV care and treatment through the hospital and an outpatient clinic[31] (http://shch.hopeworldwide.org/index.htm).

Table 64.1 Internet sources of information on international HIV treatment

Availability	Sources of information
Antiretroviral treatment guidelines	
US, British, and WHO guidelines are widely available. Country-specific guidelines are difficult to find as many countries are still drafting them and those that have completed the process often do not post them publicly.	**World Health Organization** www.who.int/3by5/en. The site has all of the WHO treatment guidelines for resource-poor countries plus supporting material. **AIDS Info** *Produced by US Department of Health and Human Services (DHHS)* (www.aidsinfo.nih.gov). This US government site has the latest versions of federally approved HIV treatment and prevention guidelines. Slide sets of these guidelines can be found on the AIDS Education and Training Centers National Resource Center website: www.aids-etc.org/aidsetc?page=et-02-00 **HIV InSite** Produced by the University of California San Francisco, Center For HIV Information (http://hivinsite.ucsf.edu/global?page=cr-00-04). HIVInSite hosts a collection of treatment guidelines from around the world. **EurasiaHealth AIDS Knowledge Network Library** Produced by American International Health Alliance (AIHA) and the World Health Organization (www.aidsknowledgehub.org). The Knowledge Hub has a large collection of resources in English and Russian, including the WHO HIV treatment and care protocols for the Commonwealth of Independent States.
Training materials and online training courses	
Currently there are few comprehensive, up-to-date, HIV curricula relevant to resource-poor settings. There are currently no complete online training courses on treatment for health workers in resource-poor countries but several are planned.	**International Training and Education Center on HIV (I-TECH)** Produced by the University of California San Francisco, Center For HIV Information (www.go2itech.org). This site hosts the Global HIV Clinical Training Materials Database which contains a comprehensive collection of HIV training curricula and tools. Most of these resources are targeted to resource-poor countries. **aidsmap** Produced by the National AIDSMAP (NAM), UK (www.aidsmap.com/en/docs/ 3F5509B5-BC9C-4C63-9AFD-EDA4EEA3B52E.asp) aidsmap has a comprehensive training course for healthcare workers in resource-poor settings that provides basic training on HIV treatment and care. Users must register to access the course, which contains a written discussion and slides.

Table 64.1 Internet sources of information on international HIV treatment—cont'd

Availability	Sources of information
	AIDS Education and Training Centers National Resource Center Produced by the University of California San Francisco, Center For HIV Information (www.aids-etc.org). This site has a large collection of treatment training material created for healthcare providers in the USA. **Reproductive Health Online (ReproLine®)** Produced by JHPIEGO Corporation (www.reproline.jhu.edu). The JHPIEGO site has a collection of general training material as well as training a self-paced course on reproductive health in HIV-infected clients and a multimedia course on the care of HIV-infected women in resource-poor settings. **Global AIDS Learning and Evaluation Network (GALEN) Curriculum** Produced by International Association of Physicians in AIDS Care (IAPAC) (www.iapac.org/home.asp?pid=62). This curriculum offers a detailed HIV treatment training for physicians in resource-poor countries. As of January 2005, 4 of the 15 modules were available online.
Clinician resources and ARV drug information	
While these resources are widely available online, almost none of them are targeted at clinicians in resource poor countries.	**HIV InSite** Produced by the University of California San Francisco, Center For HIV Information (http://hivinsite.ucsf.edu). This HIV information portal has an extensive collection of up-to-date, practitioner-oriented material on HIV treatment. Of note are the site's Database of Antiretroviral Drug Interactions (http://hivinsite.ucsf.edu/arvdb?page=ar-00-02), ARV Drug Profiles (http://hivinsite.ucsf.edu/InSite?page=ar-drugs), and the *HIV InSite* Knowledge Base, a comprehensive on-line textbook with 120 chapters on HIV prevention, care, treatment and policy. **aidsmap** Produced by the National AIDSMAP (NAM), UK (www.aidsmap.com). The aidsmap website provides excellent analysis of breaking HIV news and research relevant to resource-poor settings. The site also has treatment summaries on a various topics. Of note is the site's 'HIV & AIDS Treatment in Practice' newsletter (www.aidsmap.com/cms1037059.asp) for healthcare workers in resource-poor settings, which provides in-depth discussion of current treatment issues. **Johns Hopkins AIDS Service** Produced by the Johns Hopkins University (www.hopkins-aids.edu). This site has a literature review service, expert question and answer forums (http://hopkins-aids.edu/ask.html), and the Point of Care Technology Center (POC-IT) guide, which has detailed drug profiles as well as tools for diagnosing illnesses, managing therapy, and monitoring resistance (http://hopkins-hivguide.org). Users must register to access the POC-IT content. **Women, Children, and HIV** Produced by the University of California San Francisco, Center For HIV Information (www.womenchildrenhiv.org). This site has a comprehensive library of up-to-date resources on preventing and treating HIV infection in women and children in resource-poor settings, including material on VCT, PMTCT, infant feeding, clinical care of women and children living with HIV infection, and the support of orphans. The site also hosts a self-paced, electronic PMTCT training course and a library of clinical HIV images.

Table 64.1 Internet sources of information on international HIV treatment—cont'd

Availability	Sources of information

Journal articles and conference coverage

Full text journal articles are difficult to access for health officials in resource poor countries. Abstracts are widely available.

PubMed/Medline
Produced by the National Library of Medicine (www.ncbi.nlm.nih.gov/entrez/query.fcgi).
This bibliographic database provides access to journal abstracts (when available) for HIV related articles written since 1980. About 1000 new HIV citations are added each month.

International AIDS Society
(www.iasociety.org).
The site has a searchable database of abstracts from various IAS Conferences including IAS2001 (Buenos Aires), AIDS 2002 (Barcelona), IAS2003 (Paris), and AIDS 2004 (Bangkok).

aidsmap
Produced by the National AIDSMAP (NAM), UK (www.aidsmap.com).
The aidsmap website provides regular review of research findings and conference presentations relevant to resource-poor countries.

PLoS Medicine
Produced by the Public Library of Science (www.plos.org).
PLoS Medicine is a peer-reviewed open access journal that covers medical advances in all disciplines. Full text articles are available free of charge.

The Lancet
(www.thelancet.com).
The journal allows free access to full text versions for most of its articles on HIV in resource-poor settings. Users must register to gain access to articles.

The British Medical Journal
(http://bmj.bmjjournals.com).
Full text versions of most BMJ articles are available free of charge on the journal's website.

Medscape
Produced by the WebMD Corporation (www.medscape.com).
This site has conference coverage, CME activities, overviews of clinical issues, and commentary on new research. Users must register to access content.

Clinical trials

Information on clinical trials is widely available. A comprehensive list of links to trial information can be found at http://hivinsite.ucsf.edu/InSite?page=li-04-24

Agence nationale de recherches sur le sida (ANRS)
(http://www.anrs.fr).
The French government site provides information on the ANRS's activities, as well as information on obtaining financing for research, and updates on ANRS-sponsored conferences and publications.

AIDS Info
Produced by U.S. Department of Health and Human Services (DHHS) (http://aidsinfo.nih.gov/clinical_trials).
This site has a searchable database of HIV clinical trials funded by the US government. The database contains provides detailed summaries on the various studies.

HIV Prevention Trials Network
(www.hptn.org).
The site provides information on the US National Institutes of Health-sponsored network's studies as well as detailed information on the network's structure, operational tools, policies and guidelines, and information on events. See also the Adult AIDS Clinical Trials Group – AACTG (http://aactg.s-3.com) and the Pediatric AIDS Clinical Trials Group – PACTG (http://pactg.s-3.com) and the HIV Vaccine Trials Network – HVTN (www.hvtn.org) websites.

Table 64.1 Internet sources of information on international HIV treatment—cont'd

Availability	Sources of information
Country-specific in formation	
There is very good coverage of breaking HIV news about different countries. HIV statistics are also widely posted. However country-specific clinical, training and program management material can be difficult to find, particularly for resource-poor countries.	**UNAIDS** (www.unaids.org/en). UNAIDS has epidemiological information for every country in the world as well as country-specific UNAIDS reports, profiles and case studies. **HIV InSite's Countries and Regions** Produced by the University of California San Francisco, Center For HIV Information (http://hivinsite.ucsf. edu/InSite?page=Country). HIV InSite has individual resource pages for every country in the world. These pages contain HIV and health profiles, HIV statistics, policy documents, training material, links to local organizations and when available clinical guidelines. **IRIN Plus News** Produced by UN Office for the Coordination of Humanitarian Affairs (www.plusnews.org). This site has daily news stories on HIV in Africa, country profiles, job postings, and a 'treatment map' that tracks access to ART on the continent (www.plusnews.org/aids/treatment.asp). The site event updates, has information in French and English. IRIN also covers HIV stories for Asia (www.irinnews.org/ME.asp?SelectTheme=HIV_AIDS), and the Middle East (www.irinnews.org/ME.asp?SelectTheme=HIV_AIDS). There are also several regional HIV portals worth noting including: *Solidarity and Action Against The HIV Infection in India (SAATHII)* (www.saathii.org). This site provides information on advocacy, networking, research, capacity building, care, support, and treatment services in India. **YouandAIDS** Produced by the South Asia Intercountry Programme office of UNAIDS (www.youandaids.org). This site includes basic information on HIV, country information, topical resources, reference materials, and links to service organizations. **Regional Knowledge Hub for the Care and Treatment of HIV/AIDS in Eurasia** (www.aidsknowledgehub.org). This site offers online training modules, treatment protocols, networking tools, and additional relevant HIV-related treatment and care materials in English, Russian, and other regional languages. **Southern African AIDS Information Dissemination Service (SAfAIDS)** (www.safaids.org.zw). The SAfAIDS site provides documents produced by the organization, discussion forums, and links to news stories and other sources of information.
Project management tools	
HIV project management material, particularly monitoring and evaluation tools, are widely available.	**Antiretroviral Treatment Toolkit** Produced by the World HealthOrganization (www.who.int/hiv/toolkit/arv/en/index.jsp). This toolkit contains technical guidance on planning and implementing ARV treatment programs. **HIV NGO/CBO Support Toolkit** Produced by the International HIV Alliance (www.aidsalliance.org/ngosupport). This is an electronic library of resources on working with community-based organizations in initiating, implementing, and monitoring HIV/AIDS programs in resource-poor settings. The toolkit is also available in Portuguese.

Table 64.1 Internet sources of information on international HIV treatment—cont'd

Availability	Sources of information
	Synergy APDIME Toolkit Produced by Social & Scientific Systems, Inc. and the University of Washington (www.synergyaids.com/apdime/index.htm). This toolkit is a collection of resources for people managing HIV care and support programs in resource poor settings. It has training guides, worksheets, budget templates, survey instruments, and other tools. **The DELIVER Project** Produced by John Snow International (www.deliver.jsi.com). The site has an excellent collection of tools on commodity logistics and procurement. **GFATM Price Reporting Mechanism** Produced by the Global Fund to Fight AIDS, Tuberculosis and Malaria (www.theglobalfund.org/en/funds_raised/price_reporting/default.asp). The GFATM database lists the prices paid by Global Fund Principal Recipients for ARVs, anti-TB drugs, antimalarial drugs, and bed nets. **Management Sciences for Health** (http://www.msh.org). This site contains links to procurement and management tools created by the organization as well as links to its publications. The site also has a link to MSH's Manager's Electronic Resource Center (http://erc.msh.org/), which contains practical health management information and tools and The Health Manager's Toolkit (http://erc.msh.org/mainpage.cfm?file=1.0.htm&module=toolkit&language=English), which contains practical management tools.
Patient education material	
While there are many excellent HIV patient fact sheets available online, few are targeted at people living with HIV in resource-poor countries. A comprehensive listing of fact sheets can be found at: http://hivinsite.ucsf.edu/InSite?page=li-04-22	**New Mexico AIDS InfoNet** Produced by New Mexico AIDS Education and Training Center (www.aidsinfonet.org). The site contains 80 fact sheets on care and treatment topics. They are written in simple language and reviewed by a medical doctor. The material is not targeted to patients in resource-poor countries. The fact sheets are also available in Spanish. **aidsmap** Produced by the National AIDSMAP (NAM), UK (www.aidsmap.com/en/docs/E0248BED-DA7B-4AFE-832D-505DC58185EC.asp).aidsmap has a collection of patient fact sheets and booklets on a wide array of HIV treatment topics. These are targeted at a British audience.

References

1. Tassie JM, Szumilin E, Calmy A, et al. for Médecins Sans Frontières. Highly active antiretroviral therapy in resource-poor settings: the experience of Médecins Sans Frontières. AIDS 2003; 17:1995–1997.
2. Mukherjee J, Colas M, Farmer P, et al. Access to antiretroviral treatment and care: The experience of the HIV equity initiative, Cange, Haiti – Case Study Switzerland: WHO September 2003. Online. Available: www.who.int/hiv/pub/prev_care/en/Haiti_E.pdf (accessed 7 February 2007).
3. World Health Organization. Progress on global access to HIV antiretroviral therapy: An update on '3 by 5'. Geneva, Switzerland: WHO, June 2005. Online. Available: www.who.int/hiv/pub/progressreports/3by5%20Progress%20Report_E_light.pdf (accessed 7 February 2007).
4. Médecins Sans Frontières. MSF and HIV/AIDS Treatment December 2005 update. December 2005. Online. Available: www.accessmed-msf.org/documents/MSF%20and%20AIDS%20data%20sheet%20Dec%202005%20w%20logo.doc (accessed 7 February 2007).
5. Médecins Sans Frontières, MSF AIDS treatment experience: rapid expansion, emerging challenges. Médecins Sans Frontières' Campaign for Access to Essential Medicines. July 2004. Online. Available: http://aids2004.msf.org.hk/en/bkkbriefing.pdf (accessed 7 February 2007).
6. Médecins Sans Frontières South Africa, the Department of Public Health at the University of Cape Town, and the Provincial Administration of the Western Cape, South Africa; Antiretroviral Therapy in Primary Health Care: Experience of the Khayelitsha Programme in South Africa – Case Study Switzerland: WHO September 2003. Online. Available: www.who.int/hiv/pub/prev_care/en/South_Africa_E.pdf (accessed 7 February 2007).

7. Médecins Sans Frontières, Malawi. Antiretroviral therapy in primary health care: experience of the Chiradzulu Programme in Malawi – Case Study, Médecins Sans Frontières; July 2004: 3. Online. Available: www.synergyaids.com/documents/ARV_ChiradzuluCaseStudy.pdf (accessed 7 February 2007).

8. d'Adesky A-C, HIV Meds come to rural Haiti, American Foundation for AIDS Research. September 2001. Online. Available: www.aegis.com/pubs/amfar/2001/AM010902.html (accessed 7 February 2007).

9. Partners in Health. Partners in Health 2004 Annual Report. 2005. Online. Available: www.pih.org/inforesources/annual/PIH2004-annualreport.pdf (accessed 7 February 2007).

10. French Red Cross. An effective Network. Online. Available: www.croix-rouge.fr/goto/actions/sida/reseau.asp (accessed 7 February 2007).

11. The MTCT-Plus Initiative. MTCT-Plus 2005 Group Meeting Report: 13–15 March 2005 Maputo, Mozambique. Online. Available: www.mtctplus.org/pdf/Maputo%202005/meeting%20report%20FINAL.pdf (accessed 7 February 2007).

12. Abrams EJ, Rabkin M, El-Sadr WM, et al. Successful enrollment of infants and children with HIV in the MTCT-Plus Initiative. XV International AIDS Conference, 2004. Poster presentation. Abstract no. TuPeB4439. Online. Available: www.mtctplus.org/pdf/Pediatric_Enrollment.pdf (accessed 7 February 2007).

13. MTCT-Plus, MCAP Welcome. Online. Available: www.columbia-mcap.org (accessed 7 February 2007).

14. Kline M. Antiretroviral treatment for children in resource-limited settings. Presentation given International HIV/AIDS Alliance Workshop, 'Scaling up ARV treatment in resource limited settings: Perspectives on policy and practice', Cape Town, South Africa. 10–15 May, 2004. Online. Available: http://synkronweb.aidsalliance.org/graphics/secretariat/documents/news/Workshop/SA_Workshop_ART_for_children.pdf (accessed 7 February 2007).

15. Medecins du Monde. Médecins du Monde – International, Fighting AIDS. Online. Available: www.mdm-international.org/international/pages/sidapresentationan.htm (accessed 7 February 2007).

16. FHI, USAID. The treatment and care initiative Fact Sheet. April 2003. Online. Available: www.fhi.org/NR/rdonlyres/eawe74y4rkesryi3dvuxj4dmesar2kogynqlqiazdc7rmy2ozguywjl247jmehqulbkct7ayfs2ffm/TCI81903.pdf (accessed 7 January 2005).

17. Dr Mukadi Ya Diul. Scaling up ART and patient response to treatment. TAC on ART Meeting. Bangkok, Thailand: July 2004. Online. Available: www.fhi.org/NR/rdonlyres/e4g7lr7ua6f2tr4weq4j7zkoecjd4tpgwslvituyvbq6whrmflbuluta3b25vq4276qnv6csyvundm/Mukadi.ppt (accessed 7 February 2007).

18. Family Health International. Delivering antiretroviral therapy in resource-constrained settings: Lessons from Ghana, Kenya and Rwanda. August 2005. Online. Available: http://womenchildrenhiv.org/wchiv?page=cw-10-00 (accessed 7 February 2007).

19. Avert.org. PEPFAR funding for focus countries. Online. Available: www.avert.org/focus.htm (accessed 7 February 2007).

20. Family Health International. GHARP builds capacity in services to prevent mother-to-child HIV transmission. Online. Available: www.fhi.org/en/HIVAIDS/country/Guyana/res_ggharp.htm (accessed 7 February 2007).

21. Harvard School of Public Health. Harvard School of Public Health's AIDS treatment care and prevention initiative in Africa receives $107 million 5 year grant from White House for rapid antiretroviral program expansion. 23 February 2004. Online. Available: www.hsph.harvard.edu/press/releases/press02232004.html (accessed 7 February 2007).

22. Galbraith J, Mathai R. Faith-based leadership in effective HIV/AIDS program delivery: Improving access to treatment through church health institutions and parish networks in Africa, India and the Caribbean. The XVth International AIDS Conference: 2004; Abstract no. MoPeE4292.

23. Attawell K, Mundy J. Provision of antiretroviral therapy in resource-limited settings: a review of experience up to August 2003 DFID, WHO November 2003. Online. Available: www.who.int/3by5/publications/documents/en/ARTpaper_DFID_WHO.pdf (accessed 7 February 2007).

24. US Consortium to Support Antiretroviral Therapy. AIDS Relief Project Delivering Treatment, Restoring Hope, Catholic Relief Services 2004.

25. Mathai R, Foti C, Olouch P, et al. Born to live: Nationwide implementation of prevention of mother-to-child transmission (PMCT) services and ARV access in existing faith-based health networks in Kenya. The XVth International AIDS Conference: 2004; Abstract no. TuOrE1128. Online. Available: www.iasociety.org/abstract/show.asp?abstract_id=2169373 (accessed 7 February 2007).

26. Phiri S, Weigel R, Housseinipour M, et al. The Lighthouse. A centre for comprehensive HIV/AIDS treatment and care in Malawi: Case study. Switzerland: World Health Organization 2003. Online. Available: www.who.int/hiv/pub/prev_care/en/lighthouse.pdf (accessed 7 February 2007).

27. Reach Out Mbuya Parish HIV/AIDS Initiative. Quarterly Report July–September 2005. October 2005. Online. Available: www.reachoutmbuya.org/Reports/Quaterly%20Reports/Quarterly%20Report,%20July-Sept.05.%20Final.doc (accessed 7 February 2007).

28. The President's Emergency Plan for AIDS Relief (PEPFAR). Initial commitments.

29. Southern African Catholic Bishops Conference AIDS Office. Antiretroviral therapy in South African Catholic facilities. 2 July 2004.

30. Global Fund to Fight AIDS, tuberculosis, and malaria. Global fund signs major new AIDS and TB grants for India. Press Release 10 February 2004. Online. Available: www.theglobalfund.org/en/media_center/press/pr_040210.asp (accessed 7 February 2007).

31. Dhaliwal M, Ellman T. Improving access to anti-retroviral treatment in Cambodia. The Khmer HIV/AIDS NGO Alliance, The International HIV/AIDS Alliance, September 2003. Online. Available: www.synergyaids.com/documents/IHAA_ARVCambodia.pdf (accessed 7 February 2007).

CHAPTER 65

Etiology and Management of Diarrhea in HIV-infected Patients and Impact on Antiretroviral Therapy

Oluma Y. Bushen
Richard L. Guerrant

Introduction

Diarrhea is one of the most common symptoms of HIV occurring in up to 60% of patients in developed countries and up to 90% in developing countries at initial presentation. The CDC revised criteria for the diagnosis of AIDS includes HIV wasting syndrome with profound involuntary weight loss of >10% of baseline body weight plus chronic diarrhea (at least two loose stools per day for ≥30 days), cryptosporidiosis or isosporiasis of >1 month's duration or disseminated *Mycobacterium avium* complex as AIDS defining conditions.

Irrespective of the cause, chronic diarrhea increases mortality and morbidity and is an independent negative predictor of survival. The probability of developing diarrhea increases as the CD4 count declines and with counts <50 cells/mm^3 the probability of developing diarrhea increases from 49% to 96%.[1] Antiretroviral therapy significantly improves the outcome and survival in patients with chronic HIV-associated diarrhea. Patients receiving antiretroviral therapy have a significantly higher rate of successful therapeutic response for identified pathogens and treatment is associated with a significant decrease in stool frequency, increase in weight, a decrease in recurrence of diarrhea, and a longer mean survival.[2]

Among patients with diarrhea, an etiology is identified in approximately 50% of cases (Fig. 65.1). Acute diarrhea may be caused by bacteria including *Campylobacter jejuni, Clostridium difficile, Salmonella, Shigella* or enteric viruses including adenovirus, astrovirus, picornavirus and caliciviruses.[3] Patients with CD4 count <200 cells/mm^3 are more likely to experience persistent or chronic diarrhea with *Cryptosporidium, Cyclospora, Isospora, Microsporidia,* CMV and MAC playing prominent roles. *Giardia* and *Entamoeba histolytica* may cause persistent or bloody diarrhea but are less clearly associated with low CD4 counts.

Before Trimethoprim-Sulfamethoxazole (TMP-SMX) prophylaxis, HIV infection was associated with a 4-fold increased rate of diarrhea in children under 5 years old and a 7-fold increase in adults. Diarrhea being more common among individuals with low CD4-cell counts, TMP-SMX prophylaxis is associated with a significantly reduced rate of diarrhea. In one study in Uganda, TMP-SMX prophylaxis was associated with a 46% reduction in mortality, and lower rates of malaria, diarrhea and hospital admission.[4] Of 109 bacterial isolates from HIV-positive individuals before the introduction of TMP-SMX prophylaxis, 83 (76%) were resistant to TMP-SMX. The proportion of resistant pathogens differed among organisms: *Salmonella* spp 43%, *Campylobacter* spp 93%, *Shigella* spp 100%, enterotoxigenic *Escherichia coli* 84%, enteropathogenic *E. coli* 56%, and *Aeromonas* spp 64%. Of 135 bacterial isolates from stool specimens provided by HIV-positive individuals after the introduction of TMP-SMX prophylaxis, 112 (83%) were resistant to this drug combination.[4]

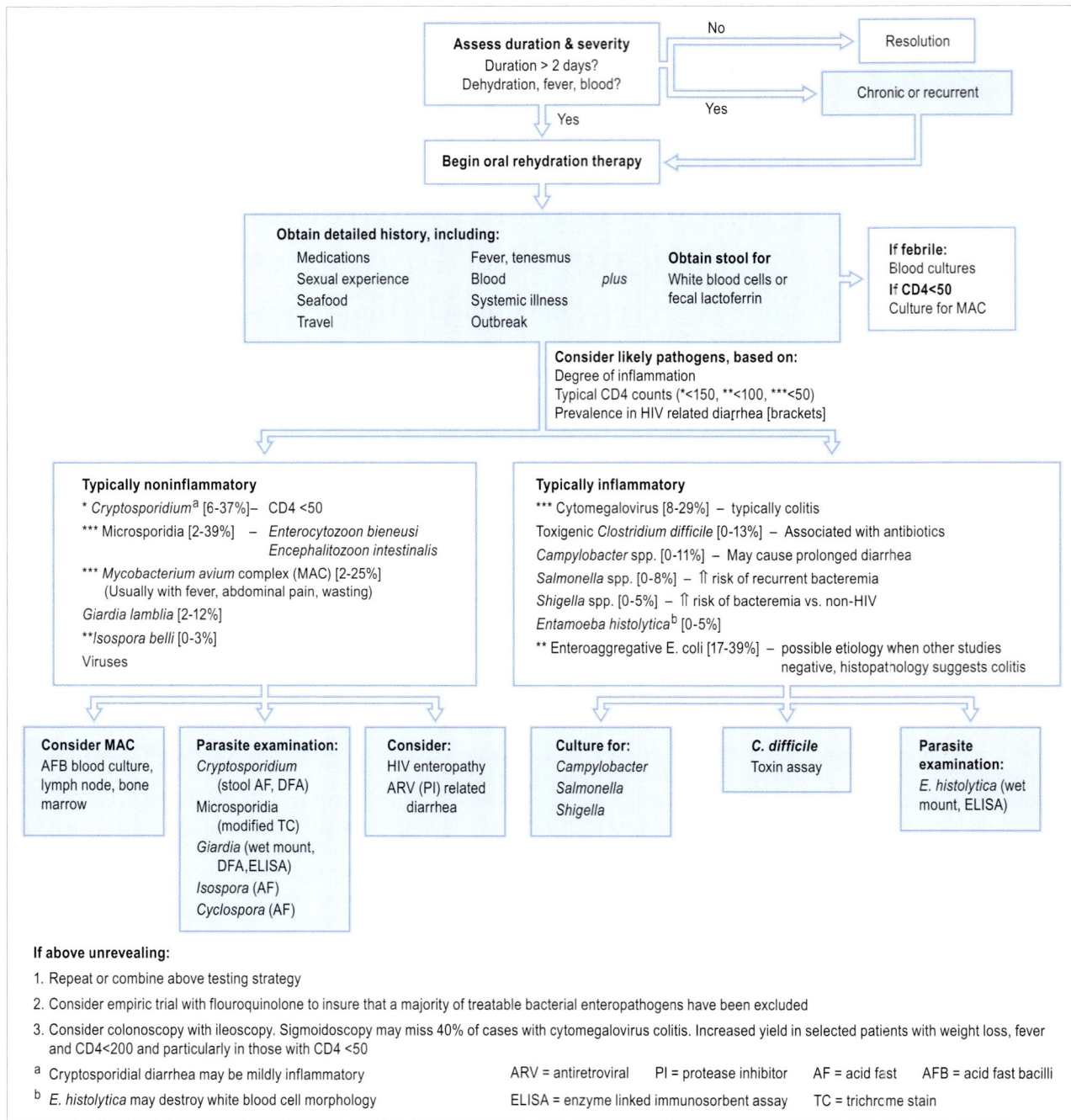

Figure 65.1 Initial approach to the diagnosis and treatment of HIV-related diarrhea.

Pathogens Associated with HIV/AIDS-related Diarrhea

Bacteria

Bacterial diarrhea may occur at any CD4 count but tend to cause recurrent attacks of enteritis and or bacteremia. Distinct from HIV-negative patients who have self-limiting enteritis, HIV-positive patients may have a severe, debilitating illness requiring prolonged and multiple courses of antimicrobial therapy.

Salmonella

Salmonellosis is estimated to be nearly 20 times more common and 5 times more often bacteremic in AIDS patients than in patients without AIDS[5] and is often life-threatening and relapsing.[6–8] In a San Francisco study, Celum and co-workers[5] found the average annual incidence of salmonellosis in men 15–60 years old with AIDS was 384 per 100 000, whereas the average annual incidence for men the same age without AIDS was only 20 per 100 000. Salmonella bacteremia was also more common in persons with AIDS (45%) than HIV-negative patients with salmonellosis (9%). Treatment is with ciprofloxacin 500 mg p.o. b.i.d. or, if the organism is susceptible, TMP-SMX (160/800 mg) b.i.d. Treatment is for 14 days unless the CD4 count is <200 or if bacteremia is present, then this should be extended to 4–6 weeks and several months if there is recurrence. The reduction in Salmonella infections after the initiation of antiretroviral therapy may be due in part to the anti-Salmonella effects of zidovudine.[9,10]

Shigella

Shigella gastroenteritis may occur among HIV-seropositive patients and may be complicated in some patients by bacteremia, though it is uncommon. While recurrent Salmonella bacteremia is common among HIV-seropositive patients, recurrent Shigella bacteremia is not. Treatment is with ciprofloxacin (500 mg b.i.d.) or, if susceptible, TMP-SMX (160/800 mg) b.i.d. for 7–10 days. Nalidixic acid, 55 mg/kg per day (pediatric) or 1 g/day (adults), ceftriaxone or azithromycin could also be used.

Campylobacter

Like Salmonella, there is an increased incidence of Campylobacter infection severity and long-term car-riage in patients with AIDS. In addition to enteritis, it can cause bacteremia which can be difficult to cure.[11,12] Treatment is with Erythromycin 500 mg p.o. b.i.d. for 5 days, but may require prolonged therapy. Long-term administration of erythromycin therapy may lead to in vivo development of resistance to this antibiotic. Ciprofloxacin may also be used but resistance develops rapidly.

Enteroaggregative E. coli

Enteroaggregative E. coli (EAggEc) cause persistent diarrhea in HIV patients and tends to occur in those with low CD4 counts. HIV-positive patients with diarrhea and EAggEc in their stool tended to lose more weight than those who were HIV-positive and had diarrhea but whose stool was negative for EAggEc.[13] Furthermore, eradication of EAggEc in these patients led to resolution of symptoms in 79%.[14] Treatment is with a fluoroquinolone like ciprofloxacin 500 mg twice daily for 7 days, or if susceptible, with TMP-SMZ (160/800 mg) twice daily, for 7 days.

Clostridium difficile

Clostridium difficile associated diarrhea is important to remember, especially because patients are often on multiple antimicrobial agents and may occur at any CD4 count. Clinical manifestations and therapeutic responses are similar in HIV-infected and non-infected individuals.[15]

Mycobacteria

Mycobacterium avium-intracellulare

MAC is ubiquitous in the environment, and disseminated infection results from recent infection rather than reactivation of previous infection. The gastrointestinal tract is an important portal of entry from which the organism may disseminate, especially to the blood, bone marrow, liver, and lymph nodes. The major risk factor for MAC infection is the severity of the immunologic deficit commonly occurring in patients with CD4 cell counts of <50/mm^3. The most common findings at diagnosis are fever, anemia, night sweats, diarrhea, and ≥10% weight loss and may account for 10–20% of chronic diarrhea in AIDS patients. Endoscopic biopsy specimens showed duodenal involvement in 88% with some having characteristic white nodules observed in some patients. Involvement of the rectum, esophagus and liver were also noted. Gastrointestinal tract involvement was associated with dissemination; in one study,

89% had bone marrow infection and 85% had bacteremia.[16]

Although the gastrointestinal tract is a major portal of entry, gut colonization is uncommon, and routine screening of stool specimens with acid-fast stains and mycobacterial cultures is not an effective method for detecting MAC. Disseminated MAC infection is most readily diagnosed by mycobacterial culture of normally sterile sites like blood, lymph node or bone marrow. For patients undergoing gastrointestinal endoscopy, MAC infection can be detected in mucosal biopsy specimens examined under light microscopy using H&E and Ziehl-Neelsen staining.

MAC prophylaxis should be initiated when CD4 count is <50/mm[3]. Treatment is with clarithromycin (500 mg b.i.d.) and ethambutol (15 mg/kg per day) and one or more of the following can be added as a third or fourth drug: rifabutin, rifampin, clofazimine, ciprofloxacin, and, in some situations, amikacin. Providing concurrent antiretroviral therapy is important in the resolution of the disease.

Viruses

Various enteric viruses may cause acute or chronic diarrhea in 15–30% of AIDS patients and may occur at any CD4 count. Specimens from patients with diarrhea were more likely to have astrovirus; picobirnavirus; caliciviruses, including small round structured viruses; and adenoviruses. Patients with diarrhea due to viruses are more likely to have a mixed viral infection.[3] Most of these viruses are hard to detect by routine laboratory methods and treatment is supportive.

CMV

Gastrointestinal involvement in disseminated CMV infection accounts for 20% of diarrhea in patients with AIDS and a CD4 count <50/mm[3]. The esophagus and colon are the most commonly identified affected parts of the GI tract. Prolonged fever and chronic diarrhea are the most common clinical presentation and the clinical spectrum varies from chronic diarrhea and abdominal pain to GI bleeding complicated by bowel obstruction, perforation, and even death. Serologic tests show low sensitivity in diagnosing CMV infection, hence the diagnosis is established by endoscopy and tissue diagnosis. The most frequent colonoscopic findings include colitis and multiple mucosal ulcers and biopsy demonstrating typical intranuclear and intracytoplasmic eosin-

ophilic inclusions. Treatment is with valganciclovir, ganciclovir or foscarnet for 3–6 weeks. Despite resolution of the symptoms, relapses usually occur and maintenance therapy and initiation of antiretroviral therapy may be considered to improve the clinical outcome.

Adenovirus

Adenoviruses are ubiquitous double-stranded DNA viruses that are best known as agents that cause respiratory tract infections in children. Several serotypes, notably types 40 and 41, have been recognized to cause diarrhea in children. Adenoviruses infect intestinal epithelial cells and elicit a marked mucosal immune response in patients with normal immunity and in patients with impaired immunity, the infection is commonly systemic. Infection can be recognized morphologically by the presence of large amphophilic-to-basophilic nuclear inclusions, with infected cells being termed *smudge cells*. Because the morphologic features of adenovirus-infected cells are not as easy to recognize as those produced by the HSV or CMV, it is likely that infection with this virus is underdiagnosed.

Protozoa

Cryptosporidium

Cryptosporidia are coccidian parasites that are 3–5 μm that are highly infectious. Patients with AIDS are prone to developing debilitating disease and can be fulminant and fatal. In a Nevada outbreak, 61 of the 2270 known HIV-infected patients in the area developed diarrhea, and 32 of these died within 6 months; this is similar to the high mortality in the Milwaukee outbreak, in which 48 of 82 infected patients with AIDS died within 1 year, with excess mortality largely attributable to the cryptosporidial illnesses.[17,18]

Cryptosporidiosis often causes chronic intermittent diarrhea, with recurring 3–30-day episodes lasting up to 14 months. Those with low CD4 lymphocyte counts are prone to develop protracted, fulminant and rapidly fatal diarrhea. In one series, cryptosporidial infection was asymptomatic in 4%, transient in 29%, chronic in 60%, or fulminant (>2 L of stool per day) in 8%. Mean survival in these patients with *Cryptosporidium* and HIV co-infection was 25 weeks in the study by Blanshard and co-workers[19] Patients who develop fulminant disease usually have <50 CD4 cells/mm[3] and sharply limited survival of only 5 weeks. Spontaneous clinical remission is associated with higher lymphocyte[20] or CD4 count.[21] Our experience in Tanzania suggests that asymptomatic cryptosporidiosis may be more common than previously reported.[22]

Extraintestinal disease due to *Cryptosporidium* has been seen in immunocompromised patients, especially those in the late stages of AIDS (CD4 <50/mm³). By far the most common site is the biliary tree, manifestations of which include sclerosing cholangitis and acalculous cholecystitis. Direct luminal spread of organisms from the duodenum is believed to be responsible. The hallmark symptom is right upper quadrant pain, which can resemble that of chronic or acute calculous cholecystitis. Patients with AIDS, especially those with CD4 counts <100/mm³, should be advised of the potentially devastating impact of cryptosporidiosis. Filters that provide the greatest assurance of oocyst removal include those that operate by reverse osmosis, those labeled as absolute 1-μm filters, and those labeled as meeting National Sanitation Foundation (NSF) standard No. 53 for cyst removal. Some patients may decide that the inconvenience of boiling or filtering (through 'absolute' 1-μm filters) all of their drinking water is worth the benefit of protecting themselves from this disease. These patients should also be advised to avoid young farm animals, especially those with diarrhea. Initiation of HAART and immune reconstitution is important in the treatment of cryptosporidiosis. Nitazoxanide is approved for use in treating *Cryptosporidium* infection in children aged <11 years. In one study, patients with documented cryptosporidial diarrhea, nitazoxanide demonstrated resolution of diarrhea and symptoms in 80% compared with 41% of the placebo group. Among 25 malnourished HIV-negative children with cryptosporidiosis, a 3-day course of therapy led, not only to clinical and parasitological improvement, but also to improved survival. Diarrhea resolved in 14 (56%) of 25 HIV-seronegative children receiving nitazoxanide, compared with five (23%) of 22 receiving placebo, and *C. parvum* was eradicated from stool by day 10 after initiation of treatment in 52% of patients receiving nitazoxanide versus only 14% of patients receiving placebo.[23] HIV-seropositive children with cryptosporidiosis, a 3-day course of nitazoxanide did not show significant efficacy in clinical or parasitological response.[24] It is suggested that a higher dose or extended duration of treatment may be required to achieve a sustained clinical and parasitological response in the immunocompromised population. Among many drugs tested, azithromycin and paromomycin have been used with relative success.

Microsporidium

Microsporidia are intracellular spore forming protozoa that include *Enterocytozoon bieneusi*, and less commonly *Encephalitozoon* (Septata) *intestinalis*, which also causes systemic infection involving the hepato-biliary tract, respiratory tract, sinuses, kidney, eye, and brain. The majority of symptomatic infections in humans occur in patients with HIV infection who are significantly immunocompromised (CD4 <100 cells/mm³). The prevalence of infections rises with increased levels of immunosuppression ranging from 7% to 50% making microsporidiosis one of the most common enteropathogens in patients with HIV infection. Microsporidia are difficult to see by light microscopy because of their small size. Their reservoir in the environment is not known. Spores shed in the feces are resistant, but when ingested, pass to the small intestine, where they attach to epithelial cells and inject a sporoplasm into the host cell where the parasite proliferates. *E. bieneusi* Type I (genotype A and B) cause most infections in HIV patients.[25] Treatment is with albendazole 400 mg orally twice daily for 4–6 weeks.[26] It is effective against most microsporidia but only partially effective against *E. bieneusi*. Other treatments that have shown varied success include nitazoxanide, atovaquone, metronidazole, azithromycin, doxycycline, thalidomide, and fumagillin. Combination antiretroviral therapy can restore immunity to microsporidia and often result in complete clinical, microbiological, and histological responses within 6 weeks.[27]

Cyclospora

The clinical manifestations of cyclosporiasis are indistinguishable from the persistent diarrhea caused by *Cryptosporidium* and are characterized by watery diarrhea associated with non-specific symptoms of cramping abdominal pain, anorexia, malaise, flatulence, nausea, vomiting, and low-grade fever. In addition, right upper quadrant pain in patients with AIDS, suggesting biliary tract involvement, has been reported. The clinical presentation of illness varies according to the immune status of the host. For normal hosts, the onset is usually acute and the disease is generally self-limited, lasting from 7 days to as long as 6 weeks. In HIV-infected patients, the onset is usually insidious and the disease tends to become more chronic and can lead to malabsorption. The treatment of choice is TMP-SMX (160/800 mg) orally twice daily to four times a day for 1 week. This treatment is equally effective in patients with AIDS, although maintenance therapy with a single dose three times a week is often needed to prevent relapses.[28]

Isospora

Isospora can cause prolonged, severe disease in immunocompromised patients. The symptoms can resemble cryptosporidiosis, with watery diarrhea and abdominal pain lasting <1 month but may last up to 6 months, associated with diffuse abdominal cramps and nausea. Disseminated disease can also occur. Isosporiasis can be treated successfully in patients with or without AIDS. The drug of choice is TMP-SMX (160 mg/800 mg) orally four times daily for 7–10 days. This treatment often provides relief within 3 days in patients with AIDS and longstanding diarrhea. Alternative agents include pyrimethamine 75 mg/day, roxithromycin 2.5 mg/kg every 12 h for 15 days and diclazuril. Maintenance therapy with TMP-SMX (160/800 mg) three times a week or Fansidar (pyrimethamine 25 mg/sulfadoxine 500 mg) once a week should be continued indefinitely in patients with AIDS, since relapses are common (50% within 1.6 months of completing the initial treatment). Pyrimethamine alone at 25 mg/day is an alternative for patients who cannot take sulfonamides.[28]

Less common protozoan pathogens and those deemed to be 'nonpathogenic' may occasionally cause diarrhea in immunocompromised patients. *Blastocystis hominis*[29] may cause persistent and/or chronic diarrhea, though this is debated.[30] Symptomatic patients should have other potential pathogens excluded. If no pathogens are found, treatment may be administered. Metronidazole has been used at 1.5 g daily for 5–10 days.[31] Other agents used include TMP-SMX,[32] tinidazole, iodoquinol, nitazoxanide, and furazolidone. Specific treatment may be justified for *Dientamoeba fragilis* if it is the only pathogen found. Treatment is with iodoquinol 650 mg t.i.d. for 20 days, metronidazole 500–750 mg t.i.d. for 10 days. Others drugs that could be used include paromomycin and tetracycline.[33] *Brachyspira aalborgi* and *Brachyspira pilosicoli* are spirochetes that may cause protracted and chronic diarrhea. *Brachyspira pilosicoli* is primarily isolated in developing countries and from homosexual men and HIV-infected individuals. There is no association with the degree of immunodeficiency and symptoms. Treatment is with metronidazole.

Drug-related Diarrhea

Since protease inhibitors became available, chronic diarrhea became identified as one of their main side-effects, although the mechanism of this adverse effect has not been elucidated. The incidence of diarrhea associated with the protease inhibitor saquinavir is 12.3–19.9%; with ritonavir, 12.8–21.6%; with indinavir, 0–4.6%; with nelfinavir, 14–32%, and with amprenavir, 33–56%. The incidence of diarrhea is greatest at the time of initiation of therapy; many patients who initially have problems will become tolerant of this adverse effect within the first several weeks. In a survey of 887 HIV-infected patients, diarrhea was reported by 31.7% of patients and was the second most common treatment-related adverse effect.[34] Patients are likely to attribute diarrhea symptoms directly to their antiretroviral therapy and this may result in 20% of missed doses.[35]

HIV Enteropathy

HIV was initially believed to cause intestinal symptoms since HIV-seropositive individuals free from intestinal pathogens commonly have diarrhea.[36] Most patients have low-volume diarrhea that either resolves spontaneously or is controlled with antimotility agents. HIV-seropositive persons who do not have recognized intestinal pathogens do have minor abnormalities of villus architecture, characteristically a mild villus atrophy associated with either crypt hypoplasia or hyperplasia.[37] These minor abnormalities are unlikely to cause diarrhea, since they occur in HIV-negative individuals and are associated either with no or with very mild malabsorption of carbohydrates.[38] However, there is a consistent increase in small-bowel permeability in HIV-seropositive individuals.[39] Bacterial overgrowth in the small intestine of HIV-seropositive patients, might produce an inflammatory response and villus atrophy.[40] This might occur because of the hypochlorhydria reported in AIDS patients[41] and may also occur in advanced AIDS without any HIV-induced defects in gastric secretion. Neither hypochlorhydria nor bacterial overgrowth is a universal finding in patients with advanced HIV infection, so these mechanisms are unlikely to have an important role in villus atrophy.[42]

HIV and Malabsorption

HIV-related chronic diarrhea is frequently accompanied by weight loss, particularly in those with more severe reductions in CD4 count. Gastrointestinal function in these patients is altered as measured by excretion of lactulose, mannitol and their ratios.

Mannitol crosses the intestinal mucosa transcellularly by passive diffusion both in the crypts and in the villi and thus provides a measure of total absorptive surface area, while lactulose is minimally absorbed in the normal intestine across paracellular tight junctions and its excretion reflects disrupted intestinal barrier function. Using these measurements, HIV positive patients with diarrhea have a lactulose excretion that is 1.5-fold higher than those without diarrhea and 3-fold higher than normal controls showing the increased permeability in these patient groups. Similarly, mannitol excretion was 32% less in HIV patients with diarrhea than those with no diarrhea and 55% less than in healthy controls. In combination, the lactulose:mannitol ratio was 3-fold higher for the HIV patients with diarrhea and 10-fold higher in healthy controls, thus signifying that there is not only disruption of the intestinal barrier function but also reduced intestinal absorptive capacity.[39,43]

Patients with HIV/AIDS may also have significant fat malabsorption[44] and vitamin B_{12} deficiency may be detected in 10–20% of patients.[45] Other deficiencies common in patients with AIDS include vitamin A and E, zinc, β-carotene, and hypoalbuminemia. In one study among HIV-infected children, vitamin A supplementation reduced diarrhea by a significant 49% and reduced diarrhea lasting 7 or more days by 56%.[46]

Drug malabsorption has been noted in patients with HIV/AIDS including antiretrovirals and antimycobacterial agents. Low levels of ARV drugs occurred in patients with diarrhea and wasting in one series and reveal that certain drugs are more prone to malabsorption than others.[47,48]

Despite the advances in highly active antiretroviral therapy, HIV-related wasting syndrome continues unabated given the lack of affordable interventions. The nutritional impact of this syndrome is greatly amplified by common enteric infections responsible for chronic disruption of intestinal barrier and absorptive functions. HIV infection induces glutamine deficiency even in asymptomatic and well-nourished patients, possibly due to the rapid turnover of immune cells and the high catabolism during infection. Oral supplementation with glutamine has shown relevant benefits in altering the course of AIDS-related wasting syndrome. Shabert and colleagues[49] showed that glutamine (40 g/day over 12 weeks), along with antioxidant nutrients (vitamin C and E, β-carotene, selenium, N-acetyl cysteine), increased body weight (3.2% versus 0.4%, $P = 0.04$) and body cell mass (i.e. lean tissue compartment containing metabolically active cell mass) in HIV+ patients with ≥5% weight loss. Based on known increased intestinal permeability documented in HIV patients,[39,43] a pilot study evaluated the effects of low doses of glutamine (4–8 g/day, over 28 days) on intestinal permeability of HIV+ patients without wasting. Although glutamine (8 g/day) showed a trend in increasing mannitol absorption (an indicator of intestinal absorptive surface area), glutamine at these low doses did not significantly improve intestinal permeability measured by lactulose/mannitol ratio.[50] This result raises yet additional unanswered questions regarding the optimal dosing and >20 g/day may be needed. Studies with the more stable alanyl-glutamine or higher doses of glutamine suggest that they may reduce diarrhea and improve antiretroviral drug absorption.[48] Glutamine derivatives in HIV-infected patients has immunoenhancing properties, induces T-lymphocyte proliferation, IL-2 production, and IL-2 receptor expression,[51,52] increase in CD4 and CD8 cells,[53] regulate phagocytic activity[52,54] and cytokine secretion[55] in macrophages, and enhance the antimicrobial activity of neutrophils.[56,57]

Conclusion

Diarrhea and malabsorption is a huge problem in patients with AIDS especially in developing areas where sanitation and safe drinking water are inadequate. Furthermore, it may be associated with malabsorption of badly needed antiretroviral drugs and may even drive antiretroviral drug resistance. All potentially treatable etiologies therefore must be sought and treated and novel approaches to repairing the widespread mucosal injury may prove critical to improved outcomes with the all-important rollout of global AIDS treatment programs.

References

1. Weber R, Ledergerber B, Zbinden R, et al. Enteric infections and diarrhea in human immunodeficiency virus-infected persons: prospective community-based cohort study. Swiss HIV Cohort Study Arch Intern Med 1999; 159:1473–1480.
2. Bini EJ, Cohen J. Impact of protease inhibitors on the outcome of human immunodeficiency virus-infected patients with chronic diarrhea. Am J Gastroenterol 1999; 94:3553–3559.
3. Grohmann GS, Glass RI, Pereira HG, et al. Enteric viruses and diarrhea in HIV-infected patients. Enteric Opportunistic Infections Working Group. N Engl J Med 1993; 329:14–20.
4. Mermin J, Lule J, Ekwaru JP, et al. Effect of co-trimoxazole prophylaxis on morbidity, mortality, CD4-cell count, and viral load in HIV infection in rural Uganda. Lancet 2004; 364:1428–1434.

5. Celum CL, Chaisson RE, Rutherford GW, et al. Incidence of salmonellosis in patients with AIDS. J Infect Dis 1987; 156:998–1002.

6. Jacobs JL, Gold JW, Murray HW, et al. Salmonella infections in patients with the acquired immunodeficiency syndrome. Ann Intern Med 1985; 102:186–188.

7. Fischl MA, Dickinson GM, Sinave C, et al. Salmonella bacteremia as manifestation of acquired immunodeficiency syndrome. Arch Intern Med 1986; 146:113–115.

8. Sperber SJ, Schleupner CJ. Salmonellosis during infection with human immunodeficiency virus. Rev Infect Dis 1987; 9:925–934.

9. Keith BR, White G, Wilson HR. In vivo efficacy of zidovudine (3′-azido-3′-deoxythymidine) in experimental gram-negative-bacterial infections. Antimicrob Agents Chemother 1989; 33:479–483.

10. Casado JL, Valdezate S, Calderon C, et al. Zidovudine therapy protects against Salmonella bacteremia recurrence in human immunodeficiency virus-infected patients. J Infect Dis 1999; 179:1553–1556.

11. Perlman DM, Ampel NM, Schifman RB, et al. Persistent Campylobacter jejuni infections in patients infected with the human immunodeficiency virus (HIV). Ann Intern Med 1988; 108:540–546.

12. Bernard E, Roger PM, Carles D, et al. Diarrhea and Campylobacter infections in patients infected with the human immunodeficiency virus. J Infect Dis 1989; 159:143–144.

13. Wanke CA, Mayer H, Weber R, et al. Enteroaggregative Escherichia coli as a potential cause of diarrheal disease in adults infected with human immunodeficiency virus. J Infect Dis 1998; 178:185–190.

14. Wanke CA, Gerrior J, Blais V, et al. Successful treatment of diarrheal disease associated with enteroaggregative Escherichia coli in adults infected with human immunodeficiency virus. J Infect Dis 1998; 178:1369–1372.

15. Lu SS, Schwartz JM, Simon DM, et al. Clostridium difficile-associated diarrhea in patients with HIV positivity and AIDS: a prospective controlled study. Am J Gastroenterol 1994; 89:1226–1229.

16. Gray JR, Rabeneck L. Atypical mycobacterial infection of the gastrointestinal tract in AIDS patients. Am J Gastroenterol 1989; 84:1521–1524.

17. Goldstein ST, Juranek DD, Ravenholt O, et al. Cryptosporidiosis: an outbreak associated with drinking water despite state-of-the-art water treatment. Ann Intern Med 1996; 124:459–468.

18. Vakil NB, Schwartz SM, Buggy BP, et al. Biliary cryptosporidiosis in HIV-infected people after the waterborne outbreak of cryptosporidiosis in Milwaukee. N Engl J Med 1996; 334:19–23.

19. Blanshard C, Jackson AM, Shanson DC, et al. Cryptosporidiosis in HIV-seropositive patients. Q J Med 1992; 85:813–823.

20. McGowan I, Hawkins AS, Weller IV. The natural history of cryptosporidial diarrhoea in HIV-infected patients. AIDS 1993; 7:349–354.

21. Flanigan T, Whalen C, Turner J, et al. Cryptosporidium infection and CD4 counts. Ann Intern Med 1992; 116:840–842.

22. Houpt E, Bushen O, Sam N, et al. Short Report: Asymptomatic Cryptosporidium hominis infection among HIV-infected patients in Tanzania. Am J Trop Med Hyg 2005; 73:520–522.

23. Rossignol JF, Ayoub A, Ayers MS. Treatment of diarrhea caused by Cryptosporidium parvum: a prospective randomized, double-blind, placebo-controlled study of Nitazoxanide. J Infect Dis 2001; 184:103–106.

24. Amadi B, Mwiya M, Musuku J, et al. Effect of nitazoxanide on morbidity and mortality in Zambian children with cryptosporidiosis: a randomised controlled trial. Lancet 2002; 360:1375–1380.

25. Liguory O, Sarfati C, Derouin F, et al. Evidence of different Enterocytozoon bieneusi genotypes in patients with and without human immunodeficiency virus infection. J Clin Microbiol 2001; 39:2672–2674.

26. Molina JM, Chastang C, Goguel J, et al. Albendazole for treatment and prophylaxis of microsporidiosis due to Encephalitozoon intestinalis in patients with AIDS: a randomized double-blind controlled trial. J Infect Dis 1998; 177:1373–1377.

27. Carr A, Marriott D, Field A, et al. Treatment of HIV-1-associated microsporidiosis and cryptosporidiosis with combination antiretroviral therapy. Lancet 1998; 351:256–261.

28. Guerrant RL, Van Gilder T, Steiner TS et al. Practice guidelines for the management of infectious diarrhea. Clin Infect Dis 2001; 32:331–351.

29. Brites C, Barberino MG, Bastos MA, et al. Blastocystis hominis as a potential cause of diarrhea in AIDS patients: a Report of Six Cases in Bahia, Brazil. Braz J Infect Dis 1997; 1:91–94.

30. Albrecht H, Stellbrink HJ, Koperski K, et al. Blastocystis hominis in human immunodeficiency virus-related diarrhea. Scand J Gastroenterol 1995; 30:909–914.

31. Nigro L, Larocca L, Massarelli L, et al. A placebo-controlled treatment trial of Blastocystis hominis infection with metronidazole. J Travel Med 2003; 10:128–130.

32. Ok UZ, Girginkardesler N, Balcioglu C, et al. Effect of trimethoprim-sulfamethoxazole in Blastocystis hominis infection. Am J Gastroenterol 1999; 94:3245–3247.

33. The Medical Letter. Drugs for parasitic infections. 2004: August.

34. Bertholon DR, Rossert H, Korsia S. The patient's perspective on life with antiretroviral treatment: results of an 887-person survey. AIDS Read 1999; 9:462–469.

35. Sherman DS, Fish DN. Management of protease inhibitor-associated diarrhea. Clin Infect Dis 2000; 30:908–914.

36. Blanshard C, Gazzard BG. Natural history and prognosis of diarrhoea of unknown cause in patients with acquired immunodeficiency syndrome (AIDS). Gut 1995; 36:283–286.

37. Ullrich R, Heise W, Bergs C. et al. Effects of zidovudine treatment on the small intestinal mucosa in patients infected with the human immunodeficiency virus. Gastroenterology 1992; 102:1483–1492.

38. Keating J, Bjarnason I, Somasundaram S, et al. Intestinal absorptive capacity, intestinal permeability and jejunal histology in HIV and their relation to diarrhoea. Gut 1995; 37:623–629.

39. Lima AA, Silva TM, Gifoni AM, et al. Mucosal injury and disruption of intestinal barrier function in HIV-infected individuals with and without diarrhea and cryptosporidiosis in northeast Brazil. Am J Gastroenterol 1997; 92:1861–1866.

40. Budhraja M, Levendoglu H, Kocka F, et al. Duodenal mucosal T cell subpopulation and bacterial cultures in acquired immune deficiency syndrome. Am J Gastroenterol 1987; 82:427–431.

41. Belitsos PC, Greenson JK, Yardley JH, et al. Association of gastric hypoacidity with opportunistic enteric infections in patients with AIDS. J Infect Dis 1992; 166:277–284.

42. Sharpstone D, Gazzard B. Gastrointestinal manifestations of HIV infection. Lancet 1996; 348:379–383.

43. Tepper RE, Simon D, Brandt LJ, et al. Intestinal permeability in patients infected with the human immunodeficiency virus. Am J Gastroenterol 1994; 89:878–882.

44. Cello JP, Grendell JH, Basuk P, et al. Effect of octreotide on refractory AIDS-associated diarrhea. A prospective, multicenter clinical trial. Ann Intern Med 1991; 115:705–710.

45. Ehrenpreis ED, Carlson SJ, Boorstein HL, et al. Malabsorption and deficiency of vitamin B12 in HIV-infected patients with chronic diarrhea. Dig Dis Sci 1994; 39:2159–2162.

46. Coutsoudis A, Bobat RA, Coovadia HM, et al. The effects of vitamin A supplementation on the morbidity of children born to HIV-infected women. Am J Public Health 1995; 85:1076–1081.

47. Brantley RK, Williams KR, Silva TM, et al. AIDS-associated diarrhea and wasting in Northeast Brazil is associated with subtherapeutic plasma levels of antiretroviral medications and with both bovine and human subtypes of Cryptosporidium parvum. Braz J Infect Dis 2003; 7:16–22.

48. Bushen OY, Davenport JA, Lima AB, et al. Diarrhea and reduced levels of antiretroviral drugs: improvement with glutamine or alanyl-glutamine in a randomized controlled trial in northeast Brazil. Clin Infect Dis 2004; 38:1764–1770.

49. Shabert JK, Winslow C, Lacey JM, et al. Glutamine-antioxidant supplementation increases body cell mass in AIDS patients with weight loss: a randomized, double-blind controlled trial. Nutrition 1999; 15:860–864.

50. Noyer CM, Simon D, Borczuk A, et al. A double-blind placebo-controlled pilot study of glutamine therapy for abnormal intestinal permeability in patients with AIDS. Am J Gastroenterol 1998; 93:972–975.

51. Yaqoob P, Calder PC. Glutamine requirement of proliferating T lymphocytes. Nutrition 1997; 13:646–651.

52. Parry-Billings M, Evans J, Calder PC, et al. Does glutamine contribute to immunosuppression after major burns? Lancet 1990; 336:523–525.

53. Clark RH, Feleke G, Din M, et al. Nutritional treatment for acquired immunodeficiency virus-associated wasting using beta-hydroxy beta-methylbutyrate, glutamine, and arginine: a randomized, double-blind, placebo-controlled study. JPEN J Parenter Enteral Nutr 2000; 24:133–139.

54. Wallace C, Keast D. Glutamine and macrophage function. Metabolism 1992; 41:1016–1020.

55. Murphy C, Newsholme P. Macrophage-mediated lysis of a beta-cell line, tumour necrosis factor-alpha release from bacillus Calmette-Guerin (BCG)-activated murine macrophages and interleukin-8 release from human monocytes are dependent on extracellular glutamine concentration and glutamine metabolism. Clin Sci (Lond) 1999; 96:89–97.

56. Furukawa S, Saito H, Inoue T, et al. Supplemental glutamine augments phagocytosis and reactive oxygen intermediate production by neutrophils and monocytes from postoperative patients in vitro. Nutrition 2000; 16:323–329.

57. Saito H, Furukawa S, Matsuda T. Glutamine as an immunoenhancing nutrient. JPEN J Parenter Enteral Nutr 1999; 23:S59–S61.

CHAPTER 66

Malaria and HIV Infection

Feiko O. ter Kuile
James A. G. Whitworth

Introduction

Malaria and HIV are each responsible for a high public health burden in the tropics, particularly in sub-Saharan Africa, where an estimated 25 million individuals are infected with HIV (>60% of the infected population globally), and where malaria causes more than 300 million acute illnesses and approximately 1 million deaths annually (80–90% of the global burden) Our current understanding of the immunology of HIV and malaria suggests the potential for interaction in both directions exacerbating the effects of the two infections. Although driven by very different transmission mechanisms and dynamics, wide geographical overlap and high prevalence of both infections mean that even modest interactions lead to substantial impact in populations.[1,2] Surprisingly, until the mid-1990s, information about the relationship between HIV and malaria was scanty and it was believed that there was little association other than the programmatic link of blood safety in the face of malaria-induced anemia.[2–4] It is only recently, partly due to improved ability to assess immune compromise accurately and partly due to improved study designs, that a clearer pattern of biologic and clinical interaction has begun to emerge, although many gaps in knowledge remain.

Effect of HIV on Malaria

Malarial Immune Responses

HIV infection directly affects different compartments of the immune system, including humoral and cellular components, both of which play impor-tant protective roles against malaria. HIV infection impairs T-cell immunity resulting in a shift in T-cell function from Th1 to Th2 and loss of classical recall antigen responses (lymphocyte proliferation, IL-2 and IFN-γ production) and an inability to control infections that rely on inflammatory responses and granuloma formation. T cells are essential mediators of anti-malarial immunity through a number of mechanisms. Antibodies block invasion of sporozoites into liver cells and merozoites into red blood cells and prevent sequestration. IFN-γ + CD8$^+$ T cells and NK-T cells inhibit parasite development within hepatocytes, IFN-γ + CD4$^+$ T cells and NK cells activate macrophages to phagocytose intra-erythrocytic parasites. Antibodies neutralize the malaria toxin glycosylphosphatidylinositol (GPI) and inhibit the inflammatory cytokine cascade.[5] Therefore, HIV immunosuppression may increase susceptibility to malaria infection and the severity of its clinical consequences.

Clinical and Epidemiological Interactions

Pregnant women

The first clear indication of an effect of HIV on malaria was found in pregnant women. Pregnancy, particularly first pregnancy, increase the risk of infection with *Plasmodium falciparum*. In sub-Saharan Africa, *falciparum* malaria in pregnancy is predominantly asymptomatic and yet a major cause of severe maternal anemia and low birth weight (LBW), which in turn are important risk factors for infant mortality. Steketee and co-workers[6] reported in 1996 that HIV impairs a pregnant woman's ability to control malaria parasitemia, resulting in more frequent and higher density parasitemia than in HIV-uninfected pregnant women. This has since been confirmed in numerous other studies from sub-Saharan Africa.[7] HIV-infected pregnant women have on average a 1.65-fold increased risk of malaria parasitemia and placental malaria, and have higher parasite densities and are more likely to develop symptoms (fever) once infected. Importantly, HIV appears to aggravate the adverse effect of malaria in pregnancy placing co-infected women at much higher risk on developing severe anemia or having an adverse birth outcome than women with HIV-alone or malaria alone.[7,8] The immune mechanism involved have been reviewed recently by Ned and co-workers.[9] HIV does not appear to cause a generalized suppression of cellular immune responses against malaria, but is associated with a specific cytokine dysregulation resulting from severe impairment of the IL-12 mediated IFN-γ production by intervillous blood mononuclear cells (IVBMC), affecting the protective responses against placental malaria.[9] Some, but not all, antibody responses are also impaired, notably those to malarial variant surface antigens (VSA) expressed on infected erythrocytes which bind to chondroitin sulfate A, a key receptor for placental sequestration, and implicated in the parity-specific acquisition of antimalarial immunity.[10] Although the increased risk occurs in all pregnancies, it is particularly evident in multigravidae, suggesting that HIV affects the immune memory mechanism responsible for the parity-dependent immune responses.[7] HIV thus alters the typical gravidity specific pattern of malaria risk by shifting the burden from primarily primi- and secundi-gravidae to all pregnant women. The available evidence does not suggest that maternal HIV-1 has a consistent effect on congenital malaria in the newborn.[7]

Non-pregnant adults

Recent studies in non-pregnant adults suggest that HIV erodes whatever malaria immunity has been acquired through exposure and that this increases with the degree of HIV-associated immunosuppression. The intensity of malaria transmission and the associated degree of acquired anti-malarial immunity appear critical for determining the clinical consequences of co-infection.[11,12] In areas where malaria transmission is intense and continuous and some degree of anti-malarial immunity develops early in life, HIV-related immunosuppression increases rates of malarial parasitemia and fever, but there is no evidence of an increase in rates of severe or complicated malaria, nor of death.[1,13,14] The risks of parasitemia and malarial fever increase with decreasing

CD4 count and increasing viral load.[1,13,15] In regions of unstable transmission, pre-existing anti-malarial immunity is less well-developed and adults are more likely to become symptomatic and develop severe disease when infected with *P. falciparum*. In these regions, the impact of HIV is on disease presentation, with increased risk of complicated and severe malaria and of death.[16–18] Modeling studies suggest that appreciable HIV prevalence in a population can increase malaria transmission rates.[19]

Children

In infants, most *falciparum* infections tend to be at very low parasite density in the first 4–6 months of life and clinical malaria is uncommon until the combination of factors that provide innate protection against infection gradually wanes. Severe anemia and respiratory distress are the predominant syndromes of severe malaria in this young age group in Africa, whereas cerebral malaria is more prevalent in older children.

In contrast to pregnant women and adults, there is no evidence that HIV-1-infected infants and children have more frequent episodes of malaria parasitemia,[20–23] and some studies in infants have reported lower rates of *falciparum* malaria.[24,25] However, when infected with *P. falciparum*, HIV-infected infants and children may have difficulty clearing the parasitemia and have additional symptoms and pathology placing them at considerable greater risk of developing severe anemia than HIV-uninfected children with malaria, or HIV-infected children without malaria.[24,26]

In Kwazulu-Natal, an area of unstable malaria, HIV-infected children aged >1 year are more likely to experience severe disease, coma and death,[27] although a necropsy study from western Africa, where malaria transmission is more stable, found no association between HIV and malaria.[28] More data are required to clarify the relationship between HIV and malaria in children that take the child's HIV disease progression into account, as well as the child's age, and the maternal HIV and placental malaria status.

Effect of Malaria on HIV

Non-pregnant Adults and Children

Malaria, like many other co-infecting pathogens has been postulated to influence HIV-1 disease progression by activating T lymphocytes and immune factors such as cytokines, particularly TNF-α, that can activate HIV-1 replication. *In vitro* studies conducted using peripheral blood mononuclear cells (PBMC) from malaria-exposed (semi-immune) and non-immune donors showed that stimulation with malaria antigens and malaria pigment promotes *de novo* HIV infection, and viral reactivation and replication in cells.[29,30] A recent study in non-pregnant adults from Malawi showed that HIV-1 plasma viral loads increase significantly by about half a log during malaria episodes and remain high for up to 10 weeks after successful anti-malarial treatment.[31] The increases are greatest in those with clinical malaria (fever), high-density parasitemia and relatively well-preserved immune function as evidenced by high CD4 counts. Modeling studies suggest that appreciable malaria prevalence in a population can increase HIV transmission.[19]

One birth cohort study from western Kenya does not suggest that the low-density infections typically seen in young infants affect HIV-1 viral levels.[32] Paradoxically, another prospective study found that infants with malaria had delayed progression to AIDS and death.[24]

Pregnant Women and Mother-to-child Transmission of HIV-1

Maternal HIV-1 viral load is the single most important determinant of mother-to-child transmission (MTCT) of HIV-1. Similar to studies in non-pregnant adults with clinical malaria, *falciparum* infection in pregnancy increases HIV-1 viral concentration, both in the peripheral blood and at the local level in the placenta. The magnitude, however, is smaller (2-fold increase adjusted for degree of immunosuppression), reflecting that most malaria infections in pregnant women in Africa remain low-grade and rarely result in symptoms.[7] The question whether these degrees of malaria associated increases in viral concentrations in the placenta enhances the risk of MTCT is pivotal for sub-Saharan Africa, where few women are on antiretroviral drugs (ARVs) and uptake of MTCT preventive services has been low. Three studies to date have addressed this and have come to conflicting conclusions. All were conducted prior to the introduction of ARVs in Africa.[33-35] Placental malaria was associated with an increased risk of MTCT in Uganda (RR 2.89, 95% CI 1.12–7.52),[33] while there was no effect in Mombasa, Kenya,[35] and a significant protective effect in Kisumu, western Kenya (RR 0.44, CI 0.27–0.72, *P*<0.001).[31] Further analysis in the latter study showed that women with

high density placental malaria infection showed a significantly higher level of HIV-1 transmission (25%) compared with women with low density infections (11.5% transmission).

The differences between these studies could be due to several factors. The studies that found no, or a protective, effect of placental malaria on MTCT of HIV-1 excluded women with AIDS. They also differed in the methods used to diagnose placental malaria, which may have resulted in differential misclassification of placental infection. The apparent discrepancies may reflect the complex relationship between maternal immune responses to malaria, the severity of the malaria infection, and the degree of HIV-associated immune suppression in the host.[7] Immune responses to placental malaria in relatively immunocompetent HIV-infected women may result in an adequate balance of cytokine and chemokine responses that control both the malaria infection and HIV replication tipping the balance in the direction of a protective effect on MTCT. By contrast, in women with more advanced HIV disease and high-density infections, this may result in a degree of stimulation of HIV viral replication in the placenta that could result in a local environment that favors MTCT (Fig. 66.1).[9] This remains speculative and there remain substantial gaps in our knowledge about the precise mechanisms involved.

Treatment Issues and Programmatic Implications

Anti-malarial therapy is most effective in individuals with some acquired immunity and several studies have now shown a decreased treatment response in immuno-suppressed HIV-infected individuals treated with chloroquine, sulfadoxine-pyrimethamine (SP), and artemether-lumefantrine.[13,36-38] HIV-infected pregnant women also require more frequent dosing with intermittent preventive therapy (IPT) with SP to obtain the same preventive benefit on placental malaria and LBW as HIV-uninfected women.[39] The apparent decreased treatment response appears to be due to mainly more frequent reinfection than to recrudence.[40]

UNAIDS recommends prophylaxis to prevent opportunistic infections (OI) with the antibiotic cotrimoxazole (CTX) for certain groups of HIV-infected persons including all pregnant women after the first trimester. Initial results from studies in non-pregnant adults and children suggest that OI-prophylaxis with CTX also prevents malaria, even in

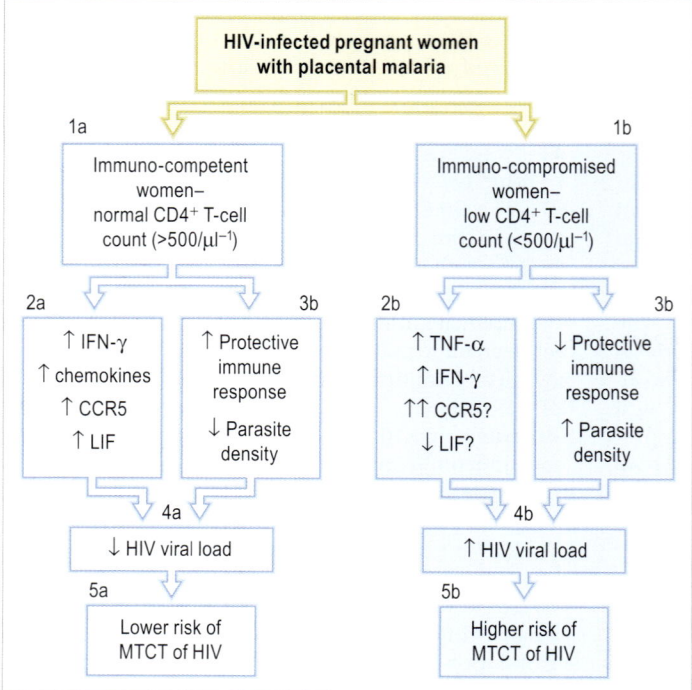

Figure 66.1 Hypothetical model of immune-factor modulation of MTCT of HIV-1 in HIV-placental-malaria co-infected mothers. HIV-infected women who are relatively immuno-competent (A) can mount protective immune responses in response to placental malaria infection, limiting both placental malaria and HIV-1 infection. Placental malaria infection can induce and sustain the production of the protective cytokine IFN-γ and chemokines such as MIP-1α, MIP-1β and RANTES that can block binding of HIV-1 to CCR5, a receptor for entry of HIV-1. At the same time, protective immune factors such as LIF that can reduce HIV-1 transmission might also be produced. Thus, relative levels of protective immune factors are at higher concentrations and can suppress viral replication and consequently MTCT.

However, women who are relatively immunocompromised (B), including those with low levels of CD4+ T cells, have a reduced ability to mount a protective immune response to limit either placental malaria or HIV-1 infection. Consequently, these women might experience high-density placental malaria infection, which can favour overproduction of cytokines such as TNF-α, which in turn further enhance HIV-1 replication resulting in higher viral load in the placenta. In this scenario, the low level of protective immune factors is overwhelmed and HIV-1 viral load is not controlled resulting in higher rates of MTCT. (Reproduced from Ned et al. 2005[9] with permission from the authors.)

areas with a moderate degree of parasite resistance to SP.[41-43] There is an urgent need to determine whether CTX prophylaxis alone provides sufficient protection against malaria in pregnant women, as SP and CTX are two similar antifolate sulfa drugs and concomitant use in HIV-infected individuals has been associated with an increased risk of severe cutaneous reactions and efficacy may be compromised because of cross-resistance.[7]

Interactions between antimalarial drugs and antiretroviral drugs (ARVs) mostly involve protease inhibitors (PIs) and non-nucleoside reverse transcriptase inhibitors (NNRTIs). PIs are not considered

for first-line therapy in most ARV treatment guidelines in sub-Saharan Africa, but they are included in second-line therapy. In patients receiving PIs (or the NNRTI delavirdine), the antimalarial drugs halofantrine, artemether and lumefantrine are best avoided because of risk of toxicity. For patients treated with other NNRTIs (nevirapine or efavirenz) lower concentrations of lumefantrine and artemether may lead to increased risk of malaria treatment failure. There is also potential for an interaction between quinine and NNRTI and PI drugs. The magnitude and clinical significance of these potential interactions needs further research.

Implications for Disease Burden

In areas like southern Africa with HIV-1 prevalence approaching 30%, population attributable fraction estimates of 20% for clinical malaria due to HIV in adults, suggest that the increased risk of clinical malaria attributable to HIV could have profound public health implications.[1] For pregnant women, the HIV-attributable proportional increase of malaria is estimated at 5.5% and 14.8% for populations with 10% and 30% HIV prevalence, respectively, corresponding to 0.57 and 1.55 million HIV-infected pregnant women respectively in sub-Saharan Africa each year.

No direct evidence has been found of an effect of HIV on malaria transmission. However, HIV infection increases asexual parasitemia, and if associated with a parallel increase in gametocyte production (this is not known), this may increase the reservoir of infection in the population, and hence transmission.[1] HIV-infected individuals are more likely to use SP and CTX, both of which increase the production of gametocytes.[44]

The effect of malaria on HIV infection is also hard to assess. There are documented transient increases in viral load but their effect on HIV progression and transmission is unknown,[45] and may not be important in public health terms, particularly in the context of ARVs. Nevertheless, it remains to be determined whether repeated episodes of malaria in areas with intense transmission lead to a more sustained cumulative effect on viral load and accelerated decline in CD4 counts, potentially shortening the time window in HIV-infected individuals until ARVs are required. If so, we would need to know whether HIV disease progression in individuals who do not yet require ARVs can be slowed down by targeted malaria control.

Modeling studies show that there is a synergistic relationship between HIV and malaria that is particularly important where the prevalence of one infection is high and the other is low.[19]

Conclusion

The effects of HIV on malaria are now well-documented in pregnant and non-pregnant adults. Malaria infection and fever rates are increased approximately 2-fold in areas of stable transmission, especially for those with low CD4 counts or high viral loads. In areas of unstable transmission, HIV is associated with more severe disease and death. Anti-malarial therapy appears to be less effective in HIV-infected individuals. In pregnant women, HIV is associated with more episodes of malaria, more fever, and more adverse birth outcomes. However, malaria upregulates HIV transcription transiently during acute episodes.

What is less clear is the effect of HIV on malaria in young children in different epidemiological settings, and particularly the effect of malaria on HIV, in terms of MTCT of HIV-1, and HIV-1 disease progression in infants and non-pregnant adults.

Notwithstanding the present gaps in our knowledge, there is a clear need to strengthen the deployment of existing malaria and HIV prevention and intervention measures. Current HIV and malaria control efforts are defined separately from one another. A more combined approach to control would be sensible, especially in rural areas with high malaria and HIV prevalence. Because of the increased risk for malaria, HIV-infected individuals need to be protected from malaria by use of insecticide-treated bednets and antimalarial chemoprophylaxis. The use of IPT could be expanded from pregnant women to all non-pregnant adults with HIV. This needs to be explored. Data are also emerging that suggest an effect of ARV and CTX on malaria parasites. A careful assessment of their impact is required. A study in Uganda has shown the large impact that can be made on malaria for those with HIV by the use of bednets, CTX and ARVs.[46] ARV use in Africa will be preferentially targeted at individuals with symptomatic and advanced HIV disease, precisely those individuals with the highest rates of malaria. The increasing use of ARV may reduce the impact of HIV on malaria, by reducing viral loads and increasing CD4 counts, therefore reducing the degree of immunocompromise. While this is an expensive intervention, this impact may prove to be valuable in terms of reducing OI and episodes of clinical malaria.

References

1. Whitworth J, Morgan D, Quigley M, et al. Effect of HIV-1 and increasing immunosuppression on malaria parasitemia and clinical episodes in adults in rural Uganda: a cohort study. Lancet 2000; 356:1051–1056.
2. Corbett EL, Steketee RW, ter Kuile FO, et al. HIV-1/AIDS and the control of other infectious diseases in Africa. Lancet 2002; 359:2177–2187.
3. Chandramohan D, Greenwood BM. Is there an interaction between human immunodeficiency virus and *Plasmodium falciparum*? Int J Epidemiol 1998; 27:296–301.
4. French N, Gilks CF. Royal Society of Tropical Medicine and Hygiene meeting at Manson House, London, 18 March 1999. Fresh from the field: some controversies in tropical medicine and hygiene. HIV and malaria, do they interact? Trans R Soc Trop Med Hyg 2000; 94:233–237.

5. Good MF, Doolan DL. Immune effector mechanisms in malaria. Curr Opin Immunol 1999; 11:412–419.
6. Steketee RW, Wirima JJ, Bloland PB, et al. Impairment of a pregnant woman's acquired ability to limit Plasmodium falciparum by infection with human immunodeficiency virus type-1. Am J Trop Med Hyg 1996; 55:S42–S49.
7. ter Kuile FO, Parise ME, Verhoeff FH, et al. The burden of co-infection with human immunodeficiency virus type 1 and malaria in pregnant women in sub-Saharan Africa. Am J Trop Med Hyg 2004; 71:S41–S54.
8. Ayisi JG, van Eijk AM, ter Kuile FO, et al. The effect of dual infection with HIV and malaria on pregnancy outcome in western Kenya. Aids 2003; 17:585–594.
9. Ned RM, Moore JM, Chaisavaneeyakorn S, et al. Modulation of immune responses during HIV-malaria co-infection in pregnancy. Trends Parasitol 2005; 21:284–291.
10. Mount AM, Mwapasa V, Elliott SR, et al. Impairment of humoral immunity to Plasmodium falciparum malaria in pregnancy by HIV infection. Lancet 2004; 363:1860–1867.
11. Hewitt K, Steketee R, Mwapasa K, et al. Interactions between HIV and malaria in non-pregnant adults: evidence and implicaitons. AIDS 2006; 20:1993–2004.
12. Laufer MK, Plowe CV. The interaction between HIV and malaria in Africa. Cur Infect Dis Rep 2007; 9:47–54.
13. French N, Nakiyingi J, Lugada E, et al. Increasing rates of malarial fever with deteriorating immune status in HIV-1-infected Ugandan adults. AIDS 2001; 15:899–906.
14. Francesconi P, Fabiani M, Dente MG, et al. HIV, malaria parasites, and acute febrile episodes in Ugandan adults: a case-control study. AIDS 2001; 15:2445–2450.
15. Patnaik P, Jere CS, Miller WC, et al. Incidence of malaria parasitemia in a cohort of rural Malawian adults according to HIV serostatus, HIV-1 RNA concentration and CD4 count. 53rd Annual Meeting of the American Society of Tropical Medicine and Hygiene, Miami, Florida: 2004.
16. Chirenda J, Siziya S, Tshimanga M. Association of HIV infection with the development of severe and complicated malaria cases at a rural hospital in Zimbabwe. Cent Afr J Med 2000; 46:5–9.
17. Cohen C, Dini L, Frean J, et al. Increase in severe malaria in HIV-positive adults in South Africa. XIVth International AIDS Conference Barcelona, Spain: 2002; Abstract No. ThPeC7602.
18. Grimwade K, French N, Mbatha DD, et al. HIV infection as a cofactor for severe falciparum malaria in adults living in a region of unstable malaria transmission in South Africa. AIDS 2004; 18:547–554.
19. Abu-Raddad LJ, Patnaik P, Kublin JG. Dual infection with HIV and malaria fuels the spread of both diseases in sub-Saharan Africa. Science 2006; 314:1603–1606.
20. Muller O, Musoke P, Sen G, et al. Pediatric HIV-1 disease in a Kampala Hospital. J Trop Pediatr 1990; 36:283–286.
21. Greenberg AE, Nsa W, Ryder RW, et al. Plasmodium Falciparum malaria and perinatally acquired human immunodeficiency virus type 1 infection in Kinshasa, Zaire. A prospective, longitudinal cohort study of 587 children. N Engl J Med 1991; 325:105–109.
22. Taha TE, Canner JK, Dallabetta GA, et al. Childhood malaria parasitemia and human immunodeficiency virus infection in Malawi. Trans R Soc Trop Med Hyg 1994; 88:164–165.
23. Jackson DJ, Klee EB, Green SD, et al. Lymphadenopathy and hepatosplenomegaly in the 1st year in children infected by HIV-1 in Zaire. Ann Trop Paediatr 1992; 12:165–168.
24. Kalyesubula I, Musoke-Mudido P, Marum L, et al. Effects of malaria infection in human immunodeficiency virus type 1-infected Ugandan children. Pediatr Infect Dis J 1997; 16:876–881.
25. Villamor E, Fataki MR, Mbise RL, et al. Malaria parasitemia in relation to HIV status and vitamin A supplementation among pre-school children. Trop Med Int Health 2003; 8:1051–1061.
26. van Eijk AM, Ayisi JG, ter Kuile FO, et al. Malaria and human immunodeficiency virus infection as risk factors for

anemia in infants in Kisumu, western Kenya. Am J Trop Med Hyg 2002; 67:44–53.
27. Grimwade K, French N, Mbatha DD, et al. Childhood malaria in a region of unstable transmission and high human immunodeficiency virus prevalence. Pediatr Infect Dis J 2003; 22:1057–1063.
28. Lucas SB, Peacock CS, Hounnou A, et al. Disease in children infected with HIV in Abidjan, Cote d'Ivoire. Br Med J 1996; 312:335–338.
29. Xiao L, Owen SM, Rudolph DL, et al. Plasmodium falciparum antigen-induced human immunodeficiency virus type 1 replication is mediated through induction of tumor necrosis factor-alpha. J Infect Dis 1998; 177:437–445.
30. Froebel K, Howard W, Schafer JR, et al. Activation by malaria antigens renders mononuclear cells susceptible to HIV infection and re-activates replication of endogenous HIV in cells from HIV-infected adults. Parasite Immunol 2004; 26:213–217.
31. Kublin JG, Patnaik P, Jere CS, et al. Effect of Plasmodium falciparum malaria on concentration of HIV-1-RNA in the blood of adults in rural Malawi: a prospective cohort study. Lancet 2005; 365:233–240.
32. Brouwer KC, Mirel LB, Yang C, et al. The effect of Plasmodium falciparum infection on HIV-1 viral load in infants. 53rd Annual Meeting of the American Society of Tropical Medicine and Hygiene, Miami Beach, Florida: 2004.
33. Brahmbhatt H, Kigozi G, Wabwire-Mangen F, et al. The effects of placental malaria on mother-to-child HIV transmission in Rakai, Uganda. AIDS 2003; 17:2539–2541.
34. Ayisi JG, van Eijk AM, Newman RD, et al. Maternal malaria and perinatal HIV transmission, western Kenya. Emerg Infect Dis 2004; 10:643–652.
35. Inion I, Mwanyumba F, Gaillard P, et al. Placental malaria and perinatal transmission of human immunodeficiency virus type 1. J Infect Dis 2003; 188:1675–1678.
36. Birku Y, Mekonnen E, Bjorkman A, et al. Delayed clearance of Plasmodium falciparum in patients with human immunodeficiency virus co-infection treated with artemisinin. Ethiop Med J 2002; 40:S17–S26.
37. Shah S, Smith E, Obonyo C, et al. The effect of HIV-infection on antimalarial treatment response: preliminary results of a 28-day drug efficacy trial in HIV-infected and HIV-uninfected adults in Siaya, Kenya. 53rd Annual Meeting of the American Society of Tropical Medicine and Hygiene, Miami Beach, Florida: 2004.
38. van Geertruyden JP, Mwananyanda L, Chalwe V, et al. Higher risk of antimalarial treatment failure in HIV positive than in HIV negative individuals with clinical malaria. 53rd Annual Meeting of the American Society of Tropical Medicine and Hygiene, Miami Beach, Florida: 2004.
39. Parise ME, Ayisi JG, Nahlen BL, et al. Efficacy of sulfadoxine-pyrimethamine for prevention of placental malaria in an area of Kenya with a high prevalence of malaria and human immunodeficiency virus infection. Am J Trop Med Hygiene 1998; 59:813–822.
40. Kamya MR, Gasasira AF, Yeka A, et al. Effect of HIV-1 infection on antimalarial treatment outcomes in Uganda: a population-based study. J Infect Dis 2006; 193:9–15.
41. Mermin J, Lule J, Ekwaru JP, et al. Effect of co-trimoxazole prophylaxis on morbidity, mortality, CD4-cell count, and viral load in HIV infection in rural Uganda. Lancet 2004; 364:1428–1434.
42. Anglaret X, Chene G, Attia A, et al. Early chemoprophylaxis with trimethoprim-sulphamethoxazole for HIV-1-infected adults in Abidjan, Cote d'Ivoire: a randomised trial. Cotrimo-CI Study Group. Lancet 1999; 353:1463–1468.
43. Watera C, Todd J, Muwonge R, et al. Feasibility and effectiveness of atrimoxazole prophylaxis in HIV-1-infected adults attending an HIV/AIDS clinica in Uganda. J AIDS 2006; 42:373–378.
44. Sowunmi A, Adedeji A, Fehintola F, et al. Effects of antifolates- co-trimoxazole and pyrimethamine-sulfadoxine on gametocytes in children with acute, symptomatic, uncomplicated, Plasmodium

falciparum malaria. 53rd Annual Meeting of the American Society of Tropical Medicine and Hygiene, Miami Beach, Florida: 2004.

45. Whitworth JA, Hewitt KA. Effect of malaria on HIV-1 progression and transmission. Lancet 2005; 365:196–197.

46. Mermin J, Ekwaru JP, Liechty CA, et al. Effect of co-trimoxazole prophylaxis, antiretroviral therapy and insecticide-treated bednets on the frequency of malaria in HIV-1-infected adults in Uganda: a prospective cohort study. Lancet 2006; 367:1256–1261.

CHAPTER 67

The Role of Unsterile Injections in the HIV Pandemic

Ernest Drucker
Cristian Apetrei
Robert Heimer
Preston Marx

Unsterile Injections: A Modern Vector for Large-scale Transmission of Blood-borne Pathogens

The nineteenth century technological innovation of medical injections evolved into mass-produced and inexpensive injection equipment by the mid-twentieth century. As this equipment became widely available, it had an enormous influence on the course of public health and medical practice worldwide. Injections permitted the use of insulin (in the 1930s); the first antibiotics to fight bacterial infections (beginning in the late 1940s) were only available in injectable form; and injections first made feasible the more efficient use of many other medications, especially biological molecules, in the succeeding decades.

But injections (like blood transfusions) are invasive medical procedures associated with a set of risks for the transmission of infectious microorganisms in human blood.[1-3] We can say now that, in addition to all their apparent benefits, injections created a set of circumstances for the large-scale transmission of blood-borne pathogens (viruses, bacteria, and parasitic organisms) in ways never before possible in human history. The development and growth of medical injecting marks the emergence of a major new vector for human infection as significant as the traditional ones of sexual, water-borne, air-borne, insect, and parasitic transmission. And because of the rapidity and massive scale of their introduction in the decades following the Second World War, injections quickly became an avenue for the movement of older pathogens to new populations and the creation and global dissemination of new ones.[4]

The biological and public health significance of this new mechanism of transmission may be measured by the probability of its facilitation of the passage of pathogens between humans and their role in epidemic spread. Unsterile injections have varying transmission efficiencies (depending on the type of injection) and many of these are equal to or greater than sexual routes. But, while the history of most human diseases is linked to the developments of civilization (e.g. village life, farming, animal herding, industrialization, urbanization), the impact of the unsterile use of invasive medical instruments and technologies has distinctive features differentiating it from the more 'natural' vectors: they are intimately wed to the global diffusion of curative and preventive medical care in the twentieth century. Furthermore, because they allow the passage of non-epidemic pathogens between humans, these technologies also constitute a new mechanism allowing viral recombination with the potential for the creation of new human pathogens. With the opening of this new, large-scale channel for the movement of blood-borne pathogens and other viral materials between individuals, it became possible for many infections that were barely communicable and much less efficiently transmitted through traditional routes (e.g. hepatitis C virus – HCV) to spread rapidly within the burgeoning populations receiving Western medical care worldwide and among those injecting illicit drugs – the other large scale opportunity in the mid-twentieth century, that allowed the transmission of blood-borne pathogens between humans.

This chapter reviews the history and current significance of injections, including their possible role in the origins of HIV and the central role they have played in the early stages of the HIV pandemic in many areas of the world and continue to play as the epidemic matures and expands.

Medical Injections: A Brief History

The history of the hypodermic syringe, over the past century, is punctuated by important manufacturing and drug developments that dramatically affected its availability, price, demand, and patterns of utilization worldwide. Following their invention in 1848, and until the end of the First World War, sterile syringes were considered precision medical instruments, individually handmade from glass and metal by skilled artisans. The cost was initially high – in 1900, syringes cost US$50 per unit (adjusted to current dollars) and even by 1920, after the considerable increases in capacity associated with the demands of the First World War, production was still very limited – only about 100 000 syringes per year worldwide. Beginning in the period between the World Wars, syringe manufacture was increasingly mechanized, using interchangeable components and mass production methods. As the number and significance of clinical applications grew, injection use outside the hospital or clinic increased, most significantly as a result of the increased injection of insulin in the USA and Europe in the 1930s and 1940s. Global production reached 2 million units per year (by 1930) and 8 million per year by 1952. Throughout this period, the unit price of injecting equipment declined steadily – by 80% between 1920 and 1950.[5-8]

The Crucial Role of Penicillin

While penicillin was first manufactured during the Second World War, it did not become generally available (especially outside of the USA and Europe) until the early 1950s. By that time, mass production of antibiotics was substantially lowering prices for these drugs and increasing their global availability.[9,10] As the efficacy of these new drugs became apparent, popular demand for injectables increased worldwide because the usual route of administration of penicillin in much of the world was, and remains, by injection. But, even with declines in the cost of antibiotics, the injection equipment needed to administer them was still relatively expensive and the safe re-use of glass syringes was still dependent on a costly infrastructure to assure sterilization. And, even at the production rate of 7 500 000 reusable syringes a year (in 1952), it was still impossible to meet the growing demand – much of it associated with the new antibiotic 'miracle drugs.'[7-10]

This increased demand for injectable medications was anticipated by the industry and led to a series of important changes in manufacturing, i.e. the development of inexpensive, disposable 'single use ' syringes. And with it, new high volume manufacturing technologies for plastic injection equipment (today a small plant with six workers can manufacture 100 million sets per year), dramatically lowering prices, and massively increasing availability worldwide. The growth in the use of injectable drugs was met by the mass production of re-usable needles and (by 1960) of the newly developed and relatively inexpensive plastic syringes. With these innovations came a 100-fold increase in global production in the period 1950–1960 (from 10 million to 1 billion units) and a 90% drop in unit price (from US$2.50 to 15 cents) – largely replacing sterilizable glass syringes with cheap, 'disposable' equipment – items never intended for re-use (Fig. 67.1).[5-8]

The Myth of Safe Injecting

Our common conception about medical injections assumes safety – the employment of sterile needles and syringes, the use of well-established injecting techniques, and adequate provision for the sterilization or disposal of contaminated equipment. Further, with the important exception of diabetics, safe injections are generally premised on the involvement of medical personnel trained in sterile techniques.

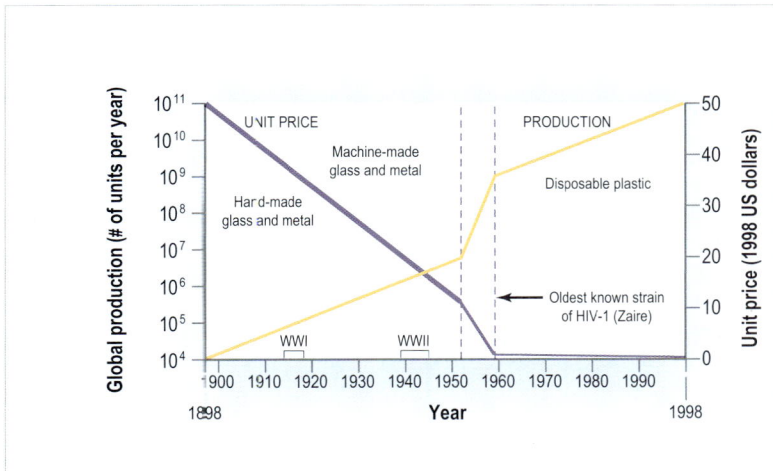

Figure 67.1 Global production and unit price of injecting equipment (1898–1998).

And, assuming that this practice is the norm (as it is in well-managed healthcare settings throughout the world), our concerns about the reduction of health risks associated with injecting generally focus on the risk of occupational exposure to health professionals, and environmental concerns about effective systems for the safe disposal of contaminated equipment, i.e. as hazardous 'medical waste.' But even in the context of modern medical practice, needle-borne transmission of disease still occurs frequently both to health workers (through injuries from contaminated sharps), and to patients through the use of inadequately sterilized equipment.[11]

The infections of particular concern are hepatitis B (HBV), hepatitis C (HCV), and the human immunodeficiency virus (HIV). In part, this is because of their ability to contaminate and survive in injecting equipment. HBV, for example, can remain infectious for periods longer than 1 week, even dried at room temperature. And the probability that a single needlestick with HBV will result in seroconversion is approximately 30%. In the global healthcare sector alone, WHO estimates that unsafe injections cause approximately 30 000 new HIV infections each year, 8 million HBV infections, and 1.2 million HCV infections worldwide every year.[12,13] For HIV and HCV, the probabilities that a single needlestick will result in seroconversion are much smaller (0.3–0.5% and 2–5%, respectively).[14] But for intravenous contamination, the efficiency increases by one or two orders of magnitude over subcutaneous or intramuscular injections with a contaminated syringe or needle.

Parameters of Transmissibility of Viruses by Unsterile Injections

Many viruses are protected in blood residues inside the used syringe. This has been best studied in the case of HIV. The duration for the survival of HIV inside syringes ranges from a few days (when the volume and viral titer are low) to 6 weeks or more when the volumes or titers are increased.[15] Most syringes used in medical care have a needle that separates from the barrel of the syringe. These syringes retain a larger volume of fluid after use and, as a result, HIV survives longer. An additional factor effecting HIV survival is temperature: higher temperatures increase the rate at which HIV loses its infectiousness.[16]

There have been two estimates made for the likelihood that a single intravenous injection with a contaminated syringe will transmit HIV-1. The first estimate, which derived from modeling studies of HIV-1 transmission among IDUs in New Haven, CT, found the probability to be between 6 and 7 per 1000 injections.[17] The second estimate, which derived from studies of seroconverters in Thailand, found the probability to be 8 per 1000 injections.[18] In these cases, it was assumed that all intravenous injections introduced some contaminated blood into the syringes.

This assumption seems warranted given ethnographic studies of intravenous drug injector practices. Injectors want to introduce the drugs directly into the blood, so they insert the needle seeking a vein. Injectors pull back on the plunger, drawing blood into the syringe. The appearance of blood indicates that the syringe is properly registered and the injector then injects. In many cases, injectors repeat the process, pulling back on the plunger allowing blood into the barrel of the syringe, and then injecting. This common practice is employed by injectors who believe that through this practice, they are getting all of the drug out of the syringe and into their blood.

On the other hand, when syringes are used exclusively for non-intravenous injection, the likelihood that they become contaminated with HIV-1 is lessened. Whereas almost all needles and syringes used for intravenous (i.v.) injection become contaminated, <5% of syringes used for intramuscular (i.m.) or subcutaneous injection (s.c.) become contaminated with virus particles.[19] The situation is even more extreme for HCV: while 95% of syringes containing residual blood from actively infected individuals were found to contain HCV, none of the nearly 100 syringes that had been used to administer medically indicated i.v. or s.c. injections were found to contain evidence of HCV particles (R. Heimer, unpublished data).

Unsterile Injections in the Developing World

The Problem of Disposables

However well suited they were to the expanding markets for injectable drugs, these cheaper 'single use' syringes were never intended for sterilization or re-use. The material from which they are fabricated, polypropylene plastic, does not maintain integrity of the seals and deforms at autoclave temperatures, and they cannot be effectively sterilized unless disassembled, heated to temperatures above 80°C, and reassembled under sterile conditions (S. Levinson, pers comm, June 2000).

Nonetheless, in much of the developing world, these new syringes flooded the market in the 1950s, adding significantly to the pool of injecting equipment already in circulation. And as more injectable medications became available (especially the antibiotics) multiple re-use quickly became common practice, re-using older injection equipment (sometimes re-sharpened by hand) often without even attempts at sterilization.[20-24] In the developing world, demand for injections far exceeded the supply of sterile equipment and, because their cost, low by western medical standards, was still prohibitive for most African societies in the 1950s, the increase in demand for injections also meant a sharp increase in unster-

ile re-use of 'disposable' equipment, both inside and outside of medical practice.

The risks of iatrogenic infections associated with unsterile injections are today recognized to be widespread throughout the developing world.[25,26] Recent surveys of World Health Organization (WHO) regional immunization programs estimate that 30% of the injections are unsterile. But immunizations accounts for only 10% of all injections to children and the rate of unsterile use outside of immunization programs likely exceeds 50%.[27,28] Under WHO auspices alone, more than 1 billion injections were performed in the developing world in 1996 (800 million for immunization; 240 million for emergency disease outbreaks). Increased usage of injections throughout the developing world is expected, as WHO plans a drive to eliminate neonatal tetanus (with 74 million women targeted in developing countries) and worldwide campaigns for hepatitis B and other new immunizations that will target 3.1 billion children under 15 years of age, by 2005.[27]

The Case of HCV in Egypt

The great potential for serious public health consequences of massive unsterile injecting were made dramatically evident in the disclosure of a large outbreak of HCV in Egypt in the 1950s, when 25% of an entire generation of 1.3 million young adults was infected with HCV through a campaign of i.v. treatment of schistosomiasis with multiple use of unsterilized syringes in a government/UN program.[1,29] The unintended side-effect of the Egyptian schistosomiasis campaign illustrates the potential public health significance of massive unsterile injecting for precipitating an explosive increase in the prevalence of (we assume) locally endemic but previously sequestered clusters of HCV; a disease that was invisible to us until quite recently. Given the poor transmissibility of HCV by the sexual route, unsterile injections are the most likely basis for launching the global pandemic of HCV. Today >400 million people are infected with HCV worldwide and the magnitude of the global HCV epidemic establishes a new model for understanding the ability of massive unsterile injecting to alter the global ecology of infectious diseases in human populations.[30,31]

The Role of Injections in HIV Epidemic Origins in Sub-Saharan Africa

In the 75 years prior to the Second World War, a network of colonial and missionary clinics was the principal base of Western medical practice in this region of Africa.[32,33] Specific practices varied, depending on the medical traditions of the French, British, or Belgian colonial powers, but most administered injectable drugs.[20,23,24,35,34] This was done on site and under medical supervision, while closely controlling access to the relatively costly drugs and injecting equipment, using sterile injecting procedures and with access to sterilization equipment on hand. There is little evidence of injection-related transmission of disease in this pre-Second World War colonial period.[35]

However, in the period following the Second World War, with independence impending across sub-Saharan Africa, Europe's control of civic affairs in the region began to weaken, including its controls on medical practice.[34,36–38] Despite substantial new investments by some colonial powers (Britain and France) in educational and administrative preparation for independence, the shrinking colonial medical care system was not quickly replaced by the newly independent, but impoverished, African states.[39,40] And, as the independent states struggled to establish medical services, the old colonial medical care system[41] was supplanted by a growing number of indigenous practitioners with varying degrees of training and minimal controls – adding many 'country clinics' utilizing Western practices, injecting equipment and medicines – where injecting equipment (most previously used and recycled) was often diverted or salvaged from the former system. These formed the basis for an 'informal' parallel system of injecting with little or no awareness of the need nor the capability for sterilization procedures.[38]

Re-use of single-use syringes in mass public health campaigns

While under colonial rule there had been some mass campaigns that involved hundreds of thousands of injections (e.g. to treat Yaws), the 1950s saw several mass campaigns to administer millions of doses of injectable antibiotics. The first UN public health project was UNICEF's yaws eradication campaign in India, Haiti and Central Africa between 1952 and 1959.[42] In Central Africa alone, there were 35 million injections associated with this campaign and in many subsequent antibiotic and anti-malaria treatment campaigns in sub-Saharan Africa, the mass administration of injectable medications by poorly trained and equipped local aids using unsterile practices became the norm.

Throughout this period and in the following decades, there was a sharp growth in the use of injections throughout sub-Saharan Africa. Injections were expected at every medical visit and for the treatment of any condition. While earlier documentation is sparse, by the mid-1960s, several studies establish that >75% of households in sub-Saharan Africa had received an injection within the previous 2-week period.[35] Ethnographic and public health surveys conducted in several parts of Africa (and India) in the 1960s found very high levels of injecting: in one study in Uganda, 80% of households owned their own syringe.[35] Considerable attention has been devoted by WHO to establishing safer injection practices in Africa.[43–46] It is clear from the experience with intravenous injectors of illicit drugs and the explosive spread of HIV ignited by this vector in many parts of the world, that large-scale transmission of HIV can be caused by unsterile injections.

Injections Involving Drug Abuse and Addiction

The unsafe use of injecting (outside of medical practice) also occurs widely in the developed world. Contaminated syringes are used and re-used for injecting illicit drugs – opiates, cocaine, amphetamines, and many performance enhancing drugs. In the USA and Europe, there are at least 3–5 million regular drug injectors who, with multiple injections each day, account for more injecting episodes per year than is associated with all the licit use of injections in these same countries.[47–49] HIV and hepatitis prevalence among these populations can be very high and often increases quickly once the virus enters the population sharing injecting equipment and drugs.[49,50] HIV prevalence among injectors can rapidly increase to 50% and beyond in just a few years.[48] HBV and HCV incidence rates can be as high as 75% per year among injectors at the beginning of epidemics.[51,52]

The differences in the likelihood of encountering a contaminated and potentially infectious syringe depend not just on how the syringe had been used, but also on how the syringe was handled after use. For instance, drug injectors in the eastern USA do not appear to routinely wash the blood out of their syringes immediately after use and the majority of syringes retain evidence of blood.[53] In contrast, the likelihood of detecting blood in syringes used by American injectors who reside on the West Coast is far lower.[54] This difference may be the result of differences in the kind of heroin injected. In the east, easily dissolvable powder heroin is the norm. In the west, the heroin is resinous and the residue may clog the syringe if the syringe is not rinsed immediately after use.[55] This difference may explain, in part, the differences in HIV prevalence among injectors on the two coasts.[56] While prevalence among injectors in New York and the surrounding areas generally exceeded 25% before the start of effective prevention programs like syringe exchange, the prevalence among injectors in the West rarely exceeded 10%.[57] In New York, HIV prevalence among drug injectors is now reutrning to 10%, a level not seen since the late 1970s.

Ominously, injection of illicit drugs has emerged as a major new trend among an ever-growing proportion of the world's developing countries, including sub-Saharan Africa, with its very high background prevalence of infection.[58] WHO now identifies more than 120 countries in which injecting drug use occurs – in the developing world among an estimated 30–50 million drug users – where the sharing of contaminated injecting equipment is central to igniting regional AIDS outbreaks.[59] But the availability of inexpensive heroin is expanding in the world far faster than the availability of sterile injecting equipment. In the context of addiction among the worlds poorest people, any price for needles is too high – in Southeast Asia a clean set of 'works' costs about the same as an entire days worth of heroin, and is harder to obtain. Unsterile injecting now accounts for the majority of incident HIV infections and 90% of the HCV infections in both the USA and Europe.[50,60]

Nosocomial Epidemics of HIV

National Case Studies in Romania, Russia, and Libya

Once HIV had spread beyond Africa (by the 1970s) nosocomial risk of transmission involving a new synergy between injections and transfusions began to appear in Eastern Europe and several years later, in Libya. The outbreaks in Eastern Europe occurred almost simultaneously in 1988–1989 in the Soviet Union and Romania, at the time of the break-up of the USSR. Both involved HIV-1 transmission to institutionalized infants and children, where nosocomial outbreaks occurred in the context of a very low prevalence of HIV infection in the adult population. At the time of these outbreaks in Eastern Europe in late

1980s, there were only 13 adult cases of AIDS reported in Romania and 71 in Russia. These events demonstrated the particular vulnerability of healthcare systems to becoming a significant locus of HIV infection independent of the general population prevalence.

The Romanian outbreak was by far the more significant, involving over 10 000 cases distributed over a 3-year period. It was first recognized in 1989, when 12 young children were diagnosed with HIV-1 infection. All identified parents tested HIV-negative. By December 1989, Romania reported 48 cases of pediatric AIDS to WHO; transmission was attributed to transfusion with unscreened blood.[61] In 1990, a seroepidemiological investigation was conducted of 1878 institutionalized children, 409 (22%) being diagnosed with HIV – all but three in children <5 years of age, 66% of whom were in orphanages.[62,63] Systematic testing of all institutionalized children revealed that the magnitude of this outbreak was dramatically higher than initially considered, as cases were distributed all over the country. WHO and CDC conducted screenings and concluded that, since the majority of HIV-infected children were born from uninfected mothers but had histories of hospitalization and/or were institutionalized, the outbreak had a nosocomial nature.[64,65] But HIV-1 prevalence in blood donors from Romania at that time was very low, making it difficult to explain the relatively uniform distribution of the pediatric AIDS cases in all geographic regions of Romania and attributing it solely to blood transfusions.[63,66]

Over the next few years, the evolution of this outbreak was also unexpected: the pediatric AIDS continued to accumulate in children from orphanages, not only as a consequence of the progression to AIDS of already infected children, but also because of new seroconversions. Therefore, this 'HIV outbreak' among very young children was difficult to control and showed a high propensity to transmission.[67] While the outbreak is currently under control, the Romanian nosocomial AIDS epidemic still accounts for >50% of pediatric AIDS cases recorded in Europe since the beginning of epidemic.

That the Romanian nosocomial AIDS epidemic was new at the time of its discovery is known because the majority of HIV-1 infections diagnosed in 1990–1991 were in the initial stages of infection, based on clinical, serological and immunological data.[64,68] Almost 40% of these cases are still living with HIV-1 in 2005, 15 years after the first reports. Their recent occurrence, in 1990, was also supported by epidemiological evidence: the age distribution of cases, showing the highest prevalence levels in the age group of 0–4 years in 1991–1993. Although in the following years, new pediatric AIDS cases were reported, the majority of HIV-1-infected children in the nosocomial epidemic were born in 1988–1989.[64] A retrospective serological investigation revealed no seropositivity in sera collected between 1977–1988 from 116 children from orphanages and 739 adults.[69] Parallel testing of HIV-1 and hepatitis B virus (HBV) not only revealed a higher HBV prevalence but also a more equilibrated age distribution of HBV.[65,69–71] Altogether, these observations, corroborated with a decrease in the risk of receiving injection with age, were interpreted as suggesting that HIV-1 was only recently introduced in the pediatric population, whereas HBV was present for a longer period at the time of HIV-1 outbreak. Romanian Ministry of Health statistics showed the HBV epidemics preceded the HIV-1 outbreak by 4 years.[72]

Numerous reports focused on the nosocomial aspect of this outbreak.[62,64,65,68–73] The majority of HIV infections in other European children (80–95%) occur following vertical transmission from infected mother in utero, intrapartum or postpartum, through breast-feeding.[1,74–76] However, in Romania, (where 57% of mothers were tested) the prevalence of vertical transmission accounted for only 6% of pediatric AIDS cases.[65] Half of the pediatric AIDS cases in Romania came from orphanages, where the age at admission was significantly lower than at the time of HIV diagnosis, the difference being enough to allow seroconversion.[77] A statistically significant relationship was established between the risk of seropositivity and the duration of care in these institutions. Similar results were observed for hepatitis B virus infection. There was also evidence for HIV-1 parenteral transmission in association with HBV, which was reported in 50% of those with HIV-1 infections.[64,69,70,72] The prevalence of HBV infection was consistently higher than that of HIV-1, probably due to a higher infectivity and resistance of HBV and also to the endemic nature of HBV infection in Romania. In early 1990, 4.4% of the general population of Romania was tested positive for HBsAg, which also might have created the basis for HBV vertical transmission. Independent seroepidemiological evidence from a CDC investigation in 1993 pointed to parenteral transmission as being responsible for the emergence of HIV-1 in Romanian orphanages.[72] In a pilot study, 19% tested positive for HIV-1, whereas 87% were positive for HBV markers. Of these, 32% presented the marker of HBV persistency, HbsAg.[72] Two of the HIV-1-infected children were transfusion recipients, the donors being localized and tested negative. All tested

mothers in this study were shown to be HIV-1 sero-negative. The study of the medical records for 1989 have shown that in this orphanage, 810 syringes had been sterilized and that in the same timeframe, 4227 injections had been administered, thus showing that every syringe had been used at least five times between sterilizations. The mean injection number for these children was 206 lifetime injections. HIV-1-infected children received a lifetime 280 injections, whereas the HIV-1 seronegative ones received 187 ($P<0.02$) additional evidence supporting parenteral HIV-1 transmission through re-used needles and syringes. There is also molecular evidence of parenteral transmission in this outbreak. Although parenteral transmission of HIV is largely acknowledged, the transmission rate of HIV following accidental needlestick injuries is low (0.47%).[78] Numerous studies suggested that the volume of blood transmitted and thus the amount of virus is influencing HIV-1 transmission rates, which is different from the pattern of HBV transmission for which the volume of blood is not determinant for parenteral transmission.[79,80] The biological basis for this observation is that the plasma viral loads (VL) for HBV infection is significantly higher that that of HIV-1, which is also varying according to the stage of infection. HIV-1-infected pediatric patients in Romania had high VL levels, increasing the likelihood of transmission through residual blood in unsterilized syringes.[81] Moreover, the high dispersion of VL levels revealed that the 'sources' were related to a higher infectivity of the 'spreaders' rather than to the number of children in a given setting. This explained the lower prevalence of HIV-1 infection compared with that of HBV in institutionalized children.[81]

These iatrogenic outbreaks have yielded to molecular epidemiological analyses, e.g. tracing HIV-1 strains from Romanian children resulted in the characterization of a new HIV-1 group M subtype, the subtype F.[82–85]

Paradoxically, the only subtype F strains available for the time being was found in Brazil.[82] Further studies revealed a wide spread of this subtype, but at very low prevalence levels.[86–88] Conversely, in Romania, subtype F was the major viral form in all risk groups, showing that the Romanian epidemic resulted from a founder effect of subtype F, originally imported from Africa.[88] The low diversity between different strains from nosocomially-infected children from different geographical regions, suggested that a single introduction of the virus occurred in the pediatric population.[82–85,89] This introduction most likely resulted from the use of HIV-infected blood products, but was disseminated by subsequent injections. Once the initial cases occurred, the explosive spread of the virus in orphanages resulting from improper medical practices illustrates how a minor HIV-1 variant may became epidemiologically significant through founder effects. In recent years, subtype F from Romania represented a source of viral diversification in Europe.[90] The origin of subtype F was reported to be Central Africa, a region closely related economically and politically to Romania in the 1980s.[88]

Natural History of the Nosocomial Transmission of HIV-1 in Romania

The combined effect of several factors fueled nosocomial transmissions in Romania. These were: (1) A high burden of institutionalized young children favoring the rapid spread of respiratory or gastrointestinal infections; (2) chronic food shortage and malnutrition; (3) an acute shortage of medication, especially for the oral administration, which resulted in a high number of injections; (4) a shortage of needles and syringes, correlated with an improperly maintained sterilizing equipment, which resulted in the re-use of syringes between sterilizations; (5) Negligence of the medical staff. All of these conditions contributed to explosive local outbreaks following the introduction of the virus in orphanages. This demonstrates that nosocomial outbreaks have an extraordinarily rapid potential to spread if universal precautions are not applied in clinical settings.

Some 15 years after the first reports, the epidemiological pattern of HIV-1 infection in Romania has changed dramatically due to implementation of effective control measures. The number of adult cases has increased dramatically in recent years. A difference from other neighboring countries is that the epidemic in Romania is not fueled by intravenous drug use, since the number of injectors has increased only recently. Therefore, the major mode of transmission in Romania is sexual contact, which is also reflected in the new diversity profiles of the virus strains. Multiple subtypes imported from multiple sources are currently co-circulating in Romania. The regions most affected by the AIDS epidemic are those around the major Romanian cities, especially the capital (Bucharest) and the most important port (Constanta). Extensive viral diversity was reported in these regions. Subtype B is the most frequent in the northwestern regions, which have the closest contact with Western Europe. However, the major viral form is still subtype F, which has produced a strong, though relatively slow, founder effect in adult

population.[89,91] Remarkably, the nosocomial outbreak demonstrated that subtype F dominated the early epidemic in adults in Romania in the late 1980s, when HIV prevalence was extremely low.

Russia

In 1988, an HIV-1 epidemic outbreak occurred in two hospitals in Elista in the Kalmyk Republic, Russia, involving 90 children who had been hospitalized repeatedly and received i.v. and i.m. injections with unsterile needles and syringes.[92] Transmission of HIV was maintained for several months by the use of unsterile syringes. Testing more than 80 000 persons in the Kalmyk Republic failed to reveal any HIV infections, other than ones related to the nosocomial epidemic.[92] Several months after the Elista outbreak, a similar outbreak occurred in children hospitalized in Rostov-on-Don, Russia, probably as a result of admitting children from Elista.[92,93] In Rostov-on-Don, eight adults were infected during the outbreak: seven women who contracted infection from their children, through breast-feeding and one man was infected in the infectious diseases ward of one of the hospitals.[92]

Molecular characterization of virus strains involved in these two epidemics showed that the two outbreaks were produced by very similar variants of a subtype G strain.[93,94] The average interpersonal variation between nucleotide sequences of HIV strains from patients from Elista and Rostov were 5.9% and 6.6%, respectively, values which are within the range of intrapatient variation. The virus from one of the mothers infected through breast-feeding matched that of her daughter.[94,95] Altogether, these data show that the two epidemics shared a common source. Further evolution of the HIV-1 epidemic in Russia switched the diversity pattern: with the advent of an increasing number of cases in intravenous drug users, with a subtype A strain entering from Ukraine and spreading in Russia and neighboring countries.[96-99] There are currently three viral forms involved in the Russian epidemic: subtype A, subtype B, and the CRF_03 A/B recombinant.[99-102]

Libya

In 1999, a cluster of 402 HIV-1-infected children was identified in Libya. An epidemiological investigation revealed that all these children had been admitted at least once in the Al-Fateh Pediatric Hospital in Benghazi during 1998–1999. The mean number of visits was 2.14 (range 1–4 visits) for outpatients and 1.56 visits (range 1–6 visits) for hospitalized patients.[103] During the hospitalization, children had received intravenous fluids, injectable antibiotics, steroids and/or bronchodilatators. Vaccination history was investigated in a subset of these children and documented for all of them; 83% had been vaccinated against HBV during the first 6 months of life. None of these children received any blood transfusion or blood derived products. Their mothers were tested and 19 of them (4.7%) were also found to be seropositive. None of the fathers tested positive. None of the infected mothers reported antecedents of hospitalization or intravenous infusions. All of the 19 HIV-1-infected mothers breast-fed their children at the time of hospital admission. The children were reported to be co-infected with hepatitis C virus (46%) and HBV (56%). Some 22% of them were co-infected with the three viruses.[103]

Two independent studies investigated the viral diversity of the HIV-1 strains involved in this epidemic. Both reported that the outbreak was produced by a monophyletic cluster of strains belonging to the Circulating Recombinant Form 02 A/G (IbNg).[103,104] There was very low strain divergence (0–2.4%) pointing to a single introduction of a nosocomial strain in most of the cases. In a more recent study, a child receiving a transfusion in 1997 was also reported to harbor a CRF_02 strain, though more divergent than those reported from the Al-Fateh cluster, thus pointing to a potential origin of the virus in the transfusion network. Although at the time of this outbreak official reports listed only 10 cases of HIV-1 infection in Libya, unofficial data suggested that the prevalence was significantly higher. It is considered that the CRF_02 strain had been introduced to Libya during the last 10 years through immigrants from Central Africa, and thereafter spread in individual cases by sexual transmission or by contaminated blood transfusion.[104]

There are two distinguishing aspects of this epidemic: first, as in Elista, it was reported that breast-feeding of a nosocomially infected child may infect mothers; second (and different from the epidemics in Romania and Russia), the Libyan epidemic included secondary nosocomials infection of nurses acquired from children – reporting for the first time that at least two of the nurses of the Al-Fateh were seropositive with the same HIV strains as the pediatric cluster. In 2004, as this history came to light, Libya brought criminal charges against foreign health personnel working in these institutions at the time, at first even calling for the death penalty as punishment for negligence.

These three national cases show several important features common to nosocomial outbreaks of HIV:

1. In instances where rigorous public health standards and procedures are not followed, explosive nosocomial outbreaks may emerge. Blood or blood products were involved in all three outbreaks, demonstrating that a national strategy should always include blood testing, even if the prevalence of HIV infection is very low, as it was at the outset in these countries.

2. All three cases involved children, a consequence of the fact that young children are more susceptible to diseases and require more frequent hospitalization. In Romania 10 000 children were infected, i.e. >50% of all the pediatric AIDS cases reported in Europe since the beginning of pandemic were nosocomially produced in <1 year.

3. The breakdown in standard sterile procedures also exposes the medical staff to the risk of infection. i.e. poor patient procedures correlate with high occupational risk from needlesticks. Disposable devices are very useful, but without education and training of the medical staff, nosocomial epidemics cannot be controlled.

Since these outbreaks occurred in countries in which the existence of AIDS at the time was officially denied, nosocomial epidemics also demonstrate that prevention of iatrogenic spread of HIV is subject to official acknowledgement of the problem and public attitudes and awareness of AIDS risks, especially among medical professionals and healthcare workers.

Conclusion

As we know from the many inadequacies in the global response to AIDS, even widespread recognition of a problem is not the same thing as its solution. The role of unsterile injections as a powerful vector for transmission of blood-borne pathogens and their important role in the global epidemiology of many infectious diseases is now well recognized.[105] But, despite this awareness, the problem may have grown even worse in the contemporary scene.

More than 30 billion needles and syringes are now manufactured annually worldwide and about one-third of these are employed in the developing world. Thus 75% of the world's population uses only one-third of the world's needles. But far greater demand (due to the higher burden of disease in poor countries) and easy access to injections outside the medical sector virtually assures continued unsterile use. It is predictable therefore, that injections will continue to play a significant role in transmission of blood-borne pathogens in developing countries. For example, in early 2005, India reported that over 60% of injections in that country were unsterile.[106] As a consequence, there have been frequent outbreaks of hepatitis B.[107,108]

Despite widespread awareness of the risks of unsterile injecting, antedating the beginning of AIDS in the 1980s, there remains a huge discrepancy between the supply of sterile injecting equipment and global demand. There has been some attempt to introduce safer injecting equipment in immunization programs. However, each year over 800 million doses of vaccine are distributed by WHO and immunization guidelines (as recently as 1997) still proposed up to 200 re-uses of (re-sterilized) plastic syringes, despite the common lack of adequate facilities for such sterilization throughout the developing world.[109]

The economic dimension is also crucial to understanding the continued problem of unsterile medical injections in the developing world. The costs of injecting equipment and the technical support infrastructure needed for sterile injecting and safe disposal are not readily available to accompany this technology. These costs, while modest by developed world standards (e.g. injecting equipment represents <0.1% of the healthcare budget of the USA), are quite substantial for developing societies and represent a very significant expense relative to their total health budgets. And while most of the world's people do not have ready access to modern healthcare services (the best guarantor of safe injections), they do have ready access to injectable drugs, both legal and illegal. A steady stream of inexpensive injectable medications are available throughout the markets of the developing world without prescription or involvement of a health professional, where drugs that are often outdated or poorly manufactured are injected with discarded (or recycled) syringes and needles.[4,30,31]

Meanwhile the intravenous use of illicit drugs is burgeoning worldwide – responsible for igniting explosive AIDS epidemic outbreaks in many regions of the developing world and countries of Eastern Europe and the former Soviet Union.[50,51,110] Even as the problem of i.v. drug use and addiction worsens, current UN drug control policies (under the strong influence of the USA and its 'war on drugs') continue to oppose 'harm reduction' programs and syringe distribution for IVDUs.[111,112] Also, while there are some needle exchange and harm reduction programs for heroin injectors in Asia and the former USSR and a number of advocacy organizations to advance

these programs (e.g. the Center for Harm Reduction in Melbourne, the Asian Harm Reduction Network in Changmai, and the Open Society Institute's International Harm Reduction Development Program), current services are grossly inadequate for the scale of the problems. While the need to focus on this vector as a significant part of AIDS control strategies is obvious, it is still largely unmet.

Finally, in addition to the role that unsterile injecting and transfusions play in the spread of infectious diseases worldwide, they may also play an important role in the creation and emergence of new human viral pathogens. There is a growing body of evidence that unsterile injecting fosters the creation of new pathogens via the mechanisms of recombination and serial passage. It has been theorized that the massive increase in unsterile injecting and transfusions in Africa in the 1950s is the biological 'event' that allowed several weakly pathogenic simian viruses native to sub-Saharan Africa to increase in pathogenicity and complete their genetic adaptation to human hosts, emerging as epidemic strains of HIV-1 and HIV-2.[113–115] Humans who hunt and butcher monkeys are routinely exposed to simian viruses. Serial passage by unsterile injecting and transfusions may have allowed these viruses to better adapt to new human hosts species, providing a plausible and parsimonious explanation of the almost simultaneous appearance of two distinct epidemic strains of HIV in separate parts of Africa in rapid succession in the late 1950s. If this theory is correct, continued massive unsterile injecting (in addition to spreading existing blood-borne viruses) can work to significantly alter the global ecology of infectious diseases by creating new viruses.

If we are to avoid these problems, it is critical that we take measures to curtail unsterile injecting worldwide. The great challenge facing public health is to limit the current damages due to unsterile injecting (an inherently dangerous technology outside the bounds of well controlled medical practice) without losing the many benefits of the medications and immunizations that are currently the principal basis for medical injections. As soon as possible, we must replace injectable drugs with new forms of drugs that do not rely on injections, using new delivery systems that allow their safer administration, e.g. via the development and utilization of technical innovations such as pre-packed unit doses, affordable oral forms of medication, transdermal patches, and implants. Every year we fail to act in this area, drives us deeper into the troubled seas of uncontrolled epidemics of infectious diseases and risks the creation of new pathogens based on the large-scale passage of contaminated blood from person-to-person – a problem new to the human species.

Acknowledgments

Thanks to Emily Meyer for editorial assistance and Sol Levinson for advice and data on the history of injecting equipment. P.A.M. and C.A. were supported by a grant from the National Institutes of Health (AI44596), R.H. by grants from NIH(NIDA R01-DA-09945 and NIMH P30-MH-62294), and E.D. acknowledges the support of The Open Society Institute.

References

1. Frank C, Mohamed MK, Strickland GT, et al. The role of parenteral antischistosomal therapy in the spread of hepatitis C virus in Egypt. Lancet 2000; 355:887–891.
2. Helpern M. An epidemic of aestivo-autumnal and Quartan malaria among drug addicts in New York City transmitted by the use of contaminated hypodermic syringes. Publ Health Rpts 1934; 49:421–423.
3. Friedland GH, Harris C, Butkus-Small C, et al. Intravenous drug abusers and the acquired immunodeficiency syndrome (AIDS). Demographic, drug use, and needle-sharing patterns. Arch Int Med 1985; 145:1413–1417.
4. Drucker E, Alcabes PG, Marx PA. The injection century: massive unsterile injections and the emergence of human pathogens. Lancet 2001; 358:1989–1992.
5. The Echo. Franklin Lakes, NJ: Becton-Dickinson Corp; 1991; 11:1.
6. The Echo. Franklin Lakes, NJ: Becton-Dickinson Corp; 1991; 11:2.
7. The Echo. Franklin Lakes, NJ: Becton-Dickinson Corp; 1991; 11:3.
8. Frost and Sullivan Corp. US disposable needles, syringes, and related products mkt. New York: Frost and Sullivan; 1996.
9. Hayward EG. Penicillin and other antibiotics. Chemurgic Papers, No 13. New York: National Farm Chemurgic Council; 1949.
10. Hewitt WL. Penicillin: historical impact on infection control. Ann NY Acad Sci 1967; 145:212–215.
11. Cardo DM, Bell DM. Bloodborne pathogen transmission in health care workers: risks and prevention strategies. Infect Dis Clin N Am 1997; 25:144–154.
12. Hauri A, Armstrong G, Hutin Y. The global burden of disease attributable to contaminated healthcare equipment. Int J STD AIDS 2004; 15:7–16.
13. WHO. Unsafe injections practices and transmission of bloodborne pathogens. Bull WHO 1999; 77:787–819.
14. Short LJ, Bell DM. Risk of occupational infection with blood-borne pathogens in operating and delivery room settings. Am J Infect Control 1993; 21:343–350.
15. Abdala N, Stephens PC, Griffith BP, et al. Survival of human immunodeficiency virus type 1 in syringes. J Acquir Immune Defic Syndr Hum Retrovir 1999; 20:73–80.
16. Abdala N, Reyes R, Carney JM, et al. Survival of HIV-1 in syringes: Effects of temperature during storage. Subst Use Misuse 2000; 35:1–19.
17. Kaplan EH, Heimer R. A model-based estimate of HIV infectivity via needle sharing. J Acquir Immune Defic Syndr 1992; 5:1116–1118.
18. Hudgens MGIM, Longini ME, Halloran K, et al. Estimating the transmission probability of human immunodeficiency virus in injecting drug users in Thailand. J R Stat Soc Appl Stat 2001; 50(Part 1):1–14.
19. Rich JD, Dickinson BP, Carney JM, et al. The presence of HIV antibodies and absence of HIV DNA in syringes used for non-intravenous injection. AIDS 1998; 12:2345–2350.
20. Whyte SR, Geest S van der. Injections: issues and methods for anthropological research. In: Etkin NL, Tan ML, eds. Medicines: Meanings and context. Quezon City: HAIN; 1994.
21. CIBA. Health and disease in tribal societies, CIBA Foundation Symposium No. 49. Oxford: Elsevier; 1977.
22. Baily H (ed.). Pye's surgical handicraft, Vol. 1. Bristol: Wright; 1962.
23. Wyatt HV. The popularity of injections in the Third World: origins and consequences for poliomyelitis. Soc Sci Med 1984; 19:911–915.
24. Reeler AV. Injections: A fatal attraction. Soc Sci Med 1990; 31:1119–1125.
25. Simonsen L, Kane A, Lloyd J, et al. Unsafe injections in the developing world and transmission of blood borne pathogens: a review. Bull World Health Organ 1999; 77:789–800.
26. Huytin YJ, Hauri AM, Armstrong GL. Use of injections in health care settings worldwide, 2000: literature review and regional estimates. Br Med J 2003; 327:1075.
27. WHO. World Health Report 2004.
28. PHR White paper. HIV Transmission in health care settings. Cambridge, MA: Physicians for Human Rights; 2004.
29. Frank C, Mohamed MK, Strickland GT, Lavanchy D, Arthur RR, Magder LS, et al. The role of parenteral antischistosmal therapy in the spread of hepatitis C virus in Egypt. Lancet 2000; 355:887–891.
30. Madhava V, Burgess C, Drucker E. Epidemiology of chronic of hepatitis C virus infection in sub-Saharan Africa. Lancet Infect Dis 2002; 2:293–302.
31. Kermode MA. Safer Injections, fewer injections: management of needles and sharps and occupational blood exposure in rural north Indian health settings. Unpublished. PhD Dissertation, Deakin Univeristy; 2003.
32. Oliver R, Atmore A. Africa since 1800. 2nd edn. Cambridge: Cambridge University Press; 1977.
33. Alland A. Adaptation in cultural evolution: an approach to medical anthropology. NY: Columbia University; 1970.
34. Hochschild A. King Leopold's ghost. New York: Houghton Mifflin; 1998.
35. Birungi H, Asiimwe D, Whyte SR. Injection use and practices in Uganda. Geneva: WHO Action Program on Essential Drugs; 1994.
36. Whyte SR. Penicillin, battery acid and sacrifice: Cures and causes in Nyole medicine. Soc Sci Med 1982; 16:2055–2056.
37. Gumodoka B, Vos J, Berge ZA, et al. Injection practices in Mwanza region, Tanzania: prescriptions, patient demand and sterility. Trop Med Int Health 1996; 1:874–880.
38. van der Geest S. The illegal distribution of Western medicines in developing countries: pharmacists, drug peddlers, injection doctors and others: a bibliographic exploration. Med Anthrop 1982; 6:197–219.
39. Miller HM, Singh RN. Urbanization during the postcolonial days. In: Tarver JD, ed. Urbanization in Africa. Westport: Greenwood Press; 1994.
40. Hendrick R. Colonialism, health and illness in French Equatorial Africa (1885–1935). Atlanta: African Studies Association Press; 1994.
41. Quataert J, Liu TP, Hunt NR, et al. (eds). Gendered colonialisms in African history. Oxford: Blackwell; 1997.
42. UNICEF. UNICEF in Africa South of the Sahara: A historical perspective. Geneva: UNICEF; 1987.
43. Yamousssoukro Declaration, 1994. WHO/ EPI Update No. 27 94/10283.
44. Schneider WH, Drucker E. Blood transfusions in the early years of AIDS in sub-Saharan Africa. Am J Publ Health 2006; 96:984–994.
45. Brewer D, Brody S, Drucker E, et al. Mounting anomalies in the epidemiology of HIV in Africa: Cry the Beloved Paradigm. Int J STD AIDS 2003; 14:144–147.

46. Lopman BA, et al. Individual level injection history: a lack of association with HIV incidence in rural Zimbabwe. PLoS Med 2005; 2:143–145.

47. Drucker E, Nadelmann E, Newman RG, et al. Harm reduction: pragmatic drug policies for public health and safety. In: Lowinson J, Ruiz P, Millman R, Langrod J, eds. Substance abuse: A comprehensive textbook. Hagerstown, MD: Lippincott Williams and Wilkins; 2004.

48. Drucker E, Lurie P, Alcabes P, et al. Measuring harm reduction: the effects of needle and syringe exchange programs and methadone maintenance on the ecology of HIV. AIDS 1998; 12(Suppl A):S217–S230.

49. Stimson VG. The global diffusion of injecting drug use: implications for human immunodeficiency virus infection. Bull Narcotics 1993; 45:3–17.

50. Des Jarlais DC, Friedman SR, Choopanya K, et al. International epidemiology of HIV and AIDS among injecting drug users. AIDS 1992; 6:1053–1068.

51. Garfein RS, Vlahov D, Galai N, et al. Viral infections in short-term injection drug users: the prevalence of the hepatitis C, hepatitis B, human immunodeficiency, and human T-lymphotropic viruses. Am J Publ Health 1996; 85:655–661.

52. van Beek I, Dwyer R, Dore GJ, et al. Infection with HIV and hepatitis C virus among injecting drug users in a prevention setting: retrospective cohort study. Br Med J 1998; 317:433–437.

53. Heimer R, Myers SS, Cadman EC, et al. Detection by polymerase chain reaction of Human Immunodeficiency Virus type 1 proviral DNA sequences in needles of injecting drug users. J Infect Dis 1992; 165:781–782.

54. Guydish J, Clark G, Garcia D, et al. Detecting HIV antibodies in needle exchange syringes. VIIth International Conference on AIDS, Florence: 1991.

55. Clatts MC, Heimer R, Abdala N, et al. Illicit drug injection and HIV-1 transmission: heating drug solutions may inactive HIV-1. J Aquir Immune Defic Syndr 1999; 22:194–199.

56. Ciccarone D, Bourgois P. Explaining the geographical variation of HIV among injection drug users in the United States. Subst Use Misuse 2003; 38:2049–2063.

57. Kral AH, Bluthenthal RN, Booth RE, et al. HIV seroprevalence among street-recruited injection drug and crack cocaine users in 16 US municipalities. Am J Publ Health 1998; 88:108–113.

58. Beckerleg S, Telfer M, Hundt GL. The rise of injecting drug use in East Africa: A case study from Kenya. Harm Reduct J 2005; 2:12.

59. Aceijas C, Stimson GV, HIckman M, Rhodes T. Global overview of injecting drug use and HIV infection among injecting drug users. United Nations Reference Group on HIV/AIDS Prevention and Care among IDU in Developing and Transitional Countries. AIDS 2004; 18(17):2295–2303.

60. Des Jarlais DC, Hagan H, Friedman S. HIV Infection and AIDS: Epidemiology and emerging public health perspectives. In: Lowinson J, Ruiz P, Millman R, Langrod J, eds. Substance abuse: a comprehensive textbook. Hagerstown, MD: Lippincott Williams and Wilkins; 2004.

61. Anon. Acquired Immunodeficiency Syndrome (AIDS): data at 31 December 1989. Wkly Epid Rec 1990; 65:1–2.

62. Anon. Acquired Immunodeficiency Syndrome: Romania. Wkly Epid Rec 1990; 65:56–57.

63. SIDA. Situation de la region Europeene de l'OMS au 31 mars 1990 et analyse des cas transfusionnels au 31 decembre 1989. Rel Epidemiol Hebd 1990; 65:239–242.

64. Hersh BS, Popovici F, Apetrei RC, et al. Acquired immunodeficiency syndrome in Romania. Lancet 1991; 338:645–649.

65. Hersh BS, Popovici F, Zolotusca L, et al. The epidemiology of HIV and AIDS in Romania. AIDS 1991; 5(Suppl 2): S87–S92.

66. Anon. AIDS surveillance in Europe. Paris: European Centre for the Epidemiological Monitoring of AIDS; 1995.

67. Apetrei C, Buzdugan I, Mitroi I, et al. Nosocomial HIV-1 transmission and primary prevention in Romania. Lancet 1994; 344:1028–1029.

68. Zaknun D, DiFranco M, Oswald HP, et al. Association between neopterin and beta-2-microglobulin levels and HIV status in Romanian orphanage children. Wien Klin Wochenschr 1993; 105:284–288.

69. Patrascu IV, Dumitrescu O. The epidemic of human immunodeficiency virus infection in Romanian children. AIDS Res Hum Retroviruses 1993; 9:99–104.

70. Rudin C, Berger R, Tobler R, et al. HIV-1, hepatitis (A, B, and C), and measles in Romanian children. Lancet 1990; 336:1592–1593.

71. Di Franco MJ, Zaknun D, Zaknun J, et al. A prospective study of the association of serum neopterin, beta 2-microglobulin, and hepatitis B surface antigenemia with death in infants and children with HIV-1 disease. J Acquir Immune Defic Syndr 1994; 7:1079–1085.

72. Hersh BS, Popovici F, Jezek Z, et al. Risk factors for HIV infection among abandoned Romanian children. AIDS 1993; 7:1617–1624.

73. Patrascu IV, Constantinescu SN, Dublanchet A. HIV-1 infection in Romanian children. Lancet 1990; 335:672.

74. Scarlatti G. Mother-to-child transmission of HIV-1: advances and controversies of the twentieth centuries. AIDS Rev 2004; 6:67–78.

75. Mofenson LM. Advances in the prevention of vertical transmission of human immunodeficiency virus. Semin Pediatr Infect Dis 2003; 14:295–308.

76. Rousseau CM, Nduati RW, Richardson BA, et al. Association of levels of HIV-1-infected breast milk cells and risk of mother-to-child transmission. J Infect Dis 2004; 190:1880–1888.

77. Apetrei RC. Children with AIDS. World Health Forum 1990; 11:199.

78. Berkley S. Parenteral transmission of HIV in Africa. AIDS 1991; 5(Suppl 1):S87–S92.

79. Werner BG, Grady GF. Accidental hepatitis-B-surface-antigen-positive inoculations. Use of e antigen to estimate infectivity. Ann Intern Med 1982; 97:367–369.

80. Seeff LB, Wright EC, Zimmerman HJ, et al. Type B hepatitis after needle-stick exposure: prevention with hepatitis B immune globulin. First report of the Veterans Administration Cooperative Study. Ann Intern Med 1978; 88:285–293.

81. Apetrei C, Descamps D, Panzaru C, et al. Plasma HIV-1 load and nosocomial transmission in Romanian children. AIDS 1995; 9:977.

82. Dumitrescu O, Kalish ML, Kliks SC, et al. Characterization of human immunodeficiency virus type 1 isolates from children in Romania: identification of a new envelope subtype. J Infect Dis 1994; 169:281–288.

83. Holm-Hansen C, Grothues D, Rustad S, et al. Characterization of HIV type 1 from Romanian children: lack of correlation between V3 loop amino acid sequence and syncytium formation in MT-2 cells. AIDS Res Hum Retroviruses 1995; 11:597–603.

84. Apetrei C, Loussert-Ajaka I, Collin G, et al. HIV type 1 subtype F sequences in Romanian children and adults. AIDS Res Hum Retroviruses 1997; 13:363–365.

85. Bandea CI, Ramos A, Pieniazek D, et al. Epidemiologic and evolutionary relationships between Romanian and Brazilian HIV-subtype F strains. Emerg Infect Dis 1995; 1:91–93.

86. Peeters M, Sharp PM. Genetic diversity of HIV-1: the moving target. AIDS 2000; 14(Suppl 3):S129–S140.

87. McCutchan FE. Understanding the genetic diversity of HIV-1. AIDS 2000; 14(Suppl 3):S31–S44.

88. Triques K, Bourgeois A, Saragosti S, et al. High diversity of HIV-1 subtype F strains in Central Africa. Virology 1999; 259:99–109.

89. Apetrei C, Descamps D, Collin G, et al. HIV type 1 diversity in northeastern Romania in 200-2001 based on phylogenic analysis of pol sequences from patient failing antiretroviral therapy. AIDS Res Hum Retroviruses 2003; 19:1155–1161.

90. Reinis M, Bruckova M, Graham RR, et al. Genetic subtypes of HIV type 1 viruses circulating in the Czech Republic. AIDS Res Hum Retroviruses 2001; 17:1305–1310.

91. Apetrei C, Necula A, Holm-Hansen C, et al. HIV-1 diversity in Romania. AIDS 1998; 12:1079–1085.

92. Pokrovskii VV, Eramova I, Deulina MO, et al. [An intrahospital outbreak of HIV infection in Elista]. Zh Mikrobiol Epidemiol Immunobiol 1990; April:17–23.

93. Bobkov A, Cheingsong-Popov R, Garaev M, et al. Identification of an env G subtype and heterogeneity of HIV-1 strains in the Russian Federation and Belarus. AIDS 1994; 8:1649–1655.

94. Bobkov A, Cheingsong-Popov R, Karasyova N, et al. Sequence analysis of the glycoprotein 120 coding region of a new human immunodeficiency virus type 1 subtype G strain from Russia. AIDS Res Hum Retroviruses 1996; 12:1385–1388.

95. Pokrovskii VV, Eramov I, Kuznetsova II, et al. [HIV transmission from child to mother during breast feeding]. Zh Mikrobiol Epidemiol Immunobiol 1990; March:23–26.

96. Bobkov A, Cheingsong-Popov R, Selimova L, et al. Genetic heterogeneity of HIV type 1 in Russia: identification of H variants and relationship with epidemiological data. AIDS Res Hum Retroviruses 1996; 12:1687–1690.

97. Bobkov A, Cheingsong-Popov R, Selimova L, et al. An HIV type 1 epidemic among injecting drug users in the former Soviet Union caused by a homogeneous subtype A strain. AIDS Res Hum Retroviruses 1997; 13:1195–1201.

98. Bobkov A, Cheingsong-Popov R, Selimova L, et al. HIV type 1 subtype E in Russia. AIDS Res Hum Retroviruses 1997; 13:725–727.

99. Bobkov A, Kazennova E, Selimova L, et al. A sudden epidemic of HIV type 1 among injecting drug users in the former Soviet Union: identification of subtype A, subtype B, and novel gagA/envB recombinants. AIDS Res Hum Retroviruses 1998; 14:669–676.

100. Bobkov A, Kazennova E, Selimova L, et al. HIV type 1 gag D/env G recombinants in Russia. AIDS Res Hum Retroviruses 1998; 14:1597–1599.

101. Bobkov A, Kazennova E, Khanina T, et al. An HIV type 1 subtype A strain of low genetic diversity continues to spread among injecting drug users in Russia: study of the new local outbreaks in Moscow and Irkutsk. AIDS Res Hum Retroviruses 2001; 17:257–261.

102. Liitsola K, Holm K, Bobkov A, et al. An AB recombinant and its parental HIV type 1 strains in the area of the former Soviet Union: low requirements for sequence identity in recombination. UNAIDS Virus Isolation Network. AIDS Res Hum Retroviruses 2000; 16:1047–1053.

103. Yerly S, Quadri R, Negro F, et al. Nosocomial outbreak of multiple bloodborne viral infections. J Infect Dis 2001; 184:369–372.

104. Visco-Comandini U, Cappiello G, Liuzzi G, et al. Monophyletic HIV type 1 CRF02-AG in a nosocomial outbreak in Benghazi, Libya. AIDS Res Hum Retroviruses 2002; 18:727–732.

105. Huytin Y. The safe injecting global network. Geneva: WHO; 2001.

106. Arora NK. Almost 63 percent of Indian injections unsafe. Report of All India Institute of Medical Sciences: Reported by Agence France Presse, 2005: (01.24.05).

107. Singh J, Gupta S, Khare S, Bhatia R, Jain DC, Sokhey J. A severe and explosive outbreak of hepatitis B in a rural population in Sirsa district, Haryana, India: unnecessary therapeutic injections were a major risk factor. Epidemiology & Infection. 2000 Dec; 125(3):693–699.

108. Singh J, Bhatia R, Patnaik SK, Khare S, Bora D, Jain DC, Sokhey J. Community studies on hepatitis B in Rajahmundry town of Andhra Pradesh, India, 1997–8: unnecessary therapeutic injections are major risk factor. Epidemiology & Infection. 2000 Oct; 125(2):367–375.

109. WHO/UNICEF. Product information sheets: Global program for vaccine and immunization. Expanded program on immunization. Geneva: WHO; 1997.

110. Rhodes T. Special issue on HIV/AIDS and in Eastern Europe and USSR. Int J Drug Policy 2004; April.

111. Drucker E. Witch-hunt. Harm Reduct J 2005; 2:3.

112. Drucker E. Appendix: An open letter to the delegates of the 48th session of the UN Commission on Narcotic Drugs (CND). Harm Reduct J 2005; 2:3. Online. Available: www.harmreductionjournal.com/content/2/1/3

113. Marx PA, Alcabes PG, Drucker E. Serial human passage of simian immune virus by unsterile injecting and the emergence of epidemic HIV in Africa. Philos Trans R Soc Lond B Biol Sci 2001; 356:911–920.

114. Weiss R (ed.). The origins of HIV and the AIDS epidemic. London: The Royal Society; 2001.

115. Marx PA, Apetrie C, Drucker E. AIDS as a Zoonosis? Confusion over the origin of the virus and the origin of the epidemic. J Med Primatol 2004; 33:220–226.

CHAPTER 68

The Economic Impact of HIV/AIDS in Developing Countries: Systematic Under-estimation

Jean-Paul Moatti

Bruno Ventelou

Introduction

This is the third decade of the global HIV/AIDS pandemic. The magnitude and long-term nature of the pandemic and its severe impact on societies and economies are indisputable. In many developing countries and a growing number of countries in 'transition' of Eastern Europe, the epidemic is now generalized with seroprevalence rates already exceeding 1% of the adult population. Adult HIV/AIDS prevalence rates of 10–20% are common in many African countries, and Botswana, Lesotho and Swaziland are close to 40%. Such figures signify the epidemic is affecting each and every rural and urban household. As the World Bank put it, 'AIDS has already reversed 30 years of hard-won social progress in some countries'.[1] It is now at the very center of a global 'development crisis,' and one that is hitting the world's poorest countries the hardest.

However, public health experts as well as economists themselves, share a common dissatisfaction towards previous economic analyses of the impacts of HIV/AIDS. These analyses are increasingly viewed as only reflecting a limited part of the picture, as underestimating the actual impact of the epidemic on economic and human development, consequently leads to a systematic under-investment in the national and international resources that are devoted to the fight against the epidemic. A growing body of evidence now allows the promoting of a better understanding of the full economic and societal dimensions of the epidemic that urgently needs to inform public policies at both national and international levels.

Within the global pandemic of HIV infection, there are many different epidemics, each with its own dynamics and each influenced by many factors including time of introduction of the virus, population density, and cultural and social issues. Within each region, the HIV epidemic also consists of a multitude of smaller ongoing epidemics, which although related, pursue their own course with different velocities. Spread of the epidemic has varied considerably between developed and developing countries, depending on the existing cultural social and behavioral patterns as well as on the risk environment. This latter concept, recently introduced by some social scientists,[2] puts the emphasis on the economic and social characteristics that make individuals and groups more or less vulnerable to the risk of contracting the virus. Higher educational attainment and social status, because they provide greater economic resources, which may facilitate behaviors and opportunities that put individuals at greater risk,[3,4] were often associated with a greater risk of HIV infection in Africa at the early phases of diffusion of the epidemic.[5] The recent pattern of new infections is however changing towards a greater burden among the less educated and poorest groups. There is increasing evidence that HIV/AIDS spreads more rapidly where there is poverty, grossly unequal distribution of income and wealth, unequal gender relations, unsustainable livelihoods, large-scale population movement, and civil disorder.[6] It is now certain that poverty contributes to HIV/AIDS epidemics and that AIDS contributes to poverty although we still do not know enough about the complex pathways of this relationship.[7] Because of this multifaceted aspect of the HIV epidemic, its economic impact may indeed vary depending on prevalence rates but also with each country's level of development, dynamic of economic growth, and many other social and institutional characteristics.

Until recently, economic research on HIV/AIDS had failed to capture many important aspects of its impact on development because it *de facto* considered the disease as a sharp exogenous shock on the economy. Indeed, the epidemic installs a continuum between a sharp short-term shock and long-term structural changes that in the absence of an appropriate response, will jeopardize the whole process of development. It is a long wave event which is superimposed on other long wave trends which already affect development, like endemic poverty, poor governance, and market and public sector failures to provide basic services in Africa and other regions, as well as the social costs of rapid transition to market economies and industrialization in many others,. The combination of these long-term trends often creates dramatic short-term situations, as illustrated by the way the HIV/AIDS epidemic fuels the current famines and food crisis in Southern Africa by having increased the vulnerability of small-scale farmers to production shocks.[8,9]

The Demographic Impact: A Public Health Catastrophe

The most obvious impact of the epidemic is on demography. Through its direct contribution to the global burden of disease,[10] as well as its strong link with the burgeoning of other infectious diseases like tuberculosis,[11,12] HIV/AIDS has put paid to the optimistic views of the early 1990s about the 'epidemiologic transition.' Such transition predicted that communicable diseases would account for only a minor part of morbidity and mortality in developing countries, as chronic diseases become more pronounced at the beginning of the twenty-first century.[13]

There is no doubt that the most direct demographic consequence of AIDS is an increase in mor-

tality.[14] AIDS has been shown to be the leading cause of adult death in Abidjan, Kinshasa, and rural communities in Uganda and Tanzania.[15] In two community-based rural studies in Mosaka and Rakai districts of Uganda, mortality among HIV-infected adults was over 130 per 1000 person-years of observation, an order of magnitude 19 times higher than among adults not infected with HIV.[16] In South Africa, without interventions to reduce HIV-related mortality, it can be predicted that by the year 2010, AIDS deaths will account for double all other causes of death combined.[17]

Hardest hit by excess HIV-related deaths are those aged 25–45 years, usually a group with low mortality. In addition, mother-to-child transmission means that HIV increases infant and more particularly child mortality: when corrected for competing causes of mortality, HIV infection caused 7.7% of under-5 deaths in sub-Saharan Africa in 1999, a significant rise from 2% in 1990. In addition, 21 out of the 39 countries of the region had HIV-specific under-5 mortality rates >10 per 1000.[18]

Because AIDS deaths are concentrated in childhood and young adulthood, their effects on life expectancy have already been substantial. Life expectancy at birth is currently 3 to >15 years lower in 16 African countries compared with the 1970–1975 period.[19] Population projections suggest that AIDS mortality will lead to further declines in a growing number of countries.[20–22] In addition, AIDS impacts population size and growth rates through the related decline in fertility rates. Although no negative population growth has been yet documented due to the HIV/AIDS epidemic, figures suggest that population growth may indeed turn negative in future for some African countries or regions.[23,24]

The Economic Impact: Contradictory Evidence?

The economic consequences of these major demographic changes related to AIDS have remained rather uncertain.[25] The current evidence on the implications of HIV/AIDS on the economy has been based on three different approaches the results of which may seem quite contradictory.

Micro-studies

Micro-studies have often described huge negative consequences of the epidemic on a certain social structure or on specific agents typically private firms, households, orphans, women, communities, etc.

A recent review of the published literature about the impact of HIV/AIDS on households identified a total of 28 studies in developing countries, mostly in Africa but also in Haiti, India, the Philippines, Sri Lanka, and Thailand.[26] Most of these studies focus on 'affected households,' i.e. households that experience illness or death of one (or more) of their members due to HIV/AIDS, and on the impact of illness and death on household finances. These impacts commonly include 'direct costs' due to medical and funeral expenditures, and 'indirect costs' due to the impact of the illness on productivity.[27,28]

In low- and middle-income countries, out-of-pocket spending represents a large share of health expenditures even in countries with well-functioning public health delivery systems. In low income countries, on average 4.0% of GDP is spent on health; 2.8% from public spending and 1.2% from private sources, but these figures are, respectively 1.5% public and 1.8% private in Africa. Therefore, health costs can represent a significant proportion of the affected households' income: in a survey carried out in South Africa, the households with at least one HIV-infected member spent on average one-third of their income on medical related expenses, whereas the national average household expenditure on healthcare was only 4% per year.[29] Deaths are also costly; the funeral rites can last for several days, necessitating *de facto* a prolonged interruption of work for the entire family concerned.* In some studies in Africa, the cost of a funeral may represent four times the total monthly household income. In a longitudinal community study in a rural area in north-west Tanzania, expenditures associated with AIDS terminal illness were higher than for other causes of death, direct medical costs were about 1.5 times higher than the funeral costs, and the sum of both costs exceeded the estimated annual household income *per capita* in this population.[30] In addition, a person who develops AIDS experiences a reduction in his productive capacity, as he regularly falls ill. The reduction in his work capacity signifies a reduction in household resources. In a survey carried out in Côte d'Ivoire among a sample of HIV-infected

patients aware of their serostatus and consulting for HIV care, 30% had lost their job since their HIV diagnosis and 81% had no health insurance coverage.[31] In the study from South Africa already mentioned, two-thirds of the affected households experienced a fall in their income, and in 40% of households, caregivers had to take time off from work and other income-generating activities or school. HIV/AIDS does not only push poor households deeper into poverty, it also pushes households that were relatively wealthy into poverty: that was the case in Zambia in two-thirds of the affected households, because monthly disposable income fell by >80% when the father died due to AIDS.

Unfortunately, it is also widely acknowledged that HIV/AIDS has a devastating impact on children. According to UNICEF,[32] 13.4 million children already have lost one or both parents to AIDS, including 11 million in sub-Saharan Africa, half of whom are between the ages of 10 and 14. The projected total number of children orphaned by the disease will nearly double to 25 million by 2010. At that point, 15–25% of the children in a dozen sub-Saharan countries will be orphans, the vast majority of them having been orphaned by HIV/AIDS. Even in countries where HIV prevalence has stabilized or fallen, like Uganda, the numbers of orphans will stay high or rise as parents already infected continue to die from the disease.

Most African businesses that have more than 10 employees have already seen at least one employee dying of HIV/AIDS, or currently employ infected workers. HIV/AIDS has been shown to have a major impact on African business in terms of reduced labor supply, especially the loss of experienced workers in their most productive years, increased absenteeism, reduced profitability, loss of international competitiveness, and other financial impacts.[33,34] In both the public and private sector, the premature death of an employee leads to the disappearance of an experienced worker, and may represent a higher loss for the firm than the direct loss due to absenteeism.[35]

Sectorial Approaches

Sectorial approaches have tried to assess the global costs of the epidemic for a whole industry, such as mining, or the agriculture commercial sector, as well as for private and public delivery of certain services. As seen in the previous 'micro' approach, they have also documented significant economic losses due to HIV/AIDS in the studied sectors.

---

*Funeral costs do not refer to the amount of the funeral in itself: HIV/AIDS does not change this value. However, the implicit cost of HIV/AIDS relates on the one hand to the repetition of funeral costs or participation in funeral costs and on the other hand to the fact that the deceased passed away sooner than would have been probable in the absence of the epidemic: the sooner the death occurs, the less time to save for funeral costs, the bigger the relative funeral cost.

These sectorial approaches were often carried out in order to assess the potential benefits of alternative policies to mitigate this impact. Indeed, this impact may vary in different productive sectors mainly for two reasons. First, the rate of prevalence is different in each productive sector. Second, the incapacity due to AIDS varies according to the precise nature of the work.

The public sector, with its concentration of skilled workers, could be particularly affected, especially the education and health sectors. Education and the Millenium Goals' international effort to enrol all children in school by 2015 are being undermined, since teachers die of AIDS nearly as rapidly as nations can train them.[36] The impact on human resources is increasingly affecting the health sector, especially in low-income countries, where the rate per 100 000 population is lower than 10 for physicians and 100 for nurses. Existing healthcare systems are already overburdened by the HIV epidemic. In Côte d'Ivoire and Uganda, 50–80% of adult hospital beds are occupied by patients with HIV-related conditions. In Swaziland, the average length of stay in hospitals is 6.0 days, but increases to 30.4 days for patients with tuberculosis associated with HIV in 80% of cases.[37] In hospital services in Nairobi, Kenya, the impact of the escalating demand for HIV/AIDS-related care was accompanied by deteriorating conditions for both HIV-positive and HIV-negative patients and increased mortality during hospital stay in the two groups.[38]

Macro-models

Macro-models have tried to measure the overall impact of the epidemic on economic development. Contrary to the two previous approaches, early mac-roeconomic studies tended to conclude that the epidemic had quite a limited impact on macroeconomic growth, even in the most affected countries.

Different studies have been conducted to attempt to measure, in terms of GDP points lost, the macroeconomic consequences of HIV/AIDS. The first studies supplied quite comparable figures for the African economies (Table 68.1).[39] On average, the authors forecasted a 1-point reduction in the rate of growth of national wealth. An estimate of the impact on the national economy of India also gave a similar 1% reduction.[40] These studies were based on an *ad hoc* modelling of the economy which permits a comparative evolution to be derived, with or without the AIDS pandemic.

Why the Macroeconomic Impact has been Under-estimated

Even a loss of circa 1% growth matters in developing countries, who desperately need very high rates of growth to match international competition. However, when confronted with the microeconomic and sectorial impacts described above, the estimates look quite modest. Policy makers may believe that a 1% loss is similar to exogenous shocks, such as the economic consequences of the terrorist attacks in the USA on September 11, 2002, that are more or less easily absorbed by most countries. The reason why these estimations were modest is precisely that the models used considered AIDS as a traditional shock on labor supply.

These projections consider that HIV-related deaths tend to reduce both total income and the number of people this income must be divided between. The resultant smaller population tends to mean that there is more capital per worker for those

Table 68.1 Reduction in GDP attributable to HIV/AIDS

Country	Average reduction in GDP (in annual growth points)	Period	Sources/authors
30 sub-Saharan African countries	[0.8; 1.4]	1990–2025	Over (1992)
Cameroon	2	1987–1991	Kambou et al. (1992)
Zambia	[1; 2]	1993–2000	Forgy (1993)
Tanzania	[0.8; 1.4]	1991–2010	Cuddington (1992)
Kenya	1.5	1996–2005	Hancock et al. (1996)
Mozambique	1	1997–2020	Wils et al. (2001)

Source: Estimations collected by Touzé and Ventelou[39] using the quoted articles, the intervals relate to the size of the impact according to the scenarios studied.

that remain.[41] If a country loses 10% of its workforce in the short term, production and consequently GDP may decrease but in a more limited proportion (for example 5% or 8%), which means that mechanically GDP *per capita* will increase. Similarly, if there is scarcity of land or capital, the productivity per worker may increase as a result of the shock. Even if macroeconomic models predicted a decline in savings and investment, which will be partly due to reallocation of resources toward medical care for the HIV-infected, the negative impact on GDP growth was limited by this supposed countervailing effect of increased labor productivity*.[42]

This quite simplistic view of how the economy functions clearly ignores some phenomena that have been notably highlighted in the recent general economic literature. The so-called theory of endogenous growth[43,44] has identified important phenomena, which play a major role in the accomplishment of sustained high rates of economic growth. First, these important mechanisms concern the influence of information and subjective expectations on the individuals' long-term economic behaviors. Second, they also concern the 'complementarities' in the accumulation of the productive factors of the national economy, i.e. the interactions between the different forms of physical capital and human capital entering the production function.

As an example of the first types of 'endogenous growth' mechanisms regarding long-term trends in adaptive economic behaviors, one key element in the economic 'success stories' of some countries in East Asia has been their very high rates of savings and investment, often in excess of 30% of income being saved. It has been shown that this savings boom in East Asia is related to the rapid increase in life expectancy and is dependent on the working population being able to foresee their retirement and engaging in savings to pay for it.[45] The HIV/AIDS epidemic definitely alters these long-term economic behaviors in a number of ways that have hardly been quantified in previous studies.

Individuals who know their serostatus will not behave the same way as individuals who ignore it. Similarly, individuals who know they can be treated

are likely to make different economic decisions from individuals who ignore the existence of treatment or whose access to treatment has been denied. Beyond the immediate consequences of income loss and diversion of the remaining income to health expenditures, affected households may develop various 'coping' strategies to deal with the long-term persistence of the disease, including migration,[46] child labor, sale of assets, and use of savings. The coping strategy to face health expenditures could be punctually to sell assets, but the anticipation of future costs may lead to permanent restrictions in consumption in order to pay for those potential expenditures.

The long-term impact may also affect households who do not count any HIV-infected member. Non-directly affected households who provide care to a sick person or take care of the family of a deceased incur costs and experience interactions with HIV/AIDS related diseases, which may alter their visions of the future. It has been shown that families fostering children who lost their parents because of AIDS have a significant reduction of their consumption but also their capital accumulation.[47] New empirical evidence about the impact of being orphaned in the context of AIDS[48,49] also stresses the importance of taking into account a longer time horizon and the related evolution of economic behaviors to accurately measure impact. The reduction in children's human capital following the loss of parents' presence seems less due to the direct associated loss in income from parental deaths than a product of associated behavioral changes. In particular, the impact of orphanage on living arrangements and school enrolment seems to depend on the degree of relatedness of the orphans to the head of the household, which takes care of them after the death of their parents.[50,51]

Moreover, in countries where the epidemic is generalized and the impacts are publicly known, it is likely that a significant portion of the population will turn objective variables – such as life expectancy or future productivity – into subjective ones, due to the presence of HIV/AIDS in their environment. In South Africa, under highly plausible hypotheses about the way consumption decisions will be affected by the fall in the average national life expectancy due to HIV/AIDS, a microsimulation study revealed that the saving rate in 2015 would be at minimum 5% lower than the rate that would have prevailed in the absence of the epidemic.[52]

The threats to regional security due to the generalization of the epidemic, that have been highlighted by a series of reports,[53] are another example of 'indirect deferred costs' the impact of which may

---

*This argument is similar to the one used by Cantor who concludes that the bubonic plague in England in 1450 led to a rise in living standards for those who survived who had higher levels of land for cultivation *per capita*. However, such comparison leads to misinterpretation because the two epidemics are quite different. The 'Black Death' was a very short-term epidemic that lasted for 3 years and only produced a short-term one-off reduction in the size of the population.

be considerable on economic activities such as tourism[54] or decisions of foreign investors.[55]

The second type of 'endogenous growth' mechanisms, that have been grossly underestimated in most studies and that have even been totally neglected in previous macroeconomic models, deal with the dynamic impact of the epidemic on transmission of human capital and its interaction with physical capital. This interaction between the two categories of capital assets must be understood in the current context of the change of paradigm concerning the relationship between health improvements and economic growth. In recent years, there has been a growing awareness that health is not only a consumption good that adds to wellbeing but also an investment good that increases the future productive power of workers and employees. The traditional interpretation of the strong observed correlation between income and health, i.e. that higher income leads to better health, has been increasingly challenged: health, as measured by life expectancy at the beginning of the period, has significant effects on subsequent growth. The landmark report on macroeconomics and health commissioned by WHO has provided compelling evidence that investment in global health spurs economic development.[56] Together with the moral argument, the direct effect of health on workers' productivity is the main mechanism put forward by this report to justify increased transfers of resources to developing countries for health spending.

However, there are additional indirect mechanisms through which health can influence productivity, because health is a complementary input in the formation of human capital. Ill-health and premature death lead to wasted investment in human capital and globally reduces the incentives to invest in the future of people. In the absence of an adequate policy response, the reduction in resources linked to HIV/AIDS can have a major impact in decreasing the productivity of education, significantly reducing human capital and its transmission and contributing to a long term decline in savings and investment.

All these considerations, to which may be added the deformation of the age-pyramid of the population due to AIDS,[57] lead to the understanding that the impact of the epidemic on growth of GDP is likely to be a lot larger than previously estimated by models that did not take these 'endogenous' effects into account. By killing mostly young adults, AIDS does more than destroy the human capital embodied in them. It weakens the whole mechanism through which human capital is accumulated and transmitted across generations, it reduces the incentives to invest in education and weakens the precious informal educational mechanisms through which *savoir-faire* are transmitted from parents to children. The cumulative effects over time may lead to what economists call 'threshold externalities',[58] and in the case of AIDS to an 'epidemiological regression trap' leading to a catastrophic deterioration of the long-term growth regime of their economies (Fig. 68.1).

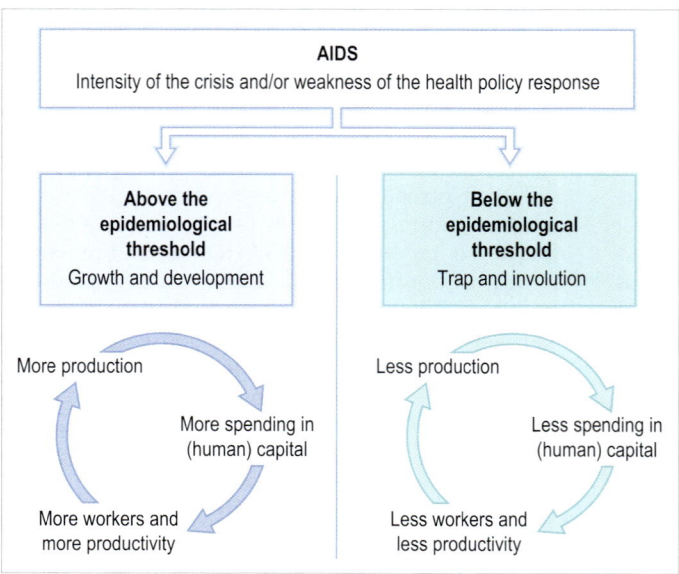

Figure 68.1 Two paths for the impact of AIDS on the economy. The basic idea underlying the figure is that of a differential impact of AIDS on economic growth, crucially depending on the level of development already attained and of the adequacy of the response. For a reasonable range of epidemiological predictions, an *involution trap* may occur, corresponding to a modification of the long-term growth regime of the economy.

The conclusions of a recent study by the World Bank,[59] which has tried for the first time to fully integrate the effect on human capital on macroeconomic predictions for South Africa, state that 'in the absence of AIDS, the counterfactual benchmark, there would have been modest growth with universal education attained with three generations. But if nothing is done to combat the epidemic, a complete economic collapse will occur within four generations', with the risk of South Africa being taken back to the level of GDP *per capita* of Kenya. Similar results, pointing out the likelihood of a catastrophic scenario in the absence of increased efforts to halt the epidemic have been obtained for the Ivory Coast and Cameroon using a comparable approach.[60] Extending this approach to predict the impact of scaling-up access to antiretroviral treatment suggests that massive investment in HIV care is a rationale choice to put economies, that are threatened by such an epidemiologic trap, back on track.[61]

Why the Impact on Human Development has been Under-estimated

While it should now be obvious that the impact of HIV/AIDS on economic growth has been strongly under-estimated, it should also be acknowledged that an emphasis on GDP to the exclusion of other aspects of human development does not capture the actual consequences of the epidemic.[62] The morbidity and mortality associated with an HIV/AIDS epidemic also affects the unpaid, non-market economic activities – what can be called non-traded socially reproductive labor and goods. These non-market activities are of prime importance in the societies of the developing world in proportions that are no longer the case in high income countries. These activities, i.e. child rearing, community participation, self-provisioning through agricultural or pastoral work, do not enter into usual economic calculations. As conceptualized by economists who call attention upon the fact that certain social relations may facilitate cooperation and trust and can be a source of value in themselves,[63,64] loss of these activities may however strongly affect the whole process of development.

The modern idea of human development characteristic of the United Nations Development Programme (UNDP) has tried to go beyond GDP alone to arrive at a more pragmatic balance between the growths of income, environmental sustainability and people's needs to be full participants in the lives

of their societies. It tries to recognize that these goals should be achieved in relation to widely varying cultural and national traditions. It also tries to incorporate the important notion of capabilities, a perspective focusing on the opportunities for choice that their economic and social environment practically offers to people.[65]

Human development has four components (UNDP): the creation of human capabilities (including improved health, knowledge, and skills to fully participate in income generation); the elimination of barriers to economic and political opportunities, enabling people to have equal access to and benefit from opportunities; people's full participation in decisions and processes affecting their lives; and intergenerational sustainability of the development process. The Human Development Index (HDI), a composite index measuring average achievement in three basic dimensions (a long and healthy life, knowledge and a decent standard of living) is an attempt, although imperfect, to better capture progress on all its major dimensions. In the 1980s, reversals in HDI were highly unusual and limited to exceptional political or war situations.* Unfortunately, since its 2003 edition, the Human Development Report shows that 21 countries[†] exhibit a decline in the value of their HDI and such decline is mainly related to the fall in life expectancy due to the HIV/AIDS epidemic. Even countries which are able to pursue progress in their absolute level of human development are however affected in that process because of HIV/AIDS: for example, Thailand in spite of successful efforts to bring the epidemic under control has fallen from 52nd in 1995 to 74th place in 2001 in HDI rankings.

The Need for Appropriate Funding

For many years, a large share of health economists working in the field of international health have tended to oppose any effort to extend access to HIV care, including antiretroviral treatment, in developing countries as an inappropriate choice by comparison with alternative use of resources for improving

---

*Between 1980 and 1990, only four countries (Dem. Rep. of Congo, Guyana, Rwanda, and Zambia) saw a drop in their HDI.
†Armenia, Belarus, Botswana, Burundi, Cameroon, Central African Republic, Congo, Dem. Rep. of Congo, Côte d'Ivoire, Kazakhstan, Kenya, Lesotho, Moldova, Russian Federation, South Africa, Swaziland, Tajikistan, Tanzania, Ukraine, Zambia, Zimbabwe.

public health. These positions have been gradually abandoned as increasing evidence supporting that antiretroviral treatment (ART) can be made a rational economic investment in middle and low income countries has been produced,[66] and as the goal of universal access to treatment for those in need has been endorsed by the international donor community and national governments. The Declaration unanimously adopted by the Special Session of the United Nations General Assembly (UNGASS) in June 2001, the advent of the Global Fund to Fight AIDS, Tuberculosis and Malaria (GFATM) in 2002, the WHO and other UN organizations' commitment to the goal of expanding access to ARVs to 3 million people in the developing world by 2005,[67] President Bush's Emergency Plan for AIDS Relief (PEPFAR) to cover two million people with ARVs by 2008 in 15 selected countries, and the G8 Summit resolution of July 2005 to pursue 'universal access' to ART, are the most spectacular examples of this trend.

In parallel, available global funding for HIV programs has significantly increased. According to UNAIDS estimates, US$6.1 billion have been available for AIDS activities from all sources in 2004 (versus only US$1.8 billion in 2001). As shown in Figure 68.2, the commitment of funds through the GFATM reveal a quite unprecedented effort in the field of international cooperation for health using a multilateral channel. The GFATM has already supported more than 300 programs in 130 countries for a cumulative total of US$8 billion: 60% of these funds have gone to African countries and the remaining 40% to other developing countries, 55% to AIDS versus 45% to the two other pandemics, and 40% for the procurement of drugs for the three diseases.

The international community is also showing increased interest in the issue of how to facilitate the production and delivery of 'global public goods for health', such as dissemination of information and promotion of technical tools to help reducing HIV-related risk behaviors, AIDS vaccines, R&D for drugs against infectious diseases such as AIDS, tuberculosis and malaria, and other health commodities that may contribute in controlling the epidemic.[68]

Estimates of the funding needs for the global fight against AIDS, however, point out that significant gaps have still to be filled.[69] The latest data, published in July 2005 by UNAIDS,[70] estimated that the funding gap between the resources available and those needed for a comprehensive response was US$4 billion in 2005 and projected gaps of, respectively US$6 billion in 2006 and US$8 billion in 2007. Of course, such exercise to appreciate global funding needs is based on many hypothetical assumptions, and government as well as international donors may indeed adapt their funding commitments in reaction to these estimates (for example, increased foreign aid for HIV care in a country may induce less national resources through the so-called fungibility mechanism between resources allocated to various Ministries, etc.). It remains however, obvious that the fight against HIV/AIDS has been chronically under-funded, and this fact has been partly legitimized by mistaken under-estimations of the impact of HIV/AIDS on economic growth and human development that need urgent revisions. A debate is currently emerging about innovative perennial funding mechanisms to guarantee the long-term sustainability of HIV programs, including antiretroviral treatment that, under existing drugs, should last for the whole

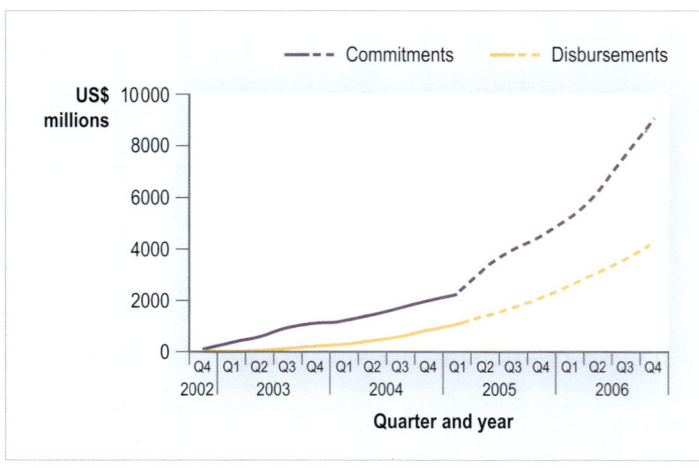

Figure 68.2 Financial aid to developing countries through the global fund against aids, tuberculosis and malaria. Actual and projected commitments and disbursements. (From GFATM 2005.)

life cycle of infected individuals: for example, the British government has launched a proposal for an International Finance Facility (IFF) in order to front load aid to help meet the internationally agreed Millennium Development Goals. The Brazilian, Chilean, French, and German governments have created an international tax, that will be based on air traffic, to guarantee long-term funding: cautious estimations report that such tax, even if it remains applied by these four countries, may bring 500 million additional US$ for international aid per year (which will mean a 50% increase in the GFATM budget currently devoted to drugs). The fight against the AIDS pandemic is clearly the primary target for experimenting these new ways, or alternative ones, to improve the financial resource flows devoted to public health and health systems in developing countries.

References

1. World Bank. Intensifying action against HIV/AIDS in Africa: responding to a development crisis. Washington: World Bank; 1999.
2. Barnett T, Whiteside A. AIDS in the twenty-first century. Disease and globalization. New York: Palgrave Macmillan; 2002.
3. Smith J, Nalagoda F, Wawer MJ, et al. Education attainment as a predictor of HIV risk in rural Uganda: results from a population-based study. Intl J STD AIDS 1999; 10:452–459.
4. Bloom SS, Urassa M, Isingo R, et al. Community effects on the risk of HIV infection in rural Tanzania. Sex Trans Infect 2002; 78:261–266.
5. Hargreaves JR, Glynn JR. Educational attainment and HIV-1 infection in developing countries: a systematic review. Trop Med Intl Hlth 2002; 7:489–498.
6. Stillwaggon E. HIV Transmission in Latin America: Comparison with Africa and policy implications. J South Afr Eco 2000; 68:985–1011.
7. Loewenson R, Whiteside A. HIV/AIDS implications for poverty reduction. United Nations Development Programme background paper. UN General Assembly Special Session on HIV/AIDS, New York: 25–27 June 2001.
8. Haddad L, Gillespie S. Effective food and nutrition policy responses to HIV/AIDS: What we know and what we need to know. J Intl Dev 2001; 13:487–511.
9. Lambrechts K, Barry G. Why is Southern Africa hungry? The roots of Southern Africa's food crisis. London: A Christian Aid Policy Briefing; 2003.
10. Murray CJL, Lopez AD. Mortality by cause in eight regions of the world: global burden of disease study. Lancet 1997; 349:1269-1276.
11. Frieden TR, Sterling TR, Munsiff SS, et al. Tuberculosis. Lancet 2003; 362:887–899.
12. Davies PDO. The world-wide increase in tuberculosis: how demographic changes, HIV infection and increasing numbers in poverty are increasing tuberculosis. Ann Med 2003; 35:235–243.
13. Jamison DT, Mosley WH. Disease control priorities in developing countries: health policy responses to epidemiological change. Am J Publ Hlth 1991; 81:15–22.
14. Caraël M, Schwartländer B, Zewdie D. Demographic impact of AIDS. Introduction. AIDS 1998; 12:S1–S2.
15. Boerma JT, Nunn AJ, Whitworth JA. Mortality impact of the AIDS epidemic: evidence from community studies in less developed countries. AIDS 1998; 12:S3–S14.
16. Sewankambo NK, Gray RH, Ahmad S, et al. Mortality associated with HIV infection in rural Rakai District, Uganda. AIDS 2000; 14:2391–2400.
17. Bradshaw D, Schneider M, Dorrington R, et al. South African cause-of-death profile in transition – 1996 and future trends. South Afr Med J 2002; 92:618–623.
18. Walker N, Schwartländer B, Bryce J. Meeting international goals in child survival and HIV/AIDS. Lancet 2002; 360:284–289.
19. United Nations Development Programme. Human Development Report 2003. Oxford: Oxford University Press; 2003.
20. US Bureau of the Census. World population profile 2000. Washington, DC: US Bureau of the Census; 2000.
21. Stover J. Modelling the demographic impact of AIDS. J Hlth Pop Nutr 2002; 20:102–103.
22. Heuveline P. HIV and population dynamics: A general model and maximum-likelihood standards for East Africa. Demography 2003; 40:217–245.
23. US Bureau of the Census. Monitoring the AIDS pandemic network. The status and trends of the HIV/AIDS epidemics in the world. Washington DC: US Bureau of the Census; 2000.
24. Mekonnen Y, Jegou R, Coutinho RA, et al. Demographic impact of AIDS in a low-fertility urban African setting: projection for Addis Ababa, Ethiopia. J Hlth Pop Nutr 2002; 20:120–129.
25. Whiteside A. Demography and economics of HIV/AIDS. Br Med Bull 2001; 58:73–88.
26. Booysen F le R, Arntz T. The methodology of HIV/AIDS impact studies: a review of current practices. Soc Sci Med 2003; 56:2391–2405.
27. Mutangadura G, Mukurazita D, Jackson H. A review of household and community responses to the HIV/AIDS epidemic in the rural areas of sub-Saharan Africa. Geneva: UNAIDS; 2000.
28. Over M. Coping with the impact of AIDS. Finance Dev 1998; March:22–24.
29. Steinberg M, Johnson S, Schierhout G, et al. Hitting home: How households cope with the impact of the HIV/AIDS epidemic. A survey of households affected by HIV/AIDS in South Africa. Washington DC: The Henry J. Kaiser Family Foundation; 2002.
30. Ngalula J, Urassa M, Mwaluko G, et al. Health service use and household expenditure during terminal illness due to AIDS in rural Tanzania. Trop Med Intl Hlth 2002; 7:873–877.
31. Msellati P, Juillet-Amar A, Prudhomme J, et al. Socio-economic and health characteristics of HIV-infected patients seeking care in relation to access to the Drug Access Initiative and to antiretroviral treatment in Côte d'Ivoire. AIDS 2003; 17:S63–S68.
32. UNICEF. Africa's orphaned generations. Washington, DC: UNICEF, 2003: Report issued in November 2003, New York.
33. Forsythe S. How does HIV/AIDS affect African businesses? In: Forsythe S, ed. State of the art: AIDS and economics. Washington, DC: International AIDS and Economics Network (IAEN); 2002: 30–37.
34. Rosen S, Simon J, Vincent JR, et al. AIDS is your business. Harv Bus Rev 2003; 81:80–87.
35. Aventin L, Huard P. The cost of AIDS to three manufacturing firms in Cote d'Ivoire. J Afr Eco 2000; 9:161–188.
36. Grassly NC, Desai K, Pegurri E, et al. The economic impact of HIV/AIDS on the education sector in Zambia. AIDS 2003; 17:1039–1044.
37. Kingdom of Swaziland. Ministry of Health and Social Welfare. Accelerating access to HIV/AIDS care in Swaziland. A partnership between the Kingdom of Swaziland, the United Nations System, and the Private sector. Project Document: September; 2000.
38. Gilks CF, Floyd K, Otieno LS, et al. Some effects of the rising case load of adult HIV-related disease on a hospital in Nairobi. J Acquir Immune Defic Syndr 1998; 18:234–240.

39. Touzé V, Ventelou B. AIDS and development, a global challenge. Rev L'OFCE 2002; 0:S153–S174.

40. Anand K, Pandav CS, Nath LM. Impact of HIV/AIDS on the national economy of India. Hlth Pol 1999; 47:195–205.

41. Bloom D, Canning D. Health as human capital and its impact on economic performance. Geneva Pap Risk Insur 2003; 28:304–315.

42. Cantor NF. In the wake of the plague: The Black Death and the world it made. New-York: The Free Press; 2001.

43. Lucas RE Jr. Some macroeconomics for the 21st century. J Eco Perspect 2000; 14:159–168.

44. Lloyd-Ellis H, Roberts J. Twin engines of growth: skills and technology as equal partners in balanced growth. J Eco Growth 2002; 7:87–115.

45. Bloom DE, Canning D, Malaney PN. Demographic change and economic growth in Asia. Pop Devt Rev 2000; 26:257–290.

46. Bronfman MN, Leyva R, Negroni MJ, et al. Mobile populations and HIV/AIDS in Central America and Mexico: research for action. AIDS 2002; 16:S42–S49.

47. Deininger K, Garcia M, Subbarao K. AIDS-induced orphanhood as a systemic shock: Magnitude, impact, and program interventions in Africa. World Dev 2003; 31:1201–1220.

48. Nyambedha EO, Wandibba S, Aagaard-Hansen J. Changing patterns of orphan care due to the HIV epidemic in western Kenya. Soc Sci Med 2003; 57:301–311.

49. Bicego G, Rutstein S, Johnson K. Dimensions of the emerging orphan crisis in sub-Saharan Africa. Soc Sci Med 2003; 56:1235–1247.

50. Case A, Paxson P, Ableidinger J. Orphans in Africa. Paper presented at the. UNAIDS Reference Group on Economics Meeting 22–23 April. Washington DC: World Bank; 2003.

51. Gertler P, Levine D, Martinez S. The presence and presents of parents: Do parents matter for more than money? UNAIDS Reference Group on Economics Meeting 22–23 April. Washington DC: World Bank; 2003.

52. Freire S. The impact of HIV/AIDS on saving behaviour in South Africa. International AIDS Economic Network Symposium on Economics of HIV/AIDS in Developing Countries, Barcelona: July 2002.

53. Eberstadt N. The future of AIDS: grim toll in Russia, China, and India. Foreign Aff 2002; 81:22–45.

54. Forsythe S. HIV/AIDS and tourism. AIDS Anal Afr 1999; 9:4–6.

55. Hemrich G, Topouzis D. Multi-sectoral responses to HIV/AIDS: Constraints and opportunities for technical co-operation. J Intl Devt 2000; 12:85–99.

56. WHO (Sachs JD, ed.). Macroeconomics and health: investing in health for economic development. Report of the Commission on Macroeconomics and Health (CMH). Geneva: World Health Organization; 2001.

57. Easterly W, Levine R. Africa's growth tragedy: policies ad ethnic divisions. Quarter J Eco 1997; 112:1203–1250.

58. Azariadis C, Drazen A. Threshold Externalities in Economic Development. Quarter J Eco 1990; 105:501–526.

59. Bell C, Devarajan S, Gersbach H. The long-run economic costs of AIDS: Theory and an application to South Africa. UNAIDS Reference Group on Economics Meeting 22–23 April. Washington DC: World Bank; 2003.

60. Drouhin N, Touzé V, Ventelou B. AIDS and economic growth in Africa: a critical assessment of the 'base-case scenario' approach. In: Moatti JP, Coriat B, Souteyrand Y, et al., eds. Economics of AIDS and access to HIV/AIDS care in developing countries. Issues and challenges. Paris: Eds ANRS; 2003.

61. Ventelou B, Couderc N. AIDS, economic growth and epidemic trap in Africa. Oxf Dev Stud 2005; 33:1–10.

62. Wehrwein P. The economic impact of AIDS in Africa. Harv AIDS Rev 2000; Winter:12–14.

63. Gui B. Beyond transactions: On the interpersonal dimension of economic reality. Ann Pub Coop Eco 2000; 71:139–169.

64. Bruni L, Sugden R. Moral canals: Trust and social capital in the work of Hume, Smith and Genovesi. Eco Philo 2000; 16:21–45.

65. Sen A. Development as freedom. New York: Albert Knopf Inc; 1999.

66. Moatti JP, N'Doye I, Hammer SM, et al. Antiretroviral treatment for HIV-infection in developing countries: an attainable new paradigm. Nat Med 2003; 9:1449–1452.

67. WHO. World Health Organization says failure to deliver AIDS medicines is a global health emergency. WHO press release. Geneva: WHO; 2003.

68. Smith R, Beaglehole R, Woodward D, et al. Global public goods for health. In: Smith R, Beaglehole R, Woodward D, Drager N, eds. Health economic and public health perspectives. New York: Oxford University Press and WHO; 2003.

69. Schwartländer B, Stover J, Walker N, et al. Resource needs for HIV/AIDS. Science 2001; 292:2434–2436.

70. UNAIDS. Resource needs for an expanded response to AIDS in low and middle income countries. Geneva: UNAIDS; 2005.

CHAPTER 69

The Long Wave of HIV/ AIDS: A Special Case of Pathogen–Host– Environment Interactions

Tony Barnett

Introduction

It offers no great insight to state that disease, and particularly communicable disease, has effects on human social and economic life. Such has been obvious from the earliest times and is indeed the basis for the development of public health medicine. We know that at the organic level, we have been shaped by communicable disease, thus the human genome reflects the 5 million year relationship between ourselves and malaria parasites. Most recently, Ewald[1] has explored the complex evolutionary history of communicable disease pathogens and their relationships with their hosts. This chapter provides a brief survey of what we know about the relationships between one very specific group of pathogens, the family of HIV-1 viruses, their particular life cycle and the results which they have for some human societies.[2-5]

HIV/AIDS: The Global Situation

In discussing the social and economic impact of HIV/AIDS it is of the utmost importance to take account of a very obvious fact that is often ignored. This is the difference between HIV seroprevalence and prevalence of AIDS. Reference is most frequently made to the former measure, while information about the latter is hard to obtain and is fraught with difficulties of interpretation given the problems of

obtaining clinical diagnoses of illness and cause of death in circumstances where clinicians may be in short supply and where an AIDS diagnosis is stigmatizing. When considering reported levels of seroprevalence, we must bear in mind that this is not an account of the present manifestation of disease related illness and death. Rather, it is a perspective on what is likely to happen in a population in the near future given the likely absence of effective antiretroviral treatments in most poor countries. Thus, a map of Africa such as that presented in Figure 69.1 is only partially a guide to impact. It has to be read as an account of both past and present and is therefore rather difficult to interpret.

In 2004, 39.4 million individuals were estimated to be living with HIV/AIDS, within the range 35.9–44.3 million individuals. Assuming that each HIV/AIDS case directly influences the lives of four other individuals, a total of more than 150 million people are currently affected by the disease. Sub-Saharan Africa is the region most troubled by HIV/AIDS – now the leading cause of adult morbidity and mortality in that region. Most, if not all, of the 25.4 million people in sub-Saharan Africa who are living with HIV/AIDS will have died by the year 2020; this in addition to the 17 million Africans already claimed by the epidemic.

HIV/AIDS is also spreading dramatically in Asia. India leads the region in absolute numbers of HIV infections, whether or not they have developed AIDS, estimated at 5.1 million, within the range 2.5–8.5 million by the end of 2003. China, too, has a

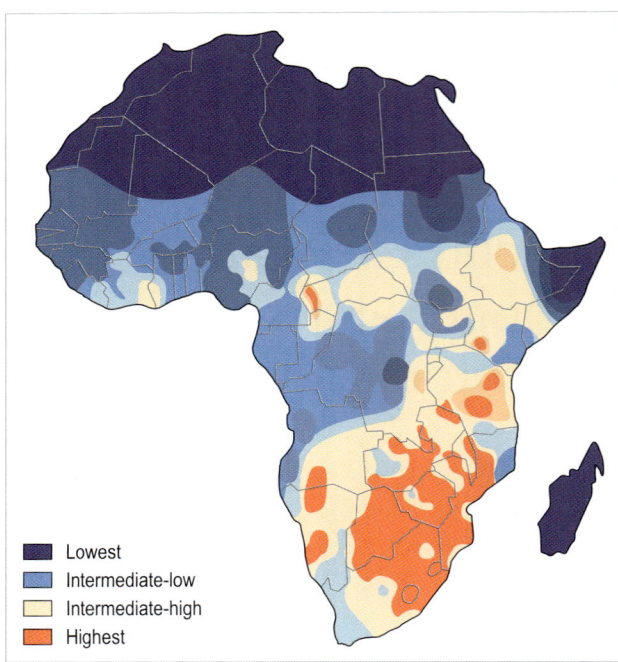

- Lowest
- Intermediate-low
- Intermediate-high
- Highest

Figure 69.1 Current adult HIV prevalence – the highest rates in southern Africa may exceed 40% of the adult population. (From: Our common interest: Report of the Commission for Africa, March 2005. Online. Available: www.commissionforafrica.org/english/report/introduction.html)

growing HIV/AIDS problem, with approximately 840 000 people with HIV infection, whether or not they have developed symptoms of AIDS, within the range 430 000–1 500 000. However, according to private estimates by Chinese specialists, China may have up to 10 million HIV infections. Asia will overtake sub-Saharan Africa in absolute numbers before 2010; by 2020 Asia could be the world's HIV/AIDS epicenter. The most recently recorded global situation is summarized in Table 69.1.[6]

Vertical Interactions

HIV is a member of the group of viruses *retroviridae*. It is also a member of the group of viruses described as *lentiviruses*. These two characteristics are the basis for much that distinguishes them from other communicable disease in terms of their implications for human social and economic life. Added to the fact that they are predominantly transmitted via human body fluids, in effect they appear most frequently as STIs, and you have the mix which makes them so significant for our social existence.

Retroviridae multiply via a process of reverse transcription, thus inserting their genetic material into that of their host. This process of reverse transcription is far from perfect and means that there is considerable room for accumulation of error in the genetic code and thus in practice enormous potential for viral mutability within the infected person over a very brief period. Given the huge numbers of viral particles produced in the early stages of infection (2×10^9), the rate of mutation and also recombination is very high indeed. The result is that it is very hard for the host to develop any meaningful and effective immune response. HIV targets the cells of the immune system and it is the slow (mean time from infection to death, 8.9 years[7,8]) destruction of this system that results in death: hence the significance of the *lentivirus* characteristic. Typical transmission globally is heterosexual and depending on local cultural, social, and economic contexts, so the potential reproductive rate of the virus can be very large indeed.[9–15] Sexual transmission is also the basis for the severe social and economic impacts observed or hypothesized in many parts of the world. An STI is inevitably incident in the most sexually active age cohorts of a population. This is usually defined as the age group 15–50, and indeed the seroprevalence and AIDS mortality patterns confirm that this is the case, although there is also evidence of MTCT, and age is not necessarily a protection against infection. The population level results of these characteristics have been modeled for some African populations, notably Botswana, although the US Bureau of the Census has noted that this 'chimney' effect on population is not necessarily generalizable to all African

Table 69.1 Global summary of the HIV/AIDS epidemic, end 2004[6]

	Estimate	Range
People newly infected with HIV in 2004 (Total)	4.9 million	4.3–6.4
Adults	4.3 million	3.7–5.7
Children <15	640 000	570 000–750 000
Total number of people living with HIV/AIDS	39.4 million	35.9–44.3
Adults	37.2 million	33.8–41.7
Women	17.6 million	16.3–19.5 million
Children <15	2.2 million	2.0–2.6
Total AIDS deaths in 2004	3.1 million	2.8–3.5
Adults	2.6 million	2.3–2.9
Children <15	510 000	460 000–600 000
Total number of AIDS deaths since the beginning of the epidemic	21.8 million	
Total number of AIDS orphans[a] since the beginning of the epidemic	14 million	
Projected total number of AIDS orphans[a] by 2010	25 million	

[a]Defined as children who lost their mother or both parents to AIDS when they were under the age of 15.

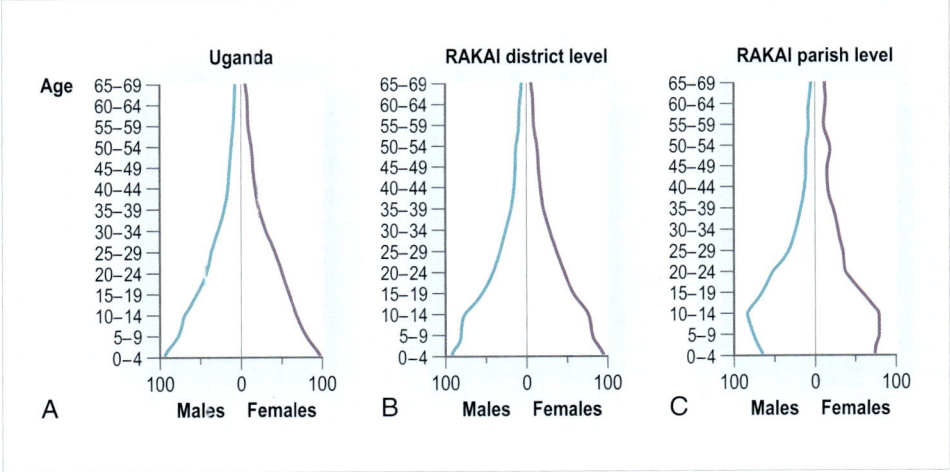

Figure 69.2 HIV/AIDS impact on population structure, Uganda 1993. (A) The age gender pyramid for all of Uganda, (B) the same for a population unit of 2–3 million people in Rakai District which at that time was among the most severely affected areas of Uganda, and (C) the population structure for parishes (population units of a few thousand) in the most affected areas of Rakai District.

populations. It is certainly not generalizable to all affected populations and indeed the base demographic structure of affected societies is an important variable in considering the potential effects of the epidemic. However, there is one piece of good evidence that shows us what had already happened to a severely infected society as early as 1991. This is the analysis by Low-Beer, Stoneburner and Mukulu of the Ugandan census data,[16] which appears in Figure 69.2. (The population effects of AIDS in this area had already been reported from smaller samples by the present author as early as 1989.[17])

Impact and Implications

There are numerous impacts of these kinds of population effects. There follows only a few of the most significant effects.

What Do We Mean by Impact?

This epidemic increases morbidity (sickness) and mortality (death) in populations at precisely those ages where normal levels of morbidity and mortality are low. This is shown in Figure 69.3. It is from these unusual events that other impacts flow. These impacts may be felt as an immediate and severe shock or they may be more complex, gradual and long-term changes. In some situations, AIDS illness and death may threaten to overwhelm communities and perhaps whole societies; in others, the shock is absorbed. Impact will occur at different levels: the household, community or nation. Vulnerability to impact is only partly determined by the numbers of people infected and where they are located in society; difference in degree will reflect differential re-source endowments. Well-resourced communities and households will be better able to cope than poor ones, and the same is true for countries.

It is useful to begin thinking about impact as a continuum between a sharp shock and slow and pro-found changes. An example of a sharp shock is the death of the main breadwinner or the main carer in a household or family. This results in immediate and marked decline in living standards and welfare. Similarly, the death of a strategically important and hard to replace individual in an organization, for example an especially skilled worker whose skills are in short supply, will have a shock impact upon the operation of that organization.

It is also relevant to think of impact as a slow but complex *series of changes* – some of them very subtle – resulting from gradual accumulation of impacts. This is illustrated by an example from the health system.

- TB is a frequent opportunistic infection associate with AIDS. It spreads to the wider population
- AIDS first affects the availability of treatment for non-AIDS illnesses in the health system
- There are additional pressures on health staff who suffer burn-out and emotional exhaustion
- Resources are constrained to the health of those who cannot gain access to care for non-AIDS illnesses suffers. TB infection rates increase in the general population
- The result is an overall reduction of people's health status
- Society bears wider costs. These are either direct costs of care or in direct costs associated with decreasing health status and consequent knock-on effects to educational attainment, social functioning, and trauma associated with the premature deaths of relatives from TB.

This example of gradual change shows how:

- cumulative and linked effects may be severe but difficult to measure over the long term and that the chain of events does not stop there
- the combination of sharp shocks and slow changes affects all areas of social reproduction, production, livelihoods, and governance.

The implication of this is that in many societies, we should probably cease to think of this as an *epidemic* and instead begin to consider it an *endemic*. Altering our thought in this way is also to stop looking for shock effects but to recognize that the nature of the affected society has altered as the disease will be part of the social, economic and cultural scene for the foreseeable future.

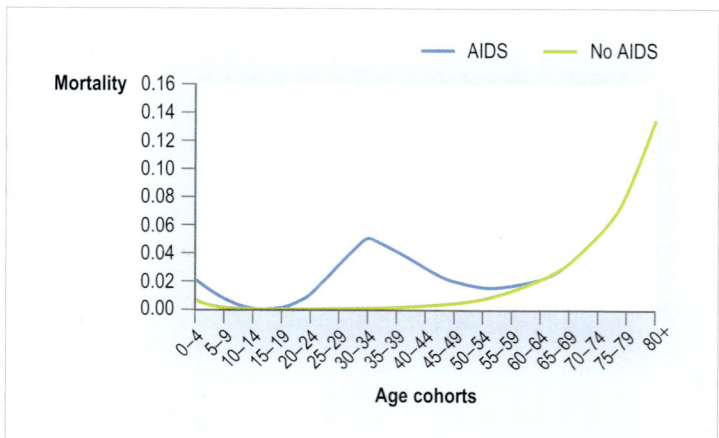

Figure 69.3 Age-specific mortality at 20% HIV seroprevalence in an African population.

Seeing Impact

The curve of HIV infection is followed by the curve of AIDS illness and death, which in turn determines the third curve, impact. In Figure 69.4, these processes are summarized in relation specifically to orphaning but this diagram can be applied to a whole range of other impacts.

For example, orphaned female children have a higher likelihood of infection, or if they are withdrawn from school, we know their children will have higher mortality rates as female education is correlated with infant and child mortality rates. Thus, AIDS impacts over three generations. So, in considering impact, we are describing some events that we can see now, mainly the shocks, and discuss-

ing other medium- and long-term events, about which we can only speculate.

Life Expectancy and Expectation of Adult Life

Figure 69.5 looks at life expectancy through the lens of some of today's 15-year-olds. These projections assume that AIDS prevention programs will be successful enough to halve the risk of becoming HIV-infected over the next 15 years. They do not take into account possible improvements in treatment or the availability of an HIV vaccine.

According to these conservative analyses, in countries where 15% of adults are currently infected,

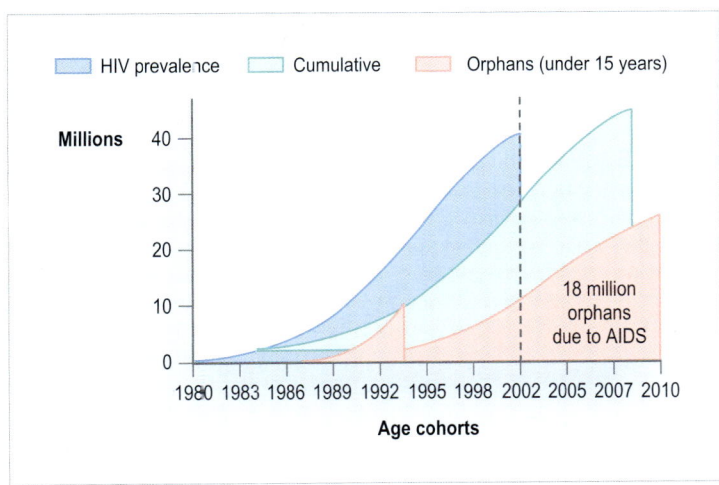

Figure 69.4 HIV prevalence, AIDS, orphans, and impacts. (Adapted from Barnett and Whiteside.[2])

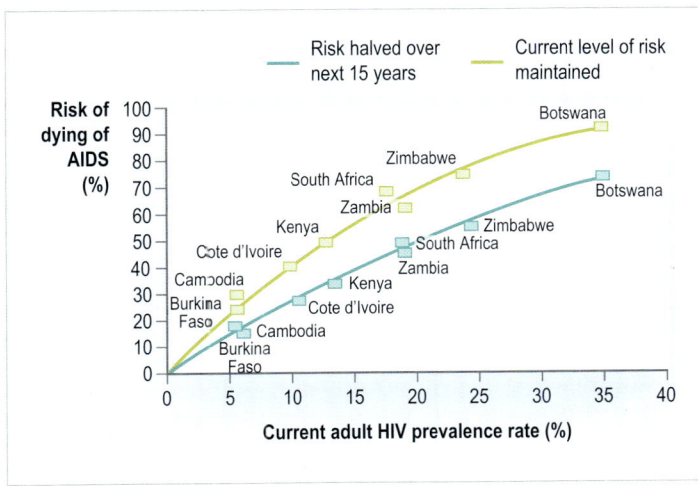

Figure 69.5 Lifetime risk of AIDS death for 15-year-old boys, assuming unchanced or halved risk of becoming infected with HIV, selected countries. (Data from Zaba B. Report on the Global HIV/AIDS epidemic. Geneva: UNAIDS; 2000: 26.)

around one-third of today's 15-year-olds will die of AIDS. Where adult prevalence rates exceed 15%, the lifetime risk of dying of AIDS is much greater. In countries such as South Africa and Zimbabwe, where one-fifth or one-quarter of the adult population is infected, AIDS is set to claim the lives of around half of all 15-year-olds. And, in Botswana, where one in three adults is already HIV-infected, the highest prevalence rate in the world – it is estimated that two-thirds of today's 15-year-old boys will die prematurely of AIDS.

Life expectancy and child mortality rates have been widely used as markers for improvements in the welfare of populations. In Botswana, life expectancy at birth is now estimated to be 36 years, instead of 71 without AIDS. Life expectancy in Botswana is estimated to drop towards 30 within the next 10 years. In Zimbabwe, life expectancy is 38 instead of 70. In fact, children born today in several southern and east African countries have life expectancies below 40. This is a disturbing picture and is even more disturbing once we consider it through the concept of expectation of years of adult life. A 15-year-old or a 20-year-old who is aware of this level of risk, through observation, education or peer group discussion or a combination of these, may well adopt a view that says it is not reasonable to plan for the future. Once an entire generation or a large part of it adopts this perspective on life, then prevention programs become hard to sustain, education has less value (as the returns will not be reaped) and there will be great societal changes. In the particular case of Botswana, such possibilities seem all-to-real when these data are considered against the very recent findings of detailed ethnographic research on orphaned children and their lives.[18]

The Impact on Rural Production, Nutrition, and Food Security

The impact of HIV/AIDS on nutrition and food security has tended to take a particular form (see below). We do not know however, how true it is of Africa in general and other world regions, where subsistence farming is a substantial part of rural people's livelihood strategies. Early research[19] used field material from a number or sites in Uganda to suggest (1) the effects of AIDS on rural production in Uganda and possibly more broadly in Africa and (2) the methods that might be employed to explore the *variability* of the impact in production systems differentiated in terms of people, climate, soils and temperature.

Since then, many studies using mainly qualitative and participatory methods have confirmed a story of an AIDS impact which runs broadly as follows: AIDS causes rural labour shortages because of excess illness and death in the productive age group, this leads to progressive decline of agricultural production and food availability as a result of reduction of cultivated land area, and shrinkage of crop and livestock portfolios accompanied by decay of rural infrastructure and overall reduced rural production and productivity and thus nutrition status of the population.

But we do not know whether and how far this story applies everywhere in Africa, or indeed in other AIDS-affected rural communities globally. It is now of the greatest importance that we culminate as clear an understanding as possible of the diversity of the AIDS impact on rural societies which depend predominantly on human labour. If we homogenize what is in reality a very diverse situation, we will create inappropriate solutions, derived from a wrong analysis. For example, one frequently proposed solution has been to meet labour shortages with a range of 'labour saving technologies' (LSTs). The problem here is that we do not have sufficient examples of successful LSTs which have been adopted in Africa in ordinary circumstances – there has been no African green revolution – far less any examples of LST innovations appropriate to the new situation consequent on the impact of AIDS.

Because of this, there is a danger that impact mitigation action could be led in the wrong direction, if based upon 'simple stories' – narratives of the epidemic and its impact that have become accepted by policy-makers, donors, opinion leaders and the research community. The situation is that, even so far into the epidemic – the third decade – we really do not have long-term evidence with the kind of detailed analyses necessary to understand the complexity and diversity of the impact of the epidemic on rural society in Africa. What we do have is a large and growing body of very uncertain 'evidence' about what has been happening. This literature has recently been reviewed by Gillespie and Kadiyala.[20] Within that 'evidence', it is hard to isolate the causal influence of HIV/AIDS from other underlying environmental and policy conditions. Indeed, the epidemic may be a tipping point factor, but in many circumstances, it may not be the sole reason for the effects that we are seeing. We are dealing with an extremely complex set of causal links and these are likely to be different or nuanced from place to place.

What we know about HIV/AIDS' impact on rural societies, nutrition, and food security can be summed up as follows: seroprevalence figures provide an insight into the future, not an account of the present; there is an impact in most societies where seroprevalence levels have been high; it is adverse in most cases, but we do not know where it is best or worst. Generalizations about the process in one place drawing on narratives derived from experience (often anecdotal) from elsewhere is unhelpful; policy responses based on general statements about 'famine,' 'labour saving technologies,' 'scaling up,' etc. are likely to waste resources and fail to meet the needs of local communities. We must also be acutely aware that the development of the disease over 8–9 years in an individual, during which time their effectiveness is compromised, may not be long enough for adoption of innovation to take place. We know that technical innovation in rural societies tends to take considerable time unless the risk involved is very small – farmers do not take chances with the unknown! In communities severely affected by AIDS, the entire dynamic of innovation and adoption may be compromised.

Conclusion

There is much that we do not know about the impact of HIV/AIDS. But we know that it is occurring, and in many forms. A general account of the situation with regard to the pathological harmony between pathogen and human society is outlined schematically in Figure 69.6. This diagram illustrates the ways in which a generalized epidemic adversely affects the potential and actual capacity for a society and economy to reproduce itself in a variety of ways, via transmission of knowledge and education, through maintenance of social and cultural patterns and via the peopling of institutions such as uniformed services, educational institutions, households in particular but also government and community infrastructure in general. Briefly, Figure 69.6 shows the following:

1. The resonance between the viral life cycle (in turquoise) and the human generational cycle (in blue). Here we see that generation 1 reproduces itself and acts as a host for the HIV pathogen. As this generation dies, it leaves orphans.

2. These orphans enter a world where the risk of infection with HIV has increased as the general epidemic curve (yellow curve) rises. In addition, as orphans, this generation is also possibly more socially, culturally, and economically exposed to infection. Thus, the pattern repeats itself, the generation reproduces, but so also does the pathogen, and a second generation of orphans is produced. This generation faces an increased risk of infection for the same reasons as did its parents – but the risk is increased as general seroprevalence rises and social exposure to sexually transmitted infections (including HIV) also increases as a result of less adequate socialization, reflecting in part the decreased expectancy of adult life of parent generation.

3. In the background is the possibility of increased viral resistance to antiretroviral medications as ARV roll out occurs under suboptimal circumstances with poor compliance and inadequate health systems. We can only

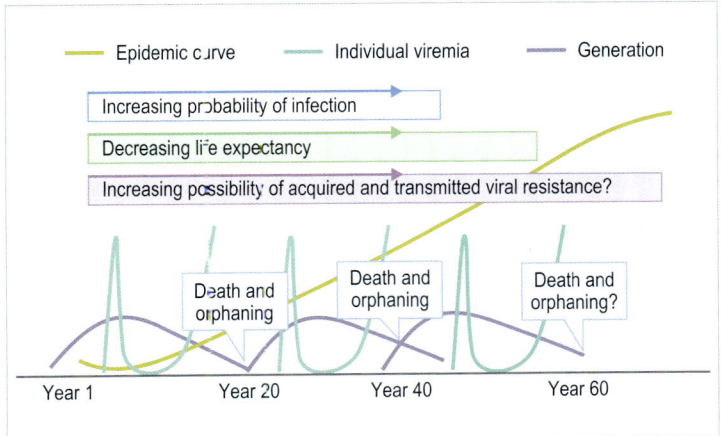

Figure 69.6 The pathological harmony between HIV and Human Society?

Epidemic curve — Individual viremia — Generation

Increasing probability of infection

Decreasing life expectancy

Increasing possibility of acquired and transmitted viral resistance?

Death and orphaning

Death and orphaning

Death and orphaning?

Year 1   Year 20   Year 40   Year 60

speculate about the significance of this development.

These then are the possibilities which might be foreseen in relation to the social, cultural and economic impact of the HIV/AIDS epidemic. In the third decade of this long wave event, we cannot be complacent.

References

1. Ewald P. Evolution of infectious disease. Oxford and New York: Oxford University Press; 1994.
2. Barnett T, Whiteside A. AIDS in the 21st century: disease and globalization, London and New York: Palgrave Macmillan; 2003.
3. Barnett T, Whiteside A, Desmond C. The social and economic impact of HIV/AIDS in poor countries: a review of studies and lessons. Progress in Development Studies 2001; 1:151–170.
4. Barnett T. HIV/AIDS impact studies II: some progress evident. Progress in Development Studies 2002; 2:219–225.
5. Barnett T, Clement C. So where have we got to and where next? Progress in Development Studies 2005; 5:1–11.
6. UNAIDS. 2004. Report on the global HIV/AIDS epidemic: 4th Global Report. Geneva: UNAIDS. Online. Available: www.unaids.org/bangkok2004/GAR2004_html/GAR2004_00_en.htm
7. Whitworth J, Shafer LA, Mahe C, et al. Survival since infection and its relation to background mortality in the Masaka general population cohort. Paper presented at meeting Empirical Evidence for the Demographic and Socioeconomic Impact of AIDS. Durban: March 2003.
8. Porter K, Zaba B. The empirical evidence for the impact of HIV on adult mortality in the developing world: data from serological studies, AIDS 2004; 18(Suppl 2):S9–S17.
9. Zulu EM, Dodoo FN, Chika-Ezeh A. Sexual risk-taking in the slums of Nairobi, Kenya: 1993–1998. Population Studies 2002; 56:311–323.
10. Dodoo FN, Sloan M, Zulu EM. Space, context and hardship: socializing children into sexual activity in Kenya Slums. 2003. In: Agyei-Mensah S, Casterline JB, eds. Fertility and reproductive health in sub-Saharan Africa: A collection of micro-demographic studies. Westport CT: Greenwood Press.
11. Taffa N, Sundby J, Holm-Hansen C, et al. HIV prevalence and socio-cultural context of sexuality among youth in Addis Ababa, Ethiopia. Ethiop J Health Dev 2002; 16:139–145.
12. Watkins S, Zulu E, Kohler H-P, et al. Introduction to social interactions and HIV/AIDS in Rural Africa. Demographic Research 2003; 19:1–28.
13. Arnfred S, ed. Re-thinking sexualities in Africa. Stockholm: Nordiska Afrikain Institutet; 2004.
14. Ssali A, Barton TG, Katongole GM, et al. Exploring sexual terminology in a vernacular. In: Rural Uganda: Lessons for health education, poster presentation. Amsterdam: International AIDS Conference; 1992.
15. Manderson L, Jolly M, eds. Sites of desire: Economies of pleasure: sexualities in Asia and the Pacific. Chicago: University of Chicago Press; 1997.
16. Low-Beer D, Stoneburner RL, Mukulu A. Empirical evidence for the severe but localised impact of AIDS on population structure. Nature Med 1997; 3:553–557.
17. Barnett T, Blaikie P, Obbo C. Community coping mechanisms in circumstances of exceptional demographic change. UEA report for UK Government's Overseas Development Administration. Norwich: Overseas Development Group; 1990.
18. Daniel M. Hidden wounds: orphanhood, expediency and cultural silence in Botswana, unpublished PhD thesis, UEA Norwich; 2005.
19. Barnett T, Blaikie P. AIDS in Africa: its present and future impact. London: Belhaven Press and Guilford Press; 1992.
20. Gillespie S, Kadiyala S. HIV/AIDS and food and nutrition security: From evidence to action. Food Policy Review 7. Washington DC: International Food Policy Research Institute; 2005.

CHAPTER 70

The Growing Problem of AIDS Orphans

Theo Sowa

The Children

April 2001. In a small town in Ethiopia, a group of teenagers take the UN special envoy for HIV/AIDS in Africa to a tiny shack tucked into a series of small winding dirt roads. Two children live in a home that consists of one and a half small, dark rooms. They have been living alone in the house since first their father, and then their mother died from AIDS-related illnesses. The eldest child helped her mother nurse her father and then did her best to nurse her mother. Since their deaths, she had been looking after her younger brother. An older woman living in a neighboring home described how the two children cook, clean, and care for themselves, adding that the only times neighbors came to the house was if they heard the children crying in the night. The neighbor showed concern for the children, but was clear that her family was in no position to take on responsibility for an extra two mouths – and through her words came an underlying fear: these were children whose parents had died from AIDS. Maryam* was 9 years old, her brother just 7 years old.

The teenagers who had taken us to meet Maryam and her brother were barely more than children themselves. A group of school children, they had formed themselves into a peer counselling and advocacy network after a school project opened their eyes to the growing numbers of HIV/AIDS orphans living in their communities. The group had no financial resources and limited human resources, but they visited, counselled and advocated on behalf of chil-

dren to the best of their ability. In the case of Maryam and her brother, they had managed to contact a large international organization that had then taken responsibility for payment of the fees to send the two children to school. This organization did not usually take on the cases of individual children and therefore agreeing to cover the school fees was a response that took them outside of their usual boundaries, but one that they felt obliged to make in the circumstances. Yet, however well meaning, however outside their immediate remit, this action could only be viewed as a totally inadequate response. Good quality education is crucial to the well-being of all children and especially orphans and vulnerable children – but it must be part of a more holistic package of responses which take into account the physical, emotional, and societal well-being of children. Where were the adults in these children's lives? Who was going to comfort Maryam on those nights when she had finished soothing her brother to sleep? Who was there to make sure that they were eating regularly, that they had proper nutrition, that their physical, emotional, and mental health and well-being was being looked after and developed? No-one was doing enough to support these children who were trying so hard to support themselves: not their neighbors, not the international organization, not their local authorities, and not civil society – national or international.

Northern Uganda, August 2003. Two VIPs are escorted around a project working with orphans*

---

*All names of children and workers have been changed where they might affect the anonymity of those concerned.

*In this chapter, the definition of 'orphan' is the UNICEF, UNAIDS, USAID definition used in the 'Children on the Brink' series of reports: any child under 18 years who has lost one or both parents.

and vulnerable children. There are numerous examples of children whose school fees are being paid by the project, children who have meals provided at school, child heads of households who are given support to return to school, community gardens to provide additional nutritious foods for the community's orphans. Yet the gaps in the care being provided become obvious when they sit down to speak to Winsome, a teenaged head of household caring for her two younger sisters and a brother. This adolescent girl had no idea of the implications of having started her own menstrual cycle and even less idea of guidance for her younger sister, other than in relation to hygiene. This became her first discussion exploring these aspects of her femininity, of her physical development and of the emotional dimensions involved – and this first exploration of these important subjects was with a stranger, however sympathetic, who lived thousands of miles away. Despite the good work being carried out by the teams from the national and international organizations partnering to cater to the needs of Winsome and other orphaned children in the area, there was clearly little recognition that the emotional and informational needs of young girls were as important as the physical, and that much more needed to be done than ensuring the provision of feminine hygiene products as part of the physical needs supplied. Yet one of the recurring themes of conversations with Ugandan and other workers in the region was a growing concern about the increasing numbers of teenage pregnancies among young orphaned girls – children having children and often without having had a family context from which to experience or learn parenting skills.

Dar Es Salaam, March 2005. An HIV/AIDS home-based care (HBC) team is working on the outskirts of Dar Es Salaam. The team is part of the outreach of a large healthcare clinic that has developed a far reaching and comprehensive HIV/AIDS prevention, care, and treatment programme. The HBC team consists of a nurse from the local clinic, a volunteer community worker and a driver, and they are accompanied on this day by a supervising nurse from the main clinic. The all-Tanzanian team are breathtakingly impressive: knowledgeable, confident, caring, and committed – attributes that have led to their complete acceptance in the sprawling labyrinth of poorly built shacks and huts that comprise the community that they are visiting on this occasion. During the first home visit, the team sit in a darkened room with a woman so dehydrated and so ill that she can barely move. While one nurse tries to give the woman some water, the team is shown the medicines the family have been given – but which their sister is unable to take because she cannot keep down food or drink. As we leave the room, Anna, the supervising nurse, tells me that the antiretrovirals (ARVs) that are now available at the clinic have arrived too late for the woman we have just visited – and yet she is better off than many because her family are caring for her as well as they can and her child has already been taken into her sister's family.

In the second home we visit are a mother and her daughter. The mother has recently started on ARVs, but when we come into the house, she looks tired and drawn. She has not taken her ARVs that morning, knowing that she must eat before taking the drugs – but there is no food in the house and no money to buy any. The nurses produce some bags of porridge meal, which the woman's 12-year-old daughter immediately begins to prepare. Mwajuma is her mother's only support. Anna says that before the mother started on the ARV treatment she was too weak to work, to take care of Mwajuma or of herself, and it was her daughter who stayed away from school, cooked, nursed her mother, and took on the responsibilities of running the household. The ARVs had not only given her mother better health and hope of an extension of life – they had provided the opportunity for Mwajuma to return to school. Yet the grinding poverty in which they lived threatened the efficacy of the treatment and of this new opportunity.

The final visit that morning was to check on the recovery of John, a young boy who had been fighting a serious infection. Both his parents had died from AIDS-related illness and his own HIV positive status had made him vulnerable to a series of infections and illnesses. Although he had shown great resilience in recovering from these over time, at 12 years old, he was the size of an average 7 or 8 year old. All of his questions for the HBC team were about when they would make him well enough to return to school. His only hope of this happening on a long-term basis was if he was placed on ARVs. Although the clinic had recently acquired the ability and resources to place a limited number of children on ARVs, the number of children who needed the treatment far outnumbered the resources available and the clinic was forced to choose who to treat and who to leave to die. John had been living with an uncle and his family in a desperately poor household since his parents' death. As Anna put it, 'Medically, we should put him on ARVs, but we know there is never enough food in the house – how can we put him on the drugs in that case?'

The Impact

The impact of HIV/AIDS on families, communities, and nations has been well documented: the physical impacts of illness and death on individuals and their families; the financial impacts of increased health-care costs and loss or reduction of household earnings; the increased food insecurity arising from the illness of farmers; the social impacts of children watching their parents die and growing up without the emotional security and guidance to which they are entitled; the stress placed on extended families attempting to absorb the large numbers of children left on their own; the political and social security of nations becoming undermined by the loss of productive workers, key societal figures, economic, and communal instability. Children have to bear these same impacts, but without the additional physical, emotional, and intellectual protection afforded by adulthood. UNICEF estimates that 15 million children under the age of 18 years have lost one or both parents to HIV/AIDS. Each one of those 15 million children is a Maryam, a Winsome, a John, a Mwajuma – children who have lost their primary carers, have lost the first people to turn to for physical, emotional, and social security, have had to adopt adult responsibilities and live through myriad psychosocial pressures. In addition to the emotional and psychological pain that loss brings, each of those children are in a category of: orphaned and vulnerable children that have been found to be the least likely to be properly nourished; the least likely to have access to education or to healthcare; the least likely to have their basic physical and psychosocial needs met; and the most likely to be subjected to physical, social, and emotional abuse, including physical violence and land grabbing.[1]

Although the impact of the pandemic has been greatest in Africa thus far, the potential numbers of orphaned and vulnerable children in India and China could far outstrip the crisis that is taking place on the African continent. Africa has the greatest percentage of children orphaned by AIDS and other causes, but Asia has a far greater absolute number of orphans.

Vulnerable Children

Children orphaned by HIV/AIDS are only a small proportion of the estimated numbers of children made vulnerable by the pandemic. Children in households where the primary caregivers are seri-ously ill, the primary earner is unable to work or where the family is stigmatized because of the presence of HIV positive people in the household are sometimes more vulnerable than children who have been orphaned and taken into extended families. On an even wider scale, the impact of HIV/AIDS on communities and nations has had a devastating effect on many societies – effects that place all children in those societies in greater vulnerability. For example, as teachers, healthcare workers and key workers become ill, unable to work, or die from AIDS-related illness, children have less access to education, to healthcare, to social services, and become more vulnerable to pressure to take part in work that is unsuitable and sometimes dangerous for them. As key adults in communities die, societies become less stable and less secure. The UN Security Council, the International Crisis Group, and numerous governments have described HIV/AIDS as a major threat to political, economic, and social security of individual nations, but also to global security.[2] As societies become less stable, all children have less access to even basic physical and human security. Thus, it is crucial that any strategies or programming to alleviate the impact of HIV/AIDS on children are comprehensive and integrated. Focusing solely on children orphaned by HIV/AIDS can stigmatize those children. As importantly, focusing only on orphans ignores the far larger numbers of children made vulnerable by the pandemic, who in certain cases can be in even more precarious circumstances than children orphaned by the pandemic. And for such programs and strategies to be effective, they must address other causes of child vulnerability, which may not always be directly AIDS related.

Children Living with HIV/AIDS

Although almost all children in the countries most affected by the HIV/AIDS pandemic find their security and healthy development compromised, those made most vulnerable are probably children living with HIV/AIDS who face the same difficulties experienced by orphans and other vulnerable children, but often also face stigma as a result of their HIV status and may have to cope with the physical effects of their status with limited, if any, medical assistance. There are an estimated 2.2 million children living with HIV/AIDS, 90% of these in Africa. Although children make up only 6% of people living with HIV/AIDS, they accounted for 13% of new infections in 2003 and for 17% of all deaths from AIDS-related illnesses[3] – just under half a million child deaths in 2003 and the same number again in 2004. Although WHO estimates that currently over 500 000 children are in urgent need of antiretroviral treatment (ART),[3] only up to 25 000 children are on ARV treatment[4] – and almost half of those are in Thailand and Brazil, although the vast majority of children in need of the treatment are in Africa. Without access to ARV and treatment for opportunistic infections, 80% of HIV-positive children die before the age of 5 years.[5]

Pediatric ART

In the recent efforts to achieve universal access to treatment for HIV/AIDS, there is no doubt that children have been marginalized. The campaigns to reduce the prices of ART for adults were successful, but the price reductions were predominantly applied to adult drugs. Pediatric formulations, where they exist, are still significantly more expensive than adult formulations – between two and four times as expensive as adult formulation. Price has proven to be a major disincentive to the inclusion of children in treatment programs and planning as governments and NGOs attempt to scale-up the roll-out of ART in developing countries.

Price is not the only disincentive. Pediatric formulations of HIV/AIDS drugs are not widely available. Where they are available, they often involve the ingestion of large quantities of unpleasant tasting syrups. In many situations where children do have access to ART, health workers find themselves breaking adult drugs into smaller pieces for use with children – a difficult situation for health workers and an almost impossible one for caregivers in stressed circumstances. An even more basic problem is the lack of readily available and affordable diagnostic tools for children, especially for infants. This includes simple tests for diagnosing HIV status in children and simple protocols and dosage guidance for the administration of ART medications for children. The current systems using age/weight/body surface area to calculate dosages are overly complicated in resource-poor settings. It is essential that such pediatric treatment issues are urgently addressed – but also that any such treatment programs are part of more comprehensive health programs for children, including treatment for opportunistic infections, nutrition and other routine child healthcare provision.

Prevention of Mother-to-Child Transmission

In 2003, 95% of new HIV infections in children were a result of mother-to-child transmission.[3] Undoubtedly, one of the most effective methods for significantly reducing new HIV infection in children is to stop this vertical transmission. The methods, pharmacology, and protocols to make this happen have been in existence for many years and in wealthy Northern countries, Prevention of Mother-to-Child Transmission (PMTCT) programs using research, effective, low-cost interventions, and triple dose ART have radically reduced mother-to-child transmission to <2% of babies.[6] However, in resource-poor developing nations, only 10% of pregnant women have access to PMTCT interventions. Governments in affected countries, international organizations and funding bodies are all aware of the potential of PMTCT programs, yet there is still no global strategy to scale-up such programs and make this life-saving intervention available routinely.

An Inadequate Response

The issue of rising numbers of children orphaned or made vulnerable by AIDS is enormous and according to UNICEF/UNAIDS, is growing. However, perhaps the real issue is not the numbers of orphaned and vulnerable children, but the inadequate response generated thus far to the whole HIV/AIDS crisis, but in particular those facets that most affect children. The inadequacies of the response to children affected by HIV/AIDS are apparent in every sphere. In 1990, less than 1 million children in sub-Saharan Africa had been orphaned through AIDS.[7] By the end of 2003, that figure had risen to 12.3 million.[8] In the intervening years, development workers, activists, academics, child rights workers, HIV/AIDS specialists, and others had all pointed to the danger of growing numbers of children orphaned by AIDS, as an almost inevitable result of the growing numbers of adults dying in the course of the pandemic. Yet responses did not even begin to match the magnitude of the crisis that was being predicted and we watched this tragedy continue to unroll.

Years of development experience has shown that the most effective work on a number of generic and child-focused development issues happens when children are fully accounted for and participate in the planning, implementation, and monitoring of programs. Yet many of the most important initiatives to counter HIV/AIDS on a global scale have failed to integrate children's concerns, needs, and rights – resulting in the marginalization at best of strategies and programs to counter the impact of HIV/AIDS on orphans and vulnerable children. It is only recently that demands for clearly child-focused strategies and implementation in prevention and care, as well as the establishment of significant and concrete goals for pediatric treatment are being made of initiatives and organizations as varied as PEPFAR, the Global Fund, national governments, UNICEF, UNAIDS, MSF, and others. The response in terms of increased funding and more programming has been marked – but on the whole, funding addressed to children orphaned and made vulnerable by AIDS is minimal in relation to overall HIV/AIDS funding and there has been limited collaboration with other child focussed initiatives. Education has been highlighted as a powerful tool in the prevention of HIV transmission among adolescents, in the protection of orphans and other vulnerable children and in the integration of vulnerable children into their communities. Yet there appears to have been a lack of strong collaboration between the efforts to ensure free, universal primary education for all children that has been ongoing for decades and efforts to provide concrete protection for orphans and vulnerable children. The payment of school fees are an element of a large number of programs that support orphans and vulnerable children, yet a global campaign to abolish school fees has not yet found resonance between the two sets of programs.

The 'Framework'

Perhaps the most significant response has been the development of 'The Framework for the Protection, Care, and Support of Orphans and Vulnerable Children Living in a World with HIV and AIDS'.[8] Now recognized by most of the key agencies, organizations, and international partners working on pediatric AIDS issues, the 'Framework' outlines five key strategies that should be at the heart of responses to children and HIV/AIDS issues:

1. Strengthening the capacity of families to protect and care for orphans and vulnerable children by prolonging the lives of parents and providing economic, psychosocial, and other support.

2. Mobilizing and supporting community-based responses to provide both immediate and long-term assistance to vulnerable households.

3. Ensuring access for orphans and vulnerable children to essential services, including education, healthcare, birth registration, and others.

4. Ensuring that governments protect the most vulnerable children through improved policy and legislation, and by channelling resources to communities.

5. Raising awareness at all levels through advocacy and social mobilization to create a supportive environment for children affected by HIV/AIDS.

The acceptance of this Framework as a guide to planning, programming and implementation by the key organizations and governments working on issues of children and HIV provides an opportunity to make concrete inroads to reducing and eliminating the impacts of HIV/AIDS on orphans and vulnerable children – but this will only happen if the Framework generates action rather than further discussion. There has been an excess of words over action for more than a decade, resulting in impoverished lives, pain, and death for millions of children. The great strengths of the Framework are its recognition and promotion of families and communities as the first lines of care and protection for all children, but especially those made vulnerable by the pandemic, plus its clarity on the importance of comprehensive, integrated interventions for children. A move away from paying lip service to these principles and towards ensuring that financial and human resources are channelled into programs that strengthen the capacity of families and vulnerable households, and promote community responses and safety nets will be an important indicator of progress. These are actions that are crucial at a time when many African children find themselves at risk of institutionalization in a variety of orphanages, children's homes and children's villages that are appearing throughout the continent in an often unthinking, *ad hoc*, unregulated and financially and emotionally expensive response to the increasing numbers of orphans on the continent.

Children do not live in a vacuum – they thrive in a caring family and social context. And they falter without that context. HIV/AIDS has put tremendous pressure on extended families and communities as they become less able to cope with huge numbers of orphans, of children growing up without a family to care for them, without adult guidance and supervision, without the physical, emotional, and social protections they need to grow into adulthood successfully. We have the scientific, medical, social, and human knowledge to put into place programs that provide good quality prevention, care, protection, and treatment for children orphaned or made vulnerable by HIV/AIDS. There can be no doubt that the possibility of saving the lives of millions of children and securing the stability of whole societies and nations should be the best possible motivation available to plan, to carry out the necessary research, to cajole, and to persuade the wide variety of actors in this field into urgent action. The question remains, does the political will exist, locally, nationally, and internationally, to put that knowledge into practice and provide the hope and the futures that children like John, Mwajuma, Winsome, and Maryam deserve.

The real problem is not simply the growing number of AIDS orphans – it is our hopelessly inadequate response.

End note

In the time since this chapter was written, much progress has been made in the area for treatment for HIV positive children, due in large part to the advocacy and pioneering work of individuals and organizations such as Stephen Lewis (UN Secretary General's Special Representative on HIV/AIDS in Africa), Medicins Sans Frontiers, the Clinton HIV/AIDS Initiative and the Global AIDS Alliance. Yet a simple, affordable and appropriate diagnostic tool for children remains an urgent and unmet need, while appropriate pediatric formulations of ARV drugs continue to be limted and scarce.

References

1. World Vision UK. More than words? World Vision UK report: 2005.
2. UN Security Council. Debate: The Impact of AIDS on Peace and Security in Africa: January 2000.
3. WHO. Improving access to appropriate paediatric ARV formulations, Geneva. Geneva: WHO; 3–4November 2004. Online. Available: www.who.int/3by5/en/finalreport4Apr.pdf
4. UNAIDS press release. UNAIDS and WHO applaud new Clinton Foundation Initiatives to increase access to treatment, Geneva. Geneva: UNAIDS; 11 April 2005.
5. Elizabeth Glaser Pediatric Aids Foundation. Experience with ARV regimens for infants/children in resource constrained settings. HEART project, Mulago Hospital, Kampala.
6. UNAIDS. AIDS epidemic update. UNAIDS Joint United Nations Programme on HIV/AIDS: December 2002.
7. UNICEF. Africa's orphaned generations: November 2003.
8. UNAIDS, UNICEF, USAID. Children on the brink: July 2004.

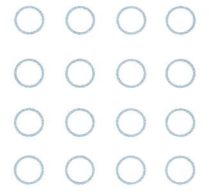

CHAPTER 71

International Funding Mechanisms for AIDS Care and Prevention

Mabel van Oranje

Introduction

HIV/AIDS, together with tuberculosis (TB) and malaria, is ravaging the lives of tens of millions across the world. AIDS constitutes not only an enormous health challenge, but is also rapidly reversing the hard-won development achievements of previous decades. It undermines hope for pulling people out of poverty and raising living standards, and in many countries jeopardizes peace and stability. There is no country, rich or poor, immune to this killer disease. Yet, as AIDS thrives in impoverished communities, stemming its spread is a linchpin in the global fight against poverty.

This chapter examines international efforts to reverse the AIDS crisis in low- and middle-income countries. In these countries, AIDS funding grew from some US$300 million in the mid-1990s to US$1.7 billion in 2002, to some US$4.7 billion in 2003,[1] and up to an estimated US$6.1 billion in 2004.[2] Most of these funds come from international donors. This chapter will first look at the three main initiatives to finance the control of AIDS: the World Bank's Multi-Country AIDS Programme (MAP), the Global Fund to Fight AIDS, Tuberculosis and Malaria (hereafter referred to as the Global Fund), and the United States (US) President's Emergency Plan for AIDS Relief (PEPFAR). Subsequently, it will examine key challenges faced by international donors: the resource gap, donor cooperation and harmonization, and programming and policy issues. Although the activities of recipient governments are an intrinsic part of the fight against the pandemic, they are not the subject of this chapter.

The Three Major Funding Mechanisms

While domestic spending by governments from affected countries and 'out-of-pocket' spending by directly affected individuals and their families is substantial, approximately two-thirds of all global AIDS funding in 2005 will be provided by international donors.[1] The fragmented international funding landscape is composed of an increasing range of global actors including bilateral donors, the European Commission, the United Nations (UN) system, the Global Fund, and the private sector including foundations and companies. In absolute terms, the total funding of all European donors is most significant. Yet, the visibility and political leverage of Europe's contribution is reduced because it flows through a multitude of bilateral channels, multilateral agencies, the Global Fund, and non-governmental organizations (NGOs).

A comprehensive assessment of the main funding mechanisms – MAP, the Global Fund, and PEPFAR – would involve looking at their operational performance, grant performance, general impact on the spread and prevalence of the disease, as well as collateral impact on broader health systems. However, given that all three funding instruments are still young and most projects started only recently, it is impossible to gauge their actual impact on AIDS and overall system effects at this moment of writing in May 2005.

Transparency is also an issue. The shortage of reliable and comprehensive data on individual projects, coverage indicators, and results achieved further complicates the picture. The information available on MAP and PEPFAR is mainly limited to an aggregate level; only for the Global Fund is it possible to easily obtain details about individual programs and disbursements to date. Of the three major funding mechanisms, only the Global Fund has been the object of various independent assessments.[3–5] Furthermore, the first comparative study of these funding mechanisms has not yet been completed.

Efforts to measure the effectiveness and impact of the three main funding mechanisms are also hampered by difficulties in attributing concrete achievements. Donor agencies are often under pressure to produce quick and easily measurable results – so-called 'deliverables'. But it is not possible to quantify impact by simply counting the number of patients receiving antiretroviral treatment (ART) from a specific donor, as the direct cost of drugs are <30% of the average costs per person for a complete treatment package.[6] It is much harder to sort out the other, indirect components of treatment, such as general clinical support for patients; training and support for healthcare personnel; medical infrastructure; and monitoring and reporting systems. Given that different aspects of an ART package are usually supported by different donors, it is often not possible or accurate to accredit specific results to one specific donor.

While attributing donor support for treatment is already difficult, measuring the results of prevention efforts – essentially, counting the number of people who did not get infected – is even more complicated. Successful prevention is usually the cumulative result of multiple, mutually reinforcing interventions and a supportive environment; not the outcome of one distinct project.

Moreover, important policy, process, and systems aspects – such as whether donor activities are part of the relevant national AIDS strategy; whether they use and strengthen existing structures; how well embedded they are in the local environment; and whether they are coordinated with other efforts – should also be taken into account when judging the performance of the major global initiatives to fight AIDS.

The World Bank's Multi-Country AIDS Program (MAP)

A total of 29 UN agencies are engaged in the fight against AIDS. Some provide funding for projects, others are involved in coordination, advocacy, and monitoring. Of the UN family, the World Bank is the most important funder of AIDS programs. In addition to its traditional funding channels – such as

loans for prevention and treatment, and the healthcare sector in general – the World Bank in 2000 initiated MAP for Africa.

This new mechanism provides funding, technical assistance, and support for knowledge exchange in countries in sub-Saharan Africa that are eligible for credits of the International Development Association (IDA). MAP's objectives are in accordance with national or sub-regional strategic AIDS plans. The country-based programs are designed to empower stakeholders with funding and decision-making authority; to involve actors at all levels – from individuals and villages, to regions and central authorities; and to encompass all sectors and the full range of AIDS prevention, care, and mitigation activities. The program provides support not only to the public sector, but also to non-traditional World Bank partners such as community organizations, NGOs, and faith-based organizations. A significant part of MAP support goes directly to small-scale, high-impact efforts by local grassroots organizations; more than 30 000 such sub-projects have been funded so far.[7]

After a slow start, the African MAP, by early May 2005, had committed approximately US$1.1 billion in credits and grants to 29 African countries and four multi-country programs. Disbursements have, however, accelerated and approximately US$440 million has been spent to date (Keith Hansen, World Bank, pers comm).[8] Under a similar program for the Caribbean, US$155 million had been committed to fight AIDS in seven countries.[9] Yet, it is difficult to obtain detailed information about the performance of specific MAP projects and a comprehensive picture of what has been achieved. Given that the World Bank often acts as donor of last resort, MAP support is frequently used for 'upstream' projects that aim to strengthen health infrastructures.

A semi-independent review, based on visits to six MAP countries and published in October 2004, found that MAP was making progress towards meeting its basic objectives, which include securing high-level political commitment to address AIDS; accelerating the national response to AIDS; formally introducing the multi-sectoral response; initiating community level action; and developing good operational plans for monitoring and evaluation.[10] The study commended MAP's flexible, open-ended, quick, client-driven, and collaborative approach – which it described as 'very innovative for the Bank.'[10] It noted, however, that this approach was not always implemented in practice.

The community-based interventions were considered the best performing component of MAP, confirming the existence of local capacity to undertake prevention, treatment, and care activities. The public-sector response was found to be generally less impressive. Yet, while the review noted that 'implementation experience of the individual MAP projects has been decidedly mixed ...,'[10] it did not evaluate individual projects but focused mainly on an aggregate level. Most of the review's findings – such as the need for better national monitoring and evaluation systems, the existence of strategic and governance issues related to national AIDS frameworks, and challenges related to health service delivery and the multi-sectoral response – apply not only to MAP, but also to national AIDS programs and to the efforts of other international donors.

The Global Fund to Fight AIDS, Tuberculosis, and Malaria

Another new funding mechanism is the Global Fund to Fight AIDS, Tuberculosis, and Malaria (the Global Fund), which has been operational since 2002. It has mobilized significant new resources and is the first multilateral instrument to support projects addressing the deadly synergy of AIDS and TB. Operating globally, the Global Fund has become a leading force in the fight against these diseases; it currently provides two-thirds of all external financing in the fight against TB, 45% in the fight against malaria, and 20% of all external support to combat AIDS.[11] The Global Fund supports programs through 5-year grants, with funding initially committed for a 2-year period.

By the end of April 2005, the Global Fund had approved 310 grants, totalling US$3.1 billion in 127 countries[12] and disbursed US$1.2 billion (Christoph Benn, the Global Fund, pers comm). Around 60% of this funding goes to sub-Saharan Africa, and 56% is earmarked for fighting AIDS.[12] Just 3 years after its inception, with 27 grants reaching the 2-year mark and the average age of grants just under 1 year, Global Fund financing had provided 130 000 people with AIDS treatment; >1 million persons with voluntary HIV testing; 335 000 patients with TB treatment; >300 000 people with malaria treatment; and >1.35 million families with bed nets to protect against malaria. It had also reached tens of millions of people through a wide range of prevention programs.[12]

The Global Fund approach to delivering assistance is innovative. This partnership between governments, the private sector, civil society, and affected communities is driven by needs on the ground. Its governance systems are open and inclusive. The Global Fund is not an implementing agency and has

no offices in affected countries; projects are designed and executed by the recipients themselves through Country Coordinating Mechanisms (CCMs). Proposals are developed at country level according to local priorities and reviewed by independent experts. Disbursements are supposed to be based on actual performance. The Global Fund attracts finances and technical assistance from a wide variety of donors – including private ones. Its procedures for decision-making and operations aim to be accountable, transparent, and participatory; from the CCMs to the board level, they include donors and recipients, governmental and non-governmental. Furthermore, the Global Fund aspires to be a flexible and responsive financing instrument with a limited bureaucracy.

Operationally, there are points of contention and failure. Grant signing and disbursements have been slow, although they are now accelerating. In a number of countries, the CCMs are dysfunctional, far from transparent, excluding civil society groups, or operating independent of relevant government structures. The absence of Global Fund field offices complicates cooperation with other donors. Issues related to procurement policies, trade-offs between efficiency and ownership, and the balance between government and non-governmental organizations as implementing partners also need to be addressed.[5] The Global Fund's board and secretariat have, however, shown great willingness to tackle these problems by re-evaluating and modifying policies and procedures. With the first series of grants reaching the end of their second year, the Global Fund will need to prove that it is indeed performance-based when deciding which grants will receive funding for their second phase (i.e. years 3 through 5), and which ones will be terminated for lack of performance.

The Global Fund is at a critical juncture. It requires at least US$2.3 billion in 2005 to pay for the 3-year renewals of successful ongoing programs and a new funding round of approximately US$1 billion. For 2006 and 2007, the needs are estimated at US$3.5 and US$3.6 billion, respectively.[13] The Fund is currently financed by voluntary contributions, with the European Commission and European Union member states jointly providing just over half of the Global Fund's needs and the USA giving up to one-third of the budget. Donor governments have long preached the importance of a funding vehicle such as the Global Fund – one that is needs-driven, relies on local input, and facilitates the merging of international funding flows. It remains to be seen, however, whether they will make good on their word and give the Global Fund sufficient means to live up to its potential.

The US President's Emergency Plan for AIDS Relief (PEPFAR)

PEPFAR is the youngest – and the only bilateral – of the three major funding mechanisms. In January 2003, the US President, George Bush, initiated this US$15 billion program, which responds to AIDS in low- and middle-income countries over a 5-year period. Most of the funds – approximately US$9 billion – will be spent bilaterally to scale-up treatment, prevention, and care activities in 15 focus countries. This description primarily focuses on those efforts. Resources are, however, also available for: ongoing bilateral programs in approximately 100 countries, research, and multilateral organizations, such as the Global Fund and the Joint United Nations Programme on HIV/AIDS (UNAIDS).

The PEPFAR focus countries: Botswana, Côte d'Ivoire, Ethiopia, Guyana, Haiti, Kenya, Mozambique, Namibia, Nigeria, Rwanda, South Africa, Tanzania, Uganda, Vietnam, and Zambia, account for approximately half of the world's infections of HIV/AIDS and almost 8 million children orphaned or made vulnerable by HIV/AIDS. This Emergency Plan aims to support treatment for 2 million people living with HIV/AIDS, prevent 7 million new HIV infections, and give support care to 10 million people infected and affected by HIV/AIDS, by 2008.[14]

In US fiscal year 2004, US$2.4 billion was committed to PEPFAR – including US$865 million to the target countries and around US$500 million to the Global Fund.[14] A March 2005 report to the US Congress stated that the Emergency Plan had in its first 8 months of operation (January–August 2004) reached, directly or indirectly, 155 000 people with treatment support and 1.2 million women with services to prevent mother-to-child transmission. PEPFAR had also supported care for more than 1.7 million people infected and affected by HIV/AIDS, including 630 200 orphans and vulnerable children, and training for more than 300 000 health workers.[14]

The centerpiece of PEPFAR's prevention strategy, the 'ABC approach', is an example of a donor-driven agenda. It earmarks a specific proportion of spending for abstinence-only programs. At issue is not only the effectiveness of the 'A' of 'abstinence' versus the 'B' of 'being faithful' or the 'C' of 'using condoms'; it is also about whether in-country experts should design programs shaped by the realities on the ground. In Africa, for example, many new infections occur among monogamous married women who are faithful and for whom abstinence is just not an option. Abstinence will also not protect the one of three South African adolescent girls whose first sexual encounter is involuntary.[15] The USA also requires non-US recipients of PEPFAR funding – except for multilateral organizations such as the Global Fund and UN agencies – to have policies explicitly opposing prostitution and sex trafficking. Taking a stance against what it considers US conditionality based on non-scientific evidence, the government of Brazil recently turned down a US$40 million US grant, because it was dependent on Brazil's condemnation of prostitution.[16]

Controversy has also arisen because of the decision by Washington policy-makers to, at least initially, favor US-manufactured brand pharmaceuticals over cheaper WHO pre-qualified generic drugs for US-funded treatment programs. Not until December 2004 and January 2005, did the US Food and Drug Administration tentatively approve PEPFAR's use of a US and a South African generic antiretroviral drug.[17]

While US-based institutions and NGOs – often religious – play an important role as implementers, over 80% of the approximately 1200 PEPFAR partners (both prime recipients of funding and sub-contractors) are indigenous organisations.[18] A guiding principle of PEPFAR is 'to build local and host-nation capacity so that national programs can achieve results, monitor and evaluate their activities, and sustain their programs for the long term.'[18] Without more detailed information about the final recipients of PEPFAR funding and the specific activities in individual countries, however, it is impossible to draw conclusions about PEPFAR's achievements in strengthening local capacity.

The USA, in absolute terms the biggest bilateral donor, deserves praise for its unprecedented commitment to the fight against AIDS as well as its attempt to move significant levels of funding quickly. But the way in which the money is being used has raised controversy and is possibly not the most effective. More program results will need to be available and evaluated before well-informed judgment can be made on whether PEPFAR is living up to its vision of turning the tide of the global pandemic.

Challenges to Effective Funding

AIDS is a fast moving target. Although efforts to combat the epidemic in poor countries have speeded up significantly, they are not keeping pace. In 2004, more than 3 million people died of AIDS and some

4.9 million became newly infected with HIV, bringing the total number of HIV-infected people to almost 40 million.[19] While around 6 million HIV-positive people in developing countries needed ART, only 700 000 persons were receiving it by the end of 2004.[20] If the world wants to stand a chance in this battle, donors must make more funding available, and increase the effectiveness of that funding by enhancing collaboration and developing comprehensive policies and programs.

The Resource Gap

A successful response to the disease requires predictability of funding levels, long-term financial commitments, and frontloading of resources. Current investments in effective prevention, treatment, and research will save millions of lives, lessen the socioeconomic impact of AIDS in poorer countries, and remove the need for increased spending on this chronic crisis in the future.

Although today's spending is 20 times what it was in 1996, it is not sufficient. To adequately respond to AIDS in low- and middle-income countries, UNAIDS estimates that US$9.7 billion will be needed in 2005 – and US$20 billion annually by 2008 – from international and domestic sources.[21] Taking into account current and expected contributions from donors, there was a 3-year shortfall (2005–2007) of at least US$8.2 billion by March 2005.[21] These amounts, which are regularly reviewed and readjusted, would allow for effective HIV prevention, AIDS treatment and care, and orphan support under current capacity limitations. Yet, they include neither resources required to scale-up healthcare systems, nor funding for R&D of desperately needed prevention technologies such as microbicides and a vaccine.

To create solid financial support, existing donors will need to multiply their efforts and consider developing new financing sources – such as increased debt relief, the International Financing Facility proposed by the UK's Chancellor, Gordon Brown, or special international taxes as suggested by the French President, Jacques Chirac. New donors – governmental and non-governmental – should also be encouraged to become active. Without a global authority to tell each donor country how much they should contribute, donors should determine and give their fair share. To optimize effectiveness, resources for the fight against AIDS must be truly additional; they cannot come at the expense of other efforts to reach the Millennium Development Goals (MDGs). Effective AIDS responses benefit from – and

often depend on – related development activities such as capacity building, infrastructure development, and poverty reduction.

While the financial shortage must be addressed, actual spending should also speed up. Donors and recipient governments have a joint responsibility for the timely disbursement of funds already committed.

Donor Cooperation and Harmonization

There are various challenges to timely and effective spending in countries heavily affected by AIDS, including lack of human and institutional capacity; the persistent negative effects of stigma and discrimination; shortfalls in political commitment; slow transfer of funds from national to local and community levels; inadequate accounting and auditing mechanisms; and inconsistent bureaucratic funding processes of the global donor community.[22] The recipients of assistance definitely bear a large share of responsibility for these bottlenecks and should address them to ensure effective use of AIDS funding.

Yet, international donors could also increase the impact of their efforts by improved cooperation and harmonization. This would require them to provide more and better information on current funding levels and activities; coordinate aid flows in support of nationally owned plans and frameworks; involve civil society and other stakeholders in program design and implementation; and streamline and harmonize donor procedures.

The lack of comparable, transparent, and current data from donor governments on their ongoing AIDS funding and future spending plans impedes donor collaboration. No one seems accountable for duplication of efforts, for reduced impact due to poor program complementarity, or for the fact that some affected countries receive disproportionately high levels of support while others receive little or nothing. To start tackling these deficiencies, funders should improve reporting on their current and planned activities.

Donors will always have different priorities and funding channels. But they need to coordinate aid flows, so that they support nationally owned plans and frameworks. All domestic stakeholders – including NGOs – should be involved in the design and implementation of national AIDS strategies. Experience on the ground shows that in countries where the response to AIDS has shown success, civil society has often played an important role in catalyzing action at the community level, influencing national plans, and holding inactive governments to account. Civil society's ability to bring AIDS to the public sphere – despite stigma, discrimination, and cultural sensitivities – is a vital complement to the actions of governments and international donors. For example, the performance of those Global Fund grants where the primary recipients come from civil society is, on the whole, better than those with governmental implementers.[23]

Streamlining and harmonization of donor procedures – such as programming, reporting, and monitoring – also enhances country capacity to use international assistance effectively. UNAIDS puts it bluntly: 'The lack of harmonization kills people.'[22] Donors need to provide resources in a coordinated way to make access as easy as possible for those who need it most. This is technically possible, but requires the political will to operate differently.

In April 2004, donors and low- and middle-income countries agreed to collaborate more effectively in scaling-up global and national AIDS responses by adopting the so-called 'Three Ones' principles.[24] To improve coordination of country-level action, they committed themselves to: one agreed AIDS action framework that provides the basis for coordinating the work of all partners and funding mechanisms; one national AIDS coordinating authority, with a broad-based multi-sectoral mandate; and one agreed country-level monitoring and evaluation system. This set of principles combines the concepts of national ownership, multi-sectorality, mainstreaming, harmonization, coherence, and clear division of tasks. If adhered to, it would help increase the effectiveness of donor spending.

At a meeting in March 2005 on implementation of the 'Three Ones', international donors repeated their commitment to improve coordination and agreed to form a Global Task Team to make specific recommendations for this purpose.[25] But, despite formal promises of cooperation and harmonization, the reality is that most donors are not systematically working together on the ground. The limited level of cooperation between the three main funding mechanisms – MAP, the Global Fund, and PEPFAR – is a case in point.

Developing Comprehensive Programs

Donor impact can also be increased by addressing policy and programming issues. Ideology – rather than pragmatism and evidence-based programming – too often determines the priorities set by donors.

An example is PEPFAR's interpretation of the ABC approach. The same is true for donor focus on 'deliverables'. It is easy to link given amounts of funding to numbers of people on antiretroviral treatment – and much more complicated to show measurable returns on investments in prevention or general support for healthcare systems. Thus, it is tempting for donors to concentrate on ART. However, it must be part of a broader approach that includes prevention, care, and mitigation.

The control of the TB and AIDS twin epidemics is another example of the need for a comprehensive approach. HIV is the most important factor behind the dramatic increase in TB in Africa; TB is the most common opportunistic infection and the number one cause of death for people living with AIDS. It is estimated that one-third of the 40 million people living with HIV/AIDS are co-infected with TB. Without proper treatment, approximately 90% of those living with HIV die within months of contracting TB.[26] Consequently, treating TB is one of the most effective means of improving and prolonging the lives of people with AIDS. Donors should expand TB treatment and prophylaxis to all dually affected persons and integrate TB treatment with HIV voluntary counselling and testing. As the two diseases form a deadly combination, donors should no longer treat TB and AIDS in isolation but support a complementary response.

When setting priorities for an all-inclusive approach to fight AIDS, donors – and recipient governments – must also have the will to address controversial aspects of the pandemic. Increased support for programs focusing on disenfranchised and marginalized people – such as injecting-drug users, sex workers, gay and bisexual men, prisoners, asylum seekers, and refugees – is crucial. For example, injecting-drug use has become the driving force behind the spread of HIV in Eastern Europe and Central Asia – which is home to the world's fastest-growing epidemic – as well as in Iran and parts of China.[27,28] Outside of Africa, more than one in every three persons newly infected with HIV is an injecting-drug user.[29] To halt the spread of AIDS in this case, donors must provide strong support for harm reduction programs, such as needle exchange and drug substitution therapy, which have proved the most effective means of reducing new infections. When necessary, donors and recipients should also confront the underlying political and legal barriers that obstruct the effective deployment of funds.

The problems of weak health systems, limited human capacity, and brain drain that prevent many affected countries from mounting effective responses should also be addressed. For example, as many nurses left Ghana in 1999 as were trained there in that year. As of 2001, only 360 of the 1200 physicians trained in Zimbabwe during the 1990s were still practicing in the country. In 2002/2003, more than 3000 nurses trained in Ghana, Kenya, Nigeria, South Africa, Zambia, and Zimbabwe registered in the UK.[30] In easing their own capacity constraints, donors are often adding to those of affected countries. AIDS needs an emergency response, but it should be complemented by investment in the human and physical resources of the health sectors of developing countries.

Finally, AIDS must be seen within the broader context of development. As the disease affects all parts of society and is especially embroiled in poverty, the international response should go beyond traditional AIDS interventions to also include support for related developmental issues such as education, nutrition, and poverty reduction strategies. In summary, a wholesale, not piecemeal, approach is needed.

Conclusion

Winning the fight against AIDS requires not only a substantial increase in funding levels, but also a more effective use of available resources – by recipients in affected countries and international donors alike.

Although it is too early to definitively judge the various new international funding mechanisms, features for the successful delivery of assistance are emerging. They include a sense of urgency, needs-driven programming, participatory processes, recipient-owned programs, performance-based funding, public-private partnerships, transparency and openness, and a willingness to address weaknesses.

Donors should tackle the shortcomings of their funding instruments, improve cooperation, harmonize their procedures, and ensure that their programming and policies match the realities and needs on the ground. These steps will not only enhance the effectiveness of the activities of individual funding agencies, but also of the collective international response against the deadly virus.

The importance of an effective and collective international response cannot be underestimated. Unchecked, the AIDS epidemic will continue to constitute an enormous health and development challenge. Failure to address the pandemic will result in falling short of the Millennium Development Goal, set out by the UN, of reversing the spread of AIDS,

TB and malaria by 2015. This will make remote any hope of reaching many of the other millennium goals in the fight against poverty.

References

1. UNAIDS. Report on the global AIDS epidemic; June 2004:131, 135.
2. UNAIDS. Resource needs for an expanded response to AIDS in low and middle income countries. Document prepared for Making the Money Work – The Three Ones in Action meeting, London; 9 March 2005.
3. Radelet S. The Global Fund to Fight AIDS, Tuberculosis and Malaria: Progress, potential, and challenges for the future – executive summary. June 2004.
4. Brugha R, Donoghue M, Starling M, et al. The Global Fund: managing great expectations. Lancet 2004; 364:95–100.
5. Bezanson KA. Replenishing the Global Fund: An independent assessment. February 2005.
6. Office of the US Global AIDS Coordinator. Engendering bold leadership: The President's emergency plan for AIDS relief. First annual report to Congress; March 2005:34.
7. Tearfund. The warriors and the faithful: 2005; 3. Online. Available: http://tilz.tearfund.org/webdocs/Website/Campaigning/Policy%20and%20research/AIDS_5_-_warriors_final.pdf
8. World Bank. Online. Available: www.worldbank.org/afr/aids/map.htm (accessed 9 May 2005).
9. World Bank. Online. Available: http://wbln0018.worldbank.org/LAC/LAC.nsf/ECADocByUnid/3AD771B69125F43A85256DE80074DA4B (accessed 9 May 2005).
10. World Bank. Interim review of the multi-country HIV/AIDS program for Africa; October 2004:ii, 5, 6.
11. The Global Fund. The resource needs of the Global Fund 2005–2007; March 2005:33.
12. The Global Fund. Investing in the future; the Global Fund at three years; March 2005:5, 7, 27.
13. The Global Fund. The resource needs of the Global Fund 2005–2007; March 2005:7.
14. Office of the US Global AIDS Coordinator. Engendering bold leadership: The President's emergency plan for AIDS relief. First Annual Report to Congress; March 2005:5, 6, 11, 12, 14.
15. UNAIDS. Violence against women and AIDS – Media backgrounder; 2 February 2004.
16. International Herald Tribune. AIDS program refuses funding over conditions. 5 May 2005.
17. Office of the US Global AIDS Coordinator. Fact Sheet. 25 January 2005.
18. Office of the US Global AIDS Coordinator. Engendering bold leadership: The President's emergency plan for AIDS relief. First Annual Report to Congress; March 2005:5, 13.
19. UNAIDS. AIDS epidemic update; November 2004:1.
20. WHO/UNAIDS/Global Fund/US Government. Joint media release. 26 January 2005.
21. UNAIDS. Resource needs for an expanded response to AIDS in low and middle income countries. Final Discussion Paper. Document prepared for Making the Money Work – The Three Ones in Action meeting, London; 9 March 2005:2, 4.
22. UNAIDS. Report on the global AIDS epidemic; June 2004:131, 147.
23. The Global Fund, Report of the Executive Director. Document prepared for the 10th Board Meeting, Geneva; 21–22 April 2005:4.
24. WHO. Online. Available: www.who.int/3by5/newsitem9/en
25. The Global Response to AIDS. Making the Money Work; the Three Ones in action. Communiqué from the high-level meeting; 9 March 2005.

26. WHO. Online. Available: www.who.int/tb/hiv/faq/en/index.html (accessed 11 May 2005).

27. UNAIDS. Report on the global AIDS epidemic; 2004:26, 84.

28. UNAIDS/WHO. Epidemological Fact Sheet on HIV/AIDS and sexually transmitted infections – Iran. Update 2004:3.

29. Wolfe D, Malinowska-Sempruch K. Illicit drug policies and the global HIV epidemic: Effects of UN and National Government approaches. New York: Open Society Institute; 2004:11.

30. Burkhalter Holly J. Physicians for human rights, human resources for health and the Global HIV/AIDS pandemic. Washington: US House International Relations Committee; 13 April 2005.

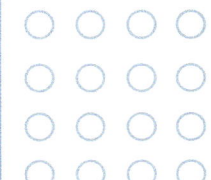

Index

Emboldened page numbers indicate chapters; *italicised* numbers indicate maps, boxes, diagrams and illustrations (there are frequently textual references on these pages also)

A

AAI (accelerated access initiative) 649, 671

AAV (adeno-associated virus) 82

AAVP (African AIDS Vaccine Program) 573, 574

abacavir (ABC) 242, 265, 521
  antiretroviral therapy *138*, 140, *142*, 145
  children and adolescents *481*, 626, *627*
  drug abuse *522*
  hypersensitivity reactions 187, *188*
  mother-to-child transmission prevention 504
  pharmacology *172*, *177*
  post-exposure prevention *716*, 717, 721
  resistance to 152, *159*, 542
  tuberculosis 350

ABC strategy (Abstinence, Be faithful, Condoms) 10, 117, *142*

ABG (arterial blood gas) 215

ABIA (Brazilian Interdisciplinary AIDS Association) 696

absolute lymphocyte count (ALC) 327

absorption, poor *see* malabsorption

ABVD 368, 468

Accelerated Access Initiative (AAI) 649, 671

access to treatment 96–7, 207
  accelerated 649, 671
  medicines 663–5
  universal *see* Brazil

acidosis 291

ACORN (Aids Research and Control Centre) 731

acquired immunity to viral infections 40–1

ACTG (Aids Clinical Trials Group) 185, 419

action stage of change 113

acupuncture 550–1

acute infection **63–74**, 76
  acute retinal necrosis (ARN) 232–3
  bacterial pneumonia 622
  clinical manifestation 66–7

diagnosis 68
management 71–2
pathophysiology 63–6
see also laboratory testing

acyclovir (Zovirax) 97
  gastrointestinal disorders 229, *252*, 254, 256, 259
  management of infections 450–1, *451*, 453, 454–5, *456*

ADC *see* AIDS dementia complex

adefovir 515
  dipivoxil *418*, 419

adeno-associated virus (AAV) 82

adenosylmethionine, S- 315

adenovirus (ADV) 82, 83, 256, 280

ADH secretion 288

adherence to antiretroviral therapy in resource-limited settings **207–13**
  barriers to 209–10
  levels of 208–9
  predictors of 208
  resource-rich settings 207–8, 210–11

adolescents 117, 483–4, 488, 631
  see also children

adrenal
  alterations in function 290
  antiretroviral and other therapies 290–1
  DHEA in HIV infection 290
  insufficiency *280*, 291
  pathology 290
  treatment considerations 291

Adult AIDS Clinical Trials Group 283

adulthood, expectations of 783–4, *783*, *785*

AFE inhibitors 596–7, *597*

affect, flattened 263

affordability of essential medicines for HIV/AIDS 664

Afghanistan 299

Africa (mainly sub-Saharan) 46, *84*, 104, 362, 415, 464, **565–75**, 589, 650
  adherence to treatment 207–9
  biology of transmission 75, 77
  cardiovascular complications 279
  children in resource-limited settings 621–2, 625, 628, 629

complementary and alternative medicine 547–8, 551
counselling 117
dermatology 237, 238, 239, 240, 241, 242, 245
diarrhea 737, 741
drug abuse *514*
drug resistance 153, 154, 704, 705, 706, 708
Eastern Europe and 587, 588
economic impact 769–73, *772*, 775n–6
essential medicines *663*, 665
fungal infections 376, 377, 378, 381, 382
global epidemiology 1, 2, 3, 4, 9–11, *10*
HAART implementation 677, 683, 686, *689*
international funding for care and prevention 794, 795, 796, 798–9
IRIS 198, 201
malaria 747–8, 750–1
malnutrition 604, 608, 609, 610
mother-to-child transmission 497, 498, *500*, *501–2*, 503, 506–7
NGOs active in HIV and Web 725n, 726, 727n, 728–30, *734*
non-sterile injections and pandemic 704, 758–9, 760, 761–3, 764
North *see* Middle East and North Africa
ocular manifestations 234
origins and diversification of HIV 15, 16, 17
orphans 78–91, 787–91
pathogen-host-environment interactions 779, *780*, 781, *782–3*
pharmacoeconomics 670, 671–4
pharmacology of antiretroviral drugs 173, 177, 178
pneumonias 309, *310–12*, 324
prevalence decline 565–6
primary neurological manifestations 261, 265

Africa (mainly sub-Saharan) (continued)
  psychiatric problems 271, 272, 273, 274
  renal complications 299, 300-2, 305, 306
  resource-poor settings 616-18, 654, 704, 705, 706, 708
  testing and counselling 118
  travel, international 560, 561, 562
  tuberculosis 333, 334, 335, 338, 339-40, 341, 350
  vaginal microbicides 595
  women and special issues 487, 488-9, 490, 491
  see also HIV-2; malnutrition; prevention in Africa
Africam diarrhea 737, 740
AG1549 (capravirine) 129
ageing, neuropathy 267
age-specific mortality 782, 783
AGF-1 288
AIDS dementia complex (ADC) 136, 261, 267, 275
  stages 264, 265
  see also HAD
AION (anterior ischemic optic neuropathy) 234-5
AITD (autoimmune thyroid diseases) 201, 289
AK602 (Aplaviroc) inhibitor 126
alanine aminotransferase 420
alanyl-glutamine 743
albendazole 256, 741
albumin, low 383
alcohol consumption/alcoholism 295, 416
alendronate 293
alitretinoin gel 470
alphavirus family 82
Alternative Medicine Care Outcomes in AIDS 549
alternative therapies 202, 538
ALVAC (canary pox) 82
AMCOA 549
AMD070 and AMD3100 inhibitors 126
amdoxovir 127-8
amebic dysentery 256
amenorrhea 295
amikacin 257, 345, 349, 358, 740
aminoglycosides 257, 328, 349
  see also amikacin; kanamycin; streptomycin
aminosalicylic acid 346, 349
amitriptyline 515, 551
amoxicillin 325, 326, 328
amoxicillin-clavulanate 325, 328
amphotericin B
  cardiovascular complications 281

dermatology 241, 244, 245
fungal infections 379, 380, 381, 382, 384, 386
  candida 368, 369, 370, 371
gastrointestinal disorders 252, 253
histoplasmosis 331
liposomal 560
penicillium marneffei infection 397
pneumonias 329, 330
travel, international 560, 561
ampicillin 257
  -sulbactam 328
amprenavir 151, 242, 360, 742
  antiretroviral therapy 139, 141, 142
  children and adolescents 481, 482
  drug abuse 521, 523
  HIV-2 643
  inhibitory quotient 543
  pharmacology 171, 172, 176, 177
  tuberculosis 351
  women 494
  see also fos-amprenavir
anabolic steroids 295, 296
anaerobes 324
anal carcinoma 258, 464
anal condyloma 258
anal fissures and fistulas 258
anal sphincter dysfunction 439
androgen therapy 296
ANECCA 627
anemia 257, 295, 327, 383, 426, 445, 607
  children 622, 624
angiomatosis see bacillary angiomatosis
angiosarcoma 430
angiotensin-converting enzyme inhibitors 304-5
Angola 547, 726
anidulafungin 370
animal studies 598, 711-12
anorectal disease 258-9
anorectal herpes infection 448-9
anorexia 289, 440, 444, 605, 611
anoscopy 259
antenatal HIV 4, 9
  mother-to-child transmission prevention 500-2
  see also pregnancy
anterior ischemic optic neuropathy (AION) 234-5
antibodies 23, 25
  anticryptococcal 382
  eliciting neutralizing 85-6
  responses to acute infection 65, 68, 69
  viral escape from 43
antihistamines 245
anti-inflammatory properties of microbicides 599
antimony 241

antipneumocystis therapy 257
antiretroviral therapy/treatment see ART; HAART; medicines; pharmacology
antiviral host factors and molecular biology of HIV 34-5
antiviral therapy/treatment for children 478-83
  breast-feeding 505
  changing 482
  initial therapy 480-2
  principles of 478-9
  resistance 482, 505-6
  therapeutic drug monitoring 483
  timing start 479, 480
  see also children in resource-limited settings
apes, HIV from see origins; SIV
aphthous stomatitis 245
aphthous ulcers 366, 493, 624
  recurrent (RAU) 216, 217, 222
Aplaviroc inhibitor 126
APOBEC3G 34-5, 34, 77, 161, 162
appendicitis 256
appetite loss 611
apraxia, dementia with 263
APRICOT study 419
aprivus see tipranavir
APV see amprenavir
Argentina 592, 733
ARGs (AIDS-restricting genes) 44, 193
  beneficial effects 194
  timing of initiative 193, 196-7
  see also IRIS
ARN (acute retinal necrosis) 232-3
ART/ARV (antiretroviral therapy/treatment) 135-48, 501, 592, 705
  acute infection 71
  adrenal 290-1
  -associated hepatotoxicity 420-1
  bone 293
  children 626, 629
  clinical application 141-4
  cornerstone agents 137, 140-1
  dermatology 238, 243
  drug pressure 163-6, 164
  experimental strategies 144
  gastrointestinal disorders 251, 255
  highly active see HAART
  immune reconstitution inflammatory syndrome 200
  induction-maintenance 144
  IRIS 198, 201
  laboratory testing 107
  'late' salvage 145-6
  in life cycle of HIV 136-7
  natural history of HIV infection 135-6
  non-suppressive 705

pancreas 292
pharmacoeconomics 668, 669, 671
pituitary 288
prevention of HIV 95, 98
primary neurological
    manifestations 261, 264–5,
    268
renal complications 304
reproductive health in men 294–5
reproductive health in
    women 295–6
susceptibility 149, 152, 154
testing and counselling 112
thyroid 289
timimg, optimal 143–4
toxic neuropathy (ATN) 266, 267
toxicity 145
tuberculosis 335, 350
unregulated 705
viral failure and management
    approaches 144–5
see also complications; drug
    resistance; new drug
    development;
    pharmacoeconomics;
    pharmacology; regimens
artemether 749, 750
artemisinine 661
arterial blood gas (ABG) 215
arthragias 297
ARV see ART/ARV
ascorbic acid (vitamin C) 608
Asia 3, 46, 84, 154, 209, 261, 299,
    577–85, 771
    Brazil compared with 701
    children in resource-limited
        settings 622, 628
    complementary and alternative
        medicine 548–9
    dermatology 241
    drug abuse 513, 514
    drug resistance in resource-poor
        settings 704, 705–6
    economic impact 771, 775
    fungal infections 376, 382, 387
    global epidemiology 2, 8–9, 11, 15,
        26
    hepatitis viral infection 415
    high-risk groups 577–82
    immune reconstitution
        inflammatory syndrome 199,
        201
    international funding for care and
        prevention 796, 798
    medicines 582–3, 663, 665
    mycobacterium avium
        complex 355, 362
    NGOs active in HIV and Web 725,
        726, 734

non-sterile injections and
    pandemic 757, 760
orphans 789–90
pathogen-host-environment
    interactions 779–80, 783
penicillium marneffei infection 394,
    395, 396, 397
pharmacoeconomics 671
pneumocystis pneumonia 309,
    313–14
prevention 91, 92, 97
psychiatric problems 272–3, 275
travel, international 555, 558, 559,
    560, 561
tuberculosis 333, 334
vaginal microbicides 595
women and special issues 487, 489
see also malnutrition
aspartate aminotransferase 420
aspergillus/aspergillus fumigatus 282,
    288, 329, 380
    aspergillosis from 217, 245, 324,
        327–8, 330
atazanavir (ATZ/ATV) 188, 360
    antiretroviral therapy 139, 141
    children and adolescents 481, 482
    drug abuse 521, 523, 524
    HIV-2 643
    inhibitory quotient 543
    pharmacology 172, 176, 177
    post-exposure prevention 716, 717,
        721
    tuberculosis 351
    women 494
atherosclerosis 281, 283
ATN (antiretroviral toxic
    neuropathy) 266, 267
atorvastatin 718
atovaquone 319, 320, 406, 407, 661, 741
atropine 256
attachment inhibitors, new 124–5
ATV/ATZ see atazanavir
Australia 1, 2, 84, 92, 273, 355, 393, 514,
    764
    essential medicines 663, 665
    fungal infections 376, 382
autoimmune thyroid diseases
    (AITD) 201, 289
autoimmunity 280
AVX754 inhibitor 127
axonal degeneration 267
azido-thymidine see AZT
azithromycin 741
    dermatology 238, 239
    essential medicines for 661
    gastrointestinal disorders 256, 257,
        258
    mycobacterium avium
        complex 358–9, 360

pneumonias 325, 326, 327, 328
    toxoplasmic encephalitis 406, 407
    travel, international 559
azoospermia 295
azotemia 300
AZT (azido-thymidine)
    Brazil 697
    children and adolescents 477, 478,
        482
    mother-to-child transmission 498,
        500, 505, 509–10, 511
    pharmacology 173, 178
aztreonam 328

B

BA see bacillary angiomatosis
babies see infants
bacillary angiomatosis (BA) 216, 238
    bartonella infections 426, 427–8,
        432–3
bacillary peliosis 425, 427, 433
bacteremia 425, 430, 433
    fever of unknown origin 428–9
    see also bartonella infections
bacterial infections 78, 281, 624
    anorectal 258
    oral 216, 217, 219–21
bacterial pneumonias 323–7, 490, 624
    pneumococcal 323–4
    see also hemophilus influenzae;
        pseudomonas aeruginosa;
        staphylococcus aureus
bactrim 515
Bahamas 501
Baltimore see urban care models in USA
Bandicoota bengalensis 394
Bangladesh 8, 577, 580
bartonella infections 425–36
    bacilliformis 430
    clinical presentation 425–9
    diagnosis 429–30
    epidemiology and
        prevention 433–4
    henselae 428–34 passim
    history 425
    quintana 425, 427, 428–34 passim
    relapse 432
    treatment 430–3
basal ganglia impairment 263
Baylor Collage of Medicine 728
B-cell receptors 40, 42, 264
BCG vaccination 352
BCH-10618 inhibitor 127
behaviour defined 275
behavioural change
    with HAD 263
    programs and sexual
        transmission 93–4

behavioural theories, testing and
counselling 112–13
belching *252*
Benin 118, 726
benzalkonium chloride 506–7, 596
benzathine penicillin 239, 259
benznidazole 560
benzodiazepines *719*
benzyl benzoate 240
Bermuda 6
betalactam and betalactamase 324, 326, *328*
BILR 355 BS 129
bioavailability of nutrients, improving 609–10
biological phenotype and disease progression 53–5
biology of HIV-1 transmission **75–80**
early target cells and virus-host dynamics 78–9
endogenous host factors 77–8
exogenous host factors 78
infecting partner 75–6
prevention 79–80
superinfection 79
viral selection 76–7
bipolar disorder 274
bisphosphonates 293
bladder dysfunction 439
blastomyces 380
blastomycosis 383, 384
bleomycin *471*
blood transfusions/blood-borne transmission 1, 9, 91–2, 415
avoiding *556*
chemistry in resource-poor settings 650, 707–8
harm reduction programs *93*, 94–5
non-sterile injections and pandemic 187
safe 94, 570, 697, 761, 763
see also DBS/DPS; drug abuse; non-sterile injections
BMD (bone marrow density) 293
BMS488043 inhibitor 23, 124–5
BMS806 *597*
bone
antiretroviral and other therapies 293
infection, bartonella *426*, 432–3
metabolism alterations 293
treatment considerations 293–4
boric acid *369*
Botswana 9, *10*, 350, 487, 674, 686, 725n
adherence to therapy 209, 210
children in resource-limited settings 621, 629
complementary and alternative medicine 547

economic impact 769, 775n
mother-to-child transmission *502*, 503
NGOs active in HIV and Web 728, 729
pathogen-host-environment interactions 780, *783*, 784
Pneumocystis pneumonia *310, 311, 312*
prevention 565, 569, 570, 573
bottom-up costing 669
brain *see* cerebral; encephalitis; encephalopathy
Brazil 6, 104, 288, *302*, 471, *501*, 560, 761, *775n*
adherence to therapy 209, 210
dermatology 239, 240
drug abuse 592
international funding 796
mycobacterium avium complex 355, 356
orphans 790
pharmacoeconomics 671, 672
pneumocystis pneumonia *313, 314*
tuberculosis *334, 335*
Brazil and universal access **695–702**
background 695–6
care and treatment 697–700
civil society 696
government 696
prevention 697
results 697, *700, 701*
breast-feeding 1, 2
alternatives to 95
biology of HIV-1 transmission 75
mother-to-child transmission prevention 498, 499, *500–2*, 505
non-sterile injections and pandemic 763
risks 11, 76, 92, 98, 505
brecanavir (GW640385, VX-385) inhibitor 131
bronchiectasis 622, *624*
bronchopneumonia 324, *325*
buffer gel *597*
buprenorphine 94, 531
drug abuse 516, *519*, 520, 521, *522*, 524
Burkina Faso *500*, 565, 569, 726, 727n
Burkitt's lymphoma 295, 464, 622
Burundi 775n
butoconazole *369*

C

C31G 596, *600*
cachexia (marasmus) 603–4
caesarean birth, elective 507

calanolide A 549–50
calcipotriene 242
Cambodia 8, 393, 573, 583–4, 671
high-risk groups 577, *578*, 580, *581*, 582
NGOs active in HIV and Web 726, 727, 728, 731
pathogen-host-environment interactions *783*
Cameroon 208–9, 306
economic impact *772*, 775
HIV-1 group M from 10, 16–17
NGOs active in HIV and Web 725n, 726
prevention 569, 573
campylobacter 440, *738*
jejuni 257
Canada *see* North America
cancer *see* malignancy
cancrum oris 245
candida/candidiasis 4, 67, 194, 253, *329*, **365–73**, 380
albicans 253, 282, 366, 367, 368, 370, 371, 372, 440
candidemia 367, *369*, 371–2
clinical manifestations 366–7
diagnosis 367–8
diet and 605
disseminated 367
dubliensis 366
endophthalmitis 228
epidemiology 365–6
erythematous *216*
gastrointestinal disorders 251, *252*, 253–4
glabrata 366, 368, 370
krusei 366, 368, 370
malnutrition *611*, 612
oesophageal 251, 253, 365, 367, *369*, 370–1
oral 215–16, *216, 217*, 624
oropharyngeal 365, 366, *369*, 370–1
penicillium marneffei infection 397
prevention 372
skin disorders 243–4
treatment 368–72
tropicalis 366
cannabis 550
cannomys badius 394
capravirine 129
capreomycin *345, 349*
Carbopol 974P 596, *600*
carcinoma *see* malignancy
cardiomyopathy 279–81, *625*
cardiovascular complications **279–86**
cardiomyopathy and congestive heart failure 279–81
coronary artery disease 282–3
endocarditis 282

neoplasms 282
pericardial disease 281
pulmonary hypertension 281–2
cardiovascular risk 184, 185, 559, 561
Caribbean/Central America 84, 91,
104, 244, 314, 590, 595, 686
dermatology 237, 240
global epidemiology 2, 3, 6
international funding for care and
prevention 794, 796
NGOs active in HIV and Web 728,
729, 730, 735, 782
prevention 91, 92, 94
travel, international 558, 559
carmustine 466
carnitine deficiency 186, 280
carpal tunnel compression 297
carrageenan 596, 597, 600
caspofungin 243
candida 252, 329, 369, 370, 371
Castleman's disease, multicentric
469
Catholicism
Catholic Medical Missions
Board 730
Catholic Relief Services
(CRS) 729–30
and condom use 697
cats and diseases 399
see also bartonella
CCD (Centers for Diseases Control and
Prevention) 623
CCLs (chemokine ligands) 55, 56, 77
CCOs (clinical cut offs) 543
CCR2 55, 56
CCR5 66, 87, 136, 166, 573
biology of HIV-1 transmission 76,
77, 78, 80
inhibitors 25, 27, 262
vaginal microbicides 595, 597
viral and host determinants of
disease progression 53, 55, 56
CD4 T-cells, numbers of 76, 87, 146,
355, 616
acute infection 63, 64, 65, 66, 67,
71–2
adherence to antiretroviral
therapy 208
antiretroviral therapy 143, 144
bartonella infections 425, 429
biology of HIV-1 transmission 76,
78–9
cardiovascular complications 282
children and adolescents 476, 477,
478, 480, 623–5, 629, 630
clinical implications of HIV
fitness 164, 165, 166, 167
drug-resistant HIV, antiretroviral
therapy of 540, 541, 542, 544

enumeration 649, 650–5, 653
fungal infections 377, 384
gastrointestinal disorders 254, 255,
256, 257, 258
hepatitis 199, 416, 419
immune response to HIV 40–4,
46
IRIS 194
laboratory testing 104, 106
loss 52–3, 136, 145
lymphocyte counts 143, 266
molecular biology of HIV and
implications for new
therapies 25, 27
neoplasia 464, 465
NRTIs 140
ocular manifestations 232
pharmacoeconomics 669, 670
pipeline technologies 655
pneumonias 324, 326–7, 328
pneumocystis 309, 315, 319
receptors 23, 136, 262
renal complications 302
resource-poor settings and
laboratories 649, 650–5, 653,
655
toxoplasmic encephalitis 400, 405,
408, 409
travel, international 556
vaginal microbicides 595–6, 597
women 494
CD8 T-cells 85, 104
acute infection 63, 64, 65, 66, 72
eliciting in responses in design of
global AIDS vaccine 82
IRIS 194
CDC (Centers for Disease Control and
Prevention) 556, 604
CDE infusional regime 466
CEA (cost-effectiveness analysis)
668
CEE see Central and Eastern Europe
cefazolin 328
cefdinir 325, 328
cefditoren 328
cefepime 328
cefotaxime 324, 325, 327, 328
cefpodoxime 325
cefprozil 325, 328
ceftazidime 328
ceftizoxime 432
ceftriaxone 258, 432
pneumonias 324, 325, 327, 328
cefuroxime 325, 328
cellulitis 515
cellulose sulfate 596, 597, 600
Center of Hope 731
Central African Republic 10, 16, 547,
775n

Central and Eastern Europe 2, 3, 8, 11,
104, 587–94, 728
children in resource-limited
settings 626, 628
drug abuse 513, 514, 592–3
dual epidemic with former Soviet
Union 588–9
economic impact 769, 775n
harm reduction programs 589–90
human rights 590–1
international funding 798
non-sterile injections and
pandemic 760–2, 763, 764
prevention 91, 92, 95
treatment 591–3
tuberculosis 334, 335, 336
vaginal microbicides 595
central nervous system and bartonella
infections 428
central reference laboratories 654–5,
656, 658
cephalosporin 432, 515
gastrointestinal disorders 257,
258–9
pneumonias 325, 326, 327,
328
cephalosporin-cefpodoxime 328
cercocebus (torquatous) atys see
mangabey
cerebral
atrophy 377
infection 262, 263
internal reward circuitry 275
leukoencephalopathy see PML
toxoplasmosis see toxoplasmic
encephalitis
cerebrovascular accident 515
cervical disorders 491–3
carcinoma 464
cervical intraepithelial neoplasia
(CIN) 491–2
ectopy 488
cesarean delivery 95
elective 507
Chagas disease 560–1
challenges for HAART in
underdeveloped countries 678–86,
678
demand-side 684–6
future 692–4
supply-side 683–4
cheilitis 218, 624
chemical prevention see microbicides
chemokine receptor 262
complex 136
inhibitors, new 125–6
ligands affecting viral load
55–7
chemotherapy, neoplasia 470–1

chest
  pain *252, 253*
  radiography 324, 327, 331, 383
chicken pox *216*
children 11, 78, **475–85**, 732
  cardiovascular complications 280
  cesarean delivery 95
  cost of treating 670
  counselling 117, 631, *632–3*
  economic impact (poverty) 769–70,
    771–2
  epidemiology 475
  HIV prevalence in 4–5, 7, 8, 9, 76
  HIV-2 in 641
  in hospitals and other
    institutions 758, 760–3
  lifetime risk of AIDS *783, 785*
  malaria 748
  management 483
  monitoring treatment 617
  natural history 475–6
  prophylaxis of other infections 483
  rarely infected with HIV-2 639
  therapeutic drugs and 177
  vertical transmission to 75
  see also adolescents; antenatal;
    antiviral therapy/treatment for
    children; breast-feeding;
    infants; mother-to-child;
    orphans; pregnancy
children in resource-limited
    settings **621–35**
  antiretroviral therapy 625–9, *627*
  clinical aspects 621–3
  diagnostic issues 623
  disease staging *623–6*
  failure of therapy and second-line
    regimens 629–30, *630*
  follow-up, monitoring and
    support 631, *632–3*
Chile *314*, 777
chimpanzee, HIV-1 from 1, 14–15, 16,
  17–18, 167
China 46, 91, 104, 209, 241, 273, 548,
  561, 584, 704, 726
  Brazil compared with 701
  complementary and alternative
    medicine 549, 550
  drug abuse 513, *514*
  essential medicines *663, 665*
  global epidemiology 8, 11
  high-risk groups 577, *578*, 580, 582
  international funding 798
  orphans 789
  pathogen-host-environment
    interactions 779–80
  penicillium marneffei infection 393,
    394
  tuberculosis 333, *334*, 336

chlamydia pneumonia 326, *328*
chlamydia trachomatis *258*
chlorhexidine 506–7
chloroquine 199, *201*, 202, 661, 749
cholesterol levels 184, 185, *283*
cholestin 550
CHOP regime (cyclophosphamide,
    doxorubicin, vincristine,
    prednisone) 465
chorioamnionitis prevention 506
chorioretinitis 437–9
chronic mental illness 271, 273–4
cidofovir (vistide) 246
  gastrointestinal disorders *252*, 254
  management of infections 438, 439,
    446, 453
  ocular manifestations 229, *230*,
    234–5
ciprofloxacin 257, 558
  diarrhea 739, 740
  mycobacterium avium
    complex 358, 362
  pneumonias 326, *328*
  travel, international *556*, 559
  tuberculosis *345, 349*
circulating recombinant forms
    (CRFs) 15
circumcision 78, 97–8, 572–3
  lack of/need for 489, 572–3
cirrhosis 419
cisapride *718, 719*
CKD (chronic kidney disease) 300
clarithromycin 257, 740
  mycobacterium avium
    complex 358–9, *360*, 361
  pneumonias 327, *328*
  toxoplasmic encephalitis *406, 407*
clindamycin 257
  dermatology 237, 242
  pneumonia 318, *319*, 325, 326, *328*
  toxoplasmic encephalitis 405, *406*,
    407
clinical features
  early 67
  fungal infections 385–6
  HIV-2 640–1
  HIV-associated dementia 263
  mycobacterium avium
    complex 356–7
  neuropathy 266
  penicillium marneffei
    infection 395–6
  renal complications 302–3
  vacuolar myelopathy 267–8
clinical implications of HIV fitness and
    virulence **161–72**
  antiretroviral drug pressure 163–6,
    164
  genetic diversity of HIV-1 161–2

  immune activation and
    virulence 162
  replicative capacity 163
clinical research and urban care models
    in USA 533
clinical trials for prevention of
    MTCT 499, *500–2*, 503–4
clofazimine 358, 359, 740
clostridium difficile 255, 257, *738*
clotrimazole 243, *252, 253, 369*, 370
CMA (cost minimization analysis) 668
CMPD167 597
CMV *see* cytomegalovirus
CNS disease
  antiretroviral drugs
    compartment 265
  HAD 262, 264
  opportunistic 267
  primary lymphoma 467
coagulopathy, disseminated
    intravascular 257
cocaine 518
  see also drug abuse
coccidioides 380
  immitis *329, 385*, 386, 394, 558
coccidiomycosis 324, *376*, 384, 385–7,
    625
  clinical manifestations 385–6
  diagnosis 386
  epidemiology 385
  microbiology 385
  travel, international 561
  treatment 386–7
cocksackie virus Group B *280*
codeine 256
cognitive changes with HAD 263, 264
cognitive motor disorder,
    HIV-associated 261, 262
  minor (MCMD) 263
cognitive theory of behaviour 112
co-incident illness 143
co-infection 66
Col-3 and neoplasia 471
colitis 255, 256, 257–8, 259
  cytomegalovirus 440, *441*
combination of drugs avoided 96,
  173
combivir 706
commercial sex workers 8, 9, 488,
  489
  Asia 577, *578, 579*, 580, *581*
  counselling 113, 118
  prevention policy in Africa 571
community interventions 93
community-based prevention programs
    in Africa 569–70
competition and essential
    medicines 664
complement receptors (CR) 336

complementary and alternative
medicine **547–54**
acupuncture 550–1
Asia 548–9
Europe 551–2
mind-body therapy 551
North America 549–51
Southern Africa 547–8
vitamins 551
complications from antiretroviral
therapy **181–91**
abacavir hypersensitivity
reactions 187, *188*
drugs 184–5
efavirenz toxicity profile 188
hematological 187
lactic acidosis and
hyperlactatemia 185–6
lipoatrophy 181, 182–4
'lipodystrophy syndrome' 181–2,
182
liver function and enzyme
abnormalities 188
monitoring and managing 185
nevirapene toxicity 189
pancreatis 186
tenofovir renal safety 187
see also cardiovascular
complications; endocrine
complications; neuropathy;
ocular complications; oral
complications; renal
complications
compound-1/compound-x 129
computed tomography *427*
concentration level of drugs *172*
condoms promoted 8, 10, 93
Africa *566*, 567, 570
Asia 580–1, 587
Brazil and Catholicism 697
harm reduction 94
insistence on difficult for
women 595
vaginal 97
condyloma, anal 258
congestive heart failure 279–81
Congo 10, *311*, 395, 775n
NGOs active in HIV and Web 726,
727
origins and diversification of
HIV 16, 17–18, 19
renal complications 299, 306
conjunctivitis 229
constipation 611
consumer and community advisory
boards in USA 534
contemplation stage of change 113
contraception 296, 495
see also condoms

co-receptor tropism 165–6
co-receptors and biological
phenotype 53–4
cornerstone agents in ARV
therapy 137, 140–1
coronary artery disease *280*, 282–3
coronaviruses 256
cortical atrophy *264*
corticosteroids 293, 305, 319
gastrointestinal disorders 254
immune reconstitution
inflammatory syndrome of
HIV 199–200, 201, 202
toxoplasmic encephalitis 405
corticosterone 290
corticotrophin-releasing hormone
(CH) 290
costs/funding 618, 668–74
in Brazil reduced 698
of care, pharmacoeconomics
and 669–70, 672
dictating choices 616–17
-effectiveness analysis 668
of illness in developing
countries 670–1
macroplanning analysis of 671–2
medicines 146, 209–10, 615, 616–17,
667–9, 790
minimization analysis 668
need for 775–7
prevention 96
of syringes and sterilization 756,
757
urban care models in USA 534–5
utility analysis 668–9
world data, interpreting 673–4
see also economic impact;
international funding
cosyntropin 291
Côte d'Ivoire *10*, 306, 569, 628,
725n
economic impact 771, 772, 775n
international funding 796
pathogen-host-environment
interactions *783*
pharmacoeconomics 670, 672
cotrimoxazole (CTX) 366, 625, 700,
749–51
Coulter XL *653*, 654
counselling 143
for children 117, 631, *632–3*
peer 117, 787
prevention 94, 95
prisoners 117, 787
targeted 93
voluntary 94
see also testing and counselling
couple, counselling 117
Coxsackie virus 280

CRAG (cryptococcal antigen) test
378–9, 381
creatine, elevated serum 306
CRFs (circulating recombinant
forms) 15
Croatia 589
Crohn's disase *258*
cross-cutting supporting
functions *680–2*
CRs (complement receptors) 336
cryotherapy 470
cryptococcal meningitis 4, 233, 275,
328, 397
children 622
fungal infections 377–8, 380–1, 383,
385, *386*
immune reconstitution
inflammatory syndrome *197*,
198–9, 201
primary neurological
manifestations 252, 261
cryptococcosis 67, *196*, *228*, 244, *281*,
375–82, *625*
clinical manifestation 377
diagnosis 377–9
disseminated 561
epidemiology and
pathogenesis 376–7
extraneural 378–9
fungal infections *329*
gastrointestinal disorders 255, 258
microbiology 375–6
non-meningeal disease 380
oral complications *216*, *217*
pneumonias 324, 328, *330*
prognosis 379
treatment 379–82, *380*
tuberculosis 195
see also cryptococcus; cryptococcal
meningitis
cryptococcus 383, 490
neoformans 282, 288, 290, 330, 375,
376, *378*, 380, 381, 397, 449, 558,
561
cryptosporidium *738*
cryptosporidium/
cryptosporidiosis 255, 256, 440,
556, *625*
CSF 262, 264, 482
CSWs *see* commercial sex workers
CT scans 264, 402, 403
CTLs (cytotoxic T-cell lymphocytes)
-based vaccines 82, 83, 85
response to infection *41*, 42, 46, 52
CTV *see* cytomegalovirus
CTX *see* cotrimoxazole
CUA (cost utility analysis) 668–9
Cunningham equation *603*, *604*
Cushing's syndrome 290–1

cutaneous bacillary angiomatosis *426*, 432
CX3CR1 56
CXCL12 56–7, 77
CXCR4 (X4) receptors 87, 136, 166, 262, 595
   biology of HIV-1 transmission 76, 77, 78
   molecular biology and implications for new therapies 25, 27
   viral and host determinants of HIV-1 disease progression 53, 55
cyanovirin 596, *597*
cyclophosphamide *465, 466*
cycloserine *345, 349*, 358
cyclospora *738*
CyFlow *653*, 654
CYP (cytochrome P450 enzymes) 174, 176
CYPA (cyclophilin A) 57
cytochrome P450 enzymes 174, 291
cytokines 290, 443
   production 262, 280
   proinflammatory 267
cytomegalovirus infections 437–47
   acute 67
   candida 367
   cardiovascular complications *280*, 282
   chorioretinitis 437–9
   colitis 440, *441*
   encephalitis 261, 262, 275, 439, 440
   endocrine complications 287, 291, 294
   gastrointestinal 251, *252, 253, 254, 255, 256, 258*, 440–1
   nervous system 438–40
   oophoritis 295
   oral complications *216, 217*
   prevention of infection 446–7
   pulmonary system 441
   radiculomyelitis 262
   retinitis 227–30, *228*, 231, 232, 442
   treatment 441–6
   ulcers 220
   ventriculitis 401
   women 490
cytoplasmic events, early 26, *27*
Cytoron *653*
cytospheres *652, 653*
cytotoxic T-cell lymphocytes *see* CTLs
cytovene *see* ganciclovir

D

D4T *see* stavudine
D30N 153
DAPD inhibitor 127–8

dapivirine *600*
dapsone 238
   pneumocystis pneumonia *319, 320*
   toxoplasmic encephalitis *406, 407, 408*
darunavir inhibitor 131, *139*, 141, *172*, 541
DBS/DPS (dried blood spot/plasma spot) technology 654, 655–6
DC *see* dendritic cells
DDC *see* dideoxycytidine; zalcitabine
DDI *see* didanosine
death rates *see* mortality
deficiency, nutritional 266
dehydroepiandrosterone (DHEA) 290
delavirdine (DLV) *150, 172*, 750
   children and adolescents *481*
   drug abuse 521, *522*
   post-exposure prevention *716, 717*, 721
   tuberculosis 350, *351*
delirium 174–5, 274–5, *274, 275*
demand-side challenges 684–6
dementia 274–5
   global 263
   subcortical 263
   ventriculoencephalitis 439–40
   see also AIDS dementia complex; HAD
demography 2, *5*, 8, 770
dendritic cells
   DC-SIGN receptor 25, 597
   impairment 43–4
   uptake of vaginal microbicides 595, 597
dengue 562
deoxycorticosterone 290
depression 208, 274, 483
dermatitis 380, *624*
   eczematous 245
   seborrheic 243
dermatology and global HIV *4*, 199, **237–47**
   skin disorders listed 237–46
design of global AIDS vaccine **81–90**
   advanced clinical trials *84*
   antibodies, eliciting neutralizing 85–6
   Cd8 T-cell responses, eliciting 82
   gene-based strategies 82
   immunogens, choice of 82–5
   immunogens, improved antibody-based 86–7
   neutralizing antibodies, eliciting 85–6
detection of virus 70–1
dexelvucitabine inhibitor 127
DFA (direct fluorescent antibody) 256
DHEA (dehydroepiandrosterone) 290

diabetes
   endocrine complications 287, 291, 292–3
   injections 756
   primary neurological manifestations 266
   renal complications 300
diagnosis
   acute infection 68
   bartonella infections 429–30
   children in resource-limited settings 623
   diagnostic testing 116
   fungal infections 367–8, 377–9
   hepatitis 417
   histoplasmosis 383–4
   HIV-associated dementia 263–4
   IRIS 194
   neuropathy 266–7
   penicillium marneffei infection 396–7
   pneumocystis pneumonia 317–18, 327
   renal complications 302–3
   toxoplasmic encephalitis 401–3, *401*
   tuberculosis 327
   vacuolar myelopathy 268
dialysis 305
diaphragms 97
diarrhea 4, 145, 188, 255, 331
   children 621, *624*
   drug-induced 258, 297
   malabsorption of food/drugs 538, 610, 742–3
   malnutrition 607, 611
   traveller's (TD) *556*, 558–9, 562
   women 494
diarrhea etiology and management **737–45**
   drug-related 742
   enteropathy, HIV 742
   infections 440, 444
   pathogens associated with 739–42
diclazuril 742
didanosine (DDL/DDI)
   antiretroviral therapy 138, 140
   cardiovascular complications 280
   children and adolescents 482
   complications 187
   endocrine complications 292
   hepatitis viral infection 420
   mother-to-child transmission prevention 505
   ocular manifestations 235
   pancreatitis 186, 543
   pharmacology *172, 173, 176, 177*
   post-exposure prevention 712, *713, 716, 717, 720, 721*

primary neurological manifestations 266
resistance to *150*, 152, 543
tuberculosis 350
dideoxycytidine (DDC) *172*, 292
dideoxynucleoside drugs 266, 267
see also didanosine; stavudine; zalcitabine
diffuse lymphocytosis syndrome *223*
dihydroergotamine *718, 719*
DILS (diffuse lymphocytosis syndrome) *223*
diphenoxylate 255
diphtheria vaccination 477, 478, 557
direct fluorescent antibody 256
direct observed therapy *see* DOT
disclosure of HIV status 114
diseases associated with HIV infection 215–474
see also bartonella ; candida; cardiovascular; cryptococcosis; dermatology; endocrine; gastrointestinal; hepatitis; herpesvirus; *Mycobacterium*; neoplasia; ocular; oral; *Penicillium*; pneumonia; primary neurological manifestations; psychiatric barriers; renal complications; toxoplasmosis; tuberculosis
disseminated mycobacterium avium complex and other mycobacterial infections *216, 324,* **355–64,** *416*
atypical infections *362*
children *625*
diagnosis 357
epidemiology 355–7
prophylaxis 361–2
therapy 358–61
distal neuropathy 440
distal sensory polyneuropathy (DSP) 186, 266
DLV *see* delavirdine
DNA
detection of toxoplasmic encephalitis 402
flap 26
HIV-DNA 623
PCR diagnosis 477
plasmid immunization 82
pro-viral 68
synthesis, interference with 267
testing 105, 107
Dominican Republic 728
dopamine antagonist effect 288
dopamine transporters, loss of 263
dorsal column sensory deficits 267
DOT (direct observed therapy) 650
-ART (antiretroviral treatment) 531

doxorubicin 280, 465, *465*, 470, *471*
doxycycline 259, 741
bartonella infections 428, 430, *431, 432*, 433
dermatology 238, 239
pneumonias *325, 326, 328*
DRI (Dietary Refernce Intake) 607
dried blood/plasma *see* DBS/DPS
dronabinol (Marinol) 297, 550
drug abuse, intravenous 5, 6, 92, 275–6, **513–26**, 573
abstinence from drugs policy, flawed 592
adherence to therapy 207, 208
Africa 571–2
Asia 577, 578–9, *578, 579,* 587
Brazil 695, 697
commonly abused drugs *see* cocaine; heroin; methamphetamine
condom provision 94
counselling 94, 113, 118
Eastern Europe 589
endocrine complications 291, 294, 295
epidemiology 513
global epidemiology of HIV/AIDS 1–2, 3, 8, 9
hepatitis 199, 415
medically supervised withdrawal 519
mental illness 520–1
needle exchange programs 94, 95, 572, 589, 697
non-sterile needles and pandemic 759–60, 764
other related factors and behaviour *514*
parenteral transmission (contaminated needles) 75
psychiatric barriers 275–6
renal complications 299
substitution programs 95, 593
treatment/therapy 516–20
interactions of drugs 521–4, *522–3*
drug resistance development 71, 107, 143, **149–59,** 450, 539
generated 150–1
to HAART 151, 154, 537, 539, 541
management of infections 443
in non-B subtypes of HIV-1 group M 153–4
protease inhibitors 153
reverse transcriptase, inhibitors of 151–3
transmission of 154–5
drug resistance in resource-poor settings **703–10**

expectations 703–4
limitation strategies 708–9
monitoring 707
public health evaluation 706–7
scaling up treatment provision 703
subtype variability 708
testing 707–8
transmission surveillance 706–7
treated populations 705–6
untreated populations 704–5
drug resistant HIV, antiretroviral therapy of **537–46**
aims of treatment 537
determinants of failure 537–9
emergence of 539
evaluating extent of 539–41
management options 541–2
systematic approach to patient 542–4
drugs, therapeutic *see* medicines
DRV *see* darunavir
DSP (distal sensory polyneuropathy) 266, 267
dual infection 79
dynabeads 652, *653*
dysentery 257
dyslipidemia 184, 185, 283, *284*, 297
dyspepsia 252, 255
dysphagia 251, *252,* 253
dysplagia *253*
dystrophy 628
see also lipodystrophy
dysuria 489

E

E. coli 257, *258*
East Timor 580
Eastern Europe *See* Central and Eastern Europe
EasyCD4 *653*
EBV *see* Epstein-Barr virus
echocardiography 281
echovirus *280*
economic evaluation of pharmacoeconomics 667–9
economic impact in developing countries **769–78**
contradictory evidence 770–2
demography 770
funding, need for 775–7
human development 775
macroeconomic 772–5
microeconomic 770–1
sectorial approaches 771–2
see also costs/funding
Ecuador 726
eczematous dermatitis 245
edema 297

education
  to avoid risk 79–80
  Brazil 697
  decline 769, 772
  dietary 609
  need for 787
  school-based prevention programs
    in Africa 569, 571–2
  school-based sex education 93–4
efavirenz (EFV) 190, 242, 265, *360, 515,*
  708
  antiretroviral therapy *138, 142,* 143,
    145, 184, 238
  children and adolescents *481,* 626,
    627, 628, 630
  drug abuse 521, *522*
  endocrine complications 294
  hepatitis viral infection 421
  malaria 750
  mother-to-child transmission
    prevention 504, *508*
  mutations 140, 153
  pharmacology *172, 173, 176, 178*
  post-exposure prevention *716, 717,*
    719, 721
  resistance to *150,* 153, 539
  toxicity profiles 188
  travel, international 560
  tuberculosis *351*
Egypt 299, 758
EIA (enzyme immunoassay) 68–9, *70,*
  417
electronic medication monitoring 207
ELISA (enzyme-linked immunosorbent
  assay) 101–2, *103,* 105, 256, 396,
  654
  resource-poor settings 656, *657*
elvucitabine inhibitor 127
Emergency Plan for AIDS Relief *see*
  PEPFAR
emtricitabine (FTC)
  antiretroviral therapy 137, *138,*
    140
  children and adolescents *481, 482,*
    630
  hepatitis viral infection *418, 419*
  pharmacology *172, 173, 178*
  post-exposure prevention *716, 717,*
    720
  resistance to 539, 541
emtriva *522*
encephalitis 275, 367
  children 622
  with dementia and
    ventriculoencephalitis 439–40
  herpes simplex virus 449–50
  primary neurological
    manifestations 261, 262
  vaccination 557
  see also toxoplasmic encephalitis

encephalopathy 280, *624*
  progressive multifocal *see* PML
endocarditis 280, 282, 367, 383, 425,
  490, *515*
endocrine complications **287–98**
  see also adrenal; bone; pancreas;
    pituitary; reproductive health;
    thyroid
endocytosis 25
endogenous economic growth
  theory 773–5
endogenous host factors 77–8
endophthalmitis 367
end-stage renal disease 299, 300, 302
energy requirements 604–5
enfuvirtide 136, *139,* 141, 166, 172, 542
  HIV-2 643
  post-exposure prevention *716, 717,*
    721
entamoeba 440
  histolytica *738*
entecavir *515*
  hepatitis viral infection *418, 419*
enteric infections 558–9
  enteritis 255–7
  enterocolitis 256, 440
  enteropathy, HIV 742
  see also diarrhea
Env (envelope protein, gp160) 23, *24,*
  53, 54, 101
  clinical implications of HIV fitness
    and virulence 165–6
  design of global AIDS vaccine 81,
    83, 85, 86, 87, 88
enzyme
  abnormalities 188
  immunoassays *see* EIA; Elisa
  induction, metabolic 175–6
  inhibition 174–5
eosinophilic folliculitis 199
epidemiology and biology of HIV
  infection 1–90, 91–2, 102, 475
  bartonella infections 433–4
  fungal 365–6, 385
  hepatitis viral infection 415–16
  HIV-2 637–9
  natural history and
    treatment **637–47**
  nosocomial (non-sterile
    injections) 760–3
  renal complications 300–2
  tuberculosis 333–6, *334*
  see also acute infection; biology of
    HIV-1 transmission; design of
    global AIDS vaccine; global
    epidemiology; immune
    response; molecular biology;
    origins and diversification;
    viral and host determinants
EPOCH regimen 466

Epstein-Barr virus (EBV) 234, *280,* 401,
  443
  neoplasia *464,* 467, 468
EQAP (external quality assessment
  program) 655
Equatorial Guinea 16
ergonovine and ergotamine *718, 719*
ertapenem 328
erythema 426, *427*
erythematous candidiasis *216*
erythromycin 257, 327, 428
  bartonella infections 425, 430, *431,*
    432, 433
  dermatology 237, 238, 239
  diarrhea 739
erythropoietin-á 280
ESGS (glomerulosclerois) 301
esophageal disorders 251–4, 259
  candidiasis 251, 253, 365, 367, *369,*
    370–1, *624*
  esophagitis 440, 449
  esophagogastroduodenoscopy
    255
ESRD (end-stage renal disease) 299,
  300, 302
essential medicines **661–6**
  access to 663–5
  competition and affordability 664
  concept and definition 660–3, *662,*
    663
  national policies of integration and
    sustainability 665
  number of 665
  politically different from other
    medicines 665–6
  rational use 665
  WHO list of 615, 661, *662*
  see also medicines
Estonia 8, 593
estrogen 294
ethambutol (myambutol) 234, 257, *515,*
  740
  mycobacterium avium
    complex 358, 359, *360,* 362
  tuberculosis 342, *343, 344, 347, 348,*
    349, 350
ethinyl estradiol 296, 494
ethionamide 345, 349, 358
Ethiopia *10,* 153, 237, 306, *312,* 565, 787,
  796
  NGOs active in HIV and Web
    725n, 726, 728
ethnic variations 178
etoposide *466, 471*
etravirine 128, 541
Europe 15, *84,* 101, 144, 166, 189, 559,
  759
  adherence to therapy 207
  Brazil compared with 698, 699
  children 622

complementary and alternative
    medicine 551-2
dermatology 238, 239, 240, 245
drug abuse 513, 514, 520, 589, 592
drug resistance in resource-poor
    settings 704, 705, 706, 708
Eastern see Central and Eastern
    Europe
economic impact 773n, 777
essential medicines 663, 665
fungal infections 376
global epidemiology 1, 2, 3, 6-8
hepatitis viral infection 415, 416,
    421
international funding for care and
    prevention 793, 795, 798
IRIS 200
mother-to-child transmission 500,
    501, 504, 506, 507
mycobacterium avium
    complex 355, 356
neoplasia 470
NGOs active in HIV and Web 727,
    728, 729, 730, 733
non-sterile injections and
    pandemic 756, 759, 760, 762
penicillium marneffei infection 393
pharmacoeconomics 669
pneumocystis pneumonia 309
prevention 92
psychiatric problems 272, 273
renal complications 299, 300, 301,
    305
resource-poor settings 655
travel, international 555, 559, 560
vaginal microbicides 599-600
women and special issues 491
see also United Kingdom
European Centre for Epidemiological
    Monitoring of AIDS 6
evolution of HIV-1 76
EVR 420
exogenous host factors 78
expenditure see costs/funding
eyes see ocular manifestations

F

FACScan, FACScalibur and
    FACScount 653, 654
failure management 693
failure of treatment see drug resistant
    HIV
famciclovir 252, 254, 256, 259, 452, 454
fat, dietary 605, 609
    fat free mass (FFM) 604, 6003
fat distribution, abnormal body 182, 183
FDC (fixed dose combinations) 649
fertility see reproductive health
fetal loss, spontaneous 296

fever 4, 562, 624
FHI (Family Health
    International) 728-9
FI see fusion inhibitors
finance
    financing obstacles of structured
        health care 684
    savings reduction and life
        expectancy 773
    see also costs/funding
fitness see replication, viral
fleas on cats as vectors see bartonella
flow cytometers 653, 654
fluconazole
    dermatology 243, 244
    drug abuse 524
    fungal infections 378, 379-80, 381,
        386, 387
        candida 368, 369, 370-1, 372
        cryptococcal 378
    gastrointestinal disorders 252, 253
    pneumonias 329, 330
    travel, international 556
flucytosine 244, 379, 380, 381, 382, 384
fluorocortisone 291
fluoroquinolone 258, 494
    diarrhea 739
    pneumonias 324, 325, 326, 327, 328
    resistance 559
fluorouracil 492
fluoxetine 288
fluticasone 291, 718
folate deficiency 607-8
folinic acid (leucovorin calcium) 256,
    405, 406
follow-up for children in resource-
    limited settings 631, 632-3
fomivirsen 230
food
    drug interaction with 176
    insecurity see malnutrition
    security and rural
        production 784-5
fortovase (FTV) 141
fos-amprenavir (Fos-An) 716, 717, 721
foscarnet (foscavir) 740
    cardiovascular complications 280
    gastrointestinal disorders 252, 254,
        256
    hepatitis viral infection 452-3
    management of infections 438, 439,
        445-6, 456
    ocular manifestations 229, 230
fosinopril 304-5
France 1, 6, 84, 241, 301, 416, 470, 669,
    759, 777
    drug abuse 592
    immune reconstitution
        inflammatory syndrome 195,
        198

international funding 797
mother-to-child transmission 500,
    504, 506
NGOs active in HIV and Web 727,
    733
penicillium marneffei
    infection 394-5
Red Cross 727
FTC see emtricitabine
fumagillin 741
funding see costs/funding; international
    funding
fungal infections **375-91**, 561, 624
    keratitis 228, 229
    pneumonias 316, 327-31, 330
    primary prophylaxis 387
    see also candida; coccidiomycosis;
        cryptococcosis; histoplasmosis
fungal oral diseases 216, 218
    see also candidiasis
fungal pneumonias
    aspergillosis 327-8, 330
    cryptococcosis 328, 330
    histoplasmosis 330-1, 330
fungal/protozoan infection 241, 257-8,
    281
    deep systemic 244
    see also cryptococcus; histoplasma;
        toxoplasma
fungibility mechanism 776
furazolidone 742
fusion inhibitors 126-7, 136, 139, 141,
    171, 172
future
    challenges to HAART
        implementation in
        resource-constrained
        settings 692-4
    no reason to plan for 784
    possibilities for IRIS 202
    see also life expectancy

G

G8 Summit 616, 776
gabapentin 267, 515
Gabon 16, 705, 727n
Gag 24, 101, 136-7, 163
    design of global AIDS vaccine 81,
        83, 85
    viral and host determinants of
        disease progression 53,
        54
galactorrhea 288
gallium scanning 316
GALT (gut associated lymphoid
    tissues) 53
Gambia 641
gamma-benzene hexachloride see
    lindane

ganciclovir (cytovene) 281, 740
   cytomegalovirus 441–5, *442, 444*
      gastrointestinal disorders *252,* 254, 256
      management of infections 438, 439, 441–5, *442, 444,* 446–7
      ocular manifestations 229, *230,* 231
garlic 538, 550, *718, 719*
gastritis and gastroenteritis 254, 257
gastroesophageal reflux disease (GERD) 251, *252,* 254
gastrointestinal disorders **251–60,** *252, 258*
gastrointestinal disorders *see* enteric infections
gastrointestinal disorders
   anorectal disease 258–9
   bacillary angiomatosis 427–8
   esophageal 251–4
   gastric 254–5
   gastrointestinal intolerance 188
   management of infections 440–1
   prevention 440–1, 443
   see also colitis; diarrhea
GDP (gross domestic product) reduction 772–3, *772*
genes, viral accessory 54–5
   see also ARGs; Nef; Vif; Vpn; Vpr
genetics
   AIDS-restricting genes (ARGs) 44
   biology of transmission 77–8
   diversity 18–19, 161–2
   gene-based strategies in design of AIDS vaccine 82
   genome of HIV provirus *24*
   of innate immunity 14
   primary neurological manifestations of HIV/AIDS 262–3
   renal complications 304
   viral genes, expression of 30–1
   see also genes
genital herpes 448
genital ulcerative disease 493
genital warts 199, 493
genotype characterisation of drug resistance 539, 540–1
gentamicin 237, 244, 326
Georgia 593
geotrichosis *217*
GERD (gastroesophageal reflux disease) 251, *252,* 254
Germany 6, *84,* 589, 777
GFATM *see* Global Fund
GH (growth hormone) *280,* 288, 297
Ghana *10,* 55, 118, 198, 573, 728, 799
giant idiopathic aphthous genital ulcers 493

giardia/giardiasis 440, *556*
   lamblia 256, *738*
gingival erythema, linear *217, 624*
gingivitis *217,* 219, 366, *624*
gliosis 264
Global Coalition on Women and AIDS (UNAIDS) 571
global
   epidemiology of HIV/AIDS **1–12**
   Asia 8–9, *26*
   burden and measurement, global 2–4
   Caribbean 2, 3, 6
   epidemic heterogeneity and reasons for 11–12
   Europe 2, 3, 6–8
   global responses 11–12
   South America 2, 3, 6
   Sub-Saharan Africa 2, 3, 9–11, *10*
   transmission 1–2
   United States 2, 3, 4–6
Global Fund to Fight AIDS, Tuberculosis and Malaria (GFATM) 11, 615, 649, 664, 703, 791, 793, 795, 798
   Eastern Europe 591, 592
   economic impact *776, 777*
Global HIV Vaccine Enterprise 97, 573
Global Program to Enhance Reproductive Health Commodity Security 570
Global Summary of HIV and AIDS epidemic 272
Global Task Team 798
glomerulonephritis 300, 301
glomerulosclerois (ESGS) 301
glucocorticoid 290
   replacement therapy 291, 294
glucose homeostasis alterations 292, 297
GLUT4 292
glutamine 743
gonadal toxicity 445
gonadotropin-releasing hormone 294
gonorrhea 258
gp41 25, *27,* 86, 87, 136, 573
gp120 binding 23, 25, *27,* 86, 87, 136, 573
gram-negative bacilli *325*
Grave's disease (GD) 289
griseofulvin 244
growth hormone (GH) *280,* 288, 297
GS9137 (JTK-303) inhibitor 130
GSK873140 inhibitor 126
Guatemala 6, 726
Guinea 565, 726
gut associated lymphoid tissues 53

Guyana 725n, 728, *775n,* 796
GW640385 (brecanavir) inhibitor 131
GW695634 129
GW873140 small-molecule antagonist 25
gynecological care *488*
gynecomastia 294

H

HAART (highly active antiretroviral therapy) 3, 4, 105, 123, 255, 264, 470, 555, 703
   cardiovascular complications 279, 282, 283
   complications of antiretroviral therapy 181, 185
   drug abuse 513, 520
   drug resistance 151, 154, 537, 539, 541
   endocrine complications 288, 289, 292, 293, 295, 297
   essential medicines 663, 665–6
   fungal infections 376, 381, 382, 384, 387
      candida 365, 367, 372
      crytococcal 377, 380
   hepatitis viral infection 415, 416, 420
   immune reconstitution inflammatory syndrome of HIV 195, 200
   implementation in resource-constrained settings **677–94**
      future 692–4
      rapid large-scale 686–92
      supply chain *678*
      see also challenges for HAART
   malnutrition 604
   management of infections 437, 440, 442
   mega- or giga- 541
   mycobacterium avium complex 355, 356
   neoplasia 463–72, *465*
   ocular manifestations 227, 228, 229, 231, 234
   pharmacoeconomics 668, 669, 671, 673
   pneumonias 323, 328
   psychiatric barriers 276
   -related metabolic syndrome 283
   renal complications 300, 302, 305, 306
   resource allocation and cost of care, impact on 669–70, 672
   scale-up 616–17
   toxoplasmic encephalitis 399, 405, 406, 407, 408, 409

travel, international 557
tuberculosis 352
women and special issues 490–1
see also antiretroviral therapy; new
    drug development; resource-
    poor settings
HAD (HIV-associated dementia) 261
clinical features 263
diagnosis 263–4
primary neurological
    manifestations 262, 263–6
treatment 264–6
Haiti 6, 84, 104, 239, 489, 686, 725n,
    759, 771, 796
NGOs active in HIV and Web
    726–7, 728, 729, 730
half-life of drugs 173
halofantrine 750
harm reduction programs 94–5, 113,
    697
Harris-Benedict equation 603, 604
Hashimoto's thyroiditis 289
HBC/HBHCT see home-based care
HBV see hepatitis B
HCV see hepatitis C
HDI (Human Development Index)
    775
health belief model of behaviour 112,
    113
health care settings/hospitals
children in 758, 760–3
HIV pandemic and 758, 760–3
infection control in 94–5
inpatients in USA 528, 532, 533
overburdened 772
reproductive 95
workers 95
Helicobacter pylori 254
hematemesis 252
hematology see blood
hematopoietic cell transplantation
    467
hematopoisis 443
hemolytic uremic syndrome 257
hemophiliacs 165, 415, 696
hemophilus influenzae 165, 282, 288,
    415, 515
pneumonias 323, 324, 325, 326
hepatic impairment 177, 188, 294
cholesterol, increased 283
liver function test 383
steatosis 185, 186
hepatitis B and A 67, 85, 106, 143, 302,
    415–23, 432, 515, 555, 759
bacillary peliosis 425, 427, 428
diagnosis 417
epidemiology 415–16
evaluation and
    management 427–18

immune reconstitution
    inflammatory syndrome 197,
    199
infection 415–16, 417, 420
natural history 416–17
non-sterile needles 757, 758, 761,
    763
testing 651
travel, international 556, 557, 562
treatment 418–21
vaccination 477, 568
see also hepatitis C
hepatitis C 197, 199, 289, 306, 415–16,
    417, 420, 543
in Egypt from non-sterile
    injections 758
from non-sterile injections 757, 758,
    763
testing 651
therapy 419–20
hepatosplenomegaly 331, 383, 427, 428,
    624
herbal medicine 176–8, 548, 549–50
heroin 513, 518, 760
see also drug abuse
herpes simplex virus
candida 367
children in resource-limited
    settings 624
clinical presentation 447–50
gastrointestinal disorders 251, 252,
    258
management of infections 439, 440,
    447–55, 449
treatment 450–5
vaginal microbicides 598
women 489
herpes simplex/herpes zoster, acute
    infection 67, 68
herpes simplex/herpes zoster
    CHECK 4, 78, 82, 166
immune reconstitution
    inflammatory syndrome 197,
    199
ophthalmicus/ocular
    manifestations 228, 229
oral 216, 217, 220
see also Kaposi's sarcoma
herpes virus 8 622
herpes zoster virus, children 624
heterogeneity of epidemic, reasons
    for 11–12
heterosexual contact see sexual
    transmission
HHE (human haplotype E) 56
highly active antiretroviral therapy see
    HAART
high-resolution computed
    tomography 316

high-risk groups in Asia 577–82
drug users 578–9
heterosexual transmission 579–82
male-to-male sex 582
histamine 254
histopathology
bartonella infections 429–30, 429
toxoplasmic encephalitis 403
histoplasma 281, 331
capsulatum 288, 329, 380, 382, 383,
    384, 394, 397, 558
histoplasmosis
clinical manifestations 384
dermatology 244–5
diagnosis 383–4
epidemiology and
    pathogenesis 382–3
fungal infections 376, 382–4
gastrointestinal 257–8
microbiology 382
oral complications 216, 217
penicillium marneffei infection 395
pneumonias 324, 330
treatment 384
see also histoplasma
HIV-1
associated vacuolar
    myelopathy 267–8
groups N and O 1, 15, 17
origins in cross-species
    transmission see chimpanzee
sub-types and recombinants, map
    of 2
HIV-1 group M subtypes 1, 15, 17, 19
drug resistance in 153–4
genetic diversity in 18–19
pandemic 13
phylogenetic tree 18, 19
HIV-2 637–47, 638
clinical features 640–1
epidemiology 637–9
interactions with HIV-1 641–2
natural history 639–40
origin see mangabey
protection against HIV-1 not
    offered by 641–2
treatment 642–3
HIVAN (HIV-associated nephropathy)
    see renal complications
HIV-associated dementia see HAD
HIV-SN (HIV-associated sensory
    neuropathy) 266–7
HLA (human leukocyte antigen) 40, 46,
    55, 77, 83, 165, 166
Hodgkin's disease 466
Hodgkin's lymphoma 216, 464, 466,
    467–8
home-based care and counselling 116,
    788

homosexuality *see* male-to-male sex
Honduras 6, 726, 729
Hong Kong 393, 579
hormone-binding globulin 289, 294
hormones *280*, 288, 289, 290, 294, 295, 489
hospitals *see* health care settings
host, biology of HIV-1 transmission from 75, 77–8
HPA *see* hypothalamic-pituitary-adrenal
HPG *see* hypothalamic-pituitary-gonadal
HPMPC *see* cidofovir
HPV (human papillomavirus) *258*
HSV *see* herpes simplex virus
human leukocyte antigen 40, 46, 55, 77, 83, 165, 166
human papillomavirus 245–6, 258, *258*, *464*, 491–2
    warts *221*
human resource priorities, testing and counselling 119–20
human rights 66, 591, 664–5
hydroxyurea 186
hyperandrogenemia 296
hyperbilirubinemia 188
hypercholesterolemia 283
hypercortisolism 290
hyperendemicity of herpes 166
hypergammaglobuliemia 280
hyperglycemia 143, 292
hyperimmune bovine colostrums 256
hyperinsulinemia 296
hyperinsulinism 280
hyperkalemia 291
hyperlactatemia 185–6
hyperlipidemia 143, 282, 283
hyperprolactinemia 288
hypersensitivity vasculitis 282
hypertension, pulmonary 281–2
hyperthyroidism 288, 290
hypertriglyceridemia 283, 292
hypoadrenalism 280
hypoalbuminemia *324*, 327
hypoandrogenism 294, 295
hypocholesterolemia 283
hypodermic syringe 756
    disposable but re-used 756, 758–9
    see also drug abuse; non-sterile injections
hypoglycemia 257, 291
hypoglycorrhachia 439
hypogonadism 294, 295, 297
hyponatremia 288, 291
hypophosphatemia 187
hypopituitarism 287

hypospermatogenesis 294
hypothalamic-pituitary axis, adrenal 291
hypothalamic-pituitary axis, gonadal 291, 294
hypothalamus activation 290
hypothyroidism *281*, 288, 289
HZO (Herpes zoster ophthalmicus) 229

idiopathic AIDS enteropathy 256
idiopathic esophageal ulcers (IEU) 251, *252*, 253, 254
IDU (injection drug use) *see* drug abuse
IDV *see* indinavir
IEU *see* idiopathic esophageal ulcers
IFN *see* interferon
IgC antibodies 101, 102
IGF-1 binding protein 288
IgG and IgM antibodies 23, 68, *69*, 101
imatinib mesylate 471–2
imidazoles 243, 244
imipenem *328*
imiquimod 246, 493
immune activation and virulence 162
immune reconstitution disease/syndrome 372, 383
immune reconstitution inflammatory syndrome *see* IRIS
immune recovery uveitis (IRU) 232
immune response to HIV **39–49**
    acquired immunity to viral infections 40–1
    reasons for failure to control HIV 42–4
    specific antiviral 51–2
    vaccines, prospects for 45–7
immune system and malnutrition 605–8
immune thrombocytopenic purpura *217*, 223
immunoassays, enzyme *see* EIA; Elisa
immunoblotting 68–9
immunodeficiency 263–4
immunogens in global AIDS vaccine design 82–7
immunoglobulins 40, 42, 264
impact of pathogen-host-environment interactions 781–5
    life expectancy and expectations of adulthood 783–4, *783*, *785*
    rural production and food security 784–5
in utero transmission 497–8
index case, biology of transmission from 75, 77–8

India 2, 8, 11, 15, 46, 196, 209, 560, 731, 771, 779
    Brazil compared with 701
    children in resource-limited settings 622
    condom use 581
    dermatology 238, 240
    drug abuse *514*
    essential medicines *663*, 665
    high-risk groups 577, *578*, 582
    non-sterile injections and pandemic 759, 764
    orphans 789
    penicillium marneffei infection 393, 394
    pharmacoeconomics 671
    pneumocystis pneumonia *313*
    prevention 91, 97
    psychiatric problems 272–3, 275
    renal complications 299
    tuberculosis 333, *334*, 336
    women and special issues 489
indinavir (IDV) 742
    antiretroviral therapy 139, 141, *142*
    children and adolescents *481*
    dermatology 238, 243
    drug abuse 521, *523*
    drug resistance 151
    endocrine complications 292, 295
    hepatitis viral infection 421
    HIV-2 643
    inhibitory quotient 543
    mycobacterium avium complex *360*
    pharmacology 172, *176*
    post-exposure prevention *716*, *717*, 721
    primary neurological manifestations 265
    tuberculosis *351*
    women 494
Indonesia 8, 584, 726
    high-risk groups 577, *578*, 580, 582
infants 476–8
    diagnosis 476–8
    immune 44
    monitoring 477
    PCP prophylaxis 478
    vaccination 477–8
    see also breast-feeding; children; mother-to-child transmission; pregnancy
Infectious Disease Society of America 283
inflammatory bowel disease 258
influenza 85
    vaccine 478, 557
    see also hemophilus influenzae

infusional chemotherapy 466
inhibitory quotient (IQ) 543
injections *see* drug abuse; non-sterile
    injections
INN (international non-proprietary
    name) of medicine 662
innate immune responses 66
innovation diffusion theory of
    behaviour 113
insulin 755
    disorders 280, 296
    -like growth factor-1 288
    resistance 184, 185, 292
integrase 26
    inhibitors 130, 136
inter partum transmission 497–8
interferon 241, 419, *420*, 515
    -á 235, 280–1, 289, 418, 469, 471
interleukins 57, 281, 289
International AIDS Conference 615
International AIDS Vaccine
    Initiative 97, 574
International Covenant on Civil and
    Political Rights 591
International Covenant on Economic,
    Social and Cultural Rights 66, 591
International Crisis Group 789
International Finance Facility (IFF) 777
international funding for care and
    prevention **793–800**
    donor cooperation and
        harmonization 797–8
    effectiveness, challenge to 796–9
    major mechanisms *see* Global Fund;
        MAP; PEPFAR
    resource gap 797
International Guidelines on HIV/AIDS
    Prevention 591
international NGOs active in HIV and
    Web 726–9
international non-proprietary name of
    medicine 662
internet and Web
    information sources *731–5*
    see also NGOs active in HIV and
        Web
interpartum period, mother-to-child
    transmission prevention *500–2*
intertrigimous infections 243–4
intestine *see* enteric infections
intraconazole 245
intracranial toxoplasmosis 233
intralesional vinblastine 470
inverase (INV) 141
investigational agents for
    neoplasia 471–2
involution trap *774*
iodine 559

iodoquinol 742
IQ (inhibitory quotient) 543
Iran 798
IRD (immune reconstitution
    disease) 372, 377
Ireland 669
IRIS (immune reconstitution
    inflammatory syndrome) **193–205**,
    350, 616
    alternative therapies 202
    children in resource-limited
        settings 629
    common clinical 197–201
    diagnosis criteria *194*
    limitations of current
        knowledge 202–3
    pathogenesis 194–5
    pathologic scenarios *194*
    in resource-limited regions 201
    risk factors 196–7
    timing 195–6
    treatment 201–3
    see also ART
iritis 229, 232
iron in diet *606, 607*
IRU (immune recovery uveitis) 232
isolation studies 402
isoniazid 362, *515*
    travel, international *556*
    tuberculosis 342, *343, 344, 347, 348,
        349,* 350, 352, 622
isospora 255, 256
    belli *738*
istoplasma *281,* 331
Italy 144, 301
itching and skin disorders 239–40
itraconazole
    dermatology 244, 245
    fungal infections 380, *384,* 387
        candida *368, 369,* 370, 371
    gastrointestinal disorders 25, 253
    histoplasmosis 331
    immune reconstitution
        inflammatory syndrome 199
    penicillium marneffei infection 397
    pneumonias *329, 330*
    travel, international *556,* 560
ivermectin 240
Ivory Coast 310, 311
    economic impact 770, 775
    mother-to-child transmission
        prevention *500, 501,* 503

J

Japan 238, 355, 393, *578*
JC virus 233
JinHunag 548

JM3100 inhibitor 126
John Hopkins AIDS Service *see* urban
    care models
JTK-303 (GS9137) inhibitor 130

K

K65R 152
K103N (EFV mutation) 140, 153
Kaletra formulation 617
kanamycin *345, 349*
Kaposi's sarcoma 4, *186,* 201, 403, 430,
    464
    -associated herpes virus
        (KSHV) 468
    candida 366
    cardiovascular complications 280,
        281, 282
    children 622, *624*
    clinical presentation and
        management 469–70
    endocrine complications 288, 291,
        294
    gastrointestinal disorders 251, *252,*
        254, 258
    management of infections 440
    neoplasia 469–70
    ocular manifestations 233, 234
    oral complications *216, 217,* 221–2,
        222
    pathogenesis 469
    pneumonias *324*
    relative risks *464*
    thyroidism 290
Kawasaki disease 283
Kazakhstan 591, 592, 593, *775n*
Kenya 84, 118, 209, 312, 749, 796
    children 11, 489, 621
    dermatology 237, 240
    economic impact *772, 775*
    global epidemiology 9, *10*
    international funding 799
    life expectancy 10–11
    NGOs active in HIV and
        Web *725n,* 726, 727, 728, 729,
        730
    pathogen-host-environment
        interactions *783*
    prevention 94, 98, 209, 565, 567,
        571, 572
    psychiatric problems 272
    women 11, 489
keratitis *228,* 229
ketoconazole 253, 387
    dermatology 238, 243
    endocrine complications 289, 291,
        293, 294
    penicillium marneffei infection 397

kidney disease *see* renal complications
klebsiella *324*
    stomatitis *217*
KMMPO5 RNase inhibitor 129
KS *see* Kaposi's sarcoma
kwashiorkor 604
Kwazulu-Natal 748
Kyrgyzstan 593

L

L-870810 inhibitor 130
laboratories
    central reference 654–5, 656, 658
    point of care 652, 654, 655–6
    regional 652, 654, 655, 656
laboratory testing 68–71, **101–9**
    detection of virus 70–1
    diagnostic 101–4
    monitoring patient health 104–5
    monitoring viral replication 105–7
    quality assurance and
        control 107–8
    serology 68–70
    viral load during primary
        infection 71
labour saving technologies 784
lactate dehydrogenase 315
lactic acidosis 185–6
lactobacilli, drug-expressing 597
lamivudine (3TC)
    antiretroviral therapy 137, *138*, 140
    children and adolescents *481*, 482
    children in resource-limited
        settings 626, 628, 630
    drug abuse *515*, *522*
    hepatitis viral infection *418*, 419
    mother-to-child transmission
        prevention 498, *500–1*, 503–7,
        509–10
    pharmacology *172*, 173, *177*
    post-exposure prevention *713*, *716*,
        717, *720*
    resistance to 152, 539, 541
    Thailand 583
    women 494, 499
lamotrigine 267
language problems 210, 263
Laos 577, *578*, 726
late targets in HIV life cycle 136–7
Latin America *84*, 104, *302*, 415, 471,
    501, 761, 777, 796
    adherence to therapy 209, 210
    dermatology 238, 239, 244, 245
    drug abuse 513, *514*
    endocrine complications 288
    essential medicines *663*, 665
    fungal infections 382, 385
    global epidemiology 2, *3*, 6

malnutrition 605
NGOs active in HIV and
    Web 725n, 726, 727, 728, *733*,
    735
orphans 790
pharmacoeconomics 671, 672
pneumocystis pneumonia 309, *314*
prevention 91, *92*, 97
psychiatric problems 271, 275
travel, international 555, 558, 559,
    560, 561
tuberculosis *334*, 335
see also Brazil; Caribbean;
    malnutrition
L-canavanine 548–9
LDH (lactate dehydrogenase) 315
lean body mass (LBM) 296, 297
lefluromide *201*, 202
legionella *324*, *325*, 327, *328*
    legionnaires' disease 326
leiomyosarcoma *464*
leishmania/leishmaniasis 240–1, *324*,
    383, 560
leprosy 241
leptospirosis 562
lesbians 489
Lesotho 9, 547, 565, 769, *775n*
leucovorin calcium 256, 405, *406*
leukocyte antigens, human 55
leukocytosis 439
leukoencephalopathy, progressive *see*
    PML
leukopenia 383
leukoplakia, hairy *216*, 217, 220–1, *220*
levofloxacin 326, *328*, 345, 349
levothyroxine 289–90
Libya: non-sterile injections 760, 762–3
life expectancy reduced 10–11, 770,
    783–4, *783*, 784, 785
    see also future; mortality
Lighthouse, The 730
lindane 240
linezolid 237, *328*
    amoxicillin *328*
lip cancer *216*
LIP (lymphocytic/lympoid interstitial
    pneumonia) 622, *624*
lipid associated AmB *369*
lipid signalling rafts 25
lipoatrophy 181, 182–4, 189, 296, 628
lipodystrophy 210, 283
    complications of antiretroviral
        therapy 181–2, *182*, 184
    endocrine complications 288,
        290–1, 292, 293, 296
lipomatosis 288
lipoprotein clearance, impaired *283*
liposomal doxo *471*
literacy problems 208, 210

Lithuania 593
liver 425
    transplantation 421
    see also hepatic; hepatitis
living standards rise for survivors
    777n
local NGOs active in HIV and
    Web 730–1
local therapies for neoplasia 470
loperamide 256, 258, 559
lopinavir (LPV) *151*, 258, *351*
    antiretroviral therapy 139, 141, *142*
    children and adolescents *481*, 482,
        626
    drug abuse 521, *523*, 524
    endocrine complications 292
    HIV-2 643
    inhibitory quotient 543
    pharmacology 172, 176
    post-exposure prevention *716*, *717*,
        721
    resistance to 539
    women 494
lovastatin *718*
LPV *see* lopinavir
LSTs (labour saving technologies) 784
LTBI (latent TB infection) 198
Ltr (long terminal repeat) 24
lumefantrine 661, 749, 750
lungs *see* pulmonary disease
luteinizing hormone (LH) 294
lymphadenopathy 291, 331, 383, 425,
    426
lymphatic system
    lymph nodes 40, 425, 595
    lymphadenopathy 4, 67
    lymphocytosis 223
    non-Hodgkin's lymphoma *216*,
        217
    structure degeneration 44
    see also CTLs; lymphocyte counts;
        T lymphocytes
lymphocyte counts 143, 319, 327
    gastrointestinal disorders 257, 258
    primary neurological
        manifestations 262, 263–4, 266
    see also CD4 T-cells
lymphocytic/lympoid interstitial
    pneumonia 622, *624*
lymphogranuloma venereum 258, 259
lymphoid interstitial pneumonitis *324*
lymphoma 222, 281, *324*, 377
    EBV-associated central nervous
        system 401
    endocrine complications 288, 294
    gastrointestinal disorders 251, *252*,
        254, 258
    plasmablastic 468
    primary effusion 468

toxoplasmic encephalitis 403
see also non-Hodgkin's lymphoma
lymphoproliferative disease 464–9
    Castleman's disease,
        multicentric 469
    plasmablastic lymphoma 468
    primary effusion lymphoma 468
    see also Hodgkin's; non-Hodgkin's
lymphpenia 420

M

M184V 155–6
MAC see disseminated mycobacterium
    avium
MAC-IRIS see mycobacterium avium
    complex
macroeconomic impact in developing
    countries 772–5
macrolide 325, 328, 515
macrophages 262, 267
macroplanning analysis of cost 671–2
maculopapular rash 189
magnetic resonance imaging 268, 402,
    427, 439
MAI (mycobacterium avium
    intracellulare) 257, 288, 294, 440
malabsorption
    of drugs 538, 742–3
    of food 605, 609–10
malaria 622, **747–53**
    disease burden implications 751
    effect on HIV 748–9
    essential medicines for 661, 664,
        749–51
    HIV's effect on 747–8
    resource-poor settings 649, 650
    travel, international 555, 558, 560,
        562
    treatment and programmatic
        implications 749
    women and 747–8, 749
    see also Global Fund
Malawi 210, 311, 487, 547, 749
    children in resource-limited
        settings 621, 622
    mother-to-child transmission
        prevention 502, 503, 506, 507
    mycobacterium avium
        complex 338, 362
    NGOs active in HIV and Web 726,
        730
    Pneumocystis pneumonia 311, 312
    prevention 579
Malaysia 238, 273, 393, 549, 578
male-to-male sex (MSM) 75, 239, 417
    Africa 571–2
    Asia 577, 578, 582
    Brazil 695

gastrointestinal disorders 255,
    258–9
global epidemiology 3, 5, 6, 7, 8, 9
management of infections 439
prevention of HIV 91, 92
Mali 237
malignancy/carcinoma 4
    anorectal 258
    esophageal 251, 252
    IRIS 201
    lymph nodes see lymphoma
    ocular (SCC) 234
    oral 216, 217, 222
    skin 246
    squamous cell 217, 233, 258
    thyroid 288
    see also Kaposi's sarcoma
malnutrition **603–13**
    basic nutritional needs 603–4
    children 622
    good practices 608–9
    immune system 605–8
    malabsorption 605, 609–10
    micronutrients 606–8, 606
    nausea 611–12
    requirements of HIV/AIDS 604–5
    side-effects leading to 609–10
    taste lost or altered 612
    thrush and oral pain 612
    see also weight loss
management of infections **437–61**
    cytomegalovirus 437–47
    herpes simplex virus 447–55
    varicella-zoster virus 455–7
    see also diarrhea etiology
Management Sciences for Health 664
mangabey, sooty, HIV-2 from 1, 14–15,
    17, 639
mania 274
MAP (Multi-Country AIDS Program of
    World Bank) 11, 615, 793, 794–5, 798
marasmus (cachexia) 603–4
Maraviroc inhibitor 125–6
marijuana 550
Marionol (dronabinol) 297, 550
Markov modelling 672, 673
mass media prevention campaigns in
    Africa 568–9
maturation inhibitors 130
MCMD (minor cognitive motor
    disorder) 263, 275
MCV see molluscum contagiosum
MDM (Médecins du Monde/Medicos
    del Munde) 728
MDRT (multidrug resistance
    therapy) 154–5, 541
measles 477, 557, 622
Médecins du Monde/Medicos del
    Munde 728

medical practice, unsafe 17–18
medicines 97, 136
    Brazil 698, 700
    choosing recipients 788
    complications from 184–5
    costs 146, 209–10, 615, 616–17,
        667–9, 790
    HAD 264
    HIV neuropathy 266–7
    non-injectable, need for 764
    ocular manifestations 229–30, 230,
        234–6
    poor adherence 144
    resistance to see drug resistance;
        drug resistant HIV
    skin 237–46 passim
    see also essential medicines; new
        drug development; nucleoside
        reverse transcriptase inhibitors
mefloquine 560
megestrol acetate 291, 292, 294, 297
melphalan 466
membranoproliferative GN 301
Memorial Sloan Kettering staging of
    ADC 264, 265, 582
memory loss 263
men
    prevalence in 4–5, 8, 76
    see also male-to-male sex
menigococcal conjugate vaccine
    478
meningitis 262, 367
    aseptic 428
    tuberculous 622
    vaccination 557
    see also cryptococcal meningitis
mental illness
    drug abuse, intravenous 520–1
    see also psychiatric barriers
Merck/HVTN 84
meropenem 328
mesangioproliferative GN 301–2
'metabolic syndrome' 184, 190
metformin 293
methadone 94, 516, 519, 520, 521, 522,
    524, 589
    illegal in Russia 589, 593
methamphetamine 518, 520
methicillin 237
methotrezate 242
methylergonovine 718, 719
metoclopramide 288
metronidazole 256, 257, 494, 741, 742
metyrapone test 291
Mexico 244, 314
    fungal infections 382, 385
    NGOs active in HIV and Web 728,
        735
    travel, international 559, 561

MHC (major histocompatibility complex) 55
micafungin 370
miconazole 369, 397
microbicides 97, 573
    see also vaginal microbicides
micronutrients 507, 606–8, 606
microsporidiosis/microsporidia 255, 256, 288, 738
    corneal 228, 229
midazolam 718, 719
Middle East and North Africa 3, 92, 415, 514, 555, 734
    non-sterile injections 760, 762–3
    pneumocystis pneumonia 311, 312
    prevention 572
    renal complications 300, 305
Mifflin-St Jeor equation 603, 604
Mildmay 730
Millennium Development Goals 772, 777, 797
miltefosine 241
mind-body therapy 551
minerals in diet 606, 607, 609, 610
minocycline 428, 432
minor cognitive motor disorder 275
mitochondrial myopathy 267
MIV150 597
MK-0518 inhibitor 130
MMR vaccine, avoiding 477
Moldova 593, 775n
molecular biology of HIV and implications for new therapies 23–38
    antiviral host factors 34–5
    assembly and budding of HIV virions 31, 32–3
    early cytoplasmic events 26, 27
    expression of viral genes 30–1
    HIV entry 23–6
    integration 28
    nuclear pore, crossing 26, 28
    replicating new virus 31
    transcriptional events 28–30, 29
molluscum contagiosum virus (MCV) 228–9, 228, 377, 624
monitoring
    children in resource-limited settings 631, 632–3
    complications 185
    drug resistance in resource-poor settings 707
    infants 477
    load (CD4 T-cell enumeration) 649, 650–5, 653
    medication 185, 207, 483
    patient health 104–5
    viral replication 105–7

monkeys, HIV from 1, 14–15, 18
    see also origins; SIV
monocytes, infected 262
mononeuritis multiplex 440
mood disorders 274
Morocco 572, 727n
morphine 572
mortality 3, 4, 565, 567
    age-specific 782, 783
    children and lifetime risk of 621, 622–3, 783, 785
    decline in Brazil 699, 701
    decline with HAART 669
    economic impact 770, 772, 774
    funeral costs 771n
    hepatitis 416
    HIV-2 640, 642
    pharmacoeconomics 672, 673
    rates per population 2, 5, 8
    total numbers 39
    toxoplasmic encephalitis 400
    see also life expectancy reduced
mother-to-child transmission, prevention of (MTCT/PMTCT) 1, 2, 102, 209, 497–512, 672, 770, 790
    Brazil 697, 701
    drug resistance 539, 705–6
    malaria 749
    nevirapine single dose 498–511, 500–2, 508–10, 539, 618
    NGOs active in HIV and Web 726, 727
    non-antiretroviral intervention 506–7
    pharmacoeconomics 672, 673
    prevention 91, 93, 95, 98
    resource-constrained guidelines 507, 509–10, 511
    risk factors 497–8
    short and long-term safety 504–5
    see also prophylactic antiretroviral intervention
mouth ulcers 366
moxifloxacin 346
Mozambique 10, 547, 772, 796
    NGOs active in HIV and Web 726, 727n, 728
MR spectroscopy 264
MRCA (most recent common ancestor) 14
MRI (magnetic resonance imaging) 268, 402, 427, 439
MSK see Memorial Sloan Kettering
Mtb see mycobacterium tuberculosis
MTCT see mother-to-child transmission
mucocutaneous infection 453
mucosal biopsy 259
multicentric Castleman's disease 469
Multi-Country AIDS Program see MAP

multidrug resistance 51, 154–5
mumps vaccine, avoiding 477
mupirocin 237
Mus musculus 394
mutations see drug resistance
mutism, akinetic 263
MVA (modified vaccinia Ankara) 82
myalgias 297
myambutol see ethambutol
Myanmar 313, 577, 578, 726
mycobacterium 440
    genavense 362
    haemophilum 362
    kansasii 324, 362
    simiae-avium 362
mycobacterium avium complex (MAC) 255, 281, 355–64, 483
    diarrhea 738
    endocrine complications 290, 291
    immune reconstitution inflammatory syndrome 195, 197, 199–200
    intracellulare (MAI) 257, 288, 294, 440
    oral complications 216, 217
    women and special issues 490
    see also disseminated mycobacterium avium
mycobacterium tuberculosis (Mtb) 288, 290, 317, 324, 333, 337–9, 514
    see also tuberculosis
mycobutin 234, 257
mycoplasma pneumonia 326, 328
mycosis 62
    penicilliosis 216, 625
    see also coccidiomycosis
myelitis 439
myelopathy, HIV-associated 261, 262
    vacuolar 267–8
myocardial infarction 281
myocarditis 279, 280

N
....

nafcillin 325, 328
nails, infections of 243–4
naltrexone 518, 520
Namibia 9, 93, 306, 547, 796
NAP (National AIDS program, Brazil) 696
naphthalene sulfonate polymer 596, 600
narcotics see drug abuse
nausea/vomiting 252, 253, 255, 611–12, 611
NCEP (National Cholesterol Education Program) 185
NCOs see non-governmental organizations

necrotizing infections 425
  retinitis 233
  stomatitis 216, 217
  ulcerative gingivitis 624
  ulcerative periodontitis 219
needles
  exchange programs 94, 95, 572,
    589, 697
  needlestick injuries rare 761
  non-sterile, pandemic and 759–60,
    764
Nef (negative effector) 24, 54, 81, 83,
  85
negative imaging, MRI 268
negative outcomes of testing and
  counselling 114–15
negative population growth 770
  see also mortality
Neisseria gonorrhea 258
nelfinavir (NFV) 141, 142, 145, 742
  children and adolescents 481
  drug abuse 521, 523
  drug resistance 153
  endocrine complications 292, 293,
    295
  gastrointestinal disorders 258
  HIV-2 643
  inhibitory quotient 543
  mother-to-child transmission 504
  mycobacterium avium complex
    360
  pharmacology 172, 176
  post-exposure prevention 716, 717,
    721
  tuberculosis 351
  women 494
neoplasia 463–74
  cardiovascular complications 280,
    282
  cervical 491–2
  chemotherapy 470–1
  epidemiology of
    malignancies 463–4
  interferon-á 471
  investigational agents 471–2
  local therapies 470
  ocular manifestations 233–4
  oral diseases 217, 221–2
  systemic therapy 470–1
  see also Kaposi's sarcoma;
    lymphoproliferative disease
Nepal 273, 559
  high-risk groups 577, 578, 579,
    580
nephropathy see renal complications
NEPs (needle exchange programs) 94,
  95, 572, 589, 697
nervous system see neurology
Netherlands 84, 196, 551–2, 589, 655,
  729

Neurologic AIDS Research
  Consortium 268
neurology
  cytomegalovirus infections 438–40
  impaired 4
  neuromuscular weakness
    syndrome 267
  neuroophthalmic
    manifestations 233–4
  neuropathy 186, 210, 233, 261,
    266–7, 515
  neuroradiologic studies of
    toxoplasmic encephalitis
    402–3
  neurosyphilis 262
  see also primary neurological
    manifestations
neutralizing antibodies, eliciting 85–6
neutropenia 367, 445, 465, 624
nevirapine (NVP) 95, 98, 150, 190, 242,
  705, 750
  antiretroviral therapy 138, 140, 142,
    145, 184–5
  children in resource-limited
    settings 626, 628–30
  drug abuse 522
  endocrine complications 296
  hepatitis viral infection 421
  mother-to-child transmission
    prevention 498–511, 500–2,
    508–10, 539, 618
  pharmacoeconomics 672
  pharmacology 172, 173, 177, 178
  post-exposure prevention 713, 716,
    717, 721
  resistance to 539
  Thailand 583
  toxicity profile 189
  tuberculosis 350, 351
  women 494
new drug development 123–33
  attachment inhibitors 124–5
  chemokine receptor
    inhibitors 125–6
  integrase inhibitors 130
  maturation inhibitors 130
  non-nucleotide reverse
    inhibitors 128–9
  nucleotide-competing reverse
    transcriptase inhibitors 129
  protease inhibitors 130
  reverse transcriptase
    inhibitors 127–8
  RNase H inhibitors 129
  see also fusion inhibitors
new therapies see molecular biology
NFV see nelfinavir
NGOs active in HIV and Web
  links 725–36
  international 726–9

internet sources of
  information 731–5
local 730–1
religious 729–30
NHL see non-Hodgkin's lymphoma
nifurtimox 560
Niger 727n
Nigeria 10, 15, 237, 341, 671, 726
  international funding 796, 799
  NGOs active in HIV and Web 729,
    730
  prevention 570, 572, 573
  renal complications 300, 301, 306
nitazoxanide 256, 741, 742
NK (natural killer) cell receptor 57
NNRTI (non-nucleoside reverse
  transcriptase inhibitors) 616, 617
  antiretroviral therapy 136, 137, 138,
    140
  children and adolescents 481,
    627
  complications 189
  hepatitis viral infection 421
  HIV-2 643
  mother-to-child transmission
    prevention 508
  new drug development 128–9
  pharmacology 171, 172
  primary neurological
    manifestations 265
  resistance to 149–50, 152–3, 539,
    541
  tuberculosis 350
  vaginal microbicides 597
  see also efavirenz; nevirapine
Nocardia 241, 323, 324, 325
nocturnal cough 252
non-antiretroviral intervention and
  mother-to-child transmission
  prevention 506–7
non-bacterial thrombotic
  endocarditis 282
non-governmental organizations
  588
  see also NGOs
non-Hodgkin's lymphoma 216, 217,
  282, 464–7, 466
  B-cell 234, 463, 464
  candida 366
  children 622, 625
  clinical management 464–6
  haematopoitec cell
    transplantation 467
  infusional chemotherapy 466
  rituximab 466–7
  systemic 464
non-infectious retinal
  microvasculopathy 227–8
non-nucleoside RTIs see NNRTIs
nonoxynol-9 596

non-sterile injections and pandemic 18, **755–67**
  in developing world 758–9
  disposables problem 758
  drug abuse and addiction 759–60
  hepatitis C in Egypt 758
  medical, history of 756–8
  myth of safe injecting 756–7
  nosocomial epidemics 760–3
  parameters of transmissibility of viruses 757–8
non-steroidal anti-inflammatory drugs 198, 201, 377
non-thyroidal illness (NTI) 288–9
North Africa see Middle East and North Africa
North America (mainly USA) 1, 2, 67, 77, *84*, 166, 583, 587
  adherence to therapy 207
  antiretroviral therapy 137
  Brazil compared with 696, 698, 699
  cardiovascular complications 279
  children and adolescents 475, *479*, 622
  complementary and alternative medicine 549–51
  dermatology 239, 240, 241, 244, 245
  diarrhea 737, 739, 740
  drug abuse *514*, 520, 589, 590, 592
  drug resistance in resource-poor settings 703, 704, 708
  economic impact 772
  endocrine complications 292–3
  essential medicines *663*, 665
  Food and Drug Administration 94, 189
  fungal infections 376, 378, 379, 380, 382, 383, 385–6, 387
  gastrointestinal disorders 256
  global epidemiology *2, 3, 4, 5,* 6
  HAART implementation 683, 686
  hepatitis viral infection 415, 416, 421
  immune reconstitution inflammatory syndrome 196, 200
  international funding for care and prevention 793, 795–6
  IRIS 196, 198, 200, 201
  laboratory testing 101–8 *passim*
  methadone use 589
  mother-to-child transmission and prevention guidelines 497, *500*, 504, 507, *508–9*
  mycobacterium avium complex 355–9, 361–2
  NGOs active in HIV and Web 727, 728, 729, *731–2*
  non-sterile injections and pandemic 756, 757, 758–60, 764

penicillium marneffei infection 393
pharmacoeconomics 669–70
pneumonias *317*, 324, 326, 327, 330
prevention *92, 93, 94,* 112, 573, 574
psychiatric problems 271, 272, 273–4
race and HIV 7
renal complications 299, 300, 302–3, *302*, 305, 306
resource-poor settings 655, 656
testing and counselling 118
travel, international 555, 557, 560, 561
treatment, barriers to 591–2
tuberculosis 333, *334*, 342, 350, *351*
vaginal microbicides 599–600
women and special issues 487, 488, 489, 490, 491, 492
  see also bartonella infections; PEPFAR; toxoplasmic encephalitis; urban care models
Norwalk virus 256, *556*
nosocomial (hospital-related) *see* health care settings
NRTIs *see* nucleoside reverse transcriptase inhibitors
NSAIDS (non-steroidal anti-inflammatory drugs) 198, 201, 377
NTI (non-thyroidal illness) 288–9
nuclear pore, crossing 26, 28
nucleic acid testing 102
nucleoside reverse transcriptase inhibitors (NRTIs) 242
  antiretroviral therapy 136, 137, *138*, 140
  children and adolescents 480, *481*
  complications of antiretroviral therapy 186, 189
  drug abuse 521
  drug resistance 149, 151, 155
  endocrine complications 292
  gastrointestinal disorders 258
  hepatitis viral infection 420, 421
  HIV-2 43
  new drug development 127–8
  pharmacology 171, 172
  primary neurological manifestations 265, 267
  tri-phosphates as active form of 538
  vaginal microbicides *597*
  see also abacavir; didanosine; emtricitabine; lamivudine; stavudine; tenofovir; zidovudine
nucleotide-competing reverse transcriptase inhibitors 129
nutrition 784–5
NVP *see* nevirapine

nystatin *369*, 370
NYVAC (New York vaccinia virus) 82

O

obesity 288
Oceania 3, *92*
octoxynol-9 596
octreotide 256
ocular manifestations **227–36**
  drugs and side-effects 229–30, *230*, 234–6
  infections 228–33, *228, 230, 231, 232*
  neuroophthalmic 233–4
  restricted movements 267
  retinal microvasculopathy 227–8, 337–8
  squamous cell carcinoma 234
  toxoplasmosis *228*, 233, 400
  varicella zoster 229–32
odynophagia 251, *252, 253*, 254
oesophageal *see* esophageal disorders
ofloxacin *346, 349*
OHL (oral hairy leukoplakia) 366, *624*
oilgospermia 295
OIs *see* opportunistic infections
onychomycosis, superficial 244
oophoritis 295
opium 256
oral complications of HIV infection **215–25**
  bacterial *217*, 219–21
  candidiasis 215–16, *216, 217*, 624
  gingivitis and periodontitis *217*, 219
  neoplastic disease *217*, 221–2
  oral hairy leukoplakia 366, *624*
  other lesions 222–3
  pain and malnutrition *611*, 612
  treatment 216–19
  ulcers *216, 217*, 222, 366, *624*
origins and diversification of HIV **13–21**
  deep roots 13–14
  genetic diversity in HIV-1 group M subtypes 18–19
  geography of 16
  HIV/SIV nomenclature 14–15
  medical practice, unsafe 17–18
  timing 17
orolabial infection 447–8
oropharyngeal candidiasis 365, 366, *369*, 370–1
orphans 11, 771, 773, *785*, **787–92**
  Africa 78–91, 787–91
  Asia 789–90
  Latin America 790
  numbers of (c. 15 million) 789

osseous bacillary angiomatosis *426*, 432–3
osteonecrosis 294
osteopenia 293
osteoporosis 291, 293, 294
otitis media 621, *624*
otorrhea *624*
ovarian function 295
oxacillin *325*, *328*

P

PA-457 inhibitor 130
paclitaxel 291, *471*
PACTG (Pediatric AIDS Clinical Trials Group) 497
Pakistan 8, 273, *578*
pan troglodytes *see* chimpanzee
Panama 244, *314*, 605
pancreas 291–3
    antiretroviral and other therapies 292
    glucose homeostasis alterations 292
    pancreatic tuberculosis 291
    pancreatitis 286, 383, 543
    pathology 291
    treatment considerations 292–3
pancytopenia 331
pandemic 13
    see also epidemiology; non-sterile injections
panhypopituitarism 287
pan-leukogating (PLG) technology 654
papillomavirus *see* human papillomavirus
Papua New Guinea 730
paracoccidioides 384
    brasiliensis 288, 558
paracoccidiomycosis 384, 561
paradoxical inflammatory response *see* IRIS
paraplegia (spastic diplegia) 263, 267
parasitic infections 256, 561
Parkinson's disease, parallels with 263, 275
paromomycin 256, 741, 742
'partial treatment' 145–6
partially suppressive regimens 542
Partners in Health (PIH) 726
pathogen-host-environment interactions **779–86**
    global situation 779–80, *781*
    vertical 780–1
    see also impact
pathogenesis
    cryptococcosis 376–7
    histoplasmosis 382–3
    Kaposi's sarcoma 469

primary neurological manifestations 262–3
    renal complications 303–4
    tuberculosis 336–7
pathophysiology of primary neurological manifestations 262–3
PCNSL (primary central nervous system lymphoma) 467
PCP *see* pneumocystis pneumonia
PCR *see* polymerase
PCS-RANTES 597
Pediatric AIDS Clinical Trials Group 497
pediatric treatment *see* children
peer
    -based programs 93
    counselling 117, 787
PEL (primary effusion lymphoma) 468
peliosis, bacillary 425, *427*, 433
pelvic inflammatory disease 491, 493–4
PEM (protein energy malnutrition) 604
penciclovir 453
penicillin 239, 259, 559
    bartonella infections 431, *432*
    history of 750
    pneumonias 324, *328*
penicilliosis 216, *625*
penicillium 241, 383, 384
    marneffei 377, 558
penicillium marneffei infection **393–8**
    clinical features 395–6
    diagnosis 396–7
    ecology and mode of transmission 394–5
    history 393
    mycology 393
    treatment 397
PENTA (Paediatric European Network for Treatment of AIDS) *479*
pentamidine 241, 281
    endocrine complications 288, 292, 293
    isethionate 318, *319*
    pneumocystis pneumonia 316, *320*
penumocystis, pneumonia jiroveci (carinii) 199–200, 257, *324*, 441
PEP *see* post-exposure prevention
PEPFAR (President's Emergency Plan for AIDS relief) 11, 165, 615, 776, 791, 793, 796, 798
peptic ulcer disease (PUD) 254
pericardial disease/pericarditis *280*, 281, 383
periodontitis/periodontal disease *216*, *217*, 219, 366, *624*
peripheral neuropathy, HIV-associated 262, 267
perirectal abscess *258*
permethrin 240

personality and psychiatric barriers 276
pertussis vaccination 477, 478
Peru *84*, 726
PET (position emission tomography) 264, 403
phaet pheun baan/phaet pheun thai 548
PharmAccess International 729
pharmacoeconomics **667–75**
    economic evaluation 667–9
    modelling 672–3
    world cost data, interpreting 673–4
    see also costs; economic impact
pharmacology of antiretroviral drugs **171–9**, 445–6
    drug transport proteins 174–6
    major drugs 171–8, *172*, *176–7*
    optimal prescribing 172–3
    traditional medicines 176–8
    see also antiretrovirals; ART/ARV; drug resistance; HAART; medicines; pharmacoeconomics
phenotype, methods of characterising drug resistance 539, 540–1
PHI (primary HIV-1 infection) 154
Philippines 577, *578*, 580, 771
phosphonoformic acid *see* foscarnet
phosphorylation, intracellular 173
phylogenetic tree *14*
physical environment, social learning theory 112
phytates 607
picornaviruses 256
PID (pelvic inflammatory disease) 491, 493–4
pigmentatiom disorders 238
pill-esophagitis 252
pimozide *718*
pipeine technologies, CD4 655
piperacillin *328*
PIs *see* protease inhibitors
pituitary 287–8
    antiretroviral therapy 288
    function changes 288
    pathology 287
    somatotropic axis 288
placenta 498
plant lectins 597
plasma viral load (PVL) and HIV-2 640, 761
plasma viral RNA 476
plasmablastic lymphoma 468
pleocytosis 439
PMBC (peripheral blood mononuclear cell) 476
PML (progressive multifocal leukoencephalopathy) 275, 401, *625*
    immune reconstitution inflammatory syndrome 200–1

PML (progressive multifocal leukoencephalopathy) *(continued)*
  ocular manifestations *228*, 233
  primary neurological manifestations 261, 262
PMPA *597, 600*
PMTCT *see* mother-to-child transmission, prevention
pneumococcal pneumonia 323–4
pneumocystis pneumonia (pneumonia jiroveci/carinii) 8, 47, 67, 228, 237, **309–20**, *315, 324*, 355, 383, 400, 490
  children and adolescents 475, 477, 621, 622, *624*
  clinical presentation *310–14*, 315
  diagnosis 317–18, 327
  endocrine complications 287, 288, 290, 291, 292
  incidence 309
  laboratory tests 315–17
  management 437, 441
  prophylaxis 319–20, *320*
  risk factors for 309
  symptoms and signs 315
  treatment 318–19, *319*
  vaccination 477, *478*
pneumonia 4, 316, **323–31**, *515*, 562
  carinii *see* pneumocystis
  children in resource-limited settings 621
  frequency 323
  jiroveci *see* pneumocystis
  lymphocytic/lympoid interstitial 622, *624*
  pneumococcal 323–4, 557
  streptoccal 559
  see also bacterial pneumonias; fungal pneumonias; streptoccus pneumonia
pneumonitis 385, 622
pneumothorax 316
PNP (purine nucleoside phosporylase) 173
point of care laboratories/PointCARE machine 652, 654, 655–6
PointCARE *653*
Poland 8, 592
polio 557
poliovirus 82
political support for prevention programs 96–7
polyarteritis nodosa 283
polycystic ovary syndrome 296
polyenes 370
polymerase/polymerase chain reaction (PCR) 24, 54, 477
  children 623
  clinical implications of HIV fitness and virulence 163, *164–5*

design of global AIDS vaccine 81, 83, 85
  laboratory testing 103–4, 105
polyradiculopathy 439
PORN (progressive outer retinal necrosis) 232–3
Portugal 1, 7, 8
posaconazol 384
position emission tomography 264, 403
post-exposure prevention 95, 98, **711–24**
  antiretroviral agents 712, *713–18*
  human studies 712
  management recommendations 718–23
  prophylaxis 711–12
postnatal transmission prevention 498
postpartum period, mother-to-child transmission prevention *500–2*
potassium hydroxide 243
potassium iodide 245
poverty 769–70
  see also economic impact
pox viruses 82
PPIs (proton-pump inhibitors) 254
praneem 597
pre-contemplation stage of change 113
prednisone *252*, 254, 305, *465*
pre-exposure prophylaxis 573
pregnancy 4, 9, 143, 177–8, 428, 505, *508–9*, 701
  and malaria 747–8, 749
  toxoplasmic encephalitis 400–1, 408–9
  see also antenatal; children; mother-to-child transmission
preintegration complex (PIC) 26
premature birth infection 76
PrEP (pre-exposure prophylaxis) 573
preparation stage of change 113
President's Emergency Plan for AIDS Relief *see* PEPFAR
prevalence of HIV infection *3*, 4, *578*
prevention **91–100**, 118–19, 618
  Asia 91, *92*, 97
  bartonella infections 433–4
  biology of HIV-1 transmission 79–80
  blood-borne transmission 94–5
  candida 372
  Eastern Europe 91, *92*, 97
  effective programs, implementing 96–7
  epidemiology 91–2
  evidence base for 92–3
  research priorities 97–8
  sexual transmission behaviour change programs 93–4
  toxoplasmic encephalitis 407–9

treatment and care linked 689–92, *690–1*
  see also international funding for care and prevention; mother-to-child transmission prevention
prevention in Africa 91, *92*, 93, 94, 95, 97, 98, **565–75**
  decline 565–6
  diagnosis and treatment 571–2
  successes 566–7
  trials 572
  see also prevention policy and actions
prevention policy and actions in Africa 567–71
  blood transfusions, safe 570
  commercial sex workers 571
  community-based programs 569–70
  condom promotion 570
  decline 565–6
  mass media campaigns 568–9
  policy and actions 567–71
  school-based programs 569
  successes 566–7
  trials *see* trials
  women and girls 570–1
  workplace programs 569
primaquine 318, 319
primary central nervous system lymphoma 467
primary effusion lymphoma (PEL) 468
primary infection 154
  skin disorders 241–2
  viral loads during 71
  see also acute infection
primary neurological manifestations **261–9**
  HIV-1 associated vacuolar myelopathy 267–8
  HIV-associated dementia 262, 263–6
  neuropathy 266–7
  pathophysiology, pathogenesis and genetics 262–3
primates (non-human) 83
  HIV from *see* origins
  see also SIV
prisoners, counselling 117–18
PRO 140 antibody 25
PRO 542 inhibitor 23, 124
PRO 2000 *597*
proctitis *258*, 259
progressive multifocal leukoencephalopathy *see* PML
progressive outer retinal necrosis 232–3
progressive resistance training 297

proguanil 661
proinflammatory cytokines 267
prolactin 288
prophylatic antiretroviral intervention
    and mother-to-child transmission
    prevention 499–506
    clinical trials 499–504, *500–2*
    mechanisms of action 499
    resistance to 505–6
    short and long-term safety of
        504–5
prophylaxis
    disseminated mycobacterium
        avium complex 361–2
    post-exposure 95, 98
    pre-exposure 573
    travel, international 558
    see also condoms
prostatitis 383
prostitution *see* commercial sex
prostratin 549–50
protease inhibitors 130, 265
    antiretroviral therapy 136–7, *138*,
        140–1
    -associated dyslipidemia *283*
    drug resistance 149, 152, 153, 155
    endocrine complications 288, 292,
        293
    gastrointestinal disorders 251, 258
    hepatitis viral infection 421
    HIV-2 643
    pharmacology 171, 172
    resistance to 539
    therapy 174–5
    tuberculosis 350
protein 609
    energy malnutrition 604, 605
    structural *see* Env; Gag; Nef; Pol;
        Rev; Tat
proteinuria 299, *300, 302, 303*, 306
protionamide *345, 349*
proton-pump inhibitors 254
proviral load and HIV-2 640
PRT (progressive resistance
    training) 297
pseudomembranous candidiasis 216
pseudomonas aeruginosa 323, *324*, 326,
    328
pseudomonas pneumonia 323
psoriasis 242
psychiatric barriers and international
    AIDS epidemic **271–7**
    chronic mental illness 271, 273–4
    delirium and dementia 274–5
    mood disorders 274
    personality and temperament 276
    substance abuse 275–6
psychological problems 483–4
psychomotor slowing/retardation 263

psychosis 263
psychosocial support for children 631,
    633
public capacity maximization *689*
PUD (peptic ulcer disease) 254
Puerto Rico 6
pulmonary disease
    cytomegalovirus infections 441
    function tests 316
    hypertension *280*, 281–2
    and toxoplasmic encephalitis 400
    tuberculosis *624*
PVL (plasma viral load) 640, 761
pyogenic granulana 430
pyrazinamide 342, *343, 344, 347, 348,
    349, 350, 515*
pyrimethamine 256, 281, 742
    sulfadoxine-pyrimethamine *408*,
        749, 750, 751
    toxoplasmic encephalitis 405, *406,
        407, 408*
pyrimidine 420

Q
....
QALY (Quality Adjusted Life
    Year) 667–8
QASI (quality control) 655
quality assurance/control
    CD4 T-cell enumeration 654–5
    laboratory testing for HIV 107–8
    medicines 664
    testing and counselling 119
    urban care models in USA 533–4
quantitative plasma RNA 477

R
....
R5 viruses 76
R5-tropic virions 25
rabies 557
radiation proctitis *258*
radiculomyelitis 261, 262
radiography *106*
    chest 324, 327, 331, 383
    pneumocystis pneumonia 35–16,
        315, 316, 317, *318*
    tuberculosis 333
radiotherapy/radiology 402–3, 470
RANTES cehmokine 25
rattus norvegicus/niditus 394
RAU (recurrent aphthous ulcers) *216,
    217, 222*
Reach Out Mbuya 730
reasoned action theory of
    behaviour 112
recombinants/recombination 162
    alpha-interferons 418
    genetic 15

human nerve growth factor 267
    viruses 1
recrudescence of infection *see* IRIS
recurrent aphthous ulcers 216, *217,
    222*
REE (Resting Energy Expenditure) 603,
    604
regimens of antiretroviral therapy
    clinical applications 141–4
    design of 137, 141–2
    overview of 137–40
regional laboratories 652, 654, 655, 656
re-infection by other partner 79
religious NGOs active in HIV and
    Web 729–30
    local 730–1
renal complications **299–307**
    clinical manifestations and
        diagnosis 302–3
    course and outcome 306
    epidemiology 300–2
    failure 257
    global health care/
        delivery 299–300
    impairment 177
    insufficiency 383
    nephritis, interstitial 300
    nephrolithiasis 188
    nephropathy *515*, 625
    nephrosclerosis 300
    pathogenesis 303–4
    replacement therapy 305–6
    safety 187
    screen *106*
    treatment 304–6
replacement therapy 289–90
replication, viral 105–7, 163, *164*, 165
    see also clinical implications of HIV
        fitness
reproductive health
    antiretroviral therapy 295–6
    family issues 296
    fertility 295, 296
    men 294–5
    services 95
    sex hormone changes 294, 295
    treatment considerations 295,
        296
    women 295–6
resistance to drugs *see* drug resistance
resource-poor settings 146, **615–20**
    Africa 616–18
    costs dictating choices 616–17
    pediatric treatment 617
    regulatory environment 617
    scale-up as catalyst for
        improvement 618–19
    see also drug resistance in resource-
        poor settings

resource-poor settings and
    laboratories **649–60**
    CD4 T-cell enumeration 649, 650–5,
        653, 655
    expensive 650, *651*
    hematology and blood
        chemistry 650
respiratory distress syndrome 400
respiratory tract infections 562, 621,
    624
    travel, international 559–60
    see also bacillary angiomatosis
Resting Energy Expenditure 603
retina
    detachment 232
    microvasculopathy 227–8, 337–8
    necrosis, acute and
        progressive 232–3
retinitis 200, 227, 228, 229–30, 383
    drugs for *230*
Retrovir 95
Rev (regulator of viral gene
    expression) 24, 81, 83
reverse transcriptase inhibitors 127–8,
    129, 136, 151–3, 155, 597
    see also nucleoside reverse
        transcriptase inhibitors
rhodococcus equi 288, *324*
ribavirin 419, 420, *420*, *515*, 543
rickettsia 562
rifabutin 234, 257, 740
    drug abuse 524
    mycobacterium avium
        complex 358, 359, 360, 362
    tuberculosis *346*, *349*, 350–1
rifampicin/rifampin 237, 257, 352,
    740
    bartonella infections *431*, *432*
    children in resource-limited
        settings *627*, 628
    drug abuse *515*, 524
    endocrine complications 289, 291
    mycobacterium avium
        complex 358, 362
    post-exposure prevention *718*
    tuberculosis 342, *343*, *344*, 347, *348*,
        349, 350
rifamycin 347, 350, 559
rifapentine 350
rifaximin 257, 559
risk
    education to avoid 79–80
    per exposure, low 75
    populations and prevention 96
    reduction theory of behaviour
        113
ritonavir (RTV) *151*, 188, 258, 360, 742
    antiretroviral therapy 136–7, *139*,
        141, *142*, 146

-boosted protease inhibitors 541
children and adolescents *481*, *482*,
    621
drug abuse 521, *523*, 534
endocrine complications 289, 291,
    292, 293, 296
hepatitis 421
pharmacology 171, *172*, 174–5, *176*,
    177
post-exposure prevention *716*, *717*,
    721
resistance to 539, 542–3
travel, international 560
tuberculosis 350, *351*
women 494
rituximab 466–7, 469
RNA 107
    drug-resistant HIV, antiretroviral
        therapy of 537
    flavovirus *see* hepatitis C
    genome 27
    pro-viral 68
    testing 105, 107
RNase H inhibitors 129
Romania 8, 95
    children in resource-limited
        settings 626, 628
    non-sterile injections and
        pandemic 760–1, 762, 763
rosiglitazone 293
rotavirus 256
roxithromycin 742
RRT (renal replacement therapy)
    305–6
RTC (routine testing and
    counselling) 116
RTIs *see* reverse transcriptase inhibitors
RTV *see* ritonavir
rubella vaccine, avoiding 477
rural production and, food
    security 784–5
Russia and Russian Federation/former
    Soviet Union 2, 8, 588, 729,
    775n
    drug abuse 591, 592, 593
    dual epidemic with Eastern
        Europe 588–9
    essential medicines 665–6
    harm reduction programs 589
    non-sterile injections and
        pandemic 760, 762, 763, 764
    vaginal microbicides 595
Rwanda *312*, *501*, 565, *775n*
    complementary and alternative
        medicine 547, 548
    international funding 796
    NGOs active in HIV and Web 726,
        727n, 728, 729
    prevention 569

S

SACBC (South African Catholic
    Bishoos Conference) 730
safety
    blood 94, 570, 697, 761, 763
    heterosexual *55*
    of injections, myth of 756–7
    mother-to-child transmission
        prevention 504–5
    renal 187
St John's wort 538, 550, *718*, 719
salivary gland disease *216*, *217*, 223
salmonella and salmonellosis 257, 258,
    558, *738*
SAM (S-adenosylmethionine) 315
same sex, counselling 118
Sanofi-Pasteur *84*
saps (secreted aspartic proteinases) 372
saquinavir (SQV) *151*, 258, *351*, 360
    antiretroviral therapy *139*, *141*, *142*,
        238
    children and adolescents *481*
    drug abuse 521, *523*
    endocrine complications 292, 295
    inhibitory quotient 543
    pharmacology *172*, 174, 175, *176*
    post-exposure prevention *716*, *717*,
        718, 719, 721
sarcoidosis 201
SCC (ocular squamous cell
    carcinoma) 234
Schering D inhibitor (SCH-D) 25, 125
schistosomiasis 562, 758
school *see* education
scleritis 229
screening 94, 112
seborrheic dermatitis 243
secreted aspartic proteinases 372
seizures 263
selenium *280*, *606*, *607*
SemiBio Ligand Catcher 655
Senegal *10*, 92, 587, 704, 727n
    adherence to therapy 208, 209, 210,
        311, *312*
    prevention 565
sepsis 257
    septic shock syndrome 331
septicemia 621
SEROCO cohort 56
serology 68–70, *106*
    bartonella infections 430
    toxoplasmic encephalitis 401–2
sex education, school-based 93–4
sex hormone changes 294, 295
sex hormone-binding globulin 294
sex workers *see* commercial sex
    workers
sexual abuse 483

sexual dysfunction 294–5
sexual transmission, heterosexual 8, 91, 469, 483, 762
  antiretroviral therapy 143
  behaviour change programs 93–4
  biology of 75, 77, 91
  safe 556
  sex workers, immune 44
  sexually transmitted infections (STI) 3
sexual transmission, homosexual see male-to-male
sexually transmitted diseases/infections (STDs/STIs) 3, 4, 555, 568
  acute infection 67, 68
  biology of HIV-1 transmission 76, 78
  Brazil 697
  control 97
  prevention 95
  screening and treatment 94
  test for 106
  travel, international 555
  women and special issues 488, 489
  see also herpes
SHBG (sex hormone-binding globulin) 294
shigella 257, 258, 440, 738
shingles see varicella zoster
SHIV (simian-human immunodeficiency) 596
side-effects of systemic ocular medication 234–5
Sierra Leone 565
sigmoidoscopy 259
sildenafil (viagra) 234, 295
silymarin 550
simian origins see origins; SIV
simian-human immunodeficiency 596, 598
simvastatin 718
Singapore 578
single nucleotide polymorphisms 56, 77
sinusitis 562, 624
SIV (simian immunodeficiency virus) 13, 14, 18, 42, 78, 82, 162, 166, 764
skin disorders 237–46, 561–2
sleep disturbance 263
SLS 596, 600
SMART study 144
SMX see trimethoprim(TMP)-sulfamethoxazole
SNPs (single nucleotide polymorphisms) 56, 77
social learning (cognitive) theory of behaviour 112

social services and urban care models in USA 531–2
somatotropic axis, pituitary 288
somostatin 256
sosporiasis 625
source partner see host
South Africa 10, 15, 84, 198, 242, 362, 615, 686, 704
  adherence to therapy 209, 210, 310, 311, 312
  Brazil compared with 695, 701
  children in resource-limited settings 621–2, 628
  economic impact 770, 771, 773, 775
  international funding 796, 799
  mother-to-child transmission prevention 500, 501, 506, 507
  NGOs active in HIV and Web 725n, 726, 727n, 728, 729, 730, 731
  pathogen-host-environment interactions 783, 784
  pharmacoeconomics 671–2, 673, 674
  prevention 565, 569, 572
  renal complications 299, 301, 302, 305
  tuberculosis 333, 334, 350
South America see Latin America
South Korea 577
South and South-East Asia 15, 84, 209, 313, 489
  children in resource-limited settings 628
  dermatology 239, 240, 241
  drug abuse 513, 514
  drug resistance in resource-poor settings 705–6
  economic impact 771, 775
  essential medicines 663, 665
  fungal infections 376, 387
  global epidemiology 2, 3, 8, 9
  international funding for care and prevention 796
  mother-to-child transmission prevention 500, 501, 503, 506
  mycobacterium avium complex 362
  NGOs active in HIV and Web 725n, 726, 728, 734
  non-sterile injections and pandemic 757, 759, 760, 763
  pathogen-host-environment interactions 783
  penicillium marneffei infection 393, 394
  pharmacoeconomics 671
  prevention 91, 92, 97, 573

psychiatric problems 272, 273, 275
  travel, international 558, 561
  tuberculosis 333, 334, 335
  women and special issues 489
  see also India; Thailand
Soviet Union, former see Russia
SP (sulfadoxine-pyrimethamine) 408, 749, 750, 751
Spain 240, 241, 305, 589, 733
sparfloxacin 358
spastic diplegia see paraplegia
SPD754 inhibitor 127
spinothalamic sensory deficits 267
SPL7013 596, 600
spleen 425
  bacillary peliosis 427, 433
  splenectomy 469
  splenomegaly 426
sporotrichosis 245
squamous cell carcinoma 217, 233, 258, 464
squamous intraepithelial neoplasia 258
SQV see saquinavir
Sri Lanka 578, 771
SSKI (potassium iodide) 245
Stanford B regimen 468
staphylococcus aureus 282, 323, 324, 325, 326, 328
  drug abuse 515
  skin infections 378–9
staphylococcus pneumonia 323, 515
STARHS technique 103, 105
statins 185, 256
stavudine (D4T)
  antiretroviral therapy 138, 140, 145
  children and adolescents 482
  children in resource-limited settings 626, 627, 628
  drug abuse 522
  hepatitis viral infection 420, 421
  low cost 146
  mother-to-child transmission prevention 504, 506, 508
  pancreatitis 186
  pharmacology 172, 173, 177
  post-exposure prevention 713, 716, 717, 720, 721
  primary neurological manifestations 265, 266, 267
  resistance to 50, 152, 543
  Thailand 583
STDs see sexually-transmitted diseases
sterilization, inadequate see non-sterile injections
steroids 243, 305, 376, 377
STI (structured treatment interruptions) 542
stibogluconate 560
stigma 210, 789

stomatitis
  aphthous 245
  necrotizing *216, 217*
streptoccus/streptoccal
  pneumonia 282, *325*, 327, *328*, 490, 559, 621
    streptococcus viridans 282
streptomycin *343, 344, 348, 349*
strongyloidis 256
  stercoralis 440
structured treatment interruptions 542
sub-Saharan Africa *see* Africa
substance users *see* drug abuse
subtypes A, B and C 77
Subutex/Suboxone *see* buprenorphine
Sudan 306
sugars in diet 609
sulfadiazine 405, *406*, 407
sulfadoxine 742
  -pyrimethamine *see* SP
sulfamethoxazole *see* trimethoprim
sulfirim 240
sulfonamide *325*, 406
super-infection and re-infection 66, 79
supply chain for HAART *678*
supply-side challenges in underdeveloped countries 683–4
support and prevention intervention 118–19
Suriname 729
susceptibility in health belief model 112
Swaziland 9, 487, 547, 730
  economic impact 769, 772, *775n*
  prevention 565, 571
Switzerland 301, 416, 463, 551, 559, 589
symptoms *see* clinical features
syphilis 68, *228*, 233, 439
  gastrointestinal disorders 258, 259, 262
  neurosyphilis 262
  skin disorders 238–9
systemic therapy for neoplasia 470–1

T

T20 inhibitor 25, 127
T-1249 inhibitor 127
T lymphocytes 78–9, 104
  see also CTLs
Taiwan *313*, 393
Tajikistan *775n*
TAK 220 small-molecule antagonist 25
Takayasu's arteritis 283
TAMs (thymidine analog mutation) 150–1, 152
Tanzania *10*, 306, 741, *775n*
  children in resource-limited settings 621

economic impact 770, 771, *772*
international funding 796
mother-to-child transmission prevention 500, 507
NGOs active in HIV and Web 725n, 727, 728, 729
orphans 788
Pneumocystis pneumonia *311, 312*
prevention 94, 97, 565, 572
target cells and virus-host dynamics 78–9
targeted, counselling 93
TASO (Aids Support Organization The) 730
taste, loss of sense of *611*
Tat (transcriptional activator) 24, 81, 83
TCA (trichloroacetic acid) 493
T-cells
  activation and endocrine complications 293
  activation and niche construction 162
  central memory (TCM) cells 41
  effector memory (TEM) cells 41
  loss mechanism 52–3
  see also CD4 T-cells; CD8 T-cells
TD (traveller's diarrhea) 558–9, 562
TDF *see* tenofovir
technologies, new laboratory *693*
telbivudine *418*, 515
telithromycin *328*
temperament and psychiatric barriers 276
tenesmus 255
tenofovir disoproxil *418*, 419
tenofovir (viread/TDF) 98
  antiretroviral therapy 137, *138*, 140, *142*
  children and adolescents *481*, 482
  complications 186, 187
  drug abuse 521, *522*
  pharmacology *172, 173, 176, 177*
  post-exposure prevention *716, 717, 720*
  renal safety 187
  resistance to *150*, 152
  vaginal microbicides *597, 600*
terbinafine 244
testicular pathology 294
testing and counselling **111–21**
  behavioural theories 112–13
  benefits of 113–14
  chemotherapy 470–1
  drug resistance in resource-poor settings 707–8
  general screening recommendations 112
  human resource priorities 119–20
  interferon-á 471

models 115–17
  negative outcomes 114–15
  quality assurance 119
  special groups 115–17
  support and prevention intervention 118–19
  voluntary *see* VCT
  see also counselling
testosterone 293, 294, 295, 296, 297
tetanus vaccination 477, 478
tetracycline *328*, 742
  bartonella infections *431, 432*
  dermatology 237, 239
tetragenesis 445
tetraglycine hydroperiodide 559
tetrahydrocannabinol 550
Thailand 15, *84*, 92, 209, *313*, 583–4, 671, 726
  children in resource-limited settings 628
  dermatology 239, 240, 241
  drug resistance 705–6
  economic impact 771, 775
  fungal infections 362, 387
  global epidemiology 8, 9
  high-risk groups 577, *578*, 579, 580, *581*, 582
  mother-to-child transmission prevention 498, *500, 501*, 503, 506
  NGOs active in HIV and Web 726, 727n, 733
  non-sterile injections and pandemic 757, 764
  orphans 790
  penicillium marneffei infection 393, 394, *395, 396*, 397
  prevention 573, 587
  psychiatric problems 273
  travel, international 559, 561
thalidomide 201, 202, 245, *252*, 377, 471, 741
T-helper cell dysfunction 280
thiabendazole 256
thioacetazone *344, 347, 348, 349*
thiocarboxanilide *600*
'third drug' 137
Three by Five initiative of WHO 11
3TC *see* lamivudine
thrombocytopenia 428, 443
thrush *see* candidiasis
thymidine analog mutation 150–1
thyroglobulin antibody 289
thyroid 288–90
  alterations in function 288–9
  antiretroviral and other therapies 289
  autoimmune diseases 201, 289
  hormone *280*

hormone-binding globulin (TBG) 289
pathology 288
peroxidase antibody 289
-stimulating hormone (TSH) 289, 290
treatment considerations 289–90
thyrotropin-releasing hormones (GnRH and TRH) 288, 289
ticarcillin 328
ticonazole 369
tinea infection 244
tinidazole 256, 257, 742
tipranavir (aprivus/TPV) 138, 172, 541
children and adolescents 481, 482
drug abuse 523, 524
new drug development 130–1
TMC114 see darunavir
TMC120 597
TMC125 (etravirine) inhibitor 128, 541
TMC278 inhibitor 128–9
TMP see trimethoprim
TNX-355 inhibitor 23, 124
tobramycin 244, 326
toll-like receptors (TLRs) 57, 336
top-down costing 669
TORO studies 124
toxicity
management of infections 443–5
to selected drugs 145, 188, 189, 190
toxoplasma gondii 280, 449, 483
endocrine complications 290, 294
mycobacterium avium complex 401, 402, 403, 407, 408, 409
see also toxoplasmic encephalitis; toxoplasmosis
toxoplasmic encephalitis 261, 287, 399–413, 622
clinical presentation 399–400
congenital, women and 400–1
diagnosis 401–3, 401
histopathology 403
maintenance 407
management 403–9, 404
prevention 407–9
primary therapy 405–7
toxoplasmosis 106, 255, 275, 281, 324, 439, 490
cerebral see toxoplasmic encephalitis
children 622, 624
endocrine complications 287, 291
fungal infections 377, 383
ocular 228, 233, 400
retinitis 228
see also toxoplasma gondii

TPV see tipranavir
trace minerals in diet 606–7, 606
traditional remedies 176–8
transcriptase, reverse, high error rate of 162
transcriptional events, molecular biology of HIV 28–30, 29
transmission of HIV
global epidemiology 1–2
main methods see blood transfusions; drug abuse, intravenous; mother-to-child; sexual transmission
women-initiated prevention 566–7, 570–1
see also biology; drug resistance; mother-to-child; sexual transmission and under Africa, Asia and Eastern Europe
transplants, kidney 305
transtheoretical theory of behaviour 112
travel, international 55–64
emerging and re-emerging infections 560–1
enteric infections 558–9
fever 562
general instructions 555–7
new HIV infections 562
parasitic infections 561
prophylaxis 558
respiratory infections 559–60
skin disorders 561–2
vaccinations 557–8
TRAx 564
treatment
Eastern Europe 591–3
HIV-2 642–3
HIV-associated dementia 264–6
neuropathy, HIV 267
renal complications 304–6
and reproductive health in men 295, 296
STD (sexually-transmitted diseases) 94
vacuolar myelopathy 268
see also antiretroviral therapy; epidemiology; pharmacoeconomics; pharmacology; substance users
treponema pallidum 258
TRH stimulation 288
trials in African prevention policy 572–4
triazolam 718, 719
trichloroacetic acid (TCA) 493
trichosporon beigelii 378
trichosporum 380
triglyceride synthesis, increased 283

TRIM (tripartite motif) protein 35, 57, 77
trimethoprim (TMP) 288, 319
trimethoprim (TMP)-sulfamethoxazole (SMX) 233, 241, 281, 292, 309, 326, 432, 477
candida 371
dermatology 237, 238, 241
diarrhea 737, 739, 741–2
gastrointestinal disorders 256, 257
pneumonias 319, 320, 325, 326, 328
toxoplasmic encephalitis 405, 406, 408
travel, international 558
trimetrexate 319
Trinidad 94, 240
trioimmune 173, 177
tri-phosphates 538
triple agent ARV therapy 137
trypanosomiasis 562
TSH (thyroid-stimulating hormone) 289, 290
TST (tuberculin skin test) 198
tuberculosis 4, 8, 11, 44, 146, 196, 316, 333–53, 439, 782
active disease 339–42, 339–40
Brazil 699–701, 700
children in resource-limited settings 622, 624, 627, 628
clinical aspects 337–42
co-infections with 617–18
cryptococcal 195
cutaneous 240
diagnosis 327
epidemiology 333–6, 334
essential medicines for 663, 664
extrapulmonary 624
gastrointestinal disorders 255
IRIS 197–8, 197, 201
luminal 257
Mtb see mycobacterium tuberculosis
mycobacterium 288, 290, 317, 324
ocular manifestations 228, 233
oral lesions 216
pancreatic 291
pathogenesis 336–7
prevention 352, 568
in prisons 590
pulmonary 624
resource-poor settings 649, 650
travel, international 555, 559–60, 562
treatment 342–51, 343–6, 348–9
see also Global Fund; mycobacterium tuberculosis
tuberculous meningitis 622
Tunisia 311, 312
typhoid 557, 562

U

UC781 *597*
Uganda 265, 301, 587, 705, 727n, 737, 749, 759
  adherence to therapy 208, 209
  children in resource-limited settings 621
  dermatology 239
  economic impact 770, 771, 772
  fungal infections 376, 377, 378
  global epidemiology 2, 9–10, *10, 311, 312*
  international funding 796
  mother-to-child transmission prevention *500, 501,* 506
  NGOs active in HIV and Web 725n, 727, 729, 730
  orphans 787–8
  pathogen-host-environment interactions *781,* 784
  pharmacoeconomics 671
  prevention 92, 97, 98, 565, 567, 569, 572, 582–3
  psychiatric problems 272, 273, 274
  tuberculosis 338, *339–40*
  women and special issues 488–9, 490
UK427–857 (Maraviroc) inhibitor 25, 125–6
Ukraine 8, 762, *775n*
  Eastern Europe and 592, 593
  NGOs active in HIV and Web 726, 728
ulcers/ulcerative
  colitis *258*
  cytomegalovirus 220
  esophagitis 253–4
  genital 493
  giant idiopathic aphthous genital 493
  idiopathic esophageal (IEU) 251, *252,* 253, 254
  mouth/aphthous/oral *216, 217, 222,* 366, 493, *624*
  peptic 254
  periodontitis, necrotizing *219*
ultrasound 296, 302–3, *303*
UNAIDS (Joint United Nations Programme on HIV/AIDS) 2, 11, 85, 96, 261
  adherence to therapy 207
  Central and Eastern Europe/former Soviet Union 588
  drug abuse 589
  economic impact 776
  Global Coalition on Women and AIDS 571
  map of global incidence *3*
  prevention 567, *568,* 572
  three Cs 115
  treatment concerns 592
underdeveloped countries *see* challenges
unemployment 771
United Kingdom 7, 8, 85, 196, 240, 301, 352, 759, *775n*
  international funding 797, 799
  NGOs active in HIV and Web 730, *731, 735*
United Nations 649, 664
  Central and Eastern Europe 588
  Children's Fund (UNICEF) 607
  Declaration of Commitment on HIV/AIDS 703
  Development Fund for Women 488
  Development Program 775
  and drug abuse 513, 590–1
  General Assembly Special Session (UNGASS) 615
  resource-poor settings 649
  Security Council 789
  UNFPA and condoms 570
  UNHCR 667
  UNICEF 667, 790, 791
  see also Global Fund; UNAIDS
United States *see* North America; urban care models
Universal Declaration of Human Rights 591
unsterile injections *see* non-sterile
urban care models in USA **527–36**
  adherence services 531
  clinical research 533
  consumer and community advisory boards 534
  financing 534–5
  inpatient *528, 532, 533*
  primary care 530–1
  quality assurance 533–4
  social services 531–2
  specialty services 531
USPSTF (US Preventative Services Task Force) 112
uveitis 233, 234
Uzbekistan 592, 593

V

V106M 153–4
vaccination 97, 324, 352, *417*
  Africa 573–4
  infants 477–8
  prospects for 39, 45–7, 79–80
  travel, international 557–8, *557*
  see also design of global AIDS vaccine
vaccinia virus 82
vacuolar myelopathy, HIV-1 associated 267–8
vaginal infections *see* vulvovaginal
vaginal microbicides **595–601**
  AFE inhibitors 596–7
  animal models 598
  clinical development 599
  delivery 598–9
  development of 597–8
  in vitro studies 597–8
  mechanism of action of 595–7
  membrane disruptive agents 596
  mother-to-child transmission 506–7
  regulatory issues 599–60
  reverse transcriptase inhibitors 597
valacyclovir (Valtrex) 229
  gastrointestinal disorders *252,* 254, 256, 259
  hepatitis viral infection 451, *452*
  management of infections 443, 454
valcyte *230*
valganciclovir *438,* 740
  gastrointestinal disorders *252,* 254, 256
  management of infections 442, 443
  ocular manifestations 229, *230*
Valtrex *see* valacyclovir
vancomycin 237, 257, *325, 328*
varicella zoster virus (shingles) 199, 261, 262, 439
  complications 455–6
  drug-resistant infection 457
  encephalitis 275
  management of infections 455–7
  ocular manifestations *228,* 229–32
  prevention 457
  primary and secondary infections 455
  treatment 457
  vaccine 478
vascular proliferated lesions 425
vasculitis 440
Vax Gen *84*
VCT (voluntary counselling and testing) 94, 115, 574, 582, 698, 726
ventricular enlargement *264*
ventriculoencephalitis 439–40
vertical pathogen-host-environment interactions 780–1
vertical transmission *see* mother-to-child
vesicular stomatitis virus 82
viagra *see* sildenafil
vicriviroc (Schering D) 25, 125

Vietnam 393, 725n, 729
    high-risk groups 577, *578*, 579, 580,
        582
    international funding 796
Vif (viral infectivity factor) 24, 54, 83,
    137, 161, 162
vinblasine, intralesional 470
vincristine *465*, *471*
vinorelbine 471, *471*
viral diseases and infections 256,
    281
    anorectal *258*
    oral *216*, *217*
    see also cytomegalovirus; herpes
viral and host determinants of HIV-1
    disease progression **51–61**
    biological phenotype 53–5
    CD4 T-cell loss mechanism 52–3
    host factors influency viral
        load 55–7
    immune response, specific
        antiviral 51–2
viral loads
    during primary infection 71
    host factors affecting 55–7
viramune 95
viread *see* tenofovir
viremia 135, 144, 417, 470
virions 25–6
    fusion 25
    new, assembly and budding of 31,
        32–3
viroptic 229
'Virtual Virus' 541
virulence of HIV
    modified as evolutionary
        strategy 166–7
    see also clinical implications of HIV
    fitness
vistide *see* cidofovir
vitamins
    D analogs 242
    B12 280 (the 12 should be
        subscript) 280
    deficiency 266, 267
    in diet *606*, 607–8, 609
    therapy 551
vitrasert *230*
vitravene *230*
vitreitis/vitritis 200, 232
VL determination technologies 655–8,
    657
voluntary counselling and testing *see*
    VCT
voriconazole and fungal infections 380,
    381–2, 384, 387, *719*
    candida *369*, 370, 371
Vpn (viral protein N) 54–5

Vpr (viral protein R) 24, 26–7, 54–5,
    83
Vpu (viral protein U) 24, 55, 83
VSV (vesicular stomatitis virus) 82,
    366, 367, 368, *369*, 371, 491, 493
    candidiasis 366, 367, 368, *369*, 371
vulvovaginal infections
    candidiasis 366, 367, 368, *369*, 371,
        491, 493
    rectovaginal fistula *625*
    see also vaginal micobicides
VX-385 (brecanavir) inhibitor 131
VZV *see* varicella zoster virus

W

warts 199, *217*, *221*, 493, *624*
wasting syndrome *see under*
    malnutrition
water in diet 609
weight loss 177, *252*, 327, 440
    cachexia 4
    combatting 610–11, *611*
    wasting syndrome 288, 296–7, 604,
        622
    see also malnutrition
West Indies *see* Caribbean basin
Western blot test 102
Whipple's Disease 257
WHO *see* World Health Organization
wild-type (WT) infections 154, 155, 165,
    539
window period 65
women 11, **487–96**, *732*
    antiretroviral treatment 494–5
    Brazil 695
    clinical manifestations 490–1
    -controlled prevention 97
    diet 607, 608
    epidemiology 487–9
    gynecologic manifestations 491–4
    hepatitis viral infection 418, 421
    HIV prevalence in 4–5, 9, 75, 566
    hormones 78
    initiated-prevention policy in
        Africa 566–7, 570–1
    and malaria 747–8, 749
    see also breast-feeding; cervical
        disorders; children; commercial
        sex workers; mother-to-child;
        pregnancy; vaginal
        microbicides; vulvovaginal
        infections
workplace-based prevention programs
    in Africa 569
World Bank 588, 664
    and Brazil 695
    economic impact 769, 775

Multi-Country AIDS Program *see*
    MAP
psychiatric barriers 272
World Food Program 569
World Health Organization 2, *731*, 776
    ARV therapy 146
    children and adolescents 479,
        623–5, 627
    definition of AIDS 4
    definition of essential medicine
        662
    drug abuse 513, 589
    drug resistance 703, 706–7
    economic impact 774
    essential medicines 615, 661, *662*
    on Europe 6
    laboratory testing 102, 108, 649
    malnutrition 610
    Model Formulary *662*
    monitoring protocol 707
    mother-to-child transmission
        prevention *509–10*
    non-sterile injections 758, 760
    pediatric immunologic
        staging *623–5*
    pharmacoeconomics 668, 673
    pneumocystis pneumonia 309,
        318
    prices 664
    psychiatric problems and Mental
        Health Consortium 271–2
    renal complications 299, 306
    resource-poor settings 649
    sexually transmitted infections
        571
    Special (Global) Programme on
        HIV/AIDS 11, 85
    Strategy for HIV Drug Resistance
        Prevention, Surveillance and
        Monitoring 706–7
    Three by Five initiative 11, 615
    treatment concerns/guidelines 592,
        617
    tuberculosis 198, 333, *334*, 335, 336,
        342, *343*, 347, 352
    website *662*
World Health Organization-UNAIDS
    HIV vaccine initiative 573
world map of HIV-1 sub-types and
    recombinants 2
World Trade Organization 671
WSW (women having sex with
    women) 489
WT *see* wild-type infections

X

x-rays *see* radiography

Y

Y181C/I (EFV mutation) 140
yaws 759
yellow fever 557–8
youth-oriented prevention 93
YRG-CARE 731

Z

Zaire 301, 770
zalcitabine (DDC) 152, 171, 186, 266
 cardiovascular complications 280
 drug abuse *522*
 hepatitis viral infection 420
 post-exposure prevention *716*, 721
Zambia *310*, 487, 506, 547, 671
 children in resource-limited
  settings 621–2, 625
 economic impact 771, *772, 775n*
 international funding 796, 799
 NGOs active in HIV and
  Web 725n, 726, 727n, 729, 730

pathogen-host-environment
 interactions *783*
prevention 571
psychiatric problems 272, 273
Zanmi Lasante 726
zidovudine (ZDV) 95, 137, 494, 705
 adverse reactions to 145
 and anemia 607
 antiretroviral therapy *138, 142,*
  238
 cardiovascular complications 280
 children and adolescents 477, *481*
 children in resource-limited
  settings 626, *627*, 628
 drug abuse 521, *522*
 endocrine complications 295
 HAD 264, 265
 hepatitis viral infection 420
 mother-to-child transmission
  prevention 497, 498, 499, *500–1,*
  503–4, 506, 507
 mutations *150*, 152
 pharmacology *172*, 173

post-exposure prevention 712, *716,*
 717, 720
renal complications 302, 304, 306
tuberculosis 350
Zimbabwe 9, *10*, 46, 153, 301, 670, *775n*
 complementary and alternative
  medicine 547, 548
 international funding 799
 mother-to-child transmission
  prevention 498, 507
 NGOs active in HIV and Web 726,
  730
 pathogen-host-environment
  interactions *783*, 784
 pneumocystis pneumonia *310, 312*
 prevention 565, 567, 569, 571, 572
zinc in diet *606*, 607, 610
zovirax *see* acyclovir
ZR59 HIV-1 sequence 17